The PDR® Pocket Guide to
PRESCRIPTION DRUGS™

A trusted name in medicine for over 60 years!

Includes important information on:
- Possible food and drug interactions
- Pregnancy-related warnings and safety
- What to avoid during treatment
- Essential contact information f
  centers
- The top 200 most com
- Photographs of mor

"An easy-to-read guide to m   ons, side effects, and efficacy....Now one can get understandable medical information that can help keep health costs down, yet give patients a fine comfort level with the medicines they take."

    —Leon G. Smith, MD
     Chairman of Medicine,
     St. Michael's Medical Center, Newark, NJ

"A must for every household where there are concerns about the safe use of medications. It is an ideal way to clarify and supplement the information provided by your health-care provider."

    —Jack M. Rosenberg, PharmD, PhD
     Professor of Pharmacy Practice and Pharmacology,
     Long Island University

THE PDR®

POCKET GUIDE

TO PRESCRIPTION DRUGS™

NINTH EDITION
FULLY REVISED AND UPDATED

Based on *Physicians' Desk Reference®*,
the Nation's Leading Drug Handbook

POCKET BOOKS
New York   London   Toronto   Sydney

Physicians' Desk Reference® and PDR® are registered trademarks of PDR
Network, LLC. The PDR® Pocket Guide to Prescription Drugs™ is a trademark of PDR Network, LLC.

Pocket Books
A Division of Simon & Schuster, Inc.
1230 Avenue of the Americas
New York, NY 10020

Copyright © 1996, 1997, 1999, 2000, 2002, 2003, 2005, 2008,
2010 by PDR Network, LLC
Published by arrangement with Thomson PDR

All rights reserved, including the right to reproduce
this book or portions thereof in any form whatsoever.
For information address Thomson Healthcare,
5 Paragon Drive, Montvale, NJ 07645.

This Pocket Books paperback edition January 2010

POCKET and colophon are registered trademarks of
Simon & Schuster, Inc.

For information about special discounts for bulk purchases,
please contact Simon & Schuster Special Sales at
1-866-506-1949 or business@simonandschuster.com.

The Simon & Schuster Speakers Bureau can bring authors to your
live event. For more information or to book an event, contact the
Simon & Schuster Speakers Bureau at 1-866-248-3049 or visit our
website at www.simonspeakers.com

Cover design by James Perales
Cover art by ShutterStock

Manufactured in the United States of America

10   9   8   7   6   5   4   3   2   1

ISBN 978-1-4391-4308-7

Publisher's Note

The drug information contained in this book is based on product labeling published in the 2009 edition of *Physicians' Desk Reference*® or supplied by the manufacturer. This information is drawn from the PDR database, which is compiled and updated on a regular basis by a staff of experienced pharmacists. While diligent efforts have been made to ensure the accuracy of each drug profile, it is essential to bear in mind that the information presented here is merely a synopsis of key points in the official product labeling, and that the complete labeling contains additional precautionary information that may be of significance in specific cases. If a profile leaves any question unanswered, be sure to consult your doctor or pharmacist for additional information.

This book does not list every possible action, adverse reaction, interaction, and precaution; and all information is presented without guarantees by the authors, consultants, and publisher, who disclaim all liability in connection with its use. This book is intended only as a reference for use in an ongoing partnership between doctor and patient in the management of the patient's health. It is not a substitute for a doctor's professional judgment, and serves only as a reminder of concerns that may need discussion. All readers are urged to consult with a doctor or other healthcare provider before beginning or discontinuing use of any prescription drug or undertaking any form of self-treatment. Brand names listed in this book are intended to represent only the more commonly used products. Inclusion of a brand name does not signify endorsement of the product; absence of a name does not imply a criticism or rejection of the product. The publisher is not advocating the use of any product described in this book, does not warrant or guarantee any of these products, and has not performed any independent analysis in connection with the product information contained herein.

Contents

The PDR® Pocket Guide to Prescription Drugs™, based on the 2009 edition of PDR®

Senior Director, Editorial & Publishing: Bette Kennedy

Director, Clinical Services: Sylvia Nashed, PharmD

Manager, Clinical Services: Nermin Shenouda, PharmD

Drug Information Specialists: Anila Patel, PharmD; Christine Sunwoo, PharmD

Manager, Editorial Services: Lori Murray

Associate Editor: Jennifer Reed

Manager, Art Department: Livio Udina

Electronic Publishing Designer: Carrie Spinelli Faeth

PDR Network, LLC

CEO: Edward Fotsch, MD

President: David Tanzer

Chief Medical Officer: Henry DePhillips, MD

Vice President, Product Management: Cy Caine

Vice President, Publishing & Operations: Valerie Berger

Vice President, Clinical Relations: Mukesh Mehta, RPh

Senior Director, Copy Sales: Bill Gaffney

Board of Medical Consultants to the 1st Edition

Younghee Limb, MD
Assistant Professor of Clinical Medicine
State University of New York, Stony Brook, NY

Gardiner Morse, MS
Editor, Harvard Health Publications, Boston, MA

Louis V. Napolitano, MD
Family Practice
Hackensack University Medical Center, Hackensack, NJ

Mark D. Ravenscraft, MD
Creve Coeur, MO

Martin I. Resnick, MD
Professor and Chairman, Department of Urology
Case Western Reserve University, Cleveland, OH

Frank Simo, MD
St. Louis, MO

Karl Singer, MD
Exeter Family Medicine Associates, Exeter, NH

Eugene W. Sweeney, MD
Department of Dermatology
Columbia Presbyterian Medical Center
New York, NY

Josephine Chaou, MD
Assistant Professor of Clinical Medicine
State University of New York, Stony Brook, NY

Caroline Marie, MS
Editor, Harvard Health Publications, Boston, MA

Laurel Kelley-Rhoden, MD
Family Practice, ...

...

John Tomasz, MD, PhD
Grove Clinic, NW ...

Martin L. Pernak, MD
Professor and Chairman, Department of Biology
Case Western Reserve University, Cleveland, OH

Frank Shao, MD
...

Karl Stamm, MD
Lecturer, Loyola Medicine Associates, Boston, MA

Eugene W. Seaman, MD
Department of Cardiology
Columbia Presbyterian Medical Center
New York, NY

Foreword

The PDR® Pocket Guide to Prescription Drugs™ strives to make the many benefits of modern pharmaceuticals—as well as their possible risks—as clear and simple as can be. *The PDR Pocket Guide* spells out why each drug is prescribed and the most important information to remember about it, then discloses its most common side effects. As a safeguard against error, it also provides you with information on standard dosage recommendations and tells what to do when you miss a dose of your medication. And to help you find all these facts as quickly as possible, it lists each medication under its familiar brand name—with a cross-reference in case the drug is dispensed generically.

Still, despite the depth and detail of the information you'll find here, *The PDR Pocket Guide* is not a replacement for your doctor's advice. Rather, it serves as a reminder of the basic instructions and caveats that may be forgotten by the time you leave your doctor's office, as well as providing you with a checklist of the problems and conditions that you must be certain the doctor knows about—facts that might call for a change in your prescription. In this way, the book is designed to serve as an aid in an ongoing dialogue between you and your doctor—a collaboration necessary for any treatment to work. Just as the doctor must tell you how and why to use a particular drug, you must tell the doctor how it affects you, reporting any reactions or drug interactions you suspect you may have. And while it's up to the doctor to devise your treatment strategy, it's up to you to make sure that the right doses are administered at the right times, and that the prescribed course of therapy is completed as planned.

Physicians' Desk Reference® has been providing doctors with the information needed for safe, effective drug therapy for more than 60 years. Designed especially for healthcare professionals, it presents the facts in a detailed, technical format approved by the Food and Drug Administration (FDA). To make the key facts buried in this wealth of data accessible to everyone, *The PDR Pocket Guide* strips away the medical shorthand and technical terminology, and presents the core of this information in a simple, standard format designed for maximum convenience and ease of use by the consumer. All the information you'll find in *The PDR Pocket Guide*'s consumer drug profiles has been extracted from the PDR database, which is updated regularly by a staff of pharmacists and drug information specialists.

Modern drug therapy is a vast and complicated field—so complicated that, for many questions about medicines, the answer varies with each patient. *The PDR Pocket Guide to Prescription Drugs* gives you general guidelines for safe drug use. But only your doctor, evaluating the unique details of your case, can give you the exact instructions best suited for you. The goal of this book is simply to alert you to the most pertinent questions to ask, and to help clarify your doctor's answers—in short, to give you the tools you need to supervise your own medical care as effectively as possible.

We wish you good health.

Robert W. Hogan, MD
Chair, Board of Medical Consultants
Family Medicine
Southern California Permanente Medical Group
Assistant Clinical Professor
Physician Assessment and Clinical Education (PACE) Program
UCSD Department of Family and Preventive Medicine
San Diego, CA

How to Use This Book

Although doctors today can often work miracles with advanced technology and sophisticated medicines, it's vital for you to take an active role in managing your health. Any medicine can prove worthless if taken improperly. Likewise, you must let your doctor know if you react badly to a drug or have a condition that makes taking it dangerous. While no book is a substitute for a visit to the doctor, this guide is designed to help you use your medications safely and effectively, and to help you determine things that deserve further discussion with your doctor.

The book is divided into two major parts. In the first, you'll find profiles of the more frequently prescribed medications. The second section has helpful references and an index of medications used to treat common diseases and disorders.

THE DRUG PROFILES

The profiles provide detailed information on the most frequently prescribed prescription drugs. Though the section covers more than 1,000 products, don't be alarmed if you don't find a profile for a prescription you've received. There are a number of specialized, yet valuable drugs that have been omitted here due to lack of space.

The products described here are listed alphabetically by the manufacturer's brand name or the generic name. Full-profile headers appear in all uppercase letters; generic cross-references are boldface lowercase. In general, the drug profiles begin with the brand name followed by the generic name for the drug. The information that follows these names is divided into 12 sections. Here's what you'll find in each.

What is this medication?
This is an overview of the major conditions for which the drug is generally prescribed.

What is the most important information I should know about this medication?
Highlighted here are key points about a drug that is especially worthwhile to know. We've placed it here for the sake of emphasis. Never regard this section as a definitive summary of the drug.

Who should not take this medication?
Some drugs can be harmful under certain conditions, which are detailed here. The most common contraindication is a hypersensitivity to the

drug itself. If you think one of these restrictions applies to you, alert your doctor immediately.

What should I tell my doctor before I take the first dose of this medication?

If you have any problems or conditions noted in this section that your doctor may be unaware of, be sure to bring them to his or her attention. Always tell your doctor about your complete medical history as well as any prescription and over-the-counter products you are taking— including dietary supplements and herbs—before starting treatment with any other medication.

What is the usual dosage?

Shown here are excerpts of the dosage guidelines your doctor uses. Depending on your condition and medical history, your doctor may prescribe a different regimen. This information is intended only as a convenient double check in case you suspect a misunderstanding or a typographical error on your prescription label. **Do not use this information to determine an exact dosage yourself, and do not change the dosage or stop taking your medication without your doctor's approval.**

How should I take this medication?

This section details special instructions, including how and when to take the drug, and any dietary restrictions that may apply.

What should I avoid while taking this medication?

This section gives advice on certain activities that should be avoided during treatment due to an increased risk of side effects or other potential problems. If you have any questions about the precautions in this section, talk to your doctor. Do not change your dosage or discontinue the drug on your own. Such a change might do more harm than good. Also remember that this is not a complete list of all possible drug precautions; always consult your doctor or pharmacist for more information.

What are possible food and drug interactions associated with this medication?

This section lists specific drugs, classes of drugs, and foods that have been known to interact with the medicine being profiled. The examples are not all-inclusive. If you're not certain whether a medication you're taking falls into one of these categories, be sure to check with your doctor or pharmacist. But never stop taking any drug without first consulting your doctor.

What are the possible side effects of this medication?

Shown here are only the most common side effects listed by the manufacturer in the drug's FDA-approved product labeling. Any drug will occasionally cause an unwanted reaction. Even the most common side effects are seen in only a small percentage of patients. Not included are side effects that can be detected only by a physician or laboratory. If you have any questions about side effects—or if you have any new or continuing symptoms—talk to your doctor.

Can I receive this medication if I am pregnant or breastfeeding?

This section will tell you whether a drug has been confirmed safe for use during pregnancy or breastfeeding, is known to be dangerous, or is part of that large group about which scientists are not really sure. With certain drugs, the small theoretical risk they pose may be overshadowed by your need for treatment.

What should I do if I miss a dose of this medication?

Here you will find advice on what to do if you forget to take a dose. For many medications, the best option is to skip the dose you missed and return to your regular dosing schedule. Never take two doses at one time.

How should I store this medication?

This section provides general storage information as well as any special requirements that may apply.

OTHER FEATURES

Drug Identification Guide

This full-color guide includes actual-sized photographs of the leading products discussed in the book, arranged alphabetically by brand name. Manufacturers occasionally change the color and shape of a product, so if a prescription does not match the photo shown here, check with your pharmacist before assuming there's been a mistake.

The Appendices

This section provides you with two important safeguards that every home should always have handy: Appendix 1 is a brief guide to safe medication use; Appendix 2 is a directory of poison control centers nationwide. In addition, Appendix 3 lists the 200 most commonly prescribed drugs in the U.S.

The Disease and Disorder Index

This index helps you quickly identify drugs available for a particular medical condition. Arranged alphabetically by ailment, it lists all the medications profiled in the book.

THE PDR®

POCKET GUIDE

TO PRESCRIPTION DRUGS™

Drug Profiles

Abacavir sulfate *See Ziagen, page 1475.*

Abacavir, lamivudine, and zidovudine *See Trizivir, page 1338.*

ABILIFY/ABILIFY DISCMELT
Generic name: Aripiprazole

What is Abilify/Abilify Discmelt?
Abilify is an antipsychotic drug used for the treatment of schizophrenia in adults and adolescents 13 to 17 years old. It is also used to treat manic and mixed episodes associated with bipolar disorder in adults and children and adolescents 10 to 17 years old. Abilify may also be used with antidepressants to treat major depressive disorder in adults.

What is the most important information I should know about Abilify/Abilify Discmelt?
Abilify is not approved for elderly patients with dementia-related psychosis due to the risk of death.

If you or a family member notices new signs of nervousness, agitation, panic attacks, sleeplessness, irritability, aggressiveness, and other mood changes on a day-to-day basis, notify your doctor right away. These signs may be associated with an increased risk of suicidal thinking. People taking antidepressants should be monitored closely for changes in mood and/or behavior. Abilify is not approved for use in pediatric patients with depression.

Hyperglycemia, or elevated blood sugar, may occur when taking Abilify. If you have diabetes, monitor your blood sugar levels carefully.

If you have kidney and/or liver disease, you should be monitored closely while taking Abilify.

Report any sudden changes in temperature, heart rate (arrhythmia), or heart palpitations to your doctor, as these may be symptoms of a serious side effect. Also report any involuntary movements, seizures, or the inability to swallow while taking Abilify.

Who should not take Abilify/Abilify Discmelt?
Elderly patients with dementia-related psychosis should not receive Abilify.

What should I tell my doctor before I take the first dose of Abilify/Abilify Discmelt?

Tell your doctor about all prescription, over-the-counter, and herbal medications you are taking before beginning treatment with Abilify. Also, talk to your doctor about your complete medical history, especially if you have diabetes, high blood pressure, heart disease, or are recovering from a heart attack.

What is the usual dosage?

The information below is based on the dosage guidelines your doctor uses. Depending on your condition and medical history, your doctor may prescribe a different regimen. Do not change the dosage or stop taking your medication without your doctor's approval.

Bipolar Disorder
Adults: The initial dose is 15 milligrams (mg) daily, which can be increased to 30 mg daily if needed. Treatment may be as long as 6 weeks.

Children and adolescents 10 to 17 years old: The recommended dose is 10 mg daily, as monotherapy or adjuvant therapy with lithium or valproate. The initial dose is usually 2 mg daily, which may be increased to 10 mg daily over a period of 4 days.

Major Depressive Disorder
Adults: The recommended starting dose as add-on treatment for people already taking an antidepressant is 2 to 5 mg daily. The dose may be increased up to 15 mg daily if necessary.

Schizophrenia
Adults: The recommended starting dose is 10 to 15 mg daily. Dosage increases, if necessary, can be made 2 weeks after therapy has started.

Adolescents 13 to 17 years old: The recommended starting dose is 10 mg daily, which may be increased to 15 mg daily if needed.

How should I take Abilify/Abilify Discmelt?

Abilify tablets should be taken as one dose, with or without food, as directed.

For the Abilify Discmelt orally disintegrating tablets, use dry hands to remove the tablet, and place the entire tablet on your tongue. Tablet disintegration occurs rapidly in saliva. Although it is recommended to take the disintegrating tablet without liquid, you may do so if needed. Do not attempt to split the tablets.

What should I avoid while taking Abilify/Abilify Discmelt?

Because Abilify has the potential to impair judgment, thinking, or motor skills, use caution when operating machinery, including automobiles, until you know how Abilify affects you.

Avoid drinking alcohol during treatment with Abilify.

Avoid rapid movements, such as quickly rising from a seated or lying position. Side effects such as dizziness and fainting have been reported with Abilify due to a sudden change in heart rate or blood pressure when changing positions quickly.

Avoid strenuous exercise, or prolonged exposure to heat, since this could contribute to a rise in core body temperature, and dehydration.

Avoid excessive sugar intake if you have diabetes, since Abilify may elevate blood sugar levels.

What are possible food and drug interactions associated with Abilify/Abilify Discmelt?

If Abilify is used with certain other drugs, the effects of either could be increased, decreased, or altered. It is especially important to check with your doctor before combining Abilify with the following: alcohol, blood pressure medication, carbamazepine, fluoxetine, ketoconazole, paroxetine, and quinidine.

What are the possible side effects of Abilify/Abilify Discmelt?

Side effects cannot be anticipated. If any develop or change in intensity, tell your doctor as soon as possible. Only your doctor can determine if it is safe for you to continue taking this drug.

Side effects may include: nausea, vomiting, constipation, headache, dizziness, nervousness, sleeplessness, restlessness, tremors

Can I receive Abilify/Abilify Discmelt if I am pregnant or breastfeeding?

The effects of Abilify during pregnancy and breastfeeding are unknown. Tell your doctor immediately if you are pregnant, plan to become pregnant, or are breastfeeding.

What should I do if I miss a dose of Abilify/Abilify Discmelt?

Since Abilify is taken once daily, take the missed dose as soon as you remember. If the next dose is within 12 hours, skip the missed dose and continue with your normal dosing schedule. Never double the dose.

How should I store Abilify/Abilify Discmelt?

Store at room temperature.

ACCOLATE
Generic name: Zafirlukast

What is Accolate?
Accolate is used for the long-term treatment of asthma in adults and children 5 years and older.

What is the most important information I should know about Accolate?
Accolate will not stop an asthma attack once it starts. You will still need to use an airway-opening medication when an attack occurs. Also, this drug may cause liver problems (see "What are the possible side effects of this medication?" for symptoms).

Who should not take Accolate?
Do not begin treatment with Accolate if you are allergic to any of its ingredients.

What should I tell my doctor before I take the first dose of Accolate?
Tell your doctor about all prescription, over-the-counter, and herbal medication you are taking before beginning treatment with Accolate. Also talk to your doctor about your complete medical history, especially if you have liver problems or you are pregnant or breastfeeding.

What is the usual dosage?
The information below is based on the dosage guidelines your doctor uses. Depending on your condition and medical history, your doctor may prescribe a different regimen. Do not change the dosage or stop taking your medication without your doctor's approval.

Adults and children 12 years and older: The recommended dose is 20 milligrams (mg) twice daily.

Children 5-11 years: The recommended dose is 10 mg twice daily.

How should I take Accolate?
A full stomach can reduce Accolate's effectiveness. You should take it at least 1 hour before or 2 hours after a meal.

What should I avoid while taking Accolate?
While taking Accolate, avoid stopping—or even cutting down on—any other asthma medication you are using unless your doctor recommends it. Accolate is not an airway-opening medication. You will still need an inhaler to stop an attack.

What are possible food and drug interactions associated with Accolate?

If Accolate is taken with certain other drugs, the effects of either could be increased, decreased, or altered. It is especially important to check with your doctor before combining Accolate with aspirin, astemizole, blood-thinning drugs, carbamazepine, cyclosporine, erythromycin, heart and blood pressure medications, phenytoin, terfenadine, theophylline, and tolbutamide.

What are the possible side effects of Accolate?

Side effects cannot be anticipated. If any develop or change in intensity, tell your doctor as soon as possible. Only your doctor can determine if it is safe for you to continue taking this drug.

Side effects may include: accidental injury, back pain, bone/joint pain, diarrhea, dizziness, fever, headache, infection, muscle pain, nausea, upset stomach, vomiting

Cases of life-threatening liver failure have been reported in people taking Accolate. Contact your doctor immediately if you develop signs of a liver problem, including flu-like symptoms, jaundice (yellowing of the skin and eyes), itching, loss of appetite, nausea, sleepiness, or stomach pain.

Can I receive Accolate if I am pregnant or breastfeeding?

The effects of Accolate during pregnancy and breastfeeding are unknown. Talk with your doctor before taking this drug if you are pregnant, plan to become pregnant, or are breastfeeding.

What should I do if I miss a dose of Accolate?

Take it as soon as you remember. If it is almost time for your next dose, skip the one you missed and go back to your regular schedule. Do not take 2 doses at once.

How should I store Accolate?

Store at room temperature, in a dark place.

ACCUPRIL

Generic name: Quinapril hydrochloride

What is Accupril?

Accupril is an ACE inhibitor used to treat high blood pressure. It can be taken alone or in combination with a thiazide diuretic such as hydrochlorothiazide. Accupril is also used in combination with other drugs to treat congestive heart failure.

What is the most important information I should know about Accupril?

When used in the second and third trimester of pregnancy, Accupril may cause severe harm or death to the fetus.

Accupril does not cure high blood pressure, but keeps it under control. This drug must be taken regularly in order to keep blood pressure in a normal range.

Who should not take Accupril?

Do not begin treatment with Accupril if you are allergic to any of its ingredients, or if you have had reactions to another ACE inhibitor.

What should I tell my doctor before I take the first dose of Accupril?

Tell your doctor about all prescription, over-the-counter, and herbal medications you are taking before beginning treatment with Accupril. Also, talk to your doctor about your complete medical history, especially if you have kidney problems or you are undergoing surgery while being treated with this drug.

What is the usual dosage?

The information below is based on the dosage guidelines your doctor uses. Depending on your condition and medical history, your doctor may prescribe a different regimen. Do not change the dosage or stop taking your medication without your doctor's approval.

High Blood Pressure
Adults: The usual starting dosage is 10-20 milligrams (mg) per day. Afterward, the dosage may range from 20-80 mg daily.

Heart Failure
Adults: The usual starting dosage is 5 mg twice daily. Afterward, the dosage may range from 20-40 mg given daily in divided doses.

How should I take Accupril?

Accupril can be taken with or without food.

What should I avoid while taking Accupril?

Avoid drinking alcohol while taking Accupril, as it may cause dizziness or fainting.

What are possible food and drug interactions associated with Accupril?

If Accupril is taken with certain other drugs, the effects of either could be increased, decreased, or altered. It is especially important to check with your doctor before combining Accupril with diuretics, lithium, magnesium, potassium-sparing diuretics, potassium supplements, salt substitutes containing potassium, and tetracycline.

What are the possible side effects of Accupril?

Side effects cannot be anticipated. If any develop or change in intensity, tell your doctor as soon as possible. Only your doctor can determine if it is safe for you to continue taking this drug.

Side effects may include: dizziness, headache, nausea, sleepiness, stomach pain, vomiting

Can I receive Accupril if I am pregnant or breastfeeding?

The effects of Accupril during the first trimester of pregnancy are unknown. Do not take Accupril during the second and third trimesters, as it may cause severe harm or death to the fetus. Talk with your doctor before taking this drug if you are pregnant, plan to become pregnant, or are breastfeeding.

What should I do if I miss a dose of Accupril?

Take the forgotten dose as soon as you remember. However, if it is almost time for your next dose, skip the one you missed and go back to your regular schedule. Never try to catch up by doubling the dose.

How should I store Accupril?

Store at room temperature away from light.

ACCURETIC

*Generic name: Quinapril hydrochloride
and hydrochlorothiazide*

What is Accuretic?

Accuretic is used to treat high blood pressure. It combines two medications, the ACE inhibitor quinapril and the diuretic hydrochlorothiazide. This medication is not used for the initial treatment of high blood pressure, but only when other medications are not sufficient.

What is the most important information I should know about Accuretic?

Accuretic may cause swelling of the face, lips, tongue or throat, arms and legs, or cause difficulty with swallowing or breathing. This drug may also cause kidney and liver problems, and should not be taken during pregnancy. Accuretic can cause severe development problems during pregnancy.

Who should not take Accuretic?
Do not begin treatment with Accuretic if you are allergic to any of its ingredients, or have had angioedema (skin swelling).

What should I tell my doctor before I take the first dose of Accuretic?
Tell your doctor about all prescription, over-the-counter, and herbal medications you are taking before beginning therapy with Accuretic. Also, talk to your doctor about your complete medical history, especially if you have diabetes, a liver problem, or will be undergoing surgery while on this drug.

What is the usual dosage?
The information below is based on the dosage guidelines your doctor uses. Depending on your condition and medical history, your doctor may prescribe a different regimen. Do not change the dosage or stop taking your medication without your doctor's approval.

Adults: The usual dosage range is 10-20 milligrams (mg) of quinapril and 12.5-25 mg of hydrochlorothiazide, taken once daily.

How should I take Accuretic?
Accuretic may be taken with or without meals.

What should I avoid while taking Accuretic?
Avoid drinking alcohol while being treated with Accuretic. This drug may cause dizziness when combined with alcohol.

What are possible food and drug interactions associated with Accuretic?
If Accuretic is taken with certain other drugs, the effects of either could be increased, decreased, or altered. It is especially important to check with your doctor before combining Accuretic with barbiturates such as phenobarbital, cholestyramine, colestipol, corticosteroids, insulin, digoxin, diuretics, lithium, painkillers, nonsteroidal anti-inflammatory drugs, norepinephrine, other high blood pressure medications, potassium-sparing diuretics, potassium supplements, salt substitutes containing potassium, and tetracycline.

What are the possible side effects of Accuretic?
Side effects cannot be anticipated. If any develop or change in intensity, tell your doctor as soon as possible. Only your doctor can determine if it is safe for you to continue taking this drug.

Side effects may include: back pain, chest pain, coughing, diarrhea, dizziness, headache, muscle aches, nausea, sleeplessness, sleepiness, sore throat, stomach pain, upset stomach, vomiting

Can I receive Accuretic if I am pregnant or breastfeeding?

The effects of Accuretic on pregnancy in the first trimester are unknown. During the second and third trimesters, Accuretic may cause severe harm to the fetus. Talk with your doctor before taking this drug if you are pregnant, plan to become pregnant, or are breastfeeding.

What should I do if I miss a dose of Accuretic?

Take it as soon as you remember. If it is almost time for your next dose, skip the one you missed and go back to your regular schedule. Never take 2 doses at the same time.

How should I store Accuretic?

Store at room temperature.

ACCUTANE
Generic name: Isotretinoin

What is Accutane?

Accutane is a medication taken by mouth to clear up the most severe form of acne, nodular acne. Accutane should only be used if other forms of treatment have not worked, including antibiotics. Accutane can only be prescribed by doctors that are registered in the iPLEDGE program, dispensed by a pharmacy that is registered with the iPLEDGE program, and given to patients who are registered in the iPLEDGE program, who understand and agree to do everything required in the program.

What is the most important information I should know about Accutane?

Accutane may cause birth defects, miscarriage, death of a baby, and early births; therefore, it can only be used by patients enrolled in the iPLEDGE program. Females should not become pregnant if they or their partners are taking Accutane. Pregnancy should be avoided 1 month before taking this drug, while taking it, and 1 month after therapy has ended.

If you get pregnant while taking Accutane, stop taking it immediately and call your doctor right away. Doctors and patients should report all cases of pregnancy to: FDA MedWatch at 1-800-FDA-1088, and the iPLEDGE pregnancy registry at 1-866-495-0654.

This drug may also cause serious mental health problems such as depression, psychosis, and suicidal thoughts. If you or a family member notices signs and symptoms of depression or psychosis, stop Accutane and call your doctor right away. You may also need follow-up mental healthcare if you had any symptoms of depression or psychosis after stopping Accutane.

Who should not take Accutane?
Do not take Accutane if you are pregnant, plan to become pregnant, or become pregnant during therapy. Also, talk to your doctor about the ingredients of this drug to make sure you are not allergic to anything in it.

What should I tell my doctor before I take the first dose of Accutane?
Tell your doctor about all prescription, over-the-counter, and herbal medications you are taking before beginning treatment with Accutane. Also, talk to your doctor about your complete medical history, especially if you have asthma, bone loss/weak bones (osteoporosis), diabetes, an eating disorder (anorexia), heart problems, liver disease, mental problems, and allergies to foods or medications.

What is the usual dosage?
The information below is based on the dosage guidelines your doctor uses. Depending on your condition and medical history, your doctor may prescribe a different regimen. Do not change the dosage or stop taking your medication without your doctor's approval.

The usual dosage of Accutane is between 0.5 to 1 milligram (mg) per kilogram (kg) per day, taken twice a day, depending on what your doctor prescribes.

How should I take Accutane?
Accutane should be taken 2 times a day with a meal, unless told otherwise by your doctor. Swallow Accutane capsules whole with a full glass of water; do not chew or suck on the capsules.

What should I avoid while taking Accutane?
While being treated with Accutane, do not breastfeed, drive at night, get pregnant, give blood, have waxing, dermabrasion, or laser procedures performed on your face, stay in sunlight and under ultraviolet light (tanning beds), take other medicines or herbal products, or share Accutane with other people.

What are possible food and drug interactions associated with Accutane?
Consult with your doctor before taking antibiotics, corticosteroids, Dilantin (phenytoin), progestin-only birth control pills (mini pills), St. John's wort, and vitamin A supplements.

What are the possible side effects of Accutane?
Side effects cannot be anticipated. If any develop or change in intensity, tell your doctor as soon as possible. Only your doctor can determine if it is safe for you to continue taking this drug.

Side effects may include: back pain, birth defects in babies, blood sugar changes, blurred vision, broken bones, chapped lips, dark urine, diarrhea, dizziness, decreased red and while blood cells, dry eyes, dry nose leading to nosebleeds, dry skin, headache, heartburn, hearing problems, joint pain, painful swallowing, lipid (fats and cholesterol in blood) problems, muscle weakness/damage, nausea/vomiting, rectal bleeding, seizures, serious mental health problems, severe stomach/chest/bowel pain, stroke, yellowing of skin/eyes, vision problems, serious allergic reactions

Can I receive Accutane if I am pregnant or breastfeeding?

Do not take Accutane if you are pregnant. Do not become pregnant if you are receiving treatment with Accutane. This drug causes severe developmental problems during pregnancy, and may result in loss of the child. Also, do not nurse while on Accutane, as the drug may pass into breast milk.

What should I do if I miss a dose of Accutane?

If you miss a dose of Accutane, skip it and continue on your regular schedule. Do not take 2 doses at the same time.

How should I store Accutane?

Store at room temperature, away from light.

Acebutolol hydrochloride See Sectral, page 1179.

ACEON

Generic name: Perindopril erbumine

What is Aceon?

Aceon is a medicine that is used to control high blood pressure. Aceon is also used for people who have a heart condition called stable coronary artery disease to lower the risk of developing a heart attack or death due to a cardiovascular event.

What is the most important information I should know about Aceon?

A possible side effect of Aceon is angioedema or swelling. If you develop any symptoms suggesting angioedema (swelling of face, extremities, eyes, lips, tongue, hoarseness or difficulty in swallowing or breathing) stop taking Aceon and contact your doctor immediately.

Lightheadedness may occur, especially during the first few days of therapy. Tell your doctor if you experience this. If you faint while taking Aceon, stop taking it and contact your doctor.

Do not use salt substitutes with potassium or potassium supplements without telling your doctor first.

Tell your doctor if you are pregnant, plan to become pregnant, or are breastfeeding while taking Aceon.

Who should not take Aceon?

Aceon should not be used in patients that are allergic to the ingredients of Aceon or are allergic to a class of blood pressure medications called ACE inhibitors. Aceon should not be used in patients that have a history of swelling of the face and hands with blood pressure medications.

What should I tell my doctor before I take the first dose of Aceon?

Tell your doctor about all prescription, over-the-counter, and herbal medication you are taking before beginning treatment with Aceon. Also, talk to your doctor about your complete medical history, especially if you have ever developed swelling or allergic reactions while taking blood pressure medications.

What is the usual dosage?

The information below is based on the dosage guidelines your doctor uses. Depending on your condition and medical history, your doctor may prescribe a different regimen. Do not change the dosage or stop taking your medication without your doctor's approval.

Stable Coronary Artery Disease
Adults: The recommended initial dose of 4 mg once daily for 2 weeks, and then increased as tolerated, to a maintenance dose of 8 mg once daily.

High Blood Pressure
Adults: The recommended initial dose is 4 mg once a day. The dosage may be titrated upward until blood pressure, when measured just before the next dose, is controlled or to a maximum of 16 mg per day. The usual maintenance dose range is 4 to 8 mg administered as a single daily dose.

The Aceon dosage may need to be adjusted for people over 65 years.

How should I take Aceon?

You should take this medicine exactly how the doctor prescribed.

What should I avoid while taking Aceon?

You should avoid becoming pregnant or breastfeeding while taking Aceon.

What are possible food and drug interactions associated with Aceon?

If Aceon is taken with certain other drugs, the effect of either medication could be increased, decreased, or altered. Aceon should be used cautiously with the following: lithium, potassium supplements, or potassium-sparing diuretics such as spironolactone, amiloride, and triamterene.

What are the possible side effects of Aceon?

Side effects cannot be anticipated. If any develop or change in intensity, tell your doctor as soon as possible. Only your doctor can determine if it is safe for you to continue taking this drug.

Side effects may include: cough, back pain, viral infection, upper extremity pain, sinusitis, heart burn, fever, ear infection, palpations

Can I receive Aceon if I am pregnant or breastfeeding?

Aceon should not be used during pregnancy. If you become pregnant while taking Aceon, stop taking this medication and contact your doctor. The effect of Aceon during breastfeeding is unknown. Tell your doctor immediately if you are pregnant, plan to become pregnant, or are breastfeeding.

What should I do if I miss a dose of Aceon?

If you miss a dose, take it with food as soon as you remember. If you do not remember until it is time for your next dose, skip the missed dose and go back to your regular schedule. Do not take two doses at the same time.

How should I store Aceon?

Store at room temperature and protect from moisture.

Acetaminophen and codeine phosphate See *Tylenol with Codeine, page 1346.*

Acetaminophen and oxycodone hydrochloride See *Percocet, page 1000.*

ACETAZOLAMIDE SODIUM

What is Acetazolamide sodium?

Acetazolamide controls fluid secretion. It is used in the treatment of glaucoma (excessive pressure in the eyes), epilepsy (for both brief and unlocalized seizures), and fluid retention due to congestive heart failure or drugs. It is also used to prevent or relieve the symptoms of acute mountain sickness in climbers attempting a rapid climb and those who feel sick even though they are making a gradual climb.

What is the most important information I should know about Acetazolamide sodium?

This drug is considered to be a sulfa drug because of its chemical properties. Although rare, severe reactions have been reported with sulfa drugs. If you develop a rash, bruises, sore throat, or fever contact your doctor immediately.

Who should not take Acetazolamide sodium?

Your doctor will not prescribe this medication for you if your sodium or potassium levels are low, or if you have kidney or liver disease, including cirrhosis. Acetazolamide should not be used as a long-term treatment for the type of glaucoma called chronic noncongestive angle-closure glaucoma.

What should I tell my doctor before I take the first dose of Acetazolamide sodium?

Tell your doctor about all prescription, over-the-counter, and herbal medication you are taking before beginning treatment with this drug. Also, talk to your doctor about your complete medical history, especially if you have emphysema or other breathing disorders, or take high doses of aspirin. The effects of combining acetazolamide with aspirin can range from loss of appetite, sluggishness, and rapid breathing to unresponsiveness; the combination can be fatal.

What is the usual dosage?

The information below is based on the dosage guidelines your doctor uses. Depending on your condition and medical history, your doctor may prescribe a different regimen. Do not change the dosage or stop taking your medication without your doctor's approval.

This medication is available in both oral and injectable form. Dosages below are for the oral form only.

Glaucoma

Adults: This medication is used as an addition to regular glaucoma treatment. Dosages for open-angle glaucoma range from 250 milligrams to 1 gram per 24 hours in 2 or more smaller doses. Your doctor will supervise your dosage and watch the effect of this medication carefully if you are using it for glaucoma. In secondary glaucoma and before surgery in acute congestive (closed-angle) glaucoma, the usual dosage is 250 milligrams every 4 hours or, in some cases, 250 milligrams twice a day. Some people may take 500 milligrams to start, and then 125 or 250 milligrams every 4 hours. The injectable form of this drug is occasionally used in acute cases.

The usual dosage of the sustained-release capsules is 1 capsule (500 milligrams) twice a day, usually in the morning and evening.

Your doctor may adjust the dosage, as needed.

Epilepsy
Adults: The daily dosage is 8 to 30 milligrams per 2.2 pounds of body weight in 2 or more doses. Typical dosage may range from 375 to 1,000 milligrams per day. Your doctor will adjust the dosage to suit your needs; acetazolamide can be used with other anticonvulsant medication.

Congestive Heart Failure
Adults: The usual starting dosage to reduce fluid retention in people with congestive heart failure is 250 milligrams to 375 milligrams per day or 5 milligrams per 2.2 pounds of body weight, taken in the morning. Acetazolamide works best when it is taken every other day—or 2 days on, 1 day off—for this condition.

Edema Due to Medication
Adults: The usual dose is 250 milligrams to 375 milligrams daily for 1 or 2 days, alternating with a day of rest.

Acute Mountain Sickness
Adults: The usual dose is 500 milligrams to 1,000 milligrams a day in 2 or more doses, using either tablets or sustained-release capsules. Doses of this medication are often begun 1 or 2 days before attempting to reach high altitudes.

How should I take Acetazolamide sodium?
Take this medication exactly as prescribed by your doctor. If you are taking acetazolamide to help in rapid ascent of a mountain, you must still come down promptly if you show signs of severe mountain sickness.

What are possible food and drug interactions associated with Acetazolamide sodium?
If acetazolamide is taken with certain other drugs, the effects of either could be increased, decreased, or altered. It is especially important to check with your doctor before combining acetazolamide with the following: amitriptyline, amphetamines such as dextroamphetamine, aspirin, cyclosporine, lithium, methenamine, oral diabetes drugs such as glyburide, and quinidine.

What are the possible side effects of Acetazolamide sodium?
Side effects cannot be anticipated. If any develop or change in intensity, inform your doctor as soon as possible. Only your doctor can determine if it is safe for you to continue taking acetazolamide.

Side effects may include: change in taste, diarrhea, increase in amount or frequency of urination, loss of appetite, nausea, ringing in the ears, tingling or pins and needles in hands or feet, vomiting

Can I receive Acetazolamide sodium if I am pregnant or breastfeeding?

The effects of acetazolamide during pregnancy have not been adequately studied. If you are pregnant or plan to become pregnant, inform your doctor immediately. Acetazolamide may appear in breast milk and could affect a nursing infant. Consult your doctor if you plan on breastfeeding.

What should I do if I miss a dose of Acetazolamide sodium?

If you miss a dose of this drug, skip it. Do not take an extra dose to make up for missed doses.

How should I store Acetazolamide sodium?

Store at room temperature.

Acetyl sulfisoxazole *See Gantrisin, page 606.*

ACIPHEX

Generic name: Rabeprazole sodium

What is AcipHex?

AcipHex is used to treat gastroesophageal reflux disease (GERD), secretion problems like Zollinger-Ellison syndrome, and with clarithromycin and amoxicillin for ulcers of the small intestine. GERD is caused by the constant backflow of stomach acid into your throat. Zollinger-Ellison syndrome occurs when the stomach begins to produce too much acid.

Also, AcipHex is sometimes combined with the antibiotics amoxicillin and clarithromycin to treat infections caused by *H. pylori,* a type of bacteria that lives in the digestive tract and is often associated with recurrent ulcers.

What is the most important information I should know about AcipHex?

To treat ulcers of the small intestine, AcipHex should not be taken with clarithromycin if you are pregnant. Clarithromycin may cause harm to the unborn child. Amoxicillin should not be taken at the same time as penicillin; this combination may have a fatal interaction.

Who should not take AcipHex?

Do not begin treatment with AcipHex if you are allergic to any of its ingredients. Also, this drug should not be used if you are already taking medications containing cisapride or pimozide.

What should I tell my doctor before I take the first dose of AcipHex?

Tell your doctor about all prescription, over-the-counter, and herbal medications you are taking before beginning treatment with AcipHex. Also, talk to your doctor about your complete medical history, especially if you have ulcers caused by *H. pylori*. Alone, AcipHex may make these ulcers worse, so an antibiotic should be prescribed to take with this drug.

What is the usual dosage?

The information below is based on the dosage guidelines your doctor uses. Depending on your condition and medical history, your doctor may prescribe a different regimen. Do not change the dosage or stop taking your medication without your doctor's approval.

Healing and Maintenance of GERD
Adults: The recommended dose is one 20 milligrams (mg) delayed-release tablet taken once daily for 4-8 weeks.

Healing of Duodenal Ulcers
Adults: The recommended dose is one 20 mg delayed-release tablet to be taken once daily after the morning meal for a period up to 4 weeks.

Treatment of Zollinger-Ellison Syndrome
Adults: The recommended dose is 60 mg once per day.

How should I take AcipHex?

AcipHex alone may be taken with or without food. All three medications (AcipHex, amoxicillin, clarithromycin) should be taken twice daily with the morning and evening meals.

What should I avoid while taking AcipHex?

Do not crush, split, or chew the tablets.

What are possible food and drug interactions associated with AcipHex?

If AcipHex is taken with certain other drugs, the effects of either could be increased, decreased, or altered. It is especially important to check with your doctor before combining AcipHex with cyclosporine, digoxin, ketoconazole, or warfarin.

What are the possible side effects of AcipHex?

Side effects cannot be anticipated. If any develop or change in intensity, tell your doctor as soon as possible. Only your doctor can determine if it is safe for you to continue taking this drug.

Side effects may include: allergic reaction, bone pain, chest pain, chills, constipation, diarrhea, dry mouth, fever, gas, leg cramps, light sensitivity, migraines, nausea, sore throat, upset stomach, vomiting

Can I receive AcipHex if I am pregnant or breastfeeding?
The effects of AcipHex during pregnancy and breastfeeding are unknown. Talk with your doctor before taking this drug if you are pregnant, plan to become pregnant, or are breastfeeding.

What should I do if I miss a dose of AcipHex?
Take it as soon as you remember. If it is almost time for your next dose, skip the one you missed and go back to your regular schedule. Do not take two doses at once.

How should I store AcipHex?
Store at room temperature, away from moisture.

Acitretin See Soriatane, page 1209.

ACLOVATE
Generic name: Alclometasone dipropionate

What is Aclovate?
Aclovate is used to treat skin problems marked by rashes and itching, such as psoriasis.

What is the most important information I should know about Aclovate?
Aclovate should not be applied to large areas of skin, or covered with a bandage or dressing. This may increase the absorption of this drug, causing a reaction in the rest of the body.

Who should not take Aclovate?
Do not begin therapy with Aclovate if you are allergic to any of its ingredients.

What should I tell my doctor before I take the first dose of Aclovate?
Tell your doctor about all prescription, over-the-counter, and herbal medications you are taking before beginning treatment with Aclovate. Also talk to your doctor about your complete medical history.

What is the usual dosage?
The information below is based on the dosage guidelines your doctor uses. Depending on your condition and medical history, your doctor may prescribe a different regimen. Do not change the dosage or stop taking your medication without your doctor's approval.

Adults and children 1 year and older: The usual dosage is given by massaging a thin film of cream or ointment over the affected area 2 or 3 times a day.

How should I take Aclovate?

Apply a thin film of Aclovate cream or ointment to the affected skin areas and massage gently until the medication disappears. Do not apply this cream or ointment to face, underarms, or groin areas, unless you are directed by your doctor to do so.

What should I avoid while taking Aclovate?

Avoid using bandages or dressings on the areas of your body treated with Aclovate.

What are possible food and drug interactions associated with Aclovate?

Check with your doctor before combining Aclovate with other more potent steroids, since this could lead to large amounts of steroid hormone circulating in your bloodstream.

What are the possible side effects of Aclovate?

Side effects cannot be anticipated. If any develop or change in intensity, tell your doctor as soon as possible. Only your doctor can determine if it is safe for you to continue taking this drug.

Side effects may include: burning sensation, color change of the skin, dryness, irritation, rash, redness

Can I receive Aclovate if I am pregnant or breastfeeding?

The effects of Aclovate during pregnancy and breastfeeding are unknown. Talk with your doctor before taking this drug if you are pregnant, plan to become pregnant, or are breastfeeding.

What should I do if I miss a dose of Aclovate?

Apply it as soon as you remember. If it is almost time for the next dose, skip the one you missed and go back to your regular schedule.

How should I store Aclovate?

Store at room temperature.

ACTIGALL
Generic name: Ursodiol

What is Actigall?

Actigall is used to help dissolve certain kinds of gallstones. It is also used to prevent gallstones in people on rapid-weight-loss diets.

What is the most important information I should know about Actigall?

Actigall is not a quick remedy. It takes months of Actigall therapy to dissolve gallstones; and there is a possibility of incomplete dissolution and recurrence of stones. Your doctor will weigh Actigall against alternative treatments and recommend the best one for you.

Actigall is most effective if your gallstones are small or "floatable" (high in cholesterol). In addition, your gallbladder must still be functioning properly.

Although Actigall is not known to cause liver damage, it is theoretically possible in some people. Your doctor may run blood tests for liver function before you start to take Actigall and again while you are taking it.

Who should not take Actigall?

Do not take this medication if you are sensitive to or have ever had an allergic reaction to ursodiol or to other bile acids.

Actigall will not dissolve certain types of gallstones. If your doctor tells you that your gallstones are calcified cholesterol stones, radio-opaque stones, or radiolucent bile pigment stones, you are not a candidate for treatment with Actigall.

Also, if you have biliary tract (liver, gallbladder, bile duct) problems or certain liver and pancreas diseases, your doctor may not be able to prescribe Actigall for you.

What should I tell my doctor before I take the first dose of Actigall?

Tell your doctor about all prescription, over-the-counter, and herbal medications you are taking before beginning treatment with Actigall. Also talk to your doctor about your complete medical history.

What is the usual dosage?

The information below is based on the dosage guidelines your doctor uses. Depending on your condition and medical history, your doctor may prescribe a different regimen. Do not change the dosage or stop taking your medication without your doctor's approval.

Dissolving Gallstones
Adults: The recommended daily dosage is 8-10 milligrams (mg) per 2.2 pounds of body weight, divided into 2 or 3 doses.

Preventing Gallstones
Adults: The usual dose in people losing weight rapidly is 300 milligrams twice a day.

How should I take Actigall?

Take Actigall exactly as prescribed; otherwise the gallstones may dissolve too slowly or not dissolve at all. During treatment, your doctor will do periodic ultrasound exams to see if your stones are dissolving.

What should I avoid while taking Actigall?

Avoid missing doses or taking extra doses.

What are possible food and drug interactions associated with Actigall?

If Actigall is taken with certain other drugs, the effects of either could be increased, decreased, or altered. It is especially important to check with your doctor before combining Actigall with the following: aluminum-based antacid medications, cholesterol-lowering medications, estrogens, and oral contraceptives.

What are the possible side effects of Actigall?

Side effects cannot be anticipated. If any develop or change in intensity, tell your doctor as soon as possible. Only your doctor can determine if it is safe for you to continue taking this drug.

Side effects may include: abdominal pain, back pain, bronchitis, constipation, coughing, diarrhea, gas, headache, indigestion, joint pain, muscle pain, nausea, sinus inflammation or infection, sore throat, upper respiratory tract infection, viral infection, vomiting

Can I receive Actigall if I am pregnant or breastfeeding?

If you are pregnant or plan to become pregnant, inform your doctor immediately. So far, there is no evidence that ursodiol can harm an unborn baby; but to be safe, the medication is not recommended during pregnancy. Caution is needed during breastfeeding; it is not known whether ursodiol taken by a nursing mother passes into her breast milk.

What should I do if I miss a dose of Actigall?

Take it as soon as you remember, or at the same time as the next dose.

How should I store Actigall?

Store at room temperature in a tightly closed container.

ACTIVELLA

Generic name: Estrogen and progestin

What is Activella?

Activella is used for hormone replacement therapy. It is used to relieve the symptoms of menopause and also to treat vaginal atrophy. In addition, Activella is prescribed to prevent osteoporosis in postmenopausal women.

What is the most important information I should know about Activella?

Because of the risk of uterine cancer, be sure to alert your doctor if you experience any abnormal vaginal bleeding. There is little, if any, increase in risk during the first year of treatment, but the odds rise substantially after 5 to 10 years.

In addition to increasing the chances of uterine cancer, estrogen replacement therapy may also raise the odds of breast cancer if taken at high doses or for long periods of time. Be sure to do a monthly self-exam of your breasts, and get regular mammograms.

Estrogen replacement therapy typically doubles the chances of gallbladder disease. Notify your doctor if you experience pain, tenderness, or swelling in your abdomen.

Estrogen replacement increases the risk of blood clots in the veins, especially during the first year of therapy. Call your doctor immediately if you experience any of the following warning signs: bulging eyes, changes in vision or speech, coughing up blood, dizziness, double vision, faintness, migraine, pains in the calves or chest, severe headache or vomiting, sudden shortness of breath, sudden vision loss, weakness or numbness of an arm or leg.

Estrogen therapy sometimes causes high blood pressure, so be sure to get periodic checkups. In women prone to high blood lipid levels, estrogen can also cause a sharp spike in triglycerides, possibly leading to pancreatitis. Fluid retention is another possibility. If it develops, it can aggravate conditions such as asthma, epilepsy, heart disease, kidney disease, and migraine.

Make sure your doctor knows if you have ever been diagnosed with depression. Treatment with hormone replacement therapy may need to be discontinued if depression recurs.

If you have diabetes, watch your blood sugar levels carefully. There's a chance that estrogen/progestin products may make diabetes worse.

Who should not take Activella?

Do not take Activella if you have any of the following: known or suspected breast cancer, any other cancer stimulated by estrogen, or a past history of breast cancer associated with estrogen use; unexplained genital bleeding; a history of blood clots or phlebitis; sensitivity to estrogen or progesterone; any reason to believe that you are pregnant.

If you've had your uterus removed, you don't need the progestin in these products, and should take a different type of hormone replacement therapy. You should also avoid Activella if you have a liver condition.

What should I tell my doctor before I take the first dose of Activella?

Tell your doctor about all prescription, over-the-counter, and herbal medications you are taking before beginning treatment with Activella. Also talk to your doctor about your complete medical history, especially if you have ever had cancer, diabetes, heart problems, gallbladder disease, depression, or if you have unexplained vaginal bleeding.

What is the usual dosage?

The information below is based on the dosage guidelines your doctor uses. Depending on your condition and medical history, your doctor may prescribe a different regimen. Do not change the dosage or stop taking your medication without your doctor's approval.

Adults: The recommended dose is one tablet daily.

How should I take Activella?

Take one tablet at the same time each day, with or without food. If you are taking the medication to relieve menopausal symptoms, your doctor will reevaluate your need for medication every 3 to 6 months.

What should I avoid while taking Activella?

Do not miss regularly scheduled checkups with your doctor while taking Activella. Be sure to have an annual gynecologic exam (including a breast exam and/or mammography).

What are possible food and drug interactions associated with Activella?

If estrogen is taken with certain other drugs, the effects of either could be increased, decreased, or altered. It is especially important to check with your doctor before combining estrogen with the following: St. John's wort, phenobarbital, carbamazepine, rifampin, erythromycin, clarithromycin, ketoconazole, itraconazole, ritonavir, and grapefruit juice.

What are the possible side effects of Activella?

Side effects cannot be anticipated. If any develop or change in intensity, tell your doctor as soon as possible. Only your doctor can determine if it is safe for you to continue taking this drug.

Side effects may include: abdominal pain, breast tenderness and enlargement, depression, enlargement of uterine fibroids, headache, nausea, nervousness, skin reddening, urinary tract infection, vaginal inflammation, vomiting

Can I receive Activella if I am pregnant or breastfeeding?

Although these medications are intended only for women who are no longer in their childbearing years, it's important to note that they should never be taken during pregnancy, since they can harm the developing baby. Additionally, estrogen decreases the quantity and quality of breast milk, and progesterone finds its way into the milk.

What should I do if I miss a dose of Activella?

Take it as soon as you remember. If it is almost time for your next dose, skip the one you missed and go back to your regular schedule. Never take 2 doses at the same time.

How should I store Activella?

Store at room temperature. Keep Activella in a tightly closed container away from moisture and light.

ACTONEL

Generic name: Risedronate sodium

What is Actonel?

Actonel is used to prevent and treat bone loss (osteoporosis) in postmenopausal women and to increase bone mass in men with the condition. Actonel is also used to prevent and treat osteoporosis in adults that is caused by treatment with steroid drugs such as prednisone. Osteoporosis can result in bone fractures. Actonel may reverse bone loss by stopping further loss of bone and increasing bone strength, although a difference may not be able to be seen or felt. Actonel helps lower the risk of fractures.

Actonel is also used to treat Paget's disease of bone in men and women.

What is the most important information I should know about Actonel?

Actonel, like all bisphosphonates, may cause problems in your stomach and esophagus (the tube that connects the mouth and the stomach), such as trouble swallowing (dysphagia), heartburn (esophagitis), and ulcers. You might feel pain in your bones, joints, or muscles. (See "What are the possible side effects of Actonel?").

You must follow the instructions exactly for Actonel to work and to lower the chance of serious side effects. (See "How should I take Actonel?")

Who should not take Actonel?

Do not take Actonel if you are allergic to any of its ingredients, have low blood calcium levels (hypocalcemia), cannot stand or sit upright for at least 30 minutes, or have kidneys that work poorly.

What should I tell my doctor before I take the first dose of Actonel?

Tell your doctor about all prescription, over-the-counter, and herbal medications you are taking to avoid a possible interaction with Actonel. Also, talk to your doctor about your complete medical history, especially if you are pregnant or planning to become pregnant, nursing or planning to nurse, or if you have kidney problems.

What is the usual dosage?

The information below is based on the dosage guidelines your doctor uses. Depending on your condition and medical history, your doctor may prescribe a different regimen. Do not change the dosage or stop taking your medication without your doctor's approval.

Prevention/Treatment of Osteoporosis

The recommended dose is one 35 milligram (mg) tablet taken once a week, one 5 mg-tablet taken daily, one 75 mg-tablet taken on 2 consecutive days for a total of 2 tablets each month, or one 150 mg-tablet taken once a month.

Treatment to Increase Bone Mass in Men with Osteoporosis

The recommended dose is one 35 mg-tablet taken once per week.

Prevention/Treatment of Glucocorticoid-Induced Osteoporosis

The recommended dose is one 5 mg-tablet taken daily.

Treatment of Paget's Disease

The recommended dose is one 30 mg-tablet taken once daily for 2 months. Retreatment may be necessary.

How should I take Actonel?

Take Actonel first thing in the morning, at least 30 minutes before you eat or drink anything other than plain water. Take Actonel while you are sitting up or standing with 6 to 8 ounces (about 1 cup) of plain water. Do not take it with coffee, tea, juice, milk, or other dairy drinks. Swallow Actonel whole. Do not chew the tablet or keep it in your mouth to melt or dissolve.

Take Actonel at least 30 minutes before lying down, eating, or drinking anything except plain water, and taking vitamins, calcium, or antacids. Take these at a different time of the day from when you take Actonel.

Take Actonel exactly as prescribed for as long as your healthcare provider tells you.

What should I avoid while taking Actonel?

Do not lie down for 30 minutes after taking the medication. Do not eat or drink anything except plain water before you take Actonel and for at least 30 minutes after you take it. Do not chew or suck on the tablet because it may irritate your mouth or throat. Foods and some vitamin supplements and medicines can stop your body from absorbing (using)

Actonel. Therefore, do not take anything other than plain water at or near the time you take Actonel.

What are possible food and drug interactions associated with Actonel?

Foods and some vitamin supplements, including calcium and antacids, and some medicines can stop your body from absorbing Actonel. (See "How should I take Actonel?")

What are the possible side effects of Actonel?

Side effects cannot be anticipated. If any develop or change in intensity, tell your doctor as soon as possible. Only your doctor can determine if it is safe for you to continue taking this drug.

Side effects may include: pain (back, chest, stomach, joints, muscles, bones), upset stomach, painful or difficult swallowing, heartburn, ulcers in your stomach and esophagus, constipation, diarrhea, gas, and headache, low calcium and other mineral disturbances, jaw bone problems (including infection and slower healing after teeth are pulled), shortlasting, mild flu-like symptoms, allergic and severe skin reactions, or eye inflammation (eye pain, redness, or sensitivity to light).

Can I receive Actonel if I am pregnant or breastfeeding?

The effects of Actonel during pregnancy and breastfeeding are unknown. Tell your doctor immediately if you are pregnant, planning to become pregnant, or are nursing.

What should I do if I miss a dose of Actonel?

If you miss a dose of your Actonel 5 mg in the morning, do not take it later in the day. Take only 1 Actonel 5 mg-tablet the next morning and continue your usual schedule of 1 tablet a day. Do not take 2 tablets on the same day.

If you miss a dose of your Actonel 35 mg in the morning, do not take it later in the day. Take only 1 Actonel 35 mg-tablet the next morning and continue your usual schedule of 1 tablet a week, as originally scheduled on your chosen day. Do not take 2 tablets on the same day.

If you miss one or both tablets of your dose of Actonel 75 mg on 2 consecutive days per month in the morning, do not take it later in the day. If the next month's scheduled doses are more than 7 days away, do the following:

If both tablets were missed, take only the first Actonel 75 mg-tablet on the morning after the day it is remembered and the second tablet on the next consecutive morning.

If only 1 tablet is missed, take the missed tablet on the morning after the day it is remembered.

Then continue your usual schedule of Actonel 75 mg on 2 consecutive days each month as originally scheduled. Do not take more than two 75 mg-tablets within 7 days.

If the next month's scheduled doses are 1 to 7 days away, wait until next month's scheduled doses and then resume taking Actonel 75 mg on 2 consecutive days each month as originally scheduled.

If you miss a dose of your Actonel 150 mg once-a-month in the morning, and the next month's scheduled dose is more than 7 days away, the missed tablet should be taken in the next morning after it is remembered. Then you should resume taking your Actonel 150 mg once-a-month as originally scheduled. Do not take more than one 150 mg-tablet within 7 days.

If you miss a dose of your Actonel 150 mg once-a-month in the morning, and the next month's scheduled dose is 1 to 7 days away, wait until next month's scheduled dose and then continue taking Actonel 150 mg once-a-month as originally scheduled.

If you are not sure what to do if you miss a dose, contact your healthcare provider.

How should I store Actonel?
Store at room temperature.

ACTONEL WITH CALCIUM
Generic name: Risedronate sodium with calcium carbonate

What is Actonel with Calcium?
Actonel is used to treat and prevent bone weakening (osteoporosis) in women going through menopause. Actonel not only stops osteoporosis, but may reverse the disease and increases bone mineral density. Actonel helps make bones stronger and less likely to fracture, especially for those over 50 and postmenopausal.

What is the most important information I should know about Actonel with Calcium?
Actonel may cause problems in your stomach and esophagus, such as trouble swallowing, heartburn, and ulcers. You might feel pain in your bones, joints, or muscles. Stop taking Actonel and tell your doctor if you experience chest pain, difficult or painful swallowing, or severe/continuing heartburn, as these may be signs of serious problems.

Who should not take Actonel with Calcium?
You should not take Actonel if you are allergic to any of the ingredients, cannot stand or sit upright for 30 minutes, if you have low blood calcium (hypocalcemia), or if you have kidney problems.

What should I tell my doctor before I take the first dose of Actonel with Calcium?

Tell your doctor about all prescription, over-the-counter, and herbal medications you are taking before beginning treatment with Actonel with calcium. Also, talk to your doctor about your complete medical history, especially if you are nursing, or are going to have surgery.

What is the usual dosage?

The information below is based on the dosage guidelines your doctor uses. Depending on your condition and medical history, your doctor may prescribe a different regimen. Do not change the dosage or stop taking your medication without your doctor's approval.

Actonel should be taken as one 35 milligram (mg) tablet orally once a week.

How should I take Actonel with Calcium?

Actonel should be taken sitting up, at least 30 minutes before the first food or drink of the day, with a full glass of water. Do not lie down for 30 minutes after taking the medication. Actonel should not be taken at the same time as other medications, including calcium.

What should I avoid while taking Actonel with Calcium?

Stop taking Actonel and tell your doctor if you experience chest pain, difficult or painful swallowing, or severe or continuing heartburn, as these may be signs of serious upper digestive problems.

What are possible food and drug interactions associated with Actonel with Calcium?

If Actonel is taken with certain other drugs, the effects of either could be increased, decreased, or altered. It is especially important to check with your doctor before combining Actonel with aluminum-, calcium-, or magnesium-containing medications

What are the possible side effects of Actonel with Calcium?

Side effects cannot be anticipated. If any develop or change in intensity, tell your doctor as soon as possible. Only your doctor can determine if it is safe for you to continue taking this drug.

Side effects may include: Back pain, bone pain, constipation, joint pain, muscle pain, stomach pain

Can I receive Actonel with Calcium if I am pregnant or breastfeeding?

The effects of Actonel during pregnancy and breastfeeding are unknown. Talk with your doctor before taking this drug if you are pregnant, plan to become pregnant, or are breastfeeding.

What should I do if I miss a dose of Actonel with Calcium?

If a dose is missed, take one tablet on the morning after you remember and return to taking one tablet once a week, as originally scheduled on your chosen day. Do not take two tablets on the same day.

How should I store Actonel with Calcium?

Store at room temperature.

ACTO*PLUS* MET

Generic name: Pioglitazone hydrochloride and
metformin hydrochloride

What is ACTO*plus* met?

ACTO*plus* met contains 2 anti-diabetic medicines, pioglitazone hydrochloride (Actos) and metformin hydrochloride (Glucophage). ACTO*plus* met is used to treat people with type 2 diabetes in conjunction with diet, exercise, and, if needed, weight reduction. ACTO*plus* met is used in patients already treated with a combination of pioglitazone and metformin, or whose diabetes is not adequately controlled with metformin alone, or who have initially responded to pioglitazone alone and require additional glycemic control.

**What is the most important information
I should know about ACTO*plus* met?**

ACTO*plus* met may cause or worsen congestive heart failure (CHF) in some people. If you have the most severe form of CHF (New York Association Class III or IV heart failure), you should not start taking ACTO*plus* met. If you have less serious CHF (New York Association Class I or II heart failure), your doctor will observe you carefully while on ACTO*plus* met therapy. If you are taking ACTO*plus* met and you develop serious CHF, your doctor will decide whether you should continue therapy.

A small number of people who have taken metformin, one of the two drugs that make up ACTO*plus* met, have developed a serious and potentially fatal condition called lactic acidosis. Lactic acidosis is caused by a buildup of lactic acid in the blood. Lactic acidosis may trigger early symptoms such as feeling very weak (malaise), muscle pain, breathing problems, increased sleepiness, abdominal distress with nausea and vomiting or diarrhea, feeling cold (especially in the arms and legs), feeling dizzy or lightheaded, having a slow or irregular heartbeat, or your medical condition suddenly changes. You have a greater risk of developing lactic acidosis with ACTO*plus* met if you have kidney or liver problems, have CHF that requires treatment with medicines, drink a lot of alcohol, get dehydrated (lose a large amount of body fluids), have certain x-ray tests using injectable dyes, have surgery, have a heart attack, severe infection or stroke, are older than 80 years old and have not had your kidney function checked. Lactic acidosis happens most often in diabetic individuals with kidney problems. People with kidney problems should not take ACTO*plus* met.

Who should not take ACTO*plus* met?

Do not take ACTO*plus* met if you have type 1 diabetes, kidney problems, acute or chronic metabolic acidosis, including diabetic ketoacidosis, or if you are hypersensitive to pioglitazone, metformin, or any other component of ACTO*plus* met.

If you are going to have an x-ray procedure with an injection of contrast dyes, or if you are planning to have surgery performed, you should temporarily discontinue taking ACTO*plus* met.

What should I tell my doctor before I take the first dose of ACTO*plus* met?

Tell your doctor about all prescription, over-the-counter, and herbal medications you are taking before beginning treatment with ACTO*plus* met. Also, talk to your doctor about your complete medical history, especially if you have a history of alcoholism, kidney or liver problems, a heart condition (especially Class III/IV heart failure), a type of diabetic eye disease called macular edema (swelling of the back of the eye), if you are pregnant or planning to become pregnant, breastfeeding, if you are a premenopausal woman not having periods regularly or at all, or a woman who has gone through menopause. Tell your doctor if you are taking insulin or oral hypoglycemic drugs.

What is the usual dosage?

The information below is based on the dosage guidelines your doctor uses. Depending on your condition and medical history, your doctor may prescribe a different regimen. Do not change the dosage or stop taking your medication without your doctor's approval.

Adults: ACTO*plus* met may be started at either the 15 milligram (mg)/500 mg or 15 mg/850 mg tablet strength once or twice daily. Your starting dose will be based on your current regimen of pioglitazone and/or metformin and will be gradually adjusted according to how you respond to the medication.

How should I take ACTO plus met?

Take ACTO*plus* met in divided doses with meals to reduce the gastrointestinal side effects associated with metformin. Take ACTO*plus* met exactly as your doctor prescribes. Follow your doctor's recommendations regarding diet, exercise, and testing your blood glucose regularly while you are taking ACTO*plus* met.

What should I avoid while taking ACTO*plus* met?
Avoid taking in too few calories, especially if you're also engaging in regular strenuous exercise, since this can result in hypoglycemia while taking ACTO*plus* met. Also, avoid drinking a lot of alcohol while taking ACTO*plus* met because this can increase your chance of getting lactic acidosis.

What are possible food and drug interactions associated with ACTO*plus* met?
If ACTO*plus* met is taken with certain other drugs, the effects of either could be increased, decreased, or altered. It is especially important to check with your doctor before combining ACTO*plus* met with: alcohol, calcium channel blocking drugs, cationic medications (eg, amiloride, digoxin, morphine, procainamide, quinidine, quinine, ranitidine, triamterene, trimethoprim, and vancomycin), corticosteroids, diuretics such as thiazides, enzyme inhibitors or enzyme inducers of CYP2C8 (such as gemfibrozil and rifampin, respectively), estrogens, insulin, isoniazid, medications containing ethanol, nicotinic acid, nifedipine, oral contraceptives, oral hypoglycemic drugs, phenothiazines, phenytoin, sympathomimetics, and thyroid products.

What are the possible side effects of ACTO*plus* met?
Side effects cannot be anticipated. If any develop or change in intensity, tell your doctor as soon as possible. Only your doctor can determine if it is safe for you to continue taking this drug.

Side effects may include: Upper respiratory tract infection, diarrhea, nausea, upset stomach, water retention, headache, urinary tract infection, sinusitis, dizziness, weight gain, cold-like symptoms, decreased levels of red blood cells (anemia), low blood sugar, liver problems, bone fractures

Symptoms of lactic acidosis (call your doctor immediately):
Dizziness or light-headedness, feeling very weak or tired (malaise), low body temperature, low blood pressure, muscle pain or tenderness, unexplained hyperventilation, slow or uneven heartbeat, stomach problems, unusual sleepiness

Can I receive ACTO*plus* met if I am pregnant or breastfeeding?
Talk to your doctor if you are pregnant, planning to become pregnant, or breastfeeding. If you are not having periods, talk to your doctor. ACTO*plus* met may increase your chances of becoming pregnant.

What should I do if I miss a dose of ACTO*plus* met?
If you miss a dose of ACTO*plus* met, take your next dose as prescribed unless told otherwise by your doctor.

How should I store ACTO*plus* met?
Store tightly closed at room temperature.

ACTOS

Generic name: Pioglitazone hydrochloride

What is ACTOS?

Actos is an oral antidiabetic drug that is used to improve glycemic control in people with type 2 diabetes. It may be used alone or with other diabetes medicine. Actos decreases insulin resistance and reduces circulating insulin levels. Actos should be used in conjunction with diet, exercise, and weight loss, if needed.

What is the most important information I should know about ACTOS?

Actos can cause fluid retention when used alone or in combination with other antidiabetic drugs, including insulin. Fluid retention may lead to or worsen heart failure. Tell your doctor if you have a history of heart problems or if you experience signs of heart failure, including rapid weight gain, fluid retention, shortness of breath, or if you feel unusually tired while taking Actos. Your doctor may also perform blood tests for liver function periodically; if you notice any unexplained nausea, vomiting, stomach pain, fatigue, loss of appetite, or dark urine, tell your doctor immediately.

Who should not take ACTOS?

Certain patients with heart failure should not start taking Actos. It should not be taken by people with active liver disease or jaundice (yellowing of the skin), people with type 1 diabetes, women who are pregnant or breastfeeding, or people who are allergic to Actos or any of its ingredients.

Actos should not be used for the treatment of diabetic ketoacidosis (a complication of diabetes in which acids called ketones build up in the blood). Actos should be used with caution in people with swelling (edema).

What should I tell my doctor before I take the first dose of ACTOS?

Tell your doctor about all prescription, over-the-counter, and herbal medications you are taking before beginning treatment with Actos. Also, talk to your doctor about your complete medical history, especially if you have congestive heart failure, liver problems, type 1 diabetes, edema (swelling), if you are being treated for diabetic ketoacidosis, have a type of diabetic eye disease called macular edema (swelling of the back of the eye), if you are pregnant or planning to become pregnant, breastfeeding, or if you are a premenopausal woman and do not have periods regularly or at all.

What is the usual dosage?

The information below is based on the dosage guidelines your doctor uses. Depending on your condition and medical history, your doctor may prescribe a different regimen. Do not change the dosage or stop taking your medication without your doctor's approval.

Adults: The usual dosage of Actos is 15 milligrams (mg) or 30 mg once a day. If you do not respond adequately to the initial dose, the dose can be increased up to 45 mg once a day.

How should I take ACTOS?

Actos is taken once a day, with or without meals.

What should I avoid while taking ACTOS?

Avoid rapidly increasing your dose without speaking to your doctor first. Avoid situations which may lead to low blood sugar, especially if you are also using insulin or other blood sugar-lowering medications. Test your blood sugar and HBA1C regularly.

What are possible food and drug interactions associated with ACTOS?

If Actos is taken with certain other drugs, the effects of either could be increased, decreased, or altered. It is especially important to check with your doctor before combining Actos with insulin or oral hypoglycemic medications.

What are the possible side effects of ACTOS?

Side effects cannot be anticipated. If any develop or change in intensity, tell your doctor as soon as possible. Only your doctor can determine if it is safe for you to continue taking this drug.

Side effects may include: new or worsened heart failure, low blood sugar (hypoglycemia), swelling (edema), weight gain, ovulation, low red blood cell count (anemia), liver problems, swelling in the back of the eye, bone fractures, upper respiratory tract infection, headache, sinus infection, muscle soreness, tooth problems, aggravated diabetes, sore throat

Can I receive ACTOS if I am pregnant or breastfeeding?

Actos should not be taken during pregnancy and breastfeeding. Tell your doctor immediately if you are pregnant, planning to become pregnant, or are breastfeeding.

If you are a premenopausal woman who is not ovulating, you should know that Actos might increase your risk of pregnancy by causing you to ovulate. Therefore, you may need to consider birth control options. However, women using oral contraceptives should talk with their health professionals, as they may be at increased risk for pregnancy if appropriate contraceptive methods or adjustments are not used.

What should I do if I miss a dose of ACTOS?

If you miss a dose of Actos on one day, take it as soon as you remember within the same day. If you miss a day, do not take a double dose the next day to make up for it. Take your next dose as prescribed unless otherwise told by your doctor.

How should I store ACTOS?

Store tightly closed at room temperature, away from moisture and humidity.

Acyclovir See Zovirax, page 1497.

Adapalene See Differin, page 415.

ADDERALL

Generic name: Amphetamine salts

What is Adderall?

Adderall is indicated for the treatment of attention-deficit/hyperactivity disorder (ADHD) and narcolepsy.

What is the most important information I should know about Adderall?

The following have been reported with the use of Adderall and other stimulant medications: heart-related problems such as sudden death in patients who have heart problems or heart defects; stroke and heart attack in adults; and increased blood pressure and heart rate. Call the doctor right away if you experience any signs of heart problems such as chest pain, shortness of breath, or fainting while taking Adderall.

Other serious side effects that have been reported include mental problems such as new or worsening behavior and thought problems; new or worsening bipolar disorder; and new or worsening aggressive behavior or hostility. It is especially important to monitor children and teenagers for any new psychotic or manic symptoms.

Who should not take Adderall?

Adderall should not be taken if you have heart disease or hardening of the arteries; have moderate to severe high blood pressure; have an overactive thyroid; have an eye disease called glaucoma; are very anxious, tense, or agitated; have a history of drug abuse; are taking or have taken within the past 14 days a type of medication called a monoamine oxidase inhibitor (MAOI); or if you are sensitive to, allergic to, or had a reaction to other stimulant medicines.

Adderall is not recommended for use in children under 3 years old.

What should I tell my doctor before I take the first dose of Adderall?

Tell your doctor about all prescription, over-the-counter, and herbal medications you are taking before beginning treatment with Adderall. Also, talk to your doctor about your complete medical history, including heart problems, heart defects, high blood pressure, or a family history of these problems; a history of mental problems or a family history of suicide, bipolar disorder, or depression; tics or Tourette's syndrome; liver or kidney problems; thyroid problems; and seizures or an abnormal brain wave test (EEG).

Tell your doctor if you are pregnant, planning to become pregnant, or breastfeeding.

What is the usual dosage?

The information below is based on the dosage guidelines your doctor uses. Depending on your condition and medical history, your doctor may prescribe a different regimen. Do not change the dosage or stop taking your medication without your doctor's approval.

Attention-Deficit/Hyperactivity Disorder
Adults and children 3 years and older: Adderall is not recommended for children under 3 years old. In children 3 to 5 years old, the usual starting dose is 2.5 milligrams (mg) daily; daily dosage may be raised in increments of 2.5 mg at weekly intervals until the optimal response is achieved.

In children 6 years and older, the usual starting dose is 5 mg once or twice daily; daily dosage may be raised in increments of 5 mg at weekly intervals until the optimal response is achieved. Only in rare cases will it be necessary to exceed a total of 40 mg per day.

Narcolepsy
Adults and children 6 years and older: The usual dose is 5 mg to 60 mg per day in divided doses, depending on individual patient response.

How should I take Adderall?

Adderall tablets are usually taken two or three times a day. The first dose is usually taken when you first wake in the morning. One or two more doses may be taken during the day, 4 to 6 hours apart. Adderall can be taken with or without food.

What should I avoid while taking Adderall?

Amphetamines may impair your ability to engage in potentially hazardous activities such as operating machinery or vehicles; use caution while taking Adderall.

What are possible food and drug interactions associated with Adderall?

If Adderall is taken with certain other drugs, the effects of either could be increased, decreased, or altered. It is especially important to check with your doctor before combining Adderall with the following: antidepressant medications (including MAOIs), blood pressure medications, blood thinners, cold or allergy medicines that contain decongestants, seizure medications, and stomach acid medications.

What are the possible side effects of Adderall?

Side effects cannot be anticipated. If any develop or change in intensity, tell your doctor as soon as possible. Only your doctor can determine if it is safe for you to continue taking this drug.

Serious side effects may include: slowing of growth (height and weight) in children; seizures, mainly in patients with a history of seizures; eyesight changes or blurred vision

Common side effects may include: headache, stomachache, trouble sleeping, decreased appetite, nervousness, dizziness

Can I receive Adderall if I am pregnant or breastfeeding?

The effects of Adderall during pregnancy and breastfeeding are unknown. Amphetamines are excreted in human milk. Mothers taking amphetamines such as Adderall should refrain from nursing. Tell your doctor immediately if you are pregnant, plan to become pregnant, or are breastfeeding.

What should I do if I miss a dose of Adderall?

Take it as soon as you remember. If it is almost time for your next dose, skip the missed dose and return to your regular schedule. Never take 2 doses at the same time.

How should I store Adderall?

Store in a cool, dry place in a tightly closed, light-resistant container.

ADDERALL XR

Generic name: Amphetamine salts, extended-release

What is Adderall XR?

Adderall XR is a once-daily central nervous system stimulant medicine used for the treatment of attention-deficit/hyperactivity disorder (ADHD). Adderall XR may help increase attention and decrease impulsiveness and hyperactivity in patients with ADHD.

What is the most important information I should know about Adderall XR?

The following have been reported with the use of Adderall XR and other stimulant medications: heart-related problems such as sudden death in patients who have heart problems or heart defects; stroke and heart attack in adults; and increased blood pressure and heart rate. Call the doctor right away if you experience any signs of heart problems such as chest pain, shortness of breath, or fainting while taking Adderall XR.

Other serious side effects that have been reported include mental problems such as new or worsening behavior and thought problems; new or worsening bipolar disorder; and new or worsening aggressive behavior or hostility. It is especially important to monitor children and teenagers for any new psychotic or manic symptoms.

Who should not take Adderall XR?

Adderall XR should not be taken if you have heart disease or hardening of the arteries; have moderate to severe high blood pressure; have an overactive thyroid; have an eye disease called glaucoma; are very anxious, tense, or agitated; have a history of drug abuse; are taking or have taken within the past 14 days a type of medication called a monoamine oxidase inhibitor (MAOI); or if you are sensitive to, allergic to, or had a reaction to other stimulant medicines.

Adderall XR is not recommended for use in children under 3 years old.

What should I tell my doctor before I take the first dose of Adderall XR?

Tell your doctor about all prescription, over-the-counter, and herbal medications you are taking before beginning treatment with Adderall XR. Also, talk to your doctor about your complete medical history, including heart problems, heart defects, high blood pressure, or a family history of these problems; a history of mental problems or a family history of suicide, bipolar disorder, or depression; tics or Tourette's syndrome; liver or kidney problems; thyroid problems; and seizures or an abnormal brain wave test (EEG).

Tell your doctor if you are pregnant, planning to become pregnant, or breastfeeding.

What is the usual dosage?

The information below is based on the dosage guidelines your doctor uses. Depending on your condition and medical history, your doctor may prescribe a different regimen. Do not change the dosage or stop taking your medication without your doctor's approval.

Adults: In adults who are either starting treatment for the first time or switching from another medication, the recommended dose is 20 milligrams (mg) a day. Patients taking divided doses of immediate-release Adderall may be switched to Adderall XR at the same total daily dose taken once a day.

Adolescents: The recommended starting dose for adolescents 13 to 17 years old is 10 mg/day. The dose may be increased to 20 mg/day after 1 week if symptoms are not adequately controlled.

Children: Children 6 years and older who are either starting treatment for the first time or switching from another medication should start with 10 milligrams (mg) once daily in the morning; daily dosage may be adjusted in increments of 5 mg or 10 mg at weekly intervals. The maximum recommended dose for children is 30 mg/day.

How should I take Adderall XR?

Take Adderall XR once a day in the morning when you first wake up. Adderall XR is an extended-release capsule that releases medicine into your body throughout the day. Swallow Adderall XR capsules whole with water or other liquids. If you or your child cannot swallow the capsule, open it and sprinkle the medicine over a spoonful of applesauce. Swallow the applesauce and medicine mixture without chewing. Follow with a drink of water or other liquid. Adderall XR may be taken with or without food.

What should I avoid while taking Adderall XR?

Amphetamines may impair your ability to engage in potentially hazardous activities such as operating machinery or vehicles; use caution while taking Adderall XR.

What are possible food and drug interactions associated with Adderall XR?

If Adderall XR is taken with certain other drugs, the effects of either could be increased, decreased, or altered. It is especially important to check with your doctor before combining Adderall XR with the following: antidepressant medications (including MAOIs), antipsychotic medications, blood pressure medications, blood thinners, cold or allergy medicines that contain decongestants, lithium, narcotic pain medications, seizure medications, and stomach acid medications.

What are the possible side effects of Adderall XR?

Side effects cannot be anticipated. If any develop or change in intensity, tell your doctor as soon as possible. Only your doctor can determine if it is safe for you to continue taking this drug.

Serious side effects may include: slowing of growth (height and weight) in children; seizures, mainly in patients with a history of seizures; eyesight changes or blurred vision

Common side effects may include: headache, stomachache, trouble sleeping, decreased appetite, nervousness, mood swings, dizziness

Can I receive Adderall XR if I am pregnant or breastfeeding?
The effects of Adderall XR during pregnancy and breastfeeding are unknown. Amphetamines are excreted in human milk. Mothers taking amphetamines such as Adderall XR should refrain from nursing. Tell your doctor immediately if you are pregnant, plan to become pregnant, or are breastfeeding.

What should I do if I miss a dose of Adderall XR?
Take it as soon as you remember. If it is almost time for your next dose, skip the missed dose and return to your regular schedule. Never take 2 doses at the same time.

How should I store Adderall XR?
Store in a cool, dry place in a tightly closed, light-resistant container.

ADIPEX-P
Generic name: Phentermine hydrochloride

What is Adipex-P?
Adipex-P, an appetite suppressant, is prescribed for short-term use as part of an overall weight reduction program that also includes dieting, exercise, and counseling. The drug is for use only by excessively overweight individuals who have a condition—such as diabetes, high blood pressure, or high cholesterol—that could lead to serious medical problems.

What is the most important information I should know about Adipex-P?
Adipex-P will lose its effect after a few weeks, and should be discontinued when this happens. If you try to boost its effectiveness by increasing the dose, you will run the risk of serious side effects and dependence on the drug.

This drug may cause primary pulmonary hypertension, symptoms of which are chest pain, shortness of breath, fainting spells, or swollen ankles.

Adipex-P may cause dependence. If you continually take too much of any appetite suppressant it can cause severe skin disorders, a pronounced inability to fall or stay asleep, irritability, hyperactivity, and personality changes.

Who should not take Adipex-P?

Do not begin treatment with Adipex-P if you are allergic to any of its ingredients. Also, do not take this drug if you have atherosclerosis (thickening of the artery wall), heart disease, high blood pressure, thyroid problems, or glaucoma.

What should I tell my doctor before I take the first dose of Adipex-P?

Tell your doctor about all prescription, over-the-counter, and herbal medications you are taking before beginning treatment with Adipex-P. Also, talk to your doctor about your complete medical history, especially if you have a history of drug dependence.

What is the usual dosage?

The information below is based on the dosage guidelines your doctor uses. Depending on your condition and medical history, your doctor may prescribe a different regimen. Do not change the dosage or stop taking your medication without your doctor's approval.

Adults and adolescents over 16 years: The usual dosage of Adipex-P is 1 capsule or tablet per day.

How should I take Adipex-P?

Take Adipex-P before breakfast or up to 2 hours after breakfast. Tablets can be broken in half, if necessary.

What should I avoid while taking Adipex-P?

Avoid driving or other hazardous activities until you know how Adipex-P affects you.

What are possible food and drug interactions associated with Adipex-P?

Adipex-P should never be combined with the weight-loss drug fenfluramine (Pondimin); very dangerous side effects could result. This drug may also react badly with alcohol. Avoid alcoholic beverages while you are taking it.

If Adipex-P is taken with certain other drugs, the effects of either can be increased, decreased, or altered. It is especially important to check with your doctor before combining Adipex-P with the following: serotonin-boosting drugs (such as SSRI antidepressants), MAO inhibitors, diabetes medications, and high blood pressure medications.

What are the possible side effects of Adipex-P?

Side effects cannot be anticipated. If any develop or change in intensity, tell your doctor as soon as possible. Only your doctor can determine if it is safe for you to continue taking this drug.

Side effects may include: changes in sex drive, constipation, diarrhea, dizziness, dry mouth, exaggerated feelings of depression or elation, headache, high blood pressure, hives, impotence, inability to fall or stay asleep, increased heart rate, overstimulation, restlessness, stomach or intestinal problems, throbbing heartbeat, tremors, unpleasant taste

Can I receive Adipex-P if I am pregnant or breastfeeding?
The effects of Adipex-P during pregnancy and breastfeeding are unknown. Talk with your doctor before taking this drug if you are pregnant, plan to become pregnant, or are breastfeeding.

What should I do if I miss a dose of Adipex-P?
Skip the missed dose completely; then take the next dose at the regularly scheduled time.

How should I store Adipex-P?
Store at room temperature.

ADVAIR DISKUS
Generic name: Fluticasone propionate and salmeterol

What is Advair Diskus?
Advair Diskus contains 2 medicines, fluticasone propionate (Flovent) and salmeterol (Serevent). Fluticasone is an inhaled corticosteroid medicine, which helps to decrease inflammation in the lungs. Inflammation in the lungs can lead to asthma symptoms. Salmeterol is a long-acting beta$_2$-agonist (LABA) medicine used in patients with asthma and chronic obstructive pulmonary disease (COPD). LABA medicines help relax the muscles around the airways in your lungs, helping to prevent symptoms such as wheezing and shortness of breath.

What is the most important information I should know about Advair Diskus?
Because long-acting beta$_2$-agonist (LABA) medicines such as salmeterol may increase the risk of asthma-related death, you should only use Advair Diskus if your asthma is not adequately controlled on other medications or the severity of your asthma warrants treatment with 2 maintenance therapies.

Advair Diskus does not relieve sudden symptoms. Always have a short-acting beta$_2$-agonist medicine with you to treat sudden symptoms.

Patients with COPD have a greater chance of developing pneumonia. Advair Diskus may increase your risk of pneumonia. Call your doctor if you experience any symptoms of pneumonia, which include an increase in mucus (sputum) production, change in mucus color, fever, chills, increased cough, or increased breathing problems.

Do not stop using Advair Diskus unless told to do so by your doctor; your symptoms may get worse.

Call you doctor if breathing problems worsen over time while taking Advair Diskus. You may need a different treatment.

Get emergency medical care if your breathing problems worsen, or if you use a short-acting beta$_2$-agonist medicine which fails to relieve your breathing problems.

Who should not take Advair Diskus?
Do not use Advair Diskus if your asthma is well controlled with another drug or you only need short-acting drugs occasionally. Do not use Advair Diskus as primary treatment of acute episodes of asthma or COPD when intensive measures are required.

Do not use Advair Diskus if you are allergic to any of its ingredients, such as milk proteins.

What should I tell my doctor before I take the first dose of Advair Diskus?
Tell your doctor about all prescription, over-the-counter, and herbal medications you are taking before beginning treatment with Advair Diskus, especially if you are taking ritonavir, an anti-HIV drug. Also, talk to your doctor about your complete medical history, especially if you have allergies to other drugs or foods, diabetes, heart problems, high blood pressure, immune system problems, liver or kidney problems, if you are pregnant or planning to become pregnant, breastfeeding, or if you have seizures, a thyroid disorder, weak bones (osteoporosis), or you are exposed to chickenpox or measles.

What is the usual dosage?
The information below is based on the dosage guidelines your doctor uses. Depending on your condition and medical history, your doctor may prescribe a different regimen. Do not change the dosage or stop taking your medication without your doctor's approval.

The usual dosage of Advair Diskus is 1 inhalation twice a day (once in the morning and once in the evening, 12 hours apart).

Do not use Advair Diskus more often or at higher doses than recommended.

How should I take Advair Diskus?
Hold the Advair Diskus in 1 hand and place the thumb of your other hand on the thumbgrip. Push your thumb away as far as it will go until you see the mouthpiece and it snaps into position. Use Advair Diskus in a level, flat position.

Slide the lever away from you as far as it will go until it clicks. Before inhaling, breathe out fully, holding the Diskus level and away from your mouth. Remember to never breath into the Advair Diskus.

Put the mouthpiece to your lips and breathe in quickly and deeply. Do not breathe in through your nose. Remove the Diskus from your mouth and hold your breath for about 10 seconds or as long as you can. Slowly breathe out.

After each dose, rinse your mouth with water and spit out. Close the Advair Diskus by placing your thumb on the thumbgrip and slide it back towards you as far as it will go; it will click shut.

What should I avoid while taking Advair Diskus?
Avoid using a spacer device with this medication.

What are possible food and drug interactions associated with Advair Diskus?
If Advair Diskus is used with certain other drugs, the effects of either could be increased, decreased, or altered. It is especially important to check with your doctor before combining Advair Diskus with ritonavir, ketoconazole, monoamine oxidase inhibitors or tricyclic antidepressants, beta-blockers, or with nonpotassium-sparing diuretics, such as loop or thiazide diuretics.

While you are taking Advair Diskus, do not use other medicines that contain a long-acting beta$_2$-agonist, or LABA. Other LABA medicines include Serevent Diskus (salmeterol xinafoate inhalation powder) or Foradil Aerolizer (formoterol fumarate inhalation powder).

What are the possible side effects of Advair Diskus?
Side effects cannot be anticipated. If any develop or change in intensity, tell your doctor as soon as possible. Only your doctor can determine if it is safe for you to continue taking this drug.

Side effects may include: serious allergic reactions, including rash, hives, facial swelling, swelling of the mouth or tongue, breathing problems. Also, increased blood pressure, fast and irregular heartbeat, chest pain, headache, tremor, nervousness, immune system effects and a greater chance of infections, lower bone mineral density, eye problems including glaucoma and cataracts, slowed growth in children, throat irritation, hoarseness and voice changes, fungal infection in the mouth and throat (thrush), cough, headache, nausea and vomiting

Can I receive Advair Diskus if I am pregnant or breastfeeding?
The effects of Advair Diskus during pregnancy and breastfeeding are unknown. Tell your doctor immediately if you are pregnant, plan to become pregnant, or are breastfeeding.

What should I do if I miss a dose of Advair Diskus?
If you miss a dose of Advair Diskus, skip that dose. Take your next dose at your usual time. Do not take 2 doses at one time.

How should I store Advair Diskus?

Store at room temperature in a dry place, away from heat and sunlight. Safely discard Advair Diskus 1 month after it is removed from the foil pouch or after the dose indicator reads "0," whichever comes first.

ADVAIR HFA

Generic name: Fluticasone propionate and salmeterol

What is Advair HFA?

Advair HFA contains 2 medicines, fluticasone propionate (Flovent) and salmeterol (Serevent). Fluticasone is an inhaled corticosteroid medicine, which helps to decrease inflammation in the lungs. Inflammation in the lungs can lead to asthma symptoms. Salmeterol is a long-acting beta$_2$-agonist (LABA) medicine used to help relax the muscles around the airways in your lungs, helping to prevent symptoms of asthma such as wheezing and shortness of breath. Advair HFA is used in the treatment of asthma and also to prevent symptoms of asthma in adults and adolescents 12 years of age and older.

What is the most important information I should know about Advair HFA?

Because long-acting beta$_2$-agonist medicines such as salmeterol may increase the risk of asthma-related death, you should only use Advair HFA if your asthma is not adequately controlled on other medications or the severity of your asthma warrants treatment with 2 maintenance therapies.

Advair HFA does not relieve sudden breathing problems. Always have a short-acting bronchodilator medicine with you to treat sudden breathing problems.

Call you doctor if breathing problems worsen over time while taking Advair HFA. You may need a different treatment.

Get emergency medical care if breathing problems worsen quickly or if you use a short-acting beta$_2$-agonist medicine, which does not relieve your breathing problems.

Who should not take Advair HFA?

Do not use Advair HFA if your asthma is well controlled with an inhaled corticosteroid alone or an inhaled corticosteroid along with occasional use of a short-acting bronchodilator.

Do not use Advair HFA as primary treatment of acute episodes of asthma when intensive measures are required.

Do not use Advair HFA if you are allergic to any of its ingredients.

What should I tell my doctor before I take the first dose of Advair HFA?

Tell your doctor about all prescription, over-the-counter, and herbal medications you are taking to avoid a possible interaction with Advair HFA.

Also, talk to your doctor about your complete medical history, especially if you have diabetes, heart problems, high blood pressure, an immune system problem, liver problems, seizures, thyroid problems, have weak bones (osteoporosis), if you are pregnant or planning to become pregnant, breastfeeding, or you are exposed to chickenpox or measles.

What is the usual dosage?
The information below is based on the dosage guidelines your doctor uses. Depending on your condition and medical history, your doctor may prescribe a different regimen. Do not change the dosage or stop taking your medication without your doctor's approval.

Adults and adolescents 12 years and older: The usual dosage is 2 inhalations twice a day (once in the morning and once in the evening, 12 hours apart).

How should I take Advair HFA?
Prime the inhaler before using it for the first time so that you will get the right amount of medicine. To prime the inhaler, take the cap off the mouthpiece and shake the inhaler well for 5 seconds. Then spray it once into the air, away from your face. Shake and spray the inhaler like this 3 more times to finish priming it. Avoid spraying in the eyes.

If you have not used your inhaler in more than 4 weeks or if you have dropped it, shake it well for 5 seconds and spray it 2 times into the air, away from your face. Shake the inhaler well for 5 seconds just before each use.

Hold the inhaler with the mouthpiece down. Breathe out through your mouth and push out as much air from your lungs as possible. Put the mouthpiece in your mouth and close your lips around it. Push the canister all the way down while you breathe in deeply and slowly through your mouth. Take your finger off the canister. After breathing in fully, take the inhaler out of your mouth and close your mouth. Hold your breath for up to 10 seconds or as long as you can, then breathe normally. Wait 30 seconds and shake the inhaler for 5 seconds and repeat the inhalation process.

Always rinse your mouth with water and spit out after you use the inhaler. Do not swallow the water. Make sure to put the cap back on the mouthpiece after every time you use the inhaler so that it snaps into place. The inhaler should be at room temperature before you use it.

What should I avoid while taking Advair HFA?
Do not change or stop any of your medicines to control or treat your asthma symptoms. Do not also use other medicines that contain a long-acting beta₂-agonist.

What are possible food and drug interactions associated with Advair HFA?

If Advair HFA is taken with certain other drugs, the effects of either could be increased, decreased, or altered. It is especially important to check with your doctor before combining Advair HFA with: beta blockers, CYP450 inhibitors such as ketoconazole and erythromycin, nonpotassium-sparing diuretics, such as loop or thiazide diuretics, monoamine oxidase inhibitors, ritonavir, an anti-HIV medicine, tricyclic antidepressants.

What are the possible side effects of Advair HFA?

Side effects cannot be anticipated. If any develop or change in intensity, tell your doctor as soon as possible. Only your doctor can determine if it is safe for you to continue taking this drug.

Side effects may include: allergic reactions including rash, hives, facial swelling, swelling of the mouth or tongue, breathing problems. Also, increased blood pressure, fast and irregular heartbeat, chest pain, headache, tremor, nervousness, immune system effects and a higher chance of infections, lower bone mineral density, eye problems including glaucoma and cataracts, slowed growth in children, throat irritation, and pneumonia

Can I receive Advair HFA if I am pregnant or breastfeeding?

The effects of Advair HFA during pregnancy and breastfeeding are unknown. Tell your doctor immediately if you are pregnant, planning to become pregnant, or are breastfeeding.

What should I do if I miss a dose of Advair HFA?

If you miss a dose of Advair HFA, skip that dose. Take your next dose at your usual time. Do not take 2 doses at one time.

How should I store Advair HFA?

Store at room temperature with the mouthpiece facing downward. Do not store near heat or open flame.

ADVICOR

Generic name: Lovastatin and niacin

What is Advicor?

Advicor is a cholesterol-lowering drug. Advicor lowers total cholesterol and LDL ("bad") cholesterol, while raising the amount of HDL ("good") cholesterol.

Advicor is a combination of two cholesterol-fighting ingredients: extended-release niacin and lovastatin. It is prescribed only when other drugs and a program of diet, exercise, and weight reduction have been unsuccessful in lowering cholesterol levels.

What is the most important information I should know about Advicor?

Although you cannot feel any symptoms of high cholesterol, it is important to take Advicor every day. The drug will be more effective if it is taken as part of a program of diet, exercise, and weight loss. All these efforts keep your cholesterol levels normal and lower your risk of heart disease.

Advicor may trigger a muscle-wasting condition that also can affect the kidneys. The risk is increased if Advicor is taken with certain drugs or grapefruit juice. Contact your doctor immediately if you experience unexplained muscle pain, tenderness, or weakness.

Who should not take Advicor?

Do not take Advicor if you are allergic to any of its ingredients.

What should I tell my doctor before I take the first dose of Advicor?

Tell your doctor about all prescription, over-the-counter, and herbal medications you are taking before beginning treatment with Advicor. Also, talk to your doctor about your complete medical history, especially if you have diabetes, liver problems, an ulcer, or you are going to have surgery while on this drug. Also tell your doctor if you consume a lot of alcohol.

What is the usual dosage?

The information below is based on the dosage guidelines your doctor uses. Depending on your condition and medical history, your doctor may prescribe a different regimen. Do not change the dosage or stop taking your medication without your doctor's approval.

Adults: The usual starting dose of Advicor is one tablet containing 500 milligrams (mg) of extended-release niacin and 20 mg of lovastatin. After 4 weeks, the dosage may be increased if necessary.

How should I take Advicor?

Take Advicor at bedtime with a low-fat snack; do not take this medication on an empty stomach. Take Advicor whole; do not break, crush, or chew tablets.

What should I avoid while taking Advicor?

Do not drink alcohol or hot drinks when taking Advicor tablets.

What are possible food and drug interactions associated with Advicor?

Advicor should not be taken with grapefruit juice. Also, talk to your doctor if you are taking high blood pressure medication, aspirin, alcohol, blood anticoagulants (coumarin), cyclosporine, danazol, itraconazole, ketoconazole, gemfibrozil, niacin, erythromycin, clarithromycin, telithromycin, nefazodone or HIV protease inhibitors, propanolol, digoxin, or diabetes medications.

What are the possible side effects of Advicor?
Side effects cannot be anticipated. If any develop or change in intensity, tell your doctor as soon as possible. Only your doctor can determine if it is safe for you to continue taking this drug.

Side effects may include: abdominal pain, back pain, diarrhea, flu-like symptoms, flushing, headache, high blood sugar, indigestion, infection, itching, muscle pain, nausea, pain, rash, vomiting, weakness

Can I receive Advicor if I am pregnant or breastfeeding?
Do not begin treatment with Advicor if you are pregnant, plan to become pregnant, or are breastfeeding. This drug may cause severe harm to your unborn baby, and may pass into your breast milk. If you become pregnant while on Advicor, immediately stop your dosage and contact your doctor.

What should I do if I miss a dose of Advicor?
Take it as soon as you remember. If it is almost time for your next dose, skip the one you missed and go back to your regular schedule. Do not take two doses at once.

How should I store Advicor?
Store at room temperature.

AEROBID
Generic name: Flunisolide

What is AeroBid?
AeroBid is prescribed for people who need long-term treatment to control and prevent the symptoms of asthma. It contains an anti-inflammatory steroid type of medication and may reduce or eliminate the need for other corticosteroids.

What is the most important information I should know about AeroBid?
AeroBid helps to reduce the likelihood of an asthma attack, but will not relieve one that has already started. To be effective as a preventive measure, it must be taken every day at regularly spaced intervals. It may be several weeks before you receive its full benefit.

Your asthma should be reasonably stable before treatment with Aero-Bid Inhaler is started. AeroBid should be started in combination with your usual dose of an oral steroid medication. After approximately 1 week, your doctor will start to withdraw gradually the oral steroid by reducing

the daily or alternate daily dose. A slow rate of reduction is very important, as some people have experienced withdrawal symptoms such as
joint and/or muscular pain, fatigue, and depression. Tell your doctor if
you lose weight or feel light-headed. You may need to take more oral
corticosteroid temporarily.

This medication is not useful when you need rapid relief of asthma
symptoms.

Transferring from steroid tablet therapy to AeroBid inhaler may produce allergic conditions that were previously controlled by the steroid
tablet therapy. These include rhinitis (inflammation of the mucous membrane of the nose), conjunctivitis (pinkeye), and eczema.

Contact your doctor immediately if you have an asthma attack that isn't
controlled by a bronchodilator while you are being treated with AeroBid.
You may need an oral steroid drug.

While you are being treated with AeroBid, particularly at higher doses,
your doctor will carefully observe you for any evidence of side effects
such as the suppression of glandular function and diminished bone
growth in children. If you have just had surgery or are under extreme
stress, your doctor will also closely monitor you.

The use of AeroBid may cause a yeast-like fungal infection of the
mouth, pharynx (throat), or larynx (voice box). If you suspect a fungal
infection, notify your doctor. Treatment with antifungal medication may
be necessary.

Also, if you have tuberculosis, a herpes infection of the eye, or any
other kind of infection, make sure the doctor knows about it. You probably should not use AeroBid.

Who should not take AeroBid?

This medication is not for treatment of prolonged, severe asthma attacks
where more intensive measures are required.

If you are allergic or sensitive to AeroBid or other steroid drugs, advise
your doctor. This medication may not be right for you.

What should I tell my doctor before
I take the first dose of AeroBid?

Tell your doctor about all prescription, over-the-counter, and herbal medications you are taking before beginning treatment with AeroBid. Also,
talk to your doctor about your complete medical history, especially if you
have an infection, have had recent surgery, or have been under extreme
stress.

What is the usual dosage?

The information below is based on the dosage guidelines your doctor
uses. Depending on your condition and medical history, your doctor
may prescribe a different regimen. Do not change the dosage or stop
taking your medication without your doctor's approval.

Adults: The recommended starting dose is 2 inhalations twice daily, in the morning and evening, for a total daily dose of 1 milligram. The daily dose should not exceed 4 inhalations twice a day, for a total daily dose of 2 milligrams.

Children 6 to 15 years old: The recommended starting dose of 2 inhalations may be used twice daily, for a total daily dose of 1 milligram.

The safety and effectiveness of this drug have not been established in children less than 6 years old.

How should I take AeroBid?
Take this medication at regular intervals, exactly as prescribed by your doctor. The basic administration technique is: 1. Place the metal cartridge inside the plastic container. 2. Remove the cap; inspect the mouthpiece for foreign objects. 3. Shake the inhaler thoroughly. 4. Tilt your head slightly and breathe out as completely as possible. 5. Hold the inhaler upright and put the plastic mouthpiece in your mouth; close your lips tightly around it. 6. Press down on the metal cartridge. At the same time, take a slow, deep breath through your mouth. 7. Hold your breath as long as you can. While holding your breath, stop pressing down on the cartridge and remove the mouthpiece from your mouth. 8. Allow at least 1 minute between inhalations. Illustrated instructions for use are available with the product.

To help reduce hoarseness, throat irritation, and mouth infection, rinse out with water after each use. If your mouth is sore or has a rash, tell your doctor.

What should I avoid while taking AeroBid?
Since the contents of this inhalant are under pressure, do not puncture the container and do not use or store the medication near heat or an open flame. Exposure to temperatures above 120 degrees may cause the container to explode.

People taking drugs such as AeroBid that suppress the immune system are more open to infection. Take extra care to avoid exposure to measles and chickenpox if you've never had them or never had shots. Such diseases can be serious or even fatal when your immune system is below par. If you are exposed, tell your doctor immediately.

What are possible food and drug interactions associated with AeroBid?
If AeroBid is taken with certain other drugs, the effects of either could be increased, decreased, or altered. Always check with your doctor before combining AeroBid with any other medication.

What are the possible side effects of AeroBid?

Side effects cannot be anticipated. If any develop or change in intensity, tell your doctor as soon as possible. Only your doctor can determine if it is safe for you to continue taking this drug.

Side effects may include: cold symptoms, diarrhea, flu, headache, infection of the upper respiratory tract, nasal congestion, nausea, sore throat, unpleasant taste, upset stomach, vomiting

Can I receive AeroBid if I am pregnant or breastfeeding?

The effects of AeroBid during pregnancy have not been adequately studied. If you are pregnant or plan to become pregnant, inform your doctor immediately. It is not known whether AeroBid appears in breast milk. If this medication is essential to your health, your doctor may advise you to discontinue breastfeeding your baby until your treatment with this medication is finished.

What should I do if I miss a dose of AeroBid?

Use it as soon as you remember. If it is almost time for your next dose, skip the one you missed and go back to your regular schedule. Do not take 2 doses at the same time.

How should I store AeroBid?

Store away from heat or cold and light. Keep away from open flames.

AFLURIA

Generic name: Influenza virus vaccine

What is Afluria?

Afluria is a vaccine that is given to people 18 years and older to protect against infection with the flu virus (specifically, influenza virus subtypes A and B).

What is the most important information I should know about Afluria?

Afluria is an inactivated vaccine that cannot cause influenza but stimulates the immune system to produce antibodies that protect against influenza.

Who should not take Afluria?

You should not receive Afluria if you are allergic to eggs, chicken protein, neomycin, or polymyxin. Afluria should not be used in people who have had a life threatening reaction to a previous influenza vaccination, or who have had an occurrence of Guillain-Barré syndrome within 6 weeks of previous influenza vaccination. You should avoid receiving the vaccine if you have poor immunity or if you are receiving immunosuppressive therapy.

What should I tell my doctor before I take the first dose of Afluria?

Do not take Afluria if you are allergic to any of its ingredients. Tell your doctor about all prescription, over-the-counter and herbal medications you are taking, as well as any vaccines you are receiving before beginning treatment with Afluria. Also, talk to your doctor about your complete medical history, especially if you have a weakened immune system, or you have a history of allergic reactions to previous vaccines.

What is the usual dosage?

The information below is based on the dosage guidelines your doctor uses. Depending on your condition and medical history, your doctor may prescribe a different regimen. Do not change the dosage or stop taking your medication without your doctor's approval.

Adults 18 years and older: The usual dosage is 0.5 mL as a single intramuscular injection.

How should I take Afluria?

Afluria should be injected by your nurse or doctor in the deltoid muscle of the upper arm.

What should I avoid while taking Afluria?

For optimal protection against the flu, avoid waiting too long before you receive the vaccine. You should get the vaccine when it becomes available each fall (in October or November), but you can also get it any time throughout the flu season (into December, January, and beyond).

What are possible food and drug interactions associated with Afluria?

If Afluria is taken with certain other drugs, the effects of either could be increased, decreased, or altered. It is especially important to check with your doctor before combining Afluria with the following: corticosteroids, cytotoxic drugs, or immunosuppressive therapies including radiation.

What are the possible side effects of Afluria?

Side effects cannot be anticipated. If any develop or change in intensity, tell your doctor as soon as possible. Only your doctor can determine if it is safe for you to continue taking this drug.

Side effects may include: fever; headaches; malaise; muscle aches; pain, redness, or swelling at the injection site

As with any other vaccine, there is a risk of allergic reactions. Signs of severe allergic reactions may include hives, difficulty breathing, and swelling of the throat. If any of these events occur, seek immediate medical attention.

Can I receive Afluria if I am pregnant or breastfeeding?
The effects of Afluria during pregnancy and breastfeeding are unknown. Tell your doctor immediately if you are pregnant, plan to become pregnant, or are breastfeeding.

What should I do if I miss a dose of Afluria?
Afluria is given as a single dose.

How should I store Afluria?
Your healthcare provider will store this medication.

AGGRENOX
Generic name: Aspirin and extended-release dipyridamole

What is Aggrenox?
Aggrenox is used to reduce the chances of a stroke in people who have had a "mini-stroke" (transient ischemic attack) or a full-scale stroke due to a blood clot blocking an artery in the brain.

What is the most important information I should know about Aggrenox?
Because of the aspirin in Aggrenox, this product cannot be used by people who have an allergy to aspirin and other nonsteroidal anti-inflammatory drugs such as Advil, Motrin, and Naprosyn, or by people who suffer asthma attacks after taking aspirin.

Who should not take Aggrenox?
Do not take Aggrenox if you are allergic to any of its ingredients, have asthma, a persistent runny nose, or nasal polyps, or if you have severe liver or kidney disease. Also, because this drug contains aspirin, it is not recommended for children and teenagers, as it may cause a dangerous brain disorder called Reye's syndrome.

What should I tell my doctor before I take the first dose of Aggrenox?
Tell your doctor about all prescription, over-the-counter, and herbal medication you are taking before beginning treatment with Aggrenox. Also, talk to your doctor about your complete medical history, especially if you

have an ulcer, stomach problems, bleeding disorders, or will be having surgery or dental work while taking this medication.

What is the usual dosage?
The information below is based on the dosage guidelines your doctor uses. Depending on your condition and medical history, your doctor may prescribe a different regimen. Do not change the dosage or stop taking your medication without your doctor's approval.

Adults: The recommended dosage is one capsule twice a day, in the morning and evening.

How should I take Aggrenox?
Aggrenox should be taken once in the morning and once in the evening. The capsule should be swallowed whole without chewing. This drug may be taken with or without food.

What are possible food and drug interactions associated with Aggrenox?
If Aggrenox is taken with certain other drugs, the effects of either could be increased, decreased, or altered. It is especially important to check with your doctor before combining Aggrenox with heart and blood pressure medications, acetazolamide, blood pressure medications classified as beta-blockers, blood-thinning drugs, gout medications, methotrexate, nonsteroidal anti-inflammatory drugs, oral diabetes drugs, seizure medications, and diuretics.

If you suffer from the muscle disease myasthenia gravis, treatment with Aggrenox may interfere with your drug therapy.

What are the possible side effects of Aggrenox?
Side effects cannot be anticipated. If any develop or change in intensity, tell your doctor as soon as possible. Only your doctor can determine if it is safe for you to continue taking this drug.

Side effects may include: abdominal pain, back pain, bleeding, diarrhea, dizziness, fatigue, headache, indigestion, joint pain, nausea, pain, vomiting

Can I receive Aggrenox if I am pregnant or breastfeeding?
Do not take Aggrenox if you are pregnant, plan to become pregnant, or are breastfeeding. The aspirin in this drug may cause low birth weight, brain hemorrhages in premature births, stillbirths and neonatal death.

What should I do if I miss a dose of Aggrenox?
Take it as soon as you remember. If it is almost time for your next dose, skip the one you missed and go back to your regular schedule. Never take 2 doses at the same time.

How should I store Aggrenox?
Store at room temperature.

ALAMAST
Generic name: Pemirolast

What is Alamast?
Alamast is used to prevent itching of the eye caused by allergies. Alamast should not be used to treat contact lens-related problems. You may notice decreased itching within a few days, but frequently longer treatment (up to four weeks) is necessary.

What is the most important information I should know about Alamast?
Do not use Alamast if your eye irritation is caused by your contact lenses. Do not wear a lens if the eye is red. Alamast does not provide immediate relief. It may take a few days or as much as 4 weeks for the medication to start working.

Who should not take Alamast?
Do not begin treatment with Alamast if you are allergic to any of its ingredients.

What should I tell my doctor before I take the first dose of Alamast?
Tell your doctor about all prescription, over-the-counter, and herbal medications you are taking before beginning treatment with Alamast. Also, talk to your doctor about your complete medical history, especially if you are pregnant, plan to become pregnant, or are breastfeeding.

What is the usual dosage?
The information below is based on the dosage guidelines your doctor uses. Depending on your condition and medical history, your doctor may prescribe a different regimen. Do not change the dosage or stop taking your medication without your doctor's approval.

Adults: The recommended dosage is 1 or 2 drops in each affected eye 4 times a day. Alamast has not been evaluated in children under the age of 3.

How should I take Alamast?
Use Alamast solution only in the eyes; never swallow it. If you wear soft contact lenses, remove them before administering the eye drops and wait 10 minutes before re-inserting them.

What should I avoid while taking Alamast?

To avoid contamination, be careful to keep the dropper tip from touching the eyelid or surrounding areas when administering the medication.

What are the possible side effects of Alamast?

Side effects cannot be anticipated. If any develop or change in intensity, tell your doctor as soon as possible. Only your doctor can determine if it is safe for you to continue taking this drug.

Side effects may include: allergy, back pain, bronchitis, cold/flu symptoms, cough, dry eyes, eye discomfort, fever, headache, menstrual pain, nasal congestion, sinus inflammation, sneezing, stuffy or runny nose, temporary burning or stinging of the eyes

Can I receive Alamast if I am pregnant or breastfeeding?

The effects of Alamast during pregnancy and breastfeeding are unknown. Talk with your doctor before taking this drug if you are pregnant, plan to become pregnant, or are breastfeeding.

What should I do if I miss a dose of Alamast?

Take it as soon as you remember. If it is almost time for your next dose, skip the one you missed and go back to your regular schedule. Never take 2 doses at the same time.

How should I store Alamast?

Store at room temperature.

Albuterol sulfate See *Proventil HFA, page 1097.*

Alclometasone dipropionate See *Aclovate, page 18.*

ALCORTIN A GEL

Generic name: Hydrocortisone acetate and iodoquinol

What is Alcortin A gel?

Alcortin A is used to treat skin infections. It is an antifungal, antibacterial, and anti-inflammatory gel. Alcortin A is effective against fungi, yeast, bacteria, and the inflammation that often accompanies these infections.

What is the most important information I should know about Alcortin A gel?

Alcortin A is for external use only, and should be kept away from the eyes. Stop using Alcortin A if you have a reaction to it. Staining of the skin, hair, and fabrics may occur.

Who should not take Alcortin A gel?

Alcortin A is not recommended for use on infants or under diapers or occlusive dressings.

Alcortin A is not recommended for patients allergic to iodoquinol, hydrocortisone, acetate, aloe vera, glycine, histadine, lysine, palmitic acid, or any of the other components of this medication.

What should I tell my doctor before I take the first dose of Alcortin A gel?

Always tell your doctor about all the prescription, over-the-counter, and herbal medicines you are taking, as well as your medical history. Also, tell your doctor if you are nursing, or are going to have surgery.

What is the usual dosage?

The information below is based on the dosage guidelines your doctor uses. Depending on your condition and medical history, your doctor may prescribe a different regimen. Do not change the dosage or stop taking your medication without your doctor's approval.

Apply Alcortin A to infected skin 3 to 4 times a day or as directed by your doctor.

How should I take Alcortin A gel?

Alcortin A should be applied to the affected skin as directed by your doctor.

What should I avoid while taking Alcortin A gel?

Avoid prolonged use over large parts of your body. Also, do not cover Alcortin A-treated areas with bandages.

What are possible food and drug interactions associated with Alcortin A gel?

There are no clinically significant food or drug interactions associated with the use of Alcortin A.

What are the possible side effects of Alcortin A gel?

Side effects cannot be anticipated. If any develop or change in intensity, tell your doctor as soon as possible. Only your doctor can determine if it is safe for you to continue taking this drug.

Side effects may include: burning, irritation, itchiness, dryness, inflammation, loss of skin color (hypopigmentation), thinning of the skin (skin atrophy), stretch marks or scarring of the skin (striae), allergic skin reactions, secondary infections, rash, redness of the skin

Can I receive Alcortin A gel if I am pregnant or breastfeeding?

The effects of Alcortin A during pregnancy and breastfeeding are unknown. Talk with your doctor before taking this drug if you are pregnant, plan to become pregnant, or are breastfeeding.

What should I do if I miss a dose of Alcortin A gel?

Apply the missed dose as soon as you remember it. However, if it is almost time for your next dose, skip the one you missed and return to your regular dosing schedule. Do not double the dose.

How should I store Alcortin A gel?

Store Alcortin A at room temperature. Keep tightly closed.

ALDACTAZIDE

Generic name: Spironolactone and hydrochlorothiazide

What is Aldactazide?

Aldactazide is used in the treatment of high blood pressure and other conditions that require the elimination of excess fluid from the body. These conditions include congestive heart failure, cirrhosis of the liver, and kidney disease. Aldactazide combines two diuretic drugs that help your body produce and eliminate more urine.

What is the most important information I should know about Aldactazide?

If you have high blood pressure, you must take Aldactazide regularly for it to be effective. Since blood pressure declines gradually, it may be several weeks before you get the full benefit of Aldactazide; and you must continue taking it even if you are feeling well. Aldactazide does not cure high blood pressure; it merely keeps it under control.

Drugs such as the hydrochlorothiazide component of Aldactazide have been known to trigger gout and allergic reactions. They can also raise your blood sugar levels.

Who should not take Aldactazide?

Do not take Aldactazide if you are allergic to any of its ingredients. Also, do not take this drug if you have kidney disease or liver failure, have difficulty urinating or are unable to urinate, or have high potassium levels in your blood.

What should I tell my doctor before I take the first dose of Aldactazide?

Tell your doctor about all prescription, over-the-counter, and herbal medications you are taking before beginning treatment with Aldactazide. Also, talk to your doctor about your complete medical history, especially if you have kidney or liver problems, or lupus erythematosus (a disease that causes skin eruptions)..Your doctor should know if you are going to have surgery or dental work while on Aldactazide.

What is the usual dosage?
The information below is based on the dosage guidelines your doctor uses. Depending on your condition and medical history, your doctor may prescribe a different regimen. Do not change the dosage or stop taking your medication without your doctor's approval.

Edema (Water Retention)
Adults: The usual dosage is 100 milligrams (mg) each of spironolactone and hydrochlorothiazide daily, taken as a single dose or in divided doses. Dosage may range from 25 mg to 200 mg of each ingredient daily, depending on individual needs.

High Blood Pressure
Adults: The usual dose is 50 mg to 100 mg each of spironolactone and hydrochlorothiazide daily, in a single dose or divided into smaller doses.

What should I avoid while taking Aldactazide?
Avoid abruptly stopping Aldactazide, as it may cause your condition to worsen. Also avoid potassium supplements and foods containing high levels of potassium including salt substitutes.

What are possible food and drug interactions associated with Aldactazide?
If Aldactazide is taken with certain other drugs, the effects of either could be increased, decreased, or altered. It is especially important to check with your doctor before combining Aldactazide with ACE-inhibitor blood pressure drugs, alcohol, gout medications, barbiturates, digoxin, diuretics, insulin or oral antidiabetic drugs, lithium, narcotic drugs such as those containing codeine, nonsteroidal anti-inflammatory drugs, norepinephrine, potassium supplements, and steroids such as prednisone.

What are the possible side effects of Aldactazide?
Side effects cannot be anticipated. If any develop or change in intensity, tell your doctor as soon as possible. Only your doctor can determine if it is safe for you to continue taking this drug.

Side effects may include: breast development in males, deepening of the voice, diarrhea, dizziness, drowsiness, excessive hairiness, fever, headache, hives, irregular menstruation, lack of coordination, loss of appetite, mental confusion, muscle spasms, nausea, postmenopausal bleeding, rash, red or purple spots on skin, restlessness, sensitivity to light, severe allergic reaction, sexual dysfunction, sluggishness, stomach bleeding, stomach ulcers, tingling or pins and needles, vomiting, weakness, yellow eyes and skin

Symptoms of a change in potassium levels: dry mouth, excessive thirst, weak or irregular heartbeat, muscle pain or cramps

Can I receive Aldactazide if I am pregnant or breastfeeding?
The effects of Aldactazide during pregnancy and breastfeeding are unknown. Talk with your doctor before taking this drug if you are pregnant, plan to become pregnant, or are breastfeeding.

What should I do if I miss a dose of Aldactazide?
Take it as soon as you remember. If it is almost time for your next dose, skip the one you missed and go back to your regular schedule. Never take 2 doses at the same time.

How should I store Aldactazide?
Store at room temperature.

ALDACTONE
Generic name: Spironolactone

What is Aldactone?
Aldactone is used to control high blood pressure by flushing excess salt and water from the body. This drug is also used in the treatment of hyperaldosteronism, a condition in which the adrenal gland secretes too much aldosterone (a hormone that regulates the body's salt and potassium levels). It is also used in treating other conditions that require the elimination of excess fluid from the body such as congestive heart failure, cirrhosis of the liver, kidney disease, and unusually low potassium levels in the blood. When used for high blood pressure, Aldactone can be taken alone or with other high blood pressure medications.

What is the most important information I should know about Aldactone?
Aldactone only controls high blood pressure, it does not cure it. If you have high blood pressure, you must take Aldactone regularly for it to be effective. Since blood pressure declines gradually, it may be several weeks before you get the full benefit of Aldactone; and you must continue taking it even if you are feeling well.

Who should not take Aldactone?
Do not begin treatment with Aldactone if you are allergic to any of its ingredients. Also, do not take this drug if you have kidney disease, an

inability to urinate, difficulty urinating, or high potassium levels in your blood.

What should I tell my doctor before I take the first dose of Aldactone?

Tell your doctor about all prescription, over-the-counter, and herbal medications you are taking before beginning treatment with Aldactone. Also, talk to your doctor about your complete medical history, especially if you have kidney problems, liver disease, or you are going to have surgery or dental work while taking Aldactone.

What is the usual dosage?

The information below is based on the dosage guidelines your doctor uses. Depending on your condition and medical history, your doctor may prescribe a different regimen. Do not change the dosage or stop taking your medication without your doctor's approval.

Primary Hyperaldosteronism
Adults: The usual dosage of Aldactone is between 100 and 400 milligrams (mg) per day. In those who are not good candidates for surgery, this drug is given over the long term at the lowest effective dose.

Fluid Retention (Congestive Heart Failure, Cirrhosis of the Liver, or Kidney Disorders)
Adults: The usual starting dosage is 100 mg daily either in a single dose or divided into smaller doses.

High Blood Pressure
Adults: The usual starting dosage is 50 to 100 mg daily in a single dose or divided into smaller doses. This medication may be given with another diuretic or with other high blood pressure medications.

Potassium Loss
Adults: The usual dosage is 25 to 100 mg per day when potassium cannot be replaced with a supplement.

What should I avoid while taking Aldactone?

Avoid excessive sweating, and be sure to get enough fluids. Dehydration (loss of water in the body) can cause your blood pressure to drop significantly.

What are possible food and drug interactions associated with Aldactone?

If Aldactone is taken with certain other drugs, the effects of either could be increased, decreased, or altered. It is especially important to check with your doctor before combining Aldactone with ACE inhibitors, alcohol, barbiturates such as phenobarbital, digoxin, indomethacin, lithium, narcotic drugs such as those containing codeine, nonsteroidal anti-inflammatory drugs, norepinephrine, other diuretics, other high blood pressure medications, and steroids such as prednisone.

What are the possible side effects of Aldactone?

Side effects cannot be anticipated. If any develop or change in intensity, tell your doctor as soon as possible. Only your doctor can determine if it is safe for you to continue taking this drug.

Side effects may include: breast development in males, deepening of voice, diarrhea, drowsiness, excessive hairiness, fever, headache, hives, irregular menstruation, lack of coordination, mental confusion, post-menopausal bleeding, severe allergic reaction, sexual dysfunction, skin eruptions, sleepiness, stomach bleeding, stomach cramps, stomach inflammation, ulcers, vomiting

Symptoms of potassium level changes: dry mouth, excessive thirst, weak or irregular heartbeat, muscle pain or cramps

Can I receive Aldactone if I am pregnant or breastfeeding?

The effects of Aldactone during pregnancy and breastfeeding are unknown. Talk with your doctor before taking this drug if you are pregnant, plan to become pregnant, or are breastfeeding.

What should I do if I miss a dose of Aldactone?

Take it as soon as you remember. If it is almost time for your next dose, skip the one you missed and go back to your regular schedule. Never take 2 doses at the same time.

How should I store Aldactone?

Store at room temperature.

Alendronate sodium See Fosamax, page 597.

Alendronate sodium and cholecalciferol
See Fosamax Plus D, page 600.

Alfuzosin hydrochloride See Uroxatral, page 1360.

ALINIA

Generic name: Nitazoxanide

What is Alinia?

Alinia is used to treat diarrhea caused by the parasites *Cryptosporidium parvum* and *Giardia lambia.* The suspension is indicated for patients 1 year of age and older. The tablets are indicated for patients 12 years of age and older.

What is the most important information I should know about Alinia?

The safety and effectiveness of Alinia have not been studied in children less than 12 months old. The tablets contain a greater amount of the drug than the oral suspension and should not be used in children under 11 years old.

Who should not take Alinia?

Do not begin treatment with Alinia if you are allergic to any of its ingredients. Also, this drug should not be given to those who have kidney or liver problems or with weakened immune systems, including those with HIV or AIDS.

What should I tell my doctor before I take the first dose of Alinia?

Tell your doctor about all prescription, over-the-counter, and herbal medications you are taking before beginning treatment with Alinia. Also, talk to your doctor about your complete medical history, especially if you have diabetes (this drug contains sucrose, a type of sugar, have or had liver problems, have or had kidney problems, or you have or had bile or gallbladder problems.

What is the usual dosage?

The information below is based on the dosage guidelines your doctor uses. Depending on your condition and medical history, your doctor may prescribe a different regimen. Do not change the dosage or stop taking your medication without your doctor's approval.

Adults and children 12 years and older: 1 tablet (500 mg nitazoxanide) every 12 hours with food or 25 mL of oral suspension (500 mg nitazoxanide) every 12 hours with food.

Children 4 to 11 years: 10 mL of oral suspension (200 mg nitazoxanide) every 12 hours with food.

Children 1 to 3 years: 5 milliliters (mL) of oral suspension (100 mg nitazoxanide) every 12 hours with food.

How should I take Alinia?

Alinia should be taken with food. The amount of water needed to prepare the oral suspension is 48 mL. Tap bottle until all powder flows freely. Add approximately one-half of the total amount of water required and shake vigorously to suspend powder. Add remainder of water and again shake vigorously.

What should I avoid while taking Alinia?

Avoid taking Alinia on an empty stomach.

What are possible food and drug interactions associated with Alinia?

If Alinia is taken with certain other drugs, the effects of either could be increased, decreased, or altered. Always check with your doctor before combining Alinia with any other medication.

What are the possible side effects of Alinia?

Side effects cannot be anticipated. If any develop or change in intensity, tell your doctor as soon as possible. Only your doctor can determine if it is safe for you to continue taking this drug.

Side effects may include: constipation, diarrhea, dizziness, dry mouth, gas, headache, itchiness, leg cramps, muscle aches, nausea, sore throat, sweating, thirst

Can I receive Alinia if I am pregnant or breastfeeding?

The effects of Alinia during pregnancy and breastfeeding are unknown. Talk with your doctor before taking this drug if you are pregnant, plan to become pregnant, or are breastfeeding.

What should I do if I miss a dose of Alinia?

Take the forgotten dose with food as soon as you remember. However, if it is almost time for the next dose, skip the missed dose and return to the regular schedule. Do not take two doses at once.

How should I store Alinia?

Store at room temperature. Oral suspension may only be kept for 7 days when mixed with water.

Aliskiren *See Tekturna, page 1271.*

Aliskiren and hydrochlorothiazide *See Tekturna HCT, page 1273.*

ALLEGRA

Generic name: Fexofenadine hydrochloride

What is Allegra?

Allegra relieves the itchy, runny nose, sneezing, and itchy, red, watery eyes that come with hay fever. It is also used to relieve the itching and welts of hives.

What is the most important information I should know about Allegra?

It is important to take Allegra regularly, as your doctor prescribes—even when you start to feel better. Waiting too long between doses gives your symptoms a chance to worsen.

Who should not take Allegra?

Do not begin treatment with Allegra if you are allergic to any of its ingredients.

What should I tell my doctor before I take the first dose of Allegra?

Tell your doctor about all prescription, over-the-counter, and herbal medications you are taking before beginning treatment with Allegra. Also, talk to your doctor about your complete medical history, especially if you have liver or kidney problems, high blood pressure, diabetes, heart disease, glaucoma, thyroid disease, or symptoms of an enlarged prostate such as difficulty urinating.

What is the usual dosage?

The information below is based on the dosage guidelines your doctor uses. Depending on your condition and medical history, your doctor may prescribe a different regimen. Do not change the dosage or stop taking your medication without your doctor's approval.

Seasonal Allergies
Adults and children 12 years and older: The recommended dose is 60 milligrams (mg) twice daily or 180 mg once daily with water.

Children 6 to 11 years: The recommended dose is 30 mg twice daily with water.

Hives
Children 2 to 11 years: The recommended dose of the oral suspension is 30 mg twice daily.

Children 6 months to 11 years: The recommended dose of the oral suspension is 30 mg (5 milliliters [mL]) twice daily for patients 2 to 11 years of age and 15 mg (2.5 mL) twice daily for patients 6 months to less than 2 years of age.

How should I take Allegra?

Allegra tablets should be taken with water.

What should I avoid while taking Allegra?

Do not exceed the recommended dose as prescribed by your doctor.

What are possible food and drug interactions associated with Allegra?

Talk to your doctor if you are taking erythromycin, ketoconazole, and antacids. Also, Allegra should not be taken with fruit juices such as grapefruit, orange, or apple juice.

Allegra-D should not be taken within 2 weeks of an MAO inhibitor.

What are the possible side effects of Allegra?

Side effects cannot be anticipated. If any develop or change in intensity, tell your doctor as soon as possible. Only your doctor can determine if it is safe for you to continue taking this drug.

Side effects of Allegra may include: back pain, drowsiness, fatigue, headache, nausea, missed periods, upset stomach

Side effects of Allegra-D may include: agitation, anxiety, back pain, dizziness, dry mouth, headache, heart palpitations, indigestion, insomnia, nausea, nervousness, respiratory tract infection, stomach pain, sore throat

Can I receive Allegra if I am pregnant or breastfeeding?

The effects of Allegra during pregnancy and breastfeeding are unknown. Talk with your doctor before taking this drug if you are pregnant, plan to become pregnant, or are breastfeeding.

How should I store Allegra?

Store at room temperature.

Almotriptan malate See Axert, page 173.

ALPHAGAN P

Generic name: Brimonidine tartrate

What is Alphagan P?

Alphagan P lowers high pressure in the eye, a problem typically caused by the condition known as open-angle glaucoma. Alphagan P works in two ways: it reduces production of the liquid that fills the eyeball, and it promotes drainage of this liquid. This drug is free of the preservative benzalkonium chloride.

What is the most important information I should know about Alphagan P?

Alphagan P may have a slight effect on blood pressure. If you have severe heart disease, make sure the doctor is aware of it. Caution is warranted.

Who should not take Alphagan P?

You'll need to avoid Alphagan P if it gives you an allergic reaction, or if you're taking a medication classified as a monoamine oxidase inhibitor (MAOI).

What should I tell my doctor before I take the first dose of Alphagan P?

Tell your doctor about all prescription, over-the-counter, and herbal medications you are taking before beginning treatment with Alphagan P. Also, talk to your doctor about your complete medical history, especially if you have heart disease, circulation problems, Raynaud's disease, thromboangiitis obliterans, low blood pressure, depression, and liver or kidney problems.

What is the usual dosage?

The information below is based on the dosage guidelines your doctor uses. Depending on your condition and medical history, your doctor may prescribe a different regimen. Do not change the dosage or stop taking your medication without your doctor's approval.

Adults and children 2 years and older: The usual dose is 1 drop in the affected eye(s) 3 times daily, approximately 8 hours apart.

How should I take Alphagan P?

Alphagan P is administered with an eyedropper. If you are using other eyedrops or ointments, allow at least 5 minutes between doses of each product.

What should I avoid while taking Alphagan P?

Avoid missing regular eye checkups. Because the effect of Alphagan P may diminish over time, the doctor should check your eye pressure periodically.

Alphagan P makes some people drowsy. Do not engage in hazardous activities such as driving until you know how this drug affects you.

Alphagan P has not been studied in children less than 2 years old and should be avoided in this age group.

What are possible food and drug interactions associated with Alphagan P?

If Alphagan P is taken with certain other drugs, the effects of either could be increased, decreased, or altered. It is especially important to check with your doctor before combining Alphagan P with the following: alcohol, antidepressants, barbiturates such as phenobarbital, sleep medications, narcotic painkillers, blood pressure medications, and medications used to treat heart problems such as angina or heart failure.

Alphagan P should never be combined with MAOIs, such as the antidepressants phenelzine and tranylcypromine.

What are the possible side effects of Alphagan P?

Side effects cannot be anticipated. If any develop or change in intensity, tell your doctor as soon as possible. Only your doctor can determine if it is safe to continue using Alphagan P.

Side effects may include: eye redness or irritation, inflamed or swollen eyelids, itchy eyes, burning sensation, conjunctival folliculosis, high blood pressure, allergic reaction, oral dryness, visual disturbance

Can I receive Alphagan P if I am pregnant or breastfeeding?

Although there is no evidence that Alphagan P can cause harm, the effects of the drug during pregnancy have not been adequately studied. If you are pregnant or plan to become pregnant, inform your doctor immediately. It is not known whether Alphagan P appears in breast milk. If you are nursing, its use is not recommended.

What should I do if I miss a dose of Alphagan P?

Take the forgotten dose as soon as you remember. However, if it is almost time for your next dose, skip the one you missed and return to your regular schedule. Do not take two doses at once.

How should I store Alphagan P?

Store at room temperature.

ALPHANATE

Generic name: Antihemophilic Factor VIII (human)

What is Alphanate?

Alphanate is used to prevent and control bleeding in patients with Factor VIII deficiency due to hemophilia A or acquired Factor VIII deficiency.

What is the most important information I should know about Alphanate?

Alphanate is made from human plasma and therefore may carry a risk of transmitting viruses and other infections such as Creutzfeldt-Jacob disease.

Who should not take Alphanate?

There are no known reasons to avoid this medication.

What should I tell my doctor before I take the first dose of Alphanate?

Tell your doctor about all prescription, over-the-counter, and herbal medications you are taking before beginning treatment with Alphanate. Also, talk to your doctor about your complete medical history.

What is the usual dosage?

The information below is based on the dosage guidelines your doctor uses. Depending on your condition and medical history, your doctor may prescribe a different regimen. Do not change the dosage or stop taking your medication without your doctor's approval.

Adults: The doctor will adjust your dosage based on your condition and how you respond to the drug.

How should I take Alphanate?

Your healthcare provider will administer Alphanate intravenously (into the vein).

What should I avoid while taking Alphanate?

Avoid missing any doses as prescribed by your doctor.

What are possible food and drug interactions associated with Alphanate?

If Alphanate is used with certain other drugs, the effects of either could be increased, decreased, or altered. Always check with your doctor before combining Alphanate with any other medication.

What are the possible side effects of Alphanate?

Side effects cannot be anticipated. If any develop or change in intensity, tell your doctor as soon as possible. Only your doctor can determine if it is safe for you to continue taking this drug.

Side effects may include: allergic reactions, chills, fever, itching, increased risk of viral infections such as parvo virus and hepatitis

Signs of severe allergic reactions may include hives, difficulty breathing, and swelling of the throat. If any of these events occur, seek immediate medical attention. Massive doses of Alphanate may result in hemolytic anemia (a condition in which red blood cells get destroyed).

Can I receive Alphanate if I am pregnant or breastfeeding?

The effects of Alphanate during pregnancy and breastfeeding are unknown. Alphanate should be avoided during pregnancy and in nursing mothers.

What should I do if I miss a dose of Alphanate?

Ask your doctor for advice.

How should I store Alphanate?

Alphanate should be refrigerated but not frozen. It may be stored at room temperature for up to 2 months.

Alprazolam *See Xanax, page 1426.*

ALREX
Generic name: Loteprednol etabonate ophthalmic suspension

What is Alrex?
Alrex solution is used for the temporary relief of signs and symptoms associated with seasonal allergies (allergic conjunctivitis).

What is the most important information I should know about Alrex?
If signs and symptoms of allergic conjunctivitis do not improve after 2 days, consult with your doctor for further directions.

Be careful not to contaminate the solution, which may cause further harm to the eyes.

Do not use Alrex for more than 14 days, unless directed by your doctor.

Who should not take Alrex?
Anyone allergic to Alrex or its ingredients should not take this drug. Anyone with viral, bacterial or fungal infections of the eyes should not take Alrex.

What should I tell my doctor before I take the first dose of Alrex?
Tell your doctor about all prescription, over-the-counter, and herbal medications you are taking before beginning treatment with Alrex. Also, talk to your doctor about your complete medical history, especially if you are pregnant or plan to become pregnant. It is important to notify the doctor of previous eye infections, antibiotic use, history of glaucoma, and diabetes.

What is the usual dosage?
The information below is based on the dosage guidelines your doctor uses. Depending on your condition and medical history, your doctor may prescribe a different regimen. Do not change the dosage or stop taking your medication without your doctor's approval.

Adults: The usual dosage is 1 drop into the affected eye(s) 4 times daily.

How should I take Alrex?
Use as directed by your doctor. Before administration, wash your hands thoroughly. Shake vigorously before using. Remove cap and position yourself with head tilted back. Gently pull your lower eyelid with your index finger and administer the drops in each eye without touching the eye or eyelid. Upon administration of the drop, blink a few times and

remove the excess with a clean tissue. Repeat process for the other eye and wash your hands.

What should I avoid while taking Alrex?
Avoid wearing contact lenses.

To avoid contaminating the medication, do not allow the tip of the applicator to touch your eye, finger, or any other surface.

What are possible food and drug interactions associated with Alrex?
If Alrex is taken with certain other drugs, the effects of either could be increased, decreased, or altered. Always check with your doctor before combining Alrex with any other medication.

What are the possible side effects of Alrex?
Side effects cannot be anticipated. If any develop or change in intensity, tell your doctor as soon as possible. Only your doctor can determine if it is safe for you to continue taking this drug.

Side effects may include: blurred vision, burning of the eyes, dry eyes, discharge from the eyes, excessive tear production, itching of the eyes, light intolerance, abnormal vision

Can I receive Alrex if I am pregnant or breastfeeding?
Taking Alrex during pregnancy may be harmful to the fetus. Tell your doctor if you are pregnant or plan on becoming pregnant before beginning treatment with this drug.

The effects of Alrex during breastfeeding are unknown. Tell your doctor if you are breastfeeding or plan on breastfeeding.

What should I do if I miss a dose of Alrex?
If you miss a dose, take it as soon as you remember. If it is close to the time of your next dose, skip it and resume your scheduled dose. Do not double your dose.

How should I store Alrex?
Store upright at room temperature. Do not freeze.

ALTABAX
Generic name: Retapamulin

What is Altabax?
Altabax is a prescription medicine that belongs to a group of medicines called antibacterials. Antibacterial products work by killing disease-causing bacteria (germs) and/or keeping them from growing. Altabax is

used to treat impetigo, a skin infection anyone can get, but often seen in children. Impetigo looks like small, liquid-filled blisters that break and develop a yellowish crust. Impetigo can spread easily from one person to another.

Altabax can be used in adults and children as young as 9 months old. Altabax has not been studied in children younger than 9 months of age.

What is the most important information I should know about Altabax?

Altabax may cause severe local irritation in which case usage should be discontinued. Altabax is not intended for oral use, inside the nose, eyes, or female genital area because it has not been evaluated in these areas.

The use of Altabax may promote the growth of other infections. Appropriate measures should be taken by your healthcare provider.

Notify your healthcare professional if there is no improvement in symptoms within 3 to 4 days after starting use of Altabax. Make sure to use the medication for the full time given by the healthcare provider even if symptoms have improved in a shorter time.

Do not use this medication in children younger than 9 months of age; Altabax has not been studied in these children.

Who should not take Altabax?

Children under the age of 9 months should not be given Altabax.

What should I tell my doctor before I take the first dose of Altabax?

Tell your doctor about all prescription, over-the-counter, and herbal medications you are taking before beginning treatment with Altabax. Also, talk to your doctor about all of your medical problems, including if you: have had an allergic reaction to any medicine, are pregnant or trying to become pregnant, or are breastfeeding. It is not known if Altabax is safe for your unborn baby or if it passes into your breast milk.

What is the usual dosage?

The information below is based on the dosage guidelines your doctor uses. Depending on your condition and medical history, your doctor may prescribe a different regimen. Do not change the dosage or stop taking your medication without your doctor's approval.

A thin layer of Altabax ointment is usually applied twice a day for 5 days

How should I take Altabax?

Use a clean cotton swab to spread a thin layer of Altabax over the infected area, twice a day for 5 days. Wash your hands after applying Altabax.

If you need to spread Altabax on an infected area on you hands, keep the treated area dry. You can cover the treated area with a clean bandage or gauze if you choose. This is especially recommended for children using Altabax because it will protect the treated area and keep Altabax out of the eyes and mouth.

Altabax is for use only on the skin. Be sure to use Altabax for the full 5 days, even though the skin infection seems to be getting better. Call your doctor if there is no improvement in symptoms within 3 to 4 days after starting use of Altabax.

What should I avoid while taking Altabax?

Do not bathe, shower, or swim after applying Altabax. This could wash off the ointment.

Do not swallow or put in eyes, on mouth, lips, inside the nose, or inside the female genital area.

What are possible food and drug interactions associated with Altabax?

If Altabax is used with certain other drugs, the effects of either could be increased, decreased, or altered. It is especially important to check with your doctor before combining Altabax with ketoconazole.

What are the possible side effects of Altabax?

Side effects cannot be anticipated. If any develop or change in intensity, tell your doctor as soon as possible. Only your doctor can determine if it is safe for you to continue taking this drug.

Side effects may include: reactions at the site of application of the ointment. Inform the healthcare practitioner if the area of application worsens in irritation, redness, itching, burning, swelling, blistering, or oozing

Can I receive Altabax if I am pregnant or breastfeeding?

The effects of Altabax during pregnancy and breastfeeding are unknown. Tell your doctor immediately if you are pregnant, plan to become pregnant, or are breastfeeding.

What should I do if I miss a dose of Altabax?

If you forget to apply your dose of Altabax, apply it as soon as you remember if it is within 24 hours of your missed dose. Do not double the dose.

How should I store Altabax?

Store at room temperature. Throw away Altabax that is out of date or no longer needed.

ALTACE
Generic name: Ramipril

What is Altace?
Altace is used to reduce the risk of heart attack, stroke, and death from a heart problem. This drug is also used to help treat high blood pressure; Altace may be used alone or in combination with diuretics. Lastly, this drug is used to stabilize people after a heart attack by preventing heart failure.

What is the most important information I should know about Altace?
Blood pressure medicines called angiotensin-converting enzyme inhibitors (ACE inhibitors), such as Altace, may be associated with increased risk of birth defects if taken during early pregnancy (first three months, or first trimester).

Who should not take Altace?
Do not begin treatment with Altace if you are allergic to any of its ingredients.

What should I tell my doctor before I take the first dose of Altace?
Tell your doctor about all prescription, over-the-counter, and herbal medications you are taking before beginning treatment with Altace. Also, talk to your doctor about your complete medical history, especially if you have kidney problems, are pregnant, plan to become pregnant, or are breastfeeding.

What is the usual dosage?
The information below is based on the dosage guidelines your doctor uses. Depending on your condition and medical history, your doctor may prescribe a different regimen. Do not change the dosage or stop taking your medication without your doctor's approval.

Heart Attack, Stroke, and Related Complications
Adults: The initial dose of Altace is 2.5 milligrams (mg), once a day for 1 week, 5 mg, once a day for the next 3 weeks, and then increased as tolerated, to a dose of 10 mg, once a day.

High Blood Pressure
Adults: The usual dosage (without diuretic) is 2.5 mg once a day. The usual dosage range is 2.5 to 20 mg per day administered as a single dose or in two equally divided doses.

Heart Failure
Adults: The usual starting dosage of Altace is 2.5 mg twice daily (5 mg per day).

How should I take Altace?

Altace capsules are usually swallowed whole. The capsule can also be opened and the contents sprinkled on a small amount of apple sauce or mixed in water or apple juice.

What should I avoid while taking Altace?

Avoid becoming pregnant while being treated with Altace. Also, avoid sweating excessively—this can lead to dehydration which may cause a quick drop in blood pressure. Drink plenty of fluids to remain hydrated if you engage in strenuous activity.

What are possible food and drug interactions associated with Altace?

Talk to your doctor if you are using potassium supplements, potassium salt substitutes, potassium-sparing diuretics, or lithium.

What are the possible side effects of Altace?

Side effects cannot be anticipated. If any develop or change in intensity, tell your doctor as soon as possible. Only your doctor can determine if it is safe for you to continue taking this drug.

Side effects may include: cough, diarrhea, dizziness, fainting, low blood pressure, nausea, vomiting

Can I receive Altace if I am pregnant or breastfeeding?

Do not begin treatment with Altace if you are pregnant or suspect pregnancy. This medication can cause severe birth defects or even death to your unborn child. Altace may pass into your breast milk.

If you become pregnant while taking Altace, stop immediately and contact your doctor.

What should I do if I miss a dose of Altace?

If you forget to take a dose, take it as soon as you remember. If it is almost time for your next dose, skip the one you missed and go back to your regular schedule. Never take 2 doses at the same time.

How should I store Altace?

Store at room temperature.

AMARYL

Generic name: Glimepiride

What is Amaryl?

Amaryl is used to treat type 2 (non-insulin-dependent) diabetes when diet and exercise alone fail to control abnormally high levels of blood sugar.

Like other sulfonylureas, Amaryl lowers blood sugar by stimulating the pancreas to produce more insulin. Amaryl is often prescribed along with the insulin-boosting drug Glucophage. It may also be used with insulin and other diabetes drugs.

What is the most important information I should know about Amaryl?

Amaryl, like other diabetes medications, has caused heart problems that may lead to death. This has occurred more often than in blood sugar treatments of diet modification alone or diet modification plus insulin. This drug is not insulin, and should not be used as an insulin replacement.

The risk of low blood sugar (hypoglycemia) can be increased by missed meals, alcohol, fever, injury, infection, surgery, excessive exercise, and the addition of other diabetes medications.

Who should not take Amaryl?

Do not take Amaryl if you are allergic to any of its ingredients. Do not take this drug to correct diabetic ketoacidosis (a condition caused by insufficient insulin and marked by excessive thirst, nausea, fatigue, and fruity breath). This condition should be treated with insulin.

What should I tell my doctor before I take the first dose of Amaryl?

Tell your doctor about all prescription, over-the-counter, and herbal medications you are taking before beginning treatment with Amaryl. Also, talk to your doctor about your complete medical history, especially if you have heart problems, are pregnant, plan to become pregnant, or are breastfeeding. Insulin is recommended for diabetes treatment during pregnancy.

What is the usual dosage?

The information below is based on the dosage guidelines your doctor uses. Depending on your condition and medical history, your doctor may prescribe a different regimen. Do not change the dosage or stop taking your medication without your doctor's approval.

Adults: The usual starting dose of Amaryl as initial therapy is 1-2 milligrams (mg) once daily. The usual maintenance dose is 1 to 4 mg once daily. The maximum recommended dose is 8 mg once daily.

How should I take Amaryl?

Amaryl should be taken with breakfast or the first main meal. For mild symptoms of low blood sugar, carry pieces of hard candy or a container of juice with you.

What should I avoid while taking Amaryl?

Avoid missing regular blood glucose testing (by yourself or your doctor). Be sure to continue following a diet and exercise regimen as prescribed by your doctor.

What are possible food and drug interactions associated with Amaryl?

Talk with your doctor if you are taking other diuretics, corticosteroids, phenothiazines, thyroid products, estrogens, oral contraceptives, phenytoin, nicotinic acid, sympathomimetics, or isoniazid. Also, be sure to tell your doctor if you are taking salicylates, sulfonamides, chloramphenicol, coumarins, probenecid, monoamine oxidase inhibitors (MAOIs), aspirin, cimetidine, glimepiride, miconazole, or beta-blockers. These drug dosages may need to be adjusted, or they may interact with Amaryl.

What are the possible side effects of Amaryl?

Side effects cannot be anticipated. If any develop or change in intensity, tell your doctor as soon as possible. Only your doctor can determine if it is safe for you to continue taking this drug.

Side effects may include: blurred vision, diarrhea, dizziness, headache, itching, jaundice (yellowing of skin and eyes), muscle weakness, nausea, sensitivity to light, skin rash and eruptions, stomach pain, vomiting

Symptoms of low blood sugar: blurred vision, cold sweats, coma, dizziness, fast heartbeat, fatigue, headache, hunger, light-headedness, nausea, nervousness, pale skin, shallow breathing

Can I receive Amaryl if I am pregnant or breastfeeding?

Do not begin treatment with Amaryl if you are pregnant, plan to become pregnant, or are breastfeeding. Insulin is recommended to control diabetes during pregnancy. Also, Amaryl may pass into your breast milk.

What should I do if I miss a dose of Amaryl?

Take it as soon as you remember. If it is almost time for the next dose, skip the one you missed and go back to your regular schedule. Do not take 2 doses at the same time.

How should I store Amaryl?

Store at room temperature.

AMBIEN
Generic name: Zolpidem tartrate

What is Ambien?
Ambien is used for the short-term treatment of insomnia, which includes trouble falling asleep, waking up too early in the morning, or waking up often during the night.

What is the most important information I should know about Ambien?
Do not take Ambien if you are allergic to any of its ingredients.

Do not drive or engage in hazardous activities that require mental alertness or coordination after taking Ambien until you feel fully awake.

After you stop taking Ambien, you may experience lightheadedness, trouble sleeping, nausea, and nervousness for 1 to 2 days.

When sleep medicines are used every night for more than a few weeks, they may lose their effectiveness or cause dependence.

Call your doctor if your insomnia worsens or does not improve within 7 to 10 days of beginning treatment. This may mean that there is another condition causing your sleeping problems.

Tell your doctor if you experience abnormal thinking, mood problems, behavior changes, anxiety, or memory loss while taking this medication.

Who should not take Ambien?
Do not take Ambien if you are allergic to any of its ingredients.

What should I tell my doctor before I take the first dose of Ambien?
Tell your doctor about all prescription, over-the-counter, and herbal medications you are taking before beginning treatment with Ambien. Also, talk to your doctor about your complete medical history, especially if you have ever abused or been dependent on alcohol, prescription drugs, or street drugs. In addition, tell your doctor if you have a history of suicidal thoughts, depression, or mental illness.

What is the usual dosage?
The information below is based on the dosage guidelines your doctor uses. Depending on your condition and medical history, your doctor may prescribe a different regimen. Do not change the dosage or stop taking your medication without your doctor's approval.

Adults: The recommended dose is 10 milligrams (mg) taken immediately before bedtime. Elderly patients and those with liver problems may need to take a lower dose.

The safety and effectiveness of Ambien have not been established in children.

How should I take Ambien?

Take Ambien immediately before going to bed. Do not take Ambien with or immediately after a meal.

Do not take Ambien unless you are able to stay in bed for a full night (7-8 hours) before you must be active again.

What should I avoid while taking Ambien?

Do not drink alcohol while taking Ambien because it can increase the drug's side effects.

When you first start taking Ambien, you may be drowsy the next day. Use extreme care while doing anything that requires complete alertness, such as driving or operating machinery.

Do not take Ambien with other medications that can make you sleepy.

What are possible food and drug interactions associated with Ambien?

If Ambien is taken with certain other drugs, the effects of either could be increased, decreased, or altered. It is especially important to check with your doctor before combining Ambien with the following: alcohol, chlorpromazine, imipramine, ketoconazole, and rifampin.

What are the possible side effects of Ambien?

Side effects cannot be anticipated. If any develop or change in intensity, tell your doctor as soon as possible. Only your doctor can determine if it is safe for you to continue taking this drug.

Side effects may include: diarrhea, dizziness, drowsiness, drugged feeling

Can I receive Ambien if I am pregnant or breastfeeding?

The effects of Ambien during pregnancy are unknown. Sleep medicines may cause sedation of your unborn baby when used during the last weeks of pregnancy. Ambien should not be used if you are breastfeeding. Tell your doctor immediately if you are pregnant, planning to become pregnant, or are breastfeeding.

What should I do if I miss a dose of Ambien?

Skip the missed dose and go back to your regular dosing schedule. Do not take two doses at once. Do not take more than your total daily dose in any 24-hour period.

How should I store Ambien?

Store at room temperature.

AMBIEN CR
Generic name: Zolpidem tartrate, extended-release

What is Ambien CR?
Ambien CR belongs to a group of medicines known as sedative/hypnotics, or sleep medicines. Ambien CR is used for the short-term treatment of insomnia, which includes trouble falling asleep, waking up too early in the morning, or waking up often during the night.

What is the most important information I should know about Ambien CR?
Do not take Ambien CR if you are allergic to any of its ingredients.

Do not take Ambien CR unless you are able to stay in bed for a full night (7-8 hours) before you must be active again.

Do not drive or engage in hazardous activities that require mental alertness or coordination after taking Ambien CR until you are fully awake.

After you stop taking Ambien CR you may experience lightheadedness, trouble sleeping, nausea, or nervousness for 1 to 2 days.

When sleep medicines are used every night for more than a few weeks, they may lose their effectiveness or cause dependence.

Call your doctor if your insomnia worsens or does not improve within 7 to 10 days of beginning treatment. This may mean that there is another condition causing your sleep problems.

Tell your doctor if you experience abnormal thinking, mood problems, behavior changes, anxiety, or memory loss while taking this medication.

Who should not take Ambien CR?
Do not take Ambien CR if you are allergic to any of its ingredients.

What should I tell my doctor before I take the first dose of Ambien CR?
Tell your doctor about all prescription, over-the-counter, and herbal medications you are taking before beginning treatment with Ambien CR. Also, talk to your doctor about your complete medical history, especially if you have ever abused or been dependent on alcohol, prescription drugs, or street drugs. In addition tell your doctor if you have a history of suicidal thoughts, depression, or mental illness.

What is the usual dosage?
The information below is based on the dosage guidelines your doctor uses. Depending on your condition and medical history, your doctor may prescribe a different regimen. Do not change the dosage or stop taking your medication without your doctor's approval.

Adults: The recommended dose is 12.5 milligrams (mg) taken immediately before bedtime. Elderly patients and those with liver problems may need to take a lower dose.

The safety and effectiveness of Ambien CR have not been established in children.

How should I take Ambien CR?

Take Ambien CR immediately before going to bed. Swallow Ambien CR tablets whole. Do not divide, crush, or chew the tablets. Taking Ambien CR with or immediately after a meal may slow the medication's effects. Do not take Ambien CR unless you are able to stay in bed for a full night (7-8 hours) before you must be active again.

What should I avoid while taking Ambien CR?

Do not drink alcohol while taking Ambien CR because it can increase the drug's side effects.

Take Ambien CR exactly as prescribed. Do not take a larger dose of Ambien CR than you need.

When you first start taking Ambien CR, you may be drowsy the next day. Use extreme care while doing anything that requires complete alertness, such as driving, operating machinery, or piloting an aircraft.

Do not take Ambien CR with other medications that can make you sleepy.

What are possible food and drug interactions associated with Ambien CR?

If Ambien CR is taken with certain other drugs, the effects of either could be increased, decreased, or altered. It is especially important to check with your doctor before combining Ambien CR with the following: alcohol, chlorpromazine, imipramine, ketoconazole, rifampin, and other sedative/hypnotic drugs that slow the central nervous system, which may prolong the sedative effects of Ambien CR.

What are the possible side effects of Ambien CR?

Side effects cannot be anticipated. If any develop or change in intensity, tell your doctor as soon as possible. Only your doctor can determine if it is safe for you to continue taking this drug.

Side effects may include: daytime drowsiness, dizziness, headache, sleepiness

Can I receive Ambien CR if I am pregnant or breastfeeding?

The effects of Ambien CR during pregnancy are unknown. Sleep medicines may cause sedation of your unborn baby when used during the last weeks of pregnancy. The use of Ambien CR in nursing mothers is not recommended. Tell your doctor immediately if you are pregnant, planning to become pregnant, or are nursing.

What should I do if I miss a dose of Ambien CR?

This drug should be taken only if needed, at bedtime. If you miss a dose, skip it. Do not take an extra dose to make up for missed doses.

How should I store Ambien CR?

Store at room temperature.

Ambrisentan *See Letairis, page 716.*

AMERGE

Generic name: Naratriptan hydrochloride

What is Amerge?

Amerge is used to treat migraine headaches (but it does not prevent or reduce the number of attacks you experience).

What is the most important information I should know about Amerge?

There is a risk of heart attack associated with Amerge. If you have heart problems, talk to your doctor about other migraine treatments.

Who should not take Amerge?

Do not take Amerge if you are allergic to any of its ingredients.

Do not take Amerge if you have risk factors for heart disease such as high blood pressure, high cholesterol, are overweight, have diabetes, smoke, have a strong family history of heart disease, are postmenopausal, or a male over the age of 40.

You should not take Amerge if you have kidney or liver problems.

What should I tell my doctor before I take the first dose of Amerge?

Tell your doctor about all prescription, over-the-counter, and herbal medications you are taking before beginning treatment with Amerge. Also, talk to your doctor about your complete medical history, especially if you have heart, kidney, or liver problems, or if you have high blood pressure.

What is the usual dosage?

The information below is based on the dosage guidelines your doctor uses. Depending on your condition and medical history, your doctor may prescribe a different regimen. Do not change the dosage or stop taking your medication without your doctor's approval.

Adults: The usual dosage of Amerge is between 1 milligram (mg) and 2.5 mg taken for each migraine attack.

If your headache returns because you have only had a partial response to Amerge, speak with your doctor as he may recommend you repeat treatment 4 hours after the first dose. The maximum dose of Amerge is 5 mg a day.

How should I take Amerge?

Amerge tablets should be taken whole with fluids.

You may take it at any time after your headache starts. If you have no response to the first tablet, do not take a second tablet without first talking to your doctor. If you need more relief due to a partial response or return of your headache after the first tablet, a second tablet may be taken, but not sooner than 4 hours following the first tablet.

Do not take more than a total of 2 tablets in any 24-hour period.

If you have kidney or liver disease, take as directed by your doctor.

What should I avoid while taking Amerge?

Avoid becoming pregnant while being treated with Amerge.

What are possible food and drug interactions associated with Amerge?

If Amerge is taken with certain other drugs, the effects of either could be increased, decreased, or altered. It is especially important to check with your doctor before combining Amerge with other migraine medicines or medicines for depression, including selective serotonin reuptake inhibitors (SSRIs) or selective norepinephrine reuptake inhibitors (SNRIs).

What are the possible side effects of Amerge?

Side effects cannot be anticipated. If any develop or change in intensity, tell your doctor as soon as possible. Only your doctor can determine if it is safe for you to continue taking this drug.

Side effects may include: dizziness, drowsiness, fatigue, feeling warm, flushing, heaviness, pressure, feeling sick, tingling

Stop taking Amerge immediately and call your doctor if you have: heart throbbing, chest or throat pain or tightness, hives, shortness of breath, skin rash, skin lumps, sudden severe abdominal pain, swelling of eyelids/face/lips, wheezing, confusion, hallucinations, feeling faint, sweating, muscle spasm, difficulty walking, or diarrhea

Can I receive Amerge if I am pregnant or breastfeeding?

The effects of Amerge on pregnancy are unknown, and it may pass into breast milk. Talk to your doctor if you are pregnant, planning to become pregnant, or are nursing.

What should I do if I miss a dose of Amerge?

If you missed a dose of Amerge, take the dose as soon as possible unless it is almost time for the next dose. Do not take 2 doses at the same time.

How should I store Amerge?
Store at room temperature, away from light and heat.

Amiodarone hydrochloride See Cordarone, page 335.

AMITIZA
Generic name: Lubiprostone

What is Amitiza?
Amitiza is used to treat chronic constipation in adults when the cause is unknown. It is also used to treat irritable bowel syndrome with constipation in women 18 years and older.

What is the most important information I should know about Amitiza?
People taking Amitiza may experience difficulty breathing or shortness of breath within an hour of the first dose. However, this symptom generally resolves within 3 hours but may recur with repeated dosing.

Who should not take Amitiza?
You should not take Amitiza if you are allergic to any of its ingredients. Also avoid this drug if you have severe diarrhea or a suspected gastrointestinal obstruction.

What should I tell my doctor before I take the first dose of Amitiza?
Before you start Amitiza, tell your doctor about all prescription, over-the-counter, and herbal medication you are taking. Also talk to your doctor about your complete medical history, especially if you have symptoms of a gastrointestinal obstruction or if you are pregnant, plan to become pregnant, or are breastfeeding.

What is the usual dosage?
The information below is based on the dosage guidelines your doctor uses. Depending on your condition and medical history, your doctor may prescribe a different regimen. Do not change the dosage or stop taking your medication without your doctor's approval.

Chronic Constipation
Adults: The usual dose is 24 micrograms (mcg) taken twice daily.

Irritable Bowel Syndrome with Constipation
Women 18 years and older: The usual dose is 8 mcg taken twice daily.

How should I take Amitiza?
Take Amitiza as directed by your doctor. Take it with food and water.

What should I avoid while taking Amitiza?

To reduce symptoms of nausea, avoid taking Amitiza on an empty stomach. Report symptoms of severe nausea or diarrhea to your doctor.

What are possible food and drug interactions associated with Amitiza?

If Amitiza is used with certain other drugs, the effects of either could be increased, decreased, or altered. Always check with your doctor before combining Amitiza with any other medication.

What are the possible side effects of Amitiza?

Side effects cannot be anticipated. If any develop or change in intensity, tell your doctor as soon as possible. Only your doctor can determine if it is safe for you to continue taking this drug.

Side effects may include: nausea, diarrhea, headache, abdominal pain, gas

Can I receive Amitiza if I am pregnant or breastfeeding?

The effects of taking Amitiza during pregnancy or breastfeeding are unknown. Talk to your doctor if you are pregnant, plan to become, or are breastfeeding.

How should I store Amitiza?

Store at room temperature. Protect from extreme temperatures.

AMILORIDE AND HYDROCHLOROTHIAZIDE

What is Amiloride and hydrochlorothiazide?

Amiloride and hydrochlorothiazide is a diuretic combination used to treat high blood pressure and congestive heart failure, conditions which require the elimination of excess fluid (water) from the body.

What is the most important information I should know about Amiloride and hydrochlorothiazide?

Potassium supplements, potassium-containing salt substitutes, and other diuretics (such as triamterene) that minimize loss of potassium should not be used while you are taking amiloride and hydrochlorothiazide unless your doctor specifically says otherwise. You should also limit your consumption of potassium-rich foods such as bananas, prunes, raisins, orange juice, and whole and skim milk. Ask your doctor for advice on how much of these foods to consume.

If you are taking amiloride and hydrochlorothiazide, a complete assessment of your kidney function should be done; kidney function should continue to be monitored.

If you are taking an ACE-inhibitor type of blood pressure medication such as enalapril, this drug should be used with extreme caution.

If you have liver disease, diabetes, gout, or collagen vascular disease (lupus erythematosus), amiloride and hydrochlorothiazide should be used with caution.

If you have bronchial asthma or a history of allergies, you may be at risk for an allergic reaction to this medication.

Who should not take Amiloride and hydrochlorothiazide?

If you are unable to urinate or have serious kidney disease, or if you have high potassium levels in your blood, you should not take this medication.

If you are sensitive to or have ever had an allergic reaction to amiloride, hydrochlorothiazide or similar drugs, or if you are sensitive to other sulfonamide-derived drugs, you should not take this medication. Make sure your doctor is aware of any drug reactions you may have experienced.

What should I tell my doctor before I take the first dose of Amiloride and hydrochlorothiazide?

Tell your doctor about all prescription, over-the-counter, and herbal medications you are taking before beginning treatment with this drug. Also, talk to your doctor about your complete medical history, especially if you have kidney or liver disease, diabetes, gout, collagen vascular disease (lupus erythematosus), asthma, or allergies.

What is the usual dosage?

The information below is based on the dosage guidelines your doctor uses. Depending on your condition and medical history, your doctor may prescribe a different regimen. Do not change the dosage or stop taking your medication without your doctor's approval.

Your doctor will tailor the dosage to meet your individual requirements, taking into consideration other medical conditions you may have and other medications you may be taking.

Adults: The usual starting dose is 1 tablet per day, which may be increased to 2 tablets per day taken at the same time or separately.

How should I take Amiloride and hydrochlorothiazide?

Take this medication with food. Take Amiloride and hydrochlorothiazide exactly as prescribed by your doctor. Stopping Amiloride and hydrochlorothiazide suddenly could cause your condition to worsen.

What should I avoid while taking Amiloride and hydrochlorothiazide?

Avoid excessive sweating or becoming dehydrated. Dehydration, excessive sweating, severe diarrhea, or vomiting could deplete your fluids and cause your blood pressure to become too low. Be careful when exercising and in hot weather.

Notify your doctor or dentist that you are taking this medication if you have a medical emergency or before you have surgery.

What are possible food and drug interactions associated with Amiloride and hydrochlorothiazide?

If Amiloride and hydrochlorothiazide is taken with certain other drugs, the effects of either could be increased, decreased, or altered. It is especially important to check with your doctor before combining Amiloride and hydrochlorothiazide with the following: ACE inhibitors such as enalapril, barbiturates such as Phenobarbital, cholestyramine, colestipol, corticosteroids such as prednisone, cyclosporine, insulin, lithium, muscle relaxants such as tubocurarine, narcotics such as oxycodone, nonsteroidal anti-inflammatory drugs such as naproxen, norepinephrine, oral drugs for treating diabetes such as glyburide, other high blood pressure medications, and tacrolimus.

Amiloride and hydrochlorothiazide may increase the effects of alcohol. Avoid alcohol while taking this medication.

What are the possible side effects of Amiloride and hydrochlorothiazide?

Side effects cannot be anticipated. If any develop or change in intensity, tell your doctor as soon as possible. Only your doctor can determine if it is safe for you to continue taking this drug.

Side effects may include: diarrhea, dizziness, elevated potassium levels, fatigue, headache, irregular heartbeat, itching, leg pain, loss of appetite, nausea, rash, shortness of breath, stomach and intestinal pain, weakness

Can I receive Amiloride and hydrochlorothiazide if I am pregnant or breastfeeding?

The effects of Amiloride and hydrochlorothiazide during pregnancy have not been adequately studied. If you are pregnant or plan to become pregnant, inform your doctor immediately. Amiloride and hydrochlorothiazide appears in breast milk and could affect a nursing infant. If this medication is essential to your health, your doctor may advise you to discontinue breastfeeding until your treatment is finished.

What should I do if I miss a dose of Amiloride and hydrochlorothiazide?

Take the forgotten dose as soon as you remember. If it is almost time for your next does, skip the one you missed and go back to your regular schedule. Never take a double dose.

How should I store Amiloride and hydrochlorothiazide?

Store at room temperature. Keep this medication in the container it came in, tightly closed, and protected from moisture, light, and freezing.

AMITRIPTYLINE HYDROCHLORIDE

What is Amitriptyline hydrochloride?

Amitriptyline is used to treat depression. It is a member of the group of drugs called tricyclic antidepressants.

What is the most important information I should know about Amitriptyline hydrochloride?

Amitriptyline is not approved for use in children less than 12 years old.

Antidepressant medicines may increase suicidal thoughts or actions in some children, teenagers, and young adults when the medicine is first started. Depression and other serious mental illnesses are the most important causes of suicidal thoughts and actions. Some people may have a particularly high risk of having suicidal thoughts or actions. These include people who have (or have a family history of) bipolar disorder (also called manic-depressive illness) or suicidal thoughts or actions.

Pay close attention to any changes, especially sudden ones, in mood, behaviors, thoughts, or feelings. This is very important when an antidepressant medicine is first started or when the dose is changed.

Call the doctor right away to report new or sudden changes in mood, behavior, thoughts, or feelings. Signs to watch for include new or worsening depression, new or worsening anxiety, agitation, insomnia, hostility, panic attacks, restlessness, extreme hyperactivity, and suicidal thinking or behavior.

Keep all follow-up visits as scheduled, and call the doctor between visits as needed, especially if you have concerns about symptoms.

Do not stop taking antidepressant therapy without first consulting with your physician, as this can cause a variety of side effects.

Who should not take Amitriptyline hydrochloride?

If you are sensitive to or have ever had an allergic reaction to amitriptyline or similar drugs such as desipramine and imipramine, you should not take this medication. Make sure your doctor is aware of any drug reactions you have experienced.

Do not take amitriptyline while taking other drugs known as monoamine oxidase inhibitors (MAOIs). Drugs in this category include the antidepressants phenelzine and tranylcypromine.

Unless you are directed to do so by your doctor, do not take this medication if you are recovering from a heart attack.

Do not take this medication if you are currently taking Cisapride. Concurrent use of the two medications increases the risk for arrhythmia and irregular heart rhythm.

What should I tell my doctor before I take the first dose of Amitriptyline hydrochloride?

Tell your doctor about all prescription, over-the-counter, and herbal medications you are taking before beginning treatment with amitriptyline. Also, talk to your doctor about your complete medical history, especially if you have ever had any of the following: seizures, urinary retention, glaucoma or other chronic eye conditions, a heart or circulatory system disorder, liver problems, bipolar disorder (manic-depression), schizophrenia, or other mental illnesses. Also let your doctor know if you are receiving thyroid medication or if you have diabetes, since amitriptyline may raise or lower blood sugar levels.

Before having surgery, dental treatment, or any diagnostic procedure, tell the doctor that you are taking amitriptyline. Certain drugs used during surgery, such as anesthetics, muscle relaxants, and drugs used in certain diagnostic procedures, may react badly with amitriptyline.

What is the usual dosage?

The information below is based on the dosage guidelines your doctor uses. Depending on your condition and medical history, your doctor may prescribe a different regimen. Do not change the dosage or stop taking your medication without your doctor's approval.

Adults: The usual starting dosage is 75 milligrams (mg) per day divided into 2 or more smaller doses. Your doctor may gradually increase this dose to 150 mg per day. The total daily dose is generally never higher than 200 mg.

Alternatively, your doctor may want you to start with 50 mg to 100 mg at bedtime and may increase this bedtime dose by 25 or 50 mg, up to a total of 150 mg a day.

For long-term use, the usual dose ranges from 40 to 100 mg taken once daily, usually at bedtime.

Children 12 years and older: The usual dose is 10 mg, 3 times a day, with 20 mg taken at bedtime.

How should I take Amitriptyline hydrochloride?

Take this drug exactly as prescribed. Amitriptyline may cause dry mouth. Sucking a hard candy, chewing gum, or melting bits of ice in your mouth can provide relief.

What should I avoid while taking Amitriptyline hydrochloride?

Do not stop taking amitriptyline abruptly, especially if you have been taking large doses for a long time. Your doctor probably will want to decrease your dosage gradually. This will help prevent a possible relapse and will reduce the possibility of withdrawal symptoms.

Amitriptyline may make your skin more sensitive to sunlight. Try to stay out of the sun, wear protective clothing, and apply a sun block.

Amitriptyline may cause you to become drowsy or less alert; therefore, you should not drive or operate dangerous machinery or participate in any hazardous activity that requires full mental alertness until you know how this drug affects you.

Amitriptyline may intensify the effects of alcohol. Do not drink alcohol while taking this medication.

What are possible food and drug interactions associated with Amitriptyline hydrochloride?

If amitriptyline is taken with certain other drugs, the effects of either could be increased, decreased, or altered. It is especially important that you consult with your doctor before taking amitriptyline in combination with the following: airway-opening drugs such as albuterol and pseudo-ephedrine; antiarrhythmic drugs, such as flecainide and propafenone; antidepressants that raise serotonin levels, such as fluoxetine, paroxetine, and sertraline; other antidepressants; antihistamines such as diphenhydramine and clemastine fumarate; Antispasmodic drugs, such as dicyclomine; barbiturates such as phenobarbital; blood pressure medicines such as clonidine; cimetidine; disulfiram; estrogen-containing drugs and oral contraceptives; ethchlorvynol; MAOIs, such as phenelzine and tranylcypromine; painkillers; Parkinson's disease drugs such as benztropine and levodopa; quinidine; seizure medications such as carbamazepine and phenytoin; sleep medicines such as flurazepam and triazolam; thyroid hormones; tranquilizers such as chlorpromazine, thioridazine, alprazolam, and chlordiazepoxide; or warfarin (a blood thinner).

What are the possible side effects of Amitriptyline hydrochloride?

Side effects cannot be anticipated. If any develop or change in intensity, inform your doctor as soon as possible. Only your doctor can determine if it is safe for you to continue taking amitriptyline.

Older adults are especially liable to experience certain side effects of amitriptyline, including rapid heartbeat, constipation, dry mouth, blurred vision, sedation, and confusion, and are in greater danger of sustaining a fall.

Side effects may include: blurred vision, bone marrow depression, bowel problems, breast enlargement (in males and females), constipation, dizziness upon standing, dry mouth, hair loss, heart attack, high body temperature, problems urinating, rash, seizure, stroke, swelling of the testicles, water retention

Side effects due to a rapid decrease in dose or abrupt withdrawal include: headache, nausea, vague feeling of bodily discomfort

Side effects due to gradual dosage reduction may include: dream and sleep disturbances, irritability, restlessness

Can I receive Amitriptyline hydrochloride if I am pregnant or breastfeeding?

The effects of amitriptyline during pregnancy have not been adequately studied. If you are pregnant or planning to become pregnant, tell your doctor immediately. This medication appears in breast milk; consult your doctor before breastfeeding.

What should I do if I miss a dose of Amitriptyline hydrochloride?

If you miss a dose of this drug, skip it. Do not take an extra dose to make up for missed doses.

How should I store Amitriptyline hydrochloride?

Store at room temperature. Protect from light and excessive heat.

Amlodipine and valsartan *See Exforge, page 531.*

Amlodipine besylate *See Norvasc, page 914.*

Amlodipine besylate and atorvastatin calcium *See Caduet, page 238.*

Amlodipine besylate and benazepril hydrochloride *See Lotrel, page 767.*

Amlodipine besylate and olmesartan medoxomil *See Azor, page 189.*

Amoxicillin *See Amoxil, below.*

Amoxicillin and clavulanate potassium *See Augmentin, page 152.*

Amoxicillin, clarithromycin, and lansoprazole *See Prevpac, page 1061.*

AMOXIL

Generic name: Amoxicillin

What is Amoxil?

Amoxil, an antibiotic, is used to treat a wide variety of infections, including: gonorrhea, ear/nose/throat infections, skin infections, respiratory tract infections, and infections of the genital and urinary tract. In combination with other drugs, it is also used to treat duodenal ulcers caused by *H. pylori* bacteria.

What is the most important information I should know about Amoxil?

If you are allergic to either penicillin or cephalosporin antibiotics in any form, consult your doctor before taking Amoxil. There is a possibility that you are allergic to both types of medication; and if a reaction occurs, it could be extremely severe. If you take the drug and feel signs of a reaction, seek medical attention immediately.

You should stop using Amoxil if you experience reactions such as bruising, fever, skin rash, itching, joint pain, swollen lymph nodes, and/ or sores on the genitals. If these reactions occur, stop taking Amoxil unless your doctor advises you to continue.

Who should not take Amoxil?
You should not use Amoxil if you are allergic to penicillin or cephalosporin antibiotics.

What should I tell my doctor before I take the first dose of Amoxil?
Tell your doctor about all prescription, over-the-counter, and herbal medications you are taking before beginning treatment with Amoxil. Also, talk to your doctor about your complete medical history, especially if you have ever had asthma, hives, hay fever, or other allergies; have diabetes and need to perform urine glucose tests; or have a history of colitis (inflammatory bowel disease), diabetes, or kidney or liver disease.

What is the usual dosage?
The information below is based on the dosage guidelines your doctor uses. Depending on your condition and medical history, your doctor may prescribe a different regimen. Do not change the dosage or stop taking your medication without your doctor's approval.

Ear, Nose, Throat, Skin, Genital, and Urinary Tract Infections
Adults: For mild or moderate infections, the usual dose is 250 milligrams every 8 hours, or 500 milligrams every 12 hours. For severe infections, the usual dose is 500 milligrams every 8 hours, or 875 milligrams every 12 hours.

Lower Respiratory Tract Infections
Adults: For mild, moderate, or severe infections, the usual dose is 500 milligrams every 8 hours, or 875 milligrams every 12 hours.

Gonorrhea, Acute, Uncomplicated Anogenital, and Urethral Infections
Adults: The usual dosage is 3 grams in a single oral dose.

Ulcers
Adults: For ulcer treatment, Amoxil is combined with other medications. There are several dosage regimens available, and your doctor will choose the best one for you.

If your kidneys are severely impaired or you are undergoing hemodialysis, the doctor may have to adjust your dosage accordingly.

Children older than 3 months: Children weighing 88 pounds and over should follow the recommended adult dose schedule. Children weighing under 88 pounds will have their dosage determined by their weight.

How should I take Amoxil?

Amoxil can be taken with or without food. If you are using Amoxil suspension, shake it well before using.

Your doctor will only prescribe Amoxil to treat a bacterial infection. Amoxil will not cure a viral infection such as the common cold. It's important to take all of your medication as instructed by your doctor, even if you're feeling better in a few days. Not finishing the complete dosage of Amoxil may decrease the drug's effectiveness and increase the chances for bacterial resistance to Amoxil and similar antibiotics.

For children's dosages, the required amount of liquid medication should be placed directly on the child's tongue for swallowing. It can also be added to formula, milk, fruit juice, water, ginger ale, or cold drinks. The preparation should be taken immediately. To be certain the child is getting the full dose of medication, make sure he or she drinks the entire preparation. If your child is taking the pediatric drops, use the dropper provided to measure the dosage.

What should I avoid while taking Amoxil?

The chewable tablet form of Amoxil contains phenylalanine. If you or your child has the hereditary disease phenylketonuria, this form of Amoxil should not be used.

What are possible food and drug interactions associated with Amoxil?

If Amoxil is taken with certain other drugs, the effects of either could be increased, decreased, or altered. It is especially important to check with your doctor before combining Amoxil with the following: chloramphenicol, erythromycin, estrogen, oral contraceptives, other antibiotics including tetracycline, and probenecid.

What are the possible side effects of Amoxil?

Side effects cannot be anticipated. If any develop or change in intensity, tell your doctor as soon as possible. Only your doctor can determine if it is safe for you to continue taking this drug.

Side effects may include: agitation, anemia, anxiety, changes in behavior, colitis, confusion, convulsions, diarrhea, dizziness, hives, hyperactivity, insomnia, liver problems and jaundice, nausea, peeling skin, rash, tooth discoloration in children, vomiting

When Amoxil is used in combination with other drugs for the treatment of ulcers, the most common side effects are changes in taste sensation, diarrhea, and headache.

Can I receive Amoxil if I am pregnant or breastfeeding?

Amoxil should be used during pregnancy only when clearly needed. If you are pregnant or plan to become pregnant, inform your doctor immediately. Since Amoxil may appear in breast milk, you should consult your doctor if you plan to breastfeed your baby.

What should I do if I miss a dose of Amoxil?

Take it as soon as you remember. If it is almost time for the next dose, and you take 2 doses a day, take the one you missed and the next dose 5 to 6 hours later. If you take 3 or more doses a day, take the one you missed and the next dose 2 to 4 hours later. Then go back to your regular schedule.

How should I store Amoxil?

Amoxil suspension and pediatric drops should be stored in a tightly closed bottle. Discard any unused medication after 14 days. Refrigeration is preferable.

Store capsules at or below 68 degrees. Store chewable tablets and regular tablets at or below 77 degrees in a tightly closed container.

Amphetamine salts *See Adderall, page 34.*

Amphetamine salts, extended-release *See Adderall XR, page 36.*

AMPICILLIN

What is Ampicillin?

Ampicillin is a penicillin-like antibiotic prescribed for a wide variety of infections, including gonorrhea and other genital and urinary infections, respiratory infections, and gastrointestinal infections, as well as meningitis (inflamed membranes of the spinal cord or brain).

What is the most important information I should know about Ampicillin?

If you are allergic to either penicillin or cephalosporin antibiotics in any form, consult your doctor *before taking ampicillin.* There is a possibility that you are allergic to both types of medication; and if a reaction occurs, it could be extremely severe. If you take the drug and develop a skin reaction, diarrhea, shortness of breath, wheezing, sore throat, or fever, seek medical attention immediately.

If you have an allergic reaction, stop taking this drug and contact your doctor immediately.

After you have taken ampicillin for a long time, you may get a new infection (called a superinfection) due to an organism this medication cannot treat. Consult your doctor if your symptoms do not improve or seem to get worse.

Ampicillin sometimes causes diarrhea. Some diarrhea medications can make the diarrhea worse. Check with your doctor before taking any diarrhea remedy.

Oral contraceptives may not work properly while you are taking ampicillin. For greater certainty, use other measures while taking this drug.

If you are diabetic, be aware that ampicillin may cause a false positive in certain urine glucose tests. You should talk to your doctor about the right tests to use while you are taking ampicillin.

Who should not take Ampicillin?
You should not take ampicillin if you are allergic to penicillin or cephalosporin antibiotics.

What should I tell my doctor before I take the first dose of Ampicillin?
Tell your doctor about all prescription, over-the-counter, and herbal medications you are taking before beginning treatment with ampicillin. Also, talk to your doctor about your complete medical history, especially if you have diabetes and need to do urine glucose tests or if you are allergic to either penicillin or cephalosporin antibiotics in any form.

What is the usual dosage?
The information below is based on the dosage guidelines your doctor uses. Depending on your condition and medical history, your doctor may prescribe a different regimen. Do not change the dosage or stop taking your medication without your doctor's approval.

Unless you are being treated for gonorrhea, your doctor will have you continue to take ampicillin for 2 to 3 days after your symptoms have disappeared. Dosages are for capsules and oral suspension. Children weighing over 44 pounds should follow the adult dose schedule. Children weighing 44 pounds or less should have their dosage determined by their weight.

Infections of the Genital, Urinary, or Gastrointestinal Tracts
Adults: The usual dose is 500 milligrams, taken every 6 hours.

Gonorrhea
Adults: The usual dose is 3.5 grams in a single oral dose along with 1 gram of probenecid.

Respiratory Tract Infections
Adults: The usual dose is 250 milligrams, taken every 6 hours.

How should I take Ampicillin?
Take this medication exactly as prescribed. It works best when there is a constant amount in the body. Take your doses at evenly spaced times around the clock, and try not to miss a dose.

Take ampicillin capsules with a full glass of water, a half hour before or 2 hours after a meal. The oral suspension should be shaken well before using.

What should I avoid while taking Ampicillin?
Avoid skipping doses or not completing the full course of treatment, since this decreases antibiotic effectiveness and may increase bacterial resistance.

What are possible food and drug interactions associated with Ampicillin?
If ampicillin is taken with certain other drugs the effects of either could be increased, decreased, or altered. It is especially important to check with your doctor before combining ampicillin with any of the following: allopurinol, atenolol, chloroquine, mefloquine, and oral contraceptives.

What are the possible side effects of Ampicillin?
Side effects cannot be anticipated. If any develop or change in intensity, tell your doctor as soon as possible. Only your doctor can determine if it is safe for you to continue taking this drug.

Side effects may include: colitis (inflammation of the bowel), diarrhea, fever, itching, nausea, rash or other skin problems, sore tongue or mouth, vomiting

Can I receive Ampicillin if I am pregnant or breastfeeding?
The effects of ampicillin during pregnancy have not been adequately studied. If you are pregnant or plan to become pregnant, inform your doctor immediately. Ampicillin should be used during pregnancy only if the potential benefit justifies the potential risk to the developing baby.

Ampicillin appears in breast milk and could affect a nursing infant. If this medication is essential to your health, your doctor may advise you to stop breastfeeding until your treatment is finished.

What should I do if I miss a dose of Ampicillin?
Take it as soon as you remember. If it is almost time for the next dose, and you take 2 doses a day, take the one you missed and the next dose 5 to 6 hours later. If you take 3 or more doses a day, take the one you missed and the next dose 2 to 4 hours later. Then go back to your regular schedule. Do not take 2 doses at once.

How should I store Ampicillin?
Store capsules at room temperature in a tightly closed container. Keep the oral suspension in the refrigerator, in a tightly closed container. Discard the unused portion after 14 days.

AMRIX
Generic name: Cyclobenzaprine hydrochloride

What is Amrix?

Amrix is a muscle relaxant to be used in addition to rest and physical therapy for the relief of muscle spasms associated with acute, painful musculoskeletal conditions.

What is the most important information I should know about Amrix?

Amrix should not be taken by patients using monoamine oxidase inhibitors (MAOIs) such as isocarboxazid, selegiline, etc.) or within 14 days of stopping of MAOIs.

Amrix should not be taken by patients with heart conditions such as recent heart attack, arrhythmia, heart block conduction disturbances, or congestive heart failure.

People with hyperthyroidism should not take Amrix.

Amrix is closely related to tricyclic antidepressants such as amitriptyline and imipramine, which have been reported to produce various serious heart conditions that can lead to heart attack and stroke.

Amrix may enhance the effects of alcohol, barbiturates, and other central nervous system depressants and may impair your ability to operate machinery or drive.

Use of Amrix is not recommended in patients who have mild to moderate liver impairment or in the elderly.

Amrix should be used with caution by patients with a history of urinary retention, angle-closure glaucoma or increased intraocular pressure, and in patients taking anticholinergic medications (such as atropine, scopolamine, etc.).

Who should not take Amrix?

Amrix should not be taken by patients taking MAOIs (such as isocarboxazid, selegiline, etc.) or within 14 days of stopping of MAOIs, patients with heart conditions such as recent heart attack, arrhythmia, heart block conduction disturbances, or congestive heart failure, or by people with hyperthyroidism.

What should I tell my doctor before I take the first dose of Amrix?

Tell your doctor about all prescription, over-the-counter, and herbal medications you are taking, before beginning treatment with Amrix. Also, talk to your doctor about your complete medical history, especially if you have any heart conditions, suffer from any sort of liver problems, have glaucoma, or will need to operate machinery or perform dangerous tasks while on this medicine.

What is the usual dosage?
The information below is based on the dosage guidelines your doctor uses. Depending on your condition and medical history, your doctor may prescribe a different regimen. Do not change the dosage or stop taking your medication without your doctor's approval.

Adults: The recommended dosage for most adult patients is one 15 milligram (mg) capsule taken once daily. Some patients may require up to 30 mg a day, given as one 30-mg capsule taken once daily or two 15-mg capsule taken once daily.

How should I take Amrix?
Amrix should be taken at approximately the same time each day. Amrix should be used for only short periods, up to 2 or 3 weeks.

What should I avoid while taking Amrix?
Avoid operating dangerous machinery or driving while taking Amrix until you know how this medication affects you.

What are possible food and drug interactions associated with Amrix?
If Amrix is taken with certain other drugs, the effects of either could be increased, decreased, or altered. It is especially important to check with your doctor before combining Amrix with the following: alcohol, alprazolam, barbiturates (butabarbital, butalbital, phenobarbital, etc., diazepam, MAOIs (isocarboxazid, selegiline, etc.), guanabenz, guanethidine, reserpine, tramadol.

What are the possible side effects of Amrix?
Side effects cannot be anticipated. If any develop or change in intensity, tell your doctor as soon as possible. Only your doctor can determine if it is safe for you to continue taking this drug.

Side effects may include: drowsiness, dry mouth, headache, dizziness, blurred vision, nausea, altered taste, tremors, acne, disturbance in attention

Can I receive Amrix if I am pregnant or breastfeeding?
Amrix has not been adequately studied in human subjects, although tests on laboratory animals have shown no birth defects. Amrix should be used during pregnancy only if the possible benefits outweigh the risks.

It is not known if Amrix appears in breast milk. Talk with your doctor before taking this drug if you are pregnant, plan to become pregnant, or are breastfeeding.

What should I do if I miss a dose of Amrix?
If you miss a dose of Amrix, skip that dose. Take your next dose at your usual time. Do not take 2 doses at one time.

How should I store Amrix?
Store at room temperature away from light.

ANAFRANIL
Generic name: Clomipramine hydrochloride

What is Anafranil?
Anafranil is used to treat obsessive-compulsive disorder (OCD).

What is the most important information I should know about Anafranil?
Patients with major depressive disorder (MDD) may experience worsening of their depression and/or the emergence of suicidal ideation and behavior or unusual changes in behavior. Suicide is a known risk of depression and certain other psychiatric disorders.

During studies, seizures were the most significant risk of Anafranil use.

Who should not take Anafranil?
Do not use Anafranil if you have a history of hypersensitivity to this drug or other tricyclic antidepressants.

Anafranil should not be combined with, or taken within 14 days of, a type of drug known as a monoamine oxidase inhibitor (MAOI). In addition, Anafranil should not be used during the acute recovery period after a heart attack.

What should I tell my doctor before I take the first dose of Anafranil?
Tell your doctor about all prescription, over-the-counter, and herbal medications you are taking before beginning treatment with Anafranil. Also, talk to your doctor about your complete medical history, especially if you have ever had suicidal thoughts or behaviors; seizures; an overactive thyroid; glaucoma; urinary problems; brain tumors; impaired kidney function; or a family history of bipolar disorder, depression, or suicide.

What is the usual dosage?
The information below is based on the dosage guidelines your doctor uses. Depending on your condition and medical history, your doctor may prescribe a different regimen. Do not change the dosage or stop taking your medication without your doctor's approval.

Adults: Treatment should be initiated at a dosage of 25 milligrams (mg) daily and is gradually increased, as tolerated, to approximately 100 mg during the first two weeks up to a maximum of 250 mg daily.

Children and adolescents: The starting dose is 25 mg daily and is gradually increased during the first 2 weeks, as tolerated, up to a daily maximum of 3 mg/kg or 100 mg, whichever is smaller. The daily maximum after the titration period is 200 mg.

How should I take Anafranil?
During initial titration, Anafranil should be given in divided doses with meals in order to reduce stomach upset. After the titration period, it is best taken at bedtime to minimize daytime sedation.

What should I avoid while taking Anafranil?
Never stop taking an antidepressant without first talking to your doctor.

Because Anafranil can cause dizziness and drowsiness, avoid activities requiring mental alertness or coordination until you know how this drug affects you.

Do not drink alcohol while taking this drug.

Do not take MAOIs during or within 14 days before or after Anafranil therapy.

What are possible food and drug interactions associated with Anafranil?
If Anafranil is taken with certain other drugs, the effects of either could be increased, decreased, or altered. It is especially important to check with your doctor before combining Anafranil with the following: central nervous system medications, cimetidine, clonidine, digoxin, fluoxetine, guanethidine, phenobarbital, phenytoin, quinidine, and warfarin.

What are the possible side effects of Anafranil?
Side effects cannot be anticipated. If any develop or change in intensity, tell your doctor as soon as possible. Only your doctor can determine if it is safe for you to continue taking this drug.

Side effects may include: stomach upset, dry mouth, constipation, nausea, loss of appetite, dizziness, nervousness, sexual dysfunction, fatigue, sweating, vision changes

Can I receive Anafranil if I am pregnant or breastfeeding?
The effects of Anafranil during pregnancy are unknown. Tell your doctor immediately if you are pregnant or plan to become pregnant. Because Anafranil can pass into breast milk, it is important to consult your doctor before breastfeeding.

What should I do if I miss a dose of Anafranil?
Take it as soon as you remember. If it is almost time for your next dose, skip the missed dose and return to your regular schedule. Never take 2 doses at the same time.

How should I store Anafranil?
Store in a cool, dry place in a light-resistant container.

ANAPROX
Generic name: Naproxen sodium

What is Anaprox?
Anaprox is a non-steroidal anti-inflammatory drug (NSAID). Anaprox is used to treat pain, swelling, and inflammation from different types of arthritis, menstrual cramps, or other short-term pain.

**What is the most important information
I should know about Anaprox?**
Like other NSAIDs, this drug may increase the risk of heart attack with prolonged usage or if you already have heart disease. Anaprox should not be used right after a surgery called a coronary artery bypass graft (CABG). This drug can also cause stomach problems such as ulcers.

Who should not take Anaprox?
Do not take Anaprox right before CABG, or if you have had an asthma attack or hives. Also, do not take this medication if you are allergic to any of its ingredients.

**What should I tell my doctor before
I take the first dose of Anaprox?**
Tell your doctor about all prescription, over-the-counter, and herbal medications you are taking before beginning treatment with Anaprox. Also, talk to your doctor about your complete medical history, especially if you are pregnant or nursing.

What is the usual dosage?
The information below is based on the dosage guidelines your doctor uses. Depending on your condition and medical history, your doctor may prescribe a different regimen. Do not change the dosage or stop taking your medication without your doctor's approval.
    Your doctor will prescribe the appropriate dosage for you.

What should I avoid while taking Anaprox?
Avoid becoming pregnant or nursing without talking to your doctor first. Also, avoid beginning treatment with Anaprox if you are going to go into surgery for your heart.

What are possible food and drug interactions associated with Anaprox?

If Anaprox is taken with certain other drugs, the effects of either could be increased, decreased, or altered. It is especially important to check with your doctor before combining Anaprox with:

ACE inhibitors, antacids and sucralfat, aspirin, beta blockers, cholestyramin, coumarin-type anticoagulant, diuretics such as furosemide and thiazide, histamine-2 receptor antagonists, or H2 blocker, hydantoin, lithium, methotrexate, naproxen-containing products, oral diabetes drugs such as glyburide, other nonsteroidal anti-inflammatory drugs (NSAIDs), probenecid, sulphonylurea, warfarin.

What are the possible side effects of Anaprox?

Side effects cannot be anticipated. If any develop or change in intensity, tell your doctor as soon as possible. Only your doctor can determine if it is safe for you to continue taking this drug.

Side effects may include: Constipation, diarrhea, dizziness, gas, heartburn, nausea, stomach pain, vomiting

Contact your doctor immediately if you have: Asthma attacks, allergic reactions, blood in vomit/stool, chest pain, flu-like symptoms, heart attack, high blood pressure, itching, more fatigue than usual, nausea, shortness of breath, skin rash/blisters with fever, slurred speech, stroke, swelling of the face, throat, arms, legs or hands, weakness on one side of the body, weight gain, yellowing of the eyes or skin

Can I receive Anaprox if I am pregnant or breastfeeding?

Talk to your doctor if you are pregnant, planning to become pregnant, or are nursing. It is not recommended to begin treatment with Anaprox if you are pregnant or nursing.

How should I store Anaprox?

Store at room temperature.

Anastrozole *See Arimidex, page 125.*

ANDROGEL
Generic name: Testosterone gel

What is AndroGel?

AndroGel is a clear, colorless gel medicine used because your body does not produce enough testosterone, a condition called hypogonadism.

What is the most important information I should know about AndroGel?

Patients with benign prostatic hyperplasia (BPH) are at an increased risk for worsening signs and symptoms of BPH when being treated with AndroGel. AndroGel may also increase the risk of prostate cancer in men.

Patients should also wash their hands thoroughly after each application and cover the application site with clothing after it dries to prevent the medicine from coming in contact with others, especially women and children.

AndroGel may cause severe liver problems.

AndroGel may cause your body to retain more sodium and water than is needed, which can have serious consequences if you have heart, kidney, or liver disease.

AndroGel may worsen sleep apnea, a disorder in which your breathing pauses during sleep, especially if you have risk factors (are overweight or have chronic lung disease).

This drug should not be used by women.

This medication is inflammable and you should keep the application site away from open flames until it dries.

Who should not take AndroGel?

Women should not take AndroGel.

Do not use AndroGel if have had breast or prostate cancer.

Do not use AndroGel if you are allergic to any of its ingredients, including alcohol and soy products.

What should I tell my doctor before I take the first dose of AndroGel?

Tell your doctor about all prescription, over-the-counter, and herbal medications you are taking before beginning treatment with AndroGel. Also, talk to your doctor about your complete medical history, especially if you have a history of breast or prostate cancer.

What is the usual dosage?

The information below is based on the dosage guidelines your doctor uses. Depending on your condition and medical history, your doctor may prescribe a different regimen. Do not change the dosage or stop taking your medication without your doctor's approval.

Adults: The recommended starting dose of AndroGel is 5 grams (g), which delivers 5 milligrams (mg) of testosterone, applied once daily to clean, dry, intact skin of the shoulders and upper arms and/or abdomen.

How should I take AndroGel?

Apply AndroGel once a day at the same time each day, preferably in the morning (after a shower or bath).

Apply the gel to clean, dry, unbroken skin on your shoulders, upper arms or abdomen.

Do not apply AndroGel to the genitals or to skin with open wounds or irritation.

Wash your hands with soap and water immediately after you apply AndroGel; allow a few minutes for the medication to dry before putting your clothes on.

Wait 5-6 hours after applying before showering or swimming.

What should I avoid while taking AndroGel?

Avoid touching other people while you have AndroGel on your hands.

Avoid showering or swimming for 5-6 hours after application.

Avoid any open flames or smoking until the medication dries.

What are possible food and drug interactions associated with AndroGel?

If AndroGel is used with certain other drugs, the effects of either could be increased, decreased, or altered. It is especially important to check with your doctor before combining AndroGel with corticosteroids, insulin, oxyphenbutazone, propanolol, or anticoagulants (blood thinners).

What are the possible side effects of AndroGel?

Side effects cannot be anticipated. If any develop or change in intensity, tell your doctor as soon as possible. Only your doctor can determine if it is safe for you to continue taking this drug.

Side effects may include: acne, breast development/discomfort, emotional problems such as depression, sleep problems, local skin irritation, prostate enlargement, swelling

Talk to your doctor if you develop: breathing problems, difficulty urinating, nausea, prolonged or frequent erections, vomiting, yellowing of the skin or eyes

What should I do if I miss a dose of AndroGel?

If your next dose is less than 12 hours away, wait and take it then. Do not take the skipped dose. If it is more than 12 hours until your next dose, take the dose you missed. Resume your normal dosing the next day. If you miss a dose, do not double your next dose.

How should I store AndroGel?

Store at room temperature.

ANGELIQ

Generic name: Drospirenone and estradiol

What is Angeliq?

Angeliq is a medicine that contains two kinds of hormones, estrogen and progestin. Angeliq is used to reduce signs of menopause such as hot flashes, vaginal dryness, itching, or burning.

What is the most important information I should know about Angeliq?

Do not use Angeliq to prevent heart disease, heart attacks, or strokes. Using it may increase your chances of having a heart attack, stroke, breast cancer, and blood clots.

Angeliq may increase your risk of developing Alzheimer's disease. Estrogens should be used only as long as needed. You and your doctor should talk regularly about whether you still need treatment with Angeliq.

Who should not take Angeliq?

You should not take Angeliq if you have had your uterus removed, or have a history of breast cancer, blood clots, or unusual vaginal bleeding.

Do not take this drug if you are allergic to any of its ingredients, have unusual vaginal bleeding, have had kidney or liver disease or disease of your adrenal glands, had a heart attack or stroke in the past year, currently have blood clots, or if you are pregnant.

What should I tell my doctor before I take the first dose of Angeliq?

Tell your doctor about all prescription, over-the-counter, and herbal medications you are taking before beginning treatment with Angeliq. Also, talk to your doctor about your complete medical history, especially if you have asthma, epilepsy, migraines, endometriosis, lupus, high blood pressure, problems with your heart, liver, thyroid, or kidneys, have high calcium levels in your blood, or if you are breastfeeding or are going to have surgery.

What is the usual dosage?

The information below is based on the dosage guidelines your doctor uses. Depending on your condition and medical history, your doctor may prescribe a different regimen. Do not change the dosage or stop taking your medication without your doctor's approval.

Adults: Angeliq is available in a tablet containing 0.5 milligrams (mg) of drospirenone and 1 mg of estradiol. The dosage is 1 tablet daily.

How should I take Angeliq?

Take one tablet every day. Estrogens with or without progestins should be used at the lowest effective doses and only for as long as menopausal symptoms persist. You and your healthcare provider should talk regularly about whether or not you still require treatment.

What should I avoid while taking Angeliq?
If you are already using a product containing estrogen, you should stop taking that product before starting Angeliq. Avoid increasing your risk of heart disease by lowering blood pressure and cholesterol, losing weight, and avoiding tobacco use.

What are possible food and drug interactions associated with Angeliq?
Medications that increase the potassium in your blood, such as the following: angiotensin converting enzyme (ACE) inhibitors, angiotensin-II receptor antagonists, nonsteroidal anti-inflammatory drugs (NSAIDs), potassium-sparing diuretics, potassium supplements, and heparin.

What are the possible side effects of Angeliq?
Side effects cannot be anticipated. If any develop or change in intensity, tell your doctor as soon as possible. Only your doctor can determine if it is safe for you to continue taking this drug.

Side effects may include: breast pain, flulike symptoms, hair loss, headache, irregular vaginal bleeding or spotting, nausea/vomiting, stomach cramps/bloating, upper respiratory infection, vaginal discharge, increased potassium or decreased sodium levels in your blood

Can I receive Angeliq if I am pregnant or breastfeeding?
Angeliq should not be used if you are pregnant. The hormone in Angeliq can pass into your breast milk. Talk with your doctor before taking this drug if you are pregnant, plan to become pregnant, or are breastfeeding.

What should I do if I miss a dose of Angeliq?
Take the missed dose as soon as you remember it. However, if it is almost time for your next dose, skip the one you missed and return to your regular dosing schedule. Do not double the dose.

How should I store Angeliq?
Store at room temperature.

Anidulafungin *See Eraxis, page 493.*

ANSAID

Generic name: Flurbiprofen

What is Ansaid?

Ansaid, a nonsteroidal anti-inflammatory drug (NSAID), is used to relieve the inflammation, swelling, stiffness, and joint pain associated with rheumatoid arthritis and osteoarthritis (the most common form of arthritis).

What is the most important information I should know about Ansaid?

You should have frequent checkups with your doctor if you take Ansaid regularly. NSAIDs may cause an increased risk of serious cardiovascular thrombotic events, heart attack, stroke, and serious gastrointestinal adverse events including bleeding, ulceration, and perforation of the stomach or intestines.

Who should not take Ansaid?

If you are sensitive to or have ever had an allergic reaction to Ansaid, aspirin, or similar drugs such as ibuprofen, or if you have had asthma attacks caused by aspirin or other drugs of this type, you should not take this medication. Fatal attacks have occurred in people allergic to this drug. Make sure your doctor is aware of any drug reactions you have experienced.

Ansaid should not be used for the treatment of perioperative pain in the setting of coronary artery bypass graft (CABG) surgery.

What should I tell my doctor before I take the first dose of Ansaid?

Tell your doctor about all prescription, over-the-counter, and herbal medications you are taking before beginning treatment with Ansaid. Also, talk to your doctor about your complete medical history, especially if you have any allergies, are allergic to any medication, or have ulcers or gastrointestinal problems.

What is the usual dosage?

The information below is based on the dosage guidelines your doctor uses. Depending on your condition and medical history, your doctor may prescribe a different regimen. Do not change the dosage or stop taking your medication without your doctor's approval.

Adults: The usual starting dosage is a total of 200 to 300 milligrams a day, divided into 2, 3, or 4 smaller doses (usually 3 or 4 for rheumatoid arthritis). Your doctor will tailor the dose to suit your needs, but you should not take more than 100 milligrams at any one time or more than 300 milligrams in a day.

How should I take Ansaid?

Take this medication exactly as prescribed by your doctor. Your doctor may tell you to take Ansaid with food or an antacid.

What should I avoid while taking Ansaid?

Avoid alcohol and smoking during treatment with Ansaid.

What are possible food and drug interactions associated with Ansaid?

If Ansaid is taken with certain other drugs, the effects of either could be increased, decreased, or altered. It is especially important to check with your doctor before combining Ansaid with the following: antacids, aspirin, beta blockers such as the blood pressure medications atenolol and propranolol hydrochloride, blood thinners such as warfarin, cimetidine, methotrexate, oral diabetes drugs such as glyburide, ranitidine, and diuretics.

What are the possible side effects of Ansaid?

Side effects cannot be anticipated. If any develop or change in intensity, tell your doctor as soon as possible. Only your doctor can determine if it is safe for you to continue taking this drug.

Side effects may include: abdominal pain, diarrhea, general feeling of illness, headache, indigestion, nausea, swelling due to fluid retention, urinary tract infection

Can I receive Ansaid if I am pregnant or breastfeeding?

The effects of Ansaid during pregnancy have not been adequately studied. If you are pregnant or plan to become pregnant, inform your doctor immediately. In particular, you should not use Ansaid in late pregnancy, as it can affect the developing baby's circulatory system. Ansaid appears in breast milk and could affect a nursing infant. If this medication is essential to your health, your doctor may advise you to discontinue breastfeeding until your treatment is finished.

What should I do if I miss a dose of Ansaid?

Take the forgotten dose as soon as you remember. If it is almost time for your next dose, skip the one you missed and go back to your regular schedule. Never take 2 doses at the same time.

How should I store Ansaid?

Store at room temperature.

ANTACIDS

What are Antacids?
Available under a number of brand names, antacids are used to relieve the uncomfortable symptoms of acid indigestion, heartburn, gas, and sour stomach.

What is the most important information I should know about Antacids?
Do not take antacids for longer than 2 weeks or in larger than recommended doses unless directed by your doctor. If your symptoms persist, contact your doctor. Antacids should be used only for occasional relief of stomach upset.

Who should not take Antacids?
Do not take antacids if you have signs of appendicitis or an inflamed bowel; symptoms include stomach or lower abdominal pain, cramping, bloating, soreness, nausea, or vomiting.

If you are sensitive to or have ever had an allergic reaction to aluminum, calcium, magnesium, or simethicone, do not take an antacid containing these ingredients. If you are elderly and have bone problems or if you are taking care of an elderly person with Alzheimer's disease, do not use an antacid containing aluminum.

What should I tell my doctor before I take the first dose of Antacids?
Tell your doctor about all prescription, over-the-counter, and herbal medications you are taking before beginning taking an antacid. Also, talk to your doctor about your complete medical history, especially if you have drug allergies, kidney disease, or are on a sodium-restricted diet.

What is the usual dosage?
The information below is based on the dosage guidelines your doctor uses. Depending on your condition and medical history, your doctor may prescribe a different regimen. Do not change the dosage or stop taking your medication without your doctor's approval.

Adults: Take according to the directions on the product's label, or as directed by your doctor.

Children: Check with your doctor about the best product and dosage for your child.

How should I take Antacids?
Take after meals or as needed. If you take a chewable antacid tablet, chew thoroughly before swallowing so that the medicine can work faster and

be more effective. Allow lozenges to completely dissolve in your mouth. Shake liquids well before using.

What should I avoid while taking Antacids?
Avoid using antacids for more than 2 weeks unless directed to do so by your doctor.

What are possible food and drug interactions associated with Antacids?
If antacids are taken with certain other medications, the effects of either could be increased, decreased, or altered. It is especially important to check with your doctor before combining antacids with the following: cellulose sodium phosphate, isoniazid, ketoconazole, mecamylamine, methenamine, sodium polystyrene sulfonate resin, or tetracycline antibiotics.

What are the possible side effects of Antacids?
Side effects cannot be anticipated. If any develop or change in intensity, tell your doctor as soon as possible. Only your doctor can determine if it is safe for you to continue taking this drug.

Side effects may include: chalky taste, constipation, diarrhea, increased thirst, stomach cramps

Can I receive Antacids if I am pregnant or breastfeeding?
As with all medications, ask your doctor or healthcare professional whether it is safe for you to use antacids while you are pregnant or breastfeeding.

What should I do if I miss a dose of Antacids?
Take this medication only as needed or as instructed by your doctor.

How should I store Antacids?
Store at room temperature. Keep liquids tightly closed and protect from freezing.

ANTARA
Generic name: Fenofibrate

What is Antara?
Antara is used along with diet and exercise to reduce LDL ("bad") cholesterol, total cholesterol levels, and triglycerides, and increase HDL ("good") cholesterol.

What is the most important information I should know about Antara?
Antara may increase cholesterol excretion into the bile, leading to gallstones. Regular monitoring of liver function tests is required. If gallstones are found, then Antara therapy should be discontinued.

Treatment with Antara should be discontinued if an adequate response is not obtained after 2 months of therapy at the maximum daily dose.

Who should not take Antara?
Do not take Antara if you are allergic or sensitive to fenofibrate, have gallbladder disease, or have liver or severe kidney disease.

What should I tell my doctor before I take the first dose of Antara?
Tell your doctor about all prescription, over-the-counter, and herbal medication you are taking before beginning treatment with Antara. Also, talk to your doctor about your complete medical history, especially if you have liver problems, gallbladder disease, or severe kidney impairment.

What is the usual dosage?
The information below is based on the dosage guidelines your doctor uses. Depending on your condition and medical history, your doctor may prescribe a different regimen. Do not change the dosage or stop taking your medication without your doctor's approval.

Adults: For the treatment of high cholesterol, the initial dose is 130 milligrams (mg) per day. For the treatment of high triglyceride levels, the initial dose is 43-130 mg per day. Based on your response, the doctor may adjust the dosage at 4- to 8-week intervals. The maximum dose is 130 mg per day.

Adults 65 years and older: The initial dose should be limited to 43 mg per day.

Adults with kidney problems: Treatment should be started at a dose of 43 mg day, and increased only after evaluation of the effects on kidney function.

Cholesterol and triglyceride levels should be monitored periodically and consideration should be given to reducing the dosage if levels fall significantly below the targeted range.

How should I take Antara?
You should follow a diet and exercise plan as directed by your doctor. You may take Antara with or without food.

What should I avoid while taking Antara?
Do not neglect controlling your condition with diet and exercise, as directed by your doctor. Antara is meant to be used as part of a comprehensive treatment plan for improving cholesterol and triglyceride levels.

What are possible food and drug interactions associated with Antara?

If Antara is taken with certain other drugs, the effects of either could be increased, decreased, or altered. It is especially important to check with your doctor before combining Antara with the following: atorvastatin, colesevelam, colestipol, cyclosporine, dicumarol, ezetimibe, fluvastatin, lovastatin, phenindione, pravastatin, simvastatin and warfarin.

What are the possible side effects of Antara?

Side effects cannot be anticipated. If any develop or change in intensity, tell your doctor as soon as possible. Only your doctor can determine if it is safe for you to continue taking this drug.

Side effects may include: abnormal liver function tests, respiratory disorders, abdominal pain, back pain, headache, weakness, flu-like symptoms, diarrhea, nausea, constipation, runny nose

Antara may cause myopathy; signs of this condition include unexplained muscle pain, weakness, or tenderness. If you experience these symptoms, tell your doctor right away.

Can I receive Antara if I am pregnant or breastfeeding?

The effects of Antara during pregnancy and breastfeeding are unknown. Tell your doctor immediately if you are pregnant, plan to become pregnant, or are breastfeeding.

What should I do if I miss a dose of Antara?

Take the missed dose as soon as you remember. However, if it is almost time for the next dose, skip the missed dose and return to your regular dosing schedule. Do not double the dose.

How should I store Antara?

Store in a tightly sealed container in a cool, dry place, away from sunlight.

Antihemophilic Factor VIII (human) See Alphanate, page 68.

ANTIVERT

Generic name: Meclizine hydrochloride

What is Antivert?

Antivert, an antihistamine, is prescribed for the management of nausea, vomiting, and dizziness associated with motion sickness. Antivert may also be prescribed for the management of vertigo (a spinning sensation or a feeling that the ground is tilted) due to diseases affecting the vestibular system (the bony labyrinth of the ear, which contains the sensors that control your balance).

What is the most important information I should know about Antivert?

Antivert may cause you to become drowsy or less alert; therefore, driving a car or operating dangerous machinery is not recommended.

Who should not take Antivert?

If you are sensitive to or have ever had an allergic reaction to Antivert or similar drugs, do not take this medication.

What should I tell my doctor before I take the first dose of Antivert?

Tell your doctor about all prescription, over-the-counter, and herbal medications you are taking before beginning treatment with Antivert. Also, talk to your doctor about your complete medical history, especially if you have asthma, glaucoma, or an enlarged prostate gland.

What is the usual dosage?

The information below is based on the dosage guidelines your doctor uses. Depending on your condition and medical history, your doctor may prescribe a different regimen. Do not change the dosage or stop taking your medication without your doctor's approval.

Motion Sickness
Adults and children 12 and over: For protection against motion sickness, take 25 to 50 milligrams 1 hour before traveling. You may repeat the dose every 24 hours for the duration of the journey.

Vertigo
Adults and children 12 and over:
The recommended dosage is 25 to 100 milligrams per day, divided into equal, smaller doses as determined by your doctor.

The safety and effectiveness of Antivert have not been established in children under 12 years of age.

How should I take Antivert?

Take this medication exactly as prescribed by your doctor.

What should I avoid while taking Antivert?

Avoid driving or operating dangerous machinery until you know how this drug affects you.

What are possible food and drug interactions associated with Antivert?

Antivert may intensify the effects of alcohol. Do not drink alcohol while taking this medication.

If Antivert is taken with certain other drugs, the effects of either could be increased, decreased, or altered. Always check with your doctor before combining Antivert with any other medication.

What are the possible side effects of Antivert?
Side effects cannot be anticipated. If any develop or change in intensity, tell your doctor as soon as possible. Only your doctor can determine if it is safe for you to continue taking this drug.

Side effects may include: drowsiness, dry mouth

Can I receive Antivert if I am pregnant or breastfeeding?
Studies regarding the use of Antivert in pregnant women do not indicate that this drug increases the risk of abnormalities. The safety of using Antivert while breastfeeding is unknown. Tell your doctor if you are pregnant, plan to become pregnant, or are breastfeeding.

What should I do if I miss a dose of Antivert?
Take it as soon as you remember. If it is almost time for your next dose, skip the one you missed and go back to your regular schedule. Do not take 2 doses at the same time.

How should I store Antivert?
Store away from heat, light, and moisture.

APIDRA
Generic name: Insulin glulisine

What is Apidra?
Apidra is a rapid-acting insulin analog used to control high blood sugar in adults with diabetes. An insulin analog is chemically different from the insulin made by your body.

What is the most important information I should know about Apidra?
Do not change your insulin without talking to your doctor. You must test your blood sugar levels while using Apidra. Your doctor will tell you how often you should test your blood sugar level and what to do if it is high or low. Do not mix Apidra with other insulin or liquid when using a pump.

Who should not take Apidra?
Do not take Apidra if you are allergic to insulin glulisine or any of its other ingredients. Talk with your doctor about your allergies to avoid a reaction.

What should I tell my doctor before I take the first dose of Apidra?

Before taking Apidra, tell your doctor if you are taking any other medications, and if you have any kidney or liver problems. Also, talk with your doctor if you are pregnant or plan to become pregnant, or are breast-feeding.

What is the usual dosage?

The information below is based on the dosage guidelines your doctor uses. Depending on your condition and medical history, your doctor may prescribe a different regimen. Do not change the dosage or stop taking your medication without your doctor's approval.

Adults: Apidra should be injected 15 minutes before a meal or 20 minutes after starting a meal.

Take exactly as prescribed, being careful to follow your doctor's dietary and exercise recommendations. Before taking your injection, carefully read and follow the manufacturer's instructions on how to prepare your prefilled pen or syringe.

How should I take Apidra?

Inject Apidra under the skin of your upper arm, stomach area, or thigh; never inject it into a vein or muscle. If you use a pump, infuse Apidra through the skin of your stomach; do not mix with any other insulin or liquid when using a pump. Alternate injection sites within the same body area. Only use Apidra that is clear and colorless.

What are possible food and drug interactions associated with Apidra?

To avoid a reaction to Apidra, talk with your doctor about any prescription/nonprescription medications or supplements you are taking. Alcohol, including beer and wine, may affect your blood sugar levels and the way Apidra works. Talk with your doctor about lifestyle changes.

What are the possible side effects of Apidra?

Side effects may include: Hypoglycemia (low blood sugar), hyperglycemia (high blood sugar), allergy, and skin reactions

Symptoms of hypoglycemia may include: anxiety, irritability; tingling in your hands, feet, lips, or tongue; dizziness, light-headedness, or drowsiness; headache; blurred vision; fast heart beat; sweating; shaking

Symptoms of hyperglycemia may include: confusion or drowsiness, thirst, decreased appetite, nausea, vomiting, fast heart beat, increased urination

Can I receive Apidra if I am pregnant or breastfeeding?

The effects of Apidra have not been adequately studied. If you are pregnant, planning to become pregnant, or are breastfeeding, talk with your doctor about your treatment options.

What should I do if I miss a dose of Apidra?

Your doctor should tell you what to do if you miss an insulin injection or meal.

How should I store Apidra?

Store unopened vials in a refrigerator, and out of direct heat and sunlight. Throw away any overheated vials of Apidra. Once a vial is opened, it can be stored below room temperature for up to 28 days.

APLENZIN

Generic name: Bupropion hydrobromide

What is Aplenzin?

Aplenzin is used to treat adults with major depressive disorder.

What is the most important information I should know about Aplenzin?

Antidepressants can increase the risk of suicidal thinking and behavior in children and teenagers. Both adult and pediatric patients taking antidepressants should be watched closely for changes in moods or actions, especially when they first start therapy or when their dose is increased or decreased. Patients and their families should contact the doctor immediately if new symptoms develop or seem to get worse. Signs to watch for include anxiety, hostility, insomnia, restlessness, impulsive or dangerous behavior, and thoughts about suicide or dying.

Do not take this medication if you are currently taking a drug known as a monoamine oxidase inhibitor (MAOI). MAOIs can cause a very serious reaction or even death if taken at the same time as Aplenzin. You must stop taking your MAOI at least 14 days before beginning treatment with Aplenzin. Similarly, you should wait 7 days after stopping Aplenzin before starting an MAOI.

Who should not take Aplenzin?

Do not take Aplenzin if you have a seizure disorder or epilepsy; are taking Zyban or any medication containing bupropion, such as Wellbutrin (all forms); drink alcohol and abruptly stop drinking; use sedatives or benzodiazepines and you stop using them suddenly; have taken within the last 14 days medicine for depression called a monoamine oxidase inhibitor (MAOI); have had an eating disorder such as anorexia or bulimia; are allergic to bupropion, the active ingredient in Aplenzin.

What should I tell my doctor before I take the first dose of Aplenzin?

Tell your doctor about all prescription, over-the-counter, and herbal medications you are taking before beginning treatment with Aplenzin. Also, talk to your doctor about your complete medical history, especially if you have a history of kidney or liver problems, eating disorders, head injury, seizure disorder, or tumor in the spine or nervous system. Tell your doctor if you have had a heart attack, heart problems, high blood pressure, or if you are diabetic and you are taking insulin or other medicines to control blood sugars.

What is the usual dosage?

The information below is based on the dosage guidelines your doctor uses. Depending on your condition and medical history, your doctor may prescribe a different regimen. Do not change the dosage or stop taking your medication without your doctor's approval.

Adults: The usual dose is 348 milligrams taken once daily in the morning.

How should I take Aplenzin?

Do not chew or crush the tablet; swallow it whole. Take Aplenzin at the same time each day. Take your doses at least 24 hours apart. Aplenzin can be taken with or without food.

What should I avoid while taking Aplenzin?

Do not drink a lot of alcohol. If you usually drink a lot, talk with your doctor before suddenly stopping. Do not drive a car or use heavy machinery until you know how Aplenzin affects you.

What are possible food and drug interactions associated with Aplenzin?

Do not take Aplenzin within 14 days of an MAOI. Taking Aplenzin with agents that lower seizure threshold should be done with caution (antipsychotics, antidepressants, theophylline, systemic steroids, etc). There is increased risk of adverse events while using Aplenzin in patients using amantadine and levodopa.

What are the possible side effects of Aplenzin?

Side effects cannot be anticipated. If any develop or change in intensity, tell your doctor as soon as possible. Only your doctor can determine if it is safe for you to continue taking this drug.

Side effects may include: agitation, fast heartbeat, muscle pain, ringing in the ears, skin rash, sore throat, stomach pain, sweating, urinating more often, weight loss

When taking Aplenzin, some people may develop more serious side effects such as seizures; high blood pressure; unusual thoughts and behavior including delusions (believing you are someone else), hallucinations (seeing or hearing things that are not there), paranoia (feeling that people are against you); and allergic reactions (signs of severe allergic reactions may include hives, difficulty breathing, and swelling of the throat). If any of these events occur, seek immediate medical attention.

If you have nausea, take your medicine with food. If you have trouble sleeping, do not take your medicine too close to bedtime.

Can I receive Aplenzin if I am pregnant or breastfeeding?
Aplenzin should be avoided during pregnancy and breastfeeding. Talk with your doctor before taking this drug if you are pregnant, plan to become pregnant, or are breastfeeding.

What should I do if I miss a dose of Aplenzin?
Wait and take your next tablet at the regular time if you miss a dose. Never take an extra tablet to make up for the dose you forgot.

How should I store Aplenzin?
Store at room temperature out of direct light.

APTIVUS
Generic name: Tipranavir

What is Aptivus?
Aptivus is a medicine called a "protease inhibitor" that is used to treat adults with Human Immunodeficiency Virus (HIV). Aptivus blocks HIV protease, an enzyme which is needed for HIV to make more of the virus. Aptivus is always taken with Norvir (ritonavir).

Aptivus does not cure HIV or acquired immunodeficiency syndrome (AIDS). It also does not reduce the chance of passing HIV to others through sexual contact, sharing needles, or being exposed to your blood.

What is the most important information I should know about Aptivus?
People taking Aptivus together with 200 milligrams (mg) of Norvir (ritonavir) may develop bleeding in the brain that may cause death.

People taking Aptivus together with 200 mg Norvir (ritonavir) may develop severe liver disease that may cause death. If you develop any of the following symptoms of liver problems, you should stop taking Aptivus/ritonavir treatment and call your doctor right away: tiredness, general ill feeling or "flu-like" symptoms, loss of appetite, nausea, yellowing of your skin or whites of your eyes, dark urine, pale stools, or pain, ache, or sensitivity on your right side below your ribs. If you have chronic hepatitis

B or C infection, your doctor should check your blood tests more often because you have an increased risk of developing liver problems.

You should report any unusual bleeding to your doctor if you are taking Aptivus together with ritonavir.

Who should not take Aptivus?

Do not take Aptivus if you have liver problems, or if you are allergic to any of its, or Norvir's, ingredients.

What should I tell my doctor before I take the first dose of Aptivus?

Tell your doctor about all prescription, over-the-counter, and herbal medications you are taking before beginning treatment with Aptivus, especially if you are taking any medicine that increases your chance of bleeding, oral contraceptives, or hormone therapy. Also, talk to your doctor about your complete medical history, especially if you have liver problems, hemophilia, diabetes, or you are pregnant, planning to become pregnant, or nursing.

What is the usual dosage?

The information below is based on the dosage guidelines your doctor uses. Depending on your condition and medical history, your doctor may prescribe a different regimen. Do not change the dosage or stop taking your medication without your doctor's approval.

Adults: The usual dose is 500 mg (two 250-mg capsules) of Aptivus, together with 200 mg (two 100-mg capsules or 2.5 milliliters [mL] of solution) of Norvir, twice per day. Aptivus with Norvir must be used together with other anti-HIV medicines.

Children age 2 years or older: Children can take Aptivus with Norvir. The child's doctor will decide the right dose based on the child's weight or size. The dose should not be more than the recommended adult dose.

How should I take Aptivus?

Take Aptivus exactly as your doctor prescribed. You must take Aptivus at the same time with Norvir. Aptivus with Norvir must be taken with other anti-HIV medicines, Swallow the capsules whole; do not crush or chew capsules. You can take Aptivus with Norvir with or without food at the same time each day. If you begin to run low on Aptivus, contact your pharmacist immediately.

What should I avoid while taking Aptivus?

Avoid running out of Aptivus. When you are low, call your pharmacist for a refill to be sure you do not run out and skip a dose. Skipping a dose may cause the levels of HIV in your system to rise.

What are possible food and drug interactions associated with Aptivus?

If Aptivus is taken with certain other drugs, the effects of either could be increased, decreased, or altered. It is especially important to check with your doctor before combining Aptivus with the following: amiodarone, astemizole, bepridil, cisapride, ergot alkaloids (migraine medication), flecainide, fluticasone, lovastatin, midazolam, oral contraceptives, pimozide, propafenone, quinidine, terfenadine, triazolam, rifampin (may reduce virologic activity and possible resistance to Aptivus or to the class of protease inhibitors), sildenafil, vardenafil, or tadalafil, simvastatin, St. John's wort (may reduce virologic activity and possible resistance to Aptivus or to the class of protease inhibitors), and Vitamin E (if you are taking Aptivus oral solution).

What are the possible side effects of Aptivus?

Side effects cannot be anticipated. If any develop or change in intensity, tell your doctor as soon as possible. Only your doctor can determine if it is safe for you to continue taking this drug.

Side effects may include: bleeding in the brain, changes in body fat, diabetes and high blood sugar (hyperglycemia), diarrhea, fever, headache, increased blood fat (lipid) levels, increased hemophilia, liver problems, nausea, relocation of fat, skin rash in children or women taking oral contraceptives, stomach pain, tiredness, vomiting

Can I receive Aptivus if I am pregnant or breastfeeding?

Talk to your doctor if you are pregnant, planning to become pregnant, or are nursing. The effects of Aptivus on pregnancy are unknown; you should not breastfeed your child while on Aptivus. This drug may pass through your breast milk, and it is also possible to pass HIV to your child via breast milk.

What should I do if I miss a dose of Aptivus?

If you forget to take Aptivus, take the next dose together with Norvir (ritonavir), as soon as possible. Do not take a double dose to make up for a missed dose.

How should I store Aptivus?

Store Aptivus capsules in a refrigerator. Store Aptivus oral solution at room temperature. Do not refrigerate or freeze Aptivus oral solution. Once Aptivus is opened, the contents of the bottle must be used within 60 days.

ARAVA

Generic name: Leflunomide

What is Arava?

Arava is used in the treatment of rheumatoid arthritis. It reduces the pain, stiffness, inflammation, and swelling associated with this disease, improves physical function, and staves off the joint damage that ultimately results.

What is the most important information I should know about Arava?

You MUST NOT take Arava if you are pregnant; it can harm the developing baby. If you are still in your childbearing years, your doctor will want to see negative results from a pregnancy test before starting you on Arava. You'll also need to use reliable contraceptive measures as long as you take the drug.

If you become pregnant while taking Arava, your doctor will stop the drug immediately and prescribe a regimen of cholestyramine in 8-gram doses 3 times a day for 11 days. Cholestyramine helps to clear Arava from the bloodstream, possibly preventing harm to the unborn child.

Arava is potentially damaging to the liver. Your doctor will test your liver function before starting Arava therapy. If you have significant liver disease, including hepatitis, you'll be unable to take Arava. If you develop liver problems while taking the drug, your dose will have to be reduced or eliminated.

Since there is a possibility that Arava could damage your liver or cause blood problems (such as a loss of white blood cells used to fight infection or a loss of cells that help your blood clot), it is essential that your doctor conducts a monthly blood test for the first 6 months of therapy, then every 6 to 8 weeks thereafter. If you are taking Arava and the cancer drug methotrexate together you may be even more susceptible to these problems. Your doctor will need to test your blood every month. Notify your doctor promptly if any signs of a blood problem appear. Warnings include easy bruising, frequent infections, unusual fatigue, and paleness.

Lung disease (including scarring of the lung) has been reported in patients taking Arava. Symptoms may include coughing, shortness of breath, and fever. Contact your doctor immediately if you develop any new or unusual symptoms

Who should not take Arava?

Remember that you must not take Arava if you are pregnant or plan to become pregnant. You'll also need to avoid this drug if it gives you an allergic reaction.

What should I tell my doctor before I take the first dose of Arava?

Tell your doctor about all prescription, over-the-counter, and herbal medications you are taking before beginning treatment with Arava. Also, talk to your doctor about your complete medical history, especially if you have liver or kidney problems, cancer, bone marrow problems, a severe infection, AIDS, or any other immune system problem.

What is the usual dosage?

The information below is based on the dosage guidelines your doctor uses. Depending on your condition and medical history, your doctor may prescribe a different regimen. Do not change the dosage or stop taking your medication without your doctor's approval.

Adults: The recommended starting dose is one 100-milligram tablet daily for the first 3 days. If you have an increased risk for blood disorders or liver problems, your doctor may choose to eliminate the 100-milligram starting dose to reduce the risk of serious side effects.

After the first 3 days, the doctor will reduce the dose to 20 milligrams a day. If side effects appear, the dose may be further decreased to 10 milligrams a day.

How should I take Arava?

Your dosage of Arava will be decreased after the first 3 days. Never take more than your doctor prescribes.

What should I avoid while taking Arava?

Theoretically, Arava may interfere with your body's ability to fight off infection. You should avoid immunization with live vaccines while taking Arava.

What are possible food and drug interactions associated with Arava?

If Arava is taken with certain other drugs, the effects of either could be increased, decreased, or altered. It is especially important to check with your doctor before combining Arava with the following: cholestyramine, methotrexate, nonsteroidal anti-inflammatory drugs such as ibuprofen and naproxen, rifampin, and tolbutamide.

What are the possible side effects of Arava?

Side effects cannot be anticipated. If any develop or change in intensity, tell your doctor as soon as possible. Only your doctor can determine if it is safe for you to continue taking this drug.

Side effects may include: abdominal pain, back pain, bronchitis, cough, diarrhea, dizziness, hair loss, headache, high blood pressure, indigestion, itching, joint disorders, loss of appetite, mouth ulcers, nausea, rash, respiratory infection, sore throat, stomach inflammation, tendon inflammation, urinary tract infection, vomiting, weakness, weight loss

Arava has been known to cause rare but serious skin reactions. If you develop a skin rash or eruption, stop taking Arava and contact your doctor. Arava can also reduce your blood cell count.

Can I receive Arava if I am pregnant or breastfeeding?
Do not take Arava while pregnant or breastfeeding. Taken during pregnancy, the drug can cause birth defects. And although it is not known whether Arava appears in breast milk, there is good reason to suspect that it will cause serious side effects in nursing infants. Tell your doctor immediately if you are pregnant, plan to become pregnant, or are breastfeeding.

What should I do if I miss a dose of Arava?
Take it as soon as you remember. If it is almost time for your next dose, skip the one you missed and go back to your regular schedule. Do not take 2 doses at the same time.

How should I store Arava?
Store at room temperature away from light.

Arformoterol tartrate See *Brovana, page 228.*

ARICEPT
Generic name: Donepezil hydrochloride

What is Aricept?
Aricept is prescribed to provide some relief from the symptoms of early Alzheimer's disease. Aricept can temporarily improve brain function in some Alzheimer's sufferers, although it does not halt the progress of the underlying disease.

What is the most important information I should know about Aricept?
Aricept can aggravate asthma and other breathing problems, and can increase the risk of seizures. It can also slow the heartbeat, cause heartbeat irregularities, and lead to fainting episodes. Contact your doctor if any of these problems occur.

To maintain any improvement, Aricept must be taken regularly. If the drug is stopped, its benefits will soon be lost. It can take up to 3 weeks for any positive effects to appear.

Who should not take Aricept?

There are two reasons to avoid Aricept: an allergic reaction to the drug itself, or an allergy to a group of drugs known as piperidine derivatives (ask your doctor for a list of these medications).

What should I tell my doctor before I take the first dose of Aricept?

Tell your doctor about all prescription, over-the-counter, and herbal medications you are taking before beginning treatment with Aricept. Also, talk to your doctor about your complete medical history, especially if you have asthma or other breathing problems, seizures, heart problems, fainting problems, or stomach ulcers.

What is the usual dosage?

The information below is based on the dosage guidelines your doctor uses. Depending on your condition and medical history, your doctor may prescribe a different regimen. Do not change the dosage or stop taking your medication without your doctor's approval.

Adults: The usual starting dose is 5 milligrams once a day at bedtime for at least 4 to 6 weeks. Do not increase the dose during this period unless directed. The doctor may then change the dosage to 10 milligrams once a day if response to the drug warrants it.

How should I take Aricept?

Aricept should be taken once a day just before bedtime. Be sure it's taken every day. If Aricept is not taken regularly, it won't work. It can be taken with or without food.

What should I avoid while taking Aricept?

Use nonsteroidal anti-inflammatory drugs (NSAIDs) cautiously. In patients who have had stomach ulcers, and those who take NSAIDs such as ibuprofen or naproxen sodium, Aricept can make stomach side effects worse.

What are possible food and drug interactions associated with Aricept?

Aricept will increase the effects of certain anesthetics. Make sure the doctor is aware of Aricept therapy prior to any surgery.

If Aricept is taken with certain other drugs, the effects of either could be increased, decreased, or altered. It is especially important to check with your doctor before combining Aricept with the following: antispasmodic drugs such as dicyclomine hydrochloride and propantheline, bethanechol chloride, carbamazepine, dexamethasone, ketoconazole, phenobarbital, phenytoin, quinidine, and rifampin.

What are the possible side effects of Aricept?

Side effects cannot be anticipated. If any develop or change in intensity, tell your doctor as soon as possible. Only your doctor can determine if it is safe for you to continue taking this drug.

Side effects may include: diarrhea, fatigue, insomnia, loss of appetite, muscle cramps, nausea, vomiting, abnormal dreams, arthritis, bruising, depression, dizziness, fainting, frequent urination, headache, pain, sleepiness, weight loss

Can I receive Aricept if I am pregnant or breastfeeding?

Since it is not intended for women of child-bearing age, Aricept's effects during pregnancy have not been studied, and it is not known whether it appears in breast milk.

What should I do if I miss a dose of Aricept?

Make it up as soon as you remember. If it is almost time for the next dose, skip the one that was missed and go back to the regular schedule. Never double the dose.

How should I store Aricept?

Store at room temperature.

ARIMIDEX

Generic name: Anastrozole

What is Arimidex?

Arimidex is a first-line treatment of breast cancer in postmenopausal women. Arimidex is also used to treat advanced breast cancer in postmenopausal women whose disease has spread to other parts of the body following treatment with tamoxifen, another anticancer drug. Arimidex can also be prescribed along with other drugs to treat the early stages of breast cancer in postmenopausal women.

What is the most important information I should know about Arimidex?

Arimidex may increase the risk of cardiovascular events in patients with pre-existing ischemic heart disease. It may also cause a reduction in bone mineral density or raise blood cholesterol levels.

Who should not take Arimidex?

Do not take Arimidex if you are pregnant or if you have an allergic reaction to the drug.

What should I tell my doctor before I take the first dose of Arimidex?

Tell your doctor about all prescription, over-the-counter, and herbal medications you are taking before beginning treatment with Arimidex. Also, talk to your doctor about your complete medical history, especially if you have ever had heart problems, high cholesterol, or osteoporosis.

What is the usual dosage?

The information below is based on the dosage guidelines your doctor uses. Depending on your condition and medical history, your doctor may prescribe a different regimen. Do not change the dosage or stop taking your medication without your doctor's approval.

Adults: The usual dose is a 1-milligram tablet taken once a day. If Arimidex is being used as an initial treatment for advanced breast cancer, you will continue taking the medication until it no longer works against the tumor. The optimal duration of therapy for early breast cancer has not been determined.

How should I take Arimidex?

Take Arimidex exactly as directed.

What should I avoid while taking Arimidex?

Avoid becoming pregnant or nursing a baby while taking this drug.

What are possible food and drug interactions associated with Arimidex?

Certain drugs may decrease the effectiveness of Arimidex, including tamoxifen and estrogen-containing drugs. Be sure to tell your doctor about any medication you are taking.

What are the possible side effects of Arimidex?

Side effects cannot be anticipated. If any develop or change in intensity, tell your doctor as soon as possible. Only your doctor can determine if it is safe for you to continue taking this drug.

Side effects may include: coughing, diarrhea, dizziness, general aches and pains, headache, hot flashes, nausea, nerve pain, rash, shortness of breath, vomiting, water retention

Can I receive Arimidex if I am pregnant or breastfeeding?

If you are pregnant or plan to become pregnant, do not take Arimidex. In animal studies, this medication has caused severe birth defects, including incomplete bone formation and low birth weight; it could be poisonous to your unborn child. Arimidex also increases your chances of having a miscarriage or a stillborn baby. If you should accidentally become pregnant, tell your doctor immediately.

It is not known whether Arimidex passes into breast milk. Because of the potential risk to the infant, breastfeeding while using this drug is not recommended. Consult your doctor before breastfeeding.

What should I do if I miss a dose of Arimidex?
Take the forgotten dose if you remember within 12 hours. If it is almost time for your next dose, skip the one you missed and go back to your regular schedule. Never take 2 doses at once.

How should I store Arimidex?
Store at room temperature.

Aripiprazole *See Abilify/Abilify Discmelt, page 1.*

Armodafinil *See Nuvigil, page 929.*

ARMOUR THYROID
Generic name: Natural thyroid hormones

What is Armour Thyroid?
Armour Thyroid is prescribed when your thyroid gland is unable to produce enough hormone. It is also used to treat or prevent goiter (enlargement of the thyroid gland), and is given in a suppression test to diagnose an overactive thyroid.

What is the most important information I should know about Armour Thyroid?
Although Armour Thyroid will speed up your metabolism, it is not effective as a weight-loss drug and should not be used for that purpose. Too much Armour Thyroid may cause severe side effects, especially if you are also taking appetite suppressants.

Who should not take Armour Thyroid?
Do not take Armour Thyroid if you have ever had an allergic reaction to this drug; your thyroid gland is overactive; or your adrenal glands are not making enough corticosteroid hormone.

What should I tell my doctor before I take the first dose of Armour Thyroid?
Tell your doctor about all prescription, over-the-counter, and herbal medication you are taking before beginning treatment with this drug. Also, talk to your doctor about your complete medical history, especially if you are elderly and suffer from angina (chest pain due to a heart condition). Tell your doctor if you have diabetes or an underactive thyroid.

What is the usual dosage?

The information below is based on the dosage guidelines your doctor uses. Depending on your condition and medical history, your doctor may prescribe a different regimen. Do not change the dosage or stop taking your medication without your doctor's approval.

Adults: Your doctor will tailor the dosage of Armour Thyroid to meet your individual requirements, taking into consideration the status of your thyroid gland and any other medical conditions you may have.

How should I take Armour Thyroid?

Take Armour Thyroid exactly as prescribed by your doctor. There is no "typical" dosage; the amount you need to take will depend on how much thyroid hormone your body is able to produce. Take your dose at the same time every day for consistent effect.

What should I avoid while taking Armour Thyroid?

Avoid changing the dose or missing doses. Take no more or less than the amount your doctor prescribes.

What are possible food and drug interactions associated with Armour Thyroid?

If Armour Thyroid is taken with certain other drugs, the effects of either could be increased, decreased, or altered. It is especially important to check with your doctor before combining Armour Thyroid with the following: asthma medications such as theophylline, blood thinners such as warfarin sodium, cholestyramine, colestipol, estrogen preparations (including some birth control pills such as conjugated estrogens), insulin, and oral diabetes drugs such as chlorpropamide and glipizide.

What are the possible side effects of Armour Thyroid?

Side effects cannot be anticipated. If any develop or change in intensity, tell your doctor as soon as possible. Only your doctor can determine if it is safe for you to continue taking this drug.

Side effects may include: changes in appetite, diarrhea, fever, headache, increased heart rate, irritability, nausea, nervousness, sleeplessness, sweating, weight loss

Children treated with Armour Thyroid may experience temporary hair loss.

Can I receive Armour Thyroid if I am pregnant or breastfeeding?

If you need to take Armour Thyroid because of a thyroid hormone deficiency, you may continue using the medication during pregnancy, but your doctor will test you regularly and may change your dosage. Once your baby is born, you may breastfeed while continuing treatment with Armour Thyroid.

What should I do if I miss a dose of Armour Thyroid?

Take it as soon as you remember. If it is almost time for your next dose, skip the one you missed and go back to your regular schedule. Do not take 2 doses at the same time. If you miss 2 or more doses in a row, consult your doctor.

How should I store Armour Thyroid?

Store at room temperature in a tightly closed container.

ARTHROTEC

Generic name: Diclofenac sodium and misoprostol

What is Arthrotec?

Arthrotec is designed to relieve the symptoms of arthritis in people who are also prone to ulcers. It contains diclofenac, a nonsteroidal anti-inflammatory drug (NSAID) for control of the inflammation, swelling, stiffness, and joint pain associated with rheumatoid arthritis and osteoarthritis. However, since NSAIDs can cause stomach ulcers in susceptible people, Arthrotec also contains misoprostol, a synthetic prostaglandin that serves to reduce the production of stomach acid, protect the stomach lining, and thus prevent ulcers.

What is the most important information I should know about Arthrotec?

Be certain to avoid taking Arthrotec during pregnancy. It can cause a miscarriage with potentially dangerous bleeding, sometimes leading to hospitalization, surgery, infertility, and even death. Arthrotec can also deform or kill the developing baby. If you haven't passed menopause, your doctor should do a pregnancy test less than 2 weeks before your therapy begins. Once you've started taking the drug, it is vitally important that you also use reliable contraceptive measures. If you do become pregnant, stop taking Arthrotec and contact your doctor immediately.

Who should not take Arthrotec?

Remember that it is essential to avoid Arthrotec during pregnancy. You should also avoid this medication if you've ever had an allergic reaction to either of its components (diclofenac and misoprostol). Avoid it, too, if you've had a reaction to any other prostaglandin medication, or to any NSAID, including aspirin. Make sure the doctor is aware of any drug reactions you've experienced.

What should I tell my doctor before I take the first dose of Arthrotec?

Tell your doctor about all prescription, over-the-counter, and herbal medication you are taking before beginning treatment with Arthrotec. Also, talk to your doctor about your complete medical history, especially if you have kidney or liver disease, lupus or another connective tissue disease, severe vomiting or diarrhea, or you have porphyria.

What is the usual dosage?
The information below is based on the dosage guidelines your doctor uses. Depending on your condition and medical history, your doctor may prescribe a different regimen. Do not change the dosage or stop taking your medication without your doctor's approval.

Osteoarthritis
Adults: The recommended dose is 50 milligrams (mg) 3 times daily.

Rheumatoid Arthritis
Adults: The recommended dose is 50 mg 3 or 4 times daily.

If you can not tolerate the recommended dosage, your doctor can prescribe a dose of 50 or 75 mg twice daily. However, such lower dosages are less effective at preventing ulcers.

How should I take Arthrotec?
To minimize diarrhea and related side effects, take Arthrotec with meals, exactly as prescribed. Antacids containing magnesium can make Arthrotec-induced diarrhea worse. If you need an antacid, use one containing aluminum or calcium instead. Arthrotec tablets should be swallowed whole and not chewed, crushed, or dissolved.

What should I avoid while taking Arthrotec?
Do not give Arthrotec to anyone else. It has been prescribed for your specific condition, may not be the correct treatment for another person, and could be dangerous for another person, especially a woman who may be, or could become, pregnant.

What are possible food and drug interactions associated with Arthrotec?
If Arthrotec is taken with certain other drugs, the effects of either could be increased, decreased, or altered. It is especially important to check with your doctor before combining Arthrotec with the following: aspirin; blood pressure medications such as diltiazem hydrochloride, enalapril maleate, nifedipine, and propranolol hydrochloride; cyclosporine; digoxin; diuretics; glipizide; glyburide; insulin; lithium; magnesium-containing antacids; methotrexate; phenobarbital; prednisolone; and warfarin.

What are the possible side effects of Arthrotec?
Side effects cannot be anticipated. If any develop or change in intensity, tell your doctor as soon as possible. Only your doctor can determine if it is safe for you to continue taking this drug.

Side effects may include: abdominal pain, acid indigestion, diarrhea, gas, nausea

Can I receive Arthrotec if I am pregnant or breastfeeding?

Do not begin treatment with Arthrotec if you are pregnant, plan to become pregnant, or you are breastfeeding. Use reliable contraception while you are being treated with Arthrotec. This drug appears in breast milk, so your doctor may have you stop breastfeeding until your treatment with Arthrotec is finished.

What should I do if I miss a dose of Arthrotec?

If you are following a regular schedule, take the dose as soon as you remember. If it is almost time for the next one, skip the dose you missed and go back to your regular schedule. Do not take 2 doses at once.

How should I store Arthrotec?

Store at room temperature in a dry place.

ASACOL

Generic name: Mesalamine

What is Asacol?

Asacol tablets are indicated for the treatment of mildly or moderately active ulcerative colitis and for the maintenance of remission of ulcerative colitis (inflammation of the inner lining of the colon and rectum).

What is the most important information I should know about Asacol?

It is recommended that all people have their kidney function tested prior to starting Asacol and periodically while on Asacol therapy.

Who should not take Asacol?

Do not use Asacol if you are sensitive to salicylates such as aspirin or to any of the components of the Asacol tablet.

What should I tell my doctor before I take the first dose of Asacol?

Tell your doctor about all prescription, over-the-counter, and herbal medication you are taking before beginning treatment with Asacol. Also, talk to your doctor about your complete medical history, especially if you have kidney impairment or kidney disease.

What is the usual dosage?

The information below is based on the dosage guidelines your doctor uses. Depending on your condition and medical history, your doctor may prescribe a different regimen. Do not change the dosage or stop taking your medication without your doctor's approval.

For the treatment of mildly to moderately active ulcerative colitis: The usual dosage in adults is two 400 mg tablets three times a day (for a total daily dose of 2.4 grams) for 6 weeks.

For the maintenance of remission of ulcerative colitis: The recommended dosage in adults is 1.6 grams daily, taken in divided doses, for 6 months.

How should I take Asacol?
Take Asacol with a meal.

What should I avoid while taking Asacol?
Be sure to swallow the tablets whole; do not break or chew them.

What are possible food and drug interactions associated with Asacol?
If Asacol is taken with certain other drugs, the effects of either could be increased, decreased, or altered. Always check with your doctor before combining Asacol with any other medication.

What are the possible side effects of Asacol?
Side effects cannot be anticipated. If any develop or change in intensity, tell your doctor as soon as possible. Only your doctor can determine if it is safe for you to continue taking this drug.

Side effects may include: Headache, abdominal pain, nausea, diarrhea, pain (back, joint, muscle, swelling of extremities, or chest pain)

Can I receive Asacol if I am pregnant or breastfeeding?
The effects of Asacol during pregnancy and breastfeeding are unknown. Tell your doctor immediately if you are pregnant, plan to become pregnant, or are breastfeeding.

What should I do if I miss a dose of Asacol?
If you miss a dose, take the next dose as usual. Do not double your next dose. Do not try to make up the missed dose.

How should I store Asacol?
Keep the medication in a cool, dry place in a tightly sealed container. Protect from sunlight and heat.

ASMANEX TWISTHALER
Generic name: Mometasone furoate inhalation powder

What is Asmanex Twisthaler?
Asmanex Twisthaler is an asthma inhaler that has a medicine called an inhaled corticosteroid. Asmanex Twisthaler is used to prevent and control asthma symptoms for patients greater than 4 years old.

What is the most important information I should know about Asmanex Twisthaler?

Asmanex Twisthaler should not be used to treat asthma attacks and should not be used to relieve sudden asthma symptoms. Use an inhaler called albuterol if you are experiencing an asthma attack or seek medical help immediately.

Asmanex Twisthaler should not be used in children under the age of 4.

Patients who use inhaled steroid medications such as Asmanex Twisthaler may develop a fungal infection of the mouth or throat. It is very important to rinse your mouth every time after using Asmanex Twisthaler to prevent fungal infections.

Avoid coming in contact with measles, chicken pox virus, tuberculosis, or any other infections before or while using Asmanex. Contact your doctor immediately if you have been exposed.

If you took steroids by mouth and are having them decreased (tapered) or you are being switched to Asmanex, you should be followed closely by your health care professional. Death can occur. Tell your health care professional right away about any symptoms such as feeling tired or exhausted, weakness, nausea, vomiting, or symptoms of low blood pressure (such as dizziness or faintness). If you are under stress, such as with surgery, after surgery or trauma, you may need steroids by mouth again.

Patients who use inhaled steroid medicines for a long time may have an increased risk of decreased bone mass, which can affect bone strength. Talk with your health care provider about any questions about bone health.

Use your Asmanex regularly and at the same time each day, as prescribed by your health care provider. You may not get the most benefit for 1 to 2 weeks or longer after starting Asmanex. If your symptoms do not improve in that time frame or if your condition gets worse, contact your health care provider.

Who should not take Asmanex Twisthaler?

You should not use Asmanex Twisthaler if you are having an asthma attack. You should use Asmanex Twisthaler if you are under the age of 4 years old or if you are allergic to any of the ingredients of Asmanex.

What should I tell my doctor before I take the first dose of Asmanex Twisthaler?

Tell your doctor about all prescription, over-the-counter, and herbal medication you are taking before beginning treatment with Asmanex Twisthaler. Also, talk to your doctor about your complete medical history, especially if you have a history of liver disease. Tell your health care provider if you have or had TB, are exposed to anyone with chickenpox or measles, or about any other infections you had before or while using Asmanex Twisthaler.

What is the usual dosage?

The information below is based on the dosage guidelines your doctor uses. Depending on your condition and medical history, your doctor may prescribe a different regimen. Do not change the dosage or stop taking your medication without your doctor's approval.

Patients who received bronchodilators alone
Patients ≥12 years old: Recommended dose is 220 mcg once daily in the evening. Max daily dose is 440 mcg.

Patients who received inhaled corticosteroids
Recommended dose is 220 mcg once daily in the evening. Max daily dose is 440 mcg.

Patients who received oral corticosteroids
Recommended dose is 440 mcg twice daily. Max daily dose is 880 mcg.

Children 4-11 years of age: Recommended dose is 110 mcg once daily in the evening. Max daily dose is 110 mcg.

How should I take Asmanex Twisthaler?

If Asmanex Twisthaler is given only once a day, you should take it in the evening.

Make sure to record the date of pouch opening on the cap label, and throw out the inhaler 45 days after opening the foil pouch or when the dose counter reads "00" and the final dose has been inhaled, whichever comes first. The inhaler should be held upright while removing the cap. The medication should be taken as directed by your doctor. Breathe rapidly and deeply, and do not breathe out through the inhaler. The inhaler delivers your medicine as a very fine powder that you may not taste, smell, or feel. Do not take or give extra doses unless your doctor has told you to. The mouthpiece should be wiped dry and the cap replaced immediately following each inhalation. Rinse your mouth after each inhalation. The dose counter shows the doses remaining. When the dose counter indicates zero, the cap will lock and the inhaler should be thrown out.

What should I avoid while taking Asmanex Twisthaler?

You should avoid exhaling into the inhaler. You should also avoid using the Asmanex Twisthaler if you are having an asthma attack.

What are possible food and drug interactions associated with Asmanex Twisthaler?

If Asmanex Twisthaler is taken with certain other drugs, the effect of either medication could be increased, decreased, or altered. It is recommended that Asmanex Twisthaler be used with caution when combined with ketoconazole.

What are the possible side effects of Asmanex Twisthaler?

Side effects cannot be anticipated. If any develop or change in intensity, tell your doctor as soon as possible. Only your doctor can determine if it is safe for you to continue taking this drug.

Side effects may include: headache, nasal allergy symptoms, sore throat, upper respiratory tract infection, sinus infection, fungal infections in the mouth, painful menstrual periods, muscle and bone pain, back pain, upset stomach

Can I receive Asmanex Twisthaler if I am pregnant or breastfeeding?

The effects of Asmanex Twisthaler during pregnancy and breastfeeding are unknown. Tell your doctor immediately if you are pregnant, or plan to become pregnant, or are breastfeeding.

What should I do if I miss a dose of Asmanex Twisthaler?

If you miss a dose, take it as soon as you remember. If you do not remember until it is time for your next dose, skip the missed dose and go back to your regular schedule. Do not take two doses of Asmanex at the same time.

How should I store Asmanex Twisthaler?

Keep your inhaler clean and dry at all times. If the mouthpiece needs cleaning, gently wipe the mouth piece with a dry cloth or tissue as needed. Do not wash the inhaler. Avoid contact with any liquids. Store in a dry place at 25°C (77°F) [may range between 15°-30°C (59°-86°F)]. Keep your inhaler out of the reach of children.

ASPIRIN

What is Aspirin?

Aspirin is an anti-inflammatory pain medication (analgesic) that is used to relieve headaches, toothaches, and minor aches and pains, and to reduce fever. It also temporarily relieves the minor aches and pains of arthritis, muscle aches, colds, flu, and menstrual discomfort. In some patients, a small daily dose of aspirin may be used to ensure sufficient blood flow to the brain and prevent stroke. Aspirin may also be taken to decrease recurrence of a heart attack or other heart problems.

What is the most important information I should know about Aspirin?

Aspirin should not be used during the last 3 months of pregnancy unless specifically prescribed by a doctor. It may cause problems in the unborn child or complications during delivery.

Who should not take Aspirin?

Do not take aspirin if you are sensitive or allergic to it or similar products.

What should I tell my doctor before I take the first dose of Aspirin?

Tell your doctor about all prescription, over-the-counter, and herbal medication you are taking before beginning treatment with aspirin. Also, talk to your doctor about your complete medical history, especially if you have stomach problems, bleeding problems, ulcers, or chickenpox or flu symptoms.

What is the usual dosage?

The information below is based on the dosage guidelines your doctor uses. Depending on your condition and medical history, your doctor may prescribe a different regimen. Do not change the dosage or stop taking your medication without your doctor's approval.

Prevention of Heart Attack
Adults: The usual dose is 1 tablet daily. Your physician may suggest that you take a larger dose, however. If you use Halfprin low-strength tablets (162 milligrams), adjust dosage accordingly.

Prevention of Stroke
The usual dose is 1 tablet 4 times daily or 2 tablets 2 times a day.

Treatment of Minor Pain and Fever
The usual dose is 1 or 2 tablets every 3 to 4 hours up to 6 times a day.

How should I take Aspirin?

Do not take more than the recommended dose. Do not use aspirin if it has a strong, vinegar-like odor. If aspirin upsets your stomach, use of a coated or buffered brand may reduce the problem. Do not chew or crush sustained-release brands, such as Bayer time-release aspirin, or pills coated to delay breakdown of the drug, such as Ecotrin. To make them easier to swallow, take them with a full glass of water.

What should I avoid while taking Aspirin?

Avoid taking aspirin in the last trimester of pregnancy.

What are possible food and drug interactions associated with Aspirin?

If aspirin is taken with certain other drugs, the effects of either could be increased, decreased, or altered. It is especially important to check with your doctor before combining aspirin with the following: acetazolamide, ACE-inhibitor-type blood pressure medications such as captopril, anti-gout medications such as allopurinol, arthritis medications such as ibuprofen and indomethacin, blood thinners such as warfarin sodium, certain diuretics such as furosemide, diabetes medications such as glyburide, diltiazem, dipyridamole, insulin, seizure medications such as valproic acid, and steroids such as prednisone.

What are the possible side effects of Aspirin?
Side effects cannot be anticipated. If any develop or change in intensity, tell your doctor as soon as possible. Only your doctor can determine if it is safe for you to continue taking this drug.

Side effects may include: heartburn, nausea and/or vomiting, possible involvement in formation of stomach ulcers and bleeding, small amounts of blood in stool, stomach pain, stomach upset

Can I receive Aspirin if I am pregnant or breastfeeding?
The use of aspirin during pregnancy should be discussed with your doctor. Aspirin should not be used during the last 3 months of pregnancy unless specifically indicated by your doctor. It may cause problems in the fetus and complications during delivery. Aspirin may appear in breast milk and could affect a nursing infant. Ask your doctor whether it is safe to take aspirin while you are breastfeeding.

What should I do if I miss a dose of Aspirin?
Take it as soon as you remember. If it is almost time for your next dose, skip the one you missed and go back to your regular schedule. Never take 2 doses at the same time.

How should I store Aspirin?
Store at room temperature.

Aspirin and extended-release dipyridamole *See Aggrenox, page 53.*

ASTELIN
Generic name: Azelastine hydrochloride

What is Astelin?
Astelin is a prescription nasal spray medicine. Astelin is an antihistamine used to relieve symptoms of seasonal allergies in adults and children 5 years and older. Additionally, in people 12 years and older, it relieves symptoms caused by environmental irritants such as perfumes, cigarette smoke, exhaust fumes, chemical odors, and cold air. These symptoms include sneezing; itchy, runny, or stuffy nose; and postnasal drip.

What is the most important information I should know about Astelin?

Astelin may cause sleepiness, so it is not recommended to drive, operate machinery, or perform similar activities until you know how Astelin affects you.

Who should not take Astelin?

Do not take Astelin if you are allergic to any of its ingredients.

What should I tell my doctor before I take the first dose of Astelin?

Tell your doctor about all prescription, over-the-counter, and herbal medications you are taking before beginning treatment with Astelin. Also, talk to your doctor about your complete medical history, including all of your allergies, and if you are pregnant or planning to become pregnant, or are breastfeeding.

What is the usual dosage?

The information below is based on the dosage guidelines your doctor uses. Depending on your condition and medical history, your doctor may prescribe a different regimen. Do not change the dosage or stop taking your medication without your doctor's approval.

Seasonal Allergic Rhinitis
Adults and children >12 years: The recommended dose of Astelin is one or two sprays per nostril twice a day.

Children 5 years to 11 years: The recommended dose of Astelin is one spray per nostril twice a day.

Vasomotor Rhinitis
Adults and children >12 years: The recommended dose of Astelin is two sprays per nostril twice a day.

How should I take Astelin?

Before initial use, the delivery system should be primed with 4 sprays or until a fine mist appears. When 3 or more days have elapsed since the last use, the pump should be re-primed with 2 sprays or until a fine mist appears. Spray Astelin into your nose.

What should I avoid while taking Astelin?

Avoid taking Astelin with other antihistamines without talking to your doctor first. Avoid alcohol or other medicine that may cause drowsiness. Avoid spraying Astelin into your eyes.

What are possible food and drug interactions associated with Astelin?

If Astelin is taken with certain other drugs, the effects of either could be increased, decreased, or altered. It is especially important to check with your doctor before combining azelastine with the following: other antihistamines, alcohol or other CNS depressants, cimetidine, and ketoconazole.

What are the possible side effects of Astelin?

Side effects cannot be anticipated. If any develop or change in intensity, tell your doctor as soon as possible. Only your doctor can determine if it is safe for you to continue taking this drug.

Side effects may include: bitter taste, drowsiness, headache, nasal inflammation/burning

Can I receive Astelin if I am pregnant or breastfeeding?

Talk to your doctor if you are pregnant, planning to become pregnant, or are nursing, before starting treatment with Astelin. The effects of this drug are unknown on pregnancy, and it may pass into breast milk.

What should I do if I miss a dose of Astelin?

If you miss a dose of Astelin, take the missed dose as soon as you remember it. However, if it is almost time for your next dose, skip the dose you missed and return to your regular dosing schedule. Do not double the dose.

How should I store Astelin?

Store at room temperature, in an upright position. Do not store in the freezer.

ATACAND

Generic name: Candesartan cilexetil

What is Atacand?

Atacand is used to treat both high blood pressure as well as heart failure. This drug belongs to a family of medications known as angiotensin receptor blockers (ARBs). This type of medication stops a hormone called angiotensin II from attaching to your blood vessels. Angiotensin II normally causes arteries to narrow. As a result of taking Atacand, the blood vessels relax and widen, and your blood pressure is reduced.

What is the most important information I should know about Atacand?

Atacand should not be taken during pregnancy; this drug may cause severe birth defects.

Symptoms of abnormally low blood pressure, such as dizziness, light-headedness, feeling faint, or weakness, which can be severe, may occur if you take Atacand and are dehydrated or have low levels of salt in the blood.

Atacand can also cause an increase in potassium levels in your blood (hyperkalemia), especially in heart failure patients. During treatment with Atacand in patients with heart failure, monitoring of serum potassium is recommended when your doctor increases your dose and periodically thereafter.

Who should not take Atacand?
Do not take Atacand if you are allergic to any of its ingredients.

What should I tell my doctor before I take the first dose of Atacand?
Tell your doctor about all prescription, over-the-counter, and herbal medications you are taking before beginning treatment with Atacand. Also, talk to your doctor about your complete medical history, especially if you have liver or kidney problems. Tell your doctor if you are pregnant, planning to become pregnant, or are nursing.

What is the usual dosage?
The information below is based on the dosage guidelines your doctor uses. Depending on your condition and medical history, your doctor may prescribe a different regimen. Do not change the dosage or stop taking your medication without your doctor's approval.

High Blood Pressure
Adults: The usual dose of Atacand is 16 milligrams (mg) once a day. Atacand can be given once or twice daily, with a total dose equal to 8-32 mg.

Heart Failure
Adults: The usual dose of Atacand is 4 mg a day, with a target dose of 32 mg a day, which is achieved by doubling the dose at approximately 2-week intervals, as tolerated.

How should I take Atacand?
Atacand can be taken with or without food. If this drug does not make your blood pressure any better, it can be given with a diuretic, or other medications.

What should I avoid while taking Atacand?
Avoid becoming pregnant while being treated with Atacand, as this can cause severe harm to your unborn baby.

What are possible food and drug interactions associated with Atacand?

Taking Atacand with lithium may cause an increase in the concentration of lithium in the blood.

What are the possible side effects of Atacand?

Side effects cannot be anticipated. If any develop or change in intensity, tell your doctor as soon as possible. Only your doctor can determine if it is safe for you to continue taking this drug.

Side effects may include: back pain, cold symptoms, dizziness, runny/ stuffy nose, sore throat

Symptoms of abnormally low blood pressure include: dizziness, feeling faint or weak, lightheadedness

Can I receive Atacand if I am pregnant or breastfeeding?

Tell your doctor if you are pregnant, planning to become pregnant, or are nursing. Atacand should not be taken if you are pregnant, as it may cause severe birth defects. Also, this drug may pass into your breast milk.

What should I do if I miss a dose of Atacand?

If you miss a dose of Atacand, be sure to take your dose as soon as you remember. However, do not take more than your prescribed dose on any one day.

How should I store Atacand?

Store at room temperature in a tightly closed container.

ATACAND HCT

Generic name: Candesartan cilexetil and hydrochlorothiazide

What is Atacand HCT?

Atacand HCT is used to treat high blood pressure. This drug belongs to a family of medications known as angiotensin receptor blockers (ARBs). This type of medication stops a hormone called angiotensin II from attaching to your blood vessels. Angiotensin II normally causes arteries to narrow. As a result of taking Atacand HCT, the blood vessels relax and widen, and blood pressure is reduced. This medication also contains hydrochlorothiazide, a thiazide diuretic that helps to decrease high blood pressure as well.

What is the most important information I should know about Atacand HCT?

Atacand HCT should not be taken during pregnancy; this drug may cause severe birth defects.

Your blood pressure should be checked before and during Atacand HCT therapy. Atacand HCT may make the blood pressure too low, especially during the first days of use. If you faint, Atacand HCT should be stopped until you can talk to your doctor.

Who should not take Atacand HCT?
Do not take Atacand HCT if you are allergic to any of its ingredients.

Atacand HCT contains hydrochlorothiazide, so you should not take it if you have anuria (absence of urine formation), or if you are allergic to other sulfonamide-derived drugs.

What should I tell my doctor before I take the first dose of Atacand HCT?
Tell your doctor about all prescription, over-the-counter, and herbal medications you are taking before beginning treatment with Atacand HCT. Also, talk to your doctor about your complete medical history, especially if you are pregnant, planning to become pregnant, or are nursing.

What is the usual dosage?
The information below is based on the dosage guidelines your doctor uses. Depending on your condition and medical history, your doctor may prescribe a different regimen. Do not change the dosage or stop taking your medication without your doctor's approval.

Adults: The usual dosage of Atacand HCT is 16 milligrams (mg) once a day. Atacand HCT can be given once or twice daily, with a total dosage equal to 8-32 mg.

Hydrochlorothiazide is effective in doses of 12.5 mg to 50 mg once daily.

How should I take Atacand HCT?
Atacand HCT can be taken with or without food. If this drug does not make your blood pressure any better, it can be given with other medications.

What should I avoid while taking Atacand HCT?
Avoid becoming pregnant while being treated with Atacand HCT, as this can cause severe harm to your unborn baby.

Avoid excessive sweating and inadequate fluid intake, as this could cause a further decrease in your blood pressure.

Avoid taking potassium supplements or salt substitutes containing potassium without talking to your doctor first.

What are possible food and drug interactions associated with Atacand HCT?
If Atacand HCT is taken with certain other drugs, the effects of either could be increased, decreased, or altered. It is especially important to

check with your doctor before combining Atacand HCT with the following: alcohol, antidiabetic drugs, barbiturates, cholestyramine and colestipol resins, corticosteroids, lithium, narcotics, nondepolarizing muscle relaxants such as tubocurarine, nonsteroidal anti-inflammatory drugs (NSAIDs), pressor amines such as norepinephrine, and other high blood pressure medications.

What are the possible side effects of Atacand HCT?

Side effects cannot be anticipated. If any develop or change in intensity, tell your doctor as soon as possible. Only your doctor can determine if it is safe for you to continue taking this drug.

Side effects may include: back pain, cold symptoms, dizziness, electrolyte imbalances (increase/decrease in calcium, potassium, magnesium), headache, flu symptoms, upper respiratory infection

Symptoms of abnormally low blood pressure include: dizziness, feeling faint or weak, lightheadedness

Can I receive Atacand HCT if I am pregnant or breastfeeding?

Tell your doctor if you are pregnant, planning to become pregnant, or are nursing. Atacand HCT should not be taken if you are pregnant, as it may cause severe deformities and malformations to your child's face and limbs. Also, this drug may pass into your breast milk.

What should I do if I miss a dose of Atacand HCT?

If you miss a dose of Atacand HCT, be sure to take your dose as soon as you remember. However, do not take more than your prescribed dose on any one day.

How should I store Atacand HCT?

Store at room temperature in a tightly closed container.

Atazanavir sulphate See Reyataz, page 1148.

Atenolol See Tenormin, page 1280.

Atenolol and chlorthalidone See Tenoretic, page 1278.

ATIVAN

Generic name: Lorazepam

What is Ativan?

Ativan is an antianxiety agent, belonging to the drug class of benzodiazepines. Ativan is used for the management of anxiety disorders or for the short-term relief of the symptoms of anxiety or anxiety associated with depressive symptoms.

What is the most important information I should know about Ativan?

Patients with acute narrow-angle glaucoma should not take Ativan.

Patients with a primary depressive disorder or psychosis should not take Ativan, since pre-existing depression may emerge or worsen during use of benzodiazepines.

Use of benzodiazepines, including Ativan, whether used alone or in combination with other central nervous system depressants, may lead to potentially fatal respiratory depression.

Prolonged or excessive use of Ativan or other benzodiazepines may lead to physical and psychological dependence.

Patients taking Ativan may have a decreased tolerance for alcohol and other central nervous system depressants. Use caution when operating a vehicle or other machinery.

Who should not take Ativan?

Patients with acute narrow-angle glaucoma should not take Ativan, nor should patients with a primary depressive disorder unless they are being treated with antidepressants.

Elderly patients, as well as patients with liver or kidney diseases, should start on a low dose to minimize side effects, and should be monitored closely.

What should I tell my doctor before I take the first dose of Ativan?

Tell your doctor about all prescription, over-the-counter, and herbal medications you are taking before beginning treatment with Ativan. Also, talk to your doctor about your complete medical history, especially if you have been diagnosed with depression, acute narrow-angle glaucoma, liver or kidney disease, respiratory disorders, or cardiovascular disorders.

What is the usual dosage?

The information below is based on the dosage guidelines your doctor uses. Depending on your condition and medical history, your doctor may prescribe a different regimen. Do not change the dosage or stop taking your medication without your doctor's approval.

Adults: For anxiety, most patients require an initial dose of 2 mg to 3 mg daily, divided in two to three doses.

For insomnia due to anxiety, a single daily dose of 2 mg to 4 mg may be given at bedtime.

For elderly patients, an initial dose of 1 mg to 2 mg per day in divided doses is recommended to reduce side effects.

The dose of Ativan may be increased gradually as needed, with the higher portion of the daily dose taken at bedtime.

How should I take Ativan?

Take Ativan exactly as directed, with the larger portion of the daily dose taken at bedtime. Do not take more than the prescribed dose, as serious side effects may occur.

What should I avoid while taking Ativan?

Avoid operating dangerous machinery, including motor vehicles, as Ativan may cause drowsiness.

Avoid alcohol and other central nervous system depressants, as this can cause serious respiratory disorders.

Do not stop taking this medication without first consulting your doctor.

What are possible food and drug interactions associated with Ativan?

If Ativan is used with certain other drugs, the effects of either could be increased, decreased, or altered. It is especially important to check with your doctor before combining Ativan with the following: alcohol, anticonvulsants, antidepressants, antihistamines, clozapine, and probenecid.

What are the possible side effects of Ativan?

Side effects cannot be anticipated. If any develop or change in intensity, tell your doctor as soon as possible. Only your doctor can determine if it is safe for you to continue taking this drug.

Side effects may include: sedation, dizziness, weakness, unsteadiness, dose-dependant respiratory depression, fatigue, amnesia

Can I receive Ativan if I am pregnant or breastfeeding?

Because the use of these drugs is rarely a matter of urgency, the use of Ativan during pregnancy should be avoided. Ativan has been detected in human breast milk, therefore, it should not be administered to breastfeeding women, unless the expected benefit to the woman outweighs the potential risk to the infant.

What should I do if I miss a dose of Ativan?

Skip the dose and continue with your normal dosing schedule; never double the dose.

How should I store Ativan?

Store at room temperature.

Atomoxetine hydrochloride *See Strattera, page 1226.*

Atorvastatin calcium *See Lipitor, page 750.*

ATRALIN
Generic name: Tretinoin

What is Atralin?
Atralin is a gel used to treat acne.

What is the most important information I should know about Atralin?
Do not allow anyone else to use this medicine. Do not use it for a condition not prescribed by your doctor.

Who should not take Atralin?
Do not use Atralin if you have eczema, are allergic to fish, or are pregnant or breastfeeding.

What should I tell my doctor before I take the first dose of Atralin?
Tell your doctor about all prescription, over-the-counter, and herbal medications you are taking before beginning treatment with Atralin. Also, talk to your doctor about your complete medical history, especially if have eczema, fish allergies, or you are pregnant or breastfeeding.

What is the usual dosage?
The information below is based on the dosage guidelines your doctor uses. Depending on your condition and medical history, your doctor may prescribe a different regimen. Do not change the dosage or stop taking your medication without your doctor's approval.

Adults: The usual dose is once daily at bedtime.

How should I take Atralin?
Apply Atralin gel once daily before bedtime to skin where acne lesions appear, using a thin layer to cover the entire effected area. Keep the gel away from your mouth, eyes, the creases of your nose, and mucous membranes.

What should I avoid while taking Atralin?
Avoid unprotected exposure to light including sun lamps. Use a sunscreen when outside, and avoid extreme weather conditions such as wind or cold temperatures.

What are possible food and drug interactions associated with Atralin?
If Atralin is used with certain other drugs, the effects of either could be increased, decreased, or altered. It is especially important to check with

your doctor before combining Atralin gel with medicated soaps or other topical skin medications.

What are the possible side effects of Atralin?
Side effects cannot be anticipated. If any develop or change in intensity, tell your doctor as soon as possible. Only your doctor can determine if it is safe for you to continue taking this drug.

Side effects may include: skin irritation, such as dryness, burning, redness, and excessive flaking or peeling

Can I receive Atralin if I am pregnant or breastfeeding?
Atralin should be avoided during pregnancy and breastfeeding. Talk with your doctor before using this drug if you are pregnant, plan to become pregnant, or are breastfeeding.

What should I do if I miss a dose of Atralin?
Skip the missed dose and return to your regular dosing schedule. Do not double the dose of your next application.

How should I store Atralin?
Store at room temperature.

ATRIPLA
Generic name: Efavirenz, emtricitabine, and tenofovir disoproxil fumarate

What is Atripla?
Atripla is an anti-HIV medication that contains Sustiva, Emtriva, and Viread. Atripla helps stop HIV replication in the body and raises T-cell levels, which allows your immune system to improve. Having less HIV in your blood lowers the chance of death or infections that can happen when your immune system is weak.

What is the most important information I should know about Atripla?
Atripla does not cure HIV/AIDS.

Atripla does not reduce the risk of passing HIV/AIDS to others through sexual contact, sharing needles, or being exposed to your blood.

Some people who have taken medicine like Atripla, which contains nucleoside analogs, have developed a serious condition called lactic acidosis (a buildup of an acid in the blood). Lactic acidosis can be a medical emergency and may need to be treated in the hospital.

Some people who have taken medicines like Atripla have developed serious liver problems, called hepatotoxicity, with liver enlargements (hepatomegaly) and fat in the liver (steatosis).

You have a higher chance of getting lactic acidosis or liver problems if you are female; very overweight (obese); or have been taking nucleoside analog-containing medicines, like Atripla, for a long time.

If you have hepatitis B virus (HBV) infection and stop taking Atripla, you may get a "flare-up" of your hepatitis. A "flare-up" is when the disease suddenly returns to a worse state than it was in before.

Who should not take Atripla?
Do not take Atripla if you are allergic to it or any of its ingredients.

What should I tell my doctor before I take the first dose of Atripla?
Tell your doctor about all prescription, over-the-counter, and herbal medications you are taking before beginning therapy with Atripla. Also, talk to your doctor about your complete medical history, especially if you have/had seizures; ever had mental illness or used drugs or alcohol; have/had bone, liver (including Hepatitis B), or kidney problems (including kidney dialysis treatment). Your doctor should also know if you are pregnant, plan to become pregnant, or are nursing.

What is the usual dosage?
The information below is based on the dosage guidelines your doctor uses. Depending on your condition and medical history, your doctor may prescribe a different regimen. Do not change the dosage or stop taking your medication without your doctor's approval.

Adults: The usual adult dose of Atripla is one tablet once per day. Atripla should not be used in children under the age of 18.

How should I take Atripla?
Atripla should be taken with water on an empty stomach. Your dose could be taken at bedtime to make some side effects less bothersome.

When your Atripla supply runs low, get more from your healthcare provider or pharmacy. This is very important because if the medicine is stopped for even a short time, the amount of HIV in your blood may increase. The HIV may develop resistance to Atripla and may become harder to treat.

What should I avoid while taking Atripla?
Do not get pregnant or breastfeed while taking Atripla. If you do become pregnant, contact your doctor right away.

Avoid sharing needles or other injection equipment. Do not share personal items that can have blood or bodily fluids on them, like toothbrushes or razor blades. Do not have sex without protection.

What are possible food and drug interactions associated with Atripla?

The following medicines may cause serious and life-threatening side effects when taken with Atripla: bepridil, cisapride, midazolam, pimozide, triazolam, and ergot medications.

Due to similarities between emtricitabine and lamivudine, Atripla should not be taken with drugs that contain lamivudine.

Voriconazole should not be taken with Atripla since it may lose its effect or may increase the chance of having side effects.

Also, do not take Atripla with St. John's wort, as it may decrease Atripla levels and lead to increased levels of viral load and possible resistance to Atripla or cross-resistance to other anti-HIV medications.

These medicines may need to be replaced with another medicine when taken with Atripla: clarithromycin, itraconazole, and saquinavir.

These medicines may need to have their dose changed when taken with Atripla: calcium channel blockers such as diltiazem or verapamil; indinavir; rifabutin; rifampin; sertraline; statins such as atorvastatin, pravastatin sodium, or simvastatin.

The following medicines may result in more side effects when taken with Atripla and you may need to be monitored more carefully if you take: atazanavir sulfate, didanosine, lopinavir/ritonavir (Kaletra), tenofovir DF.

If you take medicines for seizures such as carbamazepine, phenobarbital, or phenytoin, your doctor may want to switch you to another medicine or check drug levels in your blood from time to time.

What are the possible side effects of Atripla?

Side effects cannot be anticipated. If any develop or change in intensity, tell your doctor as soon as possible. Only your doctor can determine if it is safe for you to continue taking this drug.

Side effects may include: lactic acidosis, serious liver problems, flare-ups of HBV infection, serious psychiatric problems, kidney problems, changes in bone mineral density (thinning bones), changes in body fat, skin discoloration, diarrhea, dizziness, drowsiness, gas, headache, rash, tiredness, trouble concentrating, trouble sleeping, unusual dreams, upset stomach, vomiting

Symptoms of lactic acidosis include: cold feeling in arms and legs, dizzy/light-headedness, fast/irregular heartbeat, muscle pain, stomach pain with nausea and vomiting, tired/weak feeling, trouble breathing

Symptoms of liver problems include: dark urine, skin/whites of eyes turn yellow (jaundice), light-colored bowel movements, loss of appetite, nausea, lower stomach area pain

Can I receive Atripla if I am pregnant or breastfeeding?

Do not begin treatment with Atripla if you are pregnant, planning to become pregnant, or are nursing. Atripla is hazardous to an unborn baby if taken within the first trimester of development. This drug will pass through your breast milk; therefore, do not breastfeed while being treated with Atripla.

What should I do if I miss a dose of Atripla?
Do not miss a dose of Atripla. If you forget to take Atripla, take the missed dose right away, unless it is almost time for your next dose. Do not double the next dose; carry on with your regular dosing schedule.

How should I store Atripla?
Store at room temperature. Keep Atripla in its original container, which should be tightly closed.

ATROVENT
Generic name: Ipratropium bromide

What is Atrovent?
Atrovent inhalation aerosol and solution are prescribed for long-term treatment of bronchial spasms (wheezing) associated with chronic obstructive pulmonary disease, including chronic bronchitis and emphysema. When inhaled, Atrovent opens the air passages, allowing more oxygen to reach the lungs.

Atrovent nasal spray relieves runny nose. The 0.03% spray is used for year-round runny nose due to allergies and other causes. The 0.06% spray is prescribed for hay fever and for runny nose due to colds. The spray does not relieve nasal congestion or sneezing.

What is the most important information I should know about Atrovent?
Atrovent inhalation aerosol and solution are not for initial use in acute attacks of bronchial spasm when fast action is needed.

Who should not take Atrovent?
If you are sensitive to or have ever had an allergic reaction to Atrovent or any of its ingredients, or to soybeans, soy lecithin, or peanuts, you should not take this medication.

You should also avoid Atrovent if you are allergic to drugs based on atropine. Make sure your doctor is aware of any drug reactions you have experienced.

What should I tell my doctor before I take the first dose of Atrovent?
Tell your doctor about all prescription, over-the-counter, and herbal medication you are taking before beginning treatment with Atrovent. Also, talk to your doctor about your complete medical history, especially if you

have narrow-angle glaucoma (high pressure inside the eye), an enlarged prostate, or obstruction in the neck of the bladder.

What is the usual dosage?
The information below is based on the dosage guidelines your doctor uses. Depending on your condition and medical history, your doctor may prescribe a different regimen. Do not change the dosage or stop taking your medication without your doctor's approval.

Adults: (Aerosol or solution) The usual starting dose is 2 inhalations, 4 times per day. Additional inhalations may be taken, but the total should not exceed 12 in 24 hours. Not for use in children under 12. (Nasal spray 0.03%) The usual dose is 2 sprays in each nostril 2 or 3 times a day. Not for use in children under 6.

Runny Nose Due to Colds
Adults: (Nasal spray 0.06%) The usual dose is 2 sprays in each nostril 3 or 4 times a day.

Children age 5 and older: (Nasal Spray 0.06%) The recommended dose for children age 5 to 11 is 2 sprays in each nostril 3 times a day. Do not use for more than 4 days and do not give it to children under 5.

Runny Nose due to Hay Fever
The usual dose for adults and children 5 and over is 2 sprays in each nostril 4 times a day. This medication can be used safely for hay fever for up to 3 weeks.

How should I take Atrovent?
Atrovent inhalation aerosol and solution are not intended for occasional use. To get the most benefit from this drug, you must use it consistently throughout your course of treatment, as prescribed by your doctor.

To take the inhalation aerosol, insert the metal canister in the special Atrovent mouthpiece and shake well. Holding the canister upside down, exhale deeply through the mouth, enclose the mouthpiece with your lips, and inhale slowly through the mouth while firmly pressing once on the base of the upended canister. Hold your breath for 10 seconds then exhale. Wait 15 seconds and repeat. Test spray the canister 3 times whenever it has not been used for 24 hours.

What should I avoid while taking Atrovent?
Be careful to avoid spraying the medication in your eyes.

What are possible food and drug interactions associated with Atrovent?
If Atrovent is taken with certain other drugs, the effects of either could be increased, decreased, or altered. It is especially important to check

with your doctor before combining Atrovent with the following: atropine sulfate, hyoscyamine sulfate, phenobarbital, and scopolamine hydrobromide.

What are the possible side effects of Atrovent?
Side effects cannot be anticipated. If any develop or change in intensity, tell your doctor as soon as possible. Only your doctor can determine if it is safe for you to continue taking this drug.

Side effects may include (Inhalation Aerosol and Solution): blurred vision, breathlessness, bronchitis, cough, dizziness, dry mouth, headache, irritation from aerosol, nausea, nervousness, rash, stomach and intestinal upset, wheezing, worsening of symptoms

Side effects may include (Nasal Spray): blurred vision, change in taste, conjunctivitis ("pinkeye"), cough, diarrhea, dizziness, dry mouth/throat, eye irritation, headache, hoarseness, increased runny nose or nasal inflammation, inflamed nasal ulcers, nasal congestion, nasal dryness, nasal irritation/itching/burning, nasal tumors, nausea, nosebleed, pain, posterior nasal drip, pounding heartbeat, ringing in the ears, sinus inflammation, skin rash, sneezing, sore throat, swollen nose, thirst, upper respiratory infection

Can I receive Atrovent if I am pregnant or breastfeeding?
The effects of Atrovent during pregnancy and breastfeeding are unknown. Tell your doctor immediately if you are pregnant, plan to become pregnant, or are breastfeeding.

What should I do if I miss a dose of Atrovent?
Take it as soon as you remember. If it is almost time for your next dose, skip the one you missed and go back to your regular schedule. Do not take 2 doses at once.

How should I store Atrovent?
All forms of Atrovent may be stored at room temperature. Do not freeze.
Keep the inhalation aerosol away from heat and flame; the canister could burst. Discard after 200 sprays. Keep the nasal spray tightly closed.

AUGMENTIN
Generic name: Amoxicillin and clavulanate potassium

What is Augmentin?
Augmentin is used in the treatment of lower respiratory, middle ear, sinus, skin, and urinary tract infections that are caused by certain specific bacteria. These bacteria produce a chemical enzyme called beta lactamase that makes some infections particularly difficult to treat.

Augmentin ES-600, a stronger, oral-suspension form of the drug, is prescribed for certain stubborn ear infections that previous treatment has failed to clear up in children two and under, or those attending day care.

Augmentin XR is an extended-release form of the drug used to treat pneumonia and sinus infections.

What is the most important information I should know about Augmentin?

If you are allergic to either penicillin or cephalosporin antibiotics in any form, consult your doctor *before taking Augmentin*. You may be allergic to it, and if a reaction occurs, it could be extremely severe. If you take the drug and feel signs of a reaction, seek medical attention immediately.

Who should not take Augmentin?

If you are sensitive to or have ever had an allergic reaction to any penicillin medication, do not take this drug.

Also avoid taking Augmentin if it has ever given you liver problems or yellowing of the skin and eyes. Additionally, do not take Augmentin XR if you have severe kidney problems or need dialysis.

What should I tell my doctor before I take the first dose of Augmentin?

Tell your doctor about all prescription, over-the-counter, and herbal medication you are taking before beginning treatment with Augmentin. Also, talk to your doctor about your complete medical history, especially if you have a liver, kidney or blood disorder; or if you have diabetes.

What is the usual dosage?

The information below is based on the dosage guidelines your doctor uses. Depending on your condition and medical history, your doctor may prescribe a different regimen. Do not change the dosage or stop taking your medication without your doctor's approval.

Adults: The usual adult dose is one 500-milligram (mg) tablet every 12 hours or one 250-mg tablet every 8 hours. For more severe infections and infections of the respiratory tract, the dose should be one 875-mg tablet every 12 hours or one 500-mg tablet every 8 hours. It is essential that you take this medicine according to your doctor's directions.

The total daily dose of Augmentin XR is 4000 mg of amoxicillin and 250 mg of clavulanate potassium, given in divided doses every 12 hours for 10 days (for sinus infections) or for 7 to 10 days (for pneumonia).

Children older than 3 months: For middle ear infections, sinus inflammation, lower respiratory tract infections, and more severe infections, the usual dose of the 200- or 400-mg suspension is 45 mg per 2.2 pounds per day, in 2 doses, every 12 hours, and of the 125- or 250-mg suspension, 40 mg per 2.2 pounds per day, in 3 doses, every 8 hours.

For less severe infections, the usual dose is 25 mg of the 200- or 400-mg suspension for each 2.2 pounds of weight per day, divided into 2 doses, every 12 hours, or 20 mg of the 125- or 250-mg suspension per 2.2 pounds per day, divided into 3 doses, every 8 hours.

The usual dosage of Augmentin ES-600 oral suspension is 90 mg per 2.2 pounds of body weight per day, divided into 2 doses taken every 12 hours. Treatment lasts 10 days.

Children weighing 88 pounds or more will take the adult dosage of standard Augmentin.

Less than 3 months: Children in this age group take 30 milligrams per 2.2 pounds of body weight per day, divided into 2 doses and taken every 12 hours.

How should I take Augmentin?

Augmentin should be taken every 8 or 12 hours, depending on the dosage strength. It may be taken with or without food, but taking it with meals or snacks will help prevent stomach upset. However, the extended-release form, Augmentin XR, should always be taken with food to improve absorption.

Your doctor will only prescribe Augmentin to treat a bacterial infection; it will not cure a viral infection, such as the common cold. It's important to take the full dosage schedule of Augmentin, even if you're feeling better in a few days. Not completing the full dosage schedule may decrease the drug's effectiveness and increase the chances that the bacteria may become resistant to Augmentin and similar antibiotics.

Shake the suspension well. Use a dosing spoon or medicine dropper to give a child the medication; rinse the spoon or dropper after each use.

What should I avoid while taking Augmentin?

To prevent bacterial resistance, avoid missing doses and not completing the full dosage schedule as your doctor has prescribed.

What are possible food and drug interactions associated with Augmentin?

If Augmentin is taken with certain other drugs, the effects of either could be increased, decreased, or altered. It is especially important to check with your doctor before combining Augmentin with the following: allopurinol, birth control pills, and probenecid.

What are the possible side effects of Augmentin?

Side effects cannot be anticipated. If any develop or change in intensity, tell your doctor as soon as possible. Only your doctor can determine if it is safe for you to continue taking this drug.

Side effects may include: diarrhea/loose stools, nausea, skin rashes and hives

Can I receive Augmentin if I am pregnant or breastfeeding?

The effects of Augmentin during pregnancy and breastfeeding are unknown. Tell your doctor immediately if you are pregnant, plan to become pregnant, or are breastfeeding.

What should I do if I miss a dose of Augmentin?

Take it as soon as you remember. If it is almost time for the next dose, and you take 2 doses a day, take the one you missed and the next dose 5 to 6 hours later. If you take 3 doses a day, take the one you missed and the next dose 2 to 4 hours later. Then go back to your regular schedule.

How should I store Augmentin?

Store the suspension under refrigeration and discard after 10 days. Store tablets away from heat, light, and moisture.

AVALIDE

Generic name: Irbesartan and hydrochlorothiazide

What is Avalide?

Avalide is a combination medication used to treat high blood pressure. One component, irbesartan, belongs to a class of blood pressure medications that prevents the hormone angiotensin II from constricting the blood vessels, thereby allowing blood to flow more freely and keeping blood pressure down. The other component, hydrochlorothiazide, is a diuretic that increases the output of urine, removing excess fluid from the body and thus lowering blood pressure.

What is the most important information I should know about Avalide?

When used in the second and third trimesters of pregnancy, Avalide can cause injury and even death to the unborn child. Stop taking Avalide as soon as you know you are pregnant. If you know you are pregnant or plan to become pregnant, tell your doctor immediately.

Who should not take Avalide?

If Avalide gives you an allergic reaction, you'll be unable to use it. You should also avoid it if you have an allergy to sulfa drugs, and if you're unable to urinate.

What should I tell my doctor before I take the first dose of Avalide?

Tell your doctor about all prescription, over-the-counter, and herbal medication you are taking before beginning treatment with Avalide. Also, talk to your doctor about your complete medical history, especially if you have liver or kidney disease, diabetes, gout, or lupus erythematosus.

What is the usual dosage?

The information below is based on the dosage guidelines your doctor uses. Depending on your condition and medical history, your doctor may prescribe a different regimen. Do not change the dosage or stop taking your medication without your doctor's approval.

Adults: The usual starting dose of Avalide is 1 lower-strength tablet daily.

It will take 2 to 4 weeks for Avalide to reach its maximum effectiveness. If your blood pressure does not respond to the initial dosage, your doctor may increase the dosage to 1 higher-strength tablet or 2 lower-strength tablets taken once a day.

How should I take Avalide?

Avalide can be taken with or without food.

What should I avoid while taking Avalide?

Avoid becoming dedhydrated while taking Avalide. Inadequate fluid intake or loss of fluids may result in low blood pressure, leading to lightheadedness or fainting. Seek medical attention if symptoms of hypersensitivity reactions, electrolyte imbalance (dry mouth, thirst, weakness, lethargy), lightheadedness, or fainting occur.

What are possible food and drug interactions associated with Avalide?

If Avalide is taken with certain other drugs, the effects of either could be increased, decreased, or altered. It is especially important to check with your doctor before combining Avalide with the following: alcohol; adrenocorticotropic hormone (ACTH); barbiturates such as phenobarbital and secobarbital; cholestyramine; colestipol; insulin; lithium; narcotic painkillers such as acetaminophen, codeine phosphate, meperidine hydrochloride, and oxycodone hydrochloride; nonsteroidal anti-inflammatory drugs such as ibuprofen and naproxen sodium; other blood pressure medications such as atenolol and nifedipine; oral diabetes drugs such as chlorpropamide, glipizide, and glyburide; and steroids such as prednisone.

What are the possible side effects of Avalide?

Side effects cannot be anticipated. If any develop or change in intensity, tell your doctor as soon as possible. Only your doctor can determine if it is safe for you to continue taking this drug.

Side effects may include: dizziness, fatigue, influenza, muscle and bone pain, nausea, swelling due to water retention, vomiting

Can I receive Avalide if I am pregnant or breastfeeding?

When used in the second and third trimesters of pregnancy, Avalide can cause injury and even death to the unborn child. Stop taking Avalide as soon as you know you are pregnant. If you know you are pregnant or plan to become pregnant, tell your doctor immediately.

Avalide appears in breast milk and can affect the nursing infant. If this medication is essential to your health, your doctor may advise you to stop breastfeeding while you are taking Avalide.

What should I do if I miss a dose of Avalide?
Take it as soon as you remember. If it is almost time for your next dose, skip the one you missed and go back to your regular schedule. Never take 2 doses at the same time.

How should I store Avalide?
Store at room temperature.

AVANDAMET
Generic name: Rosiglitazone maleate and metformin hydrochloride

What is Avandamet?
Avandamet is an oral medication used to control blood sugar levels in people with type 2 (non-insulin-dependent) diabetes. It contains two drugs commonly used to lower blood sugar, rosiglitazone and metformin. Avandamet replaces the need to take these two drugs separately. It is also used when treatment with metformin hydrochloride alone doesn't work. Avandamet is not, however, meant to take the place of weight loss or diet and exercise. You should continue to follow the regimen your doctor recommends.

What is the most important information I should know about Avandamet?
Avandamet could cause a very rare—but potentially fatal—side effect known as lactic acidosis. It is caused by a buildup of lactic acid in the blood. The problem is most likely to occur in people whose liver or kidneys are not working well, and in those who have multiple medical problems, take several medications, or have congestive heart failure. The risk also is higher if you are an older adult or drink alcohol. Lactic acidosis is a medical emergency that must be treated in a hospital.

Who should not take Avandamet?
You should not use Avandamet if you need to take medicine for congestive heart failure.

Do not take Avandamet if you have ever had an allergic reaction to rosiglitazone or metformin. Also, do not begin treatment with Avandamet if you have metabolic or diabetic ketoacidosis (a life-threatening medical emergency caused by insufficient insulin and marked by excessive thirst, nausea, fatigue, pain below the breastbone, and fruity breath). You should not use Avandamet if you have type 1 (insulin-dependent) diabetes, or if you are already taking insulin.

What should I tell my doctor before I take the first dose of Avandamet?

Tell your doctor about all prescription, over-the-counter, and herbal medication you are taking before beginning treatment with Avandamet. Also, talk to your doctor about your complete medical history, especially if you have heart or kidney problems, or you are going to have a surgical procedure.

What is the usual dosage?

The information below is based on the dosage guidelines your doctor uses. Depending on your condition and medical history, your doctor may prescribe a different regimen. Do not change the dosage or stop taking your medication without your doctor's approval.

Inadequately controlled on metformin therapy alone
Adults: The recommended daily starting dose is 4 milligrams (mg) of rosiglitazone plus the dose of metformin you are already taking.

Inadequately controlled on rosiglitazone therapy alone
Adults: The recommended daily starting dose is 1000 mg of metformin plus the dose of rosiglitazone you are already taking.

Combination therapy taking separate doses of rosiglitazone and metformin
Adults: The usual starting dose of Avandamet is based on your current doses of rosiglitazone and metformin.

Increasing dose of Avandamet
Adults: The daily dose of Avandamet may be increased by increments of 4 mg of rosiglitazone and/or 500 mg of metformin, up to a maximum daily dose of 8 mg of rosiglitazone and 2000 mg of metformin.

How should I take Avandamet?

Do not take more or less of this medication than directed by your doctor. Avandamet should be taken in divided doses with meals to reduce the possibility of nausea or diarrhea, especially during the first few weeks of therapy. Avandamet may start to work within the first week or two after you begin taking it, but it can take up to 3 months before the drug's full effects are seen. Be sure to check your blood sugar as your doctor recommends.

What should I avoid while taking Avandamet?

Avoid drinking too much alcohol while taking Avandamet.

What are possible food and drug interactions associated with Avandamet?

If Avandamet is taken with certain other drugs, the effects of either could be increased, decreased, or altered. It is especially important to check with your doctor before combining Avandamet with the following: alcohol; amiloride; calcium channel blockers (heart medications) such as nifedipine and verapamil hydrochloride; cimetidine; decongestant, airway-opening drugs such as Albuterol sulfate and pseudoephedrine; hydrochloride; digoxin; estrogens such as conjugated estrogens; furosemide; isoniazid, a drug used for tuberculosis; morphine; niacin; nifedipine; oral contraceptives; phenytoin; procainamide; quinidine; quinine; ranitidine; steroids such as prednisone; thyroid hormones such as levothyroxine; tranquilizers such as chlorpromazine; triamterene; trimethoprim; vancomycin; and water pills (diuretics) such as amiloride, and hydrochlorothiazide.

What are the possible side effects of Avandamet?

Side effects cannot be anticipated. If any develop or change in intensity, tell your doctor as soon as possible. Only your doctor can determine if it is safe for you to continue taking this drug.

Side effects may include: accidental injury, anemia, back pain, diarrhea, fatigue, headache, joint pain, nausea, sinus inflammation, swelling, upper respiratory infection, upset stomach, viral infection

Symptoms of lactic acidosis may include: dizziness, extreme weakness or tiredness, light-headedness, low body temperature, slow or irregular heartbeat, rapid breathing or trouble breathing, sleepiness, unexpected or unusual stomach discomfort (especially after you have been taking Avandamet for a while), unusual muscle pain

Can I receive Avandamet if I am pregnant or breastfeeding?

The effects of Avandamet during pregnancy and breastfeeding are unknown. Tell your doctor immediately if you are pregnant, plan to become pregnant, or are breastfeeding.

What should I do if I miss a dose of Avandamet?

Take the forgotten dose as soon as you remember. However, if it is almost time for your next dose, skip the one you missed and return to your regular schedule. Do not take two doses at once.

How should I store Avandamet?

Store at room temperature in a tight, light-resistant container.

AVANDARYL
Generic name: Rosiglitazone maleate and glimepiride

What is Avandaryl?
Avandaryl contains 2 medicines: rosiglitazone maleate (Avandia) and glimepiride (Amaryl). Avandaryl is used for the treatment of type 2 diabetes mellitus in conjunction with diet and exercise. Glimepiride can help your body release more of its own insulin. Rosiglitazone can help your body respond better to the insulin made in your body. Type 2 diabetes occurs when there is a buildup of sugar in the blood, which may lead to serious health conditions.

What is the most important information I should know about Avandaryl?
Full diabetic therapy should include diet and weight management, through proper eating habits and exercise.

Rosiglitazone, one of the medicines in Avandaryl, can cause heart failure or make it worse. After starting Avandaryl therapy and after dose increases, your doctor should follow up with you carefully to see if you develop any signs and symptoms of heart failure. You should not use Avandaryl if you have severe heart failure.

Who should not take Avandaryl?
Do not take Avandaryl if you are allergic/have had an allergic reaction to any of its ingredients.

Do not take Avandaryl if you have had diabetic ketoacidosis; this condition should be treated with insulin.

Certain patients with heart failure should not start taking Avandaryl.

You should not take this medication if you have type 1 diabetes.

This medication is not recommended for children under the age of 18.

What should I tell my doctor before I take the first dose of Avandaryl?
Talk to your doctor about all of your medical conditions, especially if you have heart, liver or kidney problems, have a diabetic eye condition called macular edema (swelling in the back of the eye), are menopausal, pregnant or planning to become pregnant, or are breastfeeding. Also, keep your doctor informed of all prescription, over-the-counter, and herbal medications you are taking.

What is the usual dosage?
The information below is based on the dosage guidelines your doctor uses. Depending on your condition and medical history, your doctor may prescribe a different regimen. Do not change the dosage or stop taking your medication without your doctor's approval.

Adults: The usual starting dose of Avandaryl is 4 milligrams (mg)/1 mg or 4 mg/2 mg once daily.

How should I take Avandaryl?

Take the recommended dose orally, with your first meal of the day.

Test your blood sugar regularly as told by your doctor.

It is important to stay on your recommended diet, lose excess weight, and get regular exercise while taking Avandaryl.

What should I avoid while taking Avandaryl?

Inform your doctor if you get sick, injured, or have surgery while on Avandaryl. This drug may not properly control your blood sugar levels during these times.

What are possible food and drug interactions associated with Avandaryl?

Avandaryl may react with thiazides and other diuretics, corticosteroids, phenothiazines, thyroid products, estrogens, oral contraceptives, phenytoin, nicotinic acid sympathomimetics, and isoniazid, and can produce hyperglycemia (high blood sugar).

Concurrent use with oral miconazole and oral hypoglycemic agents may lead to hypoglycemia (low blood sugar).

Inhibitors of CYP2C8 such as gemfibrozil may increase the effects of Avandaryl and this may lead to hypoglycemia and other side effects. Inducers of CYP2C8 such as rifampin may decrease how Avandaryl works in your body.

What are the possible side effects of Avandaryl?

Side effects cannot be anticipated. If any develop or change in intensity, tell your doctor as soon as possible. Only your doctor can determine if it is safe for you to continue taking this drug.

Side effects may include: cold-like symptoms, abnormal ovulation, dizziness, fractures (usually in the hand, upper arm, or foot) in females, heart problems, liver or kidney problems, low or high blood sugar, low red blood cell count (anemia), swelling, weight gain

Can I receive Avandaryl if I am pregnant or breastfeeding?

Avandaryl should not be used during pregnancy. It is recommended to have a stable blood sugar level during pregnancy; talk with your doctor about beginning insulin therapy if you are pregnant or planning to become pregnant.

What should I do if I miss a dose of Avandaryl?

If you miss a dose of Avandaryl, take it as soon as you remember. If it is already time for your next dose, do not take double.

How should I store Avandaryl?
Avandaryl should be stored in its original container at room temperature.

AVANDIA
Generic name: Rosiglitazone maleate

What is Avandia?
Avandia is used to treat adults with type 2 diabetes, in conjunction with diet and exercise. This drug helps your body become more sensitive to the insulin that you make; it does not increase the amount of insulin you produce. Avandia may be used alone or in combination with other anti-diabetic drugs.

What is the most important information I should know about Avandia?
Avandia may cause fluid retention (when your body keeps extra fluid), swelling (edema), and weight gain. These severe side effects may cause heart failure or make other heart problems worse. You should not take Avandia if you have severe heart failure. If you have heart failure with symptoms and even if these symptoms are not severe, Avandia may not be the right medication for you. Other drugs like Avandia, taken at the same time, may increase the chances of heart failure as well.

Call you doctor if you experience any of the following symptoms of heart failure:

Swelling or fluid retention, especially in the ankles or legs; shortness of breath or trouble breathing, especially when you lie down; fast increase in weight; or feeling unusually tired.

Avandia may also cause other problems related to the reduced blood flow to the heart, including chest pain (angina) or a heart attack (myocardial infarction). The risk seems to be higher in patients who take Avandia with insulin or nitrate medicines. If you have chest pain, call your doctor right away no matter what diabetes medicine you are taking. People with diabetes have a greater risk for heart problems, so it is important to work with your doctor to manage other conditions such as high blood pressure or high cholesterol.

Who should not take Avandia?
Do not begin treatment with Avandia if you are allergic to any of its ingredients. Also, do not begin treatment with this drug if you have heart or liver problems, heart failure, diabetic eye disease called macular edema, type 1 diabetes, had liver problems while taking another diabetes medicine called Rezulin, or if you are pregnant or planning to become pregnant. If you are premenopausal (in the years before menopause and experiencing irregular monthly periods), Avandia may increase your chances of becoming pregnant.

What should I tell my doctor before I take the first dose of Avandia?

Tell your doctor about all prescription, over-the-counter, and herbal medications you are taking before beginning treatment with Avandia. Also, talk to your doctor about your complete medical history, especially if you have heart or liver problems, have a type of diabetic eye disease called macular edema (swelling of the back of the eye), are pregnant or planning to become pregnant, or are breastfeeding.

What is the usual dosage?

The information below is based on the dosage guidelines your doctor uses. Depending on your condition and medical history, your doctor may prescribe a different regimen. Do not change the dosage or stop taking your medication without your doctor's approval.

Adults: The usual daily starting dose of Avandia is 4 milligrams (mg) a day taken once a day or 2 mg taken twice a day. Your doctor may adjust your dose until your blood sugar is better controlled.

How should I take Avandia?

Take Avandia with or without food.

Diet and exercise can help your body use its blood sugar better. It is important to stay on your recommended diet, lose excess weight, and get regular exercise.

Test your blood sugar regularly as told by your doctor.

What should I avoid while taking Avandia?

Avoid becoming pregnant or nursing while on Avandia. Talk to your doctor about birth control choices as Avandia may increase your chances of becoming pregnant. In addition, you should avoid taking insulin or nitrates while on therapy with Avandia.

What are possible food and drug interactions associated with Avandia?

If Avandia is taken with certain other drugs, the effects of either could be increased, decreased, or altered. It is especially important to check with your doctor before combining Avandia with the following: insulin; nitrate medicines such as nitroglycerin or isosorbide to treat a type a type of chest pain called angina; and any medicines for high blood pressure, high cholesterol, or for prevention of heart disease or stroke.

Talk with your doctor if you are taking any medication containing gemfibrozil or rifampin; a change in treatment may be necessary if you are using such drugs.

What are the possible side effects of Avandia?

Side effects cannot be anticipated. If any develop or change in intensity, tell your doctor as soon as possible. Only your doctor can determine if it is safe for you to continue taking this drug.

Side effects may include: cold-like symptoms, headache

Serious side effects may include: anemia (low red blood cell count), edema (swelling/fluid retention, shortness of breath, quick weight increase, tiredness), fractures (usually in the hand, upper arm, or foot) in females, heart failure or other heart problems such as chest pain or heart attack, liver problems (nausea, vomiting, stomach pain, unusual tiredness, loss of appetite, dark urine, yellowing of skin/eyes), low blood sugar (hypoglycemia), macular edema (a diabetic eye disease with swelling in the back of the eye), ovulation (release of egg from an ovary in a woman) leading to pregnancy, weight gain

Can I receive Avandia if I am pregnant or breastfeeding?

Talk to your doctor if you are pregnant, planning to become pregnant, or are nursing, before beginning treatment with Avandia. The effects of this drug on pregnancy are unknown, and it may pass into your breast milk.

What should I do if I miss a dose of Avandia?

If you miss a dose of Avandia, take your pill as soon as you remember, unless it is time to take your next dose. Take your next dose at the usual time. Do not take a double dose to make up for a missed dose.

How should I store Avandia?

Store at room temperature.

AVAPRO

Generic name: Irbesartan

What is Avapro?

Avapro is used to treat high blood pressure. A member of the new family of drugs called angiotensin II receptor antagonists, it works by preventing the hormone angiotensin II from narrowing the blood vessels, an action that tends to raise blood pressure. Avapro may be prescribed alone or with other blood pressure medications.

In people with type 2 diabetes and high blood pressure, Avapro is also prescribed to stave off damage to the kidneys, often delaying the need for dialysis and a kidney transplant.

What is the most important information I should know about Avapro?

You must take Avapro regularly for it to be effective. Since blood pressure declines gradually, it may be a couple of weeks before you get the full benefit of Avapro, and you must continue taking it even if you are feeling well. Avapro does not cure high blood pressure, it merely keeps it under control.

Who should not take Avapro?
Do not begin treatment with Avapro if you are allergic to any of its ingredients.

What should I tell my doctor before I take the first dose of Avapro?
Tell your doctor about all prescription, over-the-counter, and herbal medication you are taking before beginning treatment with Avapro. Also, talk to your doctor about your complete medical history, especially if you have kidney disease.

What is the usual dosage?
The information below is based on the dosage guidelines your doctor uses. Depending on your condition and medical history, your doctor may prescribe a different regimen. Do not change the dosage or stop taking your medication without your doctor's approval.

High Blood Pressure
Adults: The recommended starting dose of Avapro is 150 milligrams (mg) once a day. If your blood pressure remains elevated, your dose will be gradually increased to 300 mg once a day.

If you are being treated with hemodialysis or high doses of diuretics, you'll be started at a lower dose of 75 mg once a day.

Kidney Damage from Type 2 Diabetes
The usual dose is 300 mg once a day.

Children: For children 6 to 12 years old, the typical starting dose is 75 mg once a day. If blood pressure is still too high, the dose may be increased to 150 mg once a day. Children 13 to 16 years old are usually given the adult dosage.

How should I take Avapro?
Take your dose of Avapro around the same time every day, with or without food.

What are possible food and drug interactions associated with Avapro?
If Avapro is taken with certain other drugs, the effects of either could be increased, decreased, or altered. It is especially important to check with your doctor before combining Avapro with tolbutamide.

What are the possible side effects of Avapro?

Side effects cannot be anticipated. If any develop or change in intensity, tell your doctor as soon as possible. Only your doctor can determine if it is safe for you to continue taking this drug.

Side effects may include: diarrhea, fatigue, heartburn, respiratory tract infection

Can I receive Avapro if I am pregnant or breastfeeding?

Avapro can cause injury or even death to the unborn child when used during the last 6 months of pregnancy. As soon as you learn you're pregnant, stop taking Avapro and call your doctor.

It is not known whether Avapro appears in breast milk, but because of potential risks to the newborn, it's considered best to avoid using the drug while breastfeeding. You and your doctor should decide whether to give up nursing or discontinue Avapro.

What should I do if I miss a dose of Avapro?

Take it as soon as you remember. If it is almost time for your next dose, skip the one you missed and go back to your regular schedule. Do not take 2 doses at the same time.

How should I store Avapro?

Store at room temperature.

AVELOX

Generic name: Moxifloxacin hydrochloride

What is Avelox?

Avelox, an antibiotic, is prescribed to treat sinus and lung infections. It kills bacteria that can cause sinusitis, pneumonia, and secondary infections in chronic bronchitis. It also fights skin infections caused by staph or strep.

Avelox is a member of the quinolone family of antibiotics. Like all antibiotics, Avelox works only against bacteria. It will not cure an infection caused by a virus.

What is the most important information I should know about Avelox?

In rare cases, antibiotics can cause a serious allergic reaction. Stop taking Avelox and call your doctor immediately if you develop any of the following warning signs: skin rash, tingling, hives, shortness of breath, swelling of the face or throat, or difficulty swallowing.

Who should not take Avelox?

If you have ever had an allergic reaction to any other quinolone antibiotic, such as ciprofloxacin hydrochloride, enoxacin, levofloxacin, lomefloxacin hydrochloride, norfloxacin, ofloxacin, or you should not take Avelox.

What should I tell my doctor before I take the first dose of Avelox?

Tell your doctor about all prescription, over-the-counter, and herbal medication you are taking before beginning treatment with Avelox. Also, talk to your doctor about your complete medical history, especially if you have a heart problem, you are being treated for an abnormal heartbeat, or you have a history of convulsions or blockage of arteries in the brain. Your doctor should also know if you have convulsions.

Avelox can cause certain heart irregularities in people already prone to the problem. If you are being treated for an abnormal heartbeat, make sure the doctor is aware of it. You may have to avoid Avelox. Also tell the doctor if you or anyone in your family has a history of heart problems. If you develop palpitations or fainting spells while taking Avelox, contact your doctor immediately.

Before you take Avelox, you should tell your doctor if you have a history of convulsions or blockage of the arteries in the brain.

What is the usual dosage?

The information below is based on the dosage guidelines your doctor uses. Depending on your condition and medical history, your doctor may prescribe a different regimen. Do not change the dosage or stop taking your medication without your doctor's approval.

Acute Bacterial Sinusitis
Adults: The usual dose is one 400-milligram (mg) tablet daily for 7 to 14 days.

Acute Bacterial Infection with Chronic Bronchitis
Adults: The usual dose is one 400-mg tablet daily for 5 days.

Pneumonia
Adults: The usual dose is one 400-mg tablet daily for 7 to 14 days.

Skin Infections
Adults: The usual dose is one 400-mg tablet daily for 7 days.

How should I take Avelox?

Avelox may be taken with or without food. Your doctor will only prescribe Avelox to treat a bacterial infection; it will not cure a viral infection, such as the common cold. It's important to take the full dosage schedule of Avelox, even if you're feeling better in a few days. Not completing the full dosage schedule may decrease the drug's effectiveness and increase the chances that the bacteria may become resistant to Avelox and similar antibiotics. Be sure to drink plenty of fluids while taking Avelox.

What should I avoid while taking Avelox?

Avelox may make you dizzy or light-headed. Do not drive a car, operate machinery, or engage in activities requiring mental alertness or coordination until you know how the drug affects you.

What are possible food and drug interactions associated with Avelox?

If Avelox is taken with certain other drugs, the effects of either could be increased, decreased, or altered. It is especially important to check with your doctor before combining Avelox with the following: amiodarone; antipsychotic drugs such as chlorpromazine, haloperidol, and trifluoperazine; didanosine; erythromycin; multivitamins containing iron or zinc; antacids containing magnesium, calcium, or aluminum; nonsteroidal anti-inflammatory drugs (NSAIDs); procainamide; quinidine; Sotalol; sucralfate; tricyclic antidepressants such as amitriptyline hydrochloride, desipramine hydrochloride, and perphenazine; and warfarin.

What are the possible side effects of Avelox?

Side effects cannot be anticipated. If any develop or change in intensity, tell your doctor as soon as possible. Only your doctor can determine if it is safe for you to continue taking this drug.

Side effects may include: abdominal pain, anemia, anxiety, decreased blood pressure, diarrhea, dizziness, headache, drowsiness, insomnia, joint and muscle pain, nausea, nervousness, rapid heartbeat, rash, sweating

Can I receive Avelox if I am pregnant or breastfeeding?

The effects of Avelox during pregnancy and breastfeeding are unknown. Tell your doctor immediately if you are pregnant, plan to become pregnant, or are breastfeeding.

What should I do if I miss a dose of Avelox?

Take it as soon as you remember. If it is almost time for your next dose, skip the one you missed and go back to your regular schedule. Do not take a double dose in an effort to "catch up."

How should I store Avelox?

Store Avelox at room temperature. Avoid high humidity.

AVINZA
Generic name: Morphine sulfate, extended-release

What is Avinza?
Avinza is a modified-release formulation of morphine sulfate intended for once-daily administration. Avinza is indicated for relief of moderate to severe chronic pain that requires continuous, around-the-clock opioid therapy for a long period of time. Avinza has been shown to help people to resume their daily activities. It has also been shown to help people sleep through the night better.

What is the most important information I should know about Avinza?
Avinza is an extended-release formulation that should be taken whole. Do not chew, crush, cut, or dissolve the contents of the capsule. In addition, do not take Avinza with alcohol or with medications that contain alcohol in their formulation, as this may lead to potentially fatal doses of morphine sulfate. Also, do not take more than directed as Avinza is potentially addictive, may cause serious kidney damage, or other serious side effects.

Who should not take Avinza?
Patients with hypersensitivity to Avinza or its ingredients in this preparation should not take this medication. Patients with respiratory disease need to be assessed to see whether the benefits of Avinza clearly outweigh the risks. In addition, patients with respiratory depression in the absence of resuscitative equipment, acute or severe bronchial asthma, or impairment of the small intestines (paralytic ileus) should not be given this drug.

What should I tell my doctor before I take the first dose of Avinza?
Tell your doctor about all prescription, over-the-counter, and herbal medications you are taking before beginning treatment with Avinza. Also, talk to your doctor about your complete medical history, especially if you are pregnant or plan to become pregnant, are breastfeeding, if you have abused drugs in the past, have respiratory depression, low blood pressure (hypotension), gastrointestinal obstructions (blocked intestines), liver or kidney problems, biliary tract disease (including acute pancreatitis), Addison's disease, low thyroid levels (hypothyroidism), or prostatic hypertrophy or urethral stricture.

What is the usual dosage?
The information below is based on the dosage guidelines your doctor uses. Depending on your condition and medical history, your doctor

may prescribe a different regimen. Do not change the dosage or stop taking your medication without your doctor's approval.

Adults: Dosage is individualized for each patient based on your weight and evaluation by your doctor. Avinza is intended to be given once daily in the morning. There are 30, 60, 90, and 120 milligram (mg) capsules available for your doctor to choose from. The 60, 90, and 120 mg capsules are to be used for opioid-tolerant patients. The total maximum dose is 1600 mg/day.

How should I take Avinza?

Take the once-daily capsules whole in the morning. Do not chew, crush, cut, or dissolve the contents of the capsule; it can be taken with or without food. Do not take with alcohol or any product with alcohol in its formulation. If you have trouble swallowing the capsules, you may open them and sprinkle all of the beads on a small amount of applesauce just before swallowing. Make sure to swallow all of the beads whole.

What should I avoid while taking Avinza?

Avoid concomitant use with alcohol or products containing alcohol in their formulation. Do not drive, operate any machinery, or participate in any other possibly dangerous activities.

What are possible food and drug interactions associated with Avinza?

If Avinza is taken with certain other drugs, the effects of either could be increased, decreased, or altered. It is especially important to check with your doctor before combining Avinza with the following: adinazolam, alfentanil, alprazolam, amobarbital, anileridine, apobarbital, bromazepam, brotizolam, buprenorphrine, butabarbital, butalbital, butorphanol, carisoprodol, chloral hydrate, chlordiazepoxide, chlorpromazine, chlorzoxazone, cimetidine, clobazam, clonazepam, clorazepate, clorgyline, codeine, dantrolene, dezocine, diazepam, estazolam, ethchlorvynol, fentanyl, flunitrazepam, fluphenazine, flurazepam, halazepam, hydrocodone, hydromorphone, iproniazid, isocarboxazid, ketazolam, levorphanol, lorazepam, lormetazepam, medazepam, meperidine, mephenesin, mephobarbital, meprobamate, metaxalone, methocarbamol, methohexital, midazolam, moclobemide, morphine sulfate liposome, nalbuphine, naltrexone, nialamide, nitrazepam, nordazepam, oxazepam, oxycodone, oxymorphone, pargyline, pentazocine, pentobarbital, perphenazine, phenelzine, phenobarbital, prazepam, procarbazine, prochlorperazine, promazine, promethazine, propoxyphene, quazepam, rasagiline, remifentanil, secobarbital, selegiline, sodium oxybate, sufentanil, temazepam, thiethylperazine, thiopental, thioridazine, toloxatone, tranylcypromine, triazolam, and trifluoperazine.

What are the possible side effects of Avinza?

Side effects cannot be anticipated. If any develop or change in intensity, tell your doctor as soon as possible. Only your doctor can determine if it is safe for you to continue taking this drug.

Side effects may include: constipation, nausea, drowsiness, vomiting; itching, skin rash, headache, abdominal pain, rash, sweating, loss of appetite, dizziness, insomnia, anxiety, fever, urinary retention, depression, sexual dysfunction

Can I receive Avinza if I am pregnant or breastfeeding?

The effects of Avinza during pregnancy and breastfeeding are unknown. However, due to the potential harm to the baby, consult with your doctor if you are pregnant, intend on becoming pregnant, or are breastfeeding.

What should I do if I miss a dose of Avinza?

If you miss a dose, take it as soon as you remember. If it is close to the time of your next dose (next day), skip it and resume your scheduled dose. Do not double your dose.

How should I store Avinza?

Store at room temperature in a tight, light resistant container and away from children. Protect from light and moisture. Protect from theft.

AVODART

Generic name: Dutasteride

What is Avodart?

Avodart is a medication for the treatment of symptoms of benign prostatic hyperplasia (BPH). Avodart is used in men with an enlarged prostate to improve symptoms and to reduce the risk of a complete blockage of urine flow and the need for BPH-related surgery. It may also be used in combination with an alpha blocker called tamsulosin for the treatment of symptomatic BPH in men with an enlarged prostate.

What is the most important information I should know about Avodart?

Women should never take or handle Avodart. Women who are pregnant or may become pregnant should not handle Avodart capsules.

Men treated with Avodart should not donate blood until at least six months after their final dose to prevent transmitting the drug to a pregnant woman through a blood transfusion.

Who should not take Avodart?
Do not use Avodart if you are allergic to any of its ingredients. Women and children should not take Avodart. A woman who is pregnant or capable of becoming pregnant should not handle Avodart capsules.

What should I tell my doctor before I take the first dose of Avodart?
Tell your doctor about all prescription, over-the-counter, and herbal medications you are taking before beginning treatment with Avodart. Also, talk to your doctor about your complete medical history, especially if you have/had liver problems.

What is the usual dosage?
The information below is based on the dosage guidelines your doctor uses. Depending on your condition and medical history, your doctor may prescribe a different regimen. Do not change the dosage or stop taking your medication without your doctor's approval.

Adults: The recommended dose of Avodart is 0.5 milligrams (mg) taken orally once a day.

How should I take Avodart?
The capsules should be swallowed whole. Avodart may be administered with or without food. You may find it helpful to take Avodart at the same time every day to help you remember to take your dose.

What should I avoid while taking Avodart?
Avoid giving blood during treatment and for at least six months after treatment with Avodart. Do not allow a pregnant woman to handle Avodart capsules, as they may be hazardous to her pregnancy.

What are possible food and drug interactions associated with Avodart?
If Avodart is taken with certain other drugs, the effects of either could be increased, decreased, or altered. It is especially important to check with your doctor before combining Avodart with cytochrome P450 3A inhibitors such as ritonavir.

What are the possible side effects of Avodart?
Side effects cannot be anticipated. If any develop or change in intensity, tell your doctor as soon as possible. Only your doctor can determine if it is safe for you to continue taking this drug.

Side effects may include: decrease in sex drive, decrease in the amount of semen released during sex, hives, impotence (trouble getting or keeping an erection), itching, rash, swelling of the lips or face, swelling or tenderness of the breasts

Can I receive Avodart if I am pregnant or breastfeeding?

Women should not take Avodart. Also, avoid touching Avodart capsules if you are pregnant, planning to become pregnant, or are nursing. This drug may cause severe deformities in your unborn child.

What should I do if I miss a dose of Avodart?

If you miss a dose, you may take it later that day. Do not make up the missed dose by taking 2 doses the next day.

How should I store Avodart?

Store at room temperature.

AXERT

Generic name: Almotriptan malate

What is Axert?

Axert is a medication used to treat migraine attacks in adults. Axert belongs to a class of drugs called selective serotonin receptor agonists. Axert reduces the swelling of blood vessels that surround your brain. This swelling is associated with the headache pain of a migraine attack. Axert blocks the release of substances from nerve endings that cause more pain and other migraine symptoms, and it also interrupts the pain signals that are sent your brain. By doing all of these things, Axert helps to relieve the symptoms of your migraine.

Use Axert only for a migraine attack; do not use Axert to treat headaches that might be caused by other conditions.

What is the most important information I should know about Axert?

In very rare cases, patients taking medicines in the same class of drugs as Axert experience serious heart problems, stroke, or increased blood pressure. Tell your doctor right away if you feel tightness, pain, pressure, or heaviness in your chest, throat, neck, or jaw after you take Axert.

Cases of life-threatening serotonin syndrome have been reported during combined use of selective serotonin reuptake inhibitors (SSRIs), selective norepinephrine reuptake inhibitors (SNRIs), and triptans. Contact your doctor immediately if you experience possible signs and symptoms of serotonin syndrome, including agitation, hallucinations, sweating, fast heartbeat, nausea, vomiting, and diarrhea.

Who should not take Axert?

Do not take Axert if you have ever had heart disease, uncontrolled high blood pressure, or hemiplegic or basilar migraine. Also, if you have taken another serotonin receptor agonist or ergotamine-type medicine in the last 24 hours, do not use this drug. You should not take this drug if you have had an allergic reaction to Axert or any of its ingredients.

What should I tell my doctor before I take the first dose of Axert?

Tell your doctor about all prescription, over-the-counter, and herbal medications you are taking before beginning treatment with Axert. Also, talk to your doctor about your complete medical history, especially if you are depressed and taking medication for it, or if you are being treated for a fungal infection. You should also tell your doctor if you had/have high blood pressure; chest pain; shortness of breath; heart disease; liver or kidney problems; risk factors for heart disease such as high blood pressure, diabetes, high cholesterol, if you are overweight, smoke, have family members with heart disease, you are past menopause, or if you are a male over 40 years old; if you plan to become pregnant or are pregnant; or plan to breastfeed or are breastfeeding.

What is the usual dosage?
The information below is based on the dosage guidelines your doctor uses. Depending on your condition and medical history, your doctor may prescribe a different regimen. Do not change the dosage or stop taking your medication without your doctor's approval.

Adults: The usual dosage of Axert is a single dose of either 6.25 milligram (mg) or 12.5 mg per migraine attack, limited to 2 doses per day.

How should I take Axert?
When you have a migraine headache, take Axert as directed by your doctor. If your headache comes back after your first dose, you may take a second dose 2 hours or more after the first dose. However, if you do not experience any pain relief after a first dose, do not take a second dose without first checking with your doctor. Do not take more than two tablets in a 24-hour period.

What should I avoid while taking Axert?
Check with your doctor before you take any new medicines, including prescription and non-prescription medicines and supplements. There are some medicines that you should not take 24 hours before or 24 hours after taking Axert.

Evaluate your ability to drive or operate heavy machinery if you experience sleepiness while taking Axert.

What are possible food and drug interactions associated with Axert?
If Axert is taken with certain other drugs, the effects of either could be increased, decreased, or altered. It is especially important to check with

your doctor before combining Axert with the following: monoamine oxidase (MAO) inhibitors such as phenelzine sulfate or tranylcypromine sulfate (or if it has been less than 2 weeks since you stopped taking an MAO inhibitor); medications that may increase the effects of Axert such as ketoconazole, itraconazole, ritonavir, or erythromycin (or if it has been less than one week since you stopped taking one of these drugs); ergot-containing drugs; other serotonin receptor agonists; selective serotonin reuptake inhibitors (SSRIs) such as citalopram, escitalopram, paroxetine, fluoxetine, olanzapine/fluoxetine, sertraline, and fluvoxamine; and serotonin norepinephrine reuptake inhibitors (SNRIs) such as duloxetine and venlafaxine.

What are the possible side effects of Axert?

Side effects cannot be anticipated. If any develop or change in intensity, tell your doctor as soon as possible. Only your doctor can determine if it is safe for you to continue taking this drug.

Side effects may include: dry mouth, headache, nausea, sleepiness, tingling or burning feeling

Can I receive Axert if I am pregnant or breastfeeding?

Talk to your doctor if you are pregnant, planning to become pregnant, or are nursing. The effects of Axert on pregnancy are unknown, and it may pass into your breast milk.

What should I do if I miss a dose of Axert?

Axert should only be taken when needed. It should not be taken on a regular basis.

How should I store Axert?

Store at room temperature away from heat, light, or moisture.

AXID

Generic name: Nizatidine

What is Axid?

Axid is prescribed for the treatment of duodenal ulcers and noncancerous stomach ulcers. Full-dose therapy for these problems lasts no longer than 8 weeks. However, your doctor may prescribe Axid at a reduced dosage after a duodenal ulcer has healed. The drug is also prescribed for the heartburn and the inflammation that result when acid stomach contents flow backward into the esophagus. Axid belongs to a class of drugs known as histamine H_2 blockers.

What is the most important information I should know about Axid?

Although Axid can be used for up to 8-12 weeks, most ulcers are healed within 4 weeks of therapy.

Who should not take Axid?

If you are sensitive to or have ever had an allergic reaction to Axid or similar drugs such as Zantac, you should not take this medication. Make sure your doctor is aware of any drug reactions you have experienced.

What should I tell my doctor before I take the first dose of Axid?

Tell your doctor about all prescription, over-the-counter, and herbal medication you are taking before beginning treatment with Axid. Also, talk to your doctor about your complete medical history, especially if you kidney or stomach problems.

What is the usual dosage?

The information below is based on the dosage guidelines your doctor uses. Depending on your condition and medical history, your doctor may prescribe a different regimen. Do not change the dosage or stop taking your medication without your doctor's approval.

Active Duodenal Ulcer
Adults: The usual dose is 300 milligrams (mg) once a day at bedtime, but your doctor may have you take 150 mg twice a day.

Active Non-cancerous Stomach Ulcer
Adults: The usual dose is 150 mg twice a day or 300 mg once a day at bedtime.

Maintenance of a Healed Duodenal Ulcer
Adults: The usual dose is 150 mg once a day at bedtime.

How should I take Axid?

Take this medication exactly as prescribed by your doctor.

What are possible food and drug interactions associated with Axid?

If Axid is taken with certain other drugs, the effects of either could be increased, decreased, or altered. It is especially important to check with your doctor before combining Axid with aspirin.

What are the possible side effects of Axid?

Side effects cannot be anticipated. If any develop or change in intensity, tell your doctor as soon as possible. Only your doctor can determine if it is safe for you to continue taking this drug.

Side effects may include: abdominal pain, diarrhea, dizziness, gas, headache, indigestion, inflammation of the nose, nausea, pain, sore throat, vomiting, weakness

Can I receive Axid if I am pregnant or breastfeeding?

The effects of Axid during pregnancy and breastfeeding are unknown. Tell your doctor immediately if you are pregnant, plan to become pregnant, or are breastfeeding.

What should I do if I miss a dose of Axid?

Take it as soon as you remember. If it is almost time for your next dose, skip the one you missed and go back to your regular schedule. Do not take 2 doses at once.

How should I store Axid?

Store at room temperature.

AYGESTIN

Generic name: Norethindrone acetate

What is Aygestin?

Aygestin contains a type of hormone known as progesterone. It is used to restore menstruation in women who have stopped having menstrual cycles (also called amenorrhea). Aygestin can also help treat endometriosis, a condition where the endometrium (the lining of the uterus) doesn't shed properly and attaches to the outside of the uterus or other areas such as the ovaries or bowels. Aygestin also helps control unusual and heavy bleeding of the uterus caused by hormonal imbalance. However, the drug is not used to control bleeding caused by fibroids or cancer.

What is the most important information I should know about Aygestin?

Aygestin increases the risk of blood clots, which can lead to phlebitis, breathing problems, vision problems, or stroke. If you experience any symptoms that might suggest the onset of a clot-related disorder—pain with swelling, warmth and redness in a leg vein, coughing or shortness of breath, loss of vision or double vision, migraine, or weakness or numbness in an arm or leg—stop taking Aygestin and see your doctor immediately.

Who should not take Aygestin?

Do not take Aygestin if you have ever had an allergic reaction to it. Do not take Aygestin if you are pregnant or have had an incomplete miscarriage. Avoid it if you have ever had a blood clotting disorder or a stroke. Do not take this drug if you have breast cancer, unexplained vaginal bleeding, or severe liver disease. Aygestin should not be used to test for pregnancy.

What should I tell my doctor before I take the first dose of Aygestin?

Tell your doctor about all prescription, over-the-counter, and herbal medication you are taking before beginning treatment with Aygestin. Also, talk to your doctor about your complete medical history, especially if you have epilepsy, migraines, asthma, or a heart or kidney problem. Also, tell your doctor if you have diabetes, high cholesterol, or if you have have suffered from depression in the past.

What is the usual dosage?

The information below is based on the dosage guidelines your doctor uses. Depending on your condition and medical history, your doctor may prescribe a different regimen. Do not change the dosage or stop taking your medication without your doctor's approval.

Prevention of Abnormal Uterine Bleeding Due to Hormonal Imbalance or to Restore Menstrual Periods
Adults: The usual dose is 2.5 to 10 milligrams (mg) a day taken for 5 to 10 days during the second half of a 28-day cycle. Your period should start 3 to 7 days after you stop taking Aygestin.

Treatment of Endometriosis
Adults: The recommended starting dose is 5 mg a day for 2 weeks. The doctor may increase your dose by 2.5 mg a day every 2 weeks up to a maximum of 15 mg a day. Treatment may continue for 6 to 9 months or until intolerable breakthrough bleeding occurs.

How should I take Aygestin?

Take Aygestin as directed by your doctor.

What should I avoid while taking Aygestin?

Avoid becoming pregnant while taking Aygestin. This drug may cause harm to a developing baby.

What are possible food and drug interactions associated with Aygestin?

If Aygestin is taken with certain other drugs, the effects of either could be increased, decreased, or altered. It is especially important to check with your doctor before combining Aygestin with the following: aminoglutethimide, carbamazepine, phenobarbital, phenytoin, rifabutin, and rifampin.

What are the possible side effects of Aygestin?

Side effects cannot be anticipated. If any develop or change in intensity, tell your doctor as soon as possible. Only your doctor can determine if it is safe for you to continue taking this drug.

Side effects may include: acne, allergic reaction, blood clots, break-through menstrual bleeding, breast enlargement or tenderness, bulging eye, depression, double vision, change in menstrual flow, headache, hives, menstrual spotting, migraine, mood swings, nausea, rash with or without itchy spots, skin discoloration, sleeplessness, stopping of menstrual flow, swelling, vision loss, weight increase or decrease, yellowing of the skin or eyes

Can I receive Aygestin if I am pregnant or breastfeeding?
Do not take Aygestin if you are pregnant or trying to become pregnant, since the drug may cause harm to a developing baby.

Aygestin appears in breast milk. Because the effect of Aygestin on a nursing infant is unknown, it is best to avoid the drug while breastfeeding unless it's clearly necessary.

What should I do if I miss a dose of Aygestin?
Take it as soon as you remember. If it is almost time for your next dose, skip the one you missed and go back to your regular schedule. Never take 2 doses at the same time.

How should I store Aygestin?
Store at room temperature in a tightly closed container.

AZASITE
Generic name: Azithromycin

What is AzaSite?
AzaSite is used to treat bacterial conjunctivitis (pinkeye).

What is the most important information I should know about AzaSite?
AzaSite should be used as eyedrop only. It should not be injected.

Skipping doses or stopping too early may make the treatment less effective and allow the bacterial infection to recur.

Who should not take AzaSite?
There are no known reasons to avoid AzaSite. However, tell your doctor before taking this medication if you have a known sensitivity to azithromycin or other antibiotics.

The safety and effectiveness of this medication in children less than 1 year old have not been studied.

What should I tell my doctor before I take the first dose of AzaSite?
Tell your doctor about all prescription, over-the-counter, and herbal medications you are taking before beginning treatment with AzaSite. Also,

talk to your doctor about your complete medical history, especially if you have ever had an allergic reaction to any antibiotic.

What is the usual dosage?
The information below is based on the dosage guidelines your doctor uses. Depending on your condition and medical history, your doctor may prescribe a different regimen. Do not change the dosage or stop taking your medication without your doctor's approval.

Adults and children 1 year and older: The initial dosage is 1 drop in the affected eye twice a day, 8-12 hours apart, for the first 2 days. The dosage is then reduced to 1 drop once a day for the next 5 days.

How should I take AzaSite?
Wash your hands thoroughly before using AzaSite. Do not allow the applicator tip to touch the eye, fingers, or other surfaces.

Although it is common to feel better early in the course of therapy, it is important to use AzaSite exactly as directed by your doctor. Skipping doses or stopping too early may allow bacterial resistance to develop, causing the infection to return.

What should I avoid while taking AzaSite?
Avoid wearing contact lenses while you have pinkeye.

What are possible food and drug interactions associated with AzaSite?
Drug interaction studies have not been conducted with AzaSite. Always check with your doctor before combining AzaSite with other medications.

What are the possible side effects of AzaSite?
Side effects cannot be anticipated. If any develop or change in intensity, tell your doctor as soon as possible. Only your doctor can determine if it is safe for you to continue taking this drug.

Side effects may include: eye irritation; burning, stinging, and eye irritation upon instillation of the drops; skin irritation or rash; corneal erosion; dry eye; altered taste; nasal congestion; eye discharge; inflammation of the cornea; sinus infection

If signs of an allergic reaction occur, contact your doctor immediately.

Can I receive AzaSite if I am pregnant or breastfeeding?
AzaSite should be avoided during pregnancy and breastfeeding. Tell your doctor before taking this drug if you are pregnant, plan to become pregnant, or are breastfeeding.

What should I do if I miss a dose of AzaSite?
Ask your doctor for advice.

How should I store AzaSite?
Store the unopened bottle in the refrigerator. Once the bottle is opened, store in the refrigerator or at room temperature for up to 14 days. Throw the opened medication away after 14 days.

Azelaic acid *See Azelex, below, or Finacea, page 547.*

Azelastine hydrochloride *See Astelin, page 137.*

Azelastine hydrochloride, eye drops *See Optivar, page 944.*

AZELEX
Generic name: Azelaic acid

What is Azelex?
Azelex is a cream used to help clear up mild to moderate acne. The skin eruptions and inflammation of acne typically begin during puberty, when oily secretions increase.

What is the most important information I should know about Azelex?
You should keep using Azelex regularly, even if you see no immediate improvement. It takes up to 4 weeks for Azelex to show results.

Who should not take Azelex?
Do not begin treatment with Azelex if you are allergic to any of its ingredients.

What should I tell my doctor before I take the first dose of Azelex?
Tell your doctor about all prescription, over-the-counter, and herbal medication you are taking before beginning treatment with Azelex. Also, talk to your doctor about your complete medical history.

What is the usual dosage?
The information below is based on the dosage guidelines your doctor uses. Depending on your condition and medical history, your doctor may prescribe a different regimen. Do not change the dosage or stop taking your medication without your doctor's approval.

Adults: The usual dose is a thin film of Azelex applied twice a day.

How should I take Azelex?

Use Azelex once in the morning and again in the evening. Wash the areas to be treated and pat dry. Apply a thin film of the medication and gently but thoroughly massage it into the skin. Wash your hands afterwards. Do not put bandages or dressings over the treated areas. Avoid getting the medication in the eyes, mouth, or nose. If any of it does get into your eyes, wash it out with large amounts of water. Call your doctor if your eyes remain irritated.

What should I avoid while taking Azelex?

Avoid getting Azelex cream in your eyes. If it does come in contact with the eyes, wash your eyes with large amounts of water and talk to your doctor if eye irritation continues.

What are the possible side effects of Azelex?

Side effects cannot be anticipated. If any develop or change in intensity, tell your doctor as soon as possible. Only your doctor can determine if it is safe for you to continue taking this drug.

Side effects may include: burning, itching, stinging, tingling

Can I receive Azelex if I am pregnant or breastfeeding?

The effects of Azelex during pregnancy and breastfeeding are unknown. Tell your doctor immediately if you are pregnant, plan to become pregnant, or are breastfeeding.

What should I do if I miss a dose of Azelex?

Apply it as soon as you remember. If it is almost time for the next dose, skip the one you missed and go back to your regular schedule.

How should I store Azelex?

Store at room temperature. Protect the cream from freezing.

AZILECT

Generic name: Rasagiline

What is Azilect?

Azilect is indicated for the treatment of Parkinson's disease (PD). It can be taken alone in early stage PD, or with levodopa/carbidopa and other PD medications when more relief is needed. Azilect works by blocking the breakdown of dopamine in the brain. Azilect belongs to a group of drugs known as MAO inhibitors.

What is the most important information I should know about Azilect?

When taking Azilect, avoid foods and beverages high in tyramine (see "What are possible food and drug interactions associated with Azilect?"), as they may cause a dangerous increase in blood pressure.

All patients are advised to monitor for melanoma (skin cancer)

Who should not take Azilect?

If you have moderate to severe liver disease or a tumor of the adrenal gland, you should not take Azilect. You should not take Azilect if you are taking certain medications (see "What are possible food and drug interactions associated with Azilect?") frequently, but be sure to see a dermatologist on a regular basis.

What should I tell my doctor before I take the first dose of Azilect?

Always tell your doctor about all the prescription, over-the-counter, and herbal medicines you are taking, especially antidepressants and ciprofloxacin. Talk to your doctor about your complete medical history, especially if you are pregnant, planning to become pregnant, or are nursing. Also, tell your doctor if you are planning to have surgery.

What is the usual dosage?

The information below is based on the dosage guidelines your doctor uses. Depending on your condition and medical history, your doctor may prescribe a different regimen. Do not change the dosage or stop taking your medication without your doctor's approval.

Adults: Azilect should be administered as 1 milligram (mg) once a day if taken alone. For use with another drug such as levodopa/carbidopa, the initial dose is 0.5 mg once a day, and may be increased by your doctor to 1 mg once a day.

How should I take Azilect?

Azilect should be taken once daily with or without food. Avoid tyramine-rich foods, beverages, or dietary supplements and amines (from over-the-counter cough/cold medicines) to prevent a possibly dangerous rise in blood pressure called a hypertensive crisis.

What should I avoid while taking Azilect?

When taking Azilect, you should not have elective surgery requiring general anesthesia, and should not receive cocaine or other local anesthesia that contains ingredients that could raise blood pressure. Avoid certain foods, beverages, dietary supplements, and cold remedies to prevent a possibly dangerous rise in blood pressure called a hypertensive crisis.

What are possible food and drug interactions associated with Azilect?

Azilect should not be taken with meperidine as it could possibly result in a serious reaction such as coma or death. Azilect should also not be taken with tramadol, methadone, propoxyphene, dextromethorphan, St. John's wort, mirtazapine, or cyclobenzaprine.

Monoamine oxidase inhibitors (MAOIs), amphetamines, cold medicines containing decongestants and weight-reducing medications containing pseudoephedrine, phenylephrine, phenylpropanolamine, or ephedrine should not be taken with Azilect to avoid dangerous increases in blood pressure.

Avoid foods and beverages high in tyramine, such as aged cheeses, air-dried meats, pickled herring, yeast extract, aged red wines, tap or draft beers, sauerkraut, and soy sauce. These foods, when consumed during therapy with Azilect, may cause dangerous increases in blood pressure.

What are the possible side effects of Azilect?

Side effects cannot be anticipated. If any develop or change in intensity, tell your doctor as soon as possible. Only your doctor can determine if it is safe for you to continue taking this drug.

Side effects may include: headache, indigestion, and joint pain

Side effects when taken with levodopa may include: accidental injury, constipation, dry mouth, joint pain, low blood pressure when standing, nausea, rash, sleepiness, uncontrolled movements, vomiting, weight loss

Can I receive Azilect if I am pregnant or breastfeeding?

The effects of Azilect on pregnancy and nursing are unknown. Talk with your doctor if you are pregnant, planning to become pregnant, or are nursing.

What should I do if I miss a dose of Azilect?

If a dose is missed, just continue on your normal schedule. Do not take 2 doses of Azilect at once.

How should I store Azilect?

Store at room temperature.

Azithromycin See AzaSite, page 179, or Zithromax, page 1480.

Azithromycin, extended-release See Zmax, page 1482.

AZMACORT

Generic name: Triamcinolone acetonide

What is Azmacort?

Azmacort is used to help control and relieve asthma symptoms. But, this drug is not used to treat immediate asthma attacks (bronchospasms); for treatment of these, you must use a fast-acting inhaler.

What is the most important information I should know about Azmacort?

Fungal infections of the mouth and throat may occur when taking Azmacort. This drug may cause a bronchospasm when receiving the dosage; if this happens, a fast-acting inhaler should be used to treat the episode. It is important to use Azmacort regularly at the intervals recommended by your doctor. Azmacort is not to be used as an emergency relief medicine in the case of an asthma attack.

Who should not take Azmacort?

Do not begin treatment with Azmacort if you are allergic to any of its ingredients. This drug should not be used for the treatment of bronchospasms.

What should I tell my doctor before I take the first dose of Azmacort?

Tell your doctor about all prescription, over-the-counter, and herbal medications you are taking before beginning treatment with Azmacort. Also, talk to your doctor about your complete medical history, especially if you are pregnant, planning to become pregnant, or are nursing. Be sure to tell your doctor if you are currently taking or have been taking oral steroid therapy.

What is the usual dosage?

The information below is based on the dosage guidelines your doctor uses. Depending on your condition and medical history, your doctor may prescribe a different regimen. Do not change the dosage or stop taking your medication without your doctor's approval.

Adults: Each inhalation contains 100 micrograms (mcg) of medication. The usual recommended dose is 2 inhalations (200 mcg) given 3 to 4 times a day, or 4 inhalations (400 mcg) given twice daily. The maximum daily intake is 16 inhalations (1600 mcg).

Children 6 to 12 years: The usual recommended dose is 1 or 2 inhalations (100 to 200 mcg) given 3 to 4 times a day, or 2 to 4 inhalations (200 to 400 mcg) given twice daily. The maximum daily intake should not exceed 12 inhalations (1200 mcg).

How should I take Azmacort?

You must shake the inhaler each time before each inhalation of medication. Breathe out to empty your lungs completely before using the inhaler. Press down firmly and steadily on the metal canister while breathing in slowly and deeply through your mouth only. Do not remove the inhaler from your mouth after breathing in the medication. Hold your breath for 10 seconds with the inhaler still in your mouth, then remove the inhaler and breathe out very slowly. Wait at least one minute between each inhalation. Read all the instructions on use and care of Azmacort thoroughly.

Keep track of your Azmacort use and dispose of the canister after 240 sprays, because after 240 doses the appropriate dose may not be delivered.

What should I avoid while taking Azmacort?

If your mouth becomes sore or develops a rash, be sure to mention this to your doctor, but do not stop using your inhaler unless instructed to do so. Avoid increasing your prescribed dose if your condition does not improve without first consulting your doctor. Also, avoid using your inhaler after the expiration date on the label or box.

What are possible food and drug interactions associated with Azmacort?

If Azmacort is used with certain other drugs, the effects of either could be increased, decreased, or altered. It is especially important to check with your doctor before combining Azmacort with prednisone.

What are the possible side effects of Azmacort?

Side effects cannot be anticipated. If any develop or change in intensity, tell your doctor as soon as possible. Only your doctor can determine if it is safe for you to continue taking this drug.

Side effects may include: back pain, flu symptoms, headache, sinus infection, sore throat, weight gain

Can I receive Azmacort if I am pregnant or breastfeeding?

Talk to your doctor if you are pregnant, planning to become pregnant, or are nursing. The effects of Azmacort on pregnancy are unknown, and it may pass into breast milk.

What should I do if I miss a dose of Azmacort?

If you miss a dose of Azmacort, take the missed dose as soon as you remember. However, if it almost time for your next dose, skip the dose you missed and return to your regular dosing schedule. Do not double your dose.

How should I store Azmacort?
Keep your inhaler out of the reach of children, unless otherwise prescribed. Store Azmacort, including the metal canister, at room temperature. Protect Azmacort from freezing temperatures and direct sunlight.

AZOPT
Generic name: Brinzolamide 1% ophthalmic suspension

What is Azopt?
Azopt is an eyedrop used for the treatment of high inner eye pressure in glaucoma (open-angle) and ocular hypertension.

**What is the most important information
I should know about Azopt?**
Azopt is an eye suspension that should be used with care. It is important not to contaminate the suspension, as this may cause further harm to the eye. Also, if more than one eye suspension is used, the drugs should be spaced at least 10 minutes apart.

Notify your doctor if you have any eye surgery that may require discontinuation of this drug.

Who should not take Azopt?
If you have allergies to Azopt and its ingredients, you should not take this medication.

**What should I tell my doctor before
I take the first dose of Azopt?**
Tell your doctor about all prescription, over-the-counter, and herbal medications you are taking before beginning treatment with Azopt. In addition, tell your doctor if you are allergic to sulfur-containing products or have liver or kidney disease.

What is the usual dosage?
The information below is based on the dosage guidelines your doctor uses. Depending on your condition and medical history, your doctor may prescribe a different regimen. Do not change the dosage or stop taking your medication without your doctor's approval.

Adults: The usual dosage is one drop into the affected eye(s) three times a day.

How should I take Azopt?
Shake well before use. Before administration, wash your hands thoroughly. Remove cap and position yourself with your head tilted back.

Gently pull your lower eyelid with your index finger and administer the drops in each eye without touching the eye or eyelid. Upon administration of the drops, blink a few times and remove the excess with a clean tissue. Repeat process for the other eye and wash your hands. If you are using more than one eye drop, space them out by at least 10 minutes. You may wear contact lenses 15 minutes after administration.

What should I avoid while taking Azopt?

Avoid allowing the tip of the applicator to contact your eye, finger, or any other surface in order to avoid contamination of the product. Contamination may lead to serious damage to the eye. In addition, do not take any oral carbonic anhydrase inhibitors such as acetazolamide, dichlorphenamide, and methazolamide, which are generally taken to control seizures or treat mountain sickness.

What are possible food and drug interactions associated with Azopt?

If Azopt is taken with certain other drugs, the effects of either could be increased, decreased, or altered. It is especially important to check with your doctor before combining Azopt with the following: acetazolamide, dichlorphenamide, and methazolamide.

What are the possible side effects of Azopt?

Side effects cannot be anticipated. If any develop or change in intensity, tell your doctor as soon as possible. Only your doctor can determine if it is safe for you to continue taking this drug.

Side effects may include: blurred vision, bitter taste, dry eyes, headache, discharge from the eyes, eye pain

Can I receive Azopt if I am pregnant or breastfeeding?

The effects of Azopt on pregnancy and breastfeeding are unknown. Tell your doctor if you are pregnant, intend on becoming pregnant, or are breastfeeding.

What should I do if I miss a dose of Azopt?

If you miss a dose, take it as soon as you remember. If it is close to the time of your next dose, skip it and resume your scheduled dose. Do not double your dose.

How should I store Azopt?

Store at room temperature and away from children.

AZOR

Generic name: Amlodipine besylate and olmesartan medoxomil

What is Azor?

Azor is used alone or with other medications to treat high blood pressure.

What is the most important information I should know about Azor?

When used during the second and third trimesters of pregnancy, Azor can cause injury and even death to the developing fetus. When pregnancy is detected, Azor should be discontinued as soon as possible.

Who should not take Azor?

You should not use Azor if you are pregnant. This drug should be used with caution if you have low blood pressure or salt depletion, liver or kidney problems, have cardiovascular problems such as obstructive coronary artery disease, aortic stenosis (narrowing of the aortic valve), or congestive heart failure.

What should I tell my doctor before I take the first dose of Azor?

Tell your doctor about all prescription, over-the-counter, and herbal medications you are taking before beginning treatment with Azor. Also talk to your doctor about your complete medical history. This drug should be used with caution if you have low blood pressure or salt depletion, liver or kidney problems, or cardiovascular problems such as obstructive coronary artery, aortic stenosis (narrowing of the aortic valve), or congestive heart failure.

What is the usual dosage?

The information below is based on the dosage guidelines your doctor uses. Depending on your condition and medical history, your doctor may prescribe a different regimen. Do not change the dosage or stop taking your medication without your doctor's approval.

Adults: The usual dosage ranges from 5-10 milligrams (mg) of amlodipine and 20-40 mg of olmesartan a day.

How should I take Azor?

Take Azor exactly as prescribed by your doctor.

What should I avoid while taking Azor?

Avoid getting pregnant while on treatment with Azor.

What are possible food and drug interactions associated with Azor?

No significant drug interactions have been reported. However, you should always check with your doctor before combining Azor with any other medication.

What are the possible side effects of Azor?

Side effects cannot be anticipated. If any develop or change in intensity, tell your doctor as soon as possible. Only your doctor can determine if it is safe for you to continue taking this drug.

Side effects may include: edema (water retention), flushing, heart palpitation

Can I receive Azor if I am pregnant or breastfeeding?

Azor should be avoided during pregnancy and breastfeeding. Talk with your doctor before taking this drug if you are pregnant, plan to become pregnant, or are breastfeeding.

What should I do if I miss a dose of Azor?

Take it as soon as you remember. If it is almost time for your next dose, skip the one you missed and return to your regular schedule. Do not double the dose.

How should I store Azor?

Store at room temperature.

AZULFIDINE

Generic name: Sulfasalazine

What is Azulfidine?

Azulfidine, an anti-inflammatory medicine, is prescribed for the treatment of mild to moderate ulcerative colitis and as an added treatment in severe ulcerative colitis. This medication is also prescribed to decrease severe attacks of ulcerative colitis.

Azulfidine EN-tabs are prescribed for people with ulcerative colitis who cannot take the regular Azulfidine tablet because of symptoms of stomach and intestinal irritation such as nausea and vomiting when taking the first few doses of the drug, or for those in whom a reduction in dosage does not lessen the stomach or intestinal side effects. The EN-tabs are also prescribed for adults and children with rheumatoid arthritis who fail to get relief from salicylates (such as aspirin) or other nonsteroidal anti-inflammatory drugs (such as ibuprofen).

What is the most important information I should know about Azulfidine?

Although ulcerative colitis rarely disappears completely, the risk of recurrence can be substantially reduced by the continued use of this drug.

Who should not take Azulfidine?

If you are sensitive to or have ever had an allergic reaction to Azulfidine, salicylates (aspirin), or other sulfa drugs, you should not take this medication. Make sure your doctor is aware of any drug reactions you have experienced.

Unless you are directed to do so by your doctor, do not take Azulfidine if you have an intestinal or urinary obstruction or if you have porphyria (an inherited disorder involving the substance that gives color to the skin and iris of the eyes).

What should I tell my doctor before I take the first dose of Azulfidine?

Tell your doctor about all prescription, over-the-counter, and herbal medication you are taking before beginning treatment with Azulfidine. Also, talk to your doctor about your complete medical history, especially if you have kidney or liver damage or any blood disease.

What is the usual dosage?

The information below is based on the dosage guidelines your doctor uses. Depending on your condition and medical history, your doctor may prescribe a different regimen. Do not change the dosage or stop taking your medication without your doctor's approval.

Rheumatoid Arthritis
Adults: The usual dose of Azulfidine EN-tabs is 2 grams (g) a day, divided into smaller doses. Your doctor may have you start with a lower dose, then raise the dosage to 3 g after 12 weeks.

Children: The typical recommended daily dosage is 30 to 50 mg per 2.2 pounds of body weight, up to a maximum of 2 g, taken in 2 equally divided doses. To reduce the chance of digestive side effects and other reactions, the doctor will probably start with a fraction of the typical dose and build up to it over a period of weeks.

Ulcerative Colitis
Adults: The usual recommended initial dose of Azulfidine and Azulfidine EN-tabs is 3 to 4 g daily divided into smaller doses (intervals between nighttime doses should not exceed 8 hours). In some cases the initial dosage is set at 1 to 2 g daily to lessen side effects. As therapy continues, the dose is usually reduced to 2 g daily.

Children: The usual recommended initial dose is 40 to 60 milligrams (mg) per 2.2 pounds of body weight in each 24-hour period, divided into 3 to 6 doses. For the longer term, the dose is usually reduced to 30 mg per 2.2 pounds of body weight in each 24-hour period, divided into 4 doses.

How should I take Azulfidine?
Take this medication in evenly spaced, equal doses, as determined by your doctor, preferably after meals or with food to avoid stomach upset. Swallow Azulfidine EN-tabs whole. If you are taking Azulfidine EN-tabs for rheumatoid arthritis, it may take up to 12 weeks for relief to occur.

What should I avoid while taking Azulfidine?
Avoid becoming dehydrated. It is important that you drink plenty of fluids while taking this medication to avoid kidney stones.

What are possible food and drug interactions associated with Azulfidine?
If Azulfidine is taken with certain other drugs, the effects of either could be increased, decreased, or altered. It is especially important to check with your doctor before combining Azulfidine with the following: digoxin, folic acid (a B-complex vitamin), and methotrexate.

What are the possible side effects of Azulfidine?
Side effects cannot be anticipated. If any develop or change in intensity, tell your doctor as soon as possible. Only your doctor can determine if it is safe for you to continue taking this drug.

Side effects may include: abdominal pain, anemia, bluish skin, fever, headache, hives, inflammation of the mouth, itching, lack of appetite, nausea, rash, stomach distress, vomiting

Can I receive Azulfidine if I am pregnant or breastfeeding?
The effects of Azulfidine during pregnancy and breastfeeding are unknown. Tell your doctor immediately if you are pregnant, plan to become pregnant, or are breastfeeding.

What should I do if I miss a dose of Azulfidine?
Take it as soon as you remember. If it is almost time for your next dose, skip the one you missed and go back to your regular schedule. Do not take 2 doses at once.

How should I store Azulfidine?
Store at room temperature.

BACTRIM

Generic name: Sulfamethoxazole and trimethoprim

What is Bactrim?

Bactrim is used to treat infections caused by bacteria in different parts of the body. This drug belongs to a group of medicines called antibiotics. Bactrim works by stopping the growth of the bacteria causing the infection, but it will not work against infections caused by viruses, such as colds and flu.

What is the most important information I should know about Bactrim?

Bactrim may cause liver problems, severe skin rashes, and serious blood problems, such as anemia. Symptoms such as shortness of breath and cough are evidence of an allergic reaction to one of the ingredients in Bactrim. This drug should not be used during pregnancy or nursing, as it may pass through the womb and breast milk.

When taking Bactrim, or any other antibiotic, you may begin to feel better before you finish the complete course of medication. Do not stop taking antibiotics even if you feel better. If you stop taking your medicine, the infection may return, and it may be worse than the first time.

Who should not take Bactrim?

Do not begin treatment with Bactrim if you are allergic to any of its ingredients. Also, do not take it if you have liver or kidney disease, or any type of blood disorder/anemia. You should not receive Bactrim if you are pregnant or breastfeeding.

What should I tell my doctor before I take the first dose of Bactrim?

Tell your doctor about all prescription, over-the-counter, and herbal medications you are taking before beginning treatment with Bactrim. Also, talk to your doctor about your complete medical history, especially if you have liver or kidney disease, or if you are anemic. If you are pregnant, breastfeeding, have asthma, arthritis, or problems urinating, talk to your doctor before treatment begins. Tell your doctor about any drug allergies you may have, such as sulfa allergies.

What is the usual dosage?

The information below is based on the dosage guidelines your doctor uses. Depending on your condition and medical history, your doctor may prescribe a different regimen. Do not change the dosage or stop taking your medication without your doctor's approval.

Adults: The dosage of Bactrim depends on the type of infection you have. Talk to your doctor to get the appropriate dosage of this medication for you.

How should I take Bactrim?
Bactrim tablets should be swallowed whole (or cut in half) with a glass of water. The correct amount of Bactrim oral suspension should be measured before being given by mouth.

What should I avoid while taking Bactrim?
Avoid running out of Bactrim over the weekend or on vacation. Do not stop taking Bactrim or change your dosage without talking to your doctor.

What are possible food and drug interactions associated with Bactrim?
If Bactrim is taken with certain other drugs, the effects of either could be increased, decreased, or altered. It is especially important to check with your doctor before combining Bactrim with the following: amantadine, cyclosporine, digoxin, fluid tablets (diuretics), indomethacin, methotrexate, oral contraceptive pills, phenytoin, procainamide, pyrimethamine, rifampicin, sulphonylureas, and warfarin.

What are the possible side effects of Bactrim?
Side effects cannot be anticipated. If any develop or change in intensity, tell your doctor as soon as possible. Only your doctor can determine if it is safe for you to continue taking this drug.

Side effects may include: abdominal pain, diarrhea, nausea, vomiting

Contact your doctor immediately if you develop cough; dark urine; fever; severe and persistent headache; severe and watery diarrhea; shortness of breath; skin rash; swelling of the face and throat; vaginal infection; white, furry, sore tongue or mouth; or yellowing of your skin/eyes

Can I receive Bactrim if I am pregnant or breastfeeding?
Do not take Bactrim if you are pregnant or nursing. This drug may be passed to your child in the womb, or through your breast milk. Talk to your doctor before beginning treatment if you are pregnant, planning to become pregnant, or are nursing.

What should I do if I miss a dose of Bactrim?
Do not take an extra dose. Wait until the next dose and take your normal dose then. Do not try to make up for the dose that you missed by taking more than one dose at a time.

How should I store Bactrim?
Store at room temperature.

BACTROBAN
Generic name: Mupirocin

What is Bactroban?
Bactroban Cream and Ointment are used to treat bacterial infections that affect the skin. Bactroban Nasal Ointment is used to treat bacterial infections that affect the nostrils and may cause serious infections.

What is the most important information I should know about Bactroban?
If your skin infection does not improve within 3 to 5 days of using Bactroban, or it becomes worse, notify your doctor. Prolonged use of Bactroban, as with other antibacterial products, may result in overgrowth of other microorganisms.

Who should not take Bactroban?
Do not use Bactroban if you are sensitive to or allergic to any of the components of the product.

What should I tell my doctor before I take the first dose of Bactroban?
Tell your doctor about all prescription, over-the-counter, and herbal medications you are taking before beginning treatment with Bactroban, especially if you are using any other prescription or nonprescription medicine that is applied to the same area of skin. Also, talk to your doctor about your complete medical history.

What is the usual dosage?
The information below is based on the dosage guidelines your doctor uses. Depending on your condition and medical history, your doctor may prescribe a different regimen. Do not change the dosage or stop taking your medication without your doctor's approval.

Impetigo
Adults and children ≥2 months: Apply Bactroban Ointment three times a day to the affected area.

Children <2 months: Use and dose must be determined by your doctor.

Secondarily Infected Traumatic Skin Lesions
Adults and children ≥3 months: Apply Bactroban Cream three times a day, for 10 days.

Children <3 months: Use and dose must be determined by your doctor.

For Eradication of Nasal Colonization with Bacterial (Methicillin-Resistant S. aureus) in Adults and Health Workers
Adults and Adolescents ≥12 years: Approximately half the Bactroban Nasal Ointment from the single-use tube (about 0.25 grams) per nostril twice daily for 5 days.

Children <12 years: Safety in children under the age of 12 has not been established.

How should I take Bactroban?
Wash your hands before and after using this medication.

Before applying Bactroban, wash the affected area with soap and water. Dry thoroughly. Apply a small amount of cream or ointment. Cover the area with gauze dressing, if desired.

When using Bactroban nasal ointment, apply approximately half the ointment from the single-use tube directly into 1 nostril and the other half into the other nostril. Throw away the tube after using it. Press the sides of your nose together and gently massage after application to spread the ointment throughout the inside of the nostrils. Do not use Bactroban with other nasal products.

What should I avoid while taking Bactroban?
Avoid contact with the eyes.

Bactroban ointment should not be used in combination with other products that contain polyethylene glycol.

What are possible food and drug interactions associated with Bactroban?
If Bactroban is taken with certain other drugs, the effects of either could be increased, decreased, or altered. Check with your doctor before combining Bactroban with any drug.

What are the possible side effects of Bactroban?
Side effects cannot be anticipated. If any develop or change in intensity, tell your doctor as soon as possible. Only your doctor can determine if it is safe for you to continue taking this drug.

Side effects of Bactroban Cream may include: headache, rash, nausea

Side effects of Bactroban Ointment may include: burning, pain, stinging

Side effects of Bactroban Nasal Ointment may include: headache; runny nose; breathing problems, including congestion, sore throat, and taste changes

Can I receive Bactroban if I am pregnant or breastfeeding?
The effects of Bactroban during pregnancy and breastfeeding are unknown. Talk with your doctor before taking this drug if you are pregnant, plan to become pregnant, or are breastfeeding.

What should I do if I miss a dose of Bactroban?

Apply it as soon as you remember. If it is almost time for your next dose, skip the dose you missed and go back to your regular schedule.

How should I store Bactroban?

Store Bactroban at room temperature and away from heat and light. Keep the medicine from freezing.

Balsalazide disodium *See Colazal, page 317.*

BARACLUDE

Generic name: Entecavir

What is Baraclude?

Baraclude is a prescription medicine used for chronic infection with hepatitis B virus (HBV) in adults who also have active liver damage. Baraclude will not cure HBV. This drug may lower the amount of HBV in the body and its ability to multiply and infect new liver cells; Baraclude may improve the condition of your liver.

What is the most important information I should know about Baraclude?

Your hepatitis B virus infection may get worse or become very serious if you stop taking Baraclude. Take Baraclude exactly as prescribed and do not run out of or stop without consulting your doctor.

Baraclude may cause lactic acidosis, a build up of acid in the blood. This condition is considered an emergency and must be treated in a hospital.

Baraclude may also cause severe liver problems, such as toxicity (hepatotoxicity), liver enlargement (hepatomegaly), and fatty liver (steatosis). Also, this drug may make your hepatitis B infection worse. If you have HIV and use Baraclude at the same time, some of the HIV medications might not work as well.

Who should not take Baraclude?

Do not take Baraclude if you are allergic to any of its ingredients. Also, this drug is not recommended for children less than 16 years of age.

What should I tell my doctor before I take the first dose of Baraclude?

Tell your doctor about all prescription, over-the-counter, and herbal medications you are taking before beginning treatment with Baraclude. Also, talk to your doctor about your complete medical history, especially if you have kidney problems, are pregnant or planning to become pregnant, are breastfeeding, or if you have HIV.

What is the usual dosage?

The information below is based on the dosage guidelines your doctor uses. Depending on your condition and medical history, your doctor may prescribe a different regimen. Do not change the dosage or stop taking your medication without your doctor's approval.

Treatment Naive

Adults and adolescents >16 years: The recommended dose of Baraclude for chronic hepatitis B virus infection in treatment-naive adults and adolescents is 0.5 milligrams (mg) once daily. The oral solution provides 0.5 mg in 10 milliliters (mL) according to the dosing spoon.

With Lamivudine Therapy or Tolerance

Adults and adolescents >16 years: The recommended dose of Baraclude in adults and adolescents with a history of hepatitis B virus in the bloodstream is 1 mg once daily while receiving lamivudine. The oral solution provides 1 mg in 20 mL.

Your dose may be reduced or taken less frequently if you have kidney problems.

How should I take Baraclude?

Take Baraclude once a day on an empty stomach (at least 2 hours after a meal and at least 2 hours before the next meal) to help it work better. To help you remember to take your Baraclude, try to take it at the same time each day.

When using the oral solution, hold the dosing spoon in a vertical position and fill it gradually to the mark indicating the dose prescribed. Rinse the dosing spoon with water after each daily dose.

What should I avoid while taking Baraclude?

Avoid running out of Baraclude. Do not stop treatment without talking to your doctor. Baraclude does not stop you from spreading HBV to others; avoid unsafe sexual practices, sharing needles, and sharing personal items contaminated with blood or body fluids (toothbrushes/razor blades).

What are possible food and drug interactions associated with Baraclude?

If Baraclude is used with certain other drugs, the effects of either could be increased, decreased, or altered. It is especially important to check with your doctor before combining Baraclude with drugs that may affect how your kidneys function.

What are the possible side effects of Baraclude?

Side effects cannot be anticipated. If any develop or change in intensity, tell your doctor as soon as possible. Only your doctor can determine if it is safe for you to continue taking this drug.

Side effects may include: diarrhea, dizziness, headache, indigestion, nausea, sleepiness, tiredness, trouble sleeping, vomiting

Symptoms of lactic acidosis include: cold arms and legs, dizziness, fast or irregular heartbeat, lightheadedness, muscle pain, stomach pain with nausea/vomiting, tiredness, trouble breathing, weakness

Symptoms of liver problems include: dark urine, light-colored stool, loss of appetite, lower stomach pain, nausea, yellow skin/eyes

Can I receive Baraclude if I am pregnant or breastfeeding?
Talk to your doctor if you are pregnant, planning to become pregnant, or are nursing, before you begin treatment with Baraclude. The effects of this drug on pregnancy are unknown, and it may pass into breast milk.

What should I do if I miss a dose of Baraclude?
If you forget to take Baraclude, take it as soon as you remember and then take your next dose at its regular time. If it is almost time for your next dose, skip the missed dose. Do not take two doses at the same time.

How should I store Baraclude?
Store Baraclude tablets in a tightly closed container, at room temperature and away from humidity.

Store Baraclude oral solution in the outer carton at room temperature; protect from light. After opening the oral solution, use it until the expiration date on the bottle and then dispose of unused medicine after the expiration date has passed.

BECLOMETHASONE

What is Beclomethasone?
Beclomethasone is a type of steroid used for respiratory problems, including relief of symptoms of bronchial asthma and hay fever, and to prevent re-growth of nasal polyps following surgical removal.

What is the most important information I should know about Beclomethasone?
Beclomethasone does not quickly open airways and it should not be used for relief of asthma when other bronchodilators and other nonsteroidal drugs prove ineffective. Do not expect immediate relief from beclomethasone and do not take higher doses in an attempt to make it work. It will help control symptoms when taken routinely.

Who should not take Beclomethasone?
Do not use beclomethasone nasal products if you have recently had nasal ulcers, nose surgery, or an injury to the nose.

Do not use if you have ever had an allergic reaction to beclomethasone or to other steroid drugs.

What should I tell my doctor before
I take the first dose of Beclomethasone?

Tell your doctor about all prescription, over-the-counter, and herbal medication you are taking before beginning treatment with beclomethasone. Also, talk to your doctor about your complete medical history, especially if you are using oral steroids, have a condition called adrenal insufficiency, have increased eye pressure due to glaucoma, liver disease, underactive thyroid, if you have tuberculosis, a herpes infection of the eye, or any untreated fungal, bacterial, viral, or parasitic infections.

What is the usual dosage?

The information below is based on the dosage guidelines your doctor uses. Depending on your condition and medical history, your doctor may prescribe a different regimen. Do not change the dosage or stop taking your medication without your doctor's approval.

Beclomethasone Oral Inhalant

Adults and children 12 years of age and older: The usual dose is 2 inhalations taken 3-4 times a day. If you have severe asthma, your doctor may advise you to start with 12-16 inhalations a day. Do not exceed 20 inhalations a day.

For the double-strength inhalation aerosol, the usual dose is 2 inhalations twice a day. If your asthma is severe, your doctor may have you start with 6-8 inhalations a day. The maximum daily dosage is 10 inhalations.

Beclomethasone Nasal Inhalation

The usual dose is 1 inhalation in each nostril 2-4 times a day. A 3-times-daily schedule is often sufficient.

Beclomethasone Nasal Spray

The usual dose is 1 or 2 inhalations in each nostril 2-4 times a day, depending on the brand. For the double strength nasal spray, the dosage is 1 or 2 inhalations in each nostril once a day.

Beclomethasone Oral Inhalant

Children 6 to 12 years of age: The usual recommended dose is 1 or 2 inhalations 3 or 4 times a day. Do not exceed 10 inhalations daily.

For the double-strength inhalation aerosol, the usual dose is 2 inhalations twice daily, with a maximum of 5 inhalations a day.

Beclomethasone Nasal Inhalation

The usual dose is 1 inhalation 3 times a day.

Beclomethasone Nasal Spray

The usual dose is 1 inhalation in each nostril 2 times a day. Some children may need 2 inhalations in each nostril twice daily until adequate control is achieved and then decrease to 1 inhalation in each nostril twice daily. The maximum dose is 2 inhalations in each nostril 2 times a day.

The dosage for the double strength nasal spray is 1 or 2 inhalations in each nostril once a day.

How should I take Beclomethasone?

Beclomethasone is prescribed in an oral inhalant or nasal spray form. Use beclomethasone only as preventive therapy and take only the dose prescribed.

It may take 1 or 2 weeks for the benefits to appear. If there is no improvement in symptoms after 3 weeks, let your doctor know.

Take this drug regularly even if you have no symptoms. Many people need multiple drugs to control asthma symptoms completely, but beclomethasone may allow other drugs to be used in smaller doses.

If you are also using a bronchodilator inhalant, take it before inhaling beclomethasone. This will improve the effect of the second drug. Take the 2 inhalations several minutes apart.

Spray the inhalation aerosol into the air 2 times before you use it for the first time and if you have not used it for more than 7 days. Use it within 6 months.

Before you use the nasal spray, press the pump 6 times or until you see a fine spray. If you don't use it for more than 4 days, reprime the pump by spraying once or until a fine spray appears.

To use the inhaler:

1. Remove the cap and hold inhaler upright.
2. Shake the inhaler thoroughly.
3. Drink some water to moisten the throat.
4. Breathe out as fully as you comfortably can. Hold the inhaler upright and close your lips around the mouthpiece, keeping your tongue below it.
5. While pressing down on the can, inhale deeply and slowly. Hold your breath as long as you can.
6. Take your finger off the can, remove the inhaler, and breathe out gently.
8. Allow at least 1 minute between inhalations.

Gargle and rinse your mouth with water after each dose to help prevent hoarseness and throat irritation. Do not swallow the water after you rinse.

What should I avoid while taking Beclomethasone?

Avoid contact with the eyes. Do not exceed recommended dosage. If you have not had chickenpox or measles, avoid exposure.

What are possible food and drug interactions associated with Beclomethasone?

If beclomethasone is taken with certain other drugs, the effects of either could be increased, decreased, or altered. Always check with your doctor before combining beclomethasone with any other drugs, herbs, or supplements.

What are the possible side effects of Beclomethasone?
Side effects cannot be anticipated. If any develop or change in intensity, tell your doctor as soon as possible. Only your doctor can determine if it is safe for you to continue taking this drug.

Side effects may include: altered or unpleasant taste and smell, headache, lightheadedness, nausea, nose or throat irritation

Less common side effects may include: allergic reactions, breathing problems, mouth or throat infections, nose infection, sore mouth or throat, skin wasting

Notify your doctor if you experience symptoms such as mental disturbances, increased bruising, weight gain, facial swelling (moon face), acne, menstrual irregularities, increased pressure in the eyes, or cataracts.

Can I receive Beclomethasone if I am pregnant or breastfeeding?
The effects of beclomethasone during pregnancy and breastfeeding are unknown. Tell your doctor immediately if you are pregnant, plan to become pregnant, or are breastfeeding.

What should I do if I miss a dose of Beclomethasone?
Take it as soon as you remember and take the remaining doses for that day at evenly spaced intervals. If it is time for your next dose, skip the one you missed. Never take 2 doses at the same time.

How should I store Beclomethasone?
Store at room temperature in a dry place, away from heat and cold. Do not puncture the container, store it near an open flame, or dispose of it in a fire or incinerator.

Benazepril hydrochloride *See Lotensin, page 763.*

Benazepril hydrochloride and hydrochlorothiazide
   See Lotensin HCT, page 765.

Bendroflumethiazide and nadolol *See Corzide, page 345.*

BENICAR
Generic name: Olmesartan medoxomil

What is Benicar?
Benicar is used to treat high blood pressure (hypertension). This drug can be used alone, or in combination with other anti-hypertension drugs.

What is the most important information I should know about Benicar?

When used in the second and third trimester of pregnancy, drugs such as Benicar can cause severe injury or death to the unborn child. If pregnancy is detected while on Benicar you should stop treatment immediately.

Who should not take Benicar?

Do not take Benicar if you are allergic to any of its ingredients.

What should I tell my doctor before I take the first dose of Benicar?

Tell your doctor about all prescription, over-the-counter, and herbal medications you are taking before beginning treatment with Benicar. Also, talk to your doctor about your complete medical history, especially if you are pregnant or planning to become pregnant. Also, talk to your doctor if you have kidney or liver problems, or if you are already on diuretics to treat your blood pressure.

What is the usual dosage?

The information below is based on the dosage guidelines your doctor uses. Depending on your condition and medical history, your doctor may prescribe a different regimen. Do not change the dosage or stop taking your medication without your doctor's approval.

Adults: The usual recommended starting dose of Benicar is 20 milligrams (mg) once daily. Your doctor may give you a higher dose depending on your needs.

How should I take Benicar?

Take Benicar exactly as your doctor tells you. You may take it once a day or twice a day, depending on your dose. You can take Benicar with or without food.

What should I avoid while taking Benicar?

Avoid becoming pregnant while taking Benicar.

Also, if you are taking other medications to treat your blood pressure, avoid standing up quickly from a seated position, as this can make you dizzy.

What are possible food and drug interactions associated with Benicar?

No significant interactions have been reported at this time. However, always tell your doctor about any medicines you take, including over-the-counter drugs, vitamins, and herbal supplements.

What are the possible side effects of Benicar?

Side effects cannot be anticipated. If any develop or change in intensity, tell your doctor as soon as possible. Only your doctor can determine if it is safe for you to continue taking this drug.

Side effects may include: aching muscles, blood in urine, chest pain, diarrhea, dizziness, flu symptoms, headache, irregular heartbeat, nasal infection, rash, sinus infection, sore throat, upset stomach

Can I receive Benicar if I am pregnant or breastfeeding?

Do not take Benicar if you are pregnant or planning to become pregnant. In the first trimester, the effects of this drug are on the unborn child unknown. During the second and third trimesters, Benicar may cause severe injury or death to the unborn baby. If pregnancy is detected while you are on this drug, treatment should be immediately stopped.

What should I do if I miss a dose of Benicar?

If you miss a dose, take it as soon as you remember. If you are taking Benicar once a day and it is within twelve hours of your next dose, skip the missed dose. If you are taking Benicar twice a day and you are within six hours of your next dose, skip the missed dose. Do not double your dose.

How should I store Benicar?

Store at room temperature.

BENICAR HCT

Generic name: Olmesartan medoxomil and hydrochlorothiazide

What is Benicar HCT?

Benicar HCT is a combination drug indicated for the treatment of high blood pressure. This combination drug is not intended to be used as initial therapy.

What is the most important information I should know about Benicar HCT?

The use of this drug during the second or third trimesters of pregnancy has been shown to cause injury and/or death to the baby. After consulting your doctor, it is important to discontinue treatment with this drug if you are or intend on becoming pregnant.

Lightheadedness may occur when you first start Benicar HCT therapy. Diarrhea, vomiting, dehydration, and excessive heat exposure and sweating may cause your blood pressure to drop rapidly and may cause dizziness and fainting. If you experience lightheadedness or a brief loss of consciousness, discontinue this medication until you notify your doctor.

Who should not take Benicar HCT?
If you are unable to produce urine (anuria) or have had a previous allergy to sulfur-containing drugs, you should not take this medication.

What should I tell my doctor before I take the first dose of Benicar HCT?
Tell your doctor about all prescription, over-the-counter, and herbal medications you are taking before beginning treatment with Benicar. Also, talk to your doctor about your complete medical history, especially if you are pregnant or plan to become pregnant.

What is the usual dosage?
The information below is based on the dosage guidelines your doctor uses. Depending on your condition and medical history, your doctor may prescribe a different regimen. Do not change the dosage or stop taking your medication without your doctor's approval.

Adults: The usual dosage for the treatment of high blood pressure is 1 tablet (20 milligrams [mg] olmesartan medoxomil/12.5 mg hydrochlorothiazide) once daily. Your doctor may give you a higher dose if your blood pressure is not stabilized.

How should I take Benicar HCT?
Take one tablet with or without food as directed.

What should I avoid while taking Benicar HCT?
Avoid becoming pregnant and nursing while taking Benicar HCT. You should avoid taking Benicar HCT if you are currently taking lithium. It is important to avoid dehydration or excessive exposure to heat and sweating. Alcohol use may increase the effects of Benicar HCT and should therefore be avoided unless you have discussed its use with your doctor.

What are possible food and drug interactions associated with Benicar HCT?
If Benicar HCT is taken with certain other drugs, the effects of either could be increased, decreased, or altered. It is especially important to check with your doctor before combining Benicar HCT with the following: alcohol; antidiabetic drugs such as insulin, metformin; barbiturates such as phenobarbital, pentobarbital; cholestyramine and colestipol resins; corticosteroids; lithium; narcotics such as morphine, oxycontin; pressor amines such as norepinephrine; skeletal muscle relaxants such as tubocurarine; and nonsteroidal anti-inflammatory drugs such as ibuprofen, naproxen.

What are the possible side effects of Benicar HCT?

Side effects cannot be anticipated. If any develop or change in intensity, tell your doctor as soon as possible. Only your doctor can determine if it is safe for you to continue taking this drug.

Side effects may include: nausea, dizziness, upper respiratory tract infection, urinary tract infection, rash, headache

Can I receive Benicar HCT if I am pregnant or breastfeeding?

The use of Benicar HCT is not recommended in women who are or may become pregnant. If you are a woman of child-bearing age, it is advisable to use contraception while taking Benicar HCT due to the potential harm to the fetus. If you are pregnant, discontinue treatment and consult with your doctor.

What should I do if I miss a dose of Benicar HCT?

If you miss a dose, take it as soon as you remember. If it is close to the time of your next dose, skip it and resume your scheduled dose. Do not double your dose.

How should I store Benicar HCT?

Store at room temperature.

BENTYL

Generic name: Dicyclomine hydrochloride

What is Bentyl?

Bentyl is used to treat functional bowel/irritable bowel syndrome (abdominal pain accompanied by diarrhea and constipation associated with stress).

What is the most important information I should know about Bentyl?

Using this drug in hot weather can result in heat prostration (fever and heat stroke due to decreased sweating). If symptoms of heat prostration occur, stop taking the drug and notify your doctor immediately.

Who should not take Bentyl?

Do not take Bentyl if you are allergic to it or any of its ingredients. Do not take this drug if you have a blockage of the urinary tract, stomach, or intestines; severe ulcerative colitis (inflammatory disease of the large intestine); reflux esophagitis (inflammation of the esophagus usually caused by the backflow of acid stomach contents); glaucoma; or myasthenia gravis (a disease characterized by long-lasting fatigue and muscle weakness).

Do not use Bentyl in infants less than 6 months of age.

What should I tell my doctor before I take the first dose of Bentyl?

Tell your doctor about all prescription, over-the-counter, and herbal medications you are taking before beginning treatment with Bentyl. Also, talk to your doctor about your complete medical history, especially if you have autonomic neuropathy (a nerve disorder); liver or kidney disease; hyperthyroidism; high blood pressure; coronary heart disease; congestive heart failure; rapid, irregular heartbeat; hiatal hernia (protrusion of part of the stomach through the diaphragm); or enlargement of the prostate gland. Tell your doctor if you are sensitive to anticholinergic drugs or if you have had an ileostomy or colostomy performed.

What is the usual dosage?

The information below is based on the dosage guidelines your doctor uses. Depending on your condition and medical history, your doctor may prescribe a different regimen. Do not change the dosage or stop taking your medication without your doctor's approval.

Adults: The usual dosage is 160 milligrams (mg) per day, divided into 4 equal doses. Since this dose is associated with a significant incidence of side effects, your doctor may recommend a starting dose of 80 mg per day, divided into 4 equal doses. If no side effects occur, your doctor will then increase the dose.

How should I take Bentyl?

Take Bentyl exactly as your doctor prescribes. The safety of Bentyl for doses above 80 mg daily, taken for periods longer than two weeks, is not known. If Bentyl is not effective within two weeks or side effects require doses below 80 mg per day, your doctor should discontinue the drug.

What should I avoid while taking Bentyl?

Bentyl may produce drowsiness or blurred vision. Avoid activities that require mental alertness, such as operating a motor vehicle or other machinery, or performing hazardous work while taking this drug.

What are possible food and drug interactions associated with Bentyl?

If Bentyl is taken with certain other drugs, the effects of either could be increased, decreased, or altered. It is especially important to check with your doctor before combining Bentyl with the following: amantadine, antiarrhythmic agents, antiglaucoma drugs, antihistamines, antipsychotic drugs, benzodiazepines, corticosteroids, MAO inhibitors, narcotic analgesics, nitrates and nitrites, sympathomimetic agents, tricyclic antidepressants, and other drugs with anticholinergic activity.

What are the possible side effects of Bentyl?

Side effects cannot be anticipated. If any develop or change in intensity, tell your doctor as soon as possible. Only your doctor can determine if it is safe for you to continue taking this drug.

Side effects may include: blurred vision, dizziness, drowsiness, dry mouth, light-headedness, nausea, nervousness, weakness

Can I receive Bentyl if I am pregnant or breastfeeding?

The effects of Bentyl during pregnancy have not been adequately studied. If you are pregnant or plan to become pregnant, notify your doctor. Do not use Bentyl if you are breastfeeding.

What should I do if I miss a dose of Bentyl?

If you miss a dose of Bentyl, take it as soon as you remember. If it is almost time for your next dose, skip the one you missed and go back to your regular schedule. Do not take two doses at once.

How should I store Bentyl?

Store at room temperature, preferably below 86°F. Keep tablets out of direct sunlight. Keep syrup away from excessive heat.

BENZACLIN

Generic name: Benzoyl peroxide and clindamycin phosphate

What is BenzaClin?

BenzaClin is used for the topical treatment of acne.

What is the most important information I should know about BenzaClin?

Although BenzaClin is applied only to the skin, some of this medication can be absorbed into the bloodstream. Once in the system, it can cause severe colitis (inflammation of the colon), which may result in death. Contact your doctor immediately if you experience colitis symptoms, including severe or bloody diarrhea and abdominal cramps.

Who should not take BenzaClin?

Do not use BenzaClin if you are allergic to any of its components or to lincomycin. Also, avoid BenzaClin if you have a history of colitis or regional enteritis (inflammation of the small intestine).

What should I tell my doctor before I take the first dose of BenzaClin?

Tell your doctor about all prescription, over-the-counter, and herbal medications you are taking before beginning treatment BenzaClin, especially if you are using any other topical acne therapy. Also, talk to your doctor about your complete medical history.

What is the usual dosage?
The information below is based on the dosage guidelines your doctor uses. Depending on your condition and medical history, your doctor may prescribe a different regimen. Do not change the dosage or stop taking your medication without your doctor's approval.

Adults and children >12 years: Apply BenzaClin twice a day, once in the morning and once in the evening, or as directed by your doctor.

The safety and effectiveness of BenzaClin have not been established in children less than 12 years of age.

How should I take BenzaClin?
Apply BenzaClin twice daily, in the morning and evening or as directed by your doctor to the affected area. Before applying BenzaClin, gently wash the affected skin, rinse with warm water, and pat dry.

Evenly spread a small amount of BenzaClin with your fingertips over the affected areas. Do not use BenzaClin more often than recommended by your doctor. Excessive use can make your skin dry or irritated.

What should I avoid while taking BenzaClin?
BenzaClin is for external use only. Avoid contact with eyes and all mucous membranes. Avoid or minimize exposure to natural or artificial sunlight (tanning beds or UVA/UVB treatment). To avoid sunburns, apply a sunscreen with SPF 15 or higher. BenzaClin may bleach hair or colored fabric; avoid getting it on your clothes.

What are possible food and drug interactions associated with BenzaClin?
If BenzaClin is taken with certain other drugs, the effects of either could be increased, decreased, or altered. It is especially important to check with your doctor before combining BenzaClin with medications containing erythromycin. Use other topical acne therapy only when directed to by your doctor, since irritation may occur.

What are the possible side effects of BenzaClin?
Side effects cannot be anticipated. If any develop or change in intensity, tell your doctor as soon as possible. Only your doctor can determine if it is safe for you to continue taking this drug.

Side effects may include: dry skin, skin irritation, sunburn

Can I receive BenzaClin if I am pregnant or breastfeeding?
The effects of BenzaClin during pregnancy and breastfeeding are unknown. Talk with your doctor before taking this drug if you are pregnant

or plan to become pregnant. Clindamycin has been reported to appear in breast milk. Because of the potential for serious adverse reactions in nursing infants, a decision should be made whether to discontinue nursing or to discontinue the drug.

What should I do if I miss a dose of BenzaClin?
If you miss a dose of BenzaClin, apply the missed dose as soon as you remember it. However, if it is almost time for your next dose, skip the dose you missed and return to your regular dosing schedule. Do not double the dose.

How should I store BenzaClin?
Store BenzaClin in a tightly closed container and at room temperature. Do not freeze.

BENZAMYCIN PAK
Generic name: Benzoyl peroxide and erythromycin

What is Benzamycin Pak?
Benzamycin Pak is used for the topical treatment of acne.

What is the most important information I should know about Benzamycin Pak?
If you experience excessive irritation stop using Benzamycin Pak and notify your doctor.

Benzamycin Pak may stain clothing and may bleach hair or colored fabric.

Who should not take Benzamycin Pak?
Do not take Benzamycin Pak if you are allergic to any of its components.

What should I tell my doctor before I take the first dose of Benzamycin Pak?
Tell your doctor about all prescription, over-the-counter, and herbal medications you are taking before beginning treatment with Benzamycin Pak. Also, talk to your doctor about your complete medical history, especially if you are using other topical acne therapy.

What is the usual dosage?
The information below is based on the dosage guidelines your doctor uses. Depending on your condition and medical history, your doctor may prescribe a different regimen. Do not change the dosage or stop taking your medication without your doctor's approval.

Adults and children >12 years: Apply Benzamycin Pak twice a day, once in the morning and once in the evening, or as directed by your doctor.

The safety and effectiveness of Benzamycin Pak have not been established in children less than 12 years of age.

How should I take Benzamycin Pak?

Apply Benzamycin Pak twice daily, morning and evening, or as directed by your physician to the affected area. Before applying Benzamycin Pak, thoroughly wash the affected skin with soap and warm water, rinse well, and pat dry.

Benzamycin Pak is dispensed in one foil pouch which contains medication in 2 separated compartments. The contents of each pouch must be mixed thoroughly in the palm of your hand prior to application. Apply the product immediately after mixing and wash your hands.

Carefully read and review instructions for use before using Benzamycin Pak.

What should I avoid while taking Benzamycin Pak?

Benzamycin Pak is for external use only. Avoid contact with eyes and all mucous membranes. Avoid or minimize exposure to natural or artificial sunlight (tanning beds or UVA/UVB treatment). Benzamycin may bleach hair or colored fabric; avoid getting it on your clothes.

What are possible food and drug interactions associated with Benzamycin Pak?

If Benzamycin Pak is taken with certain other drugs, the effects of either could be increased, decreased, or altered. It is especially important to check with your doctor before combining Benzamycin Pak with any other prescription or over-the-counter acne remedy.

What are the possible side effects of Benzamycin Pak?

Side effects cannot be anticipated. If any develop or change in intensity, tell your doctor as soon as possible. Only your doctor can determine if it is safe for you to continue taking this drug.

Side effects may include: dry skin and swelling

Can I receive Benzamycin Pak if I am pregnant or breastfeeding?

The effects of Benzamycin Pak during pregnancy and breastfeeding are unknown. It is not known whether the ingredients of Benzamycin Pak appear in breast milk after topical use. However, erythromycin is excreted in human milk if it is taken orally or by injection. Talk with your doctor before taking this drug if you are pregnant, plan to become pregnant, or are breastfeeding.

What should I do if I miss a dose of Benzamycin Pak?
If you miss a dose of Benzamycin Pak, apply the missed dose as soon as you remember it. However, if it is almost time for your next dose, skip the dose you missed and return to your regular dosing schedule. Do not double the dose.

How should I store Benzamycin Pak?
Store at room temperature away from heat and any open flame. Keep out of the reach of children.

Benzonatate See Tessalon, page 1285.

Benzoyl peroxide (4% and 8%) See Brevoxyl, page 226.

Benzoyl peroxide and clindamycin phosphate
See BenzaClin, page 208.

Benzoyl peroxide and erythromycin See Benzamycin Pak, page 210.

Betamethasone dipropionate See Diprolene, page 430.

Betaxolol hydrochloride See Betoptic S, page 214.

BETIMOL
Generic name: Timolol maleate (ophthalmic)

What is Betimol?
Betimol is an ophthalmic solution indicated for the treatment of increased inner eye pressure for those patients with glaucoma (open-angle) and ocular hypertension.

What is the most important information I should know about Betimol?
Betimol is an eye solution that should be used with care. It is important not to contaminate the solution, as that may cause further harm to the eye. Also, if you are using more than one eye solution, the drugs should be spaced at least ten minutes apart.

Notify your doctor if you have any eye surgery that may require discontinuation of this drug.

Who should not take Betimol?
Do not take this medication if you have heart failure, cardiogenic shock, sinus bradycardia, heart block (2nd or 3rd degree atrioventricular block), bronchial asthma, or chronic obstructive pulmonary disease (COPD).

What should I tell my doctor before I take the first dose of Betimol?

Tell your doctor about all prescription, over-the-counter, and herbal medications you are taking before beginning treatment with Betimol. Also, talk to your doctor about your complete medical history, especially if you are pregnant or plan to become pregnant. It is important to notify the doctor of previous eye infections, history of glaucoma, and diabetes.

What is the usual dosage?

The information below is based on the dosage guidelines your doctor uses. Depending on your condition and medical history, your doctor may prescribe a different regimen. Do not change the dosage or stop taking your medication without your doctor's approval.

Adults: The usual starting dose is one drop of Betimol (0.25%) in the affected eye twice daily. Your doctor may change the dose to one drop of Betimol (0.5%) in the affected eye twice daily if necessary.

How should I take Betimol?

Shake well before use. Before administration, wash your hands thoroughly. Remove cap and position yourself with your head tilted back. Gently pull your lower eyelid with your index finger and administer the drops in each eye without touching the eye or eyelid. Upon administration of the drops, blink a few times and remove the excess with a clean tissue. Repeat process for the other eye and wash your hands. If more than one ophthalmic drug is being used the drugs need to be spaced out by at least ten minutes. You may wear contact lenses five minutes after administration.

What should I avoid while taking Betimol?

Avoid allowing the tip of the applicator to contact the eye, finger, or any other surface in order to avoid contamination of the product. Contamination may lead to serious damage to your eye.

What are possible food and drug interactions associated with Betimol?

If Betimol is taken with certain other drugs, the effects of either could be increased, decreased, or altered. It is especially important to check with your doctor before combining Betimol with the following: alpha blockers such as prazosin, terazosin; anti-diabetes drugs such as insulin, metformin; beta blockers such as metoprolol; beta agonists such as albuterol; calcium channel blockers such as verapamil, diltiazem; digoxin; and NSAIDs such as ibuprofen, indomethacin, and naproxen.

What are the possible side effects of Betimol?

Side effects cannot be anticipated. If any develop or change in intensity, tell your doctor as soon as possible. Only your doctor can determine if it is safe for you to continue taking this drug.

Side effects may include: blurred vision, bitter taste, dry eyes, headache, discharge from the eyes, eye pain, burning of the eyes, light sensitivity, hypertension, dizziness

Can I receive Betimol if I am pregnant or breastfeeding?

The effects of Betimol on pregnancy are unknown. Tell your doctor if you are pregnant or intend on being pregnant.

The effects of Betimol during breastfeeding show potential harm to the baby. The use of Betimol should be discontinued and you should consult with your doctor.

What should I do if I miss a dose of Betimol?

If you miss a dose, take it as soon as you remember. If it is close to the time of your next dose, skip it and resume your scheduled dose. Do not double your dose.

How should I store Betimol?

Store at room temperature, away from children, and protect from light.

BETOPTIC S

Generic name: Betaxolol hydrochloride

What is Betoptic S?

Betoptic S lowers internal eye pressure and is used to treat open-angle glaucoma (high fluid pressure in the eye).

What is the most important information I should know about Betoptic S?

Although Betoptic S is applied to the eye, it may be absorbed into the bloodstream. Make sure your doctor is aware if you have diabetes, asthma, chronic obstructive pulmonary disease (COPD) or other respiratory disease, overactive thyroid, or decreased heart function.

Who should not take Betoptic S?

Do not use Betoptic S if you have 2nd or 3rd degree heart block, heart failure, cardiogenic shock (when the heart is too damaged to supply sufficient blood to the body), or slow heartbeat (sinus bradycardia). Do not use Betoptic S if you are sensitive or allergic to it.

What should I tell my doctor before I take the first dose of Betoptic S?

Tell your doctor about all prescription, over-the-counter, and herbal medications you are taking before beginning treatment with Betoptic S, especially if you are taking an oral beta-andrenergic blocking drug, catecholamine-depleting drugs such as reserpine, or psychotropic drugs.

Also, talk to your doctor about your complete medical history, especially if you have asthma or other lung disorders, diabetes, heart disease, thyroid disease, neuromuscular disorders, if you plan to undergo general anesthesia, or if you have a history of anaphylactic reaction (an extreme and potentially life-threatening allergic reaction).

What is the usual dosage?

The information below is based on the dosage guidelines your doctor uses. Depending on your condition and medical history, your doctor may prescribe a different regimen. Do not change the dosage or stop taking your medication without your doctor's approval.

Adults: The usual recommended dose is 1 to 2 drops in the affected eye(s) twice daily.

How should I take Betoptic S?

Use this medication exactly as prescribed. Shake Betoptic S well before each dose. Do not use with contact lenses in the eyes.

Betopic S may be used alone or in combination with other medications to control your internal eye pressure.

Administer Betoptic as follows: 1. Wash your hands thoroughly. 2. Gently pull your lower eyelid down to form a pocket between your eye and eyelid. 3. Hold the bottle on the bridge of your nose or on your forehead. 4. Do not touch the applicator tip to any surface, including your eye. 5. Tilt your head back and squeeze Betoptic into your eye. 6. Close your eyes gently. Keep your eyes closed for 1 to 2 minutes. 7. Wait for 5 to 10 minutes before using any other eyedrops. 8. Do not rinse the dropper.

What should I avoid while taking Betoptic S?

Do not touch dropper tip to any surface, as this may contaminate the solution.

What are possible food and drug interactions associated with Betoptic S?

If Betoptic S is taken with certain other drugs, the effects of either could be increased, decreased, or altered. It is especially important to check with your doctor before combining Betoptic S with the following: andrenergic psychotropic drugs; catecholamine-depleting drugs such as reserpine; MAO inhibitors such as phenelzine; and oral beta-blockers such as propranolol or atenolol.

What are the possible side effects of Betoptic S?

Side effects cannot be anticipated. If any develop or change in intensity, tell your doctor as soon as possible. Only your doctor can determine if it is safe for you to continue taking this drug.

Side effects may include: temporary eye discomfort, including burning, dry eyes, inflammation, itching, pain

Can I receive Betoptic S if I am pregnant or breastfeeding?

The effects of Betoptic S during pregnancy and breastfeeding are unknown. Betoptic S should be used during pregnancy only if the potential benefit justifies the potential risk to the fetus. Use Betoptic S with caution if you are breastfeeding.

What should I do if I miss a dose of Betoptic S?

Take Betoptic S as soon as you remember. If it is almost time for your next dose, skip the one you missed and go back to your regular schedule. Do not use 2 doses at once.

How should I store Betoptic S?

Store at room temperature.

BIAXIN

Generic name: Clarithromycin

What is Biaxin?

Biaxin is an antibiotic used to treat a variety of bacterial infections, including strep throat, pneumonia, sinusitis, tonsillitis, acute middle ear infections, and acute flare-ups of chronic bronchitis in adults.

Biaxin is also used to treat skin infections and when combined with lansoprazole or omeprazole and amoxicillin, duodenal ulcers caused by *H. pylori* bacteria.

Biaxin XL is the extended-release tablet form and is used for sinus inflammation, bronchitis flare-ups, and community-acquired pneumonia (see separate Biaxin XL entry).

In children, Biaxin tablets and granules are used to treat bacterial infections including sore throat and tonsillitis, pneumonia, acute middle ear infections, and skin infections.

What is the most important information I should know about Biaxin?

You should not use Biaxin if you are pregnant, except in clinical circumstances where no alternative therapy is appropriate.

Colitis has been reported with nearly all antibacterial agents, including Biaxin, and may range in severity from mild to life threatening.

Biaxin should be used only to treat or prevent infections that are proven or strongly suspected to be caused by bacteria.

Skipping doses or not completing the full course of therapy may decrease the drug's effectiveness and increase the likelihood that drug-resistant bacteria will develop.

Who should not take Biaxin?

Do not use Biaxin if you are allergic to clarithromycin, erythromycin, or any of the macrolide antibiotics. Do not take Biaxin if you are also taking astemizole, cisapride, dihydroergotamine, ergotamine, pimozide, or terfenadine.

What should I tell my doctor before I take the first dose of Biaxin?

Tell your doctor about all prescription, over-the-counter, and herbal medication you are taking before beginning treatment with Biaxin. Also, talk to your doctor about your complete medical history, especially if you have severe kidney disease or if you are pregnant or are planning on becoming pregnant.

What is the usual dosage?

The information below is based on the dosage guidelines your doctor uses. Depending on your condition and medical history, your doctor may prescribe a different regimen. Do not change the dosage or stop taking your medication without your doctor's approval.

The usual dosage for Biaxin Filmtabs (tablets) and Biaxin Granules (for oral suspension) is:

Respiratory, Ear, and Skin Infections
Adults: Your doctor will carefully tailor your individual dosage of Biaxin depending upon the type of infection and organism causing it.

The usual dose varies from 250-500 milligrams (mg) every 12 hours for 7 or 14 days.

Children: The usual recommended daily dosage, based on the child's weight, is 15 mg/kg/day, taken in divided doses, for 10 days. Biaxin is not recommended for children under 6 months of age.

Duodenal Ulcers
Adults: You can expect one of the following treatment regimens:

500 mg of Biaxin, 30 mg of omeprazole, and 1 gram (g) amoxicillin every 12 hours for 10 or 14 days.

500 mg of Biaxin, 20 mg of lansoprazole, and 1 g amoxicillin every 12 hours for 10 days. Some patients need to continue taking 20 mg of lansoprazole on a once-daily basis for an additional 18 days.

500 mg of Biaxin every 8 hours plus 40 mg of lansoprazole every

morning for 14 days. Some patients need to continue taking lansoprazole at a reduced dosage of 20 mg once a day for an additional 14 days.

500 mg of Biaxin every 8 or 12 hours plus 400 mg of ranitidine bismuth citrate every 12 hours for 14 days. Some patients need to continue taking 400 mg of ranitidine bismuth citrate every 12 hours for an additional 14 days.

Mycobacterium Avium Infections
Adults: For prevention or treatment, the recommended dose is 500 mg twice a day.

Children: For prevention or treatment, the recommended dose, based on the child's weight, is 7.5 mg/kg/day, up to 500 mg twice a day.

How should I take Biaxin?
Biaxin tablets and Biaxin granules for oral suspension can be taken with or without food.

What should I avoid while taking Biaxin?
Avoid missing any doses. Do not take Biaxin if you are also taking astemizole, cisapride, dihydroergotamine, ergotamine, pimozide, or terfenadine.

What are possible food and drug interactions associated with Biaxin?
If Biaxin is taken with certain other drugs, the effects of either could be increased, decreased, or altered. It is especially important to check with your doctor before combining Biaxin with the following: alfentanil, alprazolam, blood-thinning drugs (oral) such as warfarin, bromocriptine, carbamazepine, cholesterol-lowering drugs such as lovastatin or simvastatin, cilostazol, colchicines, cyclosporine, didanosine, digoxin, disopyramide, ergot-based migraine drugs, fluconazole, hexobarbital, methylprednisolone, midazolam, omeprazole, phenytoin, pimozide, quinidine, ranitidine, rifabutin, ritonavir, sildenafil, tacrolimus, terfenadine, theophylline, triazolam, valproate, zidovudine.

In addition, tell your doctor if you take medicines for any of the following: your immune system, cholesterol, infections, heart failure, seizures, diabetes, heartburn, or stomach ulcers.

What are the possible side effects of Biaxin?
Side effects cannot be anticipated. If any develop or change in intensity, tell your doctor as soon as possible. Only your doctor can determine if it is safe for you to continue taking this drug.

Side effects in adults may include: abdominal pain or discomfort, abnormal taste, diarrhea, headache, indigestion, nausea, rash

Side effects in children may include: abdominal pain, diarrhea, headache, rash, vomiting

Can I receive Biaxin if I am pregnant or breastfeeding?
Biaxin should not be used in pregnant women, except in clinical circumstances where no alternative therapy is appropriate.

The effects of Biaxin during pregnancy and breastfeeding are unknown. Caution should be exercised when Biaxin is administered to nursing women. Talk with your doctor before taking this drug if you are pregnant, plan to become pregnant, or are breastfeeding.

What should I do if I miss a dose of Biaxin?
If you miss a dose, take it as soon as you remember. If it is almost time for your next dose, take the dose you missed and take the next dose 5 to 6 hours later, then go back to your regular schedule.

How should I store Biaxin?
Store Biaxin at room temperature in a tightly closed container, away from light. Do not refrigerate the suspension.

BIAXIN XL
Generic name: Clarithromycin extended-release tablets

What is Biaxin XL?
Biaxin XL is an antibiotic indicated for the treatment of mild to moderate infections caused by specific organisms. In particular, it is used to treat acute maxillary sinusitis, acute bacterial exacerbation of chronic bronchitis, and community-acquired pneumonia.

What is the most important information I should know about Biaxin XL?
It is important that Biaxin XL is only used to treat bacterial infections. It does not help in the treatment of viral or fungal infections. In addition, it is imperative that you finish the medication as directed, even if you think you feel better. Due to potential harm to the baby, it is also important to note that Biaxin XL should only be used by pregnant women when other alternatives have failed.

Who should not take Biaxin XL?
Do not use Biaxin XL if you have had a previous allergic response to erythromycin or any of the macrolide antibiotics. Also, due to harmful effects when administered concomitantly, do not take Biaxin XL if you are on cisapride, pimozide, astemizole, or terfenadine.

What should I tell my doctor before I take the first dose of Biaxin XL?

Tell your doctor about all prescription, over-the-counter, and herbal medications you are taking before beginning treatment with Biaxin XL. Also, talk to your doctor about your complete medical history, especially if you are pregnant or plan to become pregnant.

What is the usual dosage?

The information below is based on the dosage guidelines your doctor uses. Depending on your condition and medical history, your doctor may prescribe a different regimen. Do not change the dosage or stop taking your medication without your doctor's approval.

Acute Maxillary Sinusitis (H. influenzae, M.catarrhalis, S. pneumoniae)
Adults: Take one 500-milligram (mg) tablet twice daily for 14 days.

Acute Exacerbation of Chronic Bronchitis (H. influenzae, H. parainfluenzae, M.catarrhalis, S. pneumoniae)
Adults: Take one 500-mg tablet twice daily for 7-14 days, as directed.

Community-Acquired Pneumonia (H. influenzae, H. parainfluenzae, M. catarrhalis, S. pneumoniae, C. pneumoniae, M. pneumoniae)
Adults: Take one 500-mg tablet twice daily for 7-14 days, as directed.

Biaxin XL formulation is not appropriate for children less than 12 years old.

How should I take Biaxin XL?

Take Biaxin XL tablets with food. Biaxin XL tablets should be swallowed whole and not chewed, crushed, or cut.

What should I avoid while taking Biaxin XL?

It is important to avoid using certain medications (see list below) with Biaxin XL. Avoid becoming pregnant while on Biaxin XL therapy. Also, avoid using Biaxin XL unless you have been properly diagnosed by your doctor with a bacterial infection that is treatable with Biaxin XL.

What are possible food and drug interactions associated with Biaxin XL?

If Biaxin XL is taken with certain other drugs, the effects of either could be increased, decreased, or altered. It is especially important to check with your doctor before combining Biaxin XL with the following: alprazolam; astemizole; bepridil; carbamazepine; cisapride; colchicine; digoxin; dihydroergotamine; eplerenone; ergoloid mesylates; ergonovine; ergotamine; HIV medications such as zidovudine, didanosine, and ritonavir; methylergonovine; methysergide; omeprazole; pimozide; ranolazine; sildenafil;

statins such as lovastatin, simvastatin; terfenadine; theophylline; thioridazine; triazolam; and ziprasidone.

What are the possible side effects of Biaxin XL?
Side effects cannot be anticipated. If any develop or change in intensity, tell your doctor as soon as possible. Only your doctor can determine if it is safe for you to continue taking this drug.

Side effects may include: diarrhea, abnormal taste, nausea, headache

Can I receive Biaxin XL if I am pregnant or breastfeeding?
The use of Biaxin XL is not recommended in women who are or may become pregnant. Biaxin XL is only used in pregnant women if and when other alternatives have failed. Talk to your doctor about whether the benefits outweigh the risks of taking Biaxin XL if you are pregnant.

What should I do if I miss a dose of Biaxin XL?
If you miss a dose, take it as soon as you remember. If it is close to the time of your next dose, skip it and resume your scheduled dose. Do not double your dose.

How should I store Biaxin XL?
Store at room temperature.

BIDIL
Generic name: Hydralazine hydrochloride and
*   isosorbide dinitrate*

What is BiDil?
BiDil is used with other medications in the treatment of heart failure in African American patients.

What is the most important information I should know about BiDil?
BiDil may cause severe low blood pressure, possibly marked by dizziness or fainting, especially when you stand or sit up quickly. If you already have low blood pressure, use BiDil with caution. Not drinking enough fluids or losing too much fluid through perspiration or vomiting may increase your likelihood of developing low blood pressure. If you faint while taking BiDil, discontinue the drug and contact your doctor.

Use caution when taking erectile dysfunction drugs because BiDil can cause an unsafe drop in blood pressure.

BiDil can cause headaches, especially when first beginning treatment. BiDil can also cause an increase in heart rate, resulting in decreased blood flow to the heart and chest pain (angina).

BiDil may be associated with lightheadedness upon standing, especially after rising from a seated position.

Who should not take BiDil?
Do not use BiDil if you are allergic to any component of this medication or if you have a known allergy to organic nitrates.

The safety and effectiveness of BiDil have not been determined in individuals younger than age 18.

What should I tell my doctor before I take the first dose of BiDil?
Tell your doctor about all prescription, over-the-counter, and herbal medication you are taking before beginning treatment with BiDil, especially if you are taking blood pressure lowering medication, or erectile dysfunction or pulmonary hypertension drugs. Also, talk to your doctor about your complete medical history, especially if you suffer from low blood pressure, are dehydrated, if you have recently had a heart attack, if you have an enlarged heart, or if you suffer chest pain due to an enlarged heart.

What is the usual dosage?
The information below is based on the dosage guidelines your doctor uses. Depending on your condition and medical history, your doctor may prescribe a different regimen. Do not change the dosage or stop taking your medication without your doctor's approval.

The initial dose of BiDil is 1 tablet 3 times a day. The maximum dose is 2 tablets 3 times a day.

How should I take BiDil?
Take your dose of BiDil exactly as directed by your doctor. Tablets may be cut in half and taken 3 times a day if intolerable side effects occur, but the dose should be increased to the recommended dose once side effects subside.

What should I avoid while taking BiDil?
Get up from bed or from a seated position slowly to avoid lightheadedness or fainting on standing. Drink plenty of fluids and avoid excessive fluid loss from sweating, diarrhea, or vomiting. Avoid using BiDil with alcohol.

What are possible food and drug interactions associated with BiDil?
If BiDil is taken with certain other drugs, the effects of either could be increased, decreased, or altered. It is especially important to check with your doctor before combining BiDil with the following: drugs that can lower blood pressure, MAO inhibitors such as phenelzine or tranylcypro-

mine, and vasodilator drugs for erectile dysfunction, such as sildenafil, tadalafil, and vardenafil.

What are the possible side effects of BiDil?

Side effects cannot be anticipated. If any develop or change in intensity, tell your doctor as soon as possible. Only your doctor can determine if it is safe for you to continue taking this drug.

Side effects may include: headache, dizziness, chest pain, lack of strength or energy, nausea, bronchitis, low blood pressure, sinusitis, rapid heart beat or palpitations, excess blood sugar, inflamed or runny nose, "needles and pins" feeling on the skin, vomiting, "lazy eye," high blood fats

Can I receive BiDil if I am pregnant or breastfeeding?

The effects of BiDil during pregnancy and breastfeeding are unknown. BiDil should be used with caution during pregnancy and only if the potential benefit justifies the potential risk to the fetus. Talk with your doctor before taking this drug if you are pregnant, plan to become pregnant, or are breastfeeding.

What should I do if I miss a dose of BiDil?

If you miss a dose take it as soon as you remember. If it is almost time for your next dose, skip the one you missed and go back to your regular schedule. Do not take 2 doses at once.

How should I store BiDil?

Store tightly closed at room temperature and keep away from light.

Bimatoprost solution *See Lumigan, page 774.*

Bismuth subsalicylate, metronidazole, and tetracycline hydrochloride *See Helidac Therapy, page 638.*

Bisoprolol fumarate *See Zebeta, page 1450.*

Bisoprolol fumarate and hydrochlorothiazide *See Ziac, page 1471.*

BONIVA
Generic name: Ibandronate sodium

What is Boniva?

Boniva is a prescription medicine used to treat or prevent osteoporosis in women after menopause. Boniva may reverse bone loss by stopping more loss of bone and increasing bone mass in most women who take it, even though they won't be able to see or feel a difference. Boniva may help lower the chances of breaking bones (fractures). For Boniva to treat or prevent osteoporosis you have to take it as prescribed; Boniva will not work if you stop taking it.

What is the most important information I should know about Boniva?

Boniva may cause serious problems in the stomach and the esophagus (the tube that connects your mouth and stomach) such as trouble swallowing, heartburn, and ulcers.

Adequate intake of calcium and vitamin D is important in all patients.

Boniva should be taken at least 60 minutes before the first food or drink (other than water) of the day and before taking any oral medication or supplementation, including calcium, antacids, or vitamins.

To reduce the potential for irritation of the esophagus, Boniva tablets should be swallowed whole with a full glass of plain water while you are standing or sitting in an upright position; you should not lie down for 60 minutes after taking Boniva.

Plain water is the only drink that should be taken with Boniva. Some mineral waters may have a higher concentration of calcium and should not be used.

The Boniva 150-mg tablet should be taken on the same date each month.

Do not chew or suck the tablet.

Who should not take Boniva?

Do not take Boniva if you have low blood calcium (hypocalcemia); cannot sit or stand up for at least 1 hour; have kidneys that work very poorly; or are allergic to ibandronate sodium or any of the other ingredients of Boniva, as well as other medications in the same class as Boniva.

What should I tell my doctor before I take the first dose of Boniva?

Tell your doctor about all prescription, over-the-counter, and herbal medications you are taking in order to prevent a possible interaction with Boniva. Also, talk to your doctor about your complete medical history, especially if you have swallowing problems or other problems with your esophagus, kidney problems, or if you are planning a dental procedure such as having a tooth pulled.

What is the usual dosage?

The information below is based on the dosage guidelines your doctor uses. Depending on your condition and medical history, your doctor may prescribe a different regimen. Do not change the dosage or stop taking your medication without your doctor's approval.

Adults: The usual dosage of Boniva is one 150-milligram (mg) tablet once a month.

How should I take Boniva?
Take Boniva first thing in the morning at least 1 hour before you eat or drink anything other than plain water, or take any other oral medicine. Take Boniva with 6 to 8 ounces (about 1 full cup) of plain water. Swallow Boniva whole. Do not chew or suck the tablet or keep it in your mouth to melt or dissolve. After you take Boniva, you must wait at least 1 hour before lying down, eating/drinking, or taking other oral medications.

What should I avoid while taking Boniva?
Avoid lying down within 1 hour of taking Boniva. Also, do not eat, drink (except plain water), or take any oral medications within 1 hour of taking Boniva.

What are possible food and drug interactions associated with Boniva?
If Boniva is taken with certain other drugs, the effects of either could be increased, decreased, or altered. It is especially important to check with your doctor before combining Boniva with the following: aspirin/nonsteroidal anti-inflammatory drugs (NSAIDS) and products containing calcium and other salts (eg, aluminum, magnesium, iron) such as antacids, supplements, or vitamins. In order for Boniva to be most effective, take it at least 1 hour before first food or drink (other than water) of the day or before you take any medications or supplements (calcium, antacids, vitamins) by mouth.

What are the possible side effects of Boniva?
Side effects cannot be anticipated. If any develop or change in intensity, tell your doctor as soon as possible. Only your doctor can determine if it is safe for you to continue taking this drug.

Side effects may include: arthritis, diarrhea, dizziness, headache, pain in extremities (arms or legs), upset stomach, vomiting

Can I receive Boniva if I am pregnant or breastfeeding?
Talk to your doctor if you are pregnant, planning to become pregnant, or are breastfeeding. The effects of Boniva on an unborn baby are unknown, and Boniva may pass into breast milk.

What should I do if I miss a dose of Boniva?
If your next scheduled Boniva day is more than 7 days away, take one Boniva 150-mg tablet in the morning following the day that you remembered that you missed a dose. Then, return to taking one Boniva 150-mg

tablet every month in the morning of your chosen day, according to your original schedule.

Do not take two 150-mg tablets within the same week. If your next scheduled Boniva day is only 1 to 7 days away, **wait** until your next scheduled day to take your tablet. Then, return to taking one Boniva 150-mg tablet every month in the morning of your chosen day, according to your original schedule.

How should I store Boniva?
Store at room temperature.

BREVOXYL
Generic name: Benzoyl peroxide (4% and 8%)

What is Brevoxyl?
Brevoxyl Gel, Brevoxyl Cleansing Lotion, and Brevoxyl Creamy are indicated for the topical treatment of mild to moderate acne (vulgaris). Brevoxyl may be used with other acne products, including antibiotics, retinoic acid products, and sulfur/salicylic acid-containing products.

What is the most important information I should know about Brevoxyl?
Brevoxyl Gel, Brevoxyl Cleansing Lotion and Brevoxyl Creamy are for external use only. Brevoxyl should be kept away from eyes. If irritation develops, stop using Brevoxyl immediately. Brevoxyl's results will not be visible until the third week of treatment; therefore, do not stop treatment without consulting your doctor.

Avoid contact with hair, fabrics, or carpeting since benzoyl peroxide will cause bleaching.

Who should not take Brevoxyl?
Patients with hypersensitivity to Brevoxyl and its ingredients should not take this medication. Do not use in children less than 12 unless you have consulted with your doctor.

What should I tell my doctor before I take the first dose of Brevoxyl?
Tell your doctor about all prescription, over-the-counter, and herbal medications you are taking before beginning treatment with Brevoxyl. Also, talk to your doctor about your complete medical history, especially if you are pregnant, intend on becoming pregnant, or are breastfeeding.

What is the usual dosage?
The information below is based on the dosage guidelines your doctor uses. Depending on your condition and medical history, your doctor

may prescribe a different regimen. Do not change the dosage or stop taking your medication without your doctor's approval.

Brevoxyl-4 and Brevoxyl-8 Gels
Adults: Apply once or twice daily to affected areas.

Brevoxyl-4 and Brevoxyl-8 Cleansing Lotions
Adults: Wash with cleansing lotion once a day for the first week and twice a day the following week.

Brevoxyl-4 and Brevoxyl-8 Creamy Washes
Adults: Wash with creamy wash once a day for the first week and twice a day the following week.

How should I take Brevoxyl?

For the Brevoxyl-4 and Brevoxyl-8 Gels, clean the affected area and pat dry. Apply as directed to affected area. Gentle cleansing of the affected areas prior to application may be beneficial.

For the Brevoxyl-4 and Brevoxyl-8 Cleansing Lotions, shake well before use. Wet skin and apply lotion, work to a full lather. Rinse thoroughly and pat dry.

For the Brevoxyl-4 and Brevoxyl-8 Creamy Washes, shake well before use. Wet skin and apply lotion, work to a full lather. Rinse thoroughly and pat dry.

What should I avoid while taking Brevoxyl?

Avoid contact with eyes and mucous membrane openings. Avoid contact with your hair, fabrics, or carpeting as Brevoxyl may cause bleaching. Also, avoid excessive sun exposure.

What are possible food and drug interactions associated with Brevoxyl?

No significant interactions have been reported at this time. However, always tell your doctor about any medicines you take, including over-the-counter drugs, vitamins, and herbal supplements.

What are the possible side effects of Brevoxyl?

Side effects cannot be anticipated. If any develop or change in intensity, tell your doctor as soon as possible. Only your doctor can determine if it is safe for you to continue taking this drug.

Side effects may include: burning or stinging of skin, redness, rash

Can I receive Brevoxyl if I am pregnant or breastfeeding?

The effects of Brevoxyl during pregnancy and breastfeeding are unknown. Tell your doctor if you are pregnant, intend on become pregnant, or are breastfeeding. Benzoyl peroxide should be used by a pregnant woman only if it is clearly needed.

What should I do if I miss a dose of Brevoxyl?
Apply the missed dose as soon as you remember it. However, if it is almost time for your next dose, skip the dose you missed and return to your regular dosing schedule. Do not double your dose.

How should I store Brevoxyl?
Store at room temperature and away from children.

Brimonidine tartrate *See Alphagan P, page 66.*

Brimonidine tartrate and timolol maleate *See Combigan, page 322.*

Brinzolamide 1% ophthalmic suspension *See Azopt, page 187.*

BROVANA
Generic name: Arformoterol tartrate

What is Brovana?
Brovana is used for long-term maintenance treatment of airway constriction that comes with having chronic obstructive pulmonary disease (COPD), which includes chronic bronchitis and emphysema.

Medications such as Brovana help the muscles around the airways in your lungs stay relaxed to prevent symptoms, such as wheezing, cough, chest tightness, and shortness of breath.

What is the most important information I should know about Brovana?
Brovana may increase the risk of an asthma-related death.

This drug is intended for long-term, daily usage; it is not for use as a rescue medication or for acute spasms of the airway (asthma attacks).

Brovana does not relieve sudden symptoms of chronic obstructive pulmonary disease (COPD); always have a short-acting medicine with you, such as an albuterol inhaler, to treat sudden symptoms.

Do not stop using Brovana unless told to do so by your healthcare provider, because your symptoms might get worse.

Brovana should not be used in children as the safety and efficacy of Brovana have not been established.

Who should not take Brovana?
Do not take Brovana if you are allergic to arformoterol or any of its other ingredients.

What should I tell my doctor before I take the first dose of Brovana?

Tell your doctor about all prescription, over-the-counter, and herbal medications you are taking to prevent a possible interaction with Brovana. Also, talk to your doctor about your complete medical history, including if you have: heart problems, high blood pressure, seizures, thyroid problems, diabetes, liver problems, or if you are pregnant or planning to become pregnant. It is not known if Brovana can harm your unborn baby. It is also not known if Brovana passes into breast milk and if it can harm your baby in that way.

What is the usual dosage?

The information below is based on the dosage guidelines your doctor uses. Depending on your condition and medical history, your doctor may prescribe a different regimen. Do not change the dosage or stop taking your medication without your doctor's approval.

Adults: The usual dosage of Brovana is 15 micrograms (mcg) twice a day, given through a nebulizer. This is also the maximum amount of Brovana that should be taken.

How should I take Brovana?

Brovana should be taken by nebulizer twice a day: once in the morning and once in the evening.

Use Brovana exactly as prescribed. One ready-to-use vial of Brovana is one dose. The usual dose of Brovana is 1 ready-to-use vial, twice a day (morning and evening) breathed in through your nebulizer machine. The 2 doses should be about 12 hours apart. Do not use more than 2 ready-to-use vials of Brovana per day.

Do not mix other medicines with Brovana in your nebulizer machine.

If you miss a dose of Brovana, just skip that dose. Take your next dose at your usual time. Do not take 2 doses at one time.

What should I avoid while taking Brovana?

While taking Brovana, avoid treatment with tricyclic antidepressants and beta-blockers.

What are possible food and drug interactions associated with Brovana?

If Brovana is used with certain other drugs, the effects of either could be increased, decreased, or altered. It is especially important to check with your doctor before combining Brovana with the following: monoamine oxidase inhibitors; tricyclic antidepressants; or a drug known to prolong QTc intervals, causing a potentially harmful reaction in the cardiovascular system.

What are the possible side effects of Brovana?

Side effects cannot be anticipated. If any develop or change in intensity, tell your doctor as soon as possible. Only your doctor can determine if it is safe for you to continue taking this drug.

Side effects may include: back pain, chest pain, diarrhea, difficulty breathing, dry mouth, fast and irregular heart beat, fluctuations in blood pressure, fluctuations in blood sugar levels, flu-like syndrome, general pain, headache, leg cramps, nervousness, rash, sinus infection, tiredness, tremor, trouble sleeping

Can I receive Brovana if I am pregnant or breastfeeding?

If you are pregnant, planning to become pregnant, or are nursing, talk to your doctor before beginning treatment with Brovana. The effects of Brovana on pregnancy are unknown; also, this drug may pass into breast milk.

What should I do if I miss a dose of Brovana?

If you miss a dose of Brovana, just skip that dose and take your next dose at your usual time. Do not take 2 doses at one time.

How should I store Brovana?

Store Brovana in a refrigerator in the protective foil pouch. Protect from light and excessive heat. Do not open a sealed pouch until you are ready to use a dose of Brovana. After opening the pouch, unused ready-to-use vials should be returned to, and stored in, the pouch. Use opened ready-to use vials right away. Brovana may be used directly from the refrigerator.

Budesonide *See Rhinocort Aqua, page 1150.*

Budesonide and formoterol *See Symbicort, page 1238.*

Budesonide inhalation powder *See Pulmicort Turbuhaler, page 1107.*

Bumetanide *See Bumex, below.*

BUMEX

Generic name: Bumetanide

What is Bumex?

Bumex is used to treat fluid retention associated with congestive heart failure and liver or kidney disease. It is also used with other drugs to treat high blood pressure.

What is the most important information I should know about Bumex?

Bumex is a powerful drug. If taken in excessive amounts, it can severely decrease the levels of water and minerals, especially potassium, your body needs to function. Your doctor should monitor your dose carefully.

Who should not take Bumex?

Do not use Bumex if you are sensitive to or allergic to this drug or to similar drugs. Do not use if you cannot produce urine, if you are dehydrated, or if you have severe liver disease.

What should I tell my doctor before I take the first dose of Bumex?

Tell your doctor about all prescription, over-the-counter, and herbal medication you are taking before beginning treatment with Bumex. Also, talk to your doctor about your complete medical history, especially if you are allergic to sulfur-containing drugs such as sulfonamides (antibacterial drugs) or if you have liver disease.

What is the usual dosage?

The information below is based on the dosage guidelines your doctor uses. Depending on your condition and medical history, your doctor may prescribe a different regimen. Do not change the dosage or stop taking your medication without your doctor's approval.

The usual total daily dose is 0.5-2 milligrams (mg) a day. If the initial dose is not adequate, your doctor may have you take a second and, possibly, a third dose at 4-5-hour intervals up to a maximum daily dose of 10 mg.

For the continuing control of fluid retention, your doctor may tell you to take Bumex every other day or for 3-4 days at a time with rest periods of 1-2 days in between.

The safety and effectiveness of Bumex has not been established in children less than 18 years of age.

How should I take Bumex?

Take Bumex in the morning after breakfast. If you take more than 1 dose a day, take the last dose no later than 6:00 PM.

What should I avoid while taking Bumex?

Bumex may make you feel dizzy, light-headed, or may cause you to faint. Avoid getting up quickly from a lying or seated position.

What are possible food and drug interactions associated with Bumex?

If Bumex is taken with certain other drugs, the effects of either could be increased, decreased, or altered. It is especially important to check with your doctor before combining Bumex with the following: blood pressure medications such as atenolol or enalapril, nonsteroidal anti-inflammatory drugs such as indomethacin, and probenecid.

Combining Bumex with certain antibiotics or cisplatin may increase the risk of hearing loss.

Because Bumex can lower potassium levels, the combination of Bumex and digoxin may increase the risk of changes in heartbeat.

The combination of Bumex with lithium may increase lithium levels in the body.

What are the possible side effects of Bumex?
Side effects cannot be anticipated. If any develop or change in intensity, tell your doctor as soon as possible. Only your doctor can determine if it is safe for you to continue taking this drug.

Side effects may include: dizziness, headache, low blood pressure, muscle cramps, nausea

Bumex can cause a loss of potassium from the body. Your doctor may recommend foods or fluids high in potassium or may want you to take a potassium supplement to help prevent potassium loss. Follow your doctor's recommendation carefully.

Signs of severe potassium loss are dry mouth, irregular heartbeat, muscle cramps or pain, unusual tiredness or weakness.

Can I receive Bumex if I am pregnant or breastfeeding?
The effects of Bumex during pregnancy and breastfeeding are unknown. Tell your doctor immediately if you are pregnant, plan to become pregnant, or are breastfeeding.

What should I do if I miss a dose of Bumex?
Take the missed dose as soon as you remember. If it is almost time for your next dose, skip the one you missed and go back to your regular schedule. Never take 2 doses at the same time.

How should I store Bumex?
Store at room temperature.

Bupropion hydrobromide See *Aplenzin, page 116, or Wellbutrin, page 1417.*

Bupropion hydrochloride (for smoking cessation)
See *Zyban, page 1499.*

Bupropion hydrochloride, extended-release
See *Wellbutrin XL, page 1421.*

Bupropion hydrochloride, sustained-release
  See *Wellbutrin SR, page 1419.*

BUSPAR
Generic name: Buspirone hydrochloride

What is BuSpar?
BuSpar is used to treat anxiety disorders or to relieve symptoms of anxiety.

What is the most important information I should know about BuSpar?
BuSpar should not be used with antidepressant drugs known as mono-amine oxidase (MAO) inhibitors such as phenelzine or tranylcypromine.

  Until you know how this medication affects you, do not drive a car or operate potentially dangerous machinery.

  During your treatment with BuSpar, avoid drinking large amounts of grapefruit juice.

Who should not take BuSpar?
Do not take BuSpar if you are sensitive or allergic to it.

  Anxiety or tension related to everyday stress usually does not require treatment with BuSpar. Discuss your symptoms thoroughly with your doctor.

  BuSpar is not recommended if you have severe kidney or liver damage.

  The safety and effectiveness of BuSpar have not been established in children younger than 18 years old.

What should I tell my doctor before I take the first dose of BuSpar?
Tell your doctor about all prescription, over-the-counter, and herbal medications you are taking before beginning treatment with BuSpar. Also, talk to your doctor about your complete medical history, especially if you use alcohol, take MAOIs, or if you have kidney or liver damage.

What is the usual dosage?
The information below is based on the dosage guidelines your doctor uses. Depending on your condition and medical history, your doctor may prescribe a different regimen. Do not change the dosage or stop taking your medication without your doctor's approval.

Adults: The recommended initial dose is 15 milligrams (mg) daily divided into two doses. Your doctor may increase the dosage by 5 mg per day every 2-3 days. The maximum daily dose is 60 mg.

How should I take BuSpar?
Take BuSpar consistently at the same time. Always take it the same way; you can choose either to take it always with food or always without food.

What should I avoid while taking BuSpar?
Avoid drinking large amounts of grapefruit juice.

Avoid driving or operating machinery until you know how this medication affects you.

What are possible food and drug interactions associated with BuSpar?
If BuSpar is taken with certain other drugs, the effects of either drug could be increased, decreased, or altered. It is especially important to check with your doctor before combining BuSpar with the following: alcohol, blood thinners such as warfarin, haloperidol, MAOIs such as phenelzine or tranylcypromine, and trazodone.

What are the possible side effects of BuSpar?
Side effects cannot be anticipated. If any develop or change in intensity, tell your doctor as soon as possible. Only your doctor can determine if it is safe for you to continue taking this drug.

Side effects may include: dizziness, excitement, headache, lightheadedness, nausea, nervousness

Can I receive BuSpar if I am pregnant or breastfeeding?
The effects of BuSpar during pregnancy and breastfeeding are unknown. Talk with your doctor before taking this drug if you are pregnant, plan to become pregnant, or are breastfeeding.

What should I do if I miss a dose of BuSpar?
Take the missed dose as soon as you remember. If it is almost time for your next dose, skip the one you missed and go back to your regular schedule. Never take two doses at the same time.

How should I store BuSpar?
Store at room temperature in a tightly closed container away from light.

Buspirone hydrochloride See BuSpar, page 233.

Butalbital, acetaminophen, and caffeine See Fioricet, page 548.

Butalbital, aspirin, and caffeine See Fiorinal, page 550.

Butalbital, codeine phosphate, aspirin, and caffeine See Fiorinal with Codeine, page 552.

BYETTA

Generic name: Exenatide

What is Byetta?

Byetta is an injectable medication used to improve blood sugar control in adults with uncontrolled type 2 diabetes. It can be used with other diabetes medications such as metformin, a sulfonylurea, a thiazolidinedione, or with a combination of these medications.

What is the most important information I should know about Byetta?

Byetta is not a substitute for insulin in people whose diabetes requires insulin treatment.

Who should not take Byetta?

Do not use Byetta if you are allergic to the drug or any of its ingredients.
   Byetta has not been studied in children.

What should I tell my doctor before I take the first dose of Byetta?

Tell your doctor about all prescription, over-the-counter, and herbal medications you are taking before beginning treatment with Byetta. Also, talk to your doctor about your complete medical history, especially if you have severe problems with your stomach or food digestion, have severe kidney disease or are on dialysis, are pregnant or planning to become pregnant, or if you are breastfeeding.

What is the usual dosage?

The information below is based on the dosage guidelines your doctor uses. Depending on your condition and medical history, your doctor may prescribe a different regimen. Do not change the dosage or stop taking your medication without your doctor's approval.

Adults: The starting dose of Byetta is 5 micrograms (mcg) per dose given 2 times a day. Based on your response, the dose of Byetta can be increased to 10 mcg given 2 times a day after 1 month of therapy.

How should I take Byetta?

Byetta comes in a prefilled pen. You must do a "New Pen Set-Up" when you first start a new prefilled Byetta pen. Inject your dose of Byetta under the skin of your upper leg, stomach area, or upper arm.
   Byetta is injected 2 times a day at any time within the 60 minutes before your morning and evening meals.
   Do not take Byetta after your meal.
   Pen needles are not included; you may need a prescription to purchase pen needles, ask your healthcare provider which needle length and gauge is best for you.

What should I avoid while taking Byetta?

Avoid using alcohol while you are taking Byetta.

What are possible food and drug interactions associated with Byetta?

Byetta slows stomach emptying and can affect medicines that need to pass through the stomach quickly. Ask your healthcare provider if the time at which you take any of your oral medicines should be changed.

What are the possible side effects of Byetta?

Side effects cannot be anticipated. If any develop or change in intensity, tell your doctor as soon as possible. Only your doctor can determine if it is safe for you to continue taking this drug.

Side effects may include: nausea, vomiting, diarrhea, dizziness, drowsiness, headache, feeling jittery, acid stomach, low blood sugar, weakness, confusion, irritability, hunger

Can I receive Byetta if I am pregnant or breastfeeding?

The effects of Byetta during pregnancy and breastfeeding are unknown. Talk with your doctor before taking this drug if you are pregnant, plan to become pregnant, or are breastfeeding.

What should I do if I miss a dose of Byetta?

If you miss a dose of Byetta, skip the dose and take your next dose at the next prescribed time. Do not take an extra dose or increase the amount of your next dose to make up for the one you missed.

How should I store Byetta?

Store Byetta in the refrigerator. Do not freeze. Throw away a used Byetta pen after 30 days even if some medicine remains in the pen. Do not store the Byetta pen with the needle attached; if the needle is left on, medicine may leak from the Byetta pen or air bubbles may form in the cartridge. Keep your Byetta pen, pen needles, and all medications out of the reach of children.

BYSTOLIC

Generic name: Nebivolol

What is Bystolic?

Bystolic is used to treat high blood pressure.

What is the most important information I should know about Bystolic?

Patients with coronary artery disease treated with Bystolic should not discontinue therapy abruptly as it may result in angina and heart attack.

Patients with history of severe allergic reactions will be more prone to allergies and may not respond to the usual dose of epinephrine used to treat these allergic episodes.

Who should not take Bystolic?
Patients with severe bradycardia (slow heart rate), heart block greater than a first degree block, cardiogenic shock, severe liver disease, and sick sinus syndrome (patients with irregular heart rate requiring a pacemaker) should not use Bystolic.

What should I tell my doctor before I take the first dose of Bystolic?
Tell your doctor about all prescription, over-the-counter, and herbal medications you are taking before beginning treatment with Bystolic. Also, talk to your doctor about your complete medical history, especially if you have preexisting bradycardia (slow heart rate), heart block greater than a first degree block, cardiogenic shock, severe liver disease, sick sinus syndrome (an irregular heart rate requiring a pacemaker), bronchospastic disorders (breathing problems), diabetes, thyrotoxicosis (increased thyroid hormone levels), peripheral vascular disease, kidney problems, or any upcoming surgery.

What is the usual dosage?
The information below is based on the dosage guidelines your doctor uses. Depending on your condition and medical history, your doctor may prescribe a different regimen. Do not change the dosage or stop taking your medication without your doctor's approval.

The recommended starting dosage of Bystolic is 5 milligrams once daily.

How should I take Bystolic?
Take Bystolic as prescribed by your doctor. It is to be taken orally with or without food.

What should I avoid while taking Bystolic?
Do not drive a car or use heavy machinery until you know how Bystolic affects you, as it may impair your ability to perform these tasks. Do not discontinue therapy abruptly.

What are possible food and drug interactions associated with Bystolic?
If Bystolic is taken with certain other drugs, the effects of either could be increased, decreased, or altered. It is especially important to check with your doctor before combining Bystolic with the following: beta-blockers, clonidine, digitalis glycosides, fluoxetine, paroxetine, propafenone, and quinidine.

What are the possible side effects of Bystolic?

Side effects cannot be anticipated. If any develop or change in intensity, tell your doctor as soon as possible. Only your doctor can determine if it is safe for you to continue taking this drug.

Side effects may include: headache, chest pain, fatigue, nausea, dizziness, insomnia (reduced sleep), abdominal pain, weakness, increased likelihood of allergic reactions (eg, hives, difficulty breathing, and swelling of the throat), reduced heart rate, reduced blood pressure, congestive heart failure, bronchospasm (constriction of air tubes), hypoglycemia (reduced glucose levels)

Can I receive Bystolic if I am pregnant or breastfeeding?

Bystolic is to be avoided during pregnancy and in nursing mothers.

What should I do if I miss a dose of Bystolic?

If you miss a dose, take the next scheduled dose only without doubling it.

How should I store Bystolic?

Store at room temperature.

CADUET

Generic name: Amlodipine besylate and atorvastatin calcium

What is Caduet?

Caduet, along with diet and exercise, is used to treat both high blood pressure and high cholesterol. Since Caduet combines two medicines (Norvasc and Lipitor), it works in two ways. First, Caduet works by relaxing your blood vessels. This lets your blood flow more easily and helps lower your blood pressure. Second, Caduet lowers "bad" cholesterol by blocking an enzyme in the liver that your body uses to make cholesterol. Less cholesterol is produced, and this results in lower levels in your blood.

What is the most important information I should know about Caduet?

Caduet may increase the frequency of heart attack in people with obstructive coronary artery disease. Treatment with this drug should be discontinued if there are signs of muscular problems, such as rhabdomyolysis (the breakdown of muscle). Therefore, any unexplained muscle pain, tenderness, or weakness, particularly if accompanied by malaise or fever, should be immediately reported to your doctor.

Who should not take Caduet?

Do not take Caduet if you are allergic to any of its ingredients. Also, you should not begin therapy with Caduet if you have liver problems.

Do not take Caduet if you are pregnant, think you may be pregnant, or are planning to become pregnant. If you get pregnant, stop taking Caduet and call your doctor right away.

Do not take Caduet if you are breastfeeding. Caduet can pass into your breast milk and may harm your baby.

What should I tell my doctor before I take the first dose of Caduet?

Tell your doctor about all prescription, over-the-counter, and herbal medications you are taking before beginning treatment with Caduet. Also, talk to your doctor about your complete medical history, especially if you have or had liver disease. Tell your doctor of any muscle aches or weakness, diabetes, thyroid problems, kidney problems, or if you drink more than 2 glasses of alcohol daily.

What is the usual dosage?

The information below is based on the dosage guidelines your doctor uses. Depending on your condition and medical history, your doctor may prescribe a different regimen. Do not change the dosage or stop taking your medication without your doctor's approval.

Adults: The dosage of Caduet is based on both effectiveness and tolerance for each individual component in the treatment of high blood pressure and high cholesterol.

Because Caduet is made up of both Norvasc and Lipitor, please see those individual entries for exact dosing.

How should I take Caduet?

Take Caduet once a day at any time of day, at about the same time each day. Do not split or crush the tablets before taking them.

What should I avoid while taking Caduet?

Avoid becoming pregnant while taking Caduet.

Do not breastfeed. Caduet can pass into your breast milk and may harm your baby.

What are possible food and drug interactions associated with Caduet?

If Caduet is used with certain other drugs, the effects of either could be increased, decreased, or altered. Because Caduet is made up of both Norvasc and Lipitor, please see those individual entries for individual drug interactions. Tell your doctor if you take medications for your immune system, infections, cholesterol, birth control, heart failure, or HIV (AIDS).

You can use nitroglycerine and Caduet together. If you take nitroglycerine for chest pain (angina), do not stop taking it while taking Caduet.

What are the possible side effects of Caduet?

Side effects cannot be anticipated. If any develop or change in intensity, tell your doctor as soon as possible. Only your doctor can determine if it is safe for you to continue taking this drug.

Side effects may include: back pain, constipation, dizziness, fatigue, headache, irregular heartbeat, liver problems, muscle problems, nausea, rash, sleepiness, stomach pain, swelling of your legs or ankles, weakness

Can I receive Caduet if I am pregnant or breastfeeding?

Do not take Caduet if you are pregnant, planning to become pregnant, or are nursing. This drug may cause severe problems in your pregnancy and may be passed into your breast milk.

What should I do if I miss a dose of Caduet?

If you miss a dose of Caduet, take it as soon as you remember. If it is almost time for your next dose, skip the missed dose and return to your normal dosing schedule. Do not take a double dose.

How should I store Caduet?

Store Caduet at room temperature.

CAFERGOT

Generic name: Ergotamine tartate and caffeine

What is Cafergot?

Cafergot is prescribed for the relief or prevention of vascular headaches—for example, migraine, migraine variants, or cluster headaches.

What is the most important information I should know about Cafergot?

The excessive use of Cafergot can lead to ergot poisoning resulting in symptoms such as headache, pain in the legs when walking, muscle pain, numbness, coldness, and abnormal paleness of the fingers and toes. If this condition is not treated, it can lead to gangrene (tissue death due to decreased blood supply).

Who should not take Cafergot?

Do not take Cafergot if you are allergic to ergotamine tartate, caffeine, or similar drugs.

What should I tell my doctor before I take the first dose of Cafergot?

Tell your doctor about all prescription, over-the-counter, and herbal medication you are taking before beginning treatment with Cafergot. Also, talk to your doctor about your complete medical history, especially if you have coronary heart disease, circulatory problems, high blood pressure, liver or kidney problems, an infection, or if you are pregnant. If you experience nausea and vomiting during attacks, making it impossible to hold medication down, your doctor may prescribe rectal suppositories.

What is the usual dosage?

The information below is based on the dosage guidelines your doctor uses. Depending on your condition and medical history, your doctor may prescribe a different regimen. Do not change the dosage or stop taking your medication without your doctor's approval.

Orally
Adults: (Take at the first sign of an attack). The total daily dose for any single attack should not exceed 6 tablets.

Rectally
Adults: The maximum dose for an individual attack is 2 suppositories.
The total weekly dose should not exceed 10 tablets or 5 suppositories.
A preventive, short-term dose may be given at bedtime to certain people, but only as prescribed by a doctor.

How should I take Cafergot?

Cafergot is available in both tablet and suppository form. Cafergot works best if you use it at the first sign of a migraine attack and before the headache actually starts.
To use the suppositories, follow these steps:

1. If the suppository feels too soft, leave it in the refrigerator for about 30 minutes or put it, still wrapped, in ice water until it hardens.
2. Remove the foil wrapper and dip the tip of the suppository in water.
3. Lie down on your side and with a finger insert the suppository into the rectum. Hold it in place for a few moments.

What should I avoid while taking Cafergot?

Do not exceed the recommended dosage of Cafergot, especially when Cafergot is used over long periods. Discontinuing Cafergot may produce withdrawal symptoms such as sudden, severe headaches.
Cafergot is effective only for migraine and migraine-type headaches. Do not use it for any other kind of headaches.

What are possible food and drug interactions associated with Cafergot?

If Cafergot is taken with certain other drugs, the effects of either could be increased, decreased, or altered. It is especially important to check with your doctor before combining Cafergot with the following: beta-blocker blood pressure medications, such as atenolol and propranolol; drugs that constrict blood vessels, such as epinephrine or pseudoephedrine; macrolide antibiotics, such as erythromycin and clarithromycin; nicotine.

What are the possible side effects of Cafergot?
Side effects cannot be anticipated. If any develop or change in intensity, tell your doctor as soon as possible. Only your doctor can determine if it is safe for you to continue taking this drug.

Side effects may include: fluid retention, high blood pressure, itching, nausea, numbness, rapid heart rate, slow heartbeat, tingling or pins and needles, vertigo, vomiting, weakness

Signs that your blood vessels are narrowing are bluish tinge to the skin, chest pain, cold arms and legs, gangrene, and muscle pains.

Although these symptoms occur most commonly with long-term therapy at relatively high doses, they have been reported with short-term or normal doses. A few people on long-term therapy have developed heart valve problems.

Can I receive Cafergot if I am pregnant or breastfeeding?
Do not take Cafergot if you are pregnant. Do not breastfeed if you are taking Cafergot.

What should I do if I miss a dose of Cafergot?
Take Cafergot only when threatened with an attack.

How should I store Cafergot?
Store at room temperature in a tightly closed container away from light. Keep suppositories away from heat.

CALAN
Generic name: Verapamil hydrochloride

What is Calan?
Calan is used to treat chest pain occurring at rest or chest pain occurring with exertion. Both kinds of chest pain are due to clogged heart arteries. Calan is also used to treat irregular heartbeat and high blood pressure.

What is the most important information
I should know about Calan?
If you have high blood pressure, you must take Calan regularly for it to be effective. Since blood pressure declines gradually, it may take several weeks before you get the full benefit of Calan. You must continue taking

Calan even if you are feeling well. Calan does not cure high blood pressure; it only keeps it under control.

Who should not take Calan?

Do not take Calan if you have low blood pressure or certain types of heart disease or heartbeat irregularities. Do not take Calan if you are allergic to any of its ingredients.

What should I tell my doctor before I take the first dose of Calan?

Tell your doctor about all prescription, over-the-counter, and herbal medication you are taking before beginning treatment with Calan. Also, talk to your doctor about your complete medical history, especially if you have any heart problems, kidney disease, liver disease, muscle weakness due to a condition known as myasthenia gravis, or rapidly progressive muscle weakness due to an inherited disorder called Duchenne's muscular dystrophy. Tell your doctor if you are also using drugs known as beta-blockers.

What is the usual dosage?

The information below is based on the dosage guidelines your doctor uses. Depending on your condition and medical history, your doctor may prescribe a different regimen. Do not change the dosage or stop taking your medication without your doctor's approval.

The dose of Calan must be individualized. In general, dosages of Calan should not exceed 480 milligrams (mg) per day.

Angina

The usual initial dose is 80-120 mg, 3 times a day. Lower doses of 40 mg 3 times a day may be used by the elderly or those with decreased liver function. Your doctor may increase the dosage either daily or weekly until the desired response is seen.

Irregular Heartbeat

The usual dose in people who are also on digitalis ranges from 240-320 mg per day divided into 3 or 4 doses.

In people who are not taking digitalis, doses range from a total of 240-480 mg per day divided into 3 or 4 doses.

High Blood Pressure

The usual dose of Calan, when used alone for high blood pressure, is 80 mg, 3 times per day. Total daily doses of 360 mg and 480 mg may be used. Smaller individuals and the elderly may take smaller doses of 40 mg 3 times per day. Any adjustment of Calan to a higher dose will be based on its effectiveness as determined by your doctor.

How should I take Calan?
Calan can be taken with or without food.

What should I avoid while taking Calan?
Try not to miss any doses. Take Calan exactly as prescribed even if you are feeling well. If the drug is not taken regularly, your condition can get worse.

Do not stop taking Calan abruptly without consulting with your doctor. A slow reduction in dose may be required.

What are possible food and drug interactions associated with Calan?
If Calan is taken with certain other drugs, the effects of either could be increased, decreased, or altered. It is especially important to check with your doctor before combining Calan with the following: ACE inhibitor-type blood pressure drugs, such as captopril or enalapril; alcohol; amiodarone; aspirin; beta-blocker-type blood pressure drugs, such as metoprolol, atenolol, and propranolol; carbamazepine; chloroquine; cimetidine; cyclosporine; dantrolene; digitalis; disopyramide; diuretics, such as furosemide and hydrochlorothiazide; erythromycin; flecainide; glipizide; grapefruit juice; imipramine; lithium; nitrates, such as isosorbide dinitrate; other high blood pressure drugs, such as prazosin; phenobarbital; phenytoin; quinidine; rifampin; ritonavir; theophylline; and vasodilator-type blood pressure drugs, such as minoxidil.

What are the possible side effects of Calan?
Side effects cannot be anticipated. If any develop or change in intensity, tell your doctor as soon as possible. Only your doctor can determine if it is safe for you to continue taking this drug.

Side effects may include: congestive heart failure, constipation, dizziness, fatigue, fluid retention, headache, low blood pressure, nausea, rash, shortness of breath, slow heartbeat, upper respiratory tract infection

Can I receive Calan if I am pregnant or breastfeeding?
The effects of Calan during pregnancy and breastfeeding are unknown. Tell your doctor immediately if you are pregnant, plan to become pregnant, or are breastfeeding.

What should I do if I miss a dose of Calan?
Take it as soon as you remember. If it is almost time for your next dose, skip the one you missed and go back to your regular schedule. Never take 2 doses at the same time.

How should I store Calan?
Store at room temperature away from heat, light, and moisture.

Calcipotriene and betamethasone dipropionate ointment
See Taclonex, page 1250.

Calcitonin-salmon See Fortical Nasal Spray, page 594, or
Miacalcin, page 817.

Candesartan cilexetil See Atacand, page 139.

Candesartan cilexetil and hydrochlorothiazide
See Atacand HCT, page 141.

CAPOTEN
Generic name: Captopril hydrochloride

What is Capoten?
Capoten is used alone or with diuretics to treat high blood pressure.
Capoten is also used in combination with digitalis and diuretics for treatment of chronic heart failure. In addition, Capoten is used to improve survival in certain people who have suffered heart attacks and to treat kidney disease in diabetics.

What is the most important information I should know about Capoten?
If you have high blood pressure, you must take Capoten regularly for it to be effective. Since blood pressure declines gradually, it may be several weeks before you get the full benefit of Capoten. You must continue taking it even if you are feeling well. Capoten does not cure high blood pressure; it merely keeps it under control.

Who should not take Capoten?
Do not use Capoten if you are allergic to the product or to any other angiotensin-converting enzyme inhibitors.

What should I tell my doctor before I take the first dose of Capoten?
Tell your doctor about all prescription, over-the-counter, and herbal medication you are taking before beginning treatment with Capoten. Also, talk to your doctor about your complete medical history, especially if you are receiving bee or wasp venom to prevent an allergic reaction to stings, if you have kidney disease, or liver disease.

What is the usual dosage?
The information below is based on the dosage guidelines your doctor uses. Depending on your condition and medical history, your doctor may prescribe a different regimen. Do not change the dosage or stop taking your medication without your doctor's approval.

Hypertension
Adults: The initial dose of Capoten is 25 milligrams (mg) taken 2 or 3 times daily. If satisfactory reduction of blood pressure has not been achieved after 1 or 2 weeks, the dose may be increased to 50 mg 2 or 3 times daily. The maximum recommended daily dose is 450 mg.

Heart Failure
Adults: The usual dose is 25 mg taken 3 times a day. A daily dosage of 450 mg should not be exceeded.

After a Heart Attack
Adults: The usual starting dose is 6.25 mg, taken once, followed by 12.5 mg taken 3 times a day. Your doctor will increase the dose over the next several days to 25 mg taken 3 times a day and then, over the next several weeks, to 50 mg taken 3 times a day.

Kidney Disease in Diabetes
Adults: The usual dose is 25 mg taken 3 times a day.

How should I take Capoten?

Capoten should be taken 1 hour before meals. Take Capoten exactly as prescribed. Suddenly stopping Capoten could cause your blood pressure to increase.

What should I avoid while taking Capoten?

Capoten may cause you to become drowsy or less alert. Avoid driving or participating in any potentially hazardous activity. Avoid dehydration because this may cause a drop in blood pressure. Do not use potassium-containing salt substitutes while taking Capoten.

What are possible food and drug interactions associated with Capoten?

If Capoten is taken with certain other drugs, the effects of either could be increased, decreased, or altered. It is especially important to check with your doctor before combining Capoten with the following: allopurinol; aspirin; blood pressure drugs known as beta-blockers, such as atenolol and propranolol; cyclosporine; digoxin; diuretics such as hydrochloro-thiazide; lithium; nitroglycerin; non-steroidal anti-inflammatory drugs, such as indomethacin and piroxicam; potassium preparations; and potassium-sparing diuretics, such as amiloride or spironolactone.

What are the possible side effects of Capoten?

Side effects cannot be anticipated. If any develop or change in intensity, tell your doctor as soon as possible. Only your doctor can determine if it is safe for you to continue taking this drug.

Side effects may include: itching, loss of taste, low blood pressure, rash

Call your doctor if you have persistent, dry cough; sore throat; swelling of the face round your lips, tongue, throat, or arms and legs; yellow coloring of your skin or the whites of your eyes.

Can I receive Capoten if I am pregnant or breastfeeding?
ACE inhibitors such as Capoten have been shown to cause injury and even death to the developing baby when used in pregnancy during the second and third trimesters. If you are pregnant or plan to become pregnant, contact your doctor immediately. Capoten appears in breast milk and could affect a nursing infant. If Capoten is essential to your health, your doctor may advise you to discontinue breastfeeding until your treatment is finished.

What should I do if I miss a dose of Capoten?
Take it as soon as you remember. If it is almost time for your next dose, skip the one you missed and go back to your regular schedule. Never take 2 doses at the same time.

How should I store Capoten?
Store at room temperature in a tightly closed container, away from moisture.

CAPOZIDE
Generic name: Captopril and hydrochlorothiazide

What is Capozide?
Capozide combines a blood pressure-lowering medication (captopril) with a water pill (hydrochlorothiazide) to treat high blood pressure.

What is the most important information I should know about Capozide?
You must take Capozide regularly for it to be effective. Since blood pressure declines gradually, it may be several weeks before you get the full benefit of Capozide. Even if you are feeling well, you must continue to take Capozide. Capozide does not cure high blood pressure, it just keeps it under control.

Who should not take Capozide?
If you are sensitive to or have ever had an allergic reaction to captopril, hydrochlorothiazide, other ACE inhibitors such as enalapril or other thiazide diuretics such as chlorothiazide, or if you are sensitive to other sulfonamide-derived drugs, you should not take Capozide. If you have a history of angioedema (swelling of face, extremities, and throat) or inability to urinate, you should not take Capozide.

What should I tell my doctor before I take the first dose of Capozide?

Tell your doctor about all prescription, over-the-counter, and herbal medication you are taking before beginning treatment with Capozide. Also, talk to your doctor about your complete medical history, especially if you have chronic heart failure, a connective tissue disease called lupus erythematosus, kidney disease, liver disease, or if you are on dialysis.

What is the usual dosage?

The information below is based on the dosage guidelines your doctor uses. Depending on your condition and medical history, your doctor may prescribe a different regimen. Do not change the dosage or stop taking your medication without your doctor's approval.

Adults: Dosages of Capozide are always individualized, and your doctor will determine what combination works best for you. This medication can be used with other blood pressure medications such as beta-blockers. Dosages are also adjusted for people with decreased kidney function.

The initial dose is one 25 milligram/15 milligram (mg) tablet, once a day. If this is not effective, your doctor may adjust the dosage upward every 6 weeks. In general, the daily dose of captopril should not exceed 150 mg. The maximum recommended daily dose of hydrochlorothiazide is 50 mg.

How should I take Capozide?

Take Capozide one hour before meals. Take this medication exactly as prescribed.

What should I avoid while taking Capozide?

Do not stop taking Capozide unless instructed by your doctor. Stopping Capozide suddenly can cause your blood pressure to increase.

Patients with heart failure should not increase their physical activity too quickly.

Do not use potassium-sparing diuretics, potassium supplements or potassium-containing salt substitutes without talking to your doctor.

What are possible food and drug interactions associated with Capozide?

If Capozide is taken with certain other drugs, the effects of either could be increased, decreased, or altered. It is especially important to check with your doctor before combining Capozide with the following: alcohol; antigout drugs such as allopurinol; barbiturates; calcium; digoxin; cholestyramine; colestipol; corticosteroids, such as prednisone; diabetes drugs, such as glyburide or insulin; diazoxide; lithium; MAO inhibitors, such as phenelzine; methenamine; narcotics; nitroglycerin; nonsteroidal anti-inflammmatory drugs, such as naproxen; norepinephrine; oral blood thinners, such as warfarin; other blood pressure drugs, such as prazosin or terazosin; potassium-sparing diuretics, such as spironolactone; potassium supplements; probenecid; and sulfinpyrazone.

What are the possible side effects of Capozide?

Side effects cannot be anticipated. If any develop or change in intensity, tell your doctor as soon as possible. Only your doctor can determine if it is safe for you to continue taking this drug.

Side effects may include: itching, loss of taste, low blood pressure, rash

If you develop swelling of the face around your lips, tongue, or throat (or of your arms and legs), or have difficulty swallowing, stop taking Capozide and contact your doctor immediately. You may need emergency treatment.

If you notice a yellow coloring to your skin or the whites of your eyes (jaundice), stop taking the drug and notify your doctor immediately. Also, if you develop a sore throat; dry, persistent cough; excessive sweating; dehydration; severe diarrhea; or vomiting; contact your doctor immediately.

Can I receive Capozide if I am pregnant or breastfeeding?

If you are pregnant discontinue use of Capozide as soon as possible. If you plan to become pregnant and are taking Capozide, contact your doctor immediately. Capozide appears in breast milk. Avoid breastfeeding if you are taking Capozide.

What should I do if I miss a dose of Capozide?

Take it as soon as you remember. If it is almost time for your next dose, skip the one you missed and go back to your regular schedule. Never take 2 doses at the same time.

How should I store Capozide?

Store at room temperature in a tightly closed container away from moisture.

Captopril and hydrochlorothiazide *See Capozide, page 247.*

Captopril hydrochloride *See Capoten, page 245.*

Carbamazepine *See Tegretol, page 1268.*

Carbamazepine extended-release *See Carbatrol, page 250.*

Carbamazepine for bipolar disorder *See Equetro, page 490.*

CARBATROL
Generic name: Carbamazepine extended-release

What is Carbatrol?
Carbatrol is an extended-release formulation of carbamazepine which is indicated for treatment of seizures (partial, grand mal, mixed) and facial/head pain (trigeminal neuralgia).

What is the most important information I should know about Carbatrol?
Carbatrol has the risk of potentially dangerous side effects; it is very important to thoroughly assess the use of Carbatrol with your doctor. A detailed history and physical examination is needed to determine if you are qualified for treatment. Also, do not take Carbatrol if you have been taking a monoamine oxidase inhibitor (e.g., certain anti-depressants) within 14 days of initiating Carbatrol therapy.

Who should not take Carbatrol?
Patients with hypersensitivity to Carbatrol and its ingredients in this preparation should not take this medication. You should not take this drug if you have a previous allergic reaction to amitriptyline, desipramine, imipramine, protriptyline and nortriptyline. Also, do not take Carbatrol if you have been taking a monoamine oxidase inhibitor (eg, certain anti-depressants) within 14 days of initiating Carbatrol therapy.

What should I tell my doctor before I take the first dose of Carbatrol?
Tell your doctor about all prescription, over-the-counter, and herbal medications you are taking before beginning treatment with Carbatrol. Also, talk to your doctor about your complete medical history, especially blood disorders.

What is the usual dosage?
The information below is based on the dosage guidelines your doctor uses. Depending on your condition and medical history, your doctor may prescribe a different regimen. Do not change the dosage or stop taking your medication without your doctor's approval.

Epilepsy
Adults: The usual initial dose is 200 mg twice daily, which can be increased in weekly intervals up to 200 mg per day until optimal response is obtained. Dose should be kept at minimal effective dose, usually in the 800-1200 mg daily range.

Children under 12 years of age: Children taking total daily doses of immediate release carbamazepine of 400 mg or greater may be switched to the extended-release formulation.

Trigeminal Neuralgia
The usual initial dose is 200 mg on the first day. The dose may be increased by up to 200 mg a day every 12 hours as needed for pain relief. Do not exceed 1200 mg daily. In addition, after 3 months of therapy, a gradual dose reduction is recommended.

How should I take Carbatrol?
Carbatrol is intended for twice a day administration. Take Carbatrol at the same time with food. Do not chew, crush or cut the capsules.

What should I avoid while taking Carbatrol?
Avoid driving and operating machinery. Use contraception when having sex.

What are possible food and drug interactions associated with Carbatrol?
If Carbatrol is taken with certain other drugs, the effects of either could be increased, decreased, or altered. It is especially important to check with your doctor before combining Carbatrol with the following: acetaminophen, acetazolamide, alprazolam, amitriptyline, azole antifungals (e.g., itraconozole and ketoconozole), bupropion, buspirone, cimetidine, cisplatin, citalopram, clarithromycin, clonazepam, clozapine, cyclosporin, dalfopristin, danazol, delavirdine, desipramine, diltiazem, dicumarol, doxycycline, doxyrubicin, ethosuximide, erythromycin, felbamate, felodipine, fluoxetine, fluvoxamine, glucocorticoids, grapefruit juice, haloperidol, isoniazid, lamotrigine, levothyroxine, loratadine, lorazepam, methadone; methsuximide, midazolam, mirtazapine, nefazadone, niacinamide, nicotinamide, nortriptylline, olanzapine, oral contraceptives, oxcarbazepine, phenobarbital, phenytoin, primidone, protease inhibitors (eg, ritonavir), propoxyphene, quetiapine, quinine, quinupristin, rifampin, risperidone, theophylline, topiramate, tiagabine, tramadol, triazolam, trazodone, troleandomycin, valproate, verapamil, warfarin, ziprasidone, zileuton, and zonisamide.

What are the possible side effects of Carbatrol?
Side effects cannot be anticipated. If any develop or change in intensity, tell your doctor as soon as possible. Only your doctor can determine if it is safe for you to continue taking this drug.

Side effects may include: Blood disorders (agranulocytosis, aplastic anemia, and bone marrow suppression), rash, itching, heart disorders (edema, heart failure, hypertension, and hypotension), fever, pneumonia, urinary frequency, urinary retention, kidney impairment, impotence

Can I receive Carbatrol if I am pregnant or breastfeeding?
The use of Carbatrol is not recommended in women who are or may become pregnant. It is important to advise women of child-bearing potential

to use contraception while taking Carbatrol due to the potential harm to the baby.

In addition, Carbatrol should not be given to nursing mothers, as it may cause potential harm to the baby.

What should I do if I miss a dose of Carbatrol?
If you miss a dose, take it as soon as you remember. If it is close to the time of your next dose, skip it and resume your scheduled dose. Do not double the dose.

How should I store Carbatrol?
Store at room temperature. Protect from light and moisture.

Carbidopa and levodopa *See Sinemet CR, page 1197.*

Carbidopa, levodopa, and entacapone *See Stalevo, page 1220.*

CARDENE/CARDENE SR
Generic name: Nicardipine hydrochloride

What is Cardene/Cardene SR?
Cardene is used to treat chest pain usually caused by lack of oxygen to the heart resulting from clogged arteries, brought on by exertion. Cardene is also used to treat high blood pressure.

Cardene SR is a long-acting form of the drug and is only used to treat high blood pressure.

What is the most important information I should know about Cardene/Cardene SR?
If you have high blood pressure, you must take Cardene regularly for it to be effective. Since blood pressure declines gradually, it may take several weeks before you get the full benefit of Cardene and you must continue taking it even if you are feeling well. Cardene does not cure high blood pressure; it only keeps it under control.

Who should not take Cardene/Cardene SR?
If you have severe narrowing of the aorta resulting in obstruction of blood flow from the heart to the body, you should not take Cardene. Also, if you are sensitive to or have ever had an allergic reaction to Cardene, do not take this drug.

What should I tell my doctor before I take the first dose of Cardene/Cardene SR?
Tell your doctor about all prescription, over-the-counter, and herbal medication you are taking before beginning treatment with Cardene. Also, talk

to your doctor about your complete medical history, especially if you have chronic heart failure or liver disease. Be sure to discuss with your doctor how much exercise or exertion is safe for you.

What is the usual dosage?
The information below is based on the dosage guidelines your doctor uses. Depending on your condition and medical history, your doctor may prescribe a different regimen. Do not change the dosage or stop taking your medication without your doctor's approval.

Chest Pain
Adults: The usual starting dose is 20 milligrams (mg), 3 times a day. The usual regular dose is 20-40 mg, taken 3 times a day.

High Blood Pressure
Adults: The starting dose is usually 20 mg, 3 times a day. The usual dose ranges from 20-40 mg, taken 3 times a day.

The starting dose of Cardene SR is usually 30 mg, taken 2 times a day. The regular dose ranges from 30-60 mg, taken 2 times a day.

How should I take Cardene/Cardene SR?
Take Cardene exactly as prescribed, even if your symptoms have disappeared.

If you are taking Cardene SR, swallow the capsule whole. Do not chew, crush, or divide it.

Try not to miss any doses. If Cardene is not taken regularly, your condition may worsen.

What should I avoid while taking Cardene/Cardene SR?
Avoid driving or engaging in hazardous activities. Cardene can cause your blood pressure to become too low, making you feel lightheaded or faint.

What are possible food and drug interactions associated with Cardene/Cardene SR?
If Cardene is taken with certain other drugs, the effects of either could be increased, decreased, or altered. It is especially important to check with your doctor before combining Cardene with the following: amiodarone, cimetidine, cyclosporine, digoxin, phenytoin, and propranolol.

What are the possible side effects of Cardene/Cardene SR?
Side effects cannot be anticipated. If any develop or change in intensity, tell your doctor as soon as possible. Only your doctor can determine if it is safe for you to continue taking this drug.

Side effects may include: dizziness, flushing, headache, increased chest pain (angina), indigestion, nausea, pounding or rapid heartbeat, sleepiness, swelling of feet, weakness

Can I receive Cardene/Cardene SR if I am pregnant or breastfeeding?

The effects of Cardene during pregnancy and breastfeeding are unknown. Tell your doctor immediately if you are pregnant, plan to become pregnant, or you are breastfeeding.

What should I do if I miss a dose of Cardene/Cardene SR?

Take it as soon as you remember. If it is almost time for your next dose, skip the one you missed and go back to your regular schedule. Do not take 2 doses at the same time.

How should I store Cardene/Cardene SR?

Store at room temperature, away from light and moisture.

CARDIZEM/CARDIZEM CD/ CARDIZEM LA/CARDIZEM SR

Generic name: Diltiazem hydrochloride

What is Cardizem/Cardizem CD/Cardizem LA/Cardizem SR?

Cardizem and Cardizem CD (a controlled release form of diltiazem) are used to treat chest pain usually caused by lack of oxygen to the heart due to clogged arteries (angina). Cardizem and Cardizem LA (an extended release, once-a-day tablet form of diltiazem) are used to treat angina caused by exertion. Cardizem CD and Cardizem LA are also used to treat high blood pressure. Cardizem SR is used only for the treatment of high blood pressure.

What is the most important information I should know about Cardizem/Cardizem CD/Cardizem LA/Cardizem SR?

Cardizem does not cure high blood pressure; it only controls it. You must continue to take Cardizem regularly.

If you are taking Cardizem for chest pain, do not stop suddenly. This can lead to an increase in your attacks.

Who should not take Cardizem/Cardizem CD/Cardizem LA/ Cardizem SR?

Do not take Cardizem if you have sick sinus syndrome or types of irregular heartbeat known as second- or third-degree heart block, unless you have a ventricular pacemaker. Avoid Cardizem if you've just suffered a heart attack or have lung congestion.

Do not take Cardizem if you have low blood pressure or if you are allergic to the drug.

What should I tell my doctor before I take the first dose of Cardizem/Cardizem CD/Cardizem LA/Cardizem SR?

Tell your doctor about all prescription, over-the-counter, and herbal medication you are taking before beginning treatment with Cardizem. Also, talk to your doctor about your complete medical history, especially if you have chronic heart failure, kidney disease, or liver disease.

What is the usual dosage?

The information below is based on the dosage guidelines your doctor uses. Depending on your condition and medical history, your doctor may prescribe a different regimen. Do not change the dosage or stop taking your medication without your doctor's approval.

Cardizem
Adults: The average daily dose is 180 milligrams (mg) to 360 mg, divided into 3 or 4 smaller doses.

Cardizem CD
Adults: This is a once-a-day form of Cardizem. For high blood pressure, starting doses range from 180-240 mg. For chest pain, doses range from 120-180 mg.

Cardizem LA
Adults: This is a once-a-day form of Cardizem. For high blood pressure, when used alone, doses start at 180-240 mg and may be increased to as much as 540 mg once daily. For chest pain, the starting dose is 180 mg once daily with increases every 7-14 days if needed.

Cardizem SR
Adults: The initial dosage is 60-120 mg taken 2 times a day. The usual dose is 240-360 mg a day.

How should I take Cardizem/Cardizem CD/Cardizem LA/Cardizem SR?

Take Cardizem before meals and at bedtime. Cardizem CD, Cardizem LA, and Cardizem SR should be swallowed whole.

Take Cardizem exactly as prescribed by your doctor, even if you do not have any symptoms.

What are possible food and drug interactions associated with Cardizem/Cardizem CD/Cardizem LA/Cardizem SR?

If Cardizem is taken with certain other drugs, the effects of either could be increased, decreased, or altered. It is especially important to check with your doctor before combining Cardizem with the following: beta-blockers, such as atenolol or propranolol; carbamazepine; cimetidine; cyclosporine; digoxin; lovastatin; midazolam; rifampin; and triazolam.

What are the possible side effects of Cardizem/Cardizem CD/Cardizem LA/Cardizem SR?

Side effects cannot be anticipated. If any develop or change in intensity, tell your doctor as soon as possible. Only your doctor can determine if it is safe for you to continue taking this drug.

Side effects may include: abnormally slow heartbeat, dizziness, fatigue, fluid retention, flushing, headache, nausea, rash, weakness

Can I receive Cardizem/Cardizem CD/Cardizem LA/Cardizem SR if I am pregnant or breastfeeding?

The effects of Cardizem during pregnancy and breastfeeding are unknown. Tell you doctor immediately if you are pregnant, plan to become pregnant, or you are breastfeeding.

What should I do if I miss a dose of Cardizem/Cardizem CD/Cardizem LA/Cardizem SR?

If you forget to take a dose, take it as soon as you remember. If it is almost time for your next dose, skip the missed dose and go back to your regular schedule. Never take 2 doses at the same time.

How should I store Cardizem/Cardizem CD/Cardizem LA/Cardizem SR?

Store at room temperature away from moisture.

CARDURA

Generic name: Doxazosin mesylate

What is Cardura?

Cardura is used to treat the symptoms associated with an enlarged prostate gland (benign prostatic hypertrophy). Cardura is also used to treat high blood pressure.

What is the most important information I should know about Cardura?

If you have high blood pressure, you must take Cardura regularly for it to be effective. Since blood pressure declines gradually, it may be several weeks before you get the full benefit of Cardura. You must continue taking Cardura even if you are feeling well. Cardura does not cure blood pressure; it only keeps it under control.

Cardura can cause a sudden drop in blood pressure after the very first dose. You may feel dizzy, faint, or lightheaded, especially after you stand up from a lying or sitting position. This is more likely to occur after you've taken the first few doses or if you increase your dose, but can occur at any time while you are taking the drug. It can also occur if you stop taking the drug and then restart treatment. If you feel very dizzy, faint, or lightheaded, you should contact your doctor.

Who should not take Cardura?

Do not use Cardura if you are sensitive to or have ever had an allergic reaction to it or to drugs such as prazosin or terazosin.

What should I tell my doctor before I take the first dose of Cardura?

Tell your doctor about all prescription, over-the-counter, and herbal medications you are taking before beginning treatment with Cardura. Also, talk to your doctor about your complete medical history, especially if you have liver disease or are taking drugs that affect liver function. Prostate cancer may cause the same symptoms as an enlarged prostate gland. Prostate cancer should be ruled out before you start taking this medication.

What is the usual dosage?

The information below is based on the dosage guidelines your doctor uses. Depending on your condition and medical history, your doctor may prescribe a different regimen. Do not change the dosage or stop taking your medication without your doctor's approval.

Your Cardura dosage must be individualized.

Enlarged Prostate Gland
Adults: The starting dose of Cardura is 1 milligram (mg) daily. Depending on your response, dosage may be increased to 2 mg and then, if needed, to 4 mg or 8 mg. The maximum recommended dose is 8 mg daily.

High Blood Pressure
Adults: The initial dose is 1 mg daily. Depending on your response, dosage may be increased to 2 mg and then, if needed, to 4 mg, 8 mg, and 16 mg daily.

How should I take Cardura?

This medication can be taken with or without food. Cardura should be taken exactly as prescribed, even if you have no symptoms. Take this medication regularly otherwise your condition may worsen.

What should I avoid while taking Cardura?

Cardura can cause low blood pressure. You should avoid driving or any hazardous tasks for 24 hours after taking the first dose, after your dose has been increased, or if you stopped taking Cardura and then restarted the medication.

Cardura can cause drowsiness. Avoid participating in any activity that requires full mental alertness.

What are possible food and drug interactions associated with Cardura?
If Cardura is taken with certain other drugs, the effects of either could be increased, decreased, or altered. Always check with your doctor before combining Cardura with any other drugs, herbs, or supplements.

What are the possible side effects of Cardura?
Side effects cannot be anticipated. If any develop or change in intensity, tell your doctor as soon as possible. Only your doctor can determine if it is safe for you to continue taking this drug.

Side effects may include: dizziness, drowsiness, fatigue, headache

Side effects may increase as the dose increases.

Rarely, Cardura can cause a painful, long-lasting erection that lasts for hours. This condition can lead to impotence. Contact your doctor right away if you experience this.

Can I receive Cardura if I am pregnant or breastfeeding?
The effects of Cardura during pregnancy and breastfeeding are unknown. Talk with your doctor before taking this drug if you are pregnant or plan to become pregnant. Avoid breastfeeding if you are taking Cardura.

What should I do if I miss a dose of Cardura?
Take it as soon as you remember. If it is almost time for your next dose, skip the dose you missed and go back to your regular schedule. Never take 2 doses at the same time.

How should I store Cardura?
Store Cardura at room-temperature.

CARDURA XL
Generic name: Doxazosin mesylate, extended-release

What is Cardura XL?
Cardura XL is indicated for the treatment of the signs and symptoms of benign prostatic hyperplasia, a condition in which the prostate gland grows larger and may block the flow of urine from the bladder. The drug relieves symptoms such as weak urine stream, dribbling, incomplete emptying of the bladder, frequent urination, and burning during urination.

What is the most important information I should know about Cardura XL?
Dizziness from low blood pressure may occur within a few hours of taking Cardura XL. You should be aware that dizziness or fainting may occur,

especially within the first few doses, if your doctor increases the dose of Cardura XL, or if you miss a few doses and restart your regimen. If this happens, avoid situations such as driving, operating machinery, or performing hazardous tasks from which injury could result.

Who should not take Cardura XL?

You should not take Cardura XL if you have severe liver problems. Also, patients allergic to other quinazolines such as prazosin or terazosin; doxazosin; or any ingredients of Cardura XL should not take this medication.

What should I tell my doctor before I take the first dose of Cardura XL?

Always tell your doctor about all the prescription, over-the-counter, and herbal medicines you are taking, as well as your medical history. Also, tell your doctor if you are going to have surgery, or if you have digestive problems, constipation, or liver problems.

What is the usual dosage?

The information below is based on the dosage guidelines your doctor uses. Depending on your condition and medical history, your doctor may prescribe a different regimen. Do not change the dosage or stop taking your medication without your doctor's approval.

Adults: The usual dose of Cardura XL is 4 milligrams (mg) given once daily with breakfast. The maximum recommended dose is 8 mg daily. If Cardura XL is discontinued for several days, therapy should be restarted with the 4 mg once-daily dose.

If switching from Cardura to Cardura XL, therapy should be initiated with the lowest dose (4 mg once daily). Prior to starting therapy with Cardura XL, the final evening dose of Cardura should not be taken.

How should I take Cardura XL?

Cardura XL should be taken each day with breakfast. Swallow Cardura XL whole; do not crush, chew, divide, or cut the tablets.

What should I avoid while taking Cardura XL?

Avoid situations such as driving, operating machinery, or performing hazardous tasks while receiving initial or increased doses.

What are possible food and drug interactions associated with Cardura XL?

Caution should be taken when taking Cardura XL with atanazavir, clarithromycin, indinavir, itraconazole, ketoconazole, nefazodone, nelfinavir, ritonavir, saquinavir, telithromycin, or voriconazole.

What are the possible side effects of Cardura XL?
Side effects cannot be anticipated. If any develop or change in intensity, tell your doctor as soon as possible. Only your doctor can determine if it is safe for you to continue taking this drug.

Side effects may include: back pain, breathing problems, headache, low blood pressure/dizziness, muscle pain, muscle weakness, nausea, respiratory infection, sleepiness, stomach pain, upset stomach, urinary tract infection

Can I receive Cardura XL if I am pregnant or breastfeeding?
Women should not take Cardura XL.

What should I do if I miss a dose of Cardura XL?
If you miss a singe dose of Cardura XL, take the dose as soon as you remember it. However, if it is almost time for your next dose, skip the dose you missed and return to your regular dosing schedule. Do not double the dose. Contact your doctor if you have missed doses of Cardura XL for several days in a row.

How should I store Cardura XL?
Store at room temperature.

Carisoprodol See Soma, page 1204.

Carvedilol See Coreg, page 337.

Carvedilol phosphate, extended-release See Coreg CR, page 340.

CATAPRES
Generic name: Clonidine hydrochloride

What is Catapres?
Catapres is used alone or with other medications to treat high blood pressure.

What is the most important information I should know about Catapres?
If you have high blood pressure, you must take Catapres regularly for it to be effective. Since blood pressure declines gradually, it may be weeks before you get the full benefit of Catapres. You must continue taking it even if you are feeling well. Catapres does not cure high blood pressure; it only keeps it under control.

Do not stop taking Catapres without consulting your physician.

Catapres may cause you to become tired. You should use caution if you are using Catapres and engage in potentially hazardous activities (eg, driving, operating machinery). Using alcohol or drugs (eg, barbiturates) that may cause you to become tired may make you more tired if you combine them with Catapres.

If you are using Catapres patch and develop an allergic reaction, rash, vesicles, or severe redness at the treatment site, contact your physician. You may also develop an allergic reaction or skin rash if you discontinue using the Catapres patch and begin taking Catapres oral tablets. If you experience a mild skin irritation at the treatment site while using Catapres patch before completing the full 7 days of therapy, you may remove the Catapres patch and replace it with a new Catapres patch to a different site on your body.

If you are using the Catapres patch and it begins to loosen from your skin, use the adhesive cover that is included with the Catapres system and place it directly over the patch to ensure that the patch will stay on you for the remaining days of your dosing cycle.

Used Catapres patches will continue to contain large amounts of the drug. It is therefore important for you to keep both used and unused patches out of the reach of children and to dispose of used Catapres patches properly. Following the use of a Catapres patch, fold the adhesive side in half and discard it out of children's reach.

Who should not take Catapres?
Do not take Catapres if you have ever had an allergic reaction to it or to any of the ingredients of the transdermal patch.

What should I tell my doctor before I take the first dose of Catapres?
Tell your doctor about all prescription, over-the-counter, and herbal medication you are taking before beginning treatment with Catapres. Also, talk to your doctor about your complete medical history, especially if you have heart disease, kidney failure, had a stroke, or have recently had a heart attack.

What is the usual dosage?
The information below is based on the dosage guidelines your doctor uses. Depending on your condition and medical history, your doctor may prescribe a different regimen. Do not change the dosage or stop taking your medication without your doctor's approval.

Tablets
Adults: The usual starting dose is 0.1 milligrams (mg) taken 2 times a day. The regular dose of Catapres is determined by increasing the daily

dose by 0.1 mg at weekly intervals until the desired response is achieved. A larger portion of the increased dose can be taken at bedtime to reduce the potential side effects of drowsiness and dry mouth that may appear when you begin taking this drug.

The most common effective dosages range from 0.2 mg to 0.6 mg per day, divided into smaller doses.

Your doctor will adjust your dose according to your individual response to the medication.

Transdermal Patch
Adults: The patch comes in different strengths. Your doctor will determine which is best for you based on your blood pressure response. Apply the patch to either the outer part of your upper arm or to your chest area. The spot where the patch is applied should be hairless and not contain any cuts or bruises. The patch should be worn for 7 days and then taken off and replaced with a new patch. The new patch should not be applied to the same exact spot.

If you are using another blood pressure medication, do not stop taking it abruptly when you first begin using the patch, because the patch may take a few days to begin working. The other medication should be discontinued slowly as the patch begins to take effect.

How should I take Catapres?
Take Catapres exactly as prescribed, even if you are feeling well. Do not miss any doses. If Catapres is not taken regularly, your condition may get worse.

The Catapres patch should be put on a hairless, clean area of the outer upper arm or chest. Normally, a new patch is applied every 7 days to a new area of the skin. If the patch becomes loose, use the adhesive cover that is included with the Catapres system and place it directly over the Catapres patch to help keep the patch in place.

What should I avoid while taking Catapres?
Do not stop taking Catapres suddenly. Headache, nervousness, agitation, tremor, confusion, and rapid rise in blood pressure can occur. Your doctor should gradually reduce your dosage over several days to avoid withdrawal symptoms.

Catapres may cause drowsiness. Avoid driving, operating dangerous machinery, or participating in any hazardous activity that requires full mental alertness.

A used Catapres patch still contains enough medication to be harmful to children and pets. Fold the patch in half with the adhesive sides together and dispose of it out of the reach of children and pets.

Catapres may increase the effects of alcohol. Do not drink while taking Catapres.

What are possible food and drug interactions associated with Catapres?

If Catapres is taken with certain other drugs, the effects of either could be increased, decreased, or altered. It is especially important to check with your doctor before combining Catapres with the following: alcohol, barbiturates, beta-blocker drugs, calcium channel blockers, digitalis, sedatives, and tricyclic antidepressants.

What are the possible side effects of Catapres?

Side effects cannot be anticipated. If any develop or change in intensity, tell your doctor as soon as possible. Only your doctor can determine if it is safe for you to continue taking this drug.

Side effects may include: (Oral tablets): dry mouth, drowsiness, constipation, sedation.

(Patch): dry mouth, drowsiness, fatigue, headache, lethargy, sedation, insomnia, dizziness, impotence, dry throat, constipation, nausea, change in taste, nervousness, skin reactions at the treatment site (redness, itchiness, vesicles at the site, darkening of the skin at the site, swelling at the site, burning at the site), rash

Can I receive Catapres if I am pregnant or breastfeeding?

The effects of Catapres during pregnancy are not completely known. Notify your physician if you are pregnant or planning to become pregnant prior to beginning therapy with either Catapres tablets or patches.

Catapres is found in breast milk. Talk with your physician if you are breastfeeding and are planning to begin therapy with Catapres tablets or patches.

What should I do if I miss a dose of Catapres?

If you forget to take a Catapres tablet, take the tablet as soon as you remember it. If it is almost time for your next dose, skip the missed dose and return to your normal dosing schedule. Do not take a double dose.

Contact your physician if you have missed applying the Catapres patch at the appropriate time.

How should I store Catapres?

Store Catapres tablets at room temperature in a tightly closed container, away from light. Store Catapres patches below 86°F (30°C).

CEDAX
Generic name: Ceftibuten

What is Cedax?
Cedax is a cephalosporin antibiotic used to treat mild to moderate bacterial infections of the throat, ear, and respiratory tract in children and adults. Cedax is also used to treat acute flare-ups of chronic bronchitis in adults.

What is the most important information I should know about Cedax?
If you are allergic to either penicillin or cephalosporin antibiotics in any form, check with your doctor before taking Cedax. There is a possibility that you are allergic to both types of medication and if a reaction occurs, it could be extremely severe. If you take the drug and feel any signs of this reaction (symptoms include swelling of the face, lips, tongue, and throat; making it difficult to breathe), seek medical attention immediately.

It is also important to know that the Cedax Oral Suspension contains 1 gram of sucrose per teaspoon of suspension.

Who should not take Cedax?
If you are sensitive to or have ever had an allergic reaction to Cedax, or other cephalosporins such as cephalexin, do not take this medication.

What should I tell my doctor before I take the first dose of Cedax?
Tell your doctor about all prescription, over-the-counter, and herbal medications you are taking before beginning treatment with Cedax. Also, talk to your doctor about your complete medical history, especially if you have diabetes and are taking Cedax suspension; if you have a history of gastrointestinal disease such as inflammation of the large intestines (colitis); or if you have kidney disease.

What is the usual dosage?
The information below is based on the dosage guidelines your doctor uses. Depending on your condition and medical history, your doctor may prescribe a different regimen. Do not change the dosage or stop taking your medication without your doctor's approval.

Adults: The usual dose is 400 milligrams (mg) taken once a day, usually for a duration of 10 days. If you have serious kidney problems, your doctor may prescribe a smaller dose.

Children: Cedax oral suspension is taken once daily, for a usual duration of 10 days. The usual dose is determined by the child's weight.

22 pounds: 1 teaspoon
44 pounds: 2 teaspoons
88 pounds: 4 teaspoons

Children weighing more than 100 pounds receive the adult dose. Cedax has not been tested for treatment in infants less than 6 months old.

How should I take Cedax?

To make certain your infection is fully cleared up, take all the Cedax your doctor prescribes, even if you begin to feel better after the first few days.

Take Cedax suspension at least 2 hours before a meal or at least 1 hour after a meal. Remember to refrigerate the suspension and discard any unused medication after 14 days. Shake the suspension well.

What should I avoid while taking Cedax?

Do not stop taking Cedax before you complete the full course of therapy because doing so may lead to new infections that are more difficult to treat.

What are possible food and drug interactions associated with Cedax?

If Cedax is taken with certain other drugs, the effects of either could be increased, decreased, or altered. It is especially important to check with your doctor before combining Cedax with ranitidine.

What are the possible side effects of Cedax?

Side effects cannot be anticipated. If any develop or change in intensity, tell your doctor as soon as possible. Only your doctor can determine if it is safe for you to continue taking this drug.

Side effects in adults may include: diarrhea, headache, nausea, upset stomach

Side effects in children may include: diarrhea (especially in children under 2 years of age)

Can I receive Cedax if I am pregnant or breastfeeding?

The effects of Cedax during pregnancy and breastfeeding are unknown. Tell your doctor immediately if you are pregnant, plan to become pregnant, or are breastfeeding.

What should I do if I miss a dose of Cedax?

Take it as soon as you remember. If it is almost time for your next dose, skip the dose you missed and go back to your regular schedule. Never take 2 doses at the same time.

How should I store Cedax?

Store Cedax oral suspension in the refrigerator, and discard any unused portion after 14 days.

Store Cedax capsules at room temperature, away from moisture.

Cefadroxil monohydrate *See Duricef, page 454.*

Cefdinir *See Omnicef, page 939.*

Cefditoren *See Spectracef, page 1211.*

Cefixime *See Suprax, page 1231.*

Cefprozil *See Cefzil, page 269.*

Ceftibuten *See Cedax, page 264.*

CEFTIN

Generic name: Cefuroxime axetil

What is Ceftin?

Ceftin is a cephalosporin antibiotic used to treat mild to moderate bacterial infections. Ceftin tablets are used to treat infections of the ear, respiratory tract, sinuses, skin, throat, and urinary tract. Ceftin tablets are also used to treat gonorrhea as well as early stage Lyme disease.

Ceftin suspension is used to treat infections of the ear, throat, and skin in children 3 months to 12 years of age.

What is the most important information I should know about Ceftin?

If you are allergic to either penicillin or cephalosporin antibiotics, such as cefaclor, cefprozil, or cephalexin, consult your doctor before taking Ceftin. There is a possibility that you are allergic to both types of medication. If a reaction occurs, it could be extremely severe. If you take Ceftin and develop shortness of breath, pounding heartbeat, skin rash, or hives, seek medical attention immediately.

Who should not take Ceftin?

Do not take Ceftin if you are allergic to it or to any other cephalosporin antibiotics.

Do not take Ceftin suspension if you are a phenylketonuric. Ceftin suspension contains phenylalanine.

What should I tell my doctor before I take the first dose of Ceftin?

Tell your doctor about all prescription, over-the-counter, and herbal medications you are taking before beginning treatment with Ceftin. Also, talk to your doctor about your complete medical history, especially if you are taking blood-thinning medications; have a history of inflammation of the large intestine (colitis); kidney disease; or liver disease.

What is the usual dosage?
The information below is based on the dosage guidelines your doctor uses. Depending on your condition and medical history, your doctor may prescribe a different regimen. Do not change the dosage or stop taking your medication without your doctor's approval.

Adults and adolescents >13 years of age: The usual dose is 250 milligrams (mg) taken 2 times a day for up to 10 days. For more severe infections, the dose may be increased to 500 mg taken 2 times a day.

Bronchitis
The usual dose is 250 or 500 mg taken 2 times a day for 5-10 days.

Early Lyme Disease
The usual dose is 500 mg taken 2 times a day for 20 days.

Gonorrhea
The usual treatment is a single dose of 1 gram.

Sinus Infection
The usual dose is 250 mg taken 2 times a day for 10 days.

Skin Infection
The usual dose is 250 or 500 mg taken 2 times a day for 10 days.

Throat and Tonsil Infections
The usual dose is 250 mg taken 2 times a day for 10 days.

Urinary Tract Infections
The usual dose is 250 mg taken twice a day for 7-10 days.

Children 3 months to 12 years of age: Ceftin oral suspension may be given. Your doctor will determine the dosage based on your child's weight and the type of infection being treated. Ceftin oral suspension is given twice a day for 10 days. The maximum daily dose range is 500-1000 mg.

For children who are able to swallow tablets whole, the usual dosage for ear infection or sinus infection is 250 mg taken 2 times a day for 10 days.

Be sure to refrigerate the suspension and shake well before using.

How should I take Ceftin?
Ceftin tablets can be taken on a full or empty stomach.

Ceftin oral suspension must be taken with food. Shake the suspension well before each use.

What should I avoid while taking Ceftin?

Take Ceftin only when it is prescribed by your doctor, even if you have symptoms that are similar to those of a previous infection. Continued or prolonged use of Ceftin can lead to new infections that do not respond to Ceftin.

What are possible food and drug interactions associated with Ceftin?

If Ceftin is taken with certain other drugs, the effects of either could be increased, decreased, or altered. It is especially important to check with your doctor before combining Ceftin with the following: lomotil, probenecid, strong water pills (diuretics) such as furosemide.

What are the possible side effects of Ceftin?

Side effects cannot be anticipated. If any develop or change in intensity, tell your doctor as soon as possible. Only your doctor can determine if it is safe for you to continue taking this drug.

Side effects may include: diaper rash in infants, diarrhea, nausea, vomiting

Ceftin has also been reported to occasionally cause allergic reactions, blood disorders, inflammation of the large intestines, kidney and liver problems, yellowing of the skin and eyes, peeling skin, seizures, and severe blisters in the mouth and eyes.

Can I receive Ceftin if I am pregnant or breastfeeding?

The effects of Ceftin during pregnancy and breastfeeding are unknown. Tell your doctor immediately if you are pregnant, plan to become pregnant, or are breastfeeding.

What should I do if I miss a dose of Ceftin?

Take it as soon as you remember. If it is almost time for your next dose, skip the dose you missed and go back to the regular schedule. Do not take 2 doses at once.

How should I store Ceftin?

Store tablets at room temperature in a tightly closed container, away from moisture.

The oral suspension may be stored in the refrigerator or at room temperature. Discard any unused suspension after 10 days.

Cefuroxime axetil *See Ceftin, page 266.*

CEFZIL
Generic name: Cefprozil

What is Cefzil?
Cefzil is a cephalosporin antibiotic that is used to treat mild to moderately severe bacterial infections of the ear, respiratory tract, sinuses, skin, and throat.

What is the most important information I should know about Cefzil?
If you are allergic to penicillin or cephalosporin antibiotics in any form, consult your doctor before taking Cefzil. You may be allergic to Cefzil, and if a reaction occurs it could be extremely severe. If you take the drug and feel signs of a reaction, seek medical attention immediately.

Who should not take Cefzil?
Do not take Cefzil if you are sensitive to or have ever had an allergic reaction to this drug or to similar products.

What should I tell my doctor before I take the first dose of Cefzil?
Tell your doctor about all prescription, over-the-counter, and herbal medications you are taking before beginning treatment with Cefzil. Also, talk to your doctor about your complete medical history, especially if you are diabetic, have kidney disease, or if you take oral contraceptives.

What is the usual dosage?
The information below is based on the dosage guidelines your doctor uses. Depending on your condition and medical history, your doctor may prescribe a different regimen. Do not change the dosage or stop taking your medication without your doctor's approval.

Bronchitis
Adults (>13 years): 500 milligrams (mg) every 12 hours for 10 days.

Ear Infections
Infants and children (6 months to 12 years): 15 mg per 2.2 pounds of body weight given every 12 hours for 10 days.

Pharyngitis/Tonsillitis
Adults (>13 years): 500 mg given once a day for 10 days.

Children (2 years to 12 years): 7.5 mg per 2.2 pounds of body weight given every 12 hours for 10 days.

Sinus Infection
Adults (>13 years): 250 mg given every 12 hours for 10 days. For moderate to severe infections the dose is 500 mg given every 12 hours for 10 days.

Infants and children (6 months to 12 years): 7.5 mg per 2.2 pounds of body weight given every 12 hours for 10 days or 15 mg per 2.2 pounds of body weight given every 12 hours for 10 days.

Skin Infections

Adults (>13 years): 250 mg given every 12 hours for 10 days, or 500 mg given once daily for 10 days, or 500 mg given every 12 hours for 10 days.

Children (2 to 12 years of age): 20 mg per 2.2 pounds of body weight given once a day for 10 days.

How should I take Cefzil?

Cefzil is taken by mouth with or without food. Take Cefzil with food to avoid stomach upset.

Shake Cefzil oral suspension well before you use it.

What should I avoid while taking Cefzil?

Do not stop taking Cefzil even if you feel better. Not completing the full dosage schedule may decrease the drug's effectiveness and increase the chances that the bacteria may become resistant to Cefzil and similar antibiotics.

What are possible food and drug interactions associated with Cefzil?

If Cefzil is taken with certain other drugs, the effects of either could be increased, decreased, or altered. It is especially important to check with your doctor before combining Cefzil with the following: certain antibiotics such as amikacin, certain strong diuretics such as ethacrynic acid or furosemide, oral contraceptives, probenecid, propantheline.

What are the possible side effects of Cefzil?

Side effects cannot be anticipated. If any develop or change in intensity, tell your doctor as soon as possible. Only your doctor can determine if it is safe for you to continue taking this drug.

Side effects may include: abdominal pain, confusion, diaper rash, diarrhea, difficulty sleeping, dizziness, genital itching, headache, hives, hyperactivity, nervousness, rash, sleepiness, superinfection (additional infection), vaginal inflammation, vomiting, yellow eyes and skin

Can I receive Cefzil if I am pregnant or breastfeeding?

The effects of Cefzil during pregnancy and breastfeeding are unknown. Tell your doctor immediately if you are pregnant, plan to become pregnant, or are breastfeeding.

What should I do if I miss a dose of Cefzil?

Take it as soon as you remember. If it is almost time for your next dose, skip the dose you missed and go back to your regular schedule. Never take 2 doses at the same time.

How should I store Cefzil?

Store Cefzil tablets at room temperature. Keep the oral suspension in the refrigerator and throw away any unused portion after 14 days.

CELEBREX

Generic name: Celecoxib

What is Celebrex?

Celebrex is used to treat acute pain, menstrual cramps, pain and inflammation due to osteoarthritis, rheumatoid arthritis of the spine (ankylosing spondylitis), and rheumatoid arthritis.

Celebrex is also used to reduce the number of growths in the wall of the lower intestine and rectum (colorectal polyps) in people with a condition called familial adenomatous polyposis, an inherited tendency to develop large numbers of colorectal polyps that eventually become cancerous.

What is the most important information I should know about Celebrex?

Like other nonsteroidal anti-inflammatory drugs (NSAIDs), Celebrex could increase the risk of having a heart attack or stroke, possibly resulting in death. The risk is greater if you have heart disease or use NSAIDs for a long time.

Although Celebrex is easy on the stomach, it still poses some degree of risk, especially if you have had a stomach ulcer or gastrointestinal bleeding in the past. All NSAIDs, including Celebrex, can cause serious, and even life-threatening, ulcers and bleeding in the stomach and intestines. These side effects can happen without symptoms and may occur at any time during treatment. If you've ever had ulcers or stomach bleeding, let your doctor know. Be sure to alert your doctor if you develop any digestive problems or notice a change in your bowel movements (such as blood in the stool or black, sticky stools).

Who should not take Celebrex?

Do not take Celebrex right before or after heart bypass surgery (coronary artery bypass graft, or CABG).

Do not use Celebrex if you are allergic to it or to sulfonamide drugs such as sulfadiazine, sulfamethizole, sulfamethoxazole, or sulfisoxazole. Avoid using Celebrex if you have ever had an asthma attack, experienced face and throat swelling, or skin eruptions after taking aspirin or other NSAIDs.

Celebrex has not been studied in children less than 18 years old.

What should I tell my doctor before I take the first dose of Celebrex?

Tell your doctor about all prescription, over-the-counter, and herbal medications you are taking before beginning treatment with Celebrex. Also, talk to your doctor about your complete medical history, especially if you have had any stomach ulcers or bleeding in the past. Tell your doctor if you have asthma, heart failure, high blood pressure, if you are taking a steroid medication for your arthritis, have kidney or liver disease, or if you are prone to anemia.

What is the usual dosage?

The information below is based on the dosage guidelines your doctor uses. Depending on your condition and medical history, your doctor may prescribe a different regimen. Do not change the dosage or stop taking your medication without your doctor's approval.

The following dosages are typically reduced in half for people with moderate liver problems.

Acute Pain and Menstrual Cramps

Adults: The recommended starting dose is 400 milligrams (mg), followed by an additional 200 mg if needed on the first day. On subsequent days, the recommended dosage is 200 mg taken twice a day.

Ankylosing Spondylitis

Adults: The recommended dose is 200 mg taken once a day, or 100 mg taken twice a day. If there is no effect after 6 weeks, the doctor may increase your dose to 400 mg. If there is no effect after 6 weeks at this higher dose, other treatments should be considered.

Familial Adenomatous Polyposis

Adults: The recommended dose is 400 mg taken twice a day with food.

Osteoarthritis

Adults: The recommended dose is 200 mg, taken as a singe dose or as two 100-mg doses.

Rheumatoid Arthritis

Adults: The recommended dose is 100-200 mg taken twice a day.

Juvenile Rheumatoid Arthritis

Children >2 years of age: From 22 to 55 pounds, the dose is 50 mg twice daily. For children over 55 pounds, the dose is 100 mg twice daily.

How should I take Celebrex?

Take Celebrex exactly as prescribed. You can take it with or without food. If you have difficulty swallowing capsules, the contents of a Celebrex capsule can be added to applesauce. Carefully empty the entire contents of the capsule onto a level teaspoon of cool or room temperature applesauce and ingest immediately with water. The sprinkled capsule contents on applesauce are stable for up to 6 hours under refrigerated conditions.

What should I avoid while taking Celebrex?

Avoid taking Celebrex if you also take steroid drugs or blood thinners, smoke, drink alcohol, or if you have been using other NSAIDs for a long time.

If you are taking a steroid medication for your arthritis, do not discontinue it abruptly when you begin therapy with Celebrex.

What are possible food and drug interactions associated with Celebrex?

If Celebrex is taken with certain other drugs, the effects of either could be increased, decreased, or altered. It is especially important to check with your doctor before combining Celebrex with the following: ACE-inhibitors such as captopril, enalapril, or lisinopril; blood-thinning agents such as warfarin; fluconazole; furosemide; lithium; methotrexate; thiazide diuretics (water pills) such as hydrochlorothiazide or hydrochlorothiazide with triamterene.

If you take low-dose aspirin to protect against heart attack, you can continue taking it with Celebrex. Using aspirin increases your risk of stomach ulcers or bleeding, but Celebrex does not have aspirin's protective effect on the heart.

What are the possible side effects of Celebrex?

Side effects cannot be anticipated. If any develop or change in intensity, tell your doctor as soon as possible. Only your doctor can determine if it is safe for you to continue taking this drug.

Side effects may include: abdominal pain, diarrhea, headache, indigestion, itching, nausea, respiratory infection, sinus inflammation

Serious side effects include: heart attack, stroke, high blood pressure, kidney problems, allergic reactions, asthma attacks if you have a history of asthma

Celebrex may cause serious skin reactions such as Stevens-Johnson syndrome (marked by blisters of the eyes, mouth, and skin) and toxic epidermal necrosis (marked by large patches of red, peeling skin). If you have a skin reaction, stop taking Celebrex and seek medical attention immediately.

If you develop symptoms of liver poisoning, stop taking the drug and see your doctor immediately. Warning signs include nausea, fatigue, itching, yellowish skin, pain in the right side of the stomach, and flu-like symptoms.

Can I receive Celebrex if I am pregnant or breastfeeding?
Celebrex can harm a developing baby if taken during the third trimester. Take Celebrex during pregnancy only if the risk is justified. It is possible that Celebrex makes its way into breast milk and could cause serious reactions in a nursing infant. If Celebrex is essential to your health, your doctor may advise you to stop breastfeeding.

What should I do if I miss a dose of Celebrex?
Take it as soon as you remember. If it is almost time for your next dose, skip the dose you missed and go back to your regular schedule. Do not take 2 doses at the same time.

How should I store Celebrex?
Store Celebrex at room temperature.

Celecoxib *See Celebrex, page 271.*

CELEXA
Generic name: Citalopram hydrobromide

What is Celexa?
Celexa is a medication for the treatment of depression that persists nearly every day for at least two weeks and interferes with everyday living.

What is the most important information I should know about Celexa?
Celexa is not approved for use in children or adolescents.

Antidepressant medicines may increase suicidal thoughts or actions in some children, teenagers, and young adults when the medicine is first started. Depression and other serious mental illnesses are the most important causes of suicidal thoughts and actions. Some people may have a particularly high risk of having suicidal thoughts or actions. These include people who have (or have a family history of) bipolar disorder (also called manic-depressive illness) or suicidal thoughts or actions.

Pay close attention to any changes, especially sudden changes, in mood, behaviors, thoughts, or feelings. This is very important when an antidepressant medicine is first started or when the dose is changed.

Call the doctor right away to report new or sudden changes in mood, behavior, thoughts, or feelings. Signs to watch for include new or worsening depression, new or worsening anxiety, agitation, insomnia, hostility, panic attacks, restlessness, extreme hyperactivity, and suicidal thinking or behavior.

Keep all follow-up visits as scheduled, and call the doctor between visits as needed, especially if you have concerns about symptoms.

Who should not take Celexa?
Do not take Celexa if you are taking pimozide or a monoamine oxidase inhibitor (MAOI) or if you have stopped taking an MAOI in the last 14 days.

Do not take if you are allergic to Celexa or any of its components.

What should I tell my doctor before I take the first dose of Celexa?
Tell your doctor about all prescription, over-the-counter, and herbal medications you are taking before beginning treatment with Celexa. Also, talk to your doctor about your complete medical history, especially if you are taking MAOIs or other antidepressants, migraine drugs known as triptans, or tramadol. Tell your doctor if you have heart disease, high blood pressure, kidney or liver disease, or have ever had seizures.

What is the usual dosage?
The information below is based on the dosage guidelines your doctor uses. Depending on your condition and medical history, your doctor may prescribe a different regimen. Do not change the dosage or stop taking your medication without your doctor's approval.

Adults: The recommended starting dose of Celexa tablets or oral solution is 20 milligrams (mg) taken once a day. Dosage is usually increased to 40 mg taken once a day after at least a week has passed. The maximum dose is 40 mg a day.

For older adults and individuals with liver problems, the recommended dose is 20 mg taken once a day.

How should I take Celexa?
Celexa should be taken once a day. You can take it either in the morning or in the evening with or without food.

What should I avoid while taking Celexa?
Use caution when driving or operating dangerous equipment until you are familiar with Celexa's effects.

Do not abruptly discontinue Celexa. Abrupt discontinuation may result in irritability, agitation, dizziness, emotional ups and downs, headache, or sleepiness.

Do not take Lexapro while you are taking Celexa, since the two drugs are similar and could have increased effects.

What are possible food and drug interactions associated with Celexa?

If Celexa is taken with certain other drugs, the effects of either could be increased, decreased, or altered. It is especially important to check with your doctor before combining Celexa with any of the following: antidepressants, carbamazepine, cimetidine, digoxin, ketoconazole, lithium, metoprolol, omeprazole, pimozide, sumatriptan, theophylline, triazolam, and warfarin.

Never combine Celexa with any drug classified as an MAOI. Drugs in this category include the antidepressants phenelzine and tranylcypromine. Celexa and MAOIs should not be taken together or within 14 days of each other. Combining these drugs with Celexa can cause serious and even fatal reactions such as high body temperature, muscle rigidity, twitching, and agitation leading to delirium and coma.

What are the possible side effects of Celexa?

Side effects cannot be anticipated. If any develop or change in intensity, tell your doctor as soon as possible. Only your doctor can determine if it is safe for you to continue taking this drug.

Side effects may include: abdominal pain, agitation, anxiety, diarrhea, drowsiness, dry mouth, ejaculation disorders, fatigue, impotence, indigestion, insomnia, loss of appetite, nausea, painful menstruation, respiratory tract infection, sinus or nasal inflammation, sweating, tremor, vomiting

Can I receive Celexa if I am pregnant or breastfeeding?

The effects of Celexa during pregnancy and breastfeeding are unknown. Tell your doctor immediately if you are pregnant, plan to become pregnant, or are breastfeeding.

What should I do if I miss a dose of Celexa?

Take it as soon as you remember. If it is almost time for your next dose, skip the dose you missed and go back to your regular schedule. Do not take two doses at the same time.

How should I store Celexa?

Store at room temperature.

CELLCEPT

Generic name: Mycophenolate mofetil

What is Cellcept?

Cellcept is indicated for the prevention of organ rejection in patients receiving kidney, heart, and liver transplants. It is used together with corticosteroids and cyclosporine.

What is the most important information I should know about Cellcept?

The use of Cellcept and other immunosuppressive drugs increases the susceptibility to infection and lymphomas. It is important that a qualified doctor follow up on the patient.

Any female of childbearing potential must use highly effective (two methods) contraception 4 weeks prior to starting Cellcept therapy and continue contraception until 6 weeks after stopping Cellcept treatment, unless abstinence is the chosen method of contraception.

Who should not take Cellcept?

Patients with hypersensitivity to Cellcept and the ingredients in this preparation should not take this medication.

What should I tell my doctor before I take the first dose of Cellcept?

Tell your doctor about all prescription, over-the-counter, and herbal medications you are taking before beginning treatment with Cellcept. Also, talk to your doctor about your complete medical history, especially if you are pregnant or plan on becoming pregnant.

What is the usual dosage?

The information below is based on the dosage guidelines your doctor uses. Depending on your condition and medical history, your doctor may prescribe a different regimen. Do not change the dosage or stop taking your medication without your doctor's approval.

Heart Transplant
Adults: The usual dose is 1.5 grams (g) given intravenously (IV) or by mouth twice daily.

Liver Transplant
Adults: The usual dose is 1 g IV twice daily, or 1.5 g taken by mouth twice daily.

Kidney Transplant
Adults: The usual dose is 1 g IV or taken by mouth twice daily.

Children (oral suspension): The usual dose is 600 milligrams (mg)/m^2 twice daily; the maximum dose is 2 g/10 milliliters (ml).

How should I take Cellcept?

Take Cellcept on an empty stomach with a full glass of water.

What should I avoid while taking Cellcept?

Due to an increased risk for infection and disease, you should avoid vaccinations (live vaccines), pregnancy, excessive sunlight, and concomitant use with azathioprine.

What are possible food and drug interactions associated with Cellcept?

If Cellcept is taken with certain other drugs, the effects of either could be increased, decreased, or altered. It is especially important to check with your doctor before combining Cellcept with the following: acyclovir, antacids such as aluminum and magnesium, cholestyramine, cyclosporine, ganciclovir, iron, live vaccines, metronidazole, norfloxacin, oral contraceptives, rifampin, sevelamer, and trimethoprim/sulfamethoxazole.

What are the possible side effects of Cellcept?

Side effects cannot be anticipated. If any develop or change in intensity, tell your doctor as soon as possible. Only your doctor can determine if it is safe for you to continue taking this drug.

Side effects may include: diarrhea, constipation, nausea, vomiting, headache, hypertension, excess fluid, leucopenia, cough, increased susceptibility to infection, pain, hyperglycemia, insomnia

Can I receive Cellcept if I am pregnant or breastfeeding?

The effects of Cellcept on pregnancy and breastfeeding are unknown. Tell your doctor if you are pregnant, plan on becoming pregnant, or are breastfeeding. Effective contraception (at least two methods) is required (beginning 4 weeks before therapy and continuing for 6 weeks after Cellcept therapy has stopped).

What should I do if I miss a dose of Cellcept?

If you miss a dose, take it as soon as you remember. If it is close to the time of your next dose, skip it and resume your scheduled dose. Do not double your dose.

How should I store Cellcept?

Store at room temperature and away from children. Protect from light and moisture.

The suspension should also be kept at room temperature. For the suspension, discard any unused portion after 60 days.

CENESTIN

Generic name: Synthetic conjugated estrogens

What is Cenestin?

This medication is indicated for use by women after menopause to reduce hot flashes, and treat dryness, itching, and burning in and around the vagina. Cenestin is a mixture of estrogen hormones. It works by replacing natural estrogens in a woman who can no longer produce enough estrogen.

What is the most important information I should know about Cenestin?

Estrogens increase the chances of getting cancer of the uterus. Report any unusual vaginal bleeding right away while you are taking estrogens. Vaginal bleeding after menopause may be a warning sign of cancer of the uterus. Your healthcare provider should check any unusual vaginal bleeding to find out the cause.

Do not use estrogens with or without progestins to prevent heart disease, heart attacks, or strokes. Using estrogens with or without progestins may increase your chances of getting heart attack, strokes, breast cancer, and blood clots (risk increases with smoking, especially for women older than 35 years of age). You and your healthcare provider should talk regularly about whether you still need treatment with Cenestin.

Cenestin may cause dizziness. These effects may be worse if you take it with alcohol or certain medicines. Use Cenestin with caution. Do not drive or perform other possibly unsafe tasks until you know how you react to it.

Cenestin may affect your blood sugar. Check blood sugar levels closely. Ask your doctor before you change the dose of your diabetes medicine.

Cenestin may cause dark skin patches on your face (melasma). Exposure to the sun may make these patches darker, and you may need to avoid prolonged sun exposure and sunlamps. Consult your doctor regarding the use of sunscreens and protective clothing.

If you wear contact lenses and you develop problems with them, contact your doctor.

If you will be having surgery or will be confined to a chair or bed for a long period of time (eg, a long plane flight), notify your doctor beforehand. Special precautions may need to be taken in these circumstances if you are taking Cenestin.

Who should not take Cenestin?

Do not start taking Cenestin if you have unusual vaginal bleeding, currently have or had certain cancers, had a stroke or heart attack in the past year, currently have or have had blood clots, and currently have or had liver problems. Also, do not take Cenestin if you are allergic to the drug or any of its ingredients, or if you think you may be pregnant.

What should I tell my doctor before I take the first dose of Cenestin?

Tell your doctor about all prescription, over-the-counter, and herbal medications you are taking before beginning treatment with Cenestin. Also, talk to your doctor about your complete medical history, especially if you have asthma; seizures; migraine; depression; diabetes; endometriosis; gallbladder disease; obesity; pancreatitis; uterine fibroids; if you smoke; have problems with your heart, liver, thyroid, kidneys; have high calcium levels in your blood; lupus; and if you plan on becoming pregnant or are breastfeeding.

What is the usual dosage?
The information below is based on the dosage guidelines your doctor uses. Depending on your condition and medical history, your doctor may prescribe a different regimen. Do not change the dosage or stop taking your medication without your doctor's approval.

Moderate to Severe Vasomotor Symptoms (such as hot flashes)
Adults: 0.45 milligram (mg)/day; may be titrated up to 1.25 mg/day. Attempts to discontinue medication should be made at 3 to 6-month intervals.

Vulvar and Vaginal Atrophy
Adults: 0.3 mg/day.

How should I take Cenestin?
Take one Cenestin tablet by mouth with food or immediately after a meal each day. Taking Cenestin with food may reduce or prevent stomach upset. Take Cenestin at the same time each day.

What should I avoid while taking Cenestin?
The use of Cenestin increases the chance of having a cardiovascular event such as a heart attack, stroke, the development of a clot in your veins, and the development of a clot in your lungs. The use of tobacco products (eg, smoking) increases the likelihood of one these events occurring. Therefore, avoid the use of tobacco products (eg, smoking) while you are taking Cenestin.

What are possible food and drug interactions associated with Cenestin?
If Cenestin is taken with certain other drugs, the effects of either could be increased, decreased, or altered. It is especially important to check with your doctor before combining Cenestin with the following: aminoglutethimide, carbamazepine, clarithromycin, levothyroxine, nafcillin, nevirapine, phenobarbital, rifampin, St. John's wort.

What are the possible side effects of Cenestin?
Side effects cannot be anticipated. If any develop or change in intensity, tell your doctor as soon as possible. Only your doctor can determine if it is safe for you to continue taking this drug.

Side effects may include: headaches, bloating, depression, diarrhea, dizziness, flu syndrome, gas, increased/decreased interest in sex, nervousness, sleeplessness, sore throat, infection, indigestion, weakness, weight changes, breast pain, irregular vaginal bleeding or spotting, stomach cramps, nausea and vomiting, hair loss

Can I receive Cenestin if I am pregnant or breastfeeding?
Tell your doctor immediately if you are pregnant, plan to become pregnant, or are breastfeeding.

Estrogens are not indicated for use during pregnancy or the immediate postpartum (after birth) period. Do not use Cenestin if you are breastfeeding a baby.

What should I do if I miss a dose of Cenestin?
If you miss a dose, take it as soon as possible. If it is almost time for your next dose, skip the missed dose and go back to your normal schedule. Do not take 2 doses at the same time.

How should I store Cenestin?
Store Cenestin at room temperature. Store away from heat, moisture, and light. Do not store in the bathroom. Keep Cenestin out of the reach of children.

Cephalexin hydrochloride *See Keflex, page 683.*

CESAMET
Generic name: Nabilone

What is Cesamet?
Cesamet is used to treat nausea and vomiting that follow chemotherapy in patients who have failed to respond adequately to other anti-nausea treatments.

What is the most important information
I should know about Cesamet?
Cesamet should be used with caution in the elderly and those with high blood pressure or heart disease. Cesamet should also be used with caution in patients with psychiatric disorders (including manic depressive illness, depression, and schizophrenia); disease symptoms may return with the use of this drug.

The effects of Cesamet may last for an indefinite time period after taking by mouth. Adverse psychiatric effects can last for 48 to 72 hours after treatment. Cesamet may cause dizziness, drowsiness, euphoria or a "high" feeling, anxiousness, depression, hallucinations, and psychosis.

Taking Cesamet for long periods of time may cause dependence or addiction. If you stop taking Cesamet suddenly, you may experience withdrawal symptoms which include anxiousness, distress, hiccups, loose stools, runny nose, sweating, and trouble sleeping.

Who should not take Cesamet?
You should not take Cesamet if you are allergic to any cannabinoids.

What should I tell my doctor before I take the first dose of Cesamet?
Tell your doctor about all the prescription, over-the-counter, and herbal medications you are taking. Also, talk to your doctor about your complete medical history, especially if you have a history of high or low blood pressure, heart disease, irregular or fast heart beat, liver or kidney problems, mental or mood disorders such as depression or bipolar disorder, a history of alcohol abuse or drug abuse or dependence, or if you are pregnant, going to become pregnant, nursing or are going to have surgery.

What is the usual dosage?
The information below is based on the dosage guidelines your doctor uses. Depending on your condition and medical history, your doctor may prescribe a different regimen. Do not change the dosage or stop taking your medication without your doctor's approval.

Adults: The usual dose of Cesamet is 1-2 milligrams (mg) two times a day, 1-3 hours before chemotherapy. The maximum daily dose is 6 mg given in divided doses three times a day.

Cesamet may be administered 2 or 3 times daily during the entire course of each cycle of chemotherapy and if needed, for 48 hours after the last dose of each cycle of chemotherapy.

How should I take Cesamet?
Take Cesamet by mouth as prescribed by your doctor.

What should I avoid while taking Cesamet?
Avoid potentially hazardous activities, such as driving or operating machinery while taking Cesamet.

If you have a history of substance abuse, including drug or alcohol abuse, Cesamet may not be for you. Do not take Cesamet with alcohol, sedatives or sleep medicines, of other drugs that affect your brain.

What are possible food and drug interactions associated with Cesamet?
If Cesamet is taken with certain other drugs, the effects of either could be increased, decreased, or altered. It is especially important to check with your doctor before combining Cesamet with the following: alcohol, amphetamines, antihistamines, atropine, barbiturates, benzodiazepines, buspirone, cocaine, disulfiram, fluoxetine, lithium, naltrexone, opioids, scopolamine, sedatives, and theophylline.

What are the possible side effects of Cesamet?

Side effects cannot be anticipated. If any develop or change in intensity, tell your doctor as soon as possible. Only your doctor can determine if it is safe for you to continue taking this drug.

Side effects may include: change in appetite, difficulty concentrating, dizziness/spinning feeling, drowsiness, dry mouth, euphoria (feeling "high"), headache, poor coordination, trouble sleeping, weakness

Can I receive Cesamet if I am pregnant or breastfeeding?

The effects of Cesamet during pregnancy and breastfeeding are unknown. Tell your doctor immediately if you are pregnant, plan to become pregnant, or are breastfeeding.

What should I do if I miss a dose of Cesamet?

If you miss a dose of Cesamet, take it as soon as you remember. If it is almost time for your next dose, skip the missed dose and go back to your regular dosing schedule. Do not double the dose.

How should I store Cesamet?

Store Cesamet at room temperature away from the reach of children.

Cetirizine hydrochloride See Zyrtec, page 1510.

Cetirizine hydrochloride and pseudoephedrine hydrochloride See Zyrtec D, page 1512.

CHANTIX

Generic name: Varenicline

What is Chantix?

Chantix is a prescription medicine to help adults stop smoking.

What is the most important information I should know about Chantix?

Your body may undergo changes if you stop smoking (with or without Chantix). These changes may alter the dosage of other medications you are taking. If you experience agitation, depressed mood, changes in behavior that are not typical of you, or if you develop suicidal behavior, stop taking Chantix and notify your doctor immediately.

Tell your doctor if you have or ever had depression before beginning Chantix therapy.

When you try to quit smoking, with or without Chantix, you may experience symptoms that may be due to nicotine withdrawal. These symptoms include the urge to smoke, depressed mood, trouble sleeping, irritability, frustration, weight gain, and others.

Who should not take Chantix?
Chantix is not recommended for children under 18 years of age. Do not take Chantix if you are allergic to any of its ingredients.

What should I tell my doctor before I take the first dose of Chantix?
Tell your doctor about all prescription, over-the-counter, and herbal medications you are taking before beginning treatment with Chantix. Also, talk to your doctor about your entire medical history, especially if you are using insulin, asthma medicine, or blood thinners. Also tell your doctor if you have ever had depression or other mental health problems, and if you have kidney problems or receive kidney dialysis, since this may require a lower dose.

What is the usual dosage?
The information below is based on the dosage guidelines your doctor uses. Depending on your condition and medical history, your doctor may prescribe a different regimen. Do not change the dosage or stop taking your medication without your doctor's approval.

Adults: From Day 1 to Day 3, the usual dosage of Chantix is 1 white tablet (0.5 milligram [mg]). From Day 4 to Day 7, dosage increases to 2 white tablets, one in the morning and one at night. Day 8 to the end of treatment consists of 2 blue tablets (1 mg each), once in the morning and once at night.

How should I take Chantix?
First, choose a date when you will stop smoking. Start taking Chantix 7 days before your quit date, as this lets Chantix build up in your body. You can keep smoking during this time. Be sure to stop smoking on your quit date, and continue to take Chantix as directed.

Take Chantix after eating and with a full glass of water.

What should I avoid while taking Chantix?
Avoid smoking after the seventh day of taking Chantix.

Use caution when driving or operating machinery until you know how quitting smoking with Chantix may affect you.

What are the possible side effects of Chantix?
Side effects cannot be anticipated. If any develop or change in intensity, tell your doctor as soon as possible. Only your doctor can determine if it is safe for you to continue taking this drug.

Side effects may include: changes in dreaming or sleeping pattern, constipation, gas, nausea, vomiting

Can I receive Chantix if I am pregnant or breastfeeding?
The effects of Chantix during pregnancy and breastfeeding are unknown. Tell your doctor immediately if you are pregnant, plan to become pregnant, or are breastfeeding.

What should I do if I miss a dose of Chantix?
If you miss a dose, take it as soon as you remember. If it is close to the time for your next dose, wait and take your next regular dose. Do not take a double dose.

How should I store Chantix?
Store at room temperature.

Chlordiazepoxide hydrochloride *See Librium, page 747.*

Chlordiazepoxide hydrochloride and clidinium bromide *See Librax, page 745.*

Chlorhexidine gluconate *See Peridex, page 1009.*

Chlorothiazide *See Diuril, page 435.*

Chlorpheniramine and pseudoephedrine *See Deconamine, page 385.*

Chlorpropamide *See Diabinese, page 412.*

Chlorthalidone *See Thalitone, page 1299.*

Cholestyramine *See Questran, page 1112.*

CIALIS
Generic name: Tadalafil

What is Cialis?
Cialis is a prescription medicine taken by mouth for the treatment of erectile dysfunction (ED) in men. Cialis may help a man with ED get and keep an erection when he is sexually excited.

What is the most important information I should know about Cialis?
Cialis can cause your blood pressure to drop suddenly to an unsafe level if it is taken with some other medicines. You could get dizzy, faint, or have a heart attack or stroke.

Cialis does not cure ED, increase a man's sexual desire, serve as a male form of birth control, or protect a man or his partner from sexually transmitted diseases, including HIV.

Do not drive or perform other possibly unsafe tasks until you know how you react to this medication. Cialis may cause dizziness, drowsiness, fainting, or blurred vision. These effects may be worse if you take it with alcohol or certain medicines. Use Cialis with caution.

Do not drink large amounts of alcohol (5 drinks or more) while you take this medicine. Doing so may increase your risk of dizziness, headache, fast heartbeat, and low blood pressure.

Cialis may rarely cause a prolonged, painful erection. This could happen even when you are not having sex. If this is not treated right away, it could lead to permanent sexual problems such as impotence. Contact your doctor right away if this happens.

Cialis may uncommonly cause mild, temporary vision changes such as blurred vision, sensitivity to light, and blue/green color tint to vision. Contact your doctor if vision changes persist or are severe.

Stop sexual activity and get medical help right away if you get symptoms such as chest pain, dizziness, or nausea during sex. Sexual activity can put an extra strain on your heart, especially if your heart is already weak from a heart attack or heart disease.

Cialis is only for men over the age of 18 who have ED, including men with diabetes or who have undergone prostatectomy. Cialis is not for women or children.

Cialis must be used only under a healthcare provider's care.

Who should not take Cialis?

Do not use Cialis if you are allergic to any of its ingredients. Also, do not take this drug if you are taking nitrates, which are commonly used to treat angina (a symptom of heart disease). Cialis is not for those who have had a heart attack within the past 90 days or who had a stroke within the past 6 months. Cialis is not recommended for men who have been told to abstain from sex. Sexual activity can put an extra strain on your heart, especially if your heart is already weak from a heart attack or heart disease. Cialis is not for women or children.

What should I tell my doctor before I take the first dose of Cialis?

Tell your doctor about all prescription, over-the-counter, and herbal medications you are taking before beginning treatment with Cialis. Also, talk to your doctor about your complete medical history, especially if you have heart problems, high or low blood pressure, had a heart attack, had a stroke, are taking nitrates, have liver or kidney problems, eye disease, severe vision loss, stomach ulcers, bleeding problems, a deformed penis, or blood problems.

What is the usual dosage?

The information below is based on the dosage guidelines your doctor uses. Depending on your condition and medical history, your doctor may prescribe a different regimen. Do not change the dosage or stop taking your medication without your doctor's approval.

For Use as Needed
Adults: The usual starting dose of Cialis is 10 milligrams (mg) daily. Increase to 20 mg or decrease to 5 mg daily is based on efficacy and tolerability.

For Once-daily Use
Adults: The usual dose is 2.5 mg taken once daily without regard to timing of sexual activity. This dose may be increased to 5 mg based upon efficacy and tolerability.

How should I take Cialis?

For use as needed: Take Cialis at least 30 minutes before sexual activity, as directed by your doctor. Cialis may work for up to 36 hours after you take it.

For daily use: Take Cialis regularly at about the same time each day.

Talk with your doctor if you have questions about how you should take Cialis.

What should I avoid while taking Cialis?

Do not drink heavily; excess alcohol can increase your chances of getting a headache or getting dizzy, increasing your heart rate, or lowering your blood pressure.

Cialis may cause dizziness, drowsiness, fainting, or blurred vision. These effects may be worse if you take it with alcohol or certain medicines. Use Cialis with caution. Do not drive or perform other possibly unsafe tasks until you know how you react to this medication.

What are possible food and drug interactions associated with Cialis?

If Cialis is taken with certain other drugs, the effects of either could be increased, decreased, or altered. It is especially important to check with your doctor before combining Cialis with the following: erythromycin, grapefruit juice, HIV protease inhibitors, itraconazole, ketoconazole, nitrates, and rifampin.

What are the possible side effects of Cialis?

Side effects cannot be anticipated. If any develop or change in intensity, tell your doctor as soon as possible. Only your doctor can determine if it is safe for you to continue taking this drug.

Side effects may include: back pain, flushing, dizziness, stomach upset, headache, indigestion, muscle aches, stuffy or runny nose

Can I receive Cialis if I am pregnant or breastfeeding?
Cialis is not for women or children.

What should I do if I miss a dose of Cialis?
If you are taking Cialis as needed and you miss a dose but you still intend to engage in sexual activity, take it as soon as you remember. Continue to take it as directed by your doctor.

If you are taking Cialis daily and you miss a dose, take it as soon as possible. If it is almost time for your next dose, skip the missed dose and go back to your regular dosing schedule. Do not take 2 doses at once.

How should I store Cialis?
Store Cialis at room temperature. Store away from heat, moisture, and light. Do not store in the bathroom. Keep Cialis out of the reach of children.

Ciclopirox *See Penlac, page 993.*

Ciclopriox *See Loprox, page 761.*

CILOXAN
Generic name: Ciprofloxacin hydrochloride

What is Ciloxan?
Ciloxan is an antibiotic used in the treatment of eye infections. The ointment form of the drug is prescribed for eye inflammations. The solution can also be used to treat ulcers or sores on the cornea (the transparent covering over the pupil). Ciprofloxacin, the active ingredient, is a member of the quinolone family of antibiotics.

What is the most important information I should know about Ciloxan?
Other forms of ciprofloxacin have been known to cause allergic reactions in a few patients. These reactions can be extremely serious, leading to loss of consciousness and cardiovascular collapse. Early warning signs include a skin rash, hives, and itching. Other symptoms may include swelling of the face or throat, shortness of breath, and a tingling feeling. If you develop any of these symptoms, seek emergency help immediately.

When treating corneal ulcers with Ciloxan solution, you may notice a white buildup on the surface of the ulcer. This usually disappears within a week or two, and is no cause for concern.

Prolonged use of Ciloxan sometimes promotes the growth of germs that are unaffected by the medication. The doctor will examine your eyes for signs of this development.

The ointment form of Ciloxan may slow down healing of the cornea and cause blurred vision.

Safety and effectiveness have not been established in children under 2 years of age for Ciloxan ointment, or under 1 year of age for the solution.

Who should not take Ciloxan?

If you've ever had an allergic reaction to a quinolone antibiotic such as ciprofloxacin hydrochloride, gatifloxacin, levofloxacin, moxifloxacin hydrochloride, norfloxacin, or ofloxacin, you should not use this medication.

What should I tell my doctor before I take the first dose of Ciloxan?

Tell your doctor about all prescription, over-the-counter, and herbal medications you are taking before beginning treatment with this drug. Also, talk to your doctor about your complete medical history, especially if you are allergic to any medication.

What is the usual dosage?

The information below is based on the dosage guidelines your doctor uses. Depending on your condition and medical history, your doctor may prescribe a different regimen. Do not change the dosage or stop taking your medication without your doctor's approval.

Eye Inflammation
Ointment: Apply a ½-inch ribbon on the inner eyelid 3 times a day for the first 2 days, then 2 times a day for the next 5 days.

Solution: Apply 1 or 2 drops every 2 hours for the first 2 days, then every 4 hours for the next 5 days.

Corneal Ulcers
Solution: Apply 2 drops in the affected eye every 15 minutes for the first 6 hours, then every 30 minutes for the rest of the first day. On the second day, apply 2 drops every hour. On the third through fourteenth days, apply 2 drops every 4 hours. Treatment can continue for more than 14 days if healing doesn't occur.

How should I take Ciloxan?

Ciloxan ointment should be applied in a ribbon on the inner eyelid. Ciloxan solution is administered with an eyedropper.

What should I avoid while taking Ciloxan?

Be careful to avoid touching the dropper tip to the eye or any other surface, since this could contaminate the solution.

What are possible food and drug interactions associated with Ciloxan?

There is no information on interactions with Ciloxan. When taken internally, however, ciprofloxacin is known to interact with the following: caffeine, cyclosporine, theophylline, and warfarin.

What are the possible side effects of Ciloxan?

Side effects cannot be anticipated. If any develop or change in intensity, tell your doctor as soon as possible. Only your doctor can determine if it is safe for you to continue taking this drug.

Side effects may include: formation of crystals on the eye surface (with frequent application of solution only), eye burning or discomfort

Can I receive Ciloxan if I am pregnant or breastfeeding?

The effects of Ciloxan during pregnancy have not been adequately studied. If you are pregnant or plan to become pregnant, alert your doctor immediately. Researchers do not know whether Ciloxan makes its way into breast milk; when ciprofloxacin is taken internally, it appears in breast milk. Be cautious if using Ciloxan while nursing.

What should I do if I miss a dose of Ciloxan?

Take the forgotten dose as soon as you remember. However, if it is almost time for your next dose, skip the one you missed and return to your regular schedule. Do not take two doses at once.

How should I store Ciloxan?

Store at room temperature. Protect the solution from light.

Cimetidine *See Tagamet, page 1252.*

CIPRO

Generic name: Ciprofloxacin

What is Cipro?

Cipro is used to treat multiple types of bacterial infection, such as urinary tract infections, cystitis (inflammation of the bladder), and prostatitis (inflammation of the prostate [men]), lower respiratory tract infection, sinus infection, skin infection, bone and joint infection, abdominal infection, infectious diarrhea, and typhoid infections.

What is the most important information I should know about Cipro?

Cipro should not be used during pregnancy or nursing.

Serious and fatal reactions have occurred when Cipro and theophylline have been taken concomitantly.

Cipro should be discontinued if there are symptoms of pain, burning, tingling, numbness, or weakness in your hands, fingers, and feet.

Cipro has been associated with an increased rate of adverse events involving joints and tendons in patients less than 18 years of age. Tendons in the shoulder, hands, or the Achilles tendon (back of the ankle) may rupture, resulting in surgery and disability. Rest and avoid exercise until further instruction from your doctor if you experience pain or swelling of a tendon.

Do not drive or perform other possibly unsafe tasks until you know how you react to Cipro. It may cause drowsiness, dizziness, blurred vision, or lightheadedness. These effects may be worsened by alcohol or certain other medicines.

Be sure to take Cipro for the full course of therapy. If you do not, the medicine may not clear up your infection completely. The bacteria could also become less sensitive to Cipro or other antibiotics in the future.

Cipro may affect your blood sugar, so check your blood sugar regularly if you have diabetes. You may also be more sensitive to the sun while taking Cipro. If you get sunburned, talk to your doctor immediately.

Mild diarrhea is common with antibiotic use. However, a more serious form of diarrhea, although rare, may occur. Contact your doctor right away if you experience stomach pain or cramps, severe diarrhea, or bloody stools. Do not treat the diarrhea without first checking with your doctor.

Who should not take Cipro?
Do not take Cipro if you are allergic to any of its ingredients or to any other quinolone antibiotic like Cipro. Also, you should not take this medication if you are already taking tizanidine.

What should I tell my doctor before I take the first dose of Cipro?
Tell your doctor about all prescription, over-the-counter, and herbal medications you are taking before beginning treatment with Cipro. Also, talk to your doctor about your complete medical history, especially if you have liver or kidney problems, a history of irregular heart beat, Alzheimer's disease, brain or nervous system disorders, diarrhea, a stomach infection, seizures, inflammation of your tendons, joints problems, or skin sensitivity to the sun.

What is the usual dosage?
The information below is based on the dosage guidelines your doctor uses. Depending on your condition and medical history, your doctor may prescribe a different regimen. Do not change the dosage or stop taking your medication without your doctor's approval.

The usual dosage of Cipro is determined by the kind of infection, how severe it is, what kind of organism is infectious, your immune system, and your kidney and liver function. The usual duration of therapy is 7-14 days; however, severe and complicated infections may require longer treatment.

Acute Sinusitis
Adults: Mild/Moderate: 500 mg every 12 hours for 10 days.

Bone and Joint Infection
Adults: Mild/Moderate: 500 mg every 12 hours for 4 to 6 weeks. Severe/Complicated: 750 mg every 12 hours for 4 to 6 weeks.

Chronic Bacterial Prostatitis Infection
Adults: Mild/Moderate: 500 mg every 12 hours for 28 days.

Lower Respiratory Tract Infection
Adults: Mild/Moderate: 500 mg every 12 hours for 7 to 14 days. Severe/Complicated: 750 mg every 12 hours for 7 to 14 days.

Infectious Diarrhea
Adults: Mild/Moderate/Severe: 500 mg every 12 hours for 5 to 7 days.

Inhalational Anthrax (post-exposure)
Adults: 500 mg every 12 hours for 60 days.

Children: (I.V.) 10 mg per 2.2 pounds of body weight (maximum 400 mg per dose) every 12 hours for 60 days.

(Oral) 15 mg per 2.2 pounds of body weight (maximum 500 mg per dose) every 12 hours for 60 days.

Intra-Abdominal Infection (used with metronidazole)
Adults: Complicated: 500 mg every 12 hours for 7 to 14 days.

Skin and Skin Structure
Adults: Mild/Moderate: 500 mg every 12 hours for 7 to 14 days. Severe/Complicated: 750 mg every 12 hours for 7 to 14 days.

Typhoid Fever
Adults: Mild/Moderate: 500 mg every 12 hours for 10 days.

Urethral and Cervical Gonococcal Infections
Adults: Uncomplicated: 250 mg single dose.

Urinary Tract Infection or Pyelonephritis
Adults: Acute Uncomplicated: 250 mg every 12 hours for 3 days. Mild/Moderate: 250 mg every 12 hours for 7 to 14 days. Severe/Complicated: 500 mg every 12 hours for 7 to 14 days.

Children 1 to 17 years old: (I.V.) 6 to 10 mg per 2.2 pounds of body weight (maximum 400 mg per dose; not to be exceeded even in patients weighing more than 112 pounds) every 8 hours for 10 to 21 days. (Oral) 10 to 20 mg per 2.2 pounds of body weight (maximum 750 mg per dose; not to be exceeded even in patients weighing more than 112 pounds) every 12 hours for 10 to 21 days.

How should I take Cipro?

Cipro can be given orally (tablets or oral suspension), or administered intravenously (I.V.) in a hospital setting. Take with or without food.

Cipro should be administered at least 2 hours before or 6 hours after magnesium/aluminum antacids, or sucralfate, Videx (didanosine) chewable/buffered tablets or pediatric powder for oral solution, other highly buffered drugs, or other products containing calcium, iron or zinc.

Take Cipro with a full glass of water at the same time each day. Drink several glasses of water a day unless otherwise directed by your doctor.

What should I avoid while taking Cipro?

Avoid taking Cipro with dairy products (like milk and yogurt) and calcium-fortified juices, since they may affect the absorption of Cipro. Avoid large amounts of food or drink that have caffeine.

Also, avoid excess sunlight and artificial ultraviolet light (UV), such as tanning beds; wear sunscreen or protective clothing if outside in the sun.

Avoid driving or performing possibly unsafe tasks until you know how you react to Cipro. Avoid taking alcohol, which may worsen the effects of drowsiness, dizziness, or blurred vision.

What are possible food and drug interactions associated with Cipro?

If Cipro is taken with certain other drugs, the effects of either could be increased, decreased, or altered. It is especially important to check with your doctor before combining Cipro with the following: antacids; caffeinated food or drinks; calcium-fortified juices; cyclosporine; dairy products; didanosine; food or drink high in iron, magnesium, or zinc; glyburide; methadone; methotrexate; nonsteroidal anti-inflammatory drugs such as ibuprofen; phenytoin; tizanidine; and warfarin.

What are the possible side effects of Cipro?

Side effects cannot be anticipated. If any develop or change in intensity, tell your doctor as soon as possible. Only your doctor can determine if it is safe for you to continue taking this drug.

Side effects may include: anxiousness or nervousness, bloody stools, changes in liver function tests, diarrhea, headache, nausea and vomiting, pain or discomfort in the abdomen, vaginal yeast infection

Can I receive Cipro if I am pregnant or breastfeeding?

Cipro should not be used during pregnancy and breastfeeding. Tell your doctor immediately if you are pregnant, plan to become pregnant, or are breastfeeding.

What should I do if I miss a dose of Cipro?
Do not miss any doses. If you miss a dose of Cipro, take it as soon as you remember. If it is almost time for your next dose, skip the missed dose and go back to your regular dosing schedule. Do not double doses.

How should I store Cipro?
Store the tablets and oral suspension at or below room temperature in a tightly closed container. Store away from heat, moisture and light and out of the reach of children.

CIPRO XR
Generic name: Ciprofloxacin, extended-release

What is Cipro XR?
Cipro XR is an extended-release antibiotic used only for the treatment of urinary tract infections and acute uncomplicated pyelonephritis.

**What is the most important information
I should know about Cipro XR?**
Convulsions have been reported in patients receiving ciprofloxacin. Ciprofloxacin may cause central nervous system events, including dizziness, confusion, tremors, hallucinations, and depression. These reactions may occur following the first dose. If these reactions occur in patients receiving ciprofloxacin, the drug should be discontinued and appropriate measures need to be taken.

Ciprofloxacin should only be used to treat bacterial infections; antibiotics do not treat viral infections (eg, the common cold, flu). Do not take more than 1 Cipro XR tablet per day even if you miss a dose.

Cipro XR and ciprofloxacin immediate-release tablets are not interchangeable.

Cipro XR should be discontinued if there are symptoms of peripheral neuropathy, such as pain, burning, tingling, numbness, or weakness.

Tendons in the shoulder, hands, or the achilles tendon (back of the ankle) may rupture, resulting in surgery and disability. Cipro XR has been associated with an increased rate of adverse events involving joints and tendons in the elderly. Rest and avoid exercise until further instruction from your doctor if you experience pain or swelling of a tendon.

Do not drive or perform other possibly unsafe tasks until you know how you react to this medication. Cipro XR may cause drowsiness, dizziness, blurred vision, or lightheadedness. These effects may be worse if you take it with alcohol or certain medicines.

Be sure to use Cipro XR for the full course of treatment to ensure your infection clears up completely. Bacteria can also become less sensitive to this or other antibiotics if you don't take the entire prescription. This could make the infection harder to treat in the future.

Long-term or repeated use of Cipro XR may cause a secondary infection. Tell your doctor if signs of a second infection occur. Your medicine may need to be changed to treat this.

Cipro XR may affect your blood sugar. Check blood sugar levels closely. Ask your doctor before you change the dose of your diabetes medicine.

Cipro XR may cause you to become sunburned more easily. Avoid the sun, sunlamps, or tanning booths until you know how you react to Cipro XR. Use a sunscreen or wear protective clothing if you must be outside for more than a short time.

Mild diarrhea is common with antibiotic use. However, a more serious form of diarrhea (pseudomembranous colitis) may rarely occur. This may develop while you use the antibiotic or within several months after you stop using it. Contact your doctor right away if stomach pain or cramps, severe diarrhea, or bloody stools occur. Do not treat diarrhea without first checking with your doctor.

If you are also taking sevelamer, do not take it within 4 hours before or after taking Cipro XR.

Who should not take Cipro XR?

Do not use Cipro XR if you have a history of allergic reactions to ciprofloxacin, and any member of the quinolone class of antimicrobial agents (eg, Levaquin, Avelox) or any of the product's components.

You should also not take Cipro XR if you are taking a medication called tizanidine, since serious side effects are likely to occur.

Cipro XR is not recommended for use during pregnancy or nursing as the effects on the unborn child or nursing infant are unknown.

Cipro XR is not recommended for persons >18 years of age.

What should I tell my doctor before I take the first dose of Cipro XR?

Tell your doctor about all prescription, over-the-counter, and herbal medications you are taking before beginning treatment with Cipro XR. Also, talk to your doctor about your complete medical history, especially if you are pregnant, have a history of a brain or nervous system disorder, seizures, liver problems, kidney problems, Alzheimer's disease, inflammation of your tendons, joint problems, or a sensitivity to the sun.

What is the usual dosage?

The information below is based on the dosage guidelines your doctor uses. Depending on your condition and medical history, your doctor may prescribe a different regimen. Do not change the dosage or stop taking your medication without your doctor's approval.

Acute Uncomplicated Pyelonephritis
Adults: The recommended dosage is 1000 (milligrams) mg every 24 hours for 7 to 14 days.

Complicated Urinary Tract Infection
Adults: The recommended dosage is 1000 mg every 24 hours for 7 to 14 days.

Kidney impairment: No dosage adjustment is required for patients with uncomplicated urinary tract infections receiving 500 mg Cipro XR. In patients with complicated urinary tract infections and acute uncomplicated pyelonephritis who have a creatinine clearance of less than 30 mL/min, the dose of Cipro XR should be reduced from 1000 mg to 500 mg daily.

Elderly: No alteration of dosage is necessary for patients older than 65 years with normal kidney function. However, since some older individuals experience reduced kidney function due to their advanced age, care should be taken in dose selection for elderly patients, and kidney function monitoring may be useful in these patients.

Uncomplicated Urinary Tract Infection
Adults: The recommended dosage is 500 mg every 24 hours for 3 days.

How should I take Cipro XR?

Cipro XR should be taken once a day for 3 to 14 days depending on your infection. Take Cipro XR at approximately the same time each day. Cipro XR may be taken with or without meals. Drink plenty of water.

Swallow the Cipro XR tablet whole. Do not split, crush, or chew the tablet.

Many antacids, multivitamins, and other dietary supplements containing magnesium, calcium, aluminum, iron, or zinc can interfere with the absorption of Cipro XR and may prevent it from working. Take Cipro XR either 2 hours before or 6 hours after taking these products. If you are also taking sevelamer, do not take it within 4 hours before or after taking Cipro XR. Make sure to tell your doctor all medications and over-the-counter supplements that you are currently taking.

Avoid large amounts of food or drink containing caffeine (eg, coffee, tea, cocoa, cola, chocolate).

Avoid taking Cipro with milk or milk products (such as yogurt or calcium-enriched juice) alone; however, taking Cipro XR as part of a full meal that contains milk or milk-containing products is fine.

Be sure to use Cipro XR for the full course of treatment. If you do not, the medicine may not clear up your infection completely. The bacteria could also become less sensitive to this or other medicines. This could make the infection harder to treat in the future.

What should I avoid while taking Cipro XR?

Avoid taking Cipro XR with dairy products (such as milk or yogurt) or calcium-fortified juices alone. However, Cipro XR may be taken with a meal that contains these products.

Avoid excessive sunlight or artificial ultraviolet light while receiving Cipro XR.

Do not drive or perform other possibly unsafe tasks until you know how you react to this medication. Cipro may cause drowsiness, dizziness, blurred vision, or lightheadedness. These effects may be worse if you take it with alcohol or certain medicines.

What are possible food and drug interactions associated with Cipro XR?

If Cipro XR is taken with certain other drugs, the effects of either could be increased, decreased, or altered. It is especially important to check with your doctor before combining Cipro XR with the following: aluminum, aminophylline, caffeine, calcium, didanosine, fluvoxamine, glyburide, iron, magnesium, methotrexate, mexiletine, mirtazapine, pentoxifylline, phenytoin, probenecid, theophylline, tizanidine, warfarin, zinc.

What are the possible side effects of Cipro XR?

Side effects cannot be anticipated. If any develop or change in intensity, tell your doctor as soon as possible. Only your doctor can determine if it is safe for you to continue taking this drug.

Side effects may include: nausea, headache, restlessness, vision changes, vomiting, dizziness, diarrhea, upset stomach, rash, sensitivity to sunlight or ultraviolet light, agitation, anxiety, bloody stools, confusion, convulsions, dark urine, depression, easy bruising or bleeding, fever, hallucinations; inflammation, pain or rupture of a tendon, irregular heartbeat, muscle pain, nervousness, nightmares

Can I receive Cipro XR if I am pregnant or breastfeeding?

The effects of Cipro XR during pregnancy and breastfeeding are unknown. Tell your doctor immediately if you are pregnant, plan to become pregnant, or are breastfeeding.

What should I do if I miss a dose of Cipro XR?

If miss a dose of Cipro XR, take your pill as soon as you remember unless it is time to take your next dose. Take your next dose at the usual time. Do not take 2 doses on the same day.

How should I store Cipro XR?

Store at room temperature away from heat, moisture, and light. Do not store in the bathroom.

CIPRODEX
Generic name: Ciprofloxacin and dexamethasone

What is Ciprodex?
Ciprodex is used to treat middle ear infections with drainage through a tube in children >6 months. It is also used to treat outer ear canal infections (also known as "Swimmer's Ear") in children of the same age.

What is the most important information I should know about Ciprodex?
Ciprodex may allow the growth of other bacteria in the ear, such as yeast and fungus. If there is no improvement after 1 week of therapy, other tests should be conducted. If there is still an ear infection after the course of Ciprodex has been completed, or if there are 2 or more episodes of ear infection in 6 months, your doctor may conduct other tests to determine the cause.

Be sure to use Ciprodex for the full course of treatment. If you do not, the medicine may not clear up your infection completely or may create resistant bacteria. This could make the infection harder to treat in the future.

Do not get Ciprodex in your eyes, nose, or throat. If Ciprodex gets in your eyes, immediately flush them with cool tap water.

Talk to your doctor about how to space your doses if you are using other ear drops.

Do not use Ciprodex for other ear infections or conditions without checking with your doctor.

Who should not take Ciprodex?
Do not use Ciprodex if you are allergic to any of its ingredients or if you have a history of allergic reactions to ciprofloxacin or any member of the quinolone class of antimicrobial agents.

Ciprodex is not approved for children <6 months old.

What should I tell my doctor before I take the first dose of Ciprodex?
Tell your doctor about all prescription, over-the-counter, and herbal medications you are taking before beginning treatment with Ciprodex. Also, talk to your doctor about your complete medical history, especially if you have experienced more than 2 ear infections in the past 6 months.

What is the usual dosage?
The information below is based on the dosage guidelines your doctor uses. Depending on your condition and medical history, your doctor may prescribe a different regimen. Do not change the dosage or stop taking your medication without your doctor's approval.

Adults and children >6 years: For both middle ear infections and outer ear canal infections, the usual dosage is 4 drops per infected ear, twice a day (12 hours apart) for 1 week.

How should I take Ciprodex?

Wash your hands before and after using Ciprodex. Shake Ciprodex before each use and warm by holding the bottle in your hands for 1 to 2 minutes.

Do not take this medication by mouth or by injection. Discard unused portion after therapy is completed.

For the middle ear: Lie down with the affected ear facing up. Hold the Ciprodex dropper directly over the ear and place the appropriate number of drops into the ear. Gently press the cartilage flap covering the opening to the ear 5 times in a pumping motion. This will allow the medicine to pass into the middle ear. Keep the ear facing up for at least 1 minute so the medicine can run to the bottom of the ear canal. Switch positions and repeat on the other ear if necessary.

For the outer ear: Lie down or tilt your head so that the affected ear faces up. Gently pull the earlobe up and back to straighten the ear canal. Drop the appropriate number of drops into the ear. Keep the ear facing up for at least 60 seconds so that the medicine can run to the bottom of the ear canal. A clean cotton plug may be gently inserted into the ear canal to prevent the medicine from leaking out. Switch positions and repeat on the other ear if necessary.

What should I avoid while taking Ciprodex?

When bathing, avoid getting the infected ear(s) wet. Also, avoid swimming unless your doctor has told you otherwise. It is important that the infected ears remain clean and dry.

What are possible food and drug interactions associated with Ciprodex?

Some medicines may interact with Ciprodex. However, the risk of interaction with other medicines is low because there is a very small amount, if any, of Ciprodex absorbed into the blood. Inform your doctor of any other medications you are taking before starting treatment with Ciprodex.

What are the possible side effects of Ciprodex?

Side effects cannot be anticipated. If any develop or change in intensity, tell your doctor as soon as possible. Only your doctor can determine if it is safe for you to continue taking this drug.

Side effects may include: abnormal taste, ear congestion, ear debris, ear infection, ear pain, ear residue, irritability, pain

Can I receive Ciprodex if I am pregnant or breastfeeding?

The effects of Ciprodex during pregnancy and breastfeeding are unknown. Tell your doctor immediately if you are pregnant, plan to become pregnant, or are breastfeeding.

What should I do if I miss a dose of Ciprodex?

If you miss a dose of Ciprodex, take it as soon as possible. If it is almost time for your next dose, skip it and continue on your regular dosing schedule. Do not take 2 doses at the same time.

How should I store Ciprodex?

Store Ciprodex at room temperature, between 68° and 77° F. Store away from heat, moisture, and light. Avoid freezing. Do not store in the bathroom. Brief storage at temperatures between 59° and 86°F is permitted. Keep Ciprodex out of the reach of children.

Ciprofloxacin See Cipro, page 290.

Ciprofloxacin and dexamethasone See Ciprodex, page 298.

Ciprofloxacin hydrochloride See Ciloxan, page 288, or Proquin XR, page 1091.

Ciprofloxacin, extended-release See Cipro XR, page 294.

Citalopram hydrobromide See Celexa, page 274.

CLARINEX

Generic name: Desloratadine

What is Clarinex?

Clarinex is an antihistamine used to relieve the symptoms of seasonal and perennial allergic rhinitis, such as watery and itchy eyes, runny nose, sneezing, or hives. It works by blocking the action of histamine, which reduces the symptoms of an allergic reaction.

What is the most important information I should know about Clarinex?

If you have kidney or liver disease, your doctor should cut your starting dose in half.

Do not drive or perform other possibly unsafe tasks until you know how you react to this medication. Clarinex may cause dizziness. This effect may be worse if you take it with alcohol or certain medicines. Use Clarinex with caution.

Do not take Clarinex RediTabs if you have phenylketonuria.

Who should not take Clarinex?

Do not use Clarinex if you are allergic to this product or any of its components.

What should I tell my doctor before I take the first dose of Clarinex?

Tell your doctor about all prescription, over-the-counter, and herbal medications you are taking before beginning treatment with Clarinex. Also, talk to your doctor about your complete medical history, especially if you have kidney or liver disease, phenylketonuria (a genetic disorder in which the body cannot break down the amino acid phenylalanine), or if you have had a severe allergic reaction to loratadine in the past.

What is the usual dosage?

The information below is based on the dosage guidelines your doctor uses. Depending on your condition and medical history, your doctor may prescribe a different regimen. Do not change the dosage or stop taking your medication without your doctor's approval.

Adults and children >12 years: The usual dose is 5 milligrams (mg) taken once a day (1 tablet or 2 teaspoonfuls of syrup). If you have kidney or liver disease, the recommended dose is 5 mg taken every other day.

Children 6 to 11 years: The usual starting dose is 2.5 mg (1 teaspoonful of syrup) taken once a day. One 2.5-mg Clarinex RediTab may also be used.

Children 12 months to 5 years: The usual dose is 1.25 mg (½ teaspoonful) taken once a day. The dose should be given with a dropper that measures milliliters (mL).

Children 6 to 11 months: The usual dose is 1 mg (or 2 mL) taken once a day. The dose should be given with a dropper that measures mL.

A recommended dose has not been established for children with kidney or liver disease.

How should I take Clarinex?

Clarinex can be taken with or without food. Take Clarinex exactly as directed.

Place Clarinex RediTabs on your tongue, where they dissolve quickly. Take the RediTabs immediately after removing them from the blister pack. You can take Clarinex RediTabs with or without water.

What should I avoid while taking Clarinex?

Do not take Clarinex RediTabs if you have phenylketonuria. Do not increase the dose of Clarinex or take it more than once a day.

Do not drive or perform other possibly unsafe tasks until you know how you react to this medication. Clarinex may cause dizziness. This effect may be worse if you take it with alcohol or certain medicines.

What are possible food and drug interactions associated with Clarinex?

If Clarinex is taken with certain other drugs, the effects of either could be increased, decreased, or altered. Always check with your doctor before combining Clarinex with any other drugs, herbs, or supplements.

What are the possible side effects of Clarinex?

Side effects cannot be anticipated. If any develop or change in intensity, tell your doctor as soon as possible. Only your doctor can determine if it is safe for you to continue taking this drug.

Side effects may include: dry mouth, dizziness, headache, indigestion, muscle pain, nausea, painful menstruation, throat inflammation, fatigue, sleepiness, sore throat

Can I receive Clarinex if I am pregnant or breastfeeding?

The effects of Clarinex during pregnancy and breastfeeding are unknown. Tell your doctor immediately if you are pregnant, plan to become pregnant, or are breastfeeding.

What should I do if I miss a dose of Clarinex?

Take it as soon as you remember. If it is almost time for your next dose, skip the dose you missed and go back to your regular schedule. Never take 2 doses at the same time.

How should I store Clarinex?

Store Clarinex between 36° and 77°F in a tightly closed container. Avoid storage at above 86°F. Store away from heat, moisture, and light. Do not store in the bathroom.

Clarithromycin See Biaxin, page 216.

Clarithromycin extended-release tablets See Biaxin XL, page 219.

CLEOCIN T

Generic name: Clindamycin phosphate

What is Cleocin T?

Cleocin T is an antibiotic used to treat acne.

What is the most important information I should know about Cleocin T?

Although applied only to the skin, some of this medication could be absorbed into the bloodstream; and it has been known to cause severe—

sometimes even fatal—colitis (an inflammation of the lower bowel) when taken internally. Symptoms, which can occur a few days, weeks, or months after beginning treatment with this drug, include severe diarrhea, severe abdominal cramps, and the possibility of the passage of blood.

Use with caution if you have hay fever, asthma, or eczema.

Who should not take Cleocin T?
If you are sensitive to or have ever had an allergic reaction to Cleocin T or similar drugs, such as lincomycin, you should not use this medication. Make sure your doctor is aware of any drug reactions you have experienced.

Unless you are directed to do so by your doctor, do not take this medication if you have ever had an intestinal inflammation, ulcerative colitis, or antibiotic-associated colitis.

What should I tell my doctor before I take the first dose of Cleocin T?
Tell your doctor about all prescription, over-the-counter, and herbal medications you are taking before beginning treatment with this drug. Also, talk to your doctor about your complete medical history, especially if you have allergies, asthma, eczema, or gastrointestinal problems.

What is the usual dosage?
The information below is based on the dosage guidelines your doctor uses. Depending on your condition and medical history, your doctor may prescribe a different regimen. Do not change the dosage or stop taking your medication without your doctor's approval.

Adults and children 12 years and older: Apply a thin film of gel, solution, or lotion to the affected area 2 times a day, or use a solution pledget (application pad). Discard a pledget after you have used it once; you may use more than 1 pledget for a treatment. Do not remove the pledget from its foil container until you are ready to use it. If you are using the lotion, shake it well immediately before using.

The safety and effectiveness of Cleocin T have not been established in children less than 12 years old.

How should I take Cleocin T?
Use this medication exactly as prescribed. Excessive use of Cleocin T can cause your skin to become too dry or irritated.

What should I avoid while taking Cleocin T?
Use caution when applying this medication so as not to get it in the eyes, nose, mouth, or skin abrasions. In the event of accidental contact, rinse the affected area with cool water.

What are possible food and drug interactions associated with Cleocin T?

If you have diarrhea while taking Cleocin T, check with your doctor before taking an antidiarrhea medication, as certain drugs may cause your diarrhea to become worse. The diarrhea should not be treated with the commonly used drugs that slow movement through the intestinal tract, such as diphenoxylate hydrochloride or products containing paregoric.

What are the possible side effects of Cleocin T?

Side effects cannot be anticipated. If any develop or change in intensity, tell your doctor as soon as possible. Only your doctor can determine if it is safe for you to continue taking this drug.

Side effects may include: burning, itching, peeling skin, reddened skin, skin dryness

Can I receive Cleocin T if I am pregnant or breastfeeding?

The effects of Cleocin T during pregnancy have not been adequately studied. If you are pregnant or plan to become pregnant, inform your doctor immediately. Cleocin T may appear in breast milk and could affect a nursing infant. If this medication is essential to your health, your doctor may advise you to discontinue breastfeeding your baby until your treatment with this medication is finished.

What should I do if I miss a dose of Cleocin T?

Apply it as soon as you remember. If it is almost time for your next dose, skip the one you missed and go back to your regular schedule.

How should I store Cleocin T?

Store at room temperature. Keep from freezing. Store liquids in tightly closed containers.

CLIMARA PRO

Generic name: Estradiol and levonorgestrel transdermal system

What is Climara Pro?

Climara Pro is a medicine containing the two hormones estrogen and progestin. It is used to reduce the symptoms of menopause, such as hot flashes and osteoporosis (thin and weak bones).

What is the most important information I should know about Climara Pro?

Do not use Climara Pro (estrogen/progestin) to prevent heart disease, heart attacks, or strokes, or dementia. Using it may increase your chances of having heart attacks, strokes, breast cancer, and blood clots.

Using estrogens with progestins may increase your risk of dementia. You and your doctor should talk regularly about whether you still need treatment with this drug.

Climara Pro may cause dizziness. These effects may be worse if you take it with alcohol or certain medicines. Do not drive or perform other possibly unsafe tasks until you know how you react to it.

Talk to your doctor before you take Climara Pro if you drink more than 3 alcoholic drinks per day.

Climara Pro may cause dark skin patches on your face. Exposure to the sun may make these patches darker and you may need to avoid prolonged sun exposure and sunlamps. Consult your doctor regarding the use of sunscreens and protective clothing.

Climara Pro may increase the risk of stroke, heart attack, blood clots, high blood pressure, or similar problems. The risk may be greater if you smoke, especially if you are older than 35 years old.

Contact your doctor if vaginal bleeding of unknown cause occurs. This could be a sign of a serious condition requiring immediate medical attention. Contact your doctor if vaginal discomfort occurs or if you suspect you have developed an infection while taking Climara Pro. Follow your doctor's instructions for examining your breasts and report any lumps immediately.

If you wear contact lenses and you develop problems with them, contact your doctor.

If you will be having surgery or will be confined to a chair or bed for a long period of time (eg, a long plane flight), notify your doctor beforehand. Special precautions may need to be taken in these circumstances while you are taking Climara Pro.

Climara Pro may affect your blood sugar. Check blood sugar levels closely. Ask your doctor before you change the dose of your diabetes medicine.

Climara Pro may affect certain lab test results. Make sure laboratory personnel and your doctors know you take Climara Pro.

Grapefruit and grapefruit juice may increase the risk of side effects of this medication. Talk to your doctor before including grapefruit or grapefruit juice in your diet while you are taking Climara Pro.

Who should not take Climara Pro?
Do not use Climara Pro if you have had your uterus removed (hysterectomy) or if you have had unusual vaginal bleeding, cancer, heart attack or stroke within the year, blood clots, liver problems, or are allergic to any of the drug's ingredients.

What should I tell my doctor before I take the first dose of Climara Pro?
Tell your doctor about all prescription, over-the-counter, and herbal medications you are taking before beginning treatment with Climara Pro. Also,

talk to your doctor about your complete medical history, especially if you have a family history of breast cancer, high blood pressure, vaginal infection or womb problems, abnormal vaginal bleeding, asthma, cancer, heart disease or other heart problems, kidney or liver disease, disease of the pancreas, seizures, lupus, or low thyroid hormone levels. Also, tell your doctor if you are pregnant, plan to become pregnant, breastfeeding, will have surgery, or will be on bed rest.

What is the usual dosage?
The information below is based on the dosage guidelines your doctor uses. Depending on your condition and medical history, your doctor may prescribe a different regimen. Do not change the dosage or stop taking your medication without your doctor's approval.

Use of estrogen, alone or in combination with a progestin, should be with the lowest effective dose and for the shortest duration consistent with treatment goals and risks for the individual woman. Patients should be re-evaluated periodically as clinically appropriate (3-month to 6-month intervals) to determine if treatment is still necessary.

Adults: Climara Pro is applied weekly. The patch delivers 0.045 milligrams (mg) of estradiol per day and 0.015 mg of levonorgestrel per day. The lowest effective dose of this medication has not been determined.

Women not currently using continuous estrogen or combination estrogen/progestin therapy may start therapy with Climara Pro at any time. However, women currently using continuous estrogen or combination estrogen/progestin therapy should complete the current cycle of therapy before initiating Climara Pro therapy. Women often experience withdrawal bleeding at the completion of the cycle. The first day of this bleeding would be an appropriate time to begin therapy.

How should I take Climara Pro?
Do not open the sealed pouch containing the patch until ready to use. Open the pouch and remove the patch from the protective liner. Apply to an area of clean, dry skin on the lower stomach area below the belly button. Press the patch firmly against the skin for about 10 seconds to be sure the patch stays on. If the patch lifts up, press down to reapply. Wear only one patch at any one time.

Do not place the patch on the breast. Make sure the application site is not oily, damaged, or irritated. Avoid applying to the waistline because tight clothing may rub the patch off. Do not put the patch on areas where sitting may loosen it. Do not apply to a site that is exposed to sunlight. Contact with water while bathing, showering, or swimming will not affect the patch.

When it is time to change the patch, remove it slowly, fold in half (sticky sides together), and throw it away out of the reach of children and away from pets. Should any of the adhesive remain on the skin after removal of the patch, allow the area to dry for 15 minutes and then gently rub the area with an oil-based cream or lotion.

Apply a new patch to a different area to prevent skin irritation. Use a different site when replacing the patch and do not repeat the same site for at least 1 week. If the area around the patch becomes red, itchy, or irritated, try a new site. If the irritation continues or becomes worse, notify your doctor promptly.

What should I avoid while taking Climara Pro?
Avoid exposing the patch to sunlight for extended periods of time. Water contact and tight clothing may cause the patch to fall off. If this occurs, re-apply the same patch; if Climara Pro does not adhere, apply a new patch to a different area of the lower abdomen.

Do not eat grapefruit or drink grapefruit juice while you use Climara Pro without first speaking with your doctor.

Do not drive or perform other possibly unsafe tasks until you know how you react to Climara Pro; this medication may cause drowsiness.

What are possible food and drug interactions associated with Climara Pro?
If Climara Pro is taken with certain other drugs, the effects of either could be increased, decreased, or altered. It is especially important to check with your doctor before combining Climara Pro with the following: anticoagulants, barbiturates, corticosteroids, phenytoin, rifampin, succinylcholine, and tacrine.

What are the possible side effects of Climara Pro?
Side effects cannot be anticipated. If any develop or change in intensity, tell your doctor as soon as possible. Only your doctor can determine if it is safe for you to continue taking this drug.

Side effects may include: breast pain, hair loss, headache, irregular vaginal bleeding/spotting, nausea, stomach cramps/bloating, vomiting, calf pain or tenderness, change in vision or speech, dizziness

Can I receive Climara Pro if I am pregnant or breastfeeding?
Tell your doctor immediately if you are pregnant, plan to become pregnant, or are breastfeeding. Hormones are not indicated for use during pregnancy or immediately after birth. Increased risk of fetal reproductive tract disorders and other birth defects have been observed. Do not use during pregnancy. Use caution in breastfeeding.

What should I do if I miss a dose of Climara Pro?
If you forget to change the patch as scheduled, change it as soon as possible and go back to your regular dosing schedule. Do not use 2 doses at once.

How should I store Climara Pro?
Store at room temperature in the original sealed pouch. Store away from heat, moisture, and light. Do not store in the bathroom.

Clindamycin phosphate *See Cleocin T, page 302, or Ziana Gel, page 1477.*

Clindamycin phosphate and benzoyl peroxide
See Duac, page 446.

Clobetasol propionate *See Clobex, page 310; Clobex Spray, page 313; Olux-E, page 937; or Temovate, page 1276.*

CLOBETASOL PROPIONATE

What is clobetasol propionate?
Clobetasol is a corticosteroid indicated to treat psoriasis, skin irritation, allergic reactions, and other types of skin problems.

What is the most important information I should know about clobetasol propionate?
Clobetasol is a highly potent topical corticosteroid that has been shown to suppress the HPA (hypothalamic-pituitary-adrenal) axis at doses as low as 2g per day.

Clobetasol should not be used in the treatment of rosacea or perioral dermatitis, and should not be used on the face, groin or armpits.

Use in children under 12 years of age is not recommended.

Caution should be taken when this drug is administered to nursing mothers.

Therapy should be discontinued when control has been achieved. If no improvement is seen within 2 weeks, contact your doctor.

Who should not use clobetasol propionate?
You should not use this medicine if you have had an allergic reaction to clobetasol.

You might not be able to use this medicine if you have had an allergic reaction to other corticosteroids such as hydrocortisone, triamcinolone, or betamethasone.

What should I tell my doctor before I use the first dose of clobetasol propionate?
Tell your doctor about all prescription, over-the-counter, and herbal medication you are taking before beginning treatment with clobetasol. Also, talk to your doctor about your complete medical history, especially if you are pregnant.

What is the usual dosage?
The information below is based on the dosage guidelines your doctor uses. Depending on your condition and medical history, your doctor may prescribe a different regimen. Do not change the dosage or stop taking your medication without your doctor's approval.

Apply a thin layer of clobetasol cream or ointment to the affected areas twice daily and rub in gently and completely.

Treatment beyond 2 consecutive weeks is not recommended, and the total dosage should not exceed 50 grams per week.

How should I use clobetasol propionate?
This medication should be used as directed by the physician.

Clobetasol propionate is for external use only. Avoid contact with the eyes.

What should I avoid while using clobetasol propionate?
Do not use plastic bandages, dressings, or diapers that do not allow air to circulate to the area unless your doctor directs you to do so. The use of occlusive dressings can greatly increase the amount of drug the body absorbs.

Do not use other topical products on the treated area, unless otherwise directed by your doctor.

What are possible food and drug interactions associated with clobetasol propionate?
No significant interactions have been reported at this time. However, always tell your doctor about any medicines you take, including over-the-counter drugs, vitamins, and herbal supplements.

What are the possible side effects of clobetasol propionate?
Side effects cannot be anticipated. If any develop or change in intensity, tell your doctor as soon as possible. Only your doctor can determine if it is safe for you to continue taking this drug.

Side effects may include: burning sensation, irritation, cracking and fissuring of the skin, numbness of the finger

Can I use clobetasol propionate if I am pregnant or breastfeeding?
The effects of clobetasol during pregnancy and breastfeeding are unknown. Tell your doctor immediately if you are pregnant, plan to become pregnant, or are breastfeeding.

What should I do if I miss a dose of clobetasol propionate?
If you miss a dose or forget to use your medicine, apply it as soon as you can. If it is almost time for your next dose, wait until then to apply the

medicine and skip the missed dose. Do not apply extra medicine to make up for a missed dose.

How should I store clobetasol propionate?
Store at room temperature, away from heat, moisture, and direct light. It should not be refrigerated.

CLOBEX
Generic name: Clobetasol propionate

What is Clobex?
Clobex lotion is used for a short time to reduce the inflammation and itching of skin conditions and plaque psoriasis. Clobex shampoo is used for a short time to treat scalp psoriasis. Clobex spray is used to treat moderate to severe plaque psoriasis when symptoms affect more than 20 percent of the body.

What is the most important information I should know about Clobex?
Clobex is a highly potent topical corticosteroid that has been shown to suppress the HPA (hypothalamic-pituitary-adrenal) axis.

This medication is to be used as directed by the physician and should not be used longer than the prescribed time period. Therapy should be discontinued when control is achieved. It is for external use only.

Wash your hands before and after applying the medication, unless they are part of the treated area.

Avoid using clobetasol topical to treat skin on your face, underarms, or groin area without your doctor's advice.

Avoid getting this medication in your eyes. If contact does occur, rinse with water.

Do not use clobetasol topical on broken or infected skin. Also avoid using this medication in open wounds.

If your symptoms do not get better within 2 weeks or if they get worse, check with your doctor.

Tell your doctor or dentist that you take Clobex Spray before you receive any medical or dental care, emergency care, or surgery.

Check with your doctor before having vaccinations while using Clobex Spray.

Check with your doctor if you experience nausea, vomiting, fever, dizziness, or chest pain after you have stopped using Clobex Spray.

Contact your doctor if your condition does not improve within 2 weeks of using this medicine, or if you develop signs of a bacterial, fungal, or viral skin infection.

Who should not take Clobex?

Do not use Clobex if you are allergic to any of its ingredients or to any other corticosteroid.

Clobex is not recommended for use on anyone less than 18 years old.

What should I tell my doctor before I take the first dose of Clobex?

Tell your doctor about all prescription, over-the-counter, and herbal medications you are taking before beginning treatment with Clobex. Also, talk to your doctor about your complete medical history, especially if you have diabetes; any kind of skin infection (especially skin or scalp infection), cuts, scrapes, or reduced blood flow to your skin; if are pregnant or plan to become pregnant or are breastfeeding,.

What is the usual dosage?

The information below is based on the dosage guidelines your doctor uses. Depending on your condition and medical history, your doctor may prescribe a different regimen. Do not change the dosage or stop taking your medication without your doctor's approval.

Clobex Lotion
Adults: Apply to the affected skin area twice daily and rub in gently and completely.

Clobex Shampoo
Adults: Apply onto dry scalp once a day in a thin film to the affected areas only and leave in place for 15 minutes before lathering and rinsing.

Clobex Spray
Adults: Spray directly onto affected area twice daily and gently rub into skin. Treatment beyond 2 weeks should be limited to localized lesions that have not improved sufficiently.

How should I take Clobex?

Lotion: Apply Clobex Lotion twice a day, once in the morning and once at night or as directed by your doctor. Use only enough to cover the affected areas. Make sure your skin is clean and dry before applying Clobex Lotion.

Do not cover treated skin areas with a bandage or other covering unless your doctor has told you to. If you are treating the diaper area of a baby, do not use plastic pants or tight-fitting diapers. Covering the skin that is treated with Clobex lotion can increase the amount of medicine your skin absorbs, which may lead to unwanted side effects.

It is important to use Clobex regularly to get the most benefit.

Shampoo: Apply Clobex Shampoo on affected areas of the scalp once a day. Do not wet your hair before using Clobex Shampoo. Use only enough to cover the affected areas of your scalp. Move the hair away from the scalp so that only the affected areas are exposed. Apply a small amount of the shampoo directly onto the affected area by gently squeezing the bottle. Gently, rub Clobex Shampoo into the affected area. Leave Clobex Shampoo in place for 15 minutes before adding water, lathering and rinsing hair and scalp completely. No other shampoos are necessary. However, you can use a non-medicated shampoo on your hair after using Clobex Shampoo.

Spray: Spray Clobex directly onto affected area of skin. Gently and completely rub into skin after spraying until it is evenly distributed. Wash your hands after applying Clobex Spray, unless your hands are part of the treated area. Do not bandage or cover the treated skin area unless directed by your doctor. Do not wear tight-fitting clothes over the treated area.

What should I avoid while taking Clobex?

Do not bandage or cover your treated areas while using the lotion or spray unless your doctor tells you to do so. Do not wear tight fitting clothes over your treated skin areas. Do not use Clobex Lotion any longer than 2 weeks (14 days). Do not use Clobex Spray any longer than 4 weeks (28 days).Do not use on broken or infected skin. Also avoid using this medication in open wounds.

Do not cover your head with a shower cap or bathing cap while Clobex Shampoo is on your scalp. Do not use Clobex shampoo any longer than 4 weeks (28 days).

Do not apply any form of Clobex to your face, neck, or groin. Do not get Clobex on your lips or near your eyes. Do not use more than 50 g (50 mL or 1.75 fluid ounces) of Clobex per week. Avoid getting this medication in your eyes. If contact does occur, rinse with water.

What are possible food and drug interactions associated with Clobex?

If Clobex is taken with certain other drugs, the effects of either could be increased, decreased, or altered. It is especially important to check with your doctor before combining Clobex with other medicines.

What are the possible side effects of Clobex?

Side effects cannot be anticipated. If any develop or change in intensity, tell your doctor as soon as possible. Only your doctor can determine if it is safe for you to continue taking this drug.

Side effects may include: nausea, vomiting, fever, low blood pressure, heart attack, mild burning, stinging, itching, redness, irritation, and dry skin, thinning or softening of skin, changes in color of treated skin, muscle weakness, feeling tired, weight gain, puffiness in your face, mood changes, blurred vision, or seeing halos around lights

Can I receive Clobex if I am pregnant or breastfeeding?

The effects of Clobex during pregnancy and breastfeeding are unknown. Tell your doctor immediately if you are pregnant, plan to become pregnant, or are breastfeeding.

What should I do if I miss a dose of Clobex?

If you forget to apply Clobex at the scheduled time, use it as soon as you remember then go back to your regular schedule. If it is about time for your next dose, apply just that dose, and continue with your normal application schedule. Do not try to make up for the missed dose. If you miss several doses, tell your doctor.

How should I store Clobex?

Store Clobex Spray at room temperature. Store away from heat, moisture, and light. Do not refrigerate or freeze. Do not store in the bathroom. Store Clobex Shampoo at room temperature. Keep it tightly closed.

CLOBEX SPRAY

Generic name: Clobetasol propionate

What is Clobex Spray?

Clobex Spray is a medicine called a topical (skin use only) corticosteroid. It is used for a short time to reduce the inflammation and itching of moderate to severe plaque psoriasis.

What is the most important information I should know about Clobex Spray?

Excessive use of Clobex Spray can cause adrenal glands to shut down.

Who should not take Clobex Spray?

Do not use Clobex Spray if you are allergic to any of it ingredients, or to any other corticosteroid. Clobex Spray is not recommended for use on anyone younger than 18 years of age because their adrenal glands may shut down.

What should I tell my doctor before I take the first dose of Clobex Spray?

Always tell your doctor about all the prescription, over-the-counter, and herbal medicines you are taking, as well as your medical history. Also, tell your doctor if you are nursing, having surgery or if you think you have a skin infection. You may need another medicine to treat the skin infection before you use Clobex Spray.

What is the usual dosage?

The information below is based on the dosage guidelines your doctor uses. Depending on your condition and medical history, your doctor may prescribe a different regimen. Do not change the dosage or stop taking your medication without your doctor's approval.

Clobrex Spray is for skin use only. Apply Clobex Spray twice a day, once in the morning and once at night or as directed by your doctor.

How should I take Clobex Spray?
Make sure your skin is clean and dry before applying Clobrex Spray. Use only enough to cover the affected skin areas and rub in gently and completely. Wash your hands after using Clobex Spray.

What should I avoid while taking Clobex Spray?
Do not get Clobex Spray on your face or lips, or in or near your eyes because this might cause irritation. If you do, use a lot of water to rinse the Clobex Spray off your face, lips or out of your eyes. If your eyes keep stinging after rinsing them well with water, call your doctor.

Do not apply Clobex Spray to your groin or armpits. Do not bandage or cover your treated areas unless your doctor tells you to do so. Do not wear tight fitting clothes over your treated skin areas. Do not use Clobex Spray longer than 2 weeks for moderate to severe psoriasis or any longer than an extra 2 weeks.

What are possible food and drug interactions associated with Clobex Spray?
Combining Clobex Spray with certain medications can cause serious side effects. Tell your doctor about all medicines and skin products you use, including prescription and nonprescription drugs, cosmetics, vitamins, and herbal supplements.

What are the possible side effects of Clobex Spray?
Side effects cannot be anticipated. If any develop or change in intensity, tell your doctor as soon as possible. Only your doctor can determine if it is safe for you to continue taking this drug.

Side effects may include: Dry skin, fever, heart attack, itching, irritation, low blood pressure, mild to moderate burning, nausea, redness, skin discomfort, stinging, thinning of the skin, widening of small blood vessels in the skin, vomiting

Can I receive Clobex Spray if I am pregnant or breastfeeding?
The effects of Clobex Spray on pregnancy and nursing are unknown. Talk with your doctor if you are pregnant, planning to become pregnant, or are nursing.

How should I store Clobex Spray?
Clobex Spray should be stored at room temperature.

Clomiphene citrate *See Serophene, page 1184.*

Clomipramine hydrochloride *See Anafranil, page 99.*

Clonazepam *See Klonopin, page 694.*

Clonidine hydrochloride *See Catapres, page 260.*

Clopidogrel bisulfate *See Plavix, page 1034..*

Clorazepate dipotassium *See Tranxene, page 1320.*

Clotrimazole and betamethasone dipropionate
   See Lotrisone, page 770.

COLACE
Generic name: Docusate

What is Colace?
Colace is a stool softener that promotes easy bowel movements. Colace Microenema is used to relieve occasional constipation.

What is the most important information I should know about Colace?
Colace is for short-term relief of constipation only, unless your doctor directs otherwise. It usually takes 1-3 days for the drug to work. Some people may need to wait 4 or 5 days. Colace Microenema works in 2-15 minutes.

   The risk of loss of normal bowel function may be greater if you take Colace in high doses or for a long time. Do not take more than the recommended dose or use for longer than prescribed without checking with your doctor.

   If your symptoms do not improve within 1 week or if they get worse, check with your doctor. Also check with your doctor if you do not have a bowel movement or if you have rectal bleeding after using Colace.

   Do not take Colace with other laxatives or stool softeners, unless directed by your doctor.

   Do not use Colace if you experience stomach pain, nausea, vomiting, or rectal bleeding, except under the direction of your doctor.

   If you notice a sudden change in bowel movements that lasts for 2 weeks or more, check with your doctor.

Who should not take Colace?
Do not take Colace if you have stomach pain, nausea, vomiting, or if you have noticed a sudden change in bowel habits that has lasted more than 2 weeks.

What should I tell my doctor before I take the first dose of Colace?
Tell your doctor about all prescription, over-the-counter, and herbal medications you are taking before beginning treatment with Colace. Also, talk

to your doctor about your complete medical history, especially if you have a history of bowel obstruction, are currently taking mineral oil, if you have stomach pain, nausea, vomiting, rectal bleeding, or have noticed a sudden change in bowel habits that has lasted more than 2 weeks.

What is the usual dosage?
The information below is based on the dosage guidelines your doctor uses. Depending on your condition and medical history, your doctor may prescribe a different regimen. Do not change the dosage or stop taking your medication without your doctor's approval.

Your doctor will adjust the dosage according to your needs.

Adults and children ≥12 years: The suggested daily dosage of Colace is 50 to 360 milligrams (mg).

Children <12 years: The suggested daily dosage of Colace for children 6-12 years of age is 40 to 120 mg. For children 3 to 6 years of age, it is 20-60 mg. For children >3 years of age, it is 10 to 40 mg.

Your doctor will determine the daily dosage for children <2 years of age.

How should I take Colace?
Take the capsule form by mouth with or without food. Take Colace with a full glass of water.

Swallow Colace tablets whole; do not crush or chew the tablets. Drinking extra fluids while you are taking Colace is recommended. Check with your doctor for instructions.

Mix liquid and syrup forms with 6 to 8 ounces of milk, juice, or infant formula to prevent throat irritation. Colace liquid can also be added to an enema.

For Colace Microenema: Shake the bottle gently to make sure that the suspension is mixed. Remove the protective cap from the applicator tip. Lubricate the tip by pushing out a drop of Colace. Slowly insert the full length of the nozzle into the rectum (stop halfway for children 3-12 years of age). Squeeze out the contents of the tube. Remove the nozzle before you release your grip on the tube.

What should I avoid while taking Colace?
Do not take Colace if you are currently taking mineral oil, unless your doctor approves.

What are possible food and drug interactions associated with Colace?
If Colace is taken with certain other drugs, the effects of either could be increased, decreased, or altered. Always check with your doctor before combining Colace with any other drugs, herbs, or supplements.

What are the possible side effects of Colace?

Side effects cannot be anticipated. If any develop or change in intensity, tell your doctor as soon as possible. Only your doctor can determine if it is safe for you to continue taking this drug.

Side effects may include: bitter taste, nausea, rash, throat irritation, bloating, cramping, diarrhea, gas, irritation around the rectum, vomiting, fainting

Can I receive Colace if I am pregnant or breastfeeding?

The effects of Colace during pregnancy and breastfeeding are unknown. Tell your doctor immediately if you are pregnant, plan to become pregnant, or are breastfeeding.

What should I do if I miss a dose of Colace?

Take Colace only as needed. If you miss a dose of Colace and are taking it regularly, take it as soon as possible. If it is almost time for your next dose, skip the missed dose and go back to your regular dosing schedule. Do not take 2 doses at once.

How should I store Colace?

Store Colace at room temperature, between 68° and 77° F. Store away from heat, moisture, and light. Do not store in the bathroom. Keep in a tight, light-resistant container.

COLAZAL

Generic name: Balsalazide disodium

What is Colazal?

Colazal is used to treat the signs and symptoms of mild to moderate chronic inflammation and ulceration of the lower intestine (ulcerative colitis). Safety and effectiveness beyond 12 weeks of use have not been established.

What is the most important information I should know about Colazal?

Although there have been no reports of kidney damage from Colazal, other products containing mesalamine are known to have caused this problem. If you have kidney disease, your doctor will monitor your condition closely during treatment with Colazal. Report any problems or unusual symptoms immediately.

Do NOT take more Colazal than the recommended dose or use for longer than prescribed without checking with your doctor.

If your symptoms do not get better of if they get worse, check with your doctor.

Who should not take Colazal?

Do not take Colazal if you are allergic to the drug or any of its compo-nents, or if you are allergic to medicines such as aspirin or mesalamine.

What should I tell my doctor before
I take the first dose of Colazal?

Tell your doctor about all prescription, over-the-counter, and herbal medi-cations you are taking before beginning treatment with Colazal. Also, talk to your doctor about your complete medical history, especially if you have kidney disease, a history of kidney problems, intestinal problems, or a narrowing of the muscle that controls the emptying of the stomach (pyloric stenosis).

What is the usual dosage?

The information below is based on the dosage guidelines your doctor uses. Depending on your condition and medical history, your doctor may prescribe a different regimen. Do not change the dosage or stop taking your medication without your doctor's approval.

Adults: The usual dose is three 750-milligram (mg) capsules taken 3 times a day for 8 to 12 weeks.

Children 5 to 17 years: The usual dose is three 750-mg capsules taken 3 times a day for up to 8 weeks of treatment **OR** one 750-mg capsule 3 times a day for up to 8 weeks. Use of Colazal in the pediatric population for more than 8 weeks has not been evaluated in clinical trials.

How should I take Colazal?

Colazal can be taken by mouth with or without food. If you cannot swal-low the capsule whole, you may open it and sprinkle the contents over a spoonful of applesauce. Mix the medicine with the applesauce and swal-low the mixture right away, followed by a glass of water. You may crush or chew the medicine before swallowing if necessary. Do not store the mixture for future use. Teeth and/or tongue staining may occur in some patients who use Colazal in sprinkle form with food.

What should I avoid while taking Colazal?

Do NOT take more than the recommended dose or use for longer than prescribed without checking with your doctor.

What are possible food and drug interactions
associated with Colazal?

If Colazal is taken with certain other drugs, the effects of either could be increased, decreased, or altered. It is especially important that you check with your doctor before combining Colazal with: angiotensin-converting enzyme (ACE) inhibitors, antidiabetic drugs, meglitinide, oral antibiotics, sulfinpyrazone, sulfonylureas, or valproic acid.

What are the possible side effects of Colazal?

Side effects cannot be anticipated. If any develop or change in intensity, tell your doctor as soon as possible. Only your doctor can determine if it is safe for you to continue taking this drug.

Side effects may include: abdominal pain, diarrhea, headache, joint pain, nausea, respiratory infection, vomiting, heartburn, muscle pain, stomach pain, loss of appetite, runny or stuffy nose, dark urine, fever, yellowing of skin or eyes

Can I receive Colazal if I am pregnant or breastfeeding?

The effects of Colazal during pregnancy and breastfeeding are unknown. Tell your doctor immediately if you are pregnant, plan to become pregnant, or are breastfeeding.

What should I do if I miss a dose of Colazal?

Take it as soon as possible. If it is within 2 hours of your next dose, skip the dose you missed and go back to your regular schedule. Do not take 2 doses at once.

How should I store Colazal?

Store Colazal at room temperature, between 68° and 77°F. Brief storage between 59° and 86°F is permitted. Store in a tightly closed container. Store away from heat, moisture, and light. Do not store in the bathroom.

Colesevelam hydrochloride *See WelChol, page 1414.*

COLESTID

Generic name: Colestipol hydrochloride

What is Colestid?

Colestid is used along with dietary modification to lower high cholesterol.

What is the most important information I should know about Colestid?

Accidentally inhaling Colestid granules may cause serious effects. To avoid this, NEVER take them in their dry form. Colestid granules should always be mixed with water or other liquids BEFORE you take them.

Avoid Flavored Colestid granules if you have phenylketonuria, since it contains 18.2 milligrams of phenylalanine per 7.5-gram dose.

Do not drive or perform other possibly unsafe tasks until you know how you react to Colestid; this medication may cause dizziness or light-headedness. These effects may be worse if you take it with alcohol or certain medicines.

Follow the diet and exercise program given to you by your healthcare provider.

Do not take more than the recommended dose or use for longer than prescribed without checking with your doctor.

If severe or persistent constipation occurs, ask your doctor about taking a stool softener while you take Colestid.

If the tablet gets stuck after you swallow it, you may notice chest pressure or discomfort. If this happens, contact your doctor right away. Do not take another tablet unless your doctor tells you otherwise.

Who should not take Colestid?
You should not take Colestid if you are allergic to it or any of its components.

What should I tell my doctor before I take the first dose of Colestid?
Tell your doctor about all prescription, over-the-counter, and herbal medications you are taking before beginning treatment with Colestid. Also, talk to your doctor about your complete medical history, especially if you have a bleeding disorder, an abnormality in protein content of the blood (dysproteinemia), diabetes, heart disease, kidney or liver disease, phenylketonuria, or an underactive thyroid gland. Tell your doctor if you drink alcohol or if you suffer from constipation or hemorrhoids.

What is the usual dosage?
The information below is based on the dosage guidelines your doctor uses. Depending on your condition and medical history, your doctor may prescribe a different regimen. Do not change the dosage or stop taking your medication without your doctor's approval.

One dose (1 packet or 1 level teaspoon) of Colestid granules contains 5 grams (g) of the active drug. One dose (1 packet or 1 level scoopful) of flavored Colestid granules also contains 5 g of drug.

Adults: The usual starting dose is 1 packet or 1 level scoopful taken once or twice a day. Your doctor may increase this by 1 dose a day every month or every other month, up to 6 packets or 6 level scoopfuls taken once a day or divided into smaller doses.

If you are taking Colestid tablets, the usual starting dose is 2 g taken once or twice a day. Your doctor may increase the dose every month or every other month, to a maximum of 16 g a day, taken once a day or divided into smaller doses.

How should I take Colestid?
Colestid granules should be mixed with liquids such as carbonated beverages (may cause stomach or intestinal discomfort), flavored drinks, milk, orange juice, pineapple juice, tomato juice, or water.

Colestid may also be mixed with milk used on breakfast cereals, pulpy fruit (such as crushed peaches, pears, pineapple, or fruit cocktail), or soups with a high liquid content (such as chicken noodle or tomato).

To take Colestid granules with beverages, measure at least 3 ounces of liquid into a glass. Add the prescribed dose of Colestid to the liquid. Stir until the Colestid is completely mixed (it will not dissolve) and then drink the mixture. Pour a small amount of the beverage into the glass, swish it around, and drink it. This will ensure you have taken all the Colestid.

Never take Colestid or flavored Colestid in its dry form.

You must take Colestid tablets one at a time. Promptly swallow the tablets whole with plenty of water or another liquid. Do not chew, crush, or cut the tablets.

Take any other medicines at least 1 hour before or 4 hours after you take Colestid.

Drinking extra fluids and making sure you get enough fiber is recommended while you are taking Colestid. Check with your doctor for instructions.

Continue to take Colestid even if you feel well. Do not miss any doses.

What should I avoid while taking Colestid?

Avoid Flavored Colestid granules if you have phenylketonuria, because Flavored Colestid granules contain phenylalanine. Never take Colestid granules in their dry form.

Do not take more than the recommended dose or use for longer than prescribed without checking with your doctor.

Avoid driving or performing other possibly unsafe tasks until you know how you react to Colestid; this medication may cause dizziness or lightheadedness. These effects may be worse if you take it with alcohol or certain medicines.

What are possible food and drug interactions associated with Colestid?

Colestid may delay or reduce the absorption of other drugs. Allow as much time as possible between taking Colestid and taking other medications. Other drugs should be taken at least 1 hour before or 4 hours after taking Colestid. If Colestid is taken with certain other drugs, the effects of either could be increased, decreased, or altered. It is especially important to check with your doctor before combining Colestid with the following: chlorothiazide, digitalis, folic acid and vitamins such as A, D, and K, furosemide, gemfibrozil, hydrochlorothiazide, hydrocortisone, penicillin G, phosphate supplements, propranolol, tetracycline.

What are the possible side effects of Colestid?

Side effects cannot be anticipated. If any develop or change in intensity, tell your doctor as soon as possible. Only your doctor can determine if it is safe for you to continue taking this drug.

Side effects may include: constipation, worsening of hemorrhoids, bloating, diarrhea, gas, heartburn, indigestion, loose stools, stomach pain or cramping, vomiting

Can I receive Colestid if I am pregnant or breastfeeding?
The effects of Colestid during pregnancy and breastfeeding are unknown. Tell your doctor immediately if you are pregnant, plan to become pregnant, or are breastfeeding.

What should I do if I miss a dose of Colestid?
Take the forgotten dose as soon as you remember. If it is almost time for the next dose, skip the dose you missed and go back to your regular schedule. Never take 2 doses at once.

How should I store Colestid?
Store Colestid at room temperature. Store away from heat, moisture, and light. Do not store in the bathroom.

Colestipol hydrochloride *See Colestid, page 319.*

COMBIGAN
Generic name: Brimonidine tartrate and timolol maleate

What is Combigan?
Combigan is an eyedrop used to lower pressure in the eyes of people with glaucoma (open-angle) or ocular hypertension. Combigan contains two medications, brimonidine (an alpha agonist) and timolol (a beta-blocker).

What is the most important information I should know about Combigan?
Even though Combigan is applied externally to the eye, the medication may still be absorbed in the bloodstream and cause serious adverse reactions (see "What are the possible side effects of this medication?"). Severe respiratory reactions including death due to difficulty breathing have been reported in patients with asthma. Stimulation of the nervous system may be essential in individuals with diminished heart pumping ability. In patients without a history of cardiac failure, continued use of beta-blocking agents such as timolol over a period of time can, in some cases, lead to cardiac failure. Contact your doctor right away if you are having chest pain or discomfort; dilated neck veins; extreme fatigue; irregular breathing; an irregular heartbeat; shortness of breath; swelling of the face, fingers, feet, or lower legs; weight gain; or wheezing.

Combigan may cause changes in your blood sugar levels, or may cover up signs of low blood sugar. Check with your doctor if you have blood sugar problems or if you notice a change in the results of your blood or urine sugar tests.

If you are scheduled to have surgery or dental work, make sure the doctor or dentist knows that you are using Combigan. You may need to stop using this medication several days before having surgery.

Who should not take Combigan?

Do not take this drug if you have heart conditions such as sinus brady-cardia (slow heart rate), atrioventricular block (greater than first-degree block), cardiogenic shock, or overt cardiac failure; or if you have asthma or obstructive lung disease. Do not take Combigan if you have had a known hypersensitivity to any component of this medication in the past.

What should I tell my doctor before I take the first dose of Combigan?

Tell your doctor about all prescription, over-the-counter, and herbal medications you are taking before beginning treatment with Combigan. Also talk to your doctor about your complete medical history, especially if you have heart or breathing problems, diabetes, thyrotoxicosis (increased thyroid hormones), muscle weakness, lung problems, a history of allergic reactions, vascular insufficiency (compromised blood flow), depression, or you are scheduled to have surgery.

What is the usual dosage?

The information below is based on the dosage guidelines your doctor uses. Depending on your condition and medical history, your doctor may prescribe a different regimen. Do not change the dosage or stop taking your medication without your doctor's approval.

Adults: The recommended dosage is 1 drop in the affected eye twice a day, given 12 hours apart.

How should I take Combigan?

Take it exactly as prescribed by your doctor. Wash your hands before instilling the medication.

What should I avoid while taking Combigan?

Do not touch the dropper tip to any surface as this may contaminate the solution.

Contact lenses should be removed prior to the administration of the solution. Lenses may be reinserted 15 minutes after instilling Combigan drops.

What are possible food and drug interactions associated with Combigan?

If Combigan is used with certain other drugs, the effects of either could be increased, decreased, or altered. It is especially important to check with your doctor before combining Combigan with the following: other beta-blocking medications, blood pressure medications including beta-blockers and calcium channel blockers, digitalis, reserpine, central nervous system depressants, quinidine, and antidepressants (including selective serotonin reuptake inhibitors, monoamine oxidase inhibitors, and tricyclic antidepressants).

What are the possible side effects of Combigan?
Side effects cannot be anticipated. If any develop or change in intensity, tell your doctor as soon as possible. Only your doctor can determine if it is safe for you to continue taking this drug.

Side effects may include: eye irritation, discomfort, swelling, itching, conjunctivitis (pinkeye)

Serious systemic adverse effects may include: decreased heart rate, heart failure, heart block, asthma, difficulty breathing, lack of sleep, muscle weakness, extreme fatigue, hives, hair loss, and severe allergic reactions

Signs of severe allergic reactions may include hives, difficulty breathing, and swelling of the throat. If any of these events occur, seek immediate medical attention.

Can I receive Combigan if I am pregnant or breastfeeding?
Combigan should be avoided during pregnancy and breastfeeding. Tell your doctor immediately if you are pregnant, plan to become pregnant, or are breastfeeding.

What should I do if I miss a dose of Combigan?
If you miss a dose, apply it as soon as possible. However, if it is almost time for your next dose, skip the missed dose and go back to your regular dosing schedule. Do not double the dose.

How should I store Combigan?
Store at room temperature and protect from light.

COMBIPATCH
Generic name: Estradiol and norethindrone acetate

What is CombiPatch?
CombiPatch is used after menopause to reduce moderate to severe hot flashes; treat moderate to severe dryness, itching and burning in or around the vagina; and to treat certain conditions in which a young woman's ovaries do not produce enough estrogen naturally. If you use CombiPatch only to treat your dryness, itching and burning in or around the vagina, talk with your doctor about whether a topical vaginal product would be better for you.

What is the most important information I should know about CombiPatch?

Do not use estrogens and progestins to prevent heart disease, heart attacks, strokes or dementia. Using estrogens with progestins may increase your chances of experiencing a heart attack, stroke, breast cancer, blood clot, or dementia.

Irregular bleeding may occur, particularly in the first 6 months of therapy, but generally decreases with time and often stops completely.

Who should not take CombiPatch?

Do not use CombiPatch if you have had your uterus removed (hysterectomy). CombiPatch should not be used if you have unusual vaginal bleeding, a history of certain cancers, including cancer of the breast or uterus, a recent (in past year) history of stroke or heart attack, a history of blood clots or liver problems, or think you may be or know that you are pregnant.

CombiPatch should also be avoided if you are allergic to it or any of its ingredients.

What should I tell my doctor before I take the first dose of CombiPatch?

Tell your doctor about all prescription, over-the-counter, and herbal medications you are taking, before beginning therapy with CombiPatch. Also, talk to your doctor about your complete medical history, especially if you have had a history of cancer, kidney problems, endometriosis (severe pain and unusual bleeding during menstruation), wheezing, high blood sugar, seizures, or migraines.

What is the usual dosage?

The information below is based on the dosage guidelines your doctor uses. Depending on your condition and medical history, your doctor may prescribe a different regimen. Do not change the dosage or stop taking your medication without your doctor's approval.

Adults: The recommended starting dose is 1 patch containing 0.05 milligrams (mg) estradiol and 0.14 mg norethindrone acetate applied twice a week or every 3 to 4 days. If needed, your doctor may increase your dose to a patch containing 0.05 mg estradiol and 0.25 mg norethindrone acetate.

CombiPatch can also be used in conjunction with a 0.05 mg estradiol-only patch. The estradiol-only patch is applied twice a week for the first 14 days of a 28-day cycle, and CombiPatch is applied twice weekly for the remaining 14 days.

If you are currently taking another form of hormone replacement therapy, you should complete the current cycle before switching to CombiPatch.

How should I take CombiPatch?

Put on a new CombiPatch every 3 to 4 days, according to your doctor's instructions. It should be applied to clean, dry skin on the lower stomach; each new patch should be applied to a different area of your skin. Change the patch on the same days each week. Only one CombiPatch should be worn at any one time.

CombiPatch can be worn during bathing, swimming, or showering. Most women find that CombiPatch seldom comes off. But if a patch should fall off, the same patch may be put on a different area of the lower abdomen (make sure you are choosing a clean, dry, lotion-free area of skin). If the patch will not stick completely to your skin, put a new CombiPatch on a different area of the lower abdomen. No matter what day this happens, go back to changing the patch on the same days each week.

What should I avoid while taking CombiPatch?

Avoid exposing CombiPatch to the sun for long periods of time. Once it is in place, be sure that it is covered with clothing.

Avoid placing the patch over skin that has cuts, a rash, or other irritations.

What are possible food and drug interactions associated with CombiPatch?

If CombiPatch is taken with certain other drugs, the effects of either could be increased, decreased, or altered. It is especially important to check with your doctor before combining CombiPatch with any of the following: carbamazepine, clarithromycin, erythromycin, grapefruit juice, itraconazole, ketoconazole, phenobarbital, ritonavir, St. John's wort, thyroid medications.

What are the possible side effects of CombiPatch?

Side effects cannot be anticipated. If any develop or change in intensity, tell your doctor as soon as possible. Only your doctor can determine if it is safe for you to continue taking this drug.

Side effects may include: bloating, stomach cramps, breast pain, hair loss, headache, irregular vaginal bleeding/spotting, nausea, vomiting, yeast infection

Symptoms of serious side effects (call your doctor immediately): breast lumps, changes in speech, changes in vision, chest pain, dizziness, faintness, pain in legs, severe headache, shortness of breath, unusual vaginal bleeding, vomiting

Can I receive CombiPatch if I am pregnant or breastfeeding?

The effects of CombiPatch during pregnancy and breastfeeding are unknown. Tell your doctor immediately if you are pregnant, plan to become pregnant, or are breastfeeding.

What should I do if I miss a dose of CombiPatch?
If you are currently wearing a patch, remove it and put on a new patch in a different area of your lower stomach. Then go back to changing the patch on the same days each week.

How should I store CombiPatch?
Store at room temperature.

COMBIVENT
Generic name: Ipratropium bromide and albuterol sulfate

What is Combivent?
Combivent is a combination medication prescribed for people with chronic obstructive pulmonary disease (COPD) if they are already taking one airway-opening medication and need another.

**What is the most important information
I should know about Combivent?**
Overuse of this product can be fatal. Do not increase the dose or frequency without your doctor's approval. If you find that Combivent is becoming less effective, if your symptoms are getting worse, or if you need to use Combivent more than usual, see your doctor right away.

Who should not take Combivent?
Do not use Combivent if you are allergic to soy lecithin or related products such as soybeans and peanuts. Do not use Combivent if you are allergic to any of the ingredients in this product or if you are allergic to atropine or other similar drugs.

**What should I tell my doctor before
I take the first dose of Combivent?**
Tell your doctor about all prescription, over-the-counter, and herbal medications you are taking before beginning treatment with Combivent. Also, talk to your doctor about your complete medical history, especially if you have an eye disease that may result in loss of sight and that is characterized by rapid increases in pressure inside the eye (narrow-angle glaucoma), urinary problems, heart problems, seizures, thyroid problems, high blood sugar (diabetes), low potassium levels in your blood, and kidney or liver disease.

What is the usual dosage?
The information below is based on the dosage guidelines your doctor uses. Depending on your condition and medical history, your doctor may prescribe a different regimen. Do not change the dosage or stop taking your medication without your doctor's approval.

Adults: The usual dosage is 2 inhalations 4 times a day. You can take additional inhalations as required up to a total of 12 inhalations each 24 hours.

How should I take Combivent?

Remove the orange protective cap from the mouthpiece and shake the canister well. If you are starting a new canister, or if more than 24 hours have passed since your last dose, test-spray the canister 3 times. For best results, make sure the canister is at room temperature. Do not use near an open flame.

Exhale deeply through your mouth, then close your lips around the mouthpiece. Keep your eyes closed to protect them against an accidental spray. Inhale slowly through the mouth, and at the same time press down once on the canister's base. Hold your breath for 10 seconds, then remove the mouthpiece from your lips and exhale slowly. Wait 2 minutes, shake the canister again, and repeat.

The mouthpiece can be washed with soap and hot water. Rinse it and dry thoroughly. Keep the mouthpiece capped when not in use. Count the number of sprays and discard each canister after 200 sprays. Canisters may fail to deliver the proper dose if used for more than that amount.

What should I avoid while taking Combivent?

Avoid taking other inhaled medications without consulting with your doctor.

Avoid contact with your eyes because it can cause eye pain or discomfort, blurred vision, colored images, or high pressure in the eye.

What are possible food and drug interactions associated with Combivent?

If Combivent is taken with certain other drugs, the effects of either could be increased, decreased, or altered. It is especially important to check with your doctor before combining Combivent with any of the following: airway-opening drugs such as albuterol, fluticasone/salmeterol levalbuterol, and terbutaline, antispasmotics such as belladonna, benztropine, and hyoscyamine, beta-blocker blood pressure medications such as atenolol and propranolol, MAO inhibitors such as phenelzine and tranylcypromine, water pills (diuretics) such as furosemide and hydrochlorothiazide, tricyclic antidepressants such as doxepin, imipramine, perphenazine and protriptyline.

What are the possible side effects of Combivent?

Side effects cannot be anticipated. If any develop or change in intensity, tell your doctor as soon as possible. Only your doctor can determine if it is safe for you to continue taking this drug.

Side effects may include: bronchitis, coughing, headache, shortness of breath, upper respiratory tract infection

Combivent can cause serious allergic reactions. Symptoms include itching of the face, lips, tongue, or throat, skin rash, hives, or airway narrowing. Stop taking Combivent and call your doctor right away if you experience these symptoms.

Can I receive Combivent if I am pregnant or breastfeeding?
The effects of Combivent during pregnancy and breastfeeding are unknown. Talk with your doctor before taking this drug if you are pregnant, plan to become pregnant, or are breastfeeding.

What should I do if I miss a dose of Combivent?
Take the forgotten dose as soon as you remember. However, if it is almost time for your next dose, skip the one you missed and return to your regular schedule. Do not take 2 doses at once.

How should I store Combivent?
Store at room temperature. Protect from heat. Temperatures of 120°F can cause the canister to burst. Do not puncture the canister or discard it in an incinerator. Protect from high humidity.

COMBIVIR
Generic name: Lamivudine and zidovudine

What is Combivir?
Combivir combines lamivudine (Epivir) and zidovudine (Retrovir), two drugs used to treat HIV (human immunodeficiency virus). HIV is the virus that causes AIDS (acquired immune deficiency syndrome). Combivir is not a cure for HIV, and does not reduce the chances of spreading HIV to others.

What is the most important information I should know about Combivir?
Zidovudine, one component of Combivir, has been associated with blood toxicity and anemia; prolonged usage may cause muscle disease.

Lactic acidosis (a condition involving dangerously high levels of lactic acid in the blood) and enlarged liver have been associated with lamivudine. It may cause a severe increase in the hepatitis B virus (HBV) in people who are already infected with both HBV and HIV.

Who should not take Combivir?
Do not take Combivir if you are allergic to any of its ingredients. Also, this drug should not be given to children <12 or if you have kidney problems.

What should I tell my doctor before I take the first dose of Combivir?

Tell your doctor about all prescription, over-the-counter, and herbal medications you are taking before beginning therapy with Combivir. Also, talk to your doctor about your complete medical history, especially if you are pregnant, plan to become pregnant, or are breastfeeding. Mothers with HIV should not nurse their children, as not to spread the virus. Tell your doctor if you are having problems with your blood, muscles, kidneys, or liver (such as HBV infection).

What is the usual dosage?

The information below is based on the dosage guidelines your doctor uses. Depending on your condition and medical history, your doctor may prescribe a different regimen. Do not change the dosage or stop taking your medication without your doctor's approval.

Adults and children >12 years: The recommended dose of Combivir for adults and adolescents (>12 years of age) is 1 tablet (containing 150 milligrams [mg] of lamivudine and 300 mg of zidovudine) twice daily.

How should I take Combivir?

Take the Combivir tablets orally, with or without food.

What should I avoid while taking Combivir?

Avoid breastfeeding your child; HIV can be passed to your baby through your breast milk. Do not stop treatment without talking to your doctor first.

What are the possible side effects of Combivir?

Side effects cannot be anticipated. If any develop or change in intensity, tell your doctor as soon as possible. Only your doctor can determine if it is safe for you to continue taking this drug.

Side effects may include: abdominal pain or cramps, cough, depression, diarrhea, dizziness, fever or chills, headache, indigestion, loss of appetite, muscle and joint pain, nasal symptoms, nausea and vomiting, nerve damage, skin rashes, trouble sleeping, weakness, and fatigue

Symptoms of lactic acidosis: stomach ache, difficulty breathing, nausea and vomiting, and severe weakening of muscles in the legs and arms

Can I receive Combivir if I am pregnant or breastfeeding?

The effects of Combivir during pregnancy and breastfeeding are unknown. Tell your doctor immediately if you are pregnant, plan to become pregnant, or are breastfeeding. Also, you should not breastfeed your child if you are HIV-positive; breast milk contains the virus and can infect your baby.

What should I do if I miss a dose of Combivir?
Take it as soon as you remember. If it is almost time for your next dose, skip the one you missed and go back to your regular schedule. Do not take 2 doses at once.

How should I store Combivir?
Store at room temperature.

COMTAN
Generic name: Entacapone

What is Comtan?
Comtan is used to treat patients with Parkinson's disease. It is prescribed when doses of Sinemet (carbidopa/levodopa) begin to wear off too soon. When these medications are taken together, the patient is free from stiffness and tremors for a longer period of time.

What is the most important information I should know about Comtan?
Comtan extends the effectiveness of the combination drug carbidopa/levodopa. It is helpful only when taken with the other drug and it has no benefit when used alone.

Who should not take Comtan?
Do not use Comtan if you are allergic to it or any of its ingredients. Do not take Comtan with drugs known as monoamine oxidase inhibitors (MAOIs) such as phenelzine and tranylcypromine.

What should I tell my doctor before I take the first dose of Comtan?
Tell your doctor about all prescription, over-the-counter, and herbal medications you are taking before beginning treatment with Comtan. Also, talk to your doctor about your complete medical history, especially if you have liver disease or if you are taking MAOIs.

What is the usual dosage?
The information below is based on the dosage guidelines your doctor uses. Depending on your condition and medical history, your doctor may prescribe a different regimen. Do not change the dosage or stop taking your medication without your doctor's approval.

Adults: The recommended dose of Comtan is 200 milligrams (mg) given at the same time as carbidopa/levodopa. The maximum dose is 1600 mg per day.

If you were taking more than 800 mg of levodopa per day before starting Comtan, you will probably need a reduction in your levodopa dose once you begin taking this medication.

If you have liver disease, your doctor may need to prescribe a lower dose.

How should I take Comtan?
Comtan can be taken with or without food. Comtan should always be taken with carbidopa/levodopa.

What should I avoid while taking Comtan?
Avoid driving a car or operating complex machinery until you know how the drug affects you.

Avoid taking Comtan with other drugs that may cause you to feel sleepy.

Avoid rising rapidly after sitting or lying down because low blood pressure may occur especially at the beginning of therapy. Use caution when getting up.

Abrupt discontinuation of Comtan can cause a reappearance of Parkinson's symptoms. If you are going to discontinue the drug, it should be withdrawn slowly, under a doctor's supervision.

What are possible food and drug interactions associated with Comtan?
If Comtan is taken with certain other drugs, the effects of either could be increased, decreased, or altered. It is especially important to check with your doctor before combining Comtan with any of the following: antidepressants classified as MAOIs such as phenelzine and tranylcypromine,* bitolterol, certain antibiotics, including ampicillin and erythromycin, cholestyramine, methyldopa, isoproterenol, and probenecid.

What are the possible side effects of Comtan?
Side effects cannot be anticipated. If any develop or change in intensity, tell your doctor as soon as possible. Only your doctor can determine if it is safe for you to continue taking this drug.

Side effects may include: abdominal pain, back pain, constipation, diarrhea, discoloration of urine, dizziness, nausea, onset of new movement disorders, fatigue, vomiting

Can I receive Comtan if I am pregnant or breastfeeding?
The effects of Comtan during pregnancy and breastfeeding are unknown. Talk with your doctor before taking this drug if you are pregnant, plan to become pregnant, or are breastfeeding.

---

*Comtan can be used with a special type of MAOI called selegiline, which is used for treating Parkinson's disease.

What should I do if I miss a dose of Comtan?

Take it along with a dose of carbidopa/levodopa as soon as you remember. If it is almost time for your next dose, skip the one you missed and go back to your regular schedule. Never take 2 doses at the same time.

How should I store Comtan?

Store at room temperature.

CONCERTA

Generic name: Methylphenidate hydrochloride

What is Concerta?

Concerta is used for the treatment of attention-deficit/hyperactivity disorder (ADHD).

What is the most important information I should know about Concerta?

When given for ADHD, Concerta should be an integral part of a total treatment program that includes psychological, educational, and social measures. Symptoms of ADHD include continual problems with moderate to severe distractibility, short attention span, hyperactivity, emotional changeability, and impulsiveness.

There are reports of heart and mental problems in patients taking Concerta or other related stimulants. Some of the problems are sudden death in patients with previous heart problems, heart attacks in adults, increased blood pressure and heart rate, new or worsening symptoms of behavior problems, bipolar disorder, and aggressive or hostile behavior. Call your doctor right away if you or your child develops signs of heart problems such as chest pain, shortness of breath, or fainting while taking Concerta.

Excessive doses of Concerta over a long period of time may cause addiction. It is also possible to develop tolerance to the drug so that larger doses are needed to produce the original effect. Be sure to check with your doctor before making any change in dosage; and stop the drug only under your doctor's supervision.

There is no information regarding the safety and effectiveness of long-term treatment in children. However, slowing of growth has been seen with the long-term use of stimulants, so your doctor will monitor your child carefully while he or she is taking Concerta.

The use of Concerta in not recommended in children less than 6 years old.

Who should not take Concerta?

You should not take Concerta if you are very anxious, tense, or agitated.

Do not use Concerta if you have glaucoma, tics or Tourette's syndrome (or a family history of Tourette's), are taking or have taken within the past 14 days a medication called a monoamine oxidase inhibitor (MAOI), or if you are allergic to any component of this drug.

What should I tell my doctor before I take the first dose of Concerta?

Tell your doctor about all prescription, over-the-counter, and herbal medications you are taking before beginning treatment with Concerta. Also, talk to your doctor about your complete medical history, especially if you have ever had heart problems including heart defects; high blood pressure; mental health problems such as psychosis, mania, bipolar disorder, or depression; tics or Tourette's syndrome; seizures or an abnormal brain wave test; and stomach or intestinal problems.

What is the usual dosage?

The information below is based on the dosage guidelines your doctor uses. Depending on your condition and medical history, your doctor may prescribe a different regimen. Do not change the dosage or stop taking your medication without your doctor's approval.

Patients New to Methylphenidate
Adults: The usual starting dose is 18 milligrams (mg) once daily.

Children 6 to 12 years: The usual starting dose is 18 mg daily up to a maximum daily dose of 54 mg.

Adolescents 13 to 17 years: The usual starting dose is 18 mg daily up to a maximum daily dose of 72 mg.

Patients Currently Using Methylphenidate
Your doctor will determine the exact dose.

How should I take Concerta?

Take Concerta exactly as prescribed. Do not chew, crush, or divide the tablets. Swallow Concerta tablets whole with water or other liquids. Concerta is usually taken in the morning and can be taken with or without food.

What should I avoid while taking Concerta?

Concerta can cause side effects that may impair your vision or reactions. Be careful if you drive or do anything that requires you to be awake and alert until you know how this medication affects you.

What are possible food and drug interactions associated with Concerta?

If Concerta is taken with certain other drugs, the effects of either could be increased, decreased, or altered. It is especially important to check with your doctor before combining Concerta with any of the following: anti-depressants (especially MAOIs), antiseizure medicines, blood thinners, blood pressure medicines, and cold or allergy medicines that contain decongestants.

What are the possible side effects of Concerta?
Side effects cannot be anticipated. If any develop or change in intensity, tell your doctor as soon as possible. Only your doctor can determine if it is safe for you to continue taking this drug.

Side effects may include: heart and mental problems, slowing of growth (height and weight) in children, eyesight changes or blurred vision, decreased appetite, stomachache, insomnia, headache, muscle twitches

Can I receive Concerta if I am pregnant or breastfeeding?
The effects of Concerta during pregnancy and breastfeeding are unknown. Tell your doctor immediately if you are pregnant, plan to become pregnant, or are breastfeeding.

What should I do if I miss a dose of Concerta?
Take the missed dose as soon as you remember. If it is almost time for your next dose, skip the one you missed and return to your regular schedule. Do not take extra medicine to make up for the missed dose.

How should I store Concerta?
Store at room temperature and protect from moisture.

Conjugated estrogens *See Premarin, page 1054.*

CORDARONE
Generic name: Amiodarone hydrochloride

What is Cordarone?
Cordarone is used to treat life-threatening heartbeat conditions called ventricular arrhythmias.

What is the most important information I should know about Cordarone?
Cordarone tablets can cause serious side effects that can lead to death, including lung damage, liver damage, and worse heartbeat conditions.

Because of the possible side effects, Cordarone tablets should only be used in adults with life-threatening ventricular arrhythmias for which other treatments did not work or were not tolerated.

You may still have side effects after stopping Cordarone tablets because the medicine stays in your body months after treatment is stopped.

Who should not take Cordarone?

Do not take Cordarone tablets if you have certain heart conditions (heart block, very slow heart rate, or slow heart rate with dizziness or lightheadedness) or have an allergy to amiodarone, iodine, or any of the other ingredients in Cordarone tablets.

What should I tell my doctor before I take the first dose of Cordarone?

Tell your doctor about all prescription, over-the-counter, and herbal medications you are taking before beginning treatment with Cordarone. Also, talk to your doctor about your complete medical history, especially if you have lung or breathing problems, have a history of liver problems or thyroid problems, blood pressure problems, or are pregnant or planning to become pregnant, or are breastfeeding.

What is the usual dosage?

The information below is based on the dosage guidelines your doctor uses. Depending on your condition and medical history, your doctor may prescribe a different regimen. Do not change the dosage or stop taking your medication without your doctor's approval.

Adults: The usual starting dose is 800 to 1600 milligrams (mg) per day, divided in 1 to 2 doses and given for 1 to 3 weeks. When adequate heartbeat control is achieved, your dose may be decreased to 600 to 800 mg per day in 1 to 2 doses for 1 month.

To maintain adequate heartbeat control, the usual dose is 400 mg per day. Lower doses are recommended in certain situations and will be determined by your doctor.

How should I take Cordarone?

Keep taking your medicine until your doctor tells you to stop. Do not stop taking it because you feel better, otherwise, your condition may get worse.

You may take Cordarone with or without food. Make sure you take Cordarone tablets the same way each time.

What should I avoid while taking Cordarone?

Avoid grapefruit juice during treatment with Cordarone tablets. Avoid exposing your skin to the sun or sun lamps or becoming pregnant. Do not breastfeed while taking this medication.

What are possible food and drug interactions associated with Cordarone?

If Cordarone is taken with certain other drugs, the effects of either could be increased, decreased, or altered. It is especially important to check with your doctor before combining Cordarone with the following: antibiotics, antidepressants, blood thinners, cholesterol or bile medicines, cimetidine, cyclosporine, dextromethorphan, diabetes medicines, diuretics (water pills), HIV or AIDS medicines, narcotic pain relievers, St. John's wort.

What are the possible side effects of Cordarone?

Side effects cannot be anticipated. If any develop or change in intensity, tell your doctor as soon as possible. Only your doctor can determine if it is safe for you to continue taking this drug.

Side effects may include: vision problems (blurred vision, seeing halos, light-sensitivity), nerve problems (numbness in the hands, legs or feet, muscle weakness, uncontrolled movements), thyroid problems, skin problems, nausea and vomiting, constipation, and loss of appetite

Can I receive Cordarone if I am pregnant or breastfeeding?

Cordarone can harm your unborn baby. This medication is able to pass into your breast milk. Tell your doctor immediately if you are pregnant, plan to become pregnant, or are breastfeeding.

What should I do if I miss a dose of Cordarone?

If you miss a dose, do not take a double dose to make up for the dose you missed. Continue with your next regularly scheduled dose.

How should I store Cordarone?

Store at room temperature and protect from light. Keep Cordarone tablets in a tightly closed container.

COREG

Generic name: Carvedilol

What is Coreg?

Coreg is used, often with other medications, to treat high blood pressure. It is also used to treat patients who had a heart attack that worsened how well the heart pumps, and to treat patients with certain types of heart failure.

What is the most important information I should know about Coreg?

Coreg can cause a drop in blood pressure when you first stand up, resulting in dizziness or even fainting. If this happens, sit or lie down and notify your doctor. Taking the drug with food reduces the chance of this problem. During the first month of therapy and after a change in your dose, use caution when driving or operating dangerous machinery.

Coreg should not be used by anyone <18 years of age.

Who should not take Coreg?
Do not use Coreg if you have breathing problems, certain serious heart conditions, or liver disease. Do not take Coreg if you are allergic to it or any of its ingredients.

What should I tell my doctor before I take the first dose of Coreg?
Tell your doctor about all prescription, over-the-counter, and herbal medications you are taking before beginning treatment with Coreg. Also, talk to your doctor about your complete medical history, especially if you have lung problems, high blood sugar, thyroid problems, or liver disease.

What is the usual dosage?
The information below is based on the dosage guidelines your doctor uses. Depending on your condition and medical history, your doctor may prescribe a different regimen. Do not change the dosage or stop taking your medication without your doctor's approval.

Dosage must be individualized and closely monitored by your doctor.

Heart Failure
Adults: The recommended starting dose of Coreg is 3.125 milligrams (mg) 2 times a day for 2 weeks. If needed, your dose may be increased to 6.25, 12.5, or up to 25 mg 2 times a day, with each dose increase occurring at 2-week intervals. The maximum dose, for people weighing >187 pounds, is 50 mg twice a day.

High Blood Pressure
Adults: The recommended starting dose is 6.25 mg 2 times a day. If needed, your dose can be increased to 12.5 mg 2 times a day after 1 to 2 weeks. Your dose can be increased to 25 mg 2 times a day after another 1 to 2 weeks. Total daily dose should not exceed 50 mg.

Left Ventricular Dysfunction Following a Heart Attack
Adults: The recommended starting dose is 6.25 mg 2 times a day and may be increased after 3 to 10 days, if needed, to 12.5 mg 2 times a day, then again to the maximum dose of 25 mg 2 times a day. A lower starting dose may be used if necessary.

How should I take Coreg?
Take Coreg with food.

What should I avoid while taking Coreg?
Do not interrupt or discontinue using Coreg without speaking to your doctor. Abrupt discontinuation can lead to worsening of your symptoms. Avoid driving or hazardous tasks until you know how Coreg affects you.

What are possible food and drug interactions associated with Coreg?

If Coreg is taken with certain other drugs, the effects of either could be increased, decreased, or altered. It is especially important to check with your doctor before combining Coreg with any of the following: calcium channel blockers (such as diltiazem or verapamil), cimetidine, clonidine, cyclosporine, diabetes medications, digoxin, fluoxetine, MAO inhibitors (including the antidepressants phenelzine and tranylcypromine), paroxetine, propafenone, quinidine, reserpine, rifampin

What are the possible side effects of Coreg?

Side effects cannot be anticipated. If any develop or change in intensity, tell your doctor as soon as possible. Only your doctor can determine if it is safe for you to continue taking this drug.

Side effects may include: anemia, back pain, bronchitis, cough, diarrhea, dizziness, dry eyes, fainting, fatigue, fluid in the lungs, headache, increased blood sugar levels, increased cholesterol, joint pain, low blood pressure, nausea, pain, shortness of breath, sinus problems, slow heartbeat, swelling, upper respiratory infection, vision changes, vomiting, weakness, weight gain, wheezing

Notify your doctor if you have appetite loss, dark urine, flu-like symptoms, yellowing of the skin. You will need to be switched from Coreg.

Coreg can cover up the symptoms of low blood sugar. If you have diabetes, monitor your blood sugar regularly.

Can I receive Coreg if I am pregnant or breastfeeding?

The effects of Coreg during pregnancy and breastfeeding are unknown. Talk with your doctor before taking this drug if you are pregnant, plan to become pregnant, or are breastfeeding.

What should I do if I miss a dose of Coreg?

Take it as soon as you remember. If it is almost time for your next dose, skip the one you missed and go back to your regular schedule. Do not take 2 doses at once.

How should I store Coreg?

Store at room temperature away from light and moisture.

COREG CR
Generic name: Carvedilol phosphate, extended-release

What is Coreg CR?
Coreg CR is used to treat mild-to-severe heart failure, high blood pressure (hypertension), and/or a heart attack that reduced how well the heart pumps.

What is the most important information I should know about Coreg CR?
Coreg CR may mask the symptoms of low blood sugar or may alter blood sugar levels. If you have high blood sugar, you should report any changes in blood sugar levels to your doctor right away.

Coreg CR also may mask the symptoms of hyperthyroidism (over activity of the thyroid gland), such as a rapid heart rate.

If you are taking Coreg CR, do not suddenly stop taking it, which can lead to chest pain and, in some cases, heart attack. If your doctor decides that you should stop taking Coreg CR, he or she will slowly reduce your doses over a period of time before stopping it completely.

Who should not take Coreg CR?
Do not take Coreg CR if you are allergic to it or any of its ingredients, or if you have severe liver problems.

What should I tell my doctor before I take the first dose of Coreg CR?
Tell your doctor about all prescription, over-the-counter, and herbal medications you are taking before beginning treatment with Coreg CR. Also, talk to your doctor about your complete medical history, especially if you have severe liver impairment, breathing problems, severe slow heart rate, high blood sugar, low blood pressure, any heart problems, are pregnant, plan to become pregnant, or are breastfeeding.

What is the usual dosage?
The information below is based on the dosage guidelines your doctor uses. Depending on your condition and medical history, your doctor may prescribe a different regimen. Do not change the dosage or stop taking your medication without your doctor's approval.

Heart Failure
Adults: The recommended starting dose of Coreg CR is 10 milligrams (mg) once daily for 2 weeks. If needed, your daily dose may be increased to 20, 40, or 80 mg over successive intervals of at least 2 weeks.

Hypertension
Adults: The recommended starting dose of Coreg CR is 20 mg once daily and should be maintained for 7 to 14 days. If needed, your doctor may raise your dose every 1 or 2 weeks to a maximum of 80 mg once a day.

Left Ventricular Dysfunction Following Heart Attack
Adults: The recommended starting dose is 20 mg once a day. Your doctor may increase the dosage after 3 to 10 days to 40 mg once a day. Based on your response, your doctor may again increase the dose up to a maximum of 80 mg once a day.

How should I take Coreg CR?

Coreg CR should be taken once daily in the morning with food. The capsules should be swallowed whole and never be crushed or chewed.

If you have problems swallowing Coreg CR capsules, you may carefully open the capsule and sprinkle the beads over a spoonful of applesauce, and eat it right away. The applesauce should not be warm. Do not sprinkle the capsule beads on foods other than applesauce.

What should I avoid while taking Coreg CR?

Do not interrupt or discontinue Coreg CR treatment without speaking to your doctor. Abrupt discontinuation can lead to worsening of your symptoms. Avoid driving or hazardous tasks until you know how Coreg CR affects you.

What are possible food and drug interactions associated with Coreg CR?

If Coreg CR is taken with certain other drugs, the effects of either could be increased, decreased, or altered. It is especially important to check with your doctor before combining Coreg CR with any of the following: clonidine, cyclosporine, digoxin, diltiazem, fluoxetine, glipizide, glyburide, insulin, isocarboxazid, metformin, paroxetine, phenelzine, propafenone, reserpine, selegiline, quinide, verapamil

What are the possible side effects of Coreg CR?

Side effects cannot be anticipated. If any develop or change in intensity, tell your doctor as soon as possible. Only your doctor can determine if it is safe for you to continue taking this drug.

Side effects may include: shortness of breath, a slow heartbeat, weight gain, fatigue, low blood pressure, dizziness, faintness

Can I receive Coreg CR if I am pregnant or breastfeeding?

The effects of Coreg CR during pregnancy and breastfeeding are unknown. Tell your doctor immediately if you are pregnant, plan to become pregnant, or are breastfeeding.

What should I do if I miss a dose of Coreg CR?

Take it as soon as you remember. If it is almost time for your next dose, skip the one you missed and go back to your regular schedule. Do not take 2 doses at once.

How should I store Coreg CR?

Store the medication at room temperature.

CORGARD

Generic name: Nadolol

What is Corgard?

Corgard is used in the treatment of chest pain, usually caused by lack of oxygen to the heart due to clogged arteries. It is also used to reduce high blood pressure.

What is the most important information I should know about Corgard?

You should not stop taking Corgard suddenly. This can cause increased chest pain and even a heart attack. If needed, your dose should be gradually reduced by your doctor.

If you have high blood pressure, you must take Corgard regularly for it to be effective. Since blood pressure declines gradually, it may be several weeks before you get the full benefit of Corgard. You must continue taking it even if you are feeling well. Corgard dose not cure high blood pressure, it only keeps it under control.

Who should not take Corgard?

Do not use Corgard if you have breathing problems, certain types of heart problems, or if you are allergic to Corgard or any of its ingredients.

What should I tell my doctor before I take the first dose of Corgard?

Tell your doctor about all prescription, over-the-counter, and herbal medications you are taking before beginning treatment with Corgard. Also, talk to your doctor about your complete medical history, especially if you have breathing or heart problems, high blood sugar, kidney disease, or liver disease.

What is the usual dosage?

The information below is based on the dosage guidelines your doctor uses. Depending on your condition and medical history, your doctor may prescribe a different regimen. Do not change the dosage or stop taking your medication without your doctor's approval.

Chest Pain

Adults: The usual initial dose is 40 milligrams (mg) once daily. Your dose may be increased by 40 to 80 mg at 3- to 7-day intervals. The usual long-term dose is 40 or 80 mg once daily. Doses up to 160 or 240 mg once a day may be needed in certain patients.

High Blood Pressure
Adults: The usual initial dose is 40 mg once daily. Your dose may be gradually increased by 40 to 80 mg increments. The usual long-term dose is 40 or 80 mg once daily. Doses up to 240 or 320 mg once a day may be needed in certain patients.

If you have kidney disease your doctor may prescribe lower doses.

How should I take Corgard?
Corgard can be taken with or without food.

What should I avoid while taking Corgard?
Do not stop taking Corgard abruptly. This can cause increased chest pain and even a heart attack. Speak to your doctor before you stop taking Corgard.

Corgard may make you drowsy or less alert. Avoid driving or operating dangerous machinery or participating in any hazardous activity that requires full mental alertness until you know how Corgard affects you.

What are possible food and drug interactions associated with Corgard?
If Corgard is taken with certain other drugs, the effects of either could be increased, decreased, or altered. It is especially important to check with your doctor before combining Corgard with any of the following: blood pressure medications, diabetes medications including insulin and glyburide, epinephrine.

What are the possible side effects of Corgard?
Side effects cannot be anticipated. If any develop or change in intensity, tell your doctor as soon as possible. Only your doctor can determine if it is safe for you to continue taking this drug.

Side effects may include: change in behavior, changes in heartbeat, dizziness, mild drowsiness, slow heartbeat, weakness, fatigue

Corgard may mask the symptoms of low blood sugar or it can alter blood sugar levels. If you are diabetic, monitor your blood sugar regularly.

Can I receive Corgard if I am pregnant or breastfeeding?
The effects of Corgard during pregnancy and breastfeeding are unknown. Talk with your doctor before taking this drug if you are pregnant, plan to become pregnant, or are breastfeeding.

What should I do if I miss a dose of Corgard?
Take it as soon as you remember. If it is within 8 hours of your next scheduled dose, skip the one you missed and go back to your regular schedule. Never take 2 doses at the same time.

How should I store Corgard?
Store at room temperature away from light and heat. Keep in a tightly closed container.

CORTISPORIN OTIC
Generic name: Neomycin, polymyxin B sulfates, and hydrocortisone

What is Cortisporin Otic?
Cortisporin Otic is used in the treatment of outer ear infections.

What is the most important information I should know about Cortisporin Otic?
Cortisporin Otic's ingredient, neomycin, may cause permanent hearing loss. This particular drug may damage hair cells on an organ in the ear, leading to deafness.

Cortisporin Otic may also cause skin problems within the ear. The skin may become overly sensitive to the ingredient neomycin, leading to such problems as an outer ear infection.

Who should not take Cortisporin Otic?
Do not use Cortisporin Otic if you are allergic to any of its ingredients. Also, this drug should not be used if the outer ear infection is caused by a virus, such as herpes.

What should I tell my doctor before I take the first dose of Cortisporin Otic?
Tell your doctor about all prescription, over-the-counter, and herbal medications you are taking before beginning treatment with Cortisporin Otic. Also, talk to your doctor about your complete medical history, especially if you have had previous trauma to your ear.

What is the usual dosage?
The information below is based on the dosage guidelines your doctor uses. Depending on your condition and medical history, your doctor may prescribe a different regimen. Do not change the dosage or stop taking your medication without your doctor's approval.

Adults: The usual adult dosage of Cortisporin Otic is 4 drops in the ear, 3-4 times per day, for a maximum of 10 days.

Children: The usual children's dosage is 3 drops, 3-4 times per day.

How should I take Cortisporin Otic?
Clean and dry your ear, and shake the bottle of Coritsporin Otic well. Then, lie down on your side, with your infected ear facing upward. The prescribed number of drops should be placed in the ear; remain in this

position for 5 minutes to allow penetration of the medication. Repeat in the opposite ear if necessary.

What should I avoid while taking Cortisporin Otic?
Avoid touching the dropper to your ear or fingers; this may cause contamination of the dropper. Also, avoid using Cortisporin Otic for more than 10 days.

What are possible food and drug interactions associated with Cortisporin Otic?
If Cortisporin Otic is taken with certain other drugs, the effects of either could be increased, decreased, or altered. It is especially important to check with your doctor before combining Cortisporin Otic with the following: gentamycin, kanamycin, panomomycin, and streptomycin.

What are the possible side effects of Cortisporin Otic?
Side effects cannot be anticipated. If any develop or change in intensity, tell your doctor as soon as possible. Only your doctor can determine if it is safe for you to continue taking this drug.

Side effects may include: burning, dryness, excessive hair growth, fungal infection, inflammation of hairs in the ear, irritation, itching, skin color change, skin rashes

Can I receive Cortisporin Otic if I am pregnant or breastfeeding?
The effects of Cortisporin Otic during pregnancy and breastfeeding are unknown. Tell your doctor immediately if you are pregnant, plan to become pregnant, or are breastfeeding.

How should I store Cortisporin Otic?
Store at room temperature.

CORZIDE
Generic name: Bendroflumethiazide and nadolol

What is Corzide?
Corzide is a combination drug used to treat high blood pressure.

What is the most important information I should know about Corzide?
Do not stop taking Corzide abruptly. This can cause increased chest pain and even a heart attack. If needed, your dose should be gradually reduced by your doctor.

Corzide may mask the symptoms of low blood sugar or may alter blood sugar levels. If you have diabetes or high blood sugar, you should report any changes in blood sugar levels to your doctor right away.

You must take Corzide regularly for it to be effective. Since blood pressure declines gradually, it may be several weeks before you get the full benefit of Corzide. You must continue taking it even if you are feeling well. Corzide does not cure high blood pressure; it only keeps it under control.

Who should not take Corzide?
Do not use Corzide if you have breathing problems, slow heartbeat, certain heartbeat irregularities, active heart failure, inability to urinate, or if you are sensitive to or have ever had an allergic reaction to Corzide, its ingredients, or similar drugs.

What should I tell my doctor before I take the first dose of Corzide?
Tell your doctor about all prescription, over-the-counter, and herbal medications you are taking before beginning treatment with Corzide. Also, talk to your doctor about your complete medical history, especially if you have breathing problems, high blood sugar, lung disease, a history of long-term heart failure, kidney disease, liver disease, allergic reactions, seasonal allergies, or thyroid problems.

What is the usual dosage?
The information below is based on the dosage guidelines your doctor uses. Depending on your condition and medical history, your doctor may prescribe a different regimen. Do not change the dosage or stop taking your medication without your doctor's approval.

Adults: The usual dose is 1 Corzide 40/5 milligram (mg) tablet daily. If necessary, you may need 1 Corzide 80/5 mg tablet daily. If you have kidney problems, you may be prescribed a lower dose or take it less frequently. If Corzide fails to bring your blood pressure under control, your doctor may gradually add another high blood pressure drug.

How should I take Corzide?
Corzide may be taken with or without food. Take it exactly as prescribed even if you do not have any symptoms.

What should I avoid while taking Corzide?
Try not to miss any doses. Corzide should not be stopped suddenly. This can cause increased chest pain and even a heart attack.

Corzide may intensify the effects of alcohol. Do not drink alcoholic beverages while taking Corzide.

What are possible food and drug interactions associated with Corzide?
If Corzide is taken with any other drug, the effects of either could be increased, decreased, or altered. It is especially important to check with your doctor before combining Corzide with any of the following: alcohol,

amphotericin B, antidepressant drugs known as MAO inhibitors (such as phenelzine or tranylcypromine), antigout drugs, barbiturates, blood thinners, calcium salts, blood pressure medications (such as chlorothiazide or hydralazine/reserpine/hydrochlorothiazide or enalapril), cholestyramine, colestipol, corticosteroids, diabetes drugs, diazoxide, digoxin, epinephrine, lithium, methenamine, narcotics such as morphine, nonsteroidal anti-inflammatory drugs such as naproxen, reserpine, sulfinpyrazone

What are the possible side effects of Corzide?

Side effects cannot be anticipated. If any develop or change in intensity, tell your doctor as soon as possible. Only your doctor can determine if it is safe for you to continue taking this drug.

Side effects may include: breathing problems, changes in heartbeat, cold hands and feet, dizziness, fatigue, low blood pressure, low potassium levels (symptoms include dry mouth, excessive thirst, weakness, drowsiness, restlessness, weak or irregular heartbeat, muscle pain or cramps, diminished urination, and upset stomach)

Can I receive Corzide if I am pregnant or breastfeeding?

The effects of Corzide during pregnancy and breastfeeding are unknown. Talk with your doctor before taking this drug if you are pregnant, plan to become pregnant, or are breastfeeding.

What should I do if I miss a dose of Corzide?

Take it as soon as you remember. If it is within 8 hours of your next scheduled dose, skip the one you missed and go back to your regular schedule. Never take 2 doses at the same time.

How should I store Corzide?

Store at room temperature, away from heat, in a tightly closed container.

COSOPT

*Generic name: Dorzolamide hydrochloride
    and timolol maleate*

What is Cosopt?

Cosopt is a medicine for lowering pressure in the eye in people with open-angle glaucoma. It is often used when another eye drop medication alone is not adequate to control eye pressure.

What is the most important information I should know about Cosopt?

Eye medications, if handled improperly, can become contaminated by common bacteria known to cause eye infections. Serious damage to the eye and subsequent loss of vision may result from using contaminated eye medications. If you think your medication may be contaminated, or if you develop an eye infection, contact your doctor immediately.

Do not share this medication with anyone else.

Who should not take Cosopt?
Do not take Cosopt if you are allergic to it or any of its ingredients. Also, do not use this drug if you have breathing or lung problems, a slow or irregular heart beat, or heart failure.

What should I tell my doctor before I take the first dose of Cosopt?
Tell your doctor about all prescription, over-the-counter, and herbal medications you are taking before beginning treatment with Cosopt. Also, talk to your doctor about your complete medical history, especially if you are pregnant or planning to become pregnant, breastfeeding, or have a history of breathing or lung problems, high blood sugar, thyroid problems, and kidney or liver problems. Also, tell your doctor if you develop an eye infection, develop a red or swollen eye or eyelid, receive an eye injury and develop new or worsening eye symptoms, or if you plan on having any type of surgery.

What is the usual dosage?
The information below is based on the dosage guidelines your doctor uses. Depending on your condition and medical history, your doctor may prescribe a different regimen. Do not change the dosage or stop taking your medication without your doctor's approval.

Adults: The usual dose of Cosopt is 1 drop in the morning and 1 drop in the evening in the affected eye(s).

How should I take Cosopt?
If you are using Cosopt with another eyedrop, the eyedrops should be used at least 10 minutes apart.

To take Cosopt, tilt your head back and pull your lower eyelid down slightly to form a pocket between your eyelid and your eye. Invert the bottle, and press lightly with the thumb or index finger over the "Finger Push Area" until a single drop is dispensed into the eye.

What should I avoid while taking Cosopt?
Do not allow the tip of the bottle to touch the eye or areas around the eye to prevent the contamination of your medicine. Contamination may cause eye infections leading to serious damage to the eye, even loss of vision.

What are possible food and drug interactions associated with Cosopt?
If Cosopt is taken with certain other drugs, the effects of either could be increased, decreased, or altered. It is especially important to check with

your doctor before combining Cosopt with any of the following: beta-blockers such as propranolol, calcium antagonists such as nifedipine, clonidine, digitalis in combination with calcium antagonists, injectable epinephrine, oral carbonic anhydrase inhibitors such as acetazolamide, quinidine, reserpine, selective serotonin reuptake inhibitors (SSRIs).

What are the possible side effects of Cosopt?
Side effects cannot be anticipated. If any develop or change in intensity, tell your doctor as soon as possible. Only your doctor can determine if it is safe for you to continue taking this drug.

Side effects may include: bitter or sour taste after eyedrops have been placed in the eye, blurred vision, burning and stinging, redness of the eye(s), tearing or itching

Contact your doctor immediately if you experience an irregular heartbeat and/or a slowing of your heart rate, shortness of breath, visual changes

Can I receive Cosopt if I am pregnant or breastfeeding?
The effects of Cosopt during pregnancy and breastfeeding are unknown. Tell your doctor immediately if you are pregnant, plan to become pregnant, or are breastfeeding.

What should I do if I miss a dose of Cosopt?
Take it as soon as you remember. If it is within 8 hours of your next scheduled dose, skip the one you missed and go back to your regular schedule. Never take 2 doses at the same time.

How should I store Cosopt?
Store at room temperature, away from light.

COUMADIN
Generic name: Warfarin sodium

What is Coumadin?
Coumadin is an anticoagulant (blood thinner) used to reduce clots from forming in the blood. It is also used to prevent and/or treat blood clots in the legs and lungs associated with an irregular, rapid heartbeat or those associated with heart-valve replacement. It may also be used after a heart attack to lower the risk of death, another heart attack, stroke, or blood clots moving to other parts of the body.

What is the most important information I should know about Coumadin?
The most serious risks associated with Coumadin are hemorrhage (severe bleeding resulting in the loss of a large amount of blood) in any

tissue or organ and, less frequently, the destruction of skin tissue cells (necrosis) or gangrene. The risk of hemorrhage usually depends on the dosage and length of treatment with Coumadin.

Hemorrhage and necrosis have been reported to result in death or permanent disability. Severe necrosis can lead to the removal of damaged tissue or amputation of a limb. Necrosis appears to be associated with blood clots located in the area of tissue damage and usually occurs within a few days of starting Coumadin treatment.

Who should not take Coumadin?

Coumadin should not be used for any condition where the danger of hemorrhage may be greater than the potential benefits of treatment. Unless directed to do so by your doctor, do not take Coumadin if one of the following conditions or situations applies to you: a tendency to hemorrhage; alcoholism; an abnormal blood condition; aneurysm (balloon-like swelling of a blood vessel) in the brain or heart; bleeding tendencies associated with ulceration or bleeding of the stomach, intestines, respiratory tract, or the genital or urinary system; eclampsia (a rare and serious hypertensive disorder that can occur during pregnancy) or preeclampsia; excessive bleeding of brain blood vessels; inflammation, due to bacterial infection of the membrane that lines the inside of the heart; inflammation of the sac that surrounds the heart or an escape of fluid from the heart sac; malignant hypertension (extremely elevated blood pressure that damages the inner linings of blood vessels, the heart, spleen, kidneys, and brain); pregnancy; recent or scheduled surgery of the central nervous system (brain and spinal cord) or eyes; spinal puncture or any procedure that can cause uncontrollable bleeding; threatened miscarriage; or allergy to any of the drug's ingredients.

What should I tell my doctor before I take the first dose of Coumadin?

Tell your doctor about all prescription, over-the-counter, and herbal medication you are taking before beginning treatment with Coumadin. Also, talk to your doctor about your complete medical history, especially if you have an infectious disease or intestinal disorder; a family history of blood clotting disorders; an implanted catheter; chronic heart failure; recent or scheduled dental procedures; high blood sugar (diabetes); inflammation of a blood vessel; kidney or liver disease; moderate to severe high blood pressure; moderate to severe kidney or liver dysfunction; a blood disorder called polycythemia vera; surgery or injury that leaves large raw surfaces; or trauma or injury that may result in internal bleeding.

What is the usual dosage?

The information below is based on the dosage guidelines your doctor uses. Depending on your condition and medical history, your doctor

may prescribe a different regimen. Do not change the dosage or stop taking your medication without your doctor's approval.

Adults: A common starting dose is 2 to 5 milligrams (mg) per day. Individualized daily dosage adjustments are based on the results of blood tests that determine the amount of time it takes for the blood clotting process to begin.

A long-term dose of 2 to 10 mg per day is satisfactory for most people. The duration of treatment will be determined by your doctor.

Elderly: Low starting and long-term doses are recommended for older people.

Coumadin is not approved for use in patients <18 years.

How should I take Coumadin?

Take Coumadin exactly as prescribed. Your doctor must monitor your condition on a regular basis. Be especially careful to stick to the exact dosage schedule your doctor prescribes. Try to take Coumadin the same time every day.

Carry an identification card that indicates you are taking Coumadin.

What should I avoid while taking Coumadin?

Do not take or discontinue any other medication unless directed to do so by your doctor. Avoid alcohol, salicylates such as aspirin, larger than usual amounts of foods rich in vitamin K (eg, liver, vegetable oil, egg yolks, and green leafy vegetables) that can counteract the effect of Coumadin, or any other drastic change in diet.

Avoid activities and sports that could cause an injury and bleeding.

What are possible food and drug interactions associated with Coumadin?

Coumadin can interact with a wide variety of drugs, both prescription and over-the-counter. Check with your doctor before taking any medication or vitamin product. Be extremely cautious, too, about taking any herbal remedies and supplements. A wide assortment of herbal products, including St. John's wort, coenzyme Q10, bromelain, dan-shen, dong quai, garlic, cranberry products, and gingko biloba, are known to interact with Coumadin or otherwise affect coagulation.

What are the possible side effects of Coumadin?

Side effects cannot be anticipated. If any develop or change in intensity, tell your doctor as soon as possible. Only your doctor can determine if it is safe for you to continue taking this drug.

Side effects may include: bleeding (signs and symptoms of bleeding include headache, dizziness, or weakness; bleeding from shaving or other cuts that does not stop; nosebleeds; bleeding of gums when brushing your teeth; throwing up blood; unusual bruising for unknown reasons; red or dark brown urine; red or black color in your stool; more bleeding than usual during your menstrual period or unexpected bleeding from the vagina; unusual pain or swelling

Treatment with blood thinners may increase the risk that fatty plaque will break away from the wall of an artery and lodge at another point, causing the blockage of a blood vessel. If you notice any of the following symptoms, contact your doctor immediately: Abdominal pain, abrupt and intense pain in the leg, foot or toes, blood in the urine, bluish mottling of the skin of the legs and hands, foot ulcers, gangrene, high blood pressure, muscle pain, "purple toes syndrome" (see below), rash, or thigh or back pain.

Purple toes syndrome can occur when taking Coumadin, usually 3 to 10 weeks after starting therapy. Symptoms include dark purplish or mottled color that turns white when pressure is applied and fades when you elevate your legs; pain and tenderness; and change in intensity of the color over a period of time. If any of these symptoms develop, notify your doctor immediately.

Can I receive Coumadin if I am pregnant or breastfeeding?
Do not take Coumadin if you are or may become pregnant because it can cause fatal hemorrhage in the developing baby. If you become pregnant while taking Coumadin, inform your doctor immediately. Avoid breastfeeding while you are taking Coumadin.

What should I do if I miss a dose of Coumadin?
If you forget to take a pill, tell your healthcare provider immediately. Take the missed dose as soon as possible on the same day. Do not take 2 doses at the same time.

How should I store Coumadin?
Store at room temperature in a tightly closed container away from light.

COZAAR
Generic name: Losartan potassium

What is Cozaar?
Cozaar is used to treat high blood pressure, to lower the risk of stroke if you have high blood pressure and a heart problem called left ventricular hypertrophy, or to slow the worsening of diabetic kidney disease (nephropathy).

What is the most important information I should know about Cozaar?

You must take Cozaar regularly for it to be effective. Since blood pressure declines gradually, it may be several weeks before you get the full benefit of Cozaar. You must continue taking it even if you are feeling well. Cozaar does not cure high blood pressure; it keeps it under control.

Do not take Cozaar if you are pregnant or plan to become pregnant. Cozaar can harm your unborn baby.

Cozaar is not recommended in children <6 years of age.

Who should not take Cozaar?

Do not take Cozaar if you are allergic to any of the ingredients.

What should I tell my doctor before I take the first dose of Cozaar?

Tell your doctor about all prescription, over-the-counter, and herbal medications you are taking before beginning treatment with Cozaar. Also, talk to your doctor about your complete medical history, especially if you have chronic heart failure, kidney disease, liver disease, or if you are vomiting a lot or having diarrhea.

What is the usual dosage?

The information below is based on the dosage guidelines your doctor uses. Depending on your condition and medical history, your doctor may prescribe a different regimen. Do not change the dosage or stop taking your medication without your doctor's approval.

High Blood Pressure
Adults: The usual starting dose is 50 milligrams (mg) once daily. However, Cozaar can be taken twice daily, with total daily doses ranging from 25 to 100 mg. If your blood pressure does not respond within 3 to 6 weeks, your doctor may increase your dose or add a low-dose diuretic (water pill) to your regimen.

Children >6 years: The usual recommended dose is 0.7 mg per 2.2 pounds once a day. The maximum daily dose should not exceed 50 mg, and the doses can be given in tablets or suspension (liquid form).

High Blood Pressure with Heart Problems
Adults: The usual starting dose is 50 mg once daily. A diuretic is often added and you doctor will modify your doses accordingly.

Diabetic Kidney Disease
Adults: The usual starting dose is 50 mg once daily. The doctor may increase the dose to 100 mg once a day if blood pressure remains too high.

How should I take Cozaar?

Take Cozaar exactly as prescribed by your doctor. Cozaar can be taken with or without food.

What should I avoid while taking Cozaar?

Avoid driving or operating machinery until you know how Cozaar affects you. You may feel lightheaded or faint, especially during the first few days of therapy.

Avoid excessive sweating, dehydration, severe diarrhea, or vomiting, which could make you lose too much water and cause a severe drop in blood pressure.

Do not take potassium supplements or potassium-containing salt substitutes without consulting your doctor.

What are possible food and drug interactions associated with Cozaar?

If Cozaar is taken with certain other drugs, the effects of either could be increased, decreased, or altered. It is especially important to check with your doctor before taking Cozaar with the following: diuretics (water pills) nonsteroidal anti-inflammatory drugs (NSAIDs) such as indomethacin, potassium supplements, salt substitutes containing potassium.

What are the possible side effects of Cozaar?

Side effects cannot be anticipated. If any develop or change in intensity, tell your doctor as soon as possible. Only your doctor can determine if it is safe for you to continue taking this drug.

Side effects may include: back pain, diarrhea, dizziness, low blood pressure, low blood sugar, stuffy nose, fatigue, upper respiratory infections

Can I receive Cozaar if I am pregnant or breastfeeding?

Drugs such as Cozaar can cause injury or even death to the unborn child when used in the second or third trimester of pregnancy. Stop taking Cozaar as soon as you know you are pregnant. If you are pregnant or plan to become pregnant, tell your doctor before taking Cozaar. Do not breastfeed while you are taking Cozaar.

What should I do if I miss a dose of Cozaar?

If you miss a dose, take it as soon as you remember. If it is close to your next dose, do not take the missed dose. Take the next dose at your regular time. Do not take 2 doses at once.

How should I store Cozaar?

Store at room temperature in a tightly closed container away from light.

CRESTOR

Generic name: Rosuvastatin calcium

What is Crestor?

Crestor is used to lower cholesterol levels when diet and exercise alone have failed to work. Crestor can help lower the total cholesterol count as well as harmful levels of low-density lipoprotein (LDL) cholesterol. It can also lower triglycerides, a type of fat that is carried through the bloodstream and can end up being stored as body fat.

What is the most important information I should know about Crestor?

Crestor is prescribed only if diet, exercise, and weight loss fail to lower your cholesterol levels. Crestor is meant to supplement, not replace, these lifestyle changes. To get the full benefit of Crestor, you need to stick to the diet and exercise program prescribed by your doctor.

Who should not take Crestor?

Do not take Crestor if you have liver disease, are pregnant or could become pregnant, or are breastfeeding, or if you are allergic to Crestor or any of its ingredients.

What should I tell my doctor before I take the first dose of Crestor?

Tell your doctor about all prescription, over-the-counter, and herbal medications you are taking before beginning treatment with Crestor. Also, talk to your doctor about your complete medical history, especially if you drink large amounts of alcohol, if you have kidney disease, liver disease, or thyroid problems.

What is the usual dosage?

The information below is based on the dosage guidelines your doctor uses. Depending on your condition and medical history, your doctor may prescribe a different regimen. Do not change the dosage or stop taking your medication without your doctor's approval.

Adults: The usual starting dose is 10 milligrams (mg) once a day. Your doctor may start you at 5 mg per day if your LDL cholesterol level doesn't require a high dose or if you are at risk for muscle damage. If your LDL cholesterol level is >190, the doctor may start you at 20 mg once a day. If this dose fails to lower your cholesterol, the doctor may increase your dose to 40 mg per day.

Kidney impairment: If you have severe kidney problems, the recommended starting dose is 5 mg once a day, up to a maximum of 10 mg daily.

If you have a rare genetic disorder known as homozygous familial hypercholesterolemia, which causes unusually high cholesterol levels, the doctor will probably start you at 20 mg once a day. If needed, the dose may be raised to a maximum of 40 mg a day.

If you're taking cyclosporine, the doctor will limit your dose to 5 mg once a day. If you're taking the cholesterol-lowering drug gemfibrozil, your dose must be limited to 10 mg once a day.

How should I take Crestor?
Take Crestor once a day with or without food. Swallow each tablet whole with a glass of water. If you need to take an antacid that contains aluminum and magnesium hydroxide, such as Maalox or Mylanta, be sure to take it at least 2 hours after you take Crestor.

What should I avoid while taking Crestor?
Avoid drinking alcohol while you are taking Crestor.

What are possible food and drug interactions associated with Crestor?
If you take Crestor with certain other drugs, the effects of either could be increased, decreased, or altered. It is especially important to check with your doctor before combining Crestor with any of the following: antacids, cholesterol-lowering drugs such as clofibrate or fenofibrate, cimetidine, cyclosporine, gemfibrozil, ketoconazole, niacin, oral contraceptives, Spironolactone, warfarin

What are the possible side effects of Crestor?
Side effects cannot be anticipated. If any develop or change in intensity, tell your doctor as soon as possible. Only your doctor can determine if it is safe for you to continue taking this drug.

Side effects may include: abdominal pain, constipation, diarrhea, headache, indigestion, nausea, sore throat

Serious side effects may include: signs of muscle tissue damage include unexplained muscle pain, tenderness, or weakness, especially if you also have a fever or you generally do not feel well. If you experience any of these serious side effects, contact your doctor immediately.

Crestor may be associated with abnormal lab test results, including tests for liver and thyroid function and blood sugar levels. If you're having any lab work done, let your doctor know you're taking Crestor.

Can I receive Crestor if I am pregnant or breastfeeding?
Crestor should never be used during pregnancy. If you do become pregnant, tell your doctor immediately. Do not take Crestor while you are breastfeeding.

What should I do if I miss a dose of Crestor?
Take the forgotten dose as soon as you remember. However, if it is almost time for your next dose, skip the one you missed and go back to your regular schedule. Do not take 2 doses at once.

How should I store Crestor?
Store at room temperature and protect from moisture.

CRIXIVAN

Generic name: Indinavir sulfate

What is Crixivan?

Crixivan is used for the treatment of human immunodeficiency virus (HIV).

What is the most important information I should know about Crixivan?

Crixivan is not a cure for HIV or AIDS. People taking Crixivan may still develop infections or other conditions associated with HIV. Because of this, it is very important for you to remain under the care of a doctor. Although Crixivan is not a cure for HIV or AIDS, it can help reduce your chances of getting illnesses associated with HIV. Crixivan does not reduce the risk of passing HIV to others through sexual contact or blood contamination.

It is important that you drink at least six 8-ounce glasses of liquid (preferably water) daily while taking Crixivan. If you do not drink enough liquid, you may develop kidney stones and have to temporarily stop taking Crixivan or even discontinue it altogether. Crixivan is more likely to cause kidney stones in children than in adults.

Who should not take Crixivan?

Do not take Crixivan if you are allergic to it or any of its ingredients.

What should I tell my doctor before I take the first dose of Crixivan?

Tell your doctor about all prescription, over-the-counter, and herbal medications you are taking before beginning treatment with Crixivan. Also, talk to your doctor about your complete medical history, especially if you have high blood sugar (diabetes), if your blood does not clot normally (hemophilia), high cholesterol being treated with cholesterol-lowering medicines called statins, kidney disease, or liver disease.

What is the usual dosage?

The information below is based on the dosage guidelines your doctor uses. Depending on your condition and medical history, your doctor may prescribe a different regimen. Do not change the dosage or stop taking your medication without your doctor's approval.

Adults: The recommended dose of Crixivan is 800 milligrams (mg) every 8 hours. Your doctor may lower the dose to 600 mg every 8 hours if you have liver problems. Your dose will also need adjustment if you are taking delavirdine, didanosine, itraconazole, ketoconazole, or rifabutin.

Children: Crixivan dosage is calculated according to the size and weight of the child.

How should I take Crixivan?

Take Crixivan exactly as prescribed by your doctor. It should be taken every 8 hours, every day; try to take it at the same time every day.

Take Crixivan with water or other beverages such as nonfat milk, juice, coffee, or tea. Take each dose of Crixivan without food but with water at least 1 hour before or 2 hours after a meal. If you experience stomach upset, you can take Crixivan with a light meal. Do not take Crixivan at the same time as any meals that are high in calories, fat, and protein. You must drink at least six 8-ounce glasses of liquids throughout the day, every day.

What should I avoid while taking Crixivan?

Avoid grapefruit juice and St. John's wort while taking Crixivan. Both of these can reduce the effectiveness of the drug.

What are possible food and drug interactions associated with Crixivan?

Crixivan taken with certain other drugs may result in serious or life-threatening problems. Do not take Crixivan with the following medications: alprazolam, amiodarone, astemizole, atazanavir, atorvastatin, cisapride, ergotamine-containing medications, lovastatin, midazolam, pimozide, rifampin, triazolam.

Crixivan may interact with certain other drugs, and the effects of either could be increased, decreased, or altered. It is especially important to check with your doctor before combining Crixivan with the following: antiarrhythmics such as quinidine, anticonvulsants (such as carbamazepine, phenobarbital, or phenytoin), calcium channel blockers (such as amlodipine and felodipine), cimetidine, clarithromycin, delavirdine, didanosine, efavirenz, erectile dysfunction drugs (such as sildenafil, tadalafil, or vardenafil), fluconazole, grapefruit juice, indinavir, isoniazid, itraconazole, ketoconazole, lamivudine, methadone, oral contraceptives, rifabutin, rosuvastatin, stavudine, St. John's wort, steroids such as dexamethasone, tadalafil, trimethoprim/sulfamethoxazole, zidovudine.

What are the possible side effects of Crixivan?

Side effects cannot be anticipated. If any develop or change in intensity, tell your doctor as soon as possible. Only your doctor can determine if it is safe for you to continue taking this drug.

Side effects may include: abdominal pain, acid regurgitation, anemia (low red blood cells), back pain, bladder stones, changes in taste, diarrhea, dizziness, drowsiness, dry skin, fatigue, headache, high blood sugar levels, itching, jaundice (yellowish skin or eyes, especially in children), kidney stones, liver problems, loss of appetite, nausea, pain in the side, rash, redistribution of body fat, sore throat or upper respiratory tract infection, spontaneous bleeding (in people with hemophilia), vomiting, weakness

Can I receive Crixivan if I am pregnant or breastfeeding?
The effects of Crixivan during pregnancy and breastfeeding are unknown. Talk with your doctor before taking this drug if you are pregnant, plan to become pregnant, or are breastfeeding.

What should I do if I miss a dose of Crixivan?
If you miss a dose by more than 2 hours, wait and then take the next dose at the regularly scheduled time. However, if you miss a dose by less than 2 hours, take your missed dose immediately. Then take your next dose at the regularly scheduled time. Do not take 2 doses at the same time.

How should I store Crixivan?
Store at room temperature. Keep away from moisture.

CROLOM
Generic name: Cromolyn sodium

What is Crolom?
Crolom is an eye drop that relieves the itching, tearing, discharge, and redness caused by seasonal and chronic allergies.

What is the most important information I should know about Crolom?
In order for Crolom to work properly, you must continue to use it every day at regular intervals even if your symptoms have disappeared. It can take up to 6 weeks for your condition to clear up.

Who should not take Crolom?
Do not use Crolom if you are allergic to it or any of its ingredients.

What should I tell my doctor before I take the first dose of Crolom?
Tell your doctor about all prescription, over-the-counter, and herbal medications you are taking before beginning treatment with Crolom. Also, talk to your doctor about your complete medical history, especially if you wear contact lenses.

What is the usual dosage?
The information below is based on the dosage guidelines your doctor uses. Depending on your condition and medical history, your doctor may prescribe a different regimen. Do not change the dosage or stop taking your medication without your doctor's approval.

Adults and children: Put 1 or 2 drops into each eye 4 to 6 times a day at evenly spaced intervals.

It is not known whether Crolom is safe and effective for children <4 years.

How should I take Crolom?

Use Crolom exactly as directed by your doctor. Follow the instruction sheet that comes with Crolom. Do not use more or less than required and apply it only when scheduled.

To administer Crolom, wash your hands thoroughly with soap and warm water. Tilt your head back and gently pull your lower eyelid down to form a pocket between your eye and the lid. Drop the medicine into this pocket; release the eyelid. Do not place Crolom directly over the pupil of the eye. Blink a few times to make sure the eye is covered with medication. Close the eye and use a tissue to wipe away any extra medication.

Do not touch the applicator tip to your eye or any other surface. This could lead to infection. Do not rinse the dropper.

What should I avoid while taking Crolom?

Do not wear contact lenses while suffering from allergy-induced eye irritation and while using Crolom.

What are possible food and drug interactions associated with Crolom?

If Crolom is taken with certain other drugs, the effects of either could be increased, decreased, or altered. Always check with your doctor before combining Crolom with any other drugs, herbs, or supplements.

What are the possible side effects of Crolom?

Side effects cannot be anticipated. If any develop or change in intensity, tell your doctor as soon as possible. Only your doctor can determine if it is safe for you to continue taking this drug.

Side effects may include: allergic reactions, dryness around the eye, eye irritation, inflammation of the eyelids, itchy, puffy or watery eyes, styes

Can I receive Crolom if I am pregnant or breastfeeding?

The effects of Crolom during pregnancy and breastfeeding are unknown. Talk with your doctor before taking this drug if you are pregnant, plan to become pregnant, or are breastfeeding.

What should I do if I miss a dose of Crolom?

Use it as soon as possible. Then go back to your regular schedule.

How should I store Crolom?

Store at room temperature. Keep the container tightly closed and away from light.

Cromolyn sodium *See Crolom, page 359. or*
Intal, page 664.

CUTIVATE
Generic name: Fluticasone propionate

What is Cutivate?
Cutivate cream and ointment are prescribed for relief of inflamed, itchy rashes and other inflammatory skin conditions in people ≥3 months.

What is the most important information I should know about Cutivate?
Use of Cutivate may cause hypothalamic-pituitary-adrenal (HPA) axis suppression. This drug may also cause Cushing's syndrome (high levels of cortisol in the body), high blood sugar/glucose, and glucose in the urine.

 This medication is for external use only. If you do not see any improvement of your symptoms within 2 weeks, contact your doctor.

Who should not take Cutivate?
Do not use Cutivate if you are allergic to it or any of its ingredients.

What should I tell my doctor before I take the first dose of Cutivate?
Tell your doctor about all prescription, over-the-counter, and herbal medications you are taking, before beginning treatment with Cutivate. Also, talk to your doctor about your complete medical history.

What is the usual dosage?
The information below is based on the dosage guidelines your doctor uses. Depending on your condition and medical history, your doctor may prescribe a different regimen. Do not change the dosage or stop taking your medication without your doctor's approval.

Adults and children ≥3 months: Apply a thin film of Cutivate to the affected area once or twice daily.

 The safety and efficacy of Cutivate in children <3 months has not been established; therefore, its use is not recommended.

How should I take Cutivate?
Apply a thin layer to infected areas, and rub in gently. Do not cover areas treated with Cutivate with bandages or other dressings.

What should I avoid while taking Cutivate?
Avoid applying under a child's diapers unless your doctor specifically instructs you to do so.

Do not use Cutivate on the face, underarms, or groin areas unless directed by your doctor. Do not use this drug for longer than 4 weeks.

What are the possible side effects of Cutivate?
Side effects cannot be anticipated. If any develop or change in intensity, tell your doctor as soon as possible. Only your doctor can determine if it is safe for you to continue taking this drug.

Side effects may include: burning, stinging, skin infection, itchiness, rash

Can I receive Cutivate if I am pregnant or breastfeeding?
The effects of Cutivate during pregnancy and breastfeeding are unknown. Tell your doctor immediately if you are pregnant, plan to become pregnant, or are breastfeeding.

What should I do if I miss a dose of Cutivate?
Skip the dose you missed and continue on your regular schedule.

How should I store Cutivate?
Store at room temperature.

CYCLESSA
Generic name: Desogestrel and ethinyl estradiol

What is Cyclessa?
Cyclessa is an oral contraceptive used to prevent pregnancy. This medication, a combination of female hormones, also causes changes in your cervical mucus and the uterine lining, impairing the ability of sperm to reach the uterus and fertilized eggs to attach to the uterus.

What is the most important information I should know about Cyclessa?
Cigarette smoking increases the risk of serious cardiovascular side effects from oral contraceptive use. This risk is increased if you smoke >15 cigarettes per day and is quite marked in women >35 years.

Cyclessa (like all oral contraceptives), is intended to prevent pregnancy. It does not protect against transmission of HIV (AIDS) and other sexually transmitted diseases such as chlamydia, genital herpes, genital warts, gonorrhea, hepatitis B, and syphilis.

If any of the following side effects occur while you are taking oral contraceptives, call your doctor or healthcare provider immediately; they could be an indication of a serious medical condition: breast lumps, change in mood, coughing of blood, crushing chest pain or heaviness in the chest, dark-colored urine, difficulty in sleeping, disturbances of vision or speech, dizziness or fainting, fatigue, fever, jaundice or a yellowing of the skin or eyeballs, lack of energy, light-colored bowel movements, loss of appetite, pain in the calf, severe pain or tenderness in the stomach area, sharp chest pain, sudden partial or complete loss of vision, sudden severe headache or vomiting, sudden shortness of breath, weakness or numbness in an arm or leg.

Women with a strong family history of breast cancer or who have breast nodules should be monitored with particular care. Women who are being treated for high cholesterol should be monitored closely if they choose to use oral contraceptives.

Who should not take Cyclessa?

You should not use Cyclessa if you currently have any of the following conditions: A history of blood clots in the legs or in the deep veins of your legs, lungs, or eyes; breast nodules; fibrocystic disease of the breast; an abnormal breast x-ray or mammogram; chest pain (angina pectoris); diabetes with complications of the kidneys, eyes, nerves, or blood vessels; elevated cholesterol or triglycerides; gallbladder, heart, or kidney disease; heavy smoking (15 or more cigarettes per day) and over 35 years old; high blood pressure; history of heart attack or stroke; history of scanty or irregular menstrual periods; known or suspected breast cancer or cancer of the lining of the uterus, cervix, or vagina; known or suspected pregnancy; liver tumor (benign or cancerous); mental depression; migraine or other headaches or epilepsy; unexplained vaginal bleeding (until a diagnosis is reached by your doctor); yellowing of the whites of the eyes or of the skin (jaundice) during pregnancy or during previous use of hormonal birth control of any kind (the pill, patch, vaginal ring, injection, or implant); heart valve or heart rhythm disorders that may be associated with the formation of blood blots; prolonged bed rest following major surgery; known or suspected pregnancy; active liver disease with abnormal liver function tests; or allergy to any of the ingredients in Cyclessa.

What should I tell my doctor before I take the first dose of Cyclessa?

Tell your doctor about all prescription, over-the-counter, and herbal medications you are taking before beginning Cyclessa. Also, talk to your doctor about your complete medical history, especially if you have: breast nodules, fibrocystic disease of the breast, an abnormal breast x-ray or mammogram; diabetes; elevated cholesterol or triglycerides; high blood pressure; migraine or other headaches or epilepsy; mental depression; gallbladder, liver, heart, or kidney disease; scanty or irregular menstrual periods. You should also talk to you doctor if you smoke, recently had a baby, miscarriage, or abortion, or are breastfeeding. (See "Who should not take this medication?" above.)

What is the usual dosage?

The information below is based on the dosage guidelines your doctor uses. Depending on your condition and medical history, your doctor may prescribe a different regimen. Do not change the dosage or stop taking your medication without your doctor's approval.

Adults: Take 1 tablet once a day for 28 days, then repeat. Start the first Sunday after you begin menstruating or the first day of your period.

How should I take Cyclessa?

To achieve maximum contraceptive effectiveness, Cyclessa tablets must be taken exactly as directed, at the same time every day, and at intervals not exceeding 24 hours. Cyclessa may be initiated using either a Sunday start or a Day 1 start. Take one pill at the same time every day until the pack is empty. Do not skip pills even if you are spotting or bleeding between monthly periods or feel sick to your stomach. Do not skip pills even if you do not have sex very often. When you finish the pack or switch brand of pills, start the next pack on the day after your last pill. Do not wait any days between packs.

During the first cycle of use: A woman can begin to take Cyclessa either on the first Sunday after the onset of her menstrual period (Sunday Start) or on the first day of her menstrual period (Day 1 Start). When switching from another oral contraceptive, Cyclessa should be started on the same day that a new pack of the previous oral contraceptive would have been started.

Day 1 start: Pick the label strip that starts with the first day of your period (this is the day you start bleeding or spotting, even if it is almost midnight when the bleeding begins). Place this label strip in the cycle tablet dispenser over the area that has the days of the week (starting with Sunday) imprinted in the plastic. Take the first "active" (light yellow) pill of the first pack during the first 24 hours of your period. You will not need to use a back-up method of birth control, since you are starting the pill at the beginning of your period.

Sunday start: Take the first "active" (light yellow) pill of the first pack on the first Sunday after your period starts, even if you are still bleeding. If your period begins on Sunday, start the pack that same day. Use another method of birth control as a back-up method if you have sex anytime from the Sunday you start your first pack until the next Sunday (7 days).

What should I avoid while taking Cyclessa?

Avoid smoking while taking this medication.

What are possible food and drug interactions associated with Cyclessa?

If oral contraceptives are taken with certain other drugs, the effects of either could be increased, decreased, or altered. It is especially important to check with your doctor before combining oral contraceptives with the following: acetaminophen, antibiotics, ascorbic acid (vitamin C), atorvastatin, barbiturates, carbamazepine, clofibric acid, cyclosporine, felbamate, griseofulvin, HIV protease inhibitors such as ritonavir, itraconazole, ketoconazole, morphine, oxcarbazepine, phenylbutazone, phenytoin, prednisolone, rifampin, salicylic acid, St. John's wort, temazepam, theophylline, and topiramate.

What are the possible side effects of Cyclessa?

Side effects cannot be anticipated. If any develop or change in intensity, tell your doctor as soon as possible. Only your doctor can determine if it is safe for you to continue taking this drug.

Side effects may include: abdominal pain, cramps, or bloating, aggravation of varicose veins, allergic reactions, blood clots, breast tenderness, change in appetite, dark spotting in the skin (particularly skin of the face), difficulty wearing contact lenses, dizziness, fluid retention (swelling of the fingers or ankles), headache, high blood pressure, intolerance to contact lenses, irregular vaginal bleeding, liver tumors, loss of scalp hair, menstrual flow changes, mood changes including depression, nausea, nervousness, rash, vaginal infections, vision changes, vomiting, weight gain

Can I receive Cyclessa if I am pregnant or breastfeeding?

Tell your doctor immediately if you are pregnant, plan to become pregnant, or are breastfeeding. If you are breastfeeding, consult your doctor or healthcare provider before starting oral contraceptives.

What should I do if I miss a dose of Cyclessa?

If you miss pills, you could get pregnant. This includes starting the pack late. The more pills you miss, the more likely you are to get pregnant.

If you miss 1 pill, take it the same day, even if it means taking 2 pills on the same day and continue taking 1 pill/day until the pack is finished.

If you miss 2 pills during first 2 weeks, use a back-up form of contraception for 7 days after the missed pills. Take 2 pills immediately and 2 pills the next day. Then continue taking 1 pill/day until the pack is finished.

If you miss 2 pills during the third week, use a back-up form of contraception for 7 days after the missed pills. If you normally start on Day 1, throw out the remaining pills and start a new pack on the same day. If you normally start on Sunday, keep taking 1 pill/day until Saturday and throw out the remaining pills. On Sunday, start a new pack.

If you are still not sure what to do about the pills you have missed, use a back-up method of birth control and keep taking the active pills each day until you can speak with a healthcare provider.

How should I store Cyclessa?

Store at room temperature.

Cyclobenzaprine hydrochloride See Amrix, page 97, or
Flexeril, page 559.

Cyclosporine See Restasis, page 1137.

CYCLOSPORINE

What is Cyclosporine?

Cyclosporine is given after organ transplant surgery to help prevent
rejection of organs (kidney, heart, or liver) by holding down the body's
immune system. It is also used to avoid long-term rejection in people
previously treated with other immunosuppressant drugs.

In addition to prevention of organ rejection, some brands of cyclosporine are prescribed for certain severe cases of rheumatoid arthritis and
psoriasis.

Cyclosporine is available in capsules and liquid, or as an injection.

What is the most important information
I should know about Cyclosporine?

If you take cyclosporine orally over a period of time, your doctor will
monitor your blood levels to make sure your body is receiving the correct
amount. The reason for this repeated testing is that the absorption of this
drug in the body is erratic. Constant monitoring is necessary to prevent
toxicity due to overdosing or to prevent possible organ rejection due to
underdosing. It is important to note that cyclosporine may need to be
taken by mouth for an indefinite period following surgery.

When your immune system is suppressed by cyclosporine, you are
at increased risk of infection and of certain malignancies, including skin
cancer and lymph system cancer.

High-dose cyclosporine is toxic to the liver and kidneys and may cause
serious kidney damage. Because this toxicity has symptoms similar to
those of transplant rejection, you must be monitored closely. If your body
is trying hard to reject a transplanted organ, your doctor will probably
allow the rejection to occur rather than give you a very high dose of cyclosporine.

This drug can raise blood pressure, especially in older people.

Brain disorders have developed in patients taking this drug, sometimes leading to convulsions, loss of movement, vision problems, impaired consciousness, and psychiatric disturbances. The chance of
convulsions is greater if you are taking high doses of steroid drugs,
particularly methylprednisolone. Brain-related disorders usually clear up
once cyclosporine is discontinued.

Use a barrier method of contraception, such as diaphragms or condoms, during cyclosporine therapy. Do not use oral contraceptive pills
without your doctor's approval.

Who should not take Cyclosporine?
Do not take cyclosporine if you have ever had an allergic reaction to it. Avoid taking cyclosporine for arthritis or psoriasis if you have a kidney condition, high blood pressure, or cancer. While taking the drug, you should avoid most other psoriasis treatments, including ultraviolet light, coal tar, methotrexate, and radiation.

What should I tell my doctor before I take the first dose of Cyclosporine?
Tell your doctor about all prescription, over-the-counter, and herbal medications you are taking before beginning treatment with this drug. Also, talk to your doctor about your complete medical history, especially if you have liver or kidney problems, high blood pressure, infections, or a history of cancer.

What is the usual dosage?
The information below is based on the dosage guidelines your doctor uses. Depending on your condition and medical history, your doctor may prescribe a different regimen. Do not change the dosage or stop taking your medication without your doctor's approval.

Adults and children: Your doctor will tailor the dosage based on your weight, how your body responds, and what other drugs you are taking. The dosage is generally the same for children as for adults, though somewhat higher doses are sometimes needed. Cyclosporine has been used to prevent transplant rejection in small children. It has not, however, been tested for arthritis or psoriasis in children under 18.

How should I take Cyclosporine?
Take the cyclosporine capsule or oral liquid at the same time every day. You may take the medication either with a meal or between meals, but be consistent.

To make cyclosporine oral liquid more palatable, you may mix it with certain room-temperature beverages; check with your doctor or pharmacist about which beverages are best for mixing. Use a container made of glass, not plastic. Never let the mixture stand; drink it as soon as you prepare it. To make sure you get your full dose, rinse the glass with a little more liquid and drink that too.

After you use the dosage syringe to transfer the oral solution to a glass, dry the outside of the syringe with a clean towel and put it away. Do not rinse or wash it. If you do have to clean it, make sure it is thoroughly dry before you use it again.

What should I avoid while taking Cyclosporine?
Do not try to change dosage forms without consulting your doctor.

Avoid getting immunizations while you are taking cyclosporine. The drug may make vaccinations less effective or increase your risk of contracting an illness from a live vaccine.

If taking cyclosporine for psoriasis, remember to avoid other psoriasis treatments.

You should maintain good dental hygiene and see your dentist frequently for cleaning to prevent tenderness, bleeding, and gum enlargement.

What are possible food and drug interactions associated with Cyclosporine?

If cyclosporine is taken with certain other drugs, the effects of either could be increased, decreased, or altered. It is especially important to check with your doctor before combining cyclosporine with the following: allopurinol, amiodarone, amphotericin B, atorvastatin, bromocriptine, calcium-blocking heart and blood pressure medications, carbamazepine, cimetidine, clarithromycin, colchicines, danazol, diclofenac, digoxin, erythromycin, fluconazole, fluvastatin, gentamicin, indinavir, itraconazole, ketoconazole, lovastatin, melphalan, methotrexate, methylprednisolone, metoclopramide, nafcillin, nelfinavir, nonsteroidal anti-inflammatory drugs, octreotide, orlistat, phenobarbital, phenytoin, potassium-sparing diuretics, pravastatin, prednisolone, quinupristin, ranitidine, rifampin, ritonavir, saquinavir, simvastatin, ticlopidine, tacrolimus, tobramycin, trimethoprim/sulfamethoxazole, and vancomycin.

Avoid grapefruit and grapefruit juice while taking this drug. Also avoid the antidepressant herb St. John's wort. This over-the-counter herbal remedy reduces the effect of cyclosporine and can lead to organ rejection.

What are the possible side effects of Cyclosporine?

Side effects cannot be anticipated. If any appear or change in intensity, inform your doctor immediately. Only your doctor can determine if it is safe for you to continue taking cyclosporine. The principal side effects of cyclosporine are high blood pressure, hirsutism (unusual growth of hair), kidney damage, excessive growth of the gums, and tremor.

Other side effects may include: abdominal discomfort, acne, breathing difficulty, convulsions, coughing, cramps, diarrhea, flu-like symptoms, flushing, headache, liver damage, lymph system tumor, muscle, bone, or joint pain, nasal inflammation, nausea, numbness or tingling, sinus inflammation, vomiting, wheezing

Can I receive Cyclosporine if I am pregnant or breastfeeding?

The effects of cyclosporine in pregnancy have not been adequately studied. If you are pregnant or plan to become pregnant, inform your doctor immediately. Cyclosporine should be used during pregnancy only if the benefit justifies the potential risk to the unborn child. Since cyclosporine appears in breast milk, it should not be used during breastfeeding.

What should I do if I miss a dose of Cyclosporine?

If fewer than 12 hours have passed, take it as soon as you remember. If it is almost time for the next dose, skip the one you missed and go back to your regular schedule. Do not take 2 doses at once.

How should I store Cyclosporine?

Store both the capsules and the oral solution at room temperature. Do not store the liquid in the refrigerator. Keep the liquid from freezing.

CYMBALTA

Generic name: Duloxetine hydrochloride

What is Cymbalta?

Cymbalta is used to treat major depression and diabetic neuropathy, a painful nerve disorder associated with diabetes that affects the hands, legs, and feet. Cymbalta is also used to treat generalized anxiety disorder and fibromyalgia.

What is the most important information I should know about Cymbalta?

Cymbalta is not approved for use in children or adolescents.

Antidepressant medicines may increase suicidal thoughts or actions in some children, teenagers, and young adults when the medicine is first started. Depression and other serious mental illnesses are the most important causes of suicidal thoughts and actions. Some people may have a particularly high risk of having suicidal thoughts or actions. These include people who have (or have a family history of) bipolar disorder (also called manic-depressive illness) or suicidal thoughts or actions.

Individuals being treated with antidepressants and their caregivers can help reduce the risk of suicidal thoughts and actions by doing the following:

Pay close attention to any changes, especially sudden ones, in mood, behavior, thoughts, or feelings. This is very important when an antidepressant medicine is first started or when the dose is changed.

Call the doctor right away to report new or sudden changes in mood, behavior, thoughts, or feelings. Signs to watch for include new or worsening depression, new or worsening anxiety, agitation, insomnia, hostility, panic attacks, restlessness, extreme hyperactivity, and suicidal thinking or behavior.

Keep all follow-up visits as scheduled, and call the doctor between visits as needed, especially if you have concerns about symptoms.

Who should not take Cymbalta?

Do not use Cymbalta if you are allergic to it; if you are taking a monoamine oxidase inhibitor (MAOI) or the drug thioridazine; if you have uncontrolled increased pressure in your eyes (narrow-angle glaucoma); or if you have serious kidney or liver disease or drink alcohol excessively.

What should I tell my doctor before I take the first dose of Cymbalta?

Tell your doctor about all prescription, over-the-counter, and herbal medications you are taking before beginning treatment with Cymbalta. Also, talk to your doctor about your complete medical history, especially if you have liver problems, severe kidney disease, diabetes, glaucoma, high blood pressure, a seizure disorder, bipolar disorder, or if you consume large amounts of alcohol.

What is the usual dosage?

The information below is based on the dosage guidelines your doctor uses. Depending on your condition and medical history, your doctor may prescribe a different regimen. Do not change the dosage or stop taking your medication without your doctor's approval.

Diabetic Peripheral Neuropathy, Generalized Anxiety Disorder, and Fibromyalgia
Adults: The recommended dose is 60 mg taken once daily.

Major Depression
Adults: The total daily dose ranges from 40 milligrams (mg) taken as a 20-mg capsule twice a day to 60 mg taken as a 60-mg capsule once a day or as a 30 mg capsule taken twice a day.

How should I take Cymbalta?

Cymbalta can be taken with or without food. Do not crush, chew, or open the capsule; swallow whole.

What should I avoid while taking Cymbalta?

Cymbalta may cause drowsiness and can affect judgment or motor skills. Avoid driving or operating heavy machinery until you know how this drug affects you.

What are possible food and drug interactions associated with Cymbalta?

Never take Cymbalta with the drug thioridazine.

Due to the possibility of liver damage, do not take Cymbalta if you use alcohol more than occasionally.

If Cymbalta is taken with certain other drugs, the effects of either could be increased, decreased, or altered. It is especially important to check with your doctor before combining Cymbalta with the following: antibiotics known as quinolones, such as ciprofloxacin; antidepressants known as tricyclics, including amitriptyline, nortriptyline, and imipramine; antidepressants such as fluoxetine, paroxetine, sertraline, and venlafaxine; antipsychotic medications known as phenothiazines, including chlorpromazine, fluphenazine, mesoridazine, perphenazine, and prochlorperazine; flecainide; fluvoxamine; narcotic painkillers; propafenone; quinidine; sleep inducers; and tranquilizers.

Never combine Cymbalta with any drug classified as an MAOI. Drugs in this category include the antidepressants phenelzine and tranylcypromine. Cymbalta and MAOIs should not be taken together or within 14 days of each other. Combining these drugs with Cymbalta can cause serious and even fatal reactions such as high body temperature, muscle rigidity, twitching, and agitation leading to delirium and coma.

What are the possible side effects of Cymbalta?
Side effects cannot be anticipated. If any develop or change in intensity, tell your doctor as soon as possible. Only your doctor can determine if it is safe for you to continue taking this drug.

Side effects may include: appetite changes, constipation, diarrhea, dizziness, dry mouth, fatigue, headache, insomnia, nausea, sexual difficulties, sleepiness, sweating, tremor, urinary difficulties, vomiting, weakness

Can I receive Cymbalta if I am pregnant or breastfeeding?
The effects of Cymbalta during pregnancy and breastfeeding are unknown. Talk with your doctor before taking this drug if you are pregnant or plan to become pregnant. Avoid breastfeeding while taking Cymbalta.

What should I do if I miss a dose of Cymbalta?
Take the missed dose as soon as you remember. However, if it is almost time for your next dose, skip the one you missed and return to your regular schedule. Do not take two doses at once.

How should I store Cymbalta?
Store at room temperature.

CYTOTEC
Generic name: Misoprostol

What is Cytotec?
Cytotec is used to decrease the chance of getting stomach ulcers caused by nonsteroidal anti-inflammatory drugs (NSAIDs), including aspirin.

What is the most important information I should know about Cytotec?
You must not become pregnant while using Cytotec. This drug causes uterine contractions that could lead to a miscarriage. It is vitally important to use reliable contraception while taking Cytotec.

Who should not take Cytotec?

Do not take Cytotec if you are sensitive to or have ever had an allergic reaction to it. Do not take Cytotec if you are pregnant or might become pregnant while taking it.

What should I tell my doctor before I take the first dose of Cytotec?

Tell your doctor about all prescription, over-the-counter, and herbal medications you are taking before beginning treatment with Cytotec. Also, talk to your doctor about your complete medical history, especially if you have a history of heart disease, inflammatory bowel disease, or kidney disease.

What is the usual dosage?

The information below is based on the dosage guidelines your doctor uses. Depending on your condition and medical history, your doctor may prescribe a different regimen. Do not change the dosage or stop taking your medication without your doctor's approval.

Adults: The recommended dose is 200 micrograms (mcg) 4 times daily. If you cannot tolerate this dose, your doctor may prescribe a dose of 100 mcg 4 times daily.

How should I take Cytotec?

Take Cytotec with a meal and take the last dose of the day at bedtime. You should take Cytotec for the duration of NSAID therapy, as prescribed by your doctor.

What should I avoid while taking Cytotec?

Take Cytotec exactly as prescribed. Do not give this medication to anyone else.

What are possible food and drug interactions associated with Cytotec?

If Cytotec is taken with certain other drugs, the effects of either could be increased, decreased, or altered. Always check with your doctor before combining Cytotec with any other drugs, herbs, or supplements.

What are the possible side effects of Cytotec?

Side effects cannot be anticipated. If any develop or change in intensity, tell your doctor as soon as possible. Only your doctor can determine if it is safe for you to continue taking this drug.

Side effects may include: constipation, gas, indigestion, headache, heavy menstrual bleeding, menstrual disorder, menstrual pain or cramps, paleness, spotting (light bleeding between menstrual periods), stomach or intestinal bleeding, vomiting

Abdominal cramps, diarrhea, and/or nausea may occur during the first few weeks of treatment. These symptoms may disappear as you get used to the drug. If you experience these side effects for more than 8 days or if you have severe diarrhea, cramping, or nausea, call your doctor.

Can I receive Cytotec if I am pregnant or breastfeeding?
Do not take Cytotec if you are pregnant. If you are pregnant or plan to become pregnant, inform your doctor immediately. You will need to take a pregnancy test about 2 weeks before starting to take Cytotec. To be sure you are not pregnant at the start of Cytotec treatment, your doctor may have you take your first dose on the second or third day of your menstrual period. Do not breastfeed while you are taking Cytotec.

What should I do if I miss a dose of Cytotec?
Take it as soon as you remember. If it is almost time for your next dose, skip the one you missed and go back to your regular schedule. Do not take 2 doses at once.

How should I store Cytotec?
Store at room temperature in a dry place.

DALMANE
Generic name: Flurazepam hydrochloride

What is Dalmane?
Dalmane is a hypnotic agent used to treat insomnia, which includes difficulty falling asleep, waking up frequently at night, or waking up early in the morning. Dalmane is also used to treat patients who have medical conditions requiring restful sleep.

What is the most important information I should know about Dalmane?
Do not use this medication if you are pregnant.

The failure of insomnia to remit after 7 to 10 days of treatment may indicate the presence of a primary psychiatric and/or medical illness that should be evaluated.

Due to sedative properties, avoid alcohol consumption while on Dalmane.

Tolerance and dependence may occur with the use of Dalmane.

You may experience withdrawal symptoms if you stop using Dalmane abruptly. Discontinue or change your dose only in consultation with your doctor.

Who should not take Dalmane?
Do not take Dalmane if you are pregnant, under the age of 15, or if you are allergic to it or any of its ingredients.

Elderly patients should use caution, since Dalmane may lead to oversedation, dizziness, and confusion.

What should I tell my doctor before I take the first dose of Dalmane?

Tell your doctor about all prescription, over-the-counter, and herbal medications you are taking before beginning treatment with Dalmane. Also, talk to your doctor about your complete medical history, especially if you have chronic breathing problems, liver or kidney problems, or if you are depressed or have suicidal thoughts. Advise your doctor if you are pregnant, nursing, or you are planning to become pregnant.

What is the usual dosage?

The information below is based on the dosage guidelines your doctor uses. Depending on your condition and medical history, your doctor may prescribe a different regimen. Do not change the dosage or stop taking your medication without your doctor's approval.

Adults: The usual dosage is 30 milligrams (mg) taken before bedtime. In some patients, 15 mg may be sufficient.

How should I take Dalmane?

Take Dalmane exactly as prescribed.

What should I avoid while taking Dalmane?

Avoid driving or participating in hazardous activities after taking Dalmane.

Avoid other sedatives such as alcohol or sleep aids while taking Dalmane.

What are possible food and drug interactions associated with Dalmane?

Alcohol intensifies the effects of Dalmane. Do not drink alcohol while taking Dalmane or until several days after discontinuing it.

If Dalmane is taken with certain other drugs, the effects of either could be increased, decreased, or altered. It is especially important to check with your doctor before combining Dalmane with drugs that slow or depress the central nervous system or that have hypnotic properties. Tell your doctor about all medicines you are taking or plan to take, including prescription and nonprescription medications, nutritional supplements, and herbs.

What are the possible side effects of Dalmane?

Side effects cannot be anticipated. If any develop or change in intensity, tell your doctor as soon as possible. Only your doctor can determine if it is safe for you to continue taking this drug.

Side effects may include: dizziness, drowsiness, light-headedness, staggering, falling, sedation, lethargy, disorientation, headache, heartburn, upset stomach, nausea, vomiting, diarrhea, constipation, stomach pain, nervousness, talkativeness, apprehension, irritability, weakness, palpitations, chest pains, body and joint pain, genital and urinary pain

Withdrawal symptoms may include: convulsions, tremor, abdominal and muscle cramps, vomiting and sweating

Can I receive Dalmane if I am pregnant or breastfeeding?
Do not take Dalmane if you are pregnant or planning to become pregnant. Dalmane should be discontinued prior to becoming pregnant. Consult with your doctor if you are breastfeeding or planning to breastfeed.

How should I store Dalmane?
Store at room temperature.

Darifenacin See Enablex, page 482.

Darunavir See Prezista, page 1063.

DARVOCET-N
Generic name: Propoxyphene napsylate and acetaminophen

What is Darvocet-N?
Darvocet-N is used for the relief of mild to moderate pain, with or without fever.

What is the most important information
I should know about Darvocet-N?
People who take antidepressant drugs or tranquilizers, or who use alcohol in excess, should use caution when taking this drug.

Propoxyphene, when taken in higher-than-recommended doses over long periods of time, can produce drug dependence.

Who should not take Darvocet-N?
Do not take Darvocet-N if you are suicidal or addiction prone, or if you are sensitive to or have ever had an allergic reaction to propoxyphene or acetaminophen.

What should I tell my doctor before
I take the first dose of Darvocet-N?
Tell your doctor about all prescription, over-the-counter, and herbal medications you are taking before beginning treatment with Darvocet-N. Make

sure your doctor knows if you are taking tranquilizers, sleep aids, antide-pressants, antihistamines, or any other drugs that make you sleepy. The use of these drugs with propoxyphene increases their sedative effects and may lead to overdose symptoms, including death. Also, talk to your doctor about your complete medical history, especially if you have kidney or liver problems, if you use alcohol in excess, or if you are suicidal or addiction prone.

What is the usual dosage?
The information below is based on the dosage guidelines your doctor uses. Depending on your condition and medical history, your doctor may prescribe a different regimen. Do not change the dosage or stop taking your medication without your doctor's approval.

Adults: The usual dosage is 100 milligrams (mg) of propoxyphene na-psylate and 650 mg of acetaminophen every 4 hours as needed for pain. The maximum recommended dose of propoxyphene napsylate is 600 mg per day.

Kidney or liver impairment: Patients with kidney or liver problems should receive a lower total daily dose.

How should I take Darvocet-N?
Follow your doctor's directions exactly. Do not increase the amount you take without your doctor's approval.

What should I avoid while taking Darvocet-N?
You should limit your intake of alcohol while taking this medication. Use caution while driving a vehicle or using machinery until you know how the drug affects you, as Darvocet-N can make you sleepy. Do not take more of the drug than your doctor has prescribed.

What are possible food and drug interactions associated with Darvocet-N?
The central nervous system-depressant effect of Darvocet-N is additive with that of other central nervous system (CNS) depressants, including alcohol.

If Darvocet-N is taken with certain other drugs, the effects of either could be increased, decreased, or altered. It is especially important to check with your doctor before combining Darvocet-N with the following: alcohol, anticonvulsants, antidepressants, blood thinners, muscle relax-ants, sedatives, tranquilizers.

What are the possible side effects of Darvocet-N?
Side effects cannot be anticipated. If any develop or change in intensity, tell your doctor as soon as possible. Only your doctor can determine if it is safe for you to continue taking this drug.

Side effects may include: drowsiness, dizziness, nausea, vomiting, constipation, abdominal pain, skin rashes, lightheadedness, headache, weakness, hallucinations, minor visual disturbances, feelings of elation or discomfort

Liver dysfunction has been reported in association with both active components of Darvocet-N 50 and Darvocet-N 100.

Can I receive Darvocet-N if I am pregnant or breastfeeding?
Darvocet-N should not be used during pregnancy unless your doctor knows you are pregnant and specifically recommends its use. Cases of temporary dependence in the newborn have occurred when the mother has taken propoxyphene consistently in the weeks before delivery. Low levels of propoxyphene have been detected in human milk.

What should I do if I miss a dose of Darvocet-N?
If you miss a dose of the drug, skip that dose and resume your regular schedule. Do not take 2 doses at once.

How should I store Darvocet-N?
Store at room temperature.

DAYPRO
Generic name: Oxaprozin

What is Daypro?
Daypro is used to relieve the signs and symptoms of osteoarthritis, rheumatoid arthritis, and juvenile rheumatoid arthritis.

What is the most important information I should know about Daypro?
Daypro belongs to a class of medications known as nonsteroidal anti-inflammatory drugs (NSAIDs). NSAIDs may increase your risk for a potentially fatal heart attack or stroke. This risk is greater with longer use of NSAIDs and in people with heart disease. NSAIDs should never be used right before or after a heart surgery called a coronary artery bypass graft (CABG).

NSAIDs may cause ulcers and bleeding in the stomach and intestines. Ulcers and bleeding may happen without any warning symptoms and may cause death. The risk of getting an ulcer or bleeding is greater if you take medicines called "corticosteroids" or "anticoagulants," with longer NSAID use, or if you smoke, drink alcohol, are older, or have poor health.

Who should not take Daypro?
You should avoid this medication if you have a known sensitivity to Daypro or if you have had an asthma attack, hives, or other allergic reaction

to aspirin or any other NSAID. You should not take Daypro right before or after heart bypass surgery.

What should I tell my doctor before I take the first dose of Daypro?

Tell your doctor about all prescription, over-the-counter, and herbal medication you are taking before beginning treatment with Daypro. Also, talk to your doctor about your complete medical history, especially if you are at risk for heart disease or stroke, or if you have high blood pressure, fluid retention and edema, ulcers or intestinal bleeding, or kidney or liver problems. Tell your doctor if you are pregnant or breastfeeding. Women should not use NSAIDs in late pregnancy.

What is the usual dosage?

The information below is based on the dosage guidelines your doctor uses. Depending on your condition and medical history, your doctor may prescribe a different regimen. Do not change the dosage or stop taking your medication without your doctor's approval.

Osteoarthritis
Adults: The usual recommended dose is 1200 milligrams (mg) (two 600-mg caplets) once a day.

Rheumatoid Arthritis
Adults: The usual recommended dose is 1200 mg (two 600-mg caplets) once a day.

The maximum total daily dose of Daypro in adults is 1800 mg, in divided doses.

Juvenile Rheumatoid Arthritis
Children 6 to 16 years: The recommended daily dose is based on body weight. The recommended dose for patients weighing 48 to 69 pounds is 600 mg once a day; for patients weighing 70 to 119 pounds, it is 900 mg once a day; and for patients weighing ≥120 pounds, it is 1200 mg once a day.

Doses >1200 mg in children have not been studied.

How should I take Daypro?

This medication should be used exactly as prescribed. Use the lowest effective dose for the shortest duration needed.

What should I avoid while taking Daypro?

Avoid drinking alcohol or smoking while taking Daypro. Unless your doctor advises you to do so, avoid using aspirin or other anti-inflammatory medications simultaneously with Daypro. Since Daypro may cause sensitivity to sunlight, avoid prolonged or unprotected exposure to sunlight or artificial sunlamps.

What are possible food and drug interactions associated with Daypro?

If Daypro is taken with certain other drugs, the effects of either could be increased, decreased, or altered. It is especially important to check with your doctor before combining Daypro with the following: ACE inhibitors, aspirin, beta-blockers, diuretics, glyburide, lithium, H_2-receptor antagonists, methotrexate, warfarin.

What are the possible side effects of Daypro?

Side effects cannot be anticipated. If any develop or change in intensity, tell your doctor as soon as possible. Only your doctor can determine if it is safe for you to continue taking this drug.

Side effects may include: stomach pain, constipation, diarrhea, gas, heartburn, nausea, vomiting, dizziness

Serious side effects may include: heart attack, stroke, blood pressure changes, heart failure from fluid retention, liver and kidney problems, gastrointestinal ulcers or bleeding, life-threatening skin reactions, asthma attacks in people who have asthma

Get emergency help right away if you experience any of the following: shortness of breath or trouble breathing, chest pain, weakness in one part or side of your body, slurred speech, swelling of the face or throat.

Stop Daypro and call your doctor right away if you experience any of the following: nausea, feel more tired or weaker than usual, itching, your skin or eyes look yellow, stomach pain, flu-like symptoms, vomit blood, there is blood in your bowel movement or it is black and sticky, skin rash or blisters with fever, unusual weight gain, swelling of the arms and legs, hands, and feet.

Can I receive Daypro if I am pregnant or breastfeeding?

Daypro should be avoided in late pregnancy. If you are nursing, your doctor will advise you whether to discontinue Daypro or to discontinue nursing. It is not known whether Daypro passes from a nursing mother to her infant.

What should I do if I miss a dose of Daypro?

If you miss a dose, take it with food as soon as you remember. If you do not remember until it is time for your next dose, skip the missed dose and go back to your regular schedule. Do not take 2 doses of at the same time.

How should I store Daypro?

Store tightly closed at room temperature and protect from light.

DAYTRANA
Generic name: Methylphenidate patch

What is Daytrana?
Daytrana is a central nervous system stimulant used for the treatment of attention deficit hyperactivity disorder (ADHD). The active ingredient in Daytrana is delivered via an adhesive skin patch that releases the medication through clean and intact skin areas into the bloodstream.

What is the most important information I should know about Daytrana?
Daytrana is a stimulant medicine. The following have been reported with the use of Daytrana or other stimulant medicines: heart-related problems including sudden death in patients who have heart problems or heart defects; stroke and heart attack in adults; increased blood pressure and heart rate.

Remove the patch immediately and call your doctor right away if you or your child has any signs of heart problems.

Other potential problems reported with stimulant medicines include new or worsening behavior and thought problems; new or worsening bipolar disorder; and new or worsening aggressive behavior or hostility. Additional problems reported in children and teenagers include new psychotic symptoms (such as hearing voices, believing things that are not true, becoming suspicious) or new manic symptoms.

Call your doctor right away if you notice any new or worsening mental symptoms.

Abuse of Daytrana can lead to dependence. Daytrana should be given cautiously to people with a history of drug dependence or alcoholism.

Who should not take Daytrana?
Daytrana should not be used by anyone who is very anxious, tense, or agitated; has an eye problem called glaucoma; experiences tics or has Tourette's syndrome, or a family history of Tourette's syndrome; is taking or has taken within the past 14 days an antidepressant called a monoamine oxidase inhibitor (MAOI).

Daytrana is not for use in people known to be hypersensitive to methylphenidate or other components of the product, including an adhesive (glue) made of acrylic and silicone.

What should I tell my doctor before I take the first dose of Daytrana?
Tell your doctor about all prescription, over-the-counter, and herbal medications you or your child is taking before beginning treatment with Daytrana. Also talk to the doctor about all medical conditions (including a family history), especially the following: heart problems, heart defects, high blood pressure; mental problems including psychosis, mania, bipolar

disorder, or depression; tics or Tourette's syndrome; seizures or abnormal brain wave test (EEG); skin problems such as eczema or psoriasis, or any history of skin reactions to soaps, lotions, makeup, or adhesives (glues).

Talk with your doctor especially if you or your child takes antidepressants including MAOIs, antiseizure medications, blood thinners, blood pressure medications, or cold or allergy medications that contain decongestants.

What is the usual dosage?
The information below is based on the dosage guidelines your doctor uses. Depending on your condition and medical history, your doctor may prescribe a different regimen. Do not change the dosage or stop taking your medication without your doctor's approval.

Adults and children 6 years and older: The Daytrana patch should be fixed to the skin once a day for about 9 hours. Daytrana comes in four different strength patches; your doctor may adjust the dose until it is right for you or your child.

Daytrana has not been studied in children less than 6 years old.

How should I take Daytrana?
Daytrana patches should be fixed to a clean, dry area on the hip. Alternate hips each day, and make sure the application site is free of redness and irritation before applying. When applying Daytrana, press and hold the patch firmly to the skin with the palm of your hand for 30 seconds. For more information, refer to the medication guide that you will receive from the pharmacist.

What should I avoid while taking Daytrana?
Avoid applying heating pads or subjecting the patch to other external sources of heat. Exposing the patch to heat may cause too much medication to pass into the body and cause serious side effects.

Do not touch the sticky part of the patch.

Avoid applying the patch to cuts or to irritated areas of skin.

What are possible food and drug interactions associated with Daytrana?
If Daytrana is taken with other drugs, the effects of either could be increased, decreased, or altered. It is especially important to check with your doctor before combining Daytrana with antidepressants including MAOIs, antiseizure medications, blood thinners, blood pressure medications, or cold or allergy medications that contain decongestants.

What are the possible side effects of Daytrana?
Side effects cannot be anticipated. If any develop or change in intensity, tell your doctor as soon as possible. Only your doctor can determine if it is safe for you to continue taking this drug.

Side effects may include: decreased appetite, inflammation of the nasal passages, irritation (redness, itching) at site of application, nasal congestion, nausea, sadness/crying, sleeplessness, twitching, vomiting, weight loss

Other side effects of drugs of this type include: allergic reactions, blurred vision, dizziness, drowsiness, fever, growth suppression, headache, increased blood pressure, nervousness, psychosis (abnormal thinking or hallucinations)

Can I receive Daytrana if I am pregnant or breastfeeding?
The effects of using Daytrana during pregnancy and breastfeeding are unknown. If you or your child is sexually active, pregnant, or breastfeeding, talk to your doctor about the effects of Daytrana.

What should I do if I miss a dose of Daytrana?
If you forget to apply Daytrana at the correct time, apply it as soon as you remember. Remove the patch at the normally scheduled time, even if it has been less than 9 hours, to avoid side effects later in the day.

How should I store Daytrana?
Store at room temperature. Upon removal of Daytrana, fold used patches so that the adhesive side of the patch adheres to itself. Flush used patches down the toilet or dispose of them in a secure container with a lid.

DDAVP
Generic name: Desmopressin acetate

What is DDAVP?
DDAVP nasal spray, nose drops, and tablets are given to prevent or control the frequent urination and loss of water associated with diabetes insipidus (a rare condition characterized by very large quantities of diluted urine and excessive thirst). They are also used to treat frequent passage of urine and increased thirst in people with certain brain injuries, and those who have undergone surgery in the pituitary region of the brain. DDAVP nasal spray and nose drops are also prescribed to help stop some types of bedwetting.

What is the most important information I should know about DDAVP?
When taking DDAVP, elderly and young people in particular should limit their fluid intake to no more than what satisfies thirst. Although extremely rare, there is a possibility of water intoxication, in which reduced sodium levels in the blood can lead to seizures.

If you have cystic fibrosis or any other condition in which there is fluid and electrolyte imbalance, you should use DDAVP with extreme caution.

Because DDAVP may cause a rise in blood pressure, use this medication cautiously if you have high blood pressure and/or coronary artery disease. Your blood pressure could also fall temporarily.

Who should not take DDAVP?
Do not use DDAVP if you are sensitive to or have ever had an allergic reaction to any of its ingredients.

What should I tell my doctor before I take the first dose of DDAVP?
Tell your doctor about all prescription, over-the-counter, and herbal medications you are taking before beginning treatment with this drug. Also, talk to your doctor about your complete medical history, especially if you have cycstic fibrosis, heart disease, high blood pressure, or any condition that affects electrolyte levels.

What is the usual dosage?
The information below is based on the dosage guidelines your doctor uses. Depending on your condition and medical history, your doctor may prescribe a different regimen. Do not change the dosage or stop taking your medication without your doctor's approval.

Your doctor will carefully tailor your dosage to meet your individual needs. Your doctor may increase or decrease your dosage, depending on how you respond to DDAVP. Your response will be judged by how long you are able to sleep without having to get up to urinate and how much urine your kidneys produce.

How should I take DDAVP?
Use DDAVP exactly as prescribed. The DDAVP nasal spray pump bottle accurately delivers 50 doses of the medication. After the 50th dose, the amount of medication that comes out with each spray will no longer be a full dose. When this happens, throw the bottle away even if it is not completely empty.

Since the DDAVP spray bottle delivers only a standard-sized dose, those who need more or less medication should use the nose drops instead of the spray.

If nasal congestion, scars, or swelling inside the nose make it difficult to absorb DDAVP, your doctor may temporarily stop the drug or give you tablets or an injectable form. If you are switched to tablets, you should start taking them 12 hours after you last used the nasal spray or nose drops.

What should I avoid while taking DDAVP?
The spray and drops are for nasal use only; never swallow the medication or allow the liquid to run into your mouth.

What are possible food and drug interactions associated with DDAVP?

If DDAVP is taken with certain other drugs, the effects of either could be increased, decreased, or altered. It is especially important to check with your doctor before combining DDAVP with the following: any drug used to increase blood pressure, clofibrate, glyburide, and epinephrine.

What are the possible side effects of DDAVP?

Side effects cannot be anticipated. If any develop or change in intensity, tell your doctor as soon as possible. Only your doctor can determine if it is safe for you to continue taking this drug.

Too high a dosage of DDAVP nasal spray or drops may produce headache, nausea, mild abdominal cramps, stuffy nose, irritation of the nose, or flushing. These symptoms will probably disappear when the dosage is reduced. Some people have complained of nosebleed, sore throat, cough, or a cold or other upper respiratory infections after taking DDAVP nasal spray or drops.

Other potential side effects include: abdominal pain, chills, conjunctivitis (pinkeye), depression, dizziness, inability to produce tears, leg rash, nostril pain, rash, stomach or intestinal upset, swelling around the eyes, weakness

Can I receive DDAVP if I am pregnant or breastfeeding?

If you are pregnant or plan to become pregnant, inform your doctor immediately. Although DDAVP is not known to cause birth defects, it should be used with caution. DDAVP should be taken during pregnancy only if clearly needed. DDAVP is not believed to appear in breast milk. However, check with your doctor before using the drug while breastfeeding.

What should I do if I miss a dose of DDAVP?

Take the forgotten dose as soon as you remember. If you take 1 dose a day and don't remember until the next day, skip the dose. If you take DDAVP more than once a day and it is almost time for the next dose, skip the one you missed and go back to your regular schedule. Never double the dose.

How should I store DDAVP?

The drops should be stored in the refrigerator. If you are traveling, they will stay fresh at room temperature for up to 3 weeks.

The tablets and nasal spray can be kept at room temperature. Protect the tablets from heat and light.

DECONAMINE

Generic name: Chlorpheniramine and pseudoephedrine

What is Deconamine?

Deconamine is an antihistamine and decongestant used for the temporary relief of persistent runny nose, sneezing, and nasal congestion caused by upper respiratory infections (the common cold), sinus inflammation, or hay fever. It is also used to help clear nasal passages and shrink swollen membranes and to drain the sinuses and relieve sinus pressure.

What is the most important information I should know about Deconamine?

Use Deconamine with extreme caution if you have the eye condition called glaucoma, peptic ulcer or stomach obstructions, an enlarged prostate, or difficulty urinating.

Also use caution if you have bronchial asthma, emphysema, chronic lung disease, high blood pressure, heart disease, diabetes, or an overactive thyroid.

Deconamine may cause excitability, especially in children.

Who should not take Deconamine?

Do not use Deconamine if you have severe high blood pressure or severe heart disease, are taking an antidepressant drug known as an MAO inhibitor, or are sensitive to or have ever had an allergic reaction to antihistamines or decongestants.

What should I tell my doctor before I take the first dose of Deconamine?

Tell your doctor about all prescription, over-the-counter, and herbal medications you are taking before beginning treatment with this drug. Also, talk to your doctor about your complete medical history.

What is the usual dosage?

The information below is based on the dosage guidelines your doctor uses. Depending on your condition and medical history, your doctor may prescribe a different regimen. Do not change the dosage or stop taking your medication without your doctor's approval.

Deconamine Tablets
Adults and children over 12 years: The usual dosage is 1 tablet 3 or 4 times daily.

Deconamine Syrup
Adults and children over 12 years: The usual dose is 1 to 2 teaspoonfuls (5 to 10 milliliters) 3 or 4 times daily.

Children 6 to 12 years: The usual dose is one-half to 1 teaspoonful (2.5 to 5 milliliters) 3 or 4 times daily, not to exceed 4 teaspoonfuls in 24 hours.

Children 2 to 6 years: The usual dose is one-half teaspoonful (2.5 milliliters) 3 or 4 times daily, not to exceed 2 teaspoonfuls in 24 hours.

Children under 2 years: Use as directed by your doctor.

Deconamine SR Capsules
Adults and children over 12 years: The usual dose is 1 capsule every 12 hours.

Deconamine Chewable Tablets
Adults: The usual dose is 2 tablets 3 or 4 times a day.

Children 6 to 12 years: The usual dose is 1 tablet 3 or 4 times a day.

Children 2 to 6 years: The usual dose is half a tablet 3 or 4 times a day.

How should I take Deconamine?
If Deconamine makes you nervous or restless, or you have trouble sleeping, take the last dose of the day a few hours before you go to bed. Take Deconamine exactly as prescribed. Antihistamines can make your mouth and throat dry. It may help to suck on hard candy, chew gum, or melt bits of ice in your mouth.

What should I avoid while taking Deconamine?
Deconamine may cause you to become drowsy or less alert. You should not drive or operate machinery or participate in any activity that requires full mental alertness until you know how you react to Deconamine.

Alcohol increases the sedative effect of Deconamine. Avoid it while taking this medication.

What are possible food and drug interactions associated with Deconamine?
If Deconamine is taken with certain other drugs, the effects of either may be increased, decreased, or altered. It is especially important to check with your doctor before combining Deconamine with the following: antidepressant drugs such as the MAO inhibitors phenelzine and tranylcypromine, asthma medications such as albuterol, bromocriptine, mecamylamine, methyldopa, narcotic pain killers such as meperidine and oxycodone, phenytoin, reserpine, sleep aids such as secobarbital and triazolam, or tranquilizers such as alprazolam and diazepam.

What are the possible side effects of Deconamine?
Side effects cannot be anticipated. If any develop or change in intensity, tell your doctor as soon as possible. Only your doctor can determine if it is safe for you to continue taking this drug. The most common side effect is mild to moderate drowsiness.

Can I receive Deconamine if I am pregnant or breastfeeding?

The effects of Deconamine during pregnancy have not been adequately studied. If you are pregnant or plan to become pregnant, notify your doctor immediately. Deconamine appears in breast milk and could affect a nursing infant. If this medication is essential to your health, your doctor may advise you to discontinue breastfeeding until your treatment with Deconamine is finished.

What should I do if I miss a dose of Deconamine?

Take it as soon as you remember. If it is almost time for your next dose, skip the one you missed and go back to your regular schedule. Never take 2 doses at once.

How should I store Deconamine?

Store at room temperature.

DEMADEX

Generic name: Torsemide

What is Demadex?

Demadex is a diuretic (water pill) prescribed to reduce the water retention and swelling that often accompany congestive heart failure, kidney disease, and liver disease. It is also prescribed for high blood pressure, either alone or with other medications.

What is the most important information I should know about Demadex?

Demadex has been known to cause dehydration, chemical imbalances in the body, and a reduction in the volume of blood. Symptoms of these problems include dryness of the mouth, thirst, weakness, drowsiness, restlessness, muscle pain or fatigue, low blood pressure, diminished urination, rapid heartbeat, nausea, and vomiting. If any of these symptoms develop, discontinue Demadex and contact your doctor immediately.

Who should not take Demadex?

You should avoid Demadex if you have had a previous allergic reaction to the drug or to sulfonylurea drugs, which include certain diabetes medications. Do not take Demadex if you are unable to urinate.

What should I tell my doctor before I take the first dose of Demadex?

Tell your doctor about all prescription, over-the-counter, and herbal medications you are taking before beginning treatment with Demadex. Also, talk to your doctor about your complete medical history, especially if you have liver problems, high cholesterol, diabetes, hearing problems, or if you have allergies to sulfur or sulfur medications.

What is the usual dosage?
The information below is based on the dosage guidelines your doctor uses. Depending on your condition and medical history, your doctor may prescribe a different regimen. Do not change the dosage or stop taking your medication without your doctor's approval.

Congestive Heart Failure
Adults: The usual initial dose is 10 milligrams (mg) or 20 mg once a day. If this proves inadequate, your doctor may approximately double the dose until the desired response is obtained.

Chronic Kidney Failure
Adults: The usual initial dose is 20 mg once a day. If this proves inadequate, your doctor may approximately double the dose until the desired response is obtained.

Cirrhosis of the Liver
Adults: The usual initial dose is 5 or 10 mg once a day, administered along with other medications called "aldosterone antagonists" or "potassium-sparing diuretics." If this proves inadequate, your doctor will approximately double the dose until the desired response is obtained.

High Blood Pressure
Adults: The usual initial dose is 5 mg once a day. If, after 4 to 6 weeks your blood pressure is still too high, your doctor may increase the dose to 10 mg once a day. If that isn't sufficient, your doctor may add another drug to your treatment plan.

Safety and effectiveness in children have not been established.

How should I take Demadex?
Take this medication exactly as prescribed with or without food.

What are possible food and drug interactions associated with Demadex?
If Demadex is taken with certain other drugs, the effects of either could be increased, decreased, or altered. It is especially important to check with your doctor before combining Demadex with the following: aminoglycoside antibiotics, aspirin and other nonsteroidal anti-inflammatory drugs, cholestyramine, ethacrynic acid, lithium, probenecid

What are the possible side effects of Demadex?
Side effects cannot be anticipated. If any develop or change in intensity, tell your doctor as soon as possible. Only your doctor can determine if it is safe for you to continue taking this drug.

Side effects may include: headache, excessive urination, dizziness, runny nose, weakness, diarrhea, increased cough, constipation, nausea, joint pain, difficult digestion, sore throat, muscle pain, chest pain, insomnia, edema, nervousness

Can I receive Demadex if I am pregnant or breastfeeding?
The effects of Demadex during pregnancy have not been adequately studied. If you are pregnant or plan to become pregnant, inform your doctor immediately. Demadex should be used during pregnancy only if clearly needed. It is not known whether Demadex is excreted in breast milk. Consult your doctor before taking Demadex if you are breastfeeding or planning to breastfeed.

What should I do if I miss a dose of Demadex?
Take it as soon as you remember. If it is almost time for your next dose, skip the one you missed and go back to your regular schedule. Do not take 2 doses at once.

How should I store Demadex?
Store Demadex at room temperature. Do not freeze.

DEMEROL
Generic name: Meperidine hydrochloride

What is Demerol?
Demerol, a narcotic analgesic, is prescribed for the relief of moderate to severe pain.

What is the most important information I should know about Demerol?
Do not take Demerol if you are currently taking drugs known as MAO inhibitors or have used them in the previous 2 weeks. Drugs in this category include the antidepressants phenelzine and tranylcypromine. When taken with Demerol, they can cause unpredictable, severe, and occasionally fatal reactions.

You can build up tolerance to, and both mental and physical dependence on, Demerol if you take it repeatedly. Since it is possible that you could become addicted to Demerol, do not use it for any purpose other than what your doctor has prescribed it for. If you have ever had a problem with drug abuse, consult with your doctor before taking this drug.

Who should not take Demerol?
If you are sensitive to or have ever had an allergic reaction to Demerol or other narcotic painkillers, you should not use this medication. Make sure your doctor is aware of any drug reactions you have experienced.

You should not take Demerol if you are taking MAO inhibitors (such as phenelzine or trancylpromine) or if you have recently been taking MAO inhibitors within 14 days.

What should I tell my doctor before I take the first dose of Demerol?

Tell your doctor about all prescription, over-the-counter, and herbal medication you are taking before beginning treatment with this drug. Also, talk to your doctor about your complete medical history, especially if you have ever had any of the following: a severe liver or kidney disorder, head injury, sickle cell anemia, hypothyroidism (underactive thyroid gland), adrenal gland dysfunction or tumor, an enlarged prostate, a urethral stricture (narrowing of the tube leading from the bladder), a severe abdominal condition, an irregular heartbeat, a history of convulsions, or a history of drug abuse or alcoholism (including alcohol withdrawal marked by delirium tremens).

It's also important to let your doctor know if you have severe asthma attacks, frequently recurring lung disease, if you are unable to inhale or exhale extra air when needed, or if you have any pre-existing breathing difficulties.

Before having surgery, make sure the doctor knows you are taking Demerol. Combining Demerol with a general anesthetic could cause serious side effects.

What is the usual dosage?

The information below is based on the dosage guidelines your doctor uses. Depending on your condition and medical history, your doctor may prescribe a different regimen. Do not change the dosage or stop taking your medication without your doctor's approval.

Adults: The usual dosage of Demerol is 50 milligrams (mg) to 150 mg every 3 or 4 hours, determined according to your response and the severity of the pain. For older adults, the doctor may reduce the dosage.

Children: The usual dosage is 1.1 mg to 1.8 mg per 2.2 pounds of body weight, up to the adult dose taken every 3 or 4 hours, as determined by your doctor.

It's best to consult your doctor before giving Demerol to newborns or very young infants.

How should I take Demerol?

Take Demerol exactly as prescribed. Do not increase the amount or length of time you take this drug without your doctor's approval. Likewise, do not abruptly stop taking Demerol, since this could increase the risk of withdrawal symptoms.

If you are using Demerol in syrup form, take each dose in a half glass of water.

What should I avoid while taking Demerol?

Demerol may affect you both mentally and physically. You should not drive a car, operate machinery, or perform any other potentially hazardous activities until you know how the drug affects you.

Do not abruptly stop using Demerol, especially if you have been taking it for a while. Your doctor will have you gradually taper off this medication to reduce the risk of withdrawal symptoms, including restlessness, irritability, anxiety, insomnia, rapid heartbeat or breathing, increased blood pressure, or flu-like symptoms.

What are possible food and drug interactions associated with Demerol?

It's very important not to combine Demerol with any sleep medications or tranquilizers, since this combination could cause serious injury or death.

Demerol slows brain activity and intensifies the effects of alcohol. Do not drink alcohol while taking this medication.

If Demerol is taken with certain other drugs, the effects of either could be increased, decreased, or altered. It is especially important to check with your doctor before combining Demerol with the following: acyclovir, alcohol, antidepressant drugs such as amitriptyline or imipramine, buprenorphine, butorphanol, cimetidine, general anesthetics such as midazolam, major tranquilizers (phenothiazines) such as chlorpromazine and thioridazine, MAO inhibitors such as the antidepressant drugs phenelzine and tranylcypromine, muscle relaxants such as carisoprodol and chlorzoxazone, nalbuphine, other narcotic painkillers such as codeine and oxycodone, pentazocine, phenytoin, ritonavir, sedatives such as temazepam and triazolam, sleep aids such as zaleplon and zolpidem, tranquilizers such as alprazolam and diazepam.

What are the possible side effects of Demerol?

Side effects cannot be anticipated. If any develop or change in intensity, inform your doctor as soon as possible. Only your doctor can determine if it is safe for you to continue taking Demerol.

Side effects may include: Dizziness, light-headedness, nausea, sedation, sweating, vomiting

If any of these side effects occur, it may help if you lie down after taking the medication.

Can I receive Demerol if I am pregnant or breastfeeding?

Do not take Demerol if you are pregnant or planning to become pregnant unless you are directed to do so by your doctor. Demerol appears in breast milk and could affect a nursing infant. If this medication is essential to your health, your doctor may advise you to discontinue breastfeeding your baby until your treatment is finished.

What should I do if I miss a dose of Demerol?

Take it as soon as you remember. If it is almost time for your next dose, skip the one you missed and go back to your regular schedule. Never take 2 doses at once.

How should I store Demerol?

Store at room temperature and protect from heat.

DENAVIR

Generic name: Penciclovir

What is Denavir?

Denavir cream is used to treat recurrent cold sores on the lips and face. It works by interfering with the growth of the herpesvirus responsible for the sores.

What is the most important information I should know about Denavir?

You should begin applying Denavir at the first hint of a developing cold sore. The drug will not cure herpes, but it will reduce pain and may speed healing.

Check with your doctor if your cold sore does not improve or becomes worse. You could have an infection.

Who should not take Denavir?

If you have ever had an allergic reaction to any of the ingredients in Denavir, you should not use this medication.

What should I tell my doctor before I take the first dose of Denavir?

Tell your doctor about all prescription, over-the-counter, and herbal medication you are taking before beginning treatment with this drug. Also, talk to your doctor about your complete medical history, especially if you have a weak immune system.

What is the usual dosage?

The information below is based on the dosage guidelines your doctor uses. Depending on your condition and medical history, your doctor may prescribe a different regimen. Do not change the dosage or stop taking your medication without your doctor's approval.

Adults and children 12 to 17 years old: Apply cream every 2 hours, while awake, for 4 days.

The safety and effectiveness of this drug in children less than 12 years old have not been established.

How should I take Denavir?

Avoid using Denavir cream in or near the eyes; it can irritate them. Apply it only to sores on the lips and face.

Special warnings about this medication
It is not known whether Denavir is effective for people with weak immune systems.

What are possible food and drug interactions associated with Denavir?

If this medication is taken with certain other drugs, the effects of either could be increased, decreased, or altered. Always check with your doctor before combining Denavir with another medication.

What are the possible side effects of Denavir?

Reactions to Denavir are quite rare. If any develop or change in intensity, inform your doctor as soon as possible. Only your doctor can determine if it is safe for you to continue using this medication.

Side effects may include: Headache, hives, itching, numbing of the skin, pain, rash, skin discoloration, skin reaction or swelling where the cream was applied, swelling in the mouth and throat, taste or smell alteration, tingling, worsened condition

Can I receive Denavir if I am pregnant or breastfeeding?

The effects of Denavir during pregnancy have not been adequately studied. If you are pregnant or plan to become pregnant, inform your doctor immediately. Researchers do not know whether this drug will appear in breast milk after external application. For safety's sake, your doctor may advise you to discontinue breastfeeding your baby until your treatment with Denavir is finished.

What should I do if I miss a dose of Denavir?

If you miss a dose of this drug, skip it. Do not apply an extra dose of the cream to make up for missed doses.

How should I store Denavir?

Store at room temperature.

DEPAKENE

Generic name: Valproic acid

What is Depakene?

Depakene, an epilepsy medicine, is used to treat certain types of seizures and convulsions. It may be prescribed alone or with other anticonvulsant medications.

What is the most important information I should know about Depakene?

Depakene can cause serious, even fatal, liver damage, especially during the first 6 months of treatment. Children under 2 years of age are the most vulnerable, especially if they are also taking other anticonvulsant medicines and have certain other disorders such as mental retardation. The risk of liver damage decreases with age, but you should always be alert for the following symptoms: loss of seizure control, weakness, dizziness, drowsiness, a general feeling of ill health, facial swelling, loss of appetite, vomiting, and yellowing of the skin and eyes. If you suspect a liver problem, call your doctor immediately.

Depakene has been known to cause rare cases of life-threatening damage to the pancreas. This problem can develop at any time, even after years of treatment. Call your doctor immediately if any of the following warning signs appear: abdominal pain, loss of appetite, nausea, and vomiting.

Depakene has been shown to cause fetal harm due to birth defects. You should discuss the risks and benefits of this medication with your doctor, especially if it is prescribed for a condition other than seizure disorders, such as for migraine headaches.

Depakene has been shown to cause an increased level of ammonia in the blood, which is chemical waste blood. Depakene may also cause a brain disease called encephalopathy, especially in people with a condition known as urea cycle disorder (UCD), which is a genetic disorder that does not allow the proper removal of ammonia from the blood stream. Signs and symptoms of encephalopathy include altered mental state, loss of memory, personality change, increased tiredness, vomiting, and/or involuntary twitching of a muscle. Notify your doctor right away if any of these occur.

Who should not take Depakene?

You should not take Depakene if you have liver disease or your liver is not functioning properly, or if you have had an allergic reaction to it.

You should not take Depakene if you have UCD (see "What is the most important information I should know about this medication?").

What should I tell my doctor before I take the first dose of Depakene?

Tell your doctor about all prescription, over-the-counter, and herbal medication you are taking before beginning treatment with Depakene. Also, talk to your doctor about your complete medical history, especially if you have ever had any of the following: problems with your liver or pancreas, urea cycle disorders, manic episodes, migraines, or blood disorders.

This drug can also increase the effect of painkillers and anesthetics. Before any surgery or dental procedure, make sure the doctor knows you are taking Depakene.

What is the usual dosage?

The information below is based on the dosage guidelines your doctor uses. Depending on your condition and medical history, your doctor may prescribe a different regimen. Do not change the dosage or stop taking your medication without your doctor's approval.

Adults and children 10 years and older: The usual starting dose is 10 to 15 milligrams (mg) per 2.2 pounds of body weight per day. Your doctor may increase the dose at weekly intervals by 5 to 10 mg per 2.2 pounds per day until seizures are controlled or side effects become too severe. If stomach upset develops, the dose may be increased more slowly. The daily dose should not exceed 60 mg per 2.2 pounds per day.

Older adults generally are prescribed reduced starting doses, and receive dosage increases more gradually than younger people.

How should I take Depakene?

If Depakene irritates your digestive system, take it with food. To avoid irritating your mouth and throat, swallow Depakene capsules whole; do not chew them.

What should I avoid while taking Depakene?

Depakene may cause drowsiness, especially in older adults. You should not drive a car, operate heavy machinery, or engage in hazardous activity until you know how you react to the drug.

Do not abruptly stop taking this medicine without first consulting your doctor. A gradual reduction in dosage is usually required to prevent major seizures.

What are possible food and drug interactions associated with Depakene?

If this medication is taken with certain other drugs, the effects of either could be increased, decreased, or altered. It is especially important to check with your doctor before combining this drug with the following: amitriptyline, aspirin, barbiturates such as phenobarbital and secobarbital, blood-thinning drugs such as warfarin, carbamazepine, clonazepam, diazepam, ethosuximide, felbamate, lamotrigine, meropenem for injection, nortriptyline, phenytoin, primidone, rifampin, tolbutamide, topiramate, and zidovudine.

Extreme drowsiness and other serious effects may occur if Depakene is taken with alcohol or other central nervous system depressants such as alprazolam, temazepam, or triazolam.

What are the possible side effects of Depakene?

Side effects are more likely if you are taking more than one epilepsy medication, and when you are taking higher doses of Depakene. Indigestion, nausea, and vomiting are the most common side effects when you first start taking this drug.

If any side effects develop or change in intensity, inform your doctor as soon as possible. Only your doctor can determine if it is safe for you to continue taking Depakene.

Side effects may include: abdominal cramps, amnesia, breathing difficulty, depression, diarrhea, dimmed or blurred vision, drowsiness, hair loss, indigestion, infection, involuntary eye movements, loss or increase in appetite, nausea, nervousness, ringing in the ears, sleeplessness, swelling of the arms and legs due to fluid retention, throat inflammation, tremors, vomiting

Can I receive Depakene if I am pregnant or breastfeeding?
If taken during pregnancy, Depakene may harm the baby. The drug is not recommended for pregnant women unless the benefits of therapy clearly outweigh the risks. In fact, women in their childbearing years should take Depakene only if it has been shown to be essential in the control of seizures. Since Depakene appears in breast milk, nursing mothers should use it only with caution.

What should I do if I miss a dose of Depakene?
If you take 1 dose a day, take the dose you missed as soon as you remember. If you do not remember until the next day, skip the dose you missed and go back to your regular schedule.

If you take more than 1 dose a day and you remember the missed dose within 6 hours of the scheduled time, take it immediately. Take the rest of the doses for that day at equally spaced intervals. Never take 2 doses at once.

How should I store Depakene?
Store at room temperature.

DEPAKOTE
Generic name: Divalproex sodium, delayed-release

What is Depakote?
Depakote is used to treat complex partial seizures, and simple and complex absence seizures in adults and children 10 years and older with epilepsy.

Depakote is also used for the treatment of episodes associated with bipolar disorder (manic or mixed episodes with or without psychotic features). A manic episode is a period of abnormally and persistently elevated, unreserved, or irritable mood. A mixed episode is a manic episode with a major depressive episode (depressed mood, loss of interest or pleasure in nearly all activities).

In addition, Depakote is used for the prevention of migraine headaches in adults.

What is the most important information I should know about Depakote?

Women who can become pregnant should know Depakote is associated with birth defects such as spina bifida and other neural canal closure problems. Those taking Depakote during pregnancy may develop clotting abnormalities and should be monitored carefully. Additionally, an increased incidence of epilepsy in children born to mothers who took Depakote in their first 12 weeks of pregnancy has been reported. If you become pregnant while taking this drug, contact your doctor immediately.

Some people who take Depakote experience serious liver problems. Your doctor should check your liver function before you start this medication and continue frequently thereafter. If you experience malaise, weakness, tiredness, facial swelling, loss of appetite, or vomiting, inform your doctor immediately; this may be a sign of more serious liver problems.

Some people may experience pancreatitis, a serious and life-threatening inflammation of the pancreas. If you experience stomach pain, nausea, vomiting, and loss of appetite, contact your doctor immediately; this may be a sign of pancreatitis.

You may experience drowsiness when you start this medication. You should not drive or operate dangerous machinery until you know how this medication will affect you.

Elevated ammonia levels and hypothermia, an unintentional drop in body temperature, have been reported in some patients receiving Depakote. Contact your doctor immediately if you experience abnormal drowsiness and vomiting or changes in mental status.

You should not take this medication if you are allergic to it, or if you have a condition called urea cycle disorder, which may cause too much ammonia to build up in your body. Let your doctor know if you have been diagnosed with these conditions.

Some people taking Depakote may experience low blood platelet counts. Your doctor should order blood tests to check your platelets while you are taking this medication, as well as prior to surgery.

Who should not take Depakote?

Women who are pregnant, planning to become pregnant, or are nursing, should not begin treatment with Depakote.

Depakote should not be given to patients with liver disease or significant liver dysfunction.

You should not take this medication if you are allergic to it, or if you have a condition called urea cycle disorder.

What should I tell my doctor before I take the first dose of Depakote?

Tell your doctor about all prescription, over-the-counter, and herbal medications you are taking before beginning treatment with Depakote. Also, talk to your doctor about your complete medical history, especially if you have a condition called urea cycle disorder, a history of liver problems or liver disease, or have been allergic to Depakote in the past. In addition, tell your doctor if you are pregnant, planning to become pregnant, or are nursing.

What is the usual dosage?

The information below is based on the dosage guidelines your doctor uses. Depending on your condition and medical history, your doctor may prescribe a different regimen. Do not change the dosage or stop taking your medication without your doctor's approval.

Complex Partial Seizures

Adults and children 10 years and older: The usual starting dose of Depakote is 10 milligrams (mg) to 15 mg/kg/day. This dosage should be increased by 5 to 10 mg/kg per week until optimal clinical response is achieved. Usually, the optimal clinical response is achieved at a daily dose below 60 mg/kg per day.

Bipolar Disorder

Adults: The recommended starting dose of Depakote is 750 mg daily given in divided doses. The dose should increase as rapidly as possible to achieve the lowest therapeutic dose that produces the desired clinical effect. The maximum recommended dose is 60mg/kg per day.

Migraines

Adults: The recommended starting dose for Depakote is 250 mg two times a day. Some patients may benefit from doses up to 1000 mg daily.

Simple and Complex Absence Seizures

Adults and children 10 years and older: The recommended initial dose is 15 mg/kg daily, increasing by 5 to 10 mg/kg per day at one week intervals. The maximum recommended dose is 60 mg/kg daily. If the total daily dose exceeds 250 mg, it should be given in divided doses.

Due to an increased sensitivity to Depakote, elderly patients should be started on a lower dose of the drug. Dosage should be increased more slowly with regular monitoring.

How should I take Depakote?

Take Depakote only as directed by your doctor. Depakote tablets should be swallowed whole and should not be crushed or chewed. If you experience stomach irritation, you may benefit from taking Depakote with food or by slowly building up the dose from the initial low level. Try to take Depakote at the same time(s) every day.

What should I avoid while taking Depakote?
You should avoid combining Depakote with alcohol, a CNS depressant, which may increase the side effects of the drug.

You may experience drowsiness when you start this medication. Avoid driving or operating dangerous machinery until you know how this medication affects you.

What are possible food and drug interactions associated with Depakote?
If Depakote is taken with certain other drugs, the effects of either could be increased, decreased, or altered. It is especially important to check with your doctor before combining Depakote with the following: alcohol, amitryptyline, aspirin, carbamazepine, carbapenem antibiotics, diazepam, ethosuximide, lamotrigine, nortryptyline, phenobarbital, phenytoin, primidone, rifampin, topiramate, warfarin, and zidovudine.

What are the possible side effects of Depakote?
Side effects cannot be anticipated. If any develop or change in intensity, tell your doctor as soon as possible. Only your doctor can determine if it is safe for you to continue taking this drug.

Side effects may include: nausea, drowsiness, dizziness, vomiting, abdominal pain, diarrhea, increased appetite, weight gain, headache, fever, loss of appetite, constipation, flu, infection, sleepiness, nervousness

Can I receive Depakote if I am pregnant or breastfeeding?
The use of Depakote during pregnancy has been associated with birth defects such as spina bifida and other defects where the neural canal does not close normally. Women taking Depakote during pregnancy may develop clotting abnormalities and should be monitored carefully. Also, there is an incidence of epilepsy in children born to mothers who took Depakote in their first 12 weeks of pregnancy. If you become pregnant while on Depakote notify your doctor immediately.

Depakote is excreted in breast milk and may harm a nursing infant. A decision between you and your doctor should be made on whether to discontinue nursing or consider an alternative drug treatment.

What should I do if I miss a dose of Depakote?
If you missed a dose of Depakote, take the dose as soon as possible unless it is almost time for the next dose. If a dose is skipped, you should not double the next dose.

How should I store Depakote?
Store at room temperature.

DEPAKOTE ER
Generic name: Divalproex sodium, extended-release

What is Depakote ER?
Depakote is used to treat complex partial seizures, and simple and complex absence seizures in adults and children 10 years and older with epilepsy.

Depakote is also used for the treatment of episodes associated with bipolar disorder (manic or mixed episodes with or without psychotic features). A manic episode is a period of abnormally and persistently elevated, unreserved, or irritable mood. A mixed episode is a manic episode with a major depressive episode (depressed mood, loss of interest or pleasure in nearly all activities).

In addition, Depakote is for the prevention of migraine headaches in adults.

What is the most important information I should know about Depakote ER?
Women who can become pregnant should know Depakote is associated with birth defects such as spina bifida and other neural canal closure problems. Those taking Depakote during pregnancy may develop clotting abnormalities and should be monitored carefully. Additionally, an increased incidence of epilepsy in children born to mothers who took Depakote in their first 12 weeks of pregnancy has been reported. If you become pregnant while taking this drug, contact your doctor immediately.

Some people who take Depakote experience serious liver problems. Your doctor should check your liver function before you start this medication and continue frequently thereafter. If you experience malaise, weakness, tiredness, facial swelling, loss of appetite, or vomiting, inform your doctor immediately; this may be a sign of more serious liver problems.

Some people may experience pancreatitis, a serious and life-threatening inflammation of the pancreas. If you experience stomach pain, nausea, vomiting, and loss of appetite, contact your doctor immediately; this may be a sign of pancreatitis.

You may experience drowsiness when you start this medication. You should not drive or operate dangerous machinery until you know how this medication will affect you.

Elevated ammonia levels and hypothermia, an unintentional drop in body temperature, have been reported in some patients receiving Depakote ER. Contact your doctor immediately if you experience abnormal drowsiness and vomiting or changes in mental status.

You should not take this medication if you are allergic to it, or if you have a condition called urea cycle disorder, which may cause too much ammonia to build up in your body. Let your doctor know if you have been diagnosed with these conditions.

Some people taking Depakote ER may experience low blood platelet counts. Your doctor should order blood tests to check your platelets while you are taking this medication, as well as prior to surgery.

Who should not take Depakote ER?
Women who are pregnant, planning to become pregnant, or are nursing, should not begin treatment with Depakote ER.

Depakote ER should not be given to patients with liver disease or significant liver dysfunction.

You should not take this medication if you are allergic to it, or if you have a condition called urea cycle disorder.

What should I tell my doctor before I take the first dose of Depakote ER?
Tell your doctor about all prescription, over-the-counter, and herbal medications you are taking before beginning treatment with Depakote ER. Also, talk to your doctor about your complete medical history, especially if you have a condition called urea cycle disorder, a history of liver problems or liver disease, or have been allergic to Depakote ER in the past. In addition, tell your doctor if you are pregnant, planning to become pregnant, or are nursing.

What is the usual dosage?
The information below is based on the dosage guidelines your doctor uses. Depending on your condition and medical history, your doctor may prescribe a different regimen. Do not change the dosage or stop taking your medication without your doctor's approval.

Complex Partial Seizures
Adults and children 10 years and older: The usual starting dose of Depakote is 10 milligrams (mg) to 15 mg/kg/day. This dosage should be increased by 5 to 10 mg/kg per week until optimal clinical response is achieved. Usually, the optimal clinical response is achieved at a daily dose below 60 mg/kg per day.

Bipolar Disorder
Adults: The recommended starting dose of Depakote ER is 25 mg/kg given once daily. The dose should increase as rapidly as possible to achieve the lowest therapeutic dose that produces the desired clinical effect. The maximum recommended dose is 60 mg/kg per day.

Migraines
Adults: The recommended starting dose for Depakote ER is 500 mg once a day for one week. After one week, the dose should be increased to 1000 mg daily. The effective dose range for patients with migraines is 500-1000 mg daily.

Simple and Complex Absence Seizures
Adults and children 10 years and older: The recommended initial dose is
15 mg/kg daily, increasing by 5 to 10 mg/kg per day at one week intervals.
The maximum recommended dose is 60 mg/kg daily.

Due to an increased sensitivity to Depakote, elderly patients should be
started on a lower dose of the drug. Dosage should be increased more
slowly with regular monitoring.

How should I take Depakote ER?
Depakote ER tablets should be swallowed whole and should not be
crushed or chewed. If you experience stomach irritation, try taking Depakote ER with food or by slowly building up the dose from the initial
low level. Take Depakote ER only as directed by your doctor. Try to take
Depakote ER at the same time every day.

What should I avoid while taking Depakote ER?
You should avoid combining Depakote ER with alcohol, a CNS depressant, which may increase the side effects of the drug.

You may experience drowsiness when you start this medication. Avoid
driving or operating dangerous machinery until you know how this medication affects you.

What are possible food and drug interactions associated with Depakote ER?
If Depakote ER is taken with certain other drugs, the effects of either
could be increased, decreased, or altered. It is especially important to
check with your doctor before combining Depakote ER with the following:
alcohol, amitryptyline, aspirin, carbamazepine, carbapenem antibiotics,
diazepam, ethosuximide, lamotrigine, nortryptyline, phenobarbital, phenytoin, primidone, rifampin, topiramate, warfarin, and zidovudine.

What are the possible side effects of Depakote ER?
Side effects cannot be anticipated. If any develop or change in intensity,
tell your doctor as soon as possible. Only your doctor can determine if it
is safe for you to continue taking this drug.

Side effects may include: nausea, drowsiness, dizziness, vomiting, abdominal pain, diarrhea, increased appetite, weight gain, headache, fever,
loss of appetite, constipation, flu, infection, sleepiness, nervousness

Can I receive Depakote ER if I am pregnant or breastfeeding?
The use of Depakote ER during pregnancy has been associated with birth
defects such as spina bifida and other defects where the neural canal
does not close normally. Women taking Depakote ER during pregnancy
may develop clotting abnormalities and should be monitored carefully.
Also, there has been a reported incidence of epilepsy in children born to

mothers who took Depakote ER in their first 12 weeks of pregnancy. If you become pregnant while on Depakote ER, notify your doctor immediately.

Depakote ER is excreted in breast milk and may harm a nursing infant. A decision between you and your doctor should be made on whether to discontinue nursing or consider an alternative drug treatment.

What should I do if I miss a dose of Depakote ER?
If you missed a dose of Depakote ER, take the dose as soon as possible unless it is almost time for the next dose. If a dose is skipped, you should not double the next dose.

How should I store Depakote ER?
Store at room temperature.

Desipramine hydrochloride *See Norpramin, page 911.*

Desloratadine *See Clarinex, page 300.*

Desmopressin acetate *See DDAVP, page 382.*

Desogestrel and ethinyl estradiol *See Cyclessa, page 362.*

Desonide *See Verdeso, page 1383.*

Desoximetasone *See Topicort, page 1318.*

DESOXYN
Generic name: Methamphetamine hydrochloride

What is Desoxyn?
Desoxyn is used to treat attention deficit hyperactivity disorder (ADHD). This drug is given as part of a total treatment program that includes psychological, educational, and social measures.

Desoxyn also may be used for a short time as part of an overall diet plan for weight reduction. Desoxyn is given only when other weight loss drugs and weight loss programs have been unsuccessful.

What is the most important information I should know about Desoxyn?
Inform your doctor of any heart problems, heart defects, high blood pressure, or of a family history of these problems. Your doctor may check for any heart problems before prescribing Desoxyn and should monitor blood pressure and heart rate regularly while the medication is being used.

Call your doctor right away if symptoms such as chest pain, shortness of breath, or fainting occur.

Inform your doctor of any mental health problems or a family history of suicide, bipolar disorder, or depression. Call your doctor right away in the event of any new or worsening mental symptoms or problems while taking Desoxyn, especially psychotic symptoms such as visual or audible hallucinations or paranoia.

Excessive doses of this medication can produce addiction. Individuals who stop taking this medication after taking high doses for a long time may suffer withdrawal symptoms, including extreme fatigue, depression, and sleep disorders. Signs of excessive use of Desoxyn include severe skin inflammation, difficulty sleeping, irritability, hyperactivity, personality changes, and psychiatric problems.

Desoxyn is not appropriate for all children with symptoms of ADHD. Your doctor will do a complete history and evaluation before prescribing this medication. The doctor will take into account the duration and severity of the symptoms as well as your child's age.

This type of medication can affect the growth of children, so your doctor will monitor your child carefully while he or she is taking this drug. The long-term effects of this type of medication in children have not been established.

Desoxyn can lose its effectiveness in decreasing the appetite after a few weeks. If this happens, you should stop taking the medication. Do not take more than the recommended dose in an attempt to increase its effect.

Who should not take Desoxyn?

Do not take Desoxyn if you are also taking a monoamine oxidase inhibitor (MAOI) antidepressant such as phenelzine or tranylcypromine. Allow 14 days between stopping an MAOI and beginning therapy with Desoxyn.

Do not take Desoxyn if there is pre-existing glaucoma, advanced hardening of the arteries, heart disease, moderate to severe high blood pressure, thyroid problems, or allergy to this type of drug.

This medication should not be taken by anyone who suffers from tics (repeated, involuntary twitches) or Tourette's syndrome or who has a family history of these conditions.

People who are in an agitated state or who have a history of drug abuse should not take this medication.

Desoxyn should not be used to treat children whose symptoms may be caused by stress or a psychiatric disorder.

Desoxyn is not recommended for use in children younger than 6 years old in the treatment of ADHD.

What should I tell my doctor before I take the first dose of Desoxyn?

Tell your doctor about all prescription, over-the-counter, and herbal medications you are taking before beginning treatment with this drug. Also, talk to your doctor about your complete medical history, especially if you have mild high blood pressure.

What is the usual dosage?

The information below is based on the dosage guidelines your doctor uses. Depending on your condition and medical history, your doctor may prescribe a different regimen. Do not change the dosage or stop taking your medication without your doctor's approval.

Weight Loss

Adults and children 12 years and older: The usual starting dose for weight loss is 5 milligrams (mg) taken one-half hour before each meal. Treatment should not continue for longer than a few weeks. The safety and effectiveness of Desoxyn for weight loss have not been established in children under age 12.

ADHD

Children older than 6 years: The usual starting dose for ADHD is 5 mg taken once or twice a day. Your doctor may increase the dose by 5 mg a week until the desired response to the medication is achieved. The typical effective dose is 20 to 25 mg a day, usually divided into two doses.

Your doctor may periodically discontinue this drug in order to reassess the child's condition and see whether therapy is still needed.

Desoxyn should not be given to children under 6 years of age to treat attention deficit disorder; the safety and effectiveness in this age group have not been established.

How should I take Desoxyn?

Follow your doctor's directions carefully. Your doctor will prescribe the lowest effective dose of Desoxyn; never increase it without your doctor's approval. Do not take this medication late in the evening as it can cause difficulty sleeping.

What should I avoid while taking Desoxyn?

Desoxyn may affect your ability to perform potentially hazardous activities, such as operating machinery or driving a car. Also be aware that Desoxyn should not be used to combat fatigue or to replace rest.

What are possible food and drug interactions associated with Desoxyn?

If Desoxyn is taken with certain other drugs, the effects of either could be increased, decreased, or changed. It is especially important to check with your doctor before combining Desoxyn with the following: antidepressants classified as tricyclics (such as amitriptyline, imipramine, and nortriptyline) or as MAOIs (such as phenelzine or tranylcypromine); phenothiazines (such as the antipsychotic medications chlorpromazine and prochlorperazine); guanethidine; and insulin.

What are the possible side effects of Desoxyn?

Side effects cannot be anticipated. If any develop or change in intensity, inform your doctor as soon as possible. Only your doctor can determine if it is safe to continue taking Desoxyn.

Side effects may include: changes in sex drive, constipation, diarrhea, dizziness, dry mouth, euphoria, headache, hives, impaired growth, impotence, increased blood pressure, overstimulation, rapid or irregular heartbeat, restlessness, sleeplessness, stomach or intestinal problems, tremor, unpleasant taste, worsening of tics and Tourette's syndrome (severe twitching)

Can I receive Desoxyn if I am pregnant or breastfeeding?

Infants born to women taking this type of drug have a risk of prematurity and low birth weight. Drug dependence may occur in newborns when the mother has taken this drug prior to delivery. If you are pregnant or plan to become pregnant, tell your doctor immediately. Desoxyn appears in breast milk. Therefore, do not breastfeed while taking this medication.

What should I do if I miss a dose of Desoxyn?

If you miss a dose of this drug, skip it. Do not take an extra dose to make up for missed doses.

How should I store Desoxyn?

Store at room temperature and away from direct light.

Desvenlafaxine succinate *See Pristiq, page 1070.*

DETROL

Generic name: Tolterodine tartrate

What is Detrol?

Detrol treats symptoms of overactive bladder, including frequent urination, urgency (increased need to urinate), and urge incontinence (inability to control urination). The drug works by blocking the nerve impulses that prompt the bladder to contract.

What is the most important information I should know about Detrol?

In a limited number of people, Detrol causes blurred vision. Do not drive or operate machinery until you know how the drug affects you.

Who should not take Detrol?

If you suffer from urinary retention (inability to urinate normally), gastric retention (a blockage in the digestive system), or uncontrolled narrow-angle glaucoma (high pressure in the eyes), you should not take Detrol. You should also avoid this drug if it gives you an allergic reaction.

What should I tell my doctor before I take the first dose of Detrol?

Tell your doctor about all prescription, over-the-counter, and herbal medication you are taking before beginning treatment with this drug. Also, talk to your doctor about your complete medical history, especially if you have any of the following: a bladder obstruction or digestive disorder that could lead to a complete blockage; glaucoma; or a liver or kidney problem.

What is the usual dosage?

The information below is based on the dosage guidelines your doctor uses. Depending on your condition and medical history, your doctor may prescribe a different regimen. Do not change the dosage or stop taking your medication without your doctor's approval.

Adults: The usual starting dosage for Detrol is 2 milligrams (mg) twice a day.

How should I take Detrol?

Detrol can be taken with or without food. Swallow Detrol tablets whole.

What should I avoid while taking Detrol?

Detrol can cause blurred vision, dizziness, or drowsiness that may impair your mental alertness. Do not operate heavy machinery, drive an automobile, or engage in tasks that require for you to be alert, until you know how Detrol will affect you.

What are possible food and drug interactions associated with Detrol?

If you take Detrol with certain other drugs, the effects of either could be increased, decreased, or altered. It is especially important to check with your doctor before combining Detrol with any of the following: clarithromycin, cyclosporine, erythromycin antibiotics, ketoconazole, itraconazole, miconazole, and vinblastine.

What are the possible side effects of Detrol?

Side effects cannot be anticipated. If any develop or change in intensity, inform your doctor as soon as possible. Only your doctor can determine if it is safe for you to continue taking Detrol.

Side effects may include: abdominal pain, blurred vision, constipation, diarrhea, dizziness, drowsiness, dry eyes, dry mouth, fatigue, flu-like symptoms, headache, indigestion, vertigo

Can I receive Detrol if I am pregnant or breastfeeding?

The use of Detrol during pregnancy has not been adequately studied. If you are pregnant or plan to become pregnant, tell your doctor immediately. It is not known whether Detrol appears in breast milk. Use of the drug is not recommended while breastfeeding.

What should I do if I miss a dose of Detrol?

If you miss a dose of this drug, skip it. Do not take an extra dose to make up for missed doses.

How should I store Detrol?

Store at room temperature.

DETROL LA

Generic name: Tolterodine tartrate, extended-release

What is Detrol LA?

Detrol LA treats symptoms of overactive bladder, including frequent urination, urgency (increased need to urinate), and urge incontinence (inability to control urination). The drug works by blocking the nerve impulses that prompt the bladder to contract.

What is the most important information I should know about Detrol LA?

In a limited number of people, Detrol LA causes blurred vision and dizziness. Do not drive or operate machinery until you know how the drug affects you.

Who should not take Detrol LA?

If you suffer from urinary retention (inability to urinate normally), gastric retention (a blockage in the digestive system), or uncontrolled narrow-angle glaucoma (high pressure in the eyes), you should not take Detrol LA. You should also avoid this drug if it gives you an allergic reaction.

What should I tell my doctor before I take the first dose of Detrol LA?

Tell your doctor about all prescription, over-the-counter, and herbal medication you are taking before beginning treatment with this drug. Also, talk to your doctor about your complete medical history, especially if you have any of the following: a bladder obstruction or digestive disorder that could lead to a complete blockage; glaucoma; or a liver, kidney, or heart problem.

What is the usual dosage?

The information below is based on the dosage guidelines your doctor uses. Depending on your condition and medical history, your doctor

may prescribe a different regimen. Do not change the dosage or stop taking your medication without your doctor's approval.

Adults: The usual dosage of Detrol LA is 4 mg taken once a day. Your doctor may prescribe a lower or higher dose, depending on your needs.

How should I take Detrol LA?
Detrol LA can be taken with or without food. Swallow Detrol LA capsules whole.

What should I avoid while taking Detrol LA?
Detrol LA can cause blurred vision, dizziness, or drowsiness that may impair your mental alertness. Do not operate heavy machinery, drive an automobile, or engage in tasks that require for you to be alert, until you know how Detrol LA will affect you.

What are possible food and drug interactions associated with Detrol LA?
If you take Detrol LA with certain other drugs, the effects of either could be increased, decreased, or altered. It is especially important to check with your doctor before combining Detrol LA with any of the following: clarithromycin, cyclosporine, erythromycin antibiotics, ketoconazole, itraconazole, miconazole, and vinblastine.

What are the possible side effects of Detrol LA?
Side effects cannot be anticipated. If any develop or change in intensity, inform your doctor as soon as possible. Only your doctor can determine if it is safe for you to continue taking Detrol LA.

Side effects may include: abdominal pain, blurred vision, constipation, diarrhea, dizziness, drowsiness, dry eyes, dry mouth, fatigue, flu-like symptoms, headache, indigestion, vertigo

Can I receive Detrol LA if I am pregnant or breastfeeding?
The use of Detrol LA during pregnancy has not been adequately studied. If you are pregnant or plan to become pregnant, tell your doctor immediately. It is not known whether Detrol LA appears in breast milk. Use of the drug is not recommended while breastfeeding.

What should I do if I miss a dose of Detrol LA?
Take the missed dose as soon as you remember it. However, if it is almost time for your next dose, skip the one you missed and return to your regular dosing schedule. Do not double the dose.

How should I store Detrol LA?
Store at room temperature.

Dexmethylphenidate hydrochloride See *Focalin, page 583.*

Dexmethylphenidate hydrochloride, extended-release
See *Focalin XR, page 586.*

DIABETA
Generic name: Glyburide

What is Diabeta?
Diabeta is an oral medication used to help control blood sugar levels in patients who have type 2 diabetes. It belongs to a class of drugs called sulfonylureas.

What is the most important information I should know about Diabeta?
Treatment with sulfonylureas may increase the risk of death from heart and blood vessel problems compared to treatment of diabetes with diet alone or diet plus insulin. Discuss with your doctor the risks and benefits of treatment with Diabeta.

You should know the signs and symptoms of low blood sugar (hypoglycemia), which include headache, drowsiness, weakness, dizziness, fast heartbeat, sweating, tremor, and nausea.

Follow diet, medication, and exercise routines closely. Changing any of them can affect blood sugar levels.

Do not change your dose of Diabeta without first talking to your doctor.

Who should not take Diabeta?
Diabeta should not be used in patients with problems associated with diabetes (eg, diabetic ketoacidosis, diabetic coma), severe burns, severe acidosis, or type1 diabetes.

Diabeta should not be used in patients who are in the late stages of pregnancy.

What should I tell my doctor before I take the first dose of Diabeta?
Tell your doctor about all prescription, over-the-counter, and herbal medications you are taking before beginning treatment with Diabeta. Also, talk to your doctor about your complete medical history, especially if you are pregnant, plan to become pregnant, or are breastfeeding; have kidney disease; have liver disease; have thyroid disease; have a serious infection, illness, or injury, or if you need surgery.

What is the usual dosage?
The information below is based on the dosage guidelines your doctor uses. Depending on your condition and medical history, your doctor

may prescribe a different regimen. Do not change the dosage or stop taking your medication without your doctor's approval.

The initial dose is 2.5 to 5 milligrams (mg) once a day with breakfast or the first main meal. The dose should be increased by no more than 2.5 mg per day at weekly intervals.

The usual maintenance dose ranges from 1.25 to 20 mg given once a day or in divided doses.

For patients who have kidney disease, liver disease, adrenal or pituitary insufficiency, and those who are elderly, injured, or malnourished, the initial dose is 1.25 mg once a day.

For patients switching from another oral antidiabetic agent, the initial dose is 2.5-5 mg per day.

For patients switching from insulin, if you used to take more than 40 units a day, decrease the dose by half of the amount and take 5 mg of Diabeta once a day.

How should I take Diabeta?

Take Diabeta exactly as directed by your doctor. If you do not understand the instructions, ask your pharmacist, nurse, or doctor to explain them to you.

It is important to take Diabeta regularly to get the most benefit. Diabeta is usually taken before breakfast or the first main meal if it is taken once a day, or before meals if it is taken multiple times each day. Take each dose with a full glass of water.

What should I avoid while taking Diabeta?

Avoid alcohol. It lowers blood sugar and may interfere with diabetes treatment.

Do not take any prescription, over-the-counter, or herbal cough, cold, allergy, pain, or weight-loss medications without first talking to your doctor.

What are possible food and drug interactions associated with Diabeta?

If Diabeta is taken with certain other drugs, the effects of either could be increased, decreased, or altered. It is especially important to check with your doctor before combining Diabeta with the following: aspirin, Bosentan, nonsteroidal anti-inflammatory drugs (NSAIDs), and salicylates such as magnesium/choline salicylate, salsalate, choline salicylate, magnesium salicylate, or bismuth subsalicylate.

Drugs other than those listed here may also interact with Diabeta or affect your condition. Talk to your doctor or pharmacist before taking any prescription or over-the-counter medicines, including vitamins, minerals, and herbal products.

What are the possible side effects of Diabeta?
Side effects cannot be anticipated. If any develop or change in intensity, tell your doctor as soon as possible. Only your doctor can determine if it is safe for you to continue taking this drug.

Side effects may include: abdominal fullness, allergic skin reactions such as redness and itching; heartburn, low blood sugar, with symptoms such as shaking, headache, cold sweats, pale and cool skin, anxiety, difficulty concentrating; nausea

This is not a complete list of side effects that may occur. Talk to your doctor about any side effect that seems unusual or that is especially bothersome.

Can I receive Diabeta if I am pregnant or breastfeeding?
It is not known whether Diabeta will be harmful to an unborn baby. Insulin is usually the drug of choice for controlling diabetes during pregnancy. Do not take Diabeta without first talking to your doctor if you are pregnant or could become pregnant during treatment. It is not known whether Diabeta passes into breast milk. Do not take Diabeta without first talking to your doctor if you are breastfeeding a baby.

What should I do if I miss a dose of Diabeta?
Take the missed dose as soon as you remember. However, if it is almost time for the next dose, skip the missed dose and take only the next regularly scheduled dose. Do not take a double dose of this medication.

How should I store Diabeta?
Store at room temperature away from moisture and heat.

DIABINESE
Generic name: Chlorpropamide

What is Diabinese?
Diabinese is an oral antidiabetic medication used to treat type 2 (non-insulin-dependent) diabetes. Diabetes occurs when the body fails to produce enough insulin or is unable to use it properly.

What is the most important information
I should know about Diabinese?
Always remember that Diabinese is an aid to, not a substitute for, good diet and exercise. Failure to follow a sound diet and exercise plan can lead to serious complications, such as dangerously high or low blood sugar levels. Remember, too, that Diabinese is *not* an oral form of insulin, and cannot be used in place of insulin.

Who should not take Diabinese?

You should not take Diabinese if you have ever had an allergic reaction to it.

Do not take Diabinese if you are suffering from diabetic ketoacidosis (a life-threatening medical emergency caused by insufficient insulin and marked by excessive thirst, nausea, fatigue, and pain below the breastbone).

Remember, this medication is used to help treat type 2 diabetes. If you have type 1 diabetes, do not use this medication.

What should I tell my doctor before I take the first dose of Diabinese?

Tell your doctor about all prescription, over-the-counter, and herbal medication you are taking before beginning treatment with this drug. Also, talk to your doctor about your complete medical history, especially if you have heart problems.

What is the usual dosage?

The information below is based on the dosage guidelines your doctor uses. Depending on your condition and medical history, your doctor may prescribe a different regimen. Do not change the dosage or stop taking your medication without your doctor's approval.

Dosage levels are determined by each individual's needs.

Adults: Usually, an initial daily dose of 250 milligrams (mg) is recommended for stable, middle-aged, non-insulin-dependent diabetics. After 5 to 7 days, your doctor may adjust this dosage in increments of 50 to 125 mg every 3 to 5 days to achieve the best benefit. People with mild diabetes may respond well to daily doses of 100 mg or less of Diabinese, while those with severe diabetes may require 500 mg daily. Maintenance doses above 750 mg are not recommended.

Older adults and people who are malnourished, debilitated, or have kidney or liver problems usually take an initial dose of 100 to 125 mg.

How should I take Diabinese?

Ordinarily, the doctor will ask you to take a single daily dose of Diabinese each morning with breakfast. However, if this upsets your stomach, you may be instructed to take Diabinese in smaller doses throughout the day.

What should I avoid while taking Diabinese?

Avoid alcohol; excessive alcohol consumption can cause low blood sugar, breathlessness, and facial flushing.

Even people with well-controlled diabetes may find that stress, illness, surgery, or fever results in a loss of blood sugar control. If this happens, your doctor may recommend that Diabinese be discontinued temporarily and insulin used instead.

To help prevent low blood sugar levels (hypoglycemia), know the symptoms of hypoglycemia, know how exercise affects your blood sugar levels, maintain an adequate diet; and keep a source of quick-acting sugar with you all the time.

What are possible food and drug interactions associated with Diabinese?

When you take Diabinese with certain other drugs, the effects of either could be increased, decreased, or altered. It is important that you consult with your doctor before taking Diabinese with the following: anabolic steroids; aspirin in large doses; barbiturates such as secobarbital; beta-blocking blood pressure medications such as atenolol and propranolol; calcium-blocking blood pressure medications such as diltiazem and nifedipine; chloramphenicol; diuretics such as hydrochlorothiazide; epinephrine; estrogen medications; isoniazid; major tranquilizers such as chlorpromazine and thioridazine; MAO inhibitor-type antidepressants such as phenelzine and tranylcypromine; nicotinic acid; nonsteroidal anti-inflammatory agents such as ibuprofen and naproxen; oral contraceptives; phenothiazines; phenylbutazone; phenytoin; probenecid; steroids such as prednisone; sulfa drugs such as sulfamethoxazole; thyroid medications such as levothyroxine; and warfarin.

What are the possible side effects of Diabinese?

Side effects cannot be anticipated. If any develop or change in intensity, inform your doctor as soon as possible. Only your doctor can determine if it is safe for you to continue taking Diabinese.

Side effects from Diabinese are rare and seldom require discontinuation of the medication.

Side effects may include: diarrhea, hunger, itching, loss of appetite, nausea, stomach upset, vomiting

Diabinese, like all oral antidiabetic medications, can cause hypoglycemia (low blood sugar). The risk of hypoglycemia is increased by missed meals, alcohol, other medications, and excessive exercise. To avoid hypoglycemia, closely follow the dietary and exercise regimen suggested by your physician.

Symptoms of mild hypoglycemia may include: cold sweat, drowsiness, fast heartbeat, headache, nausea, nervousness

Symptoms of more severe hypoglycemia may include: coma, pale skin, seizures, shallow breathing

Contact your doctor immediately if these symptoms of severe low blood sugar occur.

Can I receive Diabinese if I am pregnant or breastfeeding?

The effects of Diabinese during pregnancy have not been adequately established. If you are pregnant or plan to become pregnant, inform your doctor immediately. Since studies suggest the importance of maintaining normal blood sugar (glucose) levels during pregnancy, your physician may prescribe injected insulin.

To minimize the risk of low blood sugar (hypoglycemia) in newborn babies, Diabinese, if prescribed during pregnancy, should be discontinued at least 1 month before the expected delivery date.

Since Diabinese appears in breast milk, it is not recommended for nursing mothers.

What should I do if I miss a dose of Diabinese?

If you miss a dose of Diabinese, take it as soon as possible. If it is almost time for your next dose, skip the missed dose and go back to your regular dosing schedule. Do not take two (2) doses at one time.

How should I store Diabinese?

Store at room temperature.

Diazepam *See Valium, page 1366.*

Diclofenac epolamine *See Flector, page 557.*

Diclofenac sodium *See Voltaren Gel, page 1406.*

Diclofenac sodium and misoprostol *See Arthrotec, page 129.*

Dicyclomine hydrochloride *See Bentyl, page 206.*

Didanosine *See Videx, page 1391.*

DIFFERIN

Generic name: Adapalene

What is Differin?

Differin is prescribed for the treatment of acne.

What is the most important information I should know about Differin?

Differin makes your skin more sensitive to sunlight. While using this product, keep your exposure to the sun at a minimum, and protect yourself with sunscreen and clothing. Never apply Differin to sunburned skin.

Who should not take Differin?

Do not use Differin if you are sensitive to adapalene or any other components of the gel.

What should I tell my doctor before I take the first dose of Differin?

Tell your doctor about all prescription, over-the-counter, and herbal medication you are taking before beginning treatment with this drug. Also, talk to your doctor about your complete medical history, especially if you have eczema or sunburned skin.

What is the usual dosage?

The information below is based on the dosage guidelines your doctor uses. Depending on your condition and medical history, your doctor may prescribe a different regimen. Do not change the dosage or stop taking your medication without your doctor's approval.

Adults and children 12 years and older: The usual dose is a thin film applied over the acne-affected area just before bedtime.

How should I take Differin?

Differin should be applied once a day at bedtime. Wash the affected areas, then apply a thin layer of the gel. Avoid eyes, lips, mouth, and nostrils. If you are using a single-use pledget, remove it from the foil just before using, and discard it after applying the medication. Do not use if the seal is broken.

Use Differin exactly as prescribed. Applying excessive amounts or using the gel more than once a day will not produce better results and may cause severe redness, peeling, and discomfort. If you have an allergic reaction or severe irritation, stop using the medication and call your doctor.

In the first few weeks of treatment, your acne may actually seem to get worse. This just means the medication is working on hidden acne sores. Continue using the product. It can take as much as 8 to 12 weeks before you start to see improvement in your condition.

What should I avoid while taking Differin?

Remember that Differin increases sensitivity to sunlight. Take measures to protect yourself from overexposure. Wind and cold weather may also be irritating. Do not apply Differin to cuts, abrasions, eczema, or sunburned skin.

What are possible food and drug interactions associated with Differin?

Avoid using Differin with any other product that can irritate the skin, such as medicated soaps and cleansers, soaps and cosmetics that have a strong drying effect, and products with high concentrations of alcohol, astringents, spices, and lime.

Special caution is necessary if you have used, or are currently using, any skin product containing sulfur, resorcinol, or salicylic acid. Do not use such a product with Differin. If you have used one of these products recently, do not begin Differin treatment until the effects of the other product have subsided.

What are the possible side effects of Differin?

Side effects cannot be anticipated. If any develop or change in intensity, inform your doctor as soon as possible. Only your doctor can determine if it is safe for you to continue using Differin.

Side effects are most likely to occur during the first 2 to 4 weeks and usually diminish with continued treatment. If side effects are severe, your doctor may advise you to reduce the frequency of use or discontinue the drug entirely. Side effects disappear when the drug is stopped.

Side effects may include: Acne flare-ups, burning, dryness, irritation, itching, redness, scaling, stinging, sunburn

Can I receive Differin if I am pregnant or breastfeeding?

The effects of Differin during pregnancy and breastfeeding have not been adequately studied. If you are pregnant or plan to become pregnant, notify your doctor immediately. It is not known whether Differin appears in breast milk. Consult your doctor if you plan on breastfeeding.

What should I do if I miss a dose of Differin?

If you miss a dose of this drug, skip it. Do not take an extra dose to make up for missed doses.

How should I store Differin?

Store at room temperature.

DIFLUCAN

Generic name: Fluconazole

What is Diflucan?

Diflucan is used to treat fungal infections called candidiasis (also known as thrush or yeast infections). These include vaginal infections, throat infections, and fungal infections elsewhere in the body, such as infections of the urinary tract, peritonitis (inflammation of the lining of the abdomen), and pneumonia. Diflucan is also prescribed to guard against candidiasis in some people receiving bone marrow transplants, and is used to treat meningitis (brain or spinal cord inflammation) caused by another type of fungus.

What is the most important information I should know about Diflucan?

Strong allergic reactions to Diflucan, although rare, have been reported. Symptoms may include hives, itching, swelling, sudden drop in blood pressure, difficulty breathing or swallowing, diarrhea, or abdominal pain. If you experience any of these symptoms, notify your doctor immediately.

Who should not take Diflucan?

Do not take Diflucan if you are sensitive to any of its ingredients or have ever had an allergic reaction to similar drugs, such as ketoconazole. Make sure your doctor is aware of any drug reactions you have experienced.

Diflucan should not be combined with cisapride or terfenadine. These combinations have been known to trigger heartbeat irregularities and other heart problems.

What should I tell my doctor before I take the first dose of Diflucan?

Tell your doctor about all prescription, over-the-counter, and herbal medication you are taking before beginning treatment with this drug. Also, talk to your doctor about your complete medical history, especially if you have liver problems, a compromised immune system, or heart problems such as irregular heartbeats caused or worsened by medicines, are pregnant, plan to become pregnant, think you might be pregnant, or are breastfeeding.

What is the usual dosage?

The information below is based on the dosage guidelines your doctor uses. Depending on your condition and medical history, your doctor may prescribe a different regimen. Do not change the dosage or stop taking your medication without your doctor's approval.

Adults: The dosage your doctor prescribes will depend on the type of infection you have as well as your body's response to the drug.

Vaginal Candidiasis
Adults: The recommended dose is 150 mg as a single oral dose.

Oropharyngeal Candidiasis
Adults: The recommended dose is 200 mg on the first day, followed by 100 mg once daily for at least 2 weeks.

Children: (Weight-based; total doses >600 mg per day are not recommended.) The recommended dose is 6 mg/ 2.2 pounds of body weight on the first day, followed by 3 mg/ 2.2 pounds of body weight once daily for at least 2 weeks.

Esophageal Candidiasis
Adults: The recommended dose is 200 mg on the first day, followed by 100 mg once daily for at least 3 weeks and should be continued for at least 2 weeks after the symptoms of infection resolve. Doses up to 400 mg per day may be prescribed.

Children: The recommended dose is 6 mg/kg on the first day, followed by 3 mg/ 2.2 pounds of body weight once daily for at least 3 weeks and should be continued for at least 2 weeks after the symptoms of infection resolve. Doses up to 12 mg/ 2.2 pounds of body weight per day may be prescribed.

Systemic Candida Infections
Adults: The recommended dose has not been established but doses up to 400 mg per day have been used.

Children: Doses of 6-12 mg/ 2.2 pounds of body weight have been used in some patients.

Urinary Tract Infections and Peritonitis
Adults: Doses of 50-200 mg have been used in some patients.

Cryptococcal Meningitis
Adults: The recommended dose is 400 mg on the first day, followed by 200 mg once daily for 10-12 weeks after the infection has cleared from your brain and spinal cord. Your doctor may prescribe 400 mg once daily depending on your response. If you have AIDS with recurring infections, the recommended dose is 200 mg once daily.

Children: The recommended dose is 12 mg/ 2.2 pounds of body weight on the first day, followed by 6 mg/ 2.2 pounds of body weight once daily for 10-12 weeks after the infection has cleared from your brain and spinal cord. Your doctor may prescribe 12 mg/ 2.2 pounds of body weight once daily depending on your child's response. If your child has AIDS with recurring infections, the recommended dose is 6 mg/ 2.2 pounds of body weight once daily.

Bone Marrow Transplant Prophylaxis
Adults: The recommended daily dose is 400 mg once daily. You may need to start therapy several days before expected decrease in white blood cells and for 7 days after the amount of white blood cells returns to a normal level.

Patients with Kidney Problems
Adults: Dose adjustments may be necessary if you have kidney problems or are on dialysis.

How should I take Diflucan?
You can take Diflucan with or without meals at any time of day. Diflucan may be taken orally or given by IV infusion. Diflucan keeps working for several days to treat the infection. Generally the symptoms start to go away after 24 hours.

Take this medication exactly as prescribed, and continue taking it for as long as your doctor instructs. You may begin to feel better after the first few days; but it takes weeks or even months of treatment to completely cure certain fungal infections.

What should I avoid while taking Diflucan?

Some medications can affect how well Diflucan works. Check with your doctor before starting any new medicines within seven days of taking Diflucan.

Avoid stopping therapy before recommended by your doctor, even if you start to feel better.

What are possible food and drug interactions associated with Diflucan?

If Diflucan is taken with certain other drugs, the effects of either could be increased, decreased, or altered. It is especially important to check with your doctor before combining Diflucan with the following: antidiabetic drugs such as glipizide, glyburide, and tolbutamide; astemizole; blood-thinning drugs such as warfarin; cisapride; cyclosporine; hydrochlorothiazide; phenytoin; rifabutin; rifampin; tacrolimus; terfenadine; theophylline; and ulcer medications.

What are the possible side effects of Diflucan?

Side effects cannot be anticipated. If any develop or change in intensity, inform your doctor as soon as possible. Only your doctor can determine if it is safe for you to continue taking Diflucan.

The most common side effect for people taking more than one dose is nausea.

For women taking a single dose to treat vaginal infection, the most common side effects are changes in taste, diarrhea, dizziness, headache, nausea and upset stomach. stomach pain

Other side effects may include: irregular heartbeat, skin rash, vomiting, serious allergic reactions, rare cases of severe liver damage

Can I receive Diflucan if I am pregnant or breastfeeding?

The effects of Diflucan during pregnancy have not been adequately studied. If you are pregnant or plan to become pregnant, inform your doctor immediately. Diflucan appears in breast milk and could affect a nursing infant. Consult your doctor if you plan to breastfeed.

What should I do if I miss a dose of Diflucan?

Take the missed dose as soon as you remember it. However, if it is almost time for your next dose, skip the one you missed and return to your regular dosing schedule. Do not double the dose.

How should I store Diflucan?

Store at room temperature. Protect from freezing. Keep out of reach of children.

Digoxin *See Lanoxin, page 705.*

DILANTIN
Generic name: Phenytoin sodium

What is Dilantin?

Dilantin is an antiepileptic drug prescribed to control grand mal seizures (a type of seizure in which the individual experiences a sudden loss of consciousness immediately followed by generalized convulsions) and temporal lobe seizures (a type of seizure caused by disease in the cortex of the temporal [side] lobe of the brain affecting smell, taste, sight, hearing, memory, and movement).

What is the most important information I should know about Dilantin?

If you have been taking Dilantin regularly, do not stop abruptly. This may precipitate prolonged or repeated epileptic seizures without any recovery of consciousness between attacks—a condition called status epilepticus that can be fatal if not treated promptly.

Who should not take Dilantin?

If you have ever had an allergic reaction to or are sensitive to phenytoin or similar epilepsy medications such as ethotoin or mephenytoin, do not take Dilantin. Make sure your doctor is aware of any drug reactions you have experienced.

What should I tell my doctor before I take the first dose of Dilantin?

Tell your doctor about all prescription, over-the-counter, and herbal medication you are taking before beginning treatment with this drug. Also, talk to your doctor about your complete medical history, especially if you have liver problems. Because Dilantin is processed by the liver, people with impaired liver function, older adults, and those who are seriously ill may show early signs of drug poisoning.

Also let the doctor know if you have diabetes. Hyperglycemia (high blood sugar) may occur in people taking Dilantin, which blocks the release of insulin. People with diabetes may experience increased blood sugar levels due to Dilantin.

If you have bone disease, be aware that abnormal softening of the bones may occur in people taking Dilantin because of the drug's interference with vitamin D metabolism.

Tell the doctor if you have dental problems. Because Dilantin can cause gingival hyperplasia (excessive formation of the gums over the teeth), it is important to practice good dental hygiene while using this drug.

Also tell the doctor if you develop a skin rash. If the rash is scale-like, characterized by reddish or purplish spots, or consists of (fluid-filled) blisters, your doctor may stop Dilantin and prescribe an alternative treatment. If the rash is more like measles, your doctor may have you stop taking Dilantin until the rash is completely gone.

What is the usual dosage?
The information below is based on the dosage guidelines your doctor uses. Depending on your condition and medical history, your doctor may prescribe a different regimen. Do not change the dosage or stop taking your medication without your doctor's approval.

Dosage is tailored to each individual's needs. Your doctor will monitor blood levels of the drug closely, particularly when switching you from one drug to another.

Standard Daily Dosage
Adults: If you have not had any previous treatment, your doctor will have you take one 100-milligram Dilantin capsule 3 times daily to start.

On a continuing basis, most adults need 1 capsule 3 to 4 times a day. Your doctor may increase that dosage to 2 capsules 3 times a day, if necessary.

Once-A-Day Dosage
Adults: If your seizures are controlled on 100-milligram Dilantin capsules 3 times daily, your doctor may allow you to take the entire 300 milligrams as a single dose once daily.

Children: The starting dose is 5 milligrams per 2.2 pounds of body weight per day, divided into 2 or 3 equal doses; the most a child should take is 300 milligrams a day. The regular daily dosage is usually 4 to 8 milligrams per 2.2 pounds. Children over 6 years of age and adolescents may need the minimum adult dose (300 milligrams per day).

How should I take Dilantin?
It is important that you strictly follow the prescribed dosage regimen and tell your doctor about any condition that makes it impossible for you to take Dilantin as prescribed.

If you are given Dilantin Oral Suspension, shake it well before using. Use the specially marked measuring spoon, a plastic syringe, or a small measuring cup to measure each dose accurately.

Swallow Dilantin Kapseals whole. Dilantin Infatabs can be either chewed thoroughly and then swallowed, or swallowed whole. The Infatabs are not to be used for once-a-day dosing.

Do not change from one form of Dilantin to another without consulting your doctor. Different products may not work the same way.

What should I avoid while taking Dilantin?
Avoid drinking alcoholic beverages while taking Dilantin.

What are possible food and drug interactions associated with Dilantin?

If Dilantin is taken with certain other drugs, the effects of either could be increased, decreased, or altered. It is especially important to check with your doctor before combining Dilantin with the following: alcohol, amiodarone, antacids containing calcium, blood-thinning drugs such as warfarin, chloramphenicol, chlordiazepoxide, cimetidine, diazepam, dicumarol, digitoxin, disulfiram, doxycycline, estrogens, ethosuximide, felbamate, fluoxetine, furosemide, isoniazid, major tranquilizers such as chlorpromazine and thioridazine, methylphenidate, molindone hydrochloride, oral contraceptives, paroxetine, phenobarbital, quinidine, reserpine, rifampin, salicylates such as aspirin, seizure medications such as carbamazepine, ethosuximide, and valproic acid, steroid drugs such as prednisone, sucralfate, sulfa drugs such as sulfisoxazole, theophylline, ticlopidine, tolbutamide, trazodone, ulcer medications such as cimetidine and ranitidine, tricyclic antidepressants (such as amitriptyline, desipramine, and others) may cause seizures in susceptible people, making a dosage adjustment of Dilantin necessary.

What are the possible side effects of Dilantin?

Side effects cannot be anticipated. If any develop or change in intensity, inform your doctor as soon as possible. Only your doctor can determine whether it is safe for you to continue taking Dilantin.

Side effects may include: Decreased coordination, involuntary eye movement, mental confusion, slurred speech

Can I receive Dilantin if I am pregnant or breastfeeding?

If you are pregnant or plan to become pregnant, inform your doctor immediately. Because of the possibility of birth defects with antiepileptic drugs such as Dilantin, you may need to discontinue the drug. Do not, however, stop taking it without first consulting your doctor. Dilantin appears in breast milk; breastfeeding is not recommended during treatment with this drug.

What should I do if I miss a dose of Dilantin?

If you take one dose a day, take the dose you missed as soon as you remember. If you do not remember until the next day, skip the missed dose and go back to your regular schedule. Do not take 2 doses at once.

If you take more than 1 dose a day, take the missed dose as soon as possible. If it is within 4 hours of your next dose, skip the one you missed and go back to your regular schedule. Do not take 2 doses at once.

If you forget to take your medication 2 or more days in a row, check with your doctor.

How should I store Dilantin?

Store at room temperature away from light and moisture.

Diltiazem hydrochloride *See Cardizem/Cardizem CD/ Cardizem LA/Cardizem SR, page 254.*

DIOVAN
Generic name: Valsartan

What is Diovan?
Diovan is an angiotensin receptor blocker. It is used in adults to lower high blood pressure, treat heart failure, and improve the chances of living longer after a heart attack. It is also used in children to treat high blood pressure.

What is the most important information I should know about Diovan?
Diovan should not be taken during pregnancy. Diovan can harm an unborn baby, causing injury and even death.

Who should not take Diovan?
Do not take Diovan if you are allergic to any of its ingredients, or if you are pregnant. Diovan is not for children under 6 years of age or children with certain kidney problems.

What should I tell my doctor before I take the first dose of Diovan?
Tell your doctor about all prescription, over-the-counter, and herbal medications you are taking, before beginning treatment with Diovan. Also, talk to your doctor about your complete medical history, especially if you are pregnant, plan to become pregnant, or nursing. This drug can cause harm to your unborn child, and should not be taken if you are going to nurse. Also, tell your doctor if you have heart, liver, or kidney problems.

What is the usual dosage?
The information below is based on the dosage guidelines your doctor uses. Depending on your condition and medical history, your doctor may prescribe a different regimen. Do not change the dosage or stop taking your medication without your doctor's approval.

High Blood Pressure
Adults: The usual dosage of Diovan is 80 milligrams (mg) or 160 mg once daily.

Children 6 to 16 years old: For children who can swallow tablets, the usual recommended starting dose is 1.3 milligram (mg)/kilogram (kg) once daily (up to 40mg total). For children who cannot swallow tablets or children for whom the calculated dosage (mg/kg) does not correspond to the available tablet strengths of Diovan, the use of a suspension is recommended. When the suspension is replaced by a tablet, the dose of valsartan may have to be increased.

Heart Failure
Adults: The recommended starting dose of Diovan is 40 mg twice daily.

Heart Attack
Adults: Diovan may be started as early as 12 hours after a heart attack. The recommended starting dose of Diovan is 20 mg twice daily.

How should I take Diovan?
Diovan may be taken with or without food. For children who cannot swallow the tablets, your pharmacist will mix this medicine as a liquid suspension. Shake the bottle of suspension well for at least 10 seconds before giving it to your child.

Carefully follow your doctor's instructions about any special diet. For treatment of high blood pressure, take Diovan once daily at the same time each day. For treatment of heart failure or after a heart attack, take Diovan twice a day at the same times each day.

What should I avoid while taking Diovan?
Avoid becoming pregnant while taking Diovan. Do not take potassium supplements or salt substitutes containing potassium while on Diovan; doing so may lead to increases in potassium levels in your body and may worsen your condition if you have heart failure.

What are possible food and drug interactions associated with Diovan?
If Diovan is taken with certain other drugs, the effects of either could be increased, decreased, or altered. It is especially important to check with your doctor before combining Diovan with the following: potassium sparing diuretics, potassium supplements or salt substitutes.

What are the possible side effects of Diovan?
Side effects cannot be anticipated. If any develop or change in intensity, tell your doctor as soon as possible. Only your doctor can determine if it is safe for you to continue taking this drug.

Side effects may include: cough, diarrhea, dizziness, flu symptoms, headache, high blood potassium, joint and back pain, low blood pressure, rash, stomach pain, tiredness, dizziness, swelling of the feet/hands, unexplained weight gain

Can I receive Diovan if I am pregnant or breastfeeding?
Talk to your doctor if you are pregnant, plan to become pregnant, or nursing. If pregnancy is detected, immediately stop taking Diovan. Diovan may pass into your breast milk and harm your baby. Speak to your doctor before or if already nursing.

What should I do if I miss a dose of Diovan?

Take the missed dose as soon as you remember. However, if it is almost time for your next dose, skip the one you missed and return to your regular dosing schedule. Do not double the dose.

How should I store Diovan?

Store the medicine in a closed container at room temperature, away from heat, moisture, and direct light. Store the bottle of suspension at room temperature for up to 30 days, or in the refrigerator for up to 75 days.

DIOVAN HCT

Generic name: Valsartan and hydrochlorothiazide

What is Diovan HCT?

Diovan HCT contains two prescription medicines in one tablet. It contains valsartan (Diovan), an angiotensin receptor blocker (ARB), and hydrochlorothiazide (HCTZ), a diuretic (water pill). Diovan HCT is used to lower high blood pressure (hypertension) in adults.

What is the most important information I should know about Diovan HCT?

If you get pregnant, stop taking Diovan HCT and call your doctor right away. Diovan HCT can harm an unborn baby, causing injury and even death. If you plan to become pregnant, talk to your doctor about other treatment options before taking Diovan HCT.

Do not use Diovan HCT to treat a condition for which it was not prescribed. Do not give Diovan HCT to other people, even if they have the same symptoms you have.

Drugs that lower blood pressure, such as Diovan HCT, lower your risk of having a stroke or heart attack.

When taking Diovan HCT, you may develop symptoms of low blood pressure, such as dizziness or feeling faint. Low blood pressure is most likely to happen if you are on a low salt diet, are receiving dialysis, have heart problems, get sick with vomiting or diarrhea, or drink alcohol. Lie down if you feel faint or dizzy and call your doctor right away.

If you have kidney disease, Diovan HCT has the potential to worsen your condition. Call you doctor if you get swelling in your feet, ankles, or hands, or if you experience unexplained weight gain. Call your doctor right away if you get an unusual skin rash.

Who should not take Diovan HCT?

Do not take Diovan HCT if you have trouble urinating (because of kidney problems) or if you are allergic to medicines that contain sulfonamides.

Do not take Diovan HCT if you are pregnant. If you get pregnant, stop taking Diovan HCT and call your doctor right away. Diovan HCT can harm an unborn child.

What should I tell my doctor before I take the first dose of Diovan HCT?

Tell your doctor about all prescription, over-the-counter, and herbal medication you are taking before beginning treatment with Diovan HCT. Also, talk to your doctor about your complete medical history, especially if you have or ever have had gallstones, a heart condition, kidney problems, liver problems, or lupus. Inform your doctor if you are pregnant or planning to become pregnant or are breastfeeding.

What is the usual dosage?
The information below is based on the dosage guidelines your doctor uses. Depending on your condition and medical history, your doctor may prescribe a different regimen. Do not change the dosage or stop taking your medication without your doctor's approval.

Diovan HCT should only be used by patients who have already tried Diovan by itself or HCTZ by itself. The starting dose of Diovan HCT is based on your previous dose of Diovan or HCTZ. Diovan HCT is a combination pill; the first number represents the number of milligrams (mg) of Diovan; the second number represents the number of mg of HCTZ: 80/12.5mg, 160/12.5mg, 160/25mg, 320/12.5mg, or 320/25mg.

The usual starting dose is Diovan HCT 160/12.5mg once daily. The dosage can be increased after 1 to 2 weeks of therapy to a maximum of one 320/25mg tablet once daily as needed to control blood pressure.

How should I take Diovan HCT?
Take Diovan HCT exactly as prescribed by your doctor. Your doctor may change your dose if needed. Diovan HCT is taken once a day, at the same time each day.

Diovan HCT can be taken with or without food.

What should I avoid while taking Diovan HCT?
Lithium should not be taken with diuretics such as hydrochlorothiazide, which is an ingredient of Diovan HCT. Diuretic agents may lead to high risk of lithium poisoning. Also avoid becoming pregnant while taking Diovan HCT.

What are possible food and drug interactions associated with Diovan HCT?
If Diovan HCT is taken with certain other drugs, the effects of either could be increased, decreased, or altered. It is especially important to check with your doctor before combining Diovan HCT with the following: alcohol; anti-diabetes medicine including insulin; aspirin; diuretics; lithium, a medicine used in some types of depression; narcotic pain medicines non-

steroidal anti-inflammatory drugs (NSAIDS); other medicines for high blood pressure or heart problems; potassium supplements or using a salt substitute containing potassium; sleeping pills; and steroids.

What are the possible side effects of Diovan HCT?
Side effects cannot be anticipated. If any develop or change in intensity, tell your doctor as soon as possible. Only your doctor can determine if it is safe for you to continue taking this drug.

Side effects may include: abdominal pain, allergic reaction, anemia, anxiety, back pain, blurred vision, confusion, constipation, cough, dehydration, depression, diarrhea, digestive problems, drowsiness, dry mouth, erectile dysfunction, fatigue, fever, flushing, gout, high potassium level (hyperkalemia), increased appetite, influenza, kidney problems, low blood pressure (hypotension), muscle cramps, muscle weakness, nasal congestion, respiratory tract infection, restlessness, sinus congestion, skin rash, sunburn, thirst, urinary tract infection, viral infection, vomiting, weakness

These are not all the side effects of Diovan HCT. For a complete list, ask your doctor or pharmacist.

Can I receive Diovan HCT if I am pregnant or breastfeeding?
If you become pregnant while taking Diovan HCT, stop taking it and call your doctor right away. Diovan HCT can harm an unborn baby, causing injury and even death. If you plan to become pregnant, talk to your doctor about other treatment options before taking Diovan HCT. Diovan HCT may pass through your breast milk and cause harm. Notify your doctor if you are nursing.

What should I do if I miss a dose of Diovan HCT?
If you miss a dose, take it as soon as you remember. If it is close to your next dose, do not take the missed dose. Just take the next dose at your regular time.

How should I store Diovan HCT?
Store at room temperature in a dry place.

DIPENTUM
Generic name: Olsalazine sodium

What is Dipentum?
Dipentum is an anti-inflammatory drug used to treat the symptoms of ulcerative colitis (chronic inflammation and ulceration of the large intestine and rectum). It is prescribed for people who cannot take sulfasalazine.

What is the most important information I should know about Dipentum?

If you have kidney disease, Dipentum could cause further damage. You'll need regular checks on your kidney function, so be sure to keep all regular appointments with your doctor.

Who should not take Dipentum?

You should not use Dipentum if you are allergic to salicylates such as aspirin.

What should I tell my doctor before I take the first dose of Dipentum?

Tell your doctor about all prescription, over-the-counter, and herbal medication you are taking before beginning treatment with this drug. Also, talk to your doctor about your complete medical history. If diarrhea occurs while taking Dipentum, contact your doctor.

What is the usual dosage?

The information below is based on the dosage guidelines your doctor uses. Depending on your condition and medical history, your doctor may prescribe a different regimen. Do not change the dosage or stop taking your medication without your doctor's approval.

Adults: The usual dose is a total of 1 gram per day, divided into 2 equal doses.

How should I take Dipentum?

Take Dipentum with food. The drug should be taken in equally divided doses.

What should I avoid while taking Dipentum?

You should avoid receiving a varicella (chicken pox) vaccine within six weeks of taking Dipentum.

What are possible food and drug interactions associated with Dipentum?

If Dipentum is taken with certain other drugs, the effects of either could be increased, decreased, or altered. It is especially important to check with your doctor before combining Dipentum with warfarin or low molecular weight heparins. You should discontinue salicylates, such as aspirin, before starting Dipentum.

What are the possible side effects of Dipentum?

Side effects cannot be anticipated. If any develop or change in intensity, inform your doctor as soon as possible. Only your doctor can determine if it is safe for you to continue taking Dipentum.

Side effects may include: blood in stool, blurred vision, chest pain, diarrhea or loose stools, shortness of breath, ringing of the ears

Rare cases of hepatitis have been reported in people taking Dipentum. Symptoms may include aching muscles, chills, fever, headache, joint pain, loss of appetite, vomiting, and yellowish skin.

Can I receive Dipentum if I am pregnant or breastfeeding?
The effects of Dipentum in pregnancy have not been adequately studied. Pregnant women should use Dipentum only if the possible gains warrant the possible risks to the unborn child. Women who breastfeed an infant should use Dipentum cautiously, because it is not known whether this drug appears in breast milk and what effect it might have on a nursing infant.

What should I do if I miss a dose of Dipentum?
If you miss a dose of this drug, skip it. Do not take an extra dose to make up for missed doses.

How should I store Dipentum?
Store at room temperature.

Diphenoxylate hydrochloride and atropine sulfate
See Lomotil, page 754.

Diphtheria, tetanus, pertussis, poliovirus vaccine
See Kinrix, page 692.

DIPROLENE
Generic name: Betamethasone dipropionate

What is Diprolene?
Diprolene, a synthetic cortisone-like steroid available in cream, gel, lotion, or ointment form, is used to treat certain itchy rashes and other inflammatory skin conditions.

What is the most important information I should know about Diprolene?
When you use Diprolene, you inevitably absorb some of the medication through your skin and into the bloodstream. Too much absorption can lead to unwanted side effects elsewhere in the body. To keep this problem to a minimum, avoid using large amounts of Diprolene over large areas, and do not cover it with airtight dressings such as plastic wrap or adhesive bandages.

Diprolene ointment should not be used in the treatment of diaper rash. The ointment should not be applied in the diaper area.

This medication should not be used on the face, underarms, or groin areas unless otherwise directed by the physician.

Use of the medication should be discontinued when control is achieved; if no improvement is seen within 2 weeks, contact your physician.

Other corticosteroid-containing products should not be used with Diprolene.

Who should not take Diprolene?

Do not use Diprolene if you are sensitive to it or any other steroid medication.

What should I tell my doctor before I take the first dose of Diprolene?

Tell your doctor about all prescription, over-the-counter, and herbal medication you are taking before beginning treatment with this drug. Also, talk to your doctor about your complete medical history.

What is the usual dosage?

The information below is based on the dosage guidelines your doctor uses. Depending on your condition and medical history, your doctor may prescribe a different regimen. Do not change the dosage or stop taking your medication without your doctor's approval.

Adults: Cream or ointment: Apply a thin film to the affected skin areas once or twice daily. Treatment should be limited to 45 grams per week. *Lotion:* Apply a few drops to the affected area once or twice daily and massage lightly until the lotion disappears. Treatment must be limited to 14 days; do not use any more than 50 milliliters per week. Gel: Apply a thin layer to the affected area once or twice daily and rub in gently and completely. Treatment must be limited to 14 days; do not use any more than 50 grams per week.

Children: Use of Diprolene is not recommended for children 12 and under. For those 13 and over, use no more than necessary to obtain results.

How should I take Diprolene?

Apply Diprolene in a thin film, exactly as prescribed by your doctor. A typical regimen is 1 or 2 applications per day. Do not use the medication for longer than prescribed. Diprolene is for use only on the skin. Be careful to keep it out of your eyes.

What should I avoid while taking Diprolene?

Once you have applied Diprolene, never cover the skin with an airtight bandage or other tight dressing.

Avoid using large amounts of Diprolene, and also avoid prolonged use. If too much of the drug is absorbed into the bloodstream, it may cause high blood sugar, sugar in the urine, and a group of symptoms called Cushing's syndrome.

What are possible food and drug interactions associated with Diprolene?
Do not use Diprolene with any other steroid-containing product. Such combinations increase the chance of absorption and side effects.

What are the possible side effects of Diprolene?
Side effects cannot be anticipated. A possible side effect of Diprolene is stinging or burning of the skin where the medication is applied.

Other side effects on the skin may include: acne-like eruptions, atrophy, "broken" capillaries (fine reddish lines), cracking or tightening, dryness, excess hair growth, infected hair follicles, inflammation, irritation, itching, prickly heat, rash, redness, sensitivity to touch

Can I receive Diprolene if I am pregnant or breastfeeding?
It is not known whether Diprolene, when applied to skin, causes any problem during pregnancy or while breastfeeding. It's considered best for pregnant women to avoid the product unless the possible benefits outweigh the potential risk. If it must be used, it should not be applied extensively, in large amounts, or for a long period of time.

What should I do if I miss a dose of Diprolene?
Apply the missed dose as soon as you remember it. However, if it is almost time for your next dose, skip the one you missed and return to your regular dosing schedule. Do not double the dose.

How should I store Diprolene?
Store at room temperature.

Dipyridamole *See Persantine, page 1011.*

Disopyramide phosphate *See Norpace, page 909.*

DITROPAN
Generic name: Oxybutynin chloride

What is Ditropan?
Ditropan and Ditropan XL, the extended-release form of the drug, treat symptoms of overactive bladder, including frequent urination, urgency (increased need to urinate), and urge incontinence (inability to control

urination). The drug works by blocking the nerve impulses that prompt the bladder to contract. Ditropan is also used to treat the urgency, frequency, leakage, incontinence, and painful or difficult urination caused by a neurogenic bladder (altered bladder function due to a nervous system abnormality).

Ditropan XL can also be prescribed for children 6 years of age and older who are suffering from urinary urge incontinence due to a neurological condition such as spina bifida.

What is the most important information I should know about Ditropan?

Ditropan can cause heat prostration (fever and heat stroke due to decreased sweating) in high temperatures. If you live in a hot climate or will be exposed to high temperatures, take appropriate precautions.

If you have an ileostomy or colostomy (an artificial opening to the bowel) and develop diarrhea while taking Ditropan, inform your doctor immediately.

Your doctor will prescribe Ditropan with caution if you have liver disease, kidney disease, digestive problems such as reflux disease, or a nervous system disorder.

Ditropan may aggravate the symptoms of overactive thyroid, heart disease or congestive heart failure, irregular or rapid heartbeat, high blood pressure, or enlarged prostate.

Who should not take Ditropan?

You should not take Ditropan if you have certain types of untreated glaucoma (excessive pressure in the eye), partial or complete blockage of the gastrointestinal tract, or paralytic ileus (obstructed bowel). Ditropan should also be avoided if you have severe colitis (inflamed colon), myasthenia gravis (abnormal muscle weakness), or urinary tract obstruction (inability to urinate). This drug is usually not prescribed for the elderly or debilitated.

Do not take this medication if you are sensitive or have ever had an allergic reaction to it. Make sure your doctor is aware of any allergic reactions you have experienced.

What should I tell my doctor before I take the first dose of Ditropan?

Tell your doctor about all prescription, over-the-counter, and herbal medications you are taking before beginning treatment with this drug. Also talk to your doctor about your complete medical history.

What is the usual dosage?

The information below is based on the dosage guidelines your doctor uses. Depending on your condition and medical history, your doctor

may prescribe a different regimen. Do not change the dosage or stop taking your medication without your doctor's approval.

Ditropan
Adults: The usual dose is one 5-milligram tablet or 1 teaspoonful of syrup taken 2 to 3 times a day, but not more than 4 times a day.

Children over 5 years of age: The usual dose is one 5-milligram tablet or 1 teaspoonful of syrup taken 2 times a day, but not more than 3 times a day. Ditropan is not recommended for children under 5.

Ditropan XL
Adults: The recommended starting dose is 5 or 10 milligrams once a day. If this proves insufficient, the doctor may increase the dose by 5 milligrams at weekly intervals, up to a maximum of 30 milligrams a day.

Children 6 years of age and older: The recommended starting dose is 5 milligrams once a day. If this proves insufficient, the doctor may increase the dose by 5-milligram increments, up to a maximum of 20 milligrams a day.

How should I take Ditropan?
Ditropan may be taken with or without food. Take it exactly as prescribed. Ditropan can make your mouth dry. Sucking hard candies or melting bits of ice in your mouth can remedy the problem. Ditropan tablets and syrup must be taken 2 or 3 times a day. Ditropan XL, a long-acting form of the drug, is available for once-a-day dosing. Ditropan XL tablets should be swallowed whole with plenty of fluid. Do not chew, crush, or break them.

After taking Ditropan XL, you may notice something like a tablet in your stool. This is not a cause for concern. The outer coating of the extended-release tablet sometimes fails to dissolve along with the contents.

What should I avoid while taking Ditropan?
Ditropan may cause drowsiness or blurred vision. Driving or operating dangerous machinery or participating in any hazardous activity that requires full mental alertness is not recommended until you know how this medication affects you.

What are possible food and drug interactions associated with Ditropan?
If Ditropan is taken with certain other drugs, the effects of either may be increased, decreased or altered. It is especially important to check with your doctor before combining Ditropan with alcohol or sedatives such as temazepam or triazolam because increased drowsiness may occur. You should also check with your doctor if you are taking any of the following: alendronate, antibiotics such as erythromycin and clarithromycin, antifungal medication, risedronate, and drugs used to treat spasms such as dicyclomine, glycopyrrolate, hyoscyamine, and propantheline.

What are the possible side effects of Ditropan?
Side effects cannot be anticipated. If any develop or change in intensity, tell your doctor as soon as possible. Only your doctor can determine if it is safe for you to continue taking this drug.

Side effects may include: constipation, decreased production of tears, decreased sweating, difficulty falling or staying asleep, dilation of the pupil of the eye, dim vision, dizziness, drowsiness, dry mouth, eye paralysis, hallucinations, impotence, inability to urinate, nausea, palpitations, rapid heartbeat, rash, restlessness, suppression of milk production, weakness

Can I receive Ditropan if I am pregnant or breastfeeding?
The effects of Ditropan during pregnancy have not been adequately studied. If you are pregnant or plan to become pregnant, inform your doctor immediately. Ditropan may appear in breast milk and could affect a nursing infant. If this medication is essential to your health, your doctor may advise you to stop breastfeeding until your treatment is finished.

What should I do if I miss a dose of Ditropan?
Take the forgotten dose as soon as you remember. If it is almost time for your next dose, skip the one you missed and go back to your regular schedule. Never take 2 doses at once.

How should I store Ditropan?
Keep this medication in a tightly closed container and store it at room temperature. Protect the syrup from direct light. Protect the extended-release tablets from moisture and humidity.

DIURIL
Generic name: Chlorothiazide

What is Diuril?
Diuril is used in the treatment of high blood pressure and other conditions that require the elimination of excess fluid (water) from the body. These conditions include congestive heart failure, cirrhosis of the liver, corticosteroid and estrogen therapy, and kidney disease. When used for high blood pressure, Diuril can be used alone or with other high blood pressure medications. Diuril contains a form of thiazide, a diuretic that prompts your body to eliminate more fluid, which helps lower blood pressure.

What is the most important information I should know about Diuril?
If you have high blood pressure, you must take Diuril regularly for it to be effective. Since blood pressure declines gradually, it may be several

weeks before you get the full benefit of Diuril; you must continue taking it even if you are feeling well. Diuril does not cure high blood pressure; it keeps it under control.

Who should not take Diuril?

If you are unable to urinate, you should not take this medication. If you are sensitive to or have ever had an allergic reaction to Diuril or other thiazide-type diuretics, or if you are sensitive to sulfa drugs, you should not take this medication.

What should I tell my doctor before I take the first dose of Diuril?

Tell your doctor about all prescription, over-the-counter, and herbal medication you are taking before beginning treatment with this drug. Also, talk to your doctor about your complete medical history, especially if you have kidney or liver problems, low potassium levels, diabetes, gout, the connective tissue disease lupus erythematosus, bronchial asthma, or a history of allergies.

In addition, you should notify your doctor or dentist that you are taking Diuril if you have a medical emergency, and before you have surgery or dental treatment.

What is the usual dosage?

The information below is based on the dosage guidelines your doctor uses. Depending on your condition and medical history, your doctor may prescribe a different regimen. Do not change the dosage or stop taking your medication without your doctor's approval.

The dosage will vary depending on your condition and how your body responds to the drug.

How should I take Diuril?

Take Diuril exactly as prescribed. Stopping Diuril suddenly could cause your condition to worsen.

What should I avoid while taking Diuril?

Avoid becoming overheated, and be careful when exercising and in hot weather. Dehydration, excessive sweating, severe diarrhea, or vomiting could deplete your body's fluids and lower your blood pressure too much.

Diuril may increase the effects of alcohol. Do not drink alcohol while taking this medication.

What are possible food and drug interactions associated with Diuril?

If Diuril is taken with certain other drugs, the effects of either may be increased, decreased, or altered. It is especially important to check with your doctor before combining Diuril with the following: barbiturates such as phenobarbital and secobarbital, cholesterol-lowering drugs such as cholestyramine and colestipol, drugs to treat diabetes such as insulin and glyburide, lithium, narcotic painkillers such as oxycodone, nonsteroidal anti-inflammatory drugs such as ibuprofen and naproxen, norepinephrine, other drugs for high blood pressure such as captopril and nifedipine, and steroids such as prednisone.

What are the possible side effects of Diuril?
Side effects cannot be anticipated. If any develop or change in intensity, inform your doctor as soon as possible. Only your doctor can determine if it is safe for you to continue taking Diuril.

Side effects may include: abdominal cramps, anemia, changes in blood sugar, constipation, diarrhea, difficulty breathing, dizziness, dizziness on standing up, fever, fluid in lungs, hypersensitivity reactions, jaundice, low potassium (leading to symptoms such as dry mouth, excessive thirst, weak or irregular heartbeat, muscle pain or cramps), nausea, rash, sensitivity to light, stomach irritation, stomach upset, vomiting

Can I receive Diuril if I am pregnant or breastfeeding?
The effects of Diuril during pregnancy have not been adequately studied. If you are pregnant or plan to become pregnant, inform your doctor immediately. Diuril appears in breast milk and could affect a nursing infant. Consult your doctor before breastfeeding.

What should I do if I miss a dose of Diuril?
Take the missed dose as soon as you remember it. However, if it is almost time for your next dose, skip the one you missed and return to your regular dosing schedule.

Do not double the dose.

How should I store Diuril?
Store at room temperature. Protect from moisture and freezing.

Divalproex sodium, delayed-release *See Depakote, page 396.*

Divalproex sodium, extended-release *See Depakote ER, page 400.*

Docusate *See Colace, page 315.*

Donepezil hydrochloride *See Aricept, page 123.*

DONNATAL

Generic ingredients: Phenobarbital, Hyoscyamine sulfate,
Atropine sulfate, Scopolamine hydrobromide

What is Donnatal?

Donnatal is a mild antispasmodic medication; it has been used with other drugs for relief of cramps and pain associated with various stomach, intestinal, and bowel disorders, including irritable bowel syndrome, acute colitis, spastic colon and duodenal ulcer (inconclusive for this indication).

What is the most important information
I should know about Donnatal?

Phenobarbital, one of the ingredients of Donnatal, can be habit-forming. If you have ever been dependent on drugs, do not take Donnatal.

Be careful in extreme temperatures; Donnatal can cause fever and heatstroke because it prevents your body from being able to sweat.

Donnatal may produce drowsiness or blurred vision; if this should occur, do not engage in activities requiring mental alertness, such as operating a motor vehicle or other machinery.

Who should not take Donnatal?

Do not take Donnatal if you suffer from the eye condition called glaucoma, diseases that block the urinary or gastrointestinal tracts, or myasthenia gravis, a condition in which the muscles become progressively paralyzed.

Also, you should not use Donnatal if you have intestinal atony (loss of strength in the intestinal muscles), unstable cardiovascular status, severe ulcerative colitis (chronic inflammation and ulceration of the bowel), or hiatal hernia (a rupture in the diaphragm above the stomach). You should also avoid Donnatal if you have acute intermittent porphyria—a disorder of the metabolism in which there is severe abdominal pain and sensitivity to light.

If you are sensitive to or have ever had an allergic reaction to Donnatal, its ingredients, or similar drugs, you should not take this medication. Also avoid Donnatal if phenobarbital makes you excited or restless, instead of calming you down. Make sure your doctor is aware of any drug reactions you have experienced.

What should I tell my doctor before
I take the first dose of Donnatal?

Tell your doctor about all prescription, over-the-counter, and herbal medication you are taking before beginning treatment with this drug. Also, talk to your doctor about your complete medical history, especially if you have ever had any of the following: high blood pressure, gastric ulcer, overactive thyroid (hyperthyroidism), irregular or rapid heartbeat, or heart, kidney, or liver disease. If you develop diarrhea, especially if you have an ileostomy or colostomy (artificial openings to the bowel), check with your doctor.

What is the usual dosage?

The information below is based on the dosage guidelines your doctor uses. Depending on your condition and medical history, your doctor may prescribe a different regimen. Do not change the dosage or stop taking your medication without your doctor's approval.

Adults: Your doctor will adjust the dosage to your needs. For tablets or capsules, the usual dosage is 1 or 2 tablets or capsules, 3 or 4 times a day. For liquid, the usual dosage is 1 or 2 teaspoonfuls, 3 or 4 times a day. For Donnatal Extentabs, the usual dosage is 1 tablet every 12 hours. Your doctor may tell you to take 1 tablet every 8 hours, if necessary.

Children: Dosage of the elixir is determined by body weight; it can be given every 4 to 6 hours. Follow your doctor's instructions carefully when giving this medication to a child.

How should I take Donnatal?

Take Donnatal one-half hour to 1 hour before meals. Use it exactly as prescribed.

What should I avoid while taking Donnatal?

Donnatal may cause you to become drowsy or less alert. You should not drive or operate dangerous machinery or participate in any hazardous activity that requires full mental alertness until you know how this drug affects you.

Donnatal can decrease sweating; to prevent heat stroke, you should avoid strenuous exercise and high temperatures.

What are possible food and drug interactions associated with Donnatal?

Donnatal may intensify the effects of alcohol. Check with your doctor before using alcohol with this medication.

Avoid taking antacids within 1 hour of a dose of Donnatal; they may reduce its effectiveness.

If Donnatal is taken with certain other drugs, the effects of either could be increased, decreased, or altered. It is especially important to check with your doctor before combining Donnatal with the following: antidepressants such as amitriptyline and imipramine; antidepressants known as MAO inhibitors, including phenelzine and tranylcypromine; antihistamines such as diphenhydramine; antispasmodic drugs such as dicyclomine; barbiturates such as secobarbital; blood-thinning drugs such as warfarin; diarrhea medications containing attapulgite; digitalis; narcotics such as oxycodone; potassium; steroids such as methylprednisolone and prednisone; and tranquilizers such as diazepam.

What are the possible side effects of Donnatal?

Side effects cannot be anticipated. If any develop or change in intensity, inform your doctor as soon as possible. Only your doctor can determine if it is safe for you to continue taking Donnatal.

Side effects may include: agitation, allergic reaction, bloated feeling, blurred vision, constipation, decreased sweating, difficulty sleeping, difficulty urinating, dilation of the pupil of the eye, dizziness, drowsiness, dry mouth, excitement, fast or fluttery heartbeat, headache, hives, impotence, muscular and bone pain, nausea, nervousness, rash, reduced sense of taste, suppression of lactation, vomiting, weakness

Can I receive Donnatal if I am pregnant or breastfeeding?

The effects of Donnatal during pregnancy and breastfeeding have not been adequately studied. If you are pregnant, plan to become pregnant, or breastfeeding, tell your doctor immediately.

What should I do if I miss a dose of Donnatal?

If you miss a dose of this drug, skip it. Do not take an extra dose to make up for missed doses.

How should I store Donnatal?

Store at room temperature and protect from light.

DORAL

Generic name: Quazepam

What is Doral?

Doral is a sleep medication taken as a short-term treatment for insomnia. Symptoms of insomnia may include difficulty falling asleep, frequent awakenings throughout the night, or very early morning awakening.

What is the most important information I should know about Doral?

Doral is potentially addictive. Over time, your body may get used to the prescribed dosage of Doral, and you will no longer derive any benefit from it. Use Doral only as prescribed.

After you stop taking Doral you may experience trouble sleeping, shakiness, sweating, stomach and muscle cramps.

Do not drive or engage in hazardous activities that require mental alertness or coordination after taking Doral until you feel fully awake.

Call your doctor if your insomnia worsens or does not improve within 7 to 10 days of beginning treatment. This may mean that there is another condition causing your sleeping problems.

Tell your doctor if you experience abnormal thinking, mood problems, behavior changes, anxiety or memory loss while taking this medication.

Who should not take Doral?

Do not take Doral if you are sensitive to it, or if you have ever had an allergic reaction to it or a similar sleep medication.

You should not take Doral if you know or suspect that you have sleep apnea (short periods of interrupted breathing that occur during sleep).

You should not take Doral if you are pregnant, planning to become pregnant, or breastfeeding.

What should I tell my doctor before I take the first dose of Doral?

Tell your doctor about all prescription, over-the-counter, and herbal medications you are taking before beginning treatment with Doral. Also, talk to your doctor about your complete medical history, especially if you have ever abused or have been dependent on alcohol, prescription or street drugs. In addition, tell your doctor if you have a history of suicidal thoughts, depression, mental illness, or if you are pregnant, planning to become pregnant, or are breastfeeding.

What is the usual dosage?

The information below is based on the dosage guidelines your doctor uses. Depending on your condition and medical history, your doctor may prescribe a different regimen. Do not change the dosage or stop taking your medication without your doctor's approval.

Adults: The initial recommended dose of Doral is 15 milligrams (mg) daily. Your doctor may later reduce this dose to 7.5 mg. Elderly patients may be more sensitive to the effects of Doral and may require a lower dose.

The safety and efficacy of Doral in children less then 18 years of age has not been established.

How should I take Doral?

Take Doral exactly as prescribed by your doctor. Take Doral immediately before going to bed. Doral should not be taken with or immediately after a meal.

Follow up with your doctor; if you respond very well, it may be possible to cut your dosage in half after the first few nights. Elderly patients may benefit from a lower dose of Doral due to a possible heightened sensitivity to the drug.

Never increase or decrease the dosage of Doral on your own. Tell your doctor right away if the medication no longer seems to be working.

Do not take Doral unless you are able to stay in bed for a full night (7-8 hours) before you must be active again.

What should I avoid while taking Doral?

Because Doral may decrease your daytime alertness, do not drive, operate dangerous machinery, or participate in hazardous activities until you know how the drug affects you. In some cases, Doral's sedative effect may last for several days after the last dose.

Do not drink alcohol while taking Doral because it can increase the drug's effects.

Do not suddenly stop taking Doral because you may experience withdrawal symptoms. Follow your doctor's advice on how to slowly decrease your intake of the drug.

Do not take Doral with other medications that can make you sleepy.

What are possible food and drug interactions associated with Doral?

If Doral is taken with certain other drugs, the effects of either could be increased, decreased, or altered. It is especially important to check with your doctor before combining Doral with the following: alcohol, alprazolam, carbamazepine, chlorpromazine, clozapine, diazepam, diphenhydramine, and phenytoin.

What are the possible side effects of Doral?

Side effects cannot be anticipated. If any develop or change in intensity, inform your doctor as soon as possible. Only your doctor can determine if it is safe for you to continue taking Doral.

Side effects may include: drowsiness, headache, dizziness, dry mouth, and upset stomach

In rare instances, Doral may cause abnormal thoughts and behavior, anxiety, memory loss, as well as getting out of bed while not fully awake and doing activities that you do not know you are doing (such as "sleep driving," talking on the phone, making and eating food, sleepwalking, and engaging in sexual activity). Call your doctor right away if you experience this or any other side effect that worries you while you are taking Doral.

Can I receive Doral if I am pregnant or breastfeeding?

Because Doral may cause harm to the unborn child, it should not be taken during pregnancy. If you want to have a baby, tell your doctor, and plan to discontinue taking Doral before getting pregnant. Babies whose mothers are taking Doral at the time of birth may experience withdrawal symptoms from the drug. Since Doral appears in breast milk, you should not take this medication if you are nursing.

What should I do if I miss a dose of Doral?

This drug should be taken only if needed, at bedtime. If you miss a dose, skip it. Do not take an extra dose to make up for missed doses.

How should I store Doral?
Store at room temperature.

DORYX
Generic name: Doxycycline hyclate

What is Doryx?
Doxycycline is a broad-spectrum tetracycline antibiotic used against a wide variety of bacterial infections, including Rocky Mountain spotted fever and other fevers caused by ticks, fleas, and lice; urinary tract infections; trachoma (chronic infections of the eye); and some gonococcal infections in adults. It is an approved treatment for inhalational anthrax. It is also used with other medications to treat severe acne and amoebic dysentery (diarrhea caused by severe parasitic infection of the intestines).

Doryx may also be taken for the prevention of malaria on foreign trips of less than 4 months' duration.

What is the most important information I should know about Doryx?
Your doctor will only prescribe Doryx to treat a bacterial infection; it will not cure a viral infection, such as the common cold.

Generally, children under 8 years old and women in the last half of pregnancy should not take this medication. It may cause developing teeth to become permanently discolored. (However, children under 8 may be given this drug for inhalational anthrax.)

As with other antibiotics, treatment with Doryx may result in a growth of bacteria that do not respond to this medication and can cause a secondary infection. An overgrowth of certain bacteria in the colon could cause mild to severe—and rarely, life-threatening—diarrhea. If you develop this symptom, call your doctor immediately.

Bulging foreheads in infants and headaches in adults have occurred. These symptoms disappeared when Doryx was discontinued.

Birth control pills that contain estrogen may not be as effective while you are taking tetracycline drugs. Ask your doctor or pharmacist if you should use another form of birth control while taking Doryx.

Doxycycline syrup (Vibramycin) contains a sulfite that may cause allergic reactions in certain people. This reaction happens more frequently to people with asthma.

Who should not take Doryx?
If you are sensitive to or have ever had an allergic reaction to Doryx or drugs of this type, you should not take this medication. Make sure your doctor is aware of any drug reactions that you have experienced.

What should I tell my doctor before I take the first dose of Doryx?

Tell your doctor about all prescription, over-the-counter, and herbal medications you are taking before beginning treatment with this drug. Also, talk to your doctor about your complete medical history.

What is the usual dosage?

The information below is based on the dosage guidelines your doctor uses. Depending on your condition and medical history, your doctor may prescribe a different regimen. Do not change the dosage or stop taking your medication without your doctor's approval.

Adults: The usual dose of oral Doryx is 200 milligrams on the first day of treatment (100 milligrams every 12 hours) followed by a maintenance dose of 100 milligrams per day. The maintenance dose may be taken as a single dose or as 50 milligrams every 12 hours.

Your doctor may prescribe 100 milligrams every 12 hours for severe infections such as chronic urinary tract infection.

Children: For children older than 8 years of age, the recommended dosage schedule for those weighing 100 pounds or less is 2 milligrams per pound of body weight, divided into 2 doses, on the first day of treatment, followed by 1 milligram per pound of body weight given as a single daily dose or divided into 2 doses on subsequent days. For more severe infections, up to 2 milligrams per pound of body weight may be used. For children over 100 pounds, the usual adult dose should be used.

For Uncomplicated Gonorrhea

The usual dose is 100 milligrams by mouth, twice a day for 7 days. An alternate, single-day treatment is 300 milligrams, followed in 1 hour by a second 300-milligram dose.

For Primary and Secondary Syphilis

The usual dose is 200 milligrams a day, divided into smaller, equal doses for 14 days.

For Inhalational Anthrax

Adults: To prevent or combat infection after exposure, the usual dose is 100 milligrams taken by mouth twice a day for 60 days. Treatment can be started intravenously, but should be switched to oral doses as soon as possible.

Children: For inhalational anthrax in children weighing less than 100 pounds, the usual dose is 1 milligram per pound of body weight twice daily for 60 days.

For Prevention of Malaria

Adults: The usual dose is 100 milligrams a day. Treatment should begin 1 to 2 days before travel to the area where malaria is found, then continue daily during travel in the area and 4 weeks after leaving.

Children: For prevention of malaria, the recommended dose is 2 milligrams per 2.2 pounds of body weight up to 100 milligrams.

How should I take Doryx?

Take Doryx with a full glass of water or other liquid to avoid irritating your throat or stomach. Doxycycline can be taken with or without food. However, if the medicine does upset your stomach, you may wish to take it with a glass of milk or after you have eaten.

Doxycycline tablets should be swallowed whole. If you have difficulty swallowing pills, you can take this medication by opening the capsule and sprinkling the entire contents onto a spoonful of cool, soft applesauce. Be careful not to spill any of the contents. If you do, you will not be able to use this dose and will have to start over with a new mixture. Swallow the mixture immediately, without chewing, followed by a cool 8-ounce glass of water. Discard the mixture if you are not able to use it immediately; do not store it to use later.

If you are taking an oral suspension form of Doryx, shake the bottle well before using. Do not use outdated Doryx.

What should I avoid while taking Doryx?

You may become more sensitive to sunlight while taking Doryx. Be careful if you are going out in the sun or using a sunlamp. If you develop a skin rash, notify your doctor immediately. Avoid missing doses. Not completing the full dosage schedule may decrease the drug's effectiveness and increase the chances that the bacteria may become resistant to Doryx and similar antibiotics. It's important to take the full dosage schedule of Doryx, even if you're feeling better in a few days.

What are possible food and drug interactions associated with Doryx?

If Doryx is taken with certain other drugs, the effects of either could be increased, decreased, or altered. It is especially important to check with your doctor before combining Doryx with the following: antacids containing aluminum, calcium, or magnesium, and iron-containing preparations; barbiturates such as phenobarbital; bismuth subsalicylate; blood-thinning medications such as warfarin; carbamazepine; oral contraceptives; penicillin; phenytoin; and sodium bicarbonate.

What are the possible side effects of Doryx?

Side effects cannot be anticipated. If any develop or change in intensity, tell your doctor as soon as possible. Only your doctor can determine if it is safe for you to continue taking this drug.

Side effects may include: angioedema (chest pain; swelling of face, around lips, tongue and throat, arms and legs; difficulty swallowing), bulging foreheads in infants, diarrhea, difficulty swallowing, discolored teeth in infants and children (more common during long-term use of tetracycline), inflammation of the tongue, loss of appetite, nausea, rash, rectal or genital itching, severe allergic reaction (hives, itching, and swelling), skin sensitivity to light, vomiting

Can I receive Doryx if I am pregnant or breastfeeding?
Doxycycline should not be used during pregnancy. Tetracycline can damage developing teeth during the last half of pregnancy. If you are pregnant or plan to become pregnant, inform your doctor immediately. Tetracyclines such as Doryx appear in breast milk and can affect a nursing infant. If this medication is essential to your health, your doctor may advise you to discontinue breastfeeding until your treatment is finished.

What should I do if I miss a dose of Doryx?
Take the forgotten dose as soon as you remember. If it is almost time for the next dose, put it off for several hours after taking the missed dose. Specifically, if you are taking one dose a day, take the next one 10 to 12 hours after the missed dose. If you are taking two doses a day, take the next one 5 to 6 hours after the missed dose. If you are taking three doses a day, take the next one 2 to 4 hours after the missed dose. Then return to your regular schedule.

How should I store Doryx?
Store at room temperature. Protect from light and excessive heat.

Dorzolamide hydrochloride and timolol maleate
See Cosopt, page 347.

Doxazosin mesylate See Cardura, page 256.

Doxazosin mesylate, extended-release See Cardura XL, page 258.

Doxycycline See Oracea, page 946.

Doxycycline hyclate See Doryx, page 443.

Drospirenone and estradiol See Angeliq, page 105.

Drospirenone and ethinyl estradiol See YAZ, page 1439.

DUAC
Generic name: Clindamycin phosphate and benzoyl peroxide

What is Duac?
Duac is indicated for the topical treatment of inflammatory acne.

What is the most important information I should know about Duac?

Duac is for external use only.

Duac may bleach hair or colored fabric.

Try to minimize sun exposure by wearing appropriate clothing.

Do not use any other topical acne preparations unless otherwise directed by your physician.

You should not use erythromycin-containing products in combination with Duac.

Orally and topically administered clindamycin has been associated with severe colitis, which may result in death.

Use of the topical formulation of clindamycin results in absorption of the antibiotic from the skin. Diarrhea, bloody diarrhea, and colitis have been reported. Colitis is usually characterized by severe persistent diarrhea and severe abdominal cramps and may be associated with the passage of blood and mucus.

Who should not take Duac?

Do not apply Duac gel if you have an allergy to Duac or its formulation. Also, do not apply Duac gel if you have a history of diarrhea (ulcerative colitis, pseudomembranous colitis, regional enteritis, or antibiotic-associated colitis).

What should I tell my doctor before I take the first dose of Duac?

Tell your doctor about all prescription, over-the-counter, and herbal medications you are taking before beginning treatment with Duac gel. Also, talk to your doctor about your complete medical history, especially if you are experiencing bowel problems.

What is the usual dosage?

The information below is based on the dosage guidelines your doctor uses. Depending on your condition and medical history, your doctor may prescribe a different regimen. Do not change the dosage or stop taking your medication without your doctor's approval.

Duac should be applied once daily, in the evening or as directed by your doctor.

How should I take Duac?

Wash the affected area gently with warm water and pat dry. Apply the topical gel on the affected area as directed.

What should I avoid while taking Duac?

Avoid exposing your eyes or other body openings to this product. In addition, avoid using other acne medications with this product unless directed to do so by your doctor.

What are possible food and drug interactions associated with Duac?

If Duac gel is taken with certain other drugs, the effects of either could be increased, decreased, or altered. It is especially important to check with your doctor before combining Duac gel with the following: erythromycin and other acne-medicine-containing products.

What are the possible side effects of Duac?

Side effects cannot be anticipated. If any develop or change in intensity, tell your doctor as soon as possible. Only your doctor can determine if it is safe for you to continue taking this drug.

Side effects may include: burning of the skin, dryness of affected area, peeling of the skin, reddening of the skin

Can I receive Duac if I am pregnant or breastfeeding?

The effects of Duac during pregnancy and breastfeeding are unknown. Talk to your healthcare provider if you are pregnant, plan to become pregnant, or are breastfeeding.

What should I do if I miss a dose of Duac?

If you miss a dose, take it as soon as you remember. If it is close to the time of your next dose, skip it and resume your scheduled dose. Do not double doses.

How should I store Duac?

Store at room temperature and away from children. Keep tube tightly closed and discard after the 60 day expiration date.

DUETACT

Generic name: Pioglitazone hydrochloride and glimepiride

What is Duetact?

Duetact is used, with diet and exercise, to help stabilize the blood sugar levels in people with type 2 diabetes who fail to control their sugar levels with other forms of therapy.

What is the most important information I should know about Duetact?

Drugs for low blood sugar should not be taken with Duetact; this can result in severe cardiovascular problems that may result in death.

Who should not take Duetact?

Do not take Duetact if you are allergic to any of its ingredients, or if you have diabetic ketoacidosis. This problem should be treated with insulin.

What should I tell my doctor before I take the first dose of Duetact?

Tell your doctor about all prescription, over-the-counter, and herbal medications you are taking to avoid an interaction with Duetact. Also, talk to your doctor about your complete medical history, especially about all of the forms of type 2 diabetic treatment you have taken.

What is the usual dosage?

The information below is based on the dosage guidelines your doctor uses. Depending on your condition and medical history, your doctor may prescribe a different regimen. Do not change the dosage or stop taking your medication without your doctor's approval.

Starting dose for people currently taking glimepiride alone: Based on the usual starting dose of pioglitazone (15 milligrams [mg] or 30 mg daily), Duetact may be taken as either a 30 mg/2 mg or 30 mg/4 mg tablet once daily.

Starting dose for people currently taking pioglitazone alone: Based on the usual starting dose of glimepiride (1 mg or 2 mg once daily), and pioglitazone 15 mg or 30 mg, Duetact may be taken as a 30 mg/2 mg tablet, once daily.

How should I take Duetact?

Duetact should be taken once a day with the first main meal of the day.

What should I avoid while taking Duetact?

Avoid getting pregnant while on Duetact. Talk to your doctor if you plan to become pregnant while on this type 2 diabetes therapy.

What are the possible side effects of Duetact?

Side effects cannot be anticipated. If any develop or change in intensity, tell your doctor as soon as possible. Only your doctor can determine if it is safe for you to continue taking this drug.

Side effects may include: diarrhea, headache, lower blood sugar, nausea, pain in legs, upper respiratory tract infection, urinary tract infection, weight gain

Can I receive Duetact if I am pregnant or breastfeeding?

Talk to your doctor if you are pregnant, planning to become pregnant, or nursing. Duetact is not recommended for pregnant women; blood sugar level should be maintained with insulin during pregnancy. Also, Duetact may pass into breast milk.

How should I store Duetact?

Store at room temperature, away from dampness.

Duloxetine hydrochloride *See Cymbalta, page 369.*

DUONEB
Generic name: Ipratropium bromide and albuterol sulfate

What is DuoNeb?
DuoNeb is a combination drug indicated for the treatment of broncho-spasm associated with chronic obstructive pulmonary disease (COPD).

What is the most important information I should know about DuoNeb?
DuoNeb is to be used with a nebulizer. You should use the inhaler in an appropriate way to achieve its full potential.

Do not exceed the recommended dose or frequency of this inhaler without consulting with your doctor.

Who should not take DuoNeb?
Do not take DuoNeb if you are allergic to any of the ingredients in DuoNeb or to atropine.

What should I tell my doctor before I take the first dose of DuoNeb?
Tell your doctor about all prescription, over-the-counter, and herbal medication you are taking before beginning treatment with DuoNeb. Also, talk to your doctor about your complete medical history, especially if you are pregnant or plan to become pregnant, have high blood pressure or heart problems, diabetes, have or have had seizures, have a thyroid problem called hyperthyroidism, have an eye problem called narrow-angle glaucoma, have liver or kidney problems, have problems urinating due to bladder-neck blockage or an enlarged prostate (men).

What is the usual dosage?
The information below is based on the dosage guidelines your doctor uses. Depending on your condition and medical history, your doctor may prescribe a different regimen. Do not change the dosage or stop taking your medication without your doctor's approval.

The usual dose is one 3 ml vial administered 4 times daily via the use of a nebulizer. An increase of 2 additional 3 ml doses may be added after consulting with your doctor.

How should I take DuoNeb?
Take the appropriate dose (3 ml) every 6 hours. DuoNeb needs to be administered via jet nebulizer that is connected to an air compressor with adequate air flow, equipped with a face mask. Use as directed by your doctor.

DuoNeb may help to open your airways for up to 5 hours after taking this medicine. If DuoNeb does not help your airway narrowing (bronchospasm) or your bronchospasm gets worse, call your doctor right away or get emergency help if needed.

What should I avoid while taking DuoNeb?
Avoid spraying DuoNeb into your eyes while using your nebulizer as it may lead to enlarged pupils, blurry vision, or eye pain. In addition, avoid using more than required without consulting with your doctor.

What are possible food and drug interactions associated with DuoNeb?
If DuoNeb is taken with certain other drugs, the effects of either could be increased, decreased, or altered. It is especially important to check with your doctor before combining DuoNeb with the following: anticholinergic agents (such as ipratropium bromide) including Parkinson's disease medicines; beta-adrenergic agents (sympathomimetics such as albuterol sulfate); beta-receptor blocking agents; diuretics; monoamine oxidase inhibitors; and tricyclic antidepressants.

What are the possible side effects of DuoNeb?
Side effects cannot be anticipated. If any develop or change in intensity, tell your doctor as soon as possible. Only your doctor can determine if it is safe for you to continue taking this drug.

Side effects may include: chest pain, diarrhea, nausea, leg cramps, lung disease, urinary tract infection, indigestion, headache, bronchitis, upper respiratory infection, cough, change in voice, blurry eyes

Can I receive DuoNeb if I am pregnant or breastfeeding?
The effects of DuoNeb during pregnancy and breastfeeding are unknown. Talk to your healthcare provider if you are pregnant, plan to become pregnant or are breastfeeding due to the potential danger during delivery and harm to the baby.

What should I do if I miss a dose of DuoNeb?
If you miss a dose, take it as soon as you remember. If it is close to the time of your next dose, skip it and resume your scheduled dose. Do not double your dose.

How should I store DuoNeb?
Store at room temperature and away from children. Keep the vials in the foil pouch to protect from light.

DURAGESIC
Generic name: Fentanyl transdermal system

What is Duragesic?
Duragesic is a thin, adhesive, rectangular patch that is worn on your skin to manage constant moderate to severe chronic pain that needs to be treated around the clock and which cannot be treated by a combination narcotic, short-acting narcotic, or non-narcotic pain treatment products. Duragesic contains fentanyl, an opioid pain medicine similar to morphine, hydromorphone, methadone, oxycodone, and oxymorphone.

What is the most important information I should know about Duragesic?
Duragesic should only be used by people who are receiving or have developed a tolerance to pain therapy with products known as opioids. One serious side effect is slow, shallow breathing, and/or difficulty in breathing, if the dose is too high.

Like all other opioids, this drug has the potential for abuse. People at increased risk for opioid abuse include those with a personal or family history of substance abuse (including drug or alcohol abuse or addiction) or mental illness (eg, major depression).

Who should not take Duragesic?
Do not take this medication if you are allergic to any of its ingredients. Duragesic should not be used if you have pain that will go away in a few days, such as pain from surgery, medical or dental procedures, or short-lasting conditions.

What should I tell my doctor before I take the first dose of Duragesic?
Tell your doctor about all prescription, over-the-counter, and herbal medications you are taking before beginning treatment with Duragesic. Also, talk to your doctor about your complete medical history, especially if you are pregnant or plan to become pregnant.

What is the usual dosage?
The information below is based on the dosage guidelines your doctor uses. Depending on your condition and medical history, your doctor may prescribe a different regimen. Do not change the dosage or stop taking your medication without your doctor's approval.

Adults: The usual Duragesic patch dosage is calculated by your doctor on an individual basis. The maximum amount of time a patch should be worn is 72 hours.

How should I take Duragesic?

Duragesic should be applied immediately upon removal from the sealed package. The patch should be applied to intact, non-irritated and non-irradiated skin on a flat surface such as the chest, back, side, or upper arm. If the area of skin needs to be cleaned, use clear water; avoid soaps, oils, lotions, alcohol or other skin irritating agents.

Press patch firmly in place with the palm of the hand for 30 seconds, making sure the contact is complete, especially around the edges.

Each Duragesic patch may be worn continuously for 72 hours. The next patch should be applied to a different skin site after removal of the previous one. If the patch falls off before 72 hours, a new patch may be applied to a different area. Used patches should be folded so that the adhesive side of the patch adheres to itself, then the patch should be flushed down the toilet immediately upon removal.

What should I avoid while taking Duragesic?

Avoid exposing the Duragesic application site to direct external heat sources, such as heating pads or electric blankets, heat lamps, saunas, hot tubs, and heated water beds, etc.

Avoid using damaged or cut Duragesic patches or if the seal is broken, do not use; these can change the amount that is absorbed and cause too much medicine to be absorbed through the skin, which can cause serious and sometimes fatal breathing problems.

Never adjust the number of patches applied without first consulting your doctor and receiving instructions.

What are possible food and drug interactions associated with Duragesic?

If Duragesic is taken with certain other drugs, the effects of either could be increased, decreased, or altered. It is especially important to check with your doctor before combining Duragesic with alcohol and CNS depressants, such as sleep medications and tranquilizers.

What are the possible side effects of Duragesic?

Side effects cannot be anticipated. If any develop or change in intensity, tell your doctor as soon as possible. Only your doctor can determine if it is safe for you to continue taking this drug.

Side effects may include: constipation/severe constipation, excessive sweating, nausea, drowsiness, vomiting, and dry mouth

Can I receive Duragesic if I am pregnant or breastfeeding?

The effects of Duragesic during pregnancy and breastfeeding are unknown. Tell your doctor immediately if you are pregnant, plan to become pregnant, or are breastfeeding.

What should I do if I miss a dose of Duragesic?

If you miss a dose of Duragesic, apply the missed dose as soon as you remember it. However, if it is almost time for your next dose, skip the one you missed and return to your regular dosing schedule. Do not double your dose.

How should I store Duragesic?

Store Duragesic patches at room temperature in a secure place out of the reach of children.

DURICEF
Generic name: Cefadroxil monohydrate

What is Duricef?

Duricef, a cephalosporin antibiotic, is used in the treatment of nose, throat, urinary tract, and skin infections that are caused by specific bacteria, including staph, strep, and *E. coli.*

What is the most important information I should know about Duricef?

If you are allergic to either penicillin or cephalosporin antibiotics in any form, consult your doctor *before taking* Duricef. An allergy to either type of medication may signal an allergy to Duricef; and if a reaction occurs, it could be extremely severe. If you take the drug and feel signs of a reaction, seek medical attention immediately.

As with other antibiotics, treatment with Duricef may result in a growth of bacteria that do not respond to this medication and can cause a secondary infection. An overgrowth of certain bacteria in the colon could cause mild to severe—and rarely, life-threatening—diarrhea. If you develop this symptom, call your doctor immediately.

Who should not take Duricef?

If you are sensitive to or have ever had an allergic reaction to a cephalosporin antibiotic, you should not take Duricef.

What should I tell my doctor before I take the first dose of Duricef?

Tell your doctor about all prescription, over-the-counter, and herbal medication you are taking before beginning treatment with this drug. Also, talk to your doctor about your complete medical history, especially if you have kidney problems or a history of gastrointestinal disease, particularly inflammation of the bowel (colitis).

If you have allergies, particularly to drugs, or often develop diarrhea when taking other antibiotics, you should tell your doctor before taking Duricef.

What is the usual dosage?

The information below is based on the dosage guidelines your doctor uses. Depending on your condition and medical history, your doctor may prescribe a different regimen. Do not change the dosage or stop taking your medication without your doctor's approval.

Urinary Tract Infections

Adults: The usual dosage for uncomplicated infections is a total of 1 to 2 grams per day in a single dose or 2 smaller doses. For all other urinary tract infections, the usual dosage is a total of 2 grams per day taken in 2 doses.

Skin and Skin Structure Infections

Adults: The usual dose is a total of 1 gram per day in a single dose or 2 smaller doses.

Throat Infections (Strep Throat and Tonsillitis)

Adults: The usual dosage is a total of 1 gram per day in a single dose or 2 smaller doses for 10 days.

Children: For urinary tract and skin infections, the usual dose is 30 milligrams per 2.2 pounds of body weight per day, divided into 2 doses and taken every 12 hours. For throat infections, the recommended dose per day is 30 milligrams per 2.2 pounds of body weight in a single dose or 2 smaller doses. In the treatment of strep throat, the dose should be taken for at least 10 days.

How should I take Duricef?

Take this medication exactly as prescribed. It is important that you finish all of it to obtain the maximum benefit. Your doctor will only prescribe Duricef to treat a bacterial infection; it will not cure a viral infection, such as the common cold. It's important to take the full dosage schedule of Duricef, even if you're feeling better in a few days. Not completing the full dosage schedule may decrease the drug's effectiveness and increase the chances that the bacteria may become resistant to Duricef and similar antibiotics.

Duricef may be taken with or without food. If the drug upsets your stomach, you may find that taking it with meals helps to relieve the problem. Shake the liquid suspension thoroughly before each use.

What are possible food and drug interactions associated with Duricef?

If this medication is taken with certain other drugs, the effects of either could be increased, decreased, or altered. Always check with your doctor before combining this drug with any other medication.

What are the possible side effects of Duricef?

Side effects cannot be anticipated. If any develop or change in intensity, inform your doctor as soon as possible. Only your doctor can determine if it is safe for you to continue taking Duricef.

Side effects may include: Diarrhea, inflammation of the bowel (colitis), nausea, redness and swelling of skin, skin rash and itching, vaginal inflammation, vomiting

Can I receive Duricef if I am pregnant or breastfeeding?

The effects of Duricef during pregnancy have not been adequately studied. If you are pregnant or plan to become pregnant, inform your doctor immediately. Duricef may appear in breast milk and could affect a nursing infant. Consult your doctor before breastfeeding.

What should I do if I miss a dose of Duricef?

If you miss a dose of this drug, skip it. Do not take an extra dose to make up for missed doses. If you miss two or more doses in a row, check with your doctor or pharmacist.

How should I store Duricef?

Store the liquid at room temperature in the refrigerator. Discard any unused medication after 14 days.

Dutasteride *See Avodart, page 171.*

DYAZIDE

Generic ingredients: Hydrochlorothiazide and triamterene

What is Dyazide?

Dyazide is a combination of diuretic drugs used in the treatment of high blood pressure and other conditions that require the elimination of excess fluid from the body.

What is the most important information I should know about Dyazide?

If you have high blood pressure, you must take Dyazide regularly for it to be effective. Since blood pressure declines gradually, it may be several weeks before you get the full benefit of Dyazide; and you must continue taking it even if you are feeling well. Dyazide does not cure high blood pressure; it merely keeps it under control.

Who should not take Dyazide?

If you are unable to urinate or have any serious kidney disease, if you have high potassium levels in your blood, or if you are taking other drugs that prevent loss of potassium, you should not take Dyazide.

If you are sensitive to or have ever had an allergic reaction to triamterene, hydrochlorothiazide, or sulfa drugs, you should not take this medication.

What should I tell my doctor before I take the first dose of Dyazide?

Tell your doctor about all prescription, over-the-counter, and herbal medications you are taking before beginning treatment with this drug. Also, talk to your doctor about your complete medical history, especially if you have any of the following: kidney disease, kidney stones, liver disease or cirrhosis of the liver, heart failure, or diabetes.

What is the usual dosage?

The information below is based on the dosage guidelines your doctor uses. Depending on your condition and medical history, your doctor may prescribe a different regimen. Do not change the dosage or stop taking your medication without your doctor's approval.

Adults: The usual dose of Dyazide is 1 or 2 capsules once daily, with appropriate monitoring of blood potassium levels by your doctor.

How should I take Dyazide?

Dyazide should be taken early in the day. To avoid stomach upset, take it with food.

What should I avoid while taking Dyazide?

When taking Dyazide, do not use potassium-containing salt substitutes. Take potassium supplements only if specifically directed to by your doctor. Your potassium level should be checked frequently.

What are possible food and drug interactions associated with Dyazide?

Dyazide should be used with caution if you are taking a type of blood pressure medication called an ACE inhibitor, such as captopril or enalapril.

If Dyazide is taken with certain other drugs, the effects of either could be increased, decreased, or altered. It is especially important to check with your doctor before combining Dyazide with the following: blood-thinning medications such as warfarin; corticosteroids such as prednisone; drugs for diabetes such as glyburide; gout medications such as allopurinol; laxatives; lithium; methenamine; nonsteroidal anti-inflammatory drugs such as diflunisal and indomethacin; other drugs that minimize potassium loss or contain potassium; other high blood pressure medications such as prazosin; salt substitutes containing potassium; and sodium polystyrene sulfonate.

What are the possible side effects of Dyazide?

Side effects cannot be anticipated. If any occur or change in intensity, inform your doctor as soon as possible. Only your doctor can determine if it is safe for you to continue taking Dyazide.

Side effects may include: abdominal pain, anemia, breathing difficulty, change in potassium level (causing symptoms such as numbness, tingling, muscle weakness, slow heart rate, shock), constipation, diabetes, diarrhea, dizziness, dizziness when standing up, dry mouth, fatigue, headache, hives, impotence, irregular heartbeat, kidney stones, muscle cramps, nausea, rash, sensitivity to light, strong allergic reaction (localized hives, itching, and swelling or, in severe cases, shock), vomiting, weakness, yellow eyes and skin

Can I receive Dyazide if I am pregnant or breastfeeding?

The effects of Dyazide during pregnancy have not been adequately studied. If you are pregnant or plan to become pregnant, inform your doctor immediately. Dyazide appears in breast milk and could affect a nursing infant. Consult your doctor before breastfeeding.

What should I do if I miss a dose of Dyazide?

If you miss a dose of this drug, skip it. Do not take an extra dose to make up for missed doses.

How should I store Dyazide?

Store at room temperature.

DYNACIN

Generic name: Minocycline hydrochloride

What is Dynacin?

Dynacin is an antibiotic used to treat various infections in adults, including the following: Rocky Mountain spotted fever and other fevers caused by ticks, fleas, and lice; urinary tract infections; respiratory tract infections; trachoma (chronic infections of the eye); and some gonococcal infections. It is also an approved treatment for inhalational anthrax. In addition, Dynacin is used with other medications to treat severe acne and amoebic dysentery (diarrhea caused by severe parasitic infection of the intestines). Dynacin may be used to treat other infections caused by susceptible bacteria.

What is the most important information I should know about Dynacin?

Generally, children under 8 years old and women in the last half of pregnancy should not take tetracycline antibiotics like Dynacin. It may cause developing teeth to become permanently discolored. Speak to your doctor if you are pregnant or plan to become pregnant before taking this medicine.

Dynacin does not treat viral infections (e.g., the common cold). Although you may feel better shortly after beginning treatment, it is important to avoid skipping doses and to continue the full course of therapy. If you do not take the medication exactly as directed, then Dynacin as well as other antibiotics may become less effective in treating your infection.

While taking Dynacin, you are more prone to developing an allergy to the sun called photosensitivity. Consequently, when exposed to direct sunlight or ultraviolet light, you may develop severe sunburn. If sunburn develops, notify your physician immediately and discontinue Dynacin.

It is important to immediately notify your physician if you develop a headache or blurred vision.

Dynacin may cause light headedness and dizziness. You should therefore use caution if driving or using hazardous machinery while taking Dynacin.

Dynacin may interact with oral contraceptives and decrease the effectiveness of them. It is therefore important to notify your physician if you are taking oral contraceptives.

Who should not take Dynacin?
Do not take Dynacin if you have an allergy to it or any other tetracycline antibiotic.

What should I tell my doctor before I take the first dose of Dynacin?
Tell your doctor about all prescription, over-the-counter, and herbal medications you are taking before beginning treatment with Dynacin. Also, talk to your doctor about your complete medical history, especially if you have kidney problems or you are pregnant or plan to become pregnant.

What is the usual dosage?
The information below is based on the dosage guidelines your doctor uses. Depending on your condition and medical history, your doctor may prescribe a different regimen. Do not change the dosage or stop taking your medication without your doctor's approval.

Children over 8 years: The usual dose is 4 milligrams (mg) per 2.2 pounds of body weight initially followed by 2 mg per 2.2 pounds of body weight every 12 hours.

Adults: The usual dosage of Dynacin is 200 mg initially followed by 100 mg every 12 hours. Two or four 50 mg tablets may be given initially followed by one 50 mg tablet four times a day. Dosage or frequency may be adjusted in patients with renal impairment.

Uncomplicated Gonococcal Infections Other Than Urethritis and Anorectal Infections in Men
Take 200 mg initially followed by 100 mg every 12 hours for a minimum of 4 days.

Uncomplicated Gonococcal Urethritis in Men
Take 100 mg every 12 hours for 5 days.

Syphilis
Take 200 mg initially followed by 100 mg every 12 hours for 10-15 days.

Meningococcal Carrier State
Take 100 mg every 12 hours for 5 days.

Mycobacterium Marinum Infections
Take 100 mg every 12 hours for 6 to 8 weeks.

Uncomplicated Urethral, Endocervical or Rectal Infection caused by Chlamydia trachomatis *or* Ureaplasma urcum
Take 100 mg every 12 hours for at least 7 days.

How should I take Dynacin?
This medication may be taken with or without food. Take with food if the medication upsets your stomach. Take with a full glass of water to reduce the risk of throat pain or irritation. It is important to finish the entire course of therapy as directed.

What should I avoid while taking Dynacin?
Avoid alcohol and excessive exposure to sunlight.

What are possible food and drug interactions associated with Dynacin?
If Dynacin is taken with certain other drugs, the effects of either could be increased, decreased, or altered. It is especially important to check with your doctor before combining Dynacin with the following: acitretin, antacids (eg, aluminum, calcium, or magnesium), anticoagulants (eg, warfarin), digoxin, isotretinoin, methoxyflurane, oral contraceptives, and penicillin.

What are the possible side effects of Dynacin?
Side effects cannot be anticipated. If any develop or change in intensity, tell your doctor as soon as possible. Only your doctor can determine if it is safe for you to continue taking this drug.

Side effects may include: nausea, vomiting, diarrhea, anorexia, rash, photosensitivity, dizziness, vertigo

Can I receive Dynacin if I am pregnant or breastfeeding?
Dynacin should not be used during pregnancy. Tetracyclines can damage developing teeth during the last half of pregnancy. If you are pregnant or plan to become pregnant, inform your doctor immediately. Tetracyclines such as Dynacin appear in breast milk and can affect a nursing infant. Consult your doctor before breastfeeding.

What should I do if I miss a dose of Dynacin?
If you miss a dose, take it as soon as you remember with food. If it is close to the time of your next dose, skip it and resume your scheduled dose. Do not double the dose.

How should I store Dynacin?
Store at room temperature and protect from light, moisture, and excessive heat.

DYNACIRC CR
Generic name: Isradipine

What is DynaCirc CR?
DynaCirc CR, a type of medication called a calcium channel blocker, is prescribed for the treatment of high blood pressure.

What is the most important information I should know about DynaCirc CR?
You must take DynaCirc CR regularly for it to be effective. Since blood pressure declines gradually, it may be several weeks before you get the full benefit of DynaCirc CR; continue taking it even if you are feeling well. DynaCirc CR does not cure high blood pressure; it works to keep it under control.

In some patients, DynaCirc CR can drop your blood pressure too low and you may feel faint or dizzy. Tell your doctor immediately if you experience these symptoms.

Some patients may experience swelling and fluid retention in the hands and feet while taking DynaCirc CR. Notify your doctor right away to determine if it is a side effect of the medicine or if it is a sign of your worsening condition if you have heart failure.

Do not be concerned if you occasionally notice something resembling a tablet in your stool. It is the empty shell coating that allows the slow release of the medicine for your body to absorb.

Who should not take DynaCirc CR?
If you are sensitive to or have ever had an allergic reaction to DynaCirc CR or any of its ingredients, you should not take this medication. Tell your doctor about any drug reactions you have experienced.

What should I tell my doctor before I take the first dose of DynaCirc CR?

Tell your doctor about all prescription, over-the-counter, and herbal medication you are taking before beginning treatment with DynaCirc CR. Also, talk to your doctor about your complete medical history, especially if you have congestive heart failure or stomach problems involving narrowing of the stomach, or if you are also taking a beta-blocking medication such as propranolol.

What is the usual dosage?

The usual starting dosage is 5 mg once a day, alone or in combination with a thiazide diuretic (water pill). Doses may be increased by 5 mg at 2-4 week intervals up to a maximum daily dose of 20 mg. The dosage will be adjusted to meet your individual needs, depending on your condition and how your body responds to the drug. Do not change the dosage or stop taking your medication without your doctor's approval.

How should I take DynaCirc CR?

Swallow the controlled-release tablet whole, without crushing, dividing or chewing it. Try not to miss any doses. If DynaCirc CR is not taken regularly, your condition may worsen.

What should I avoid while taking DynaCirc CR?

DynaCirc CR may cause your blood pressure levels to go very low and for you to develop dizziness or faintness. It is therefore important for you to become accustomed to the effects of DynaCirc CR before participating in activities that require mental alertness, such as driving.

What are possible food and drug interactions associated with DynaCirc CR?

If DynaCirc CR is taken with certain other drugs, the effects of either could be increased, decreased, or altered. It is especially important to check with your doctor before combining DynaCirc CR with beta-blocking blood pressure drugs such as propranolol or fentanyl.

What are the possible side effects of DynaCirc CR?

Side effects cannot be anticipated. If any develop or change in intensity, inform your doctor as soon as possible. Only your doctor can determine if it is safe for you to continue taking DynaCirc CR.

Side effects may include: chest pain, constipation, dizziness, fluid retention, flushing, headache, pounding heartbeat, fatigue, nausea, rash, stomach discomfort

Can I receive DynaCirc CR if I am pregnant or breastfeeding?

The effects of DynaCirc CR during pregnancy have not been adequately studied. If you are pregnant or plan to become pregnant, consult your doctor immediately. DynaCirc CR may appear in breast milk and could affect a nursing infant. Discuss your options with the doctor before breastfeeding.

What should I do if I miss a dose of DynaCirc CR?

If you miss a dose of DynaCirc CR, skip it. Do not take an extra dose to make up for missed doses.

How should I store DynaCirc CR?

Store at room temperature and protect from light, moisture, and humidity.

Echothiophate iodide *See Phospholine Iodide, page 1019.*

Efalizumab *See Raptiva, page 1119.*

Efavirenz *See Sustiva, page 1235.*

Efavirenz, emtricitabine, and tenofovir disoproxil fumarate *See Atripla, page 147.*

EFFEXOR

Generic name: Venlafaxine hydrochloride

What is Effexor?

Effexor is prescribed for the treatment of depression that interferes with daily functioning. The symptoms usually include changes in appetite, sleep habits, and mind/body coordination, decreased sex drive, increased fatigue, feelings of guilt or worthlessness, difficulty concentrating, slowed thinking, and suicidal thoughts.

What is the most important information I should know about Effexor?

Effexor is not approved for use in children or adolescents.

Antidepressants can increase the risk of suicidal thinking and behavior in children and teenagers. Both adult and pediatric patients taking antidepressants should be watched closely for changes in moods or actions, especially when they first start therapy or when their dose is increased or decreased. Patients and their families should contact the doctor immediately if new symptoms develop or seem to get worse. Signs to watch for include anxiety, hostility, insomnia, restlessness, impulsive or dangerous behavior, and thoughts about suicide or dying.

Who should not take Effexor?

Never take Effexor while taking other drugs known as monoamine oxidase inhibitors (MAOIs). Also avoid this drug if it has ever given you an allergic reaction.

What should I tell my doctor before I take the first dose of Effexor?

Tell your doctor about all prescription, over-the-counter, and herbal medication you are taking before beginning treatment with Effexor. Also, talk to your doctor about your complete medical history, especially if you have high blood pressure; heart, liver, or kidney disease; a history of seizures or mania; glaucoma; or an overactive thyroid.

What is the usual dosage?

The information below is based on the dosage guidelines your doctor uses. Depending on your condition and medical history, your doctor may prescribe a different regimen. Do not change the dosage or stop taking your medication without your doctor's approval.

Adults: The usual starting dose is 75 milligrams (mg) a day, divided into 2 or 3 smaller doses, and taken with food. If needed, your doctor may gradually increase your daily dose up to a maximum of 375 mg per day, generally divided in three divided doses.

If you have kidney or liver disease or are taking other medications, your doctor will adjust your dosage accordingly.

How should I take Effexor?

Effexor must be taken 2 or 3 times daily. Take it with food, exactly as prescribed. It may take several weeks before you begin to feel better. Your doctor should check your progress periodically.

What should I avoid while taking Effexor?

Effexor may cause you to feel drowsy or less alert and may affect your judgment. Therefore, avoid driving or operating dangerous machinery or participating in any hazardous activity that requires full mental alertness until you know how this drug affects you.

What are possible food and drug interactions associated with Effexor?

Effexor should never be combined with MAOIs such as the antidepressants phenelzine and tranylcypromine as this could cause a fatal reaction.

Avoid alcohol while taking this medication.

If you have high blood pressure or liver disease, or are elderly, check with your doctor before combining Effexor with cimetidine.

You should consult your doctor before combining Effexor with other drugs that affect the central nervous system, including lithium, migraine medications known as triptans, narcotic painkillers, sleep aids, weight-loss products such as phentermine, tranquilizers, antipsychotic medicines, and other antidepressants that affect serotonin, such as fluoxetine and paroxetine.

Effexor has been found to reduce blood levels of the HIV drug indinavir.

What are the possible side effects of Effexor?

Side effects cannot be anticipated. If any develop or change in intensity, tell your doctor as soon as possible. Only your doctor can determine if it is safe for you to continue taking this drug.

Side effects may include: abnormal ejaculation/orgasm, anxiety, blurred vision, constipation, dizziness, dry mouth, impotence, insomnia, nausea, nervousness, sleepiness, sweating, tremor, vomiting, weakness, weight loss

Can I receive Effexor if I am pregnant or breastfeeding?

The effects of Effexor during pregnancy have not been adequately studied. If you are pregnant or are planning to become pregnant, tell your doctor immediately. Effexor should be used during pregnancy only if clearly needed.

If Effexor is taken shortly before delivery, the baby may suffer withdrawal symptoms. Effexor appears in breast milk and could cause serious side effects in a nursing infant. You'll need to choose between nursing your baby or continuing your treatment with Effexor.

What should I do if I miss a dose of Effexor?

It is not necessary to make it up. Skip the missed dose and continue with your next scheduled dose. Do not take 2 doses at once.

How should I store Effexor?

Store in a tightly closed container at room temperature. Protect from excessive heat and moisture.

EFFEXOR XR
Generic name: Venlafaxine hydrochloride, extended-release

What is Effexor XR?

Effexor XR is used to treat depression, generalized anxiety disorder, and social anxiety disorder in adults. It may take several weeks for your symptoms to get better with Effexor XR.

What is the most important information I should know about Effexor XR?

Antidepressants can increase the risk of suicidal thinking and behavior in children and teenagers. Both adult and pediatric patients taking antidepressants should be watched closely for changes in moods or actions, especially when they first start therapy or when their dose is increased or decreased. Patients and their families should contact the doctor immediately if new symptoms develop or seem to get worse. Signs to watch for include anxiety, hostility, insomnia, restlessness, impulsive or dangerous behavior, and thoughts about suicide or dying.

Do not take this medication if you are currently taking a drug known as a monoamine oxidase inhibitor (MAOI). MAOIs can cause a very serious reaction or even death if taken at the same time as Effexor XR. You must stop taking your MAOI at least 14 days before beginning treatment with Effexor XR. Similarly, you should wait 7 days after stopping Effexor XR before starting an MAOI.

Effexor XR is not approved for use in pediatric patients.

Who should not take Effexor XR?
Do not take Effexor XR if you are allergic to it or any of its ingredients, or if you are currently taking an MAOI or have taken an MAOI within the last 14 days.

What should I tell my doctor before I take the first dose of Effexor XR?
Tell your doctor about all your medical problems, including suicidal thoughts, high blood pressure, heart disease, liver or kidney problems, glaucoma, seizures, or thyroid problems. Also alert your doctor if you have ever had symptoms of mania or hypomania, such as persistently elevated or irritable mood, a decreased need for sleep, racing thoughts, hyperactivity, and rapid or excessive talking.

What is the usual dosage?
The information below is based on the dosage guidelines your doctor uses. Depending on your condition and medical history, your doctor may prescribe a different regimen. Do not change the dosage or stop taking your medication without your doctor's approval.

Adults: The usual starting dose is 75 milligrams (mg) once a day. If needed, the doctor may increase your daily dose in steps of 75 mg, up to a maximum of 225 mg a day.

How should I take Effexor XR?
Effexor XR should be taken as a single dose with food at about the same time every day, either in the morning or evening. The capsule should be swallowed whole; it should not be divided, crushed, chewed, or placed in water. The capsule can also be carefully opened and its contents sprinkled onto a spoonful of applesauce. This should be swallowed immediately and followed with a glass of water. Do not chew this mixture before swallowing.

What should I avoid while taking Effexor XR?
Until you know how Effexor XR affects you, be careful doing activities that require alertness, such as driving a car or operating machinery. Also, avoid drinking alcohol while taking this drug.

What are possible food and drug interactions associated with Effexor XR?
Do not take Effexor XR if you have taken an MAOI within the last 14 days.
    Also, be sure to tell your doctor about all medicines you plan to take, including prescription and nonprescription medications, nutritional supplements, and herbs. Taking Effexor XR with certain drugs or supplements may increase the risk of serious side effects. It is especially important to check with your doctor before combining this drug with the following: any drug that affects the central nervous system, antidepressants, cimetidine, diazepam, linezolid, lithium, migraine drugs known as triptans, St. John's wort, tramadol, and tryptophan supplements.

What are the possible side effects of Effexor XR?
Side effects cannot be anticipated. If any develop or change in intensity, tell your doctor as soon as possible. Only your doctor can determine if it is safe for you to continue taking this drug.

Side effects may include: abnormal ejaculation, abnormal vision, agitation, confusion, constipation, dizziness, dry mouth, gas, loss of appetite, insomnia, nausea, nervousness, rapid heartbeat, sleepiness, sweating, tremor, yawning

Can I receive Effexor XR if I am pregnant or breastfeeding?
The effects of Effexor XR during pregnancy and breastfeeding are unknown. Talk with your doctor before taking this drug if you are pregnant, plan to become pregnant, or are breastfeeding. Newborns whose mothers took Effexor XR late in the third trimester have had problems.

What should I do if I miss a dose of Effexor XR?
If you miss a dose of Effexor XR, it can be taken later that day. Don't try to make up for the missed dose by taking 2 doses the next day.

How should I store Effexor XR?
Store at room temperature.

ELDEPRYL
Generic name: Selegiline hydrochloride

What is Eldepryl?
Eldepryl is prescribed along with levodopa/carbidopa for people with Parkinson's disease. It is used as an add-on treatment when levodopa/

carbidopa alone seems to be less effective. Eldepryl has no effect when taken by itself; it only works in combination with levodopa.

What is the most important information I should know about Eldepryl?

Eldepryl belongs to a class of drugs known as MAO inhibitors. These drugs can interact with certain foods—including aged cheeses and meats, pickled herring, beer, and wine—to cause a life-threatening surge in blood pressure. At the dose recommended for Eldepryl, this interaction is not a problem. But for safety's sake, you may want to watch your diet; and you should never take more Eldepryl than the doctor prescribed (usually 10 mg daily). Rare hypertensive reactions with selegiline at recommended doses associated with dietary influences have been reported.

Patients should be advised of the possible need to reduce levodopa dosage after the initiation of Eldepryl therapy.

If you or your family patient experiences severe headache or other atypical or unusual symptoms not previously experienced, contact your doctor immediately.

Do not drive, operate machinery, or do anything else that could be dangerous until you know how you react to Eldepryl; this drug may cause dizziness or lightheadedness. Using Eldepryl with certain other medications or with alcohol may increase these side effects.

Eldepryl may cause dizziness, lightheadedness, or fainting. Alcohol, hot weather, exercise, and fever can increase these effects. To prevent them, sit up or stand slowly, especially in the morning. Also, sit or lie down at the first sign of dizziness, lightheadedness, or weakness.

Do not become overheated in hot weather or during exercise or other activities; heatstroke may occur.

Before you begin taking any new prescription or over-the-counter medicine, check with your doctor or pharmacist. This includes medicines that contain pseudoephedrine, phenylpropanolamine, or dextromethorphan.

Follow all of these precautions for at least 4 weeks after taking the last dose of Eldepryl.

Who should not take Eldepryl?

Do not take Eldepryl if you are sensitive to or have ever had an allergic reaction to it. Do not take narcotic painkillers while you are taking Eldepryl. This may sometimes extend to other opioids as well.

What should I tell my doctor before I take the first dose of Eldepryl?

Tell your doctor about all prescription, over-the-counter, and herbal medication you are taking before beginning treatment with this drug. Also, talk to your doctor about your complete medical history especially if you have a history of mental disorders (psychosis), tardive dyskinesia (twitching of the face and tongue, involuntary movements of the arms and legs), or ulcers.

What is the usual dosage?

The information below is based on the dosage guidelines your doctor uses. Depending on your condition and medical history, your doctor may prescribe a different regimen. Do not change the dosage or stop taking your medication without your doctor's approval.

Adults: The recommended dose of Eldepryl is 10 milligrams per day divided into 2 smaller doses of 5 milligrams each, usually taken at breakfast and lunch. After 2 to 3 days of selegiline treatment, an attempt may be made to reduce the dose of levodopa/carbidopa.

How should I take Eldepryl?

Take Eldepryl with food, at breakfast and lunch.

Most people who take Eldepryl can eat a normal diet. However, if your dosage is more than 10 mg/day, serious increases in blood pressure may occur when you eat or drink some foods and drinks. Foods or drinks that may cause a reaction include aged cheeses, sour cream, red wines, beer, bologna, pepperoni, salami, summer sausage, pickled herring, liver, meat prepared with tenderizers, canned figs, raisins, bananas, avocados, soy sauce, fava beans, or yeast extracts.

Continue to use Eldepryl even if you feel well. Do not miss any doses.

What should I avoid while taking Eldepryl?

Never take Eldepryl at a higher dosage than prescribed; doing so could put you at risk for a dangerous rise in blood pressure. If you develop a severe headache or any other unusual symptoms, contact your doctor immediately.

You may suffer a severe reaction if you combine Eldepryl with tricyclic antidepressants such as amitriptyline and imipramine, or with antidepressants that affect serotonin levels, such as fluoxetine and paroxetine. Wait at least 14 days after taking Eldepryl before beginning therapy with any of these drugs. If you have been taking antidepressants such as fluoxetine and paroxetine, you should wait at least 5 weeks before taking Eldepryl. This much time is needed to clear the antidepressant completely from your system.

Do not drive, operate machinery, or do anything else that could be dangerous until you know how you react to Eldepryl; this drug may cause dizziness or lightheadedness.

Do not become overheated in hot weather or during exercise or other activities; heatstroke may occur.

Avoid standing or sitting up too quickly, especially when you first begin treatment with Eldepryl. Also, sit or lie down at the first sign of dizziness, lightheadedness, or weakness.

What are possible food and drug interactions associated with Eldepryl?

If Eldepryl is taken with certain other drugs, the effects of either could be increased, decreased, or altered. It is especially important to check with your doctor before combining Eldepryl with the following: antidepressant medications such as paroxetine, fluoxetine, and sertraline; antidepressant medications classified as tricyclics, such as amitriptyline and imipramine; antidiabetic agents such as repaglinide; anorexiants such as phentermine; bupropion; carbamazepine; cyclobenzaprine; dextromethorphan; insulin; narcotic painkillers such as meperidine, oxycodone, and codeine; sulfonylureas such as glyburide; sumatriptan; and sympathomimetics such as ephedrine and methylphenidate.

What are the possible side effects of Eldepryl?

Side effects cannot be anticipated. If any develop or change in intensity, inform your doctor as soon as possible. Only your doctor can determine if it is safe for you to continue taking this drug. Eldepryl may worsen side effects caused by your usual dosage of levodopa.

Side effects may include: abdominal pain, anxiety, changes in heart rate, confusion, dizziness, dry mouth, fainting, hallucinations, headache, lightheadedness, nausea, unusual body movements or difficulty moving, vomiting

Can I receive Eldepryl if I am pregnant or breastfeeding?

The effects of Eldepryl during pregnancy and breastfeeding have not been adequately studied. If you are pregnant, plan to become pregnant, or breastfeeding, tell your doctor immediately.

What should I do if I miss a dose of Eldepryl?

If you miss a dose of Eldepryl, take it as soon as possible. If it is almost time for your next dose, skip the missed dose and go back to your regular dosing schedule. Do not take 2 doses at once.

How should I store Eldepryl?

Store Eldepryl at room temperature, between 59 and 86 degrees F (15 and 30 degrees C). Store away from heat, moisture, and light. Do not store in the bathroom. Keep Eldepryl out of the reach of children.

ELESTRIN

Generic name: Estradiol gel

What is Elestrin?

Elestrin is a colorless gel that contains an estrogen hormone called estradiol, which is absorbed through the skin into the bloodstream. Elestrin is used after menopause to reduce moderate-to-severe hot flashes.

What is the most important information I should know about Elestrin?

Estrogens increase the chances of getting cancer of the uterus. Report any unusual vaginal bleeding right away while you are using Elestrin. Vaginal bleeding after menopause may be a warning sign of cancer of the uterus. Your healthcare provider should check any unusual vaginal bleeding to find out the cause.

Do not use estrogens with or without progestins to prevent heart disease, heart attacks, or strokes. Using estrogens with or without progestins may increase your chances of getting heart attacks, strokes, breast cancer, and blood clots.

Do not use estrogens with or without progestins to prevent dementia. Using estrogens with or without progestins may increase your risk of dementia, based on a study of women age 65 years or older.

You and your healthcare provider should talk regularly about whether you still need treatment with Elestrin.

Do not use Elestrin to treat conditions for which it was not prescribed.

If you get Elestrin in your eyes, rinse your eyes right away with warm clean water to flush out any Elestrin. Seek medical attention if needed.

Do not give Elestrin to other people, even if they have the same symptoms you have.

Who should not take Elestrin?

Estrogen products, including Elestrin, should not be used in women who have or have had certain cancers, a stroke or heart attack in the past year, currently have or have had blood clots, currently have or have had liver problems. Do not take Elestrin if there is any chance you may be pregnant.

What should I tell my doctor before I take the first dose of Elestrin?

Tell your doctor about all prescription, over-the-counter, and herbal medication you are taking before beginning treatment with Elestrin. Also, talk to your doctor about your complete medical history, especially if you have certain conditions, such as asthma (wheezing), diabetes, gallbladder disease, depression, if you had your uterus removed (hysterectomy), epilepsy (seizures), migraine, endometriosis, lupus, or problems with your heart, liver, thyroid, or kidneys, or you have high calcium levels in your blood.

Tell your doctor if you are going to have surgery or will be on bed rest. You may need to stop using Elestrin.

What is the usual dosage?

The information below is based on the dosage guidelines your doctor uses. Depending on your condition and medical history, your doctor

may prescribe a different regimen. Do not change the dosage or stop taking your medication without your doctor's approval.

Adults: *Starting dose:* 1 pump (0.87g) every day to upper arm. Apply Elestrin at the same time each day. Dosage adjustments will be made based on your response to treatment.

Start at the lowest dose and talk to your healthcare provider about how well that dose is working for you. Elestrin should be used at the lowest dose possible for your treatment and only as long as needed. You and your healthcare provider should talk regularly (for example, every 3 to 6 months) about the dose you are taking and whether you still need treatment with Elestrin.

How should I take Elestrin?

To activate the pump, unlock the pump by turning the spout on top of the bottle a quarter turn to the left or the right.

Before using the pump for the first time, prime the pump by fully depressing the spout ten (10) times. Throw away the unused gel by placing it in the trash to avoid another person or pet from accidental contact with the gel or, eating or drinking it.

After priming, the pump is ready to use. One complete pump will dispense the same amount of Elestrin each time. After each daily dose, return the spout to the locked position and replace the cap before you put it away.

Dry skin completely before applying Elestrin. You should apply your daily dose of gel to clean, dry, unbroken skin. If you take a bath or shower or use a sauna, apply Elestrin afterwards. If you go swimming, try to leave as much time as possible, at least 2 hours, between applying your Elestrin dose and going into the water.

To apply the dose, hold the pump with the tip facing the application area of the arm. For each pump depression needed, press the pump firmly and fully with a continuous motion without hesitation. Gently spread the gel using only 2 fingers. Spread and gently rub in the gel over the entire area of your upper arm and shoulder area. Allow the gel to dry for five minutes or more before dressing.

Never apply Elestrin to the breast or in or around the vagina.

Wash your hands with soap and water after applying the gel. Avoid fire, flame or smoking until the gel has dried. Elestrin contains alcohol. Alcohol-based gels are flammable.

Always move the spout into locked position and place the cap over the top of the pump after each use.

What should I avoid while taking Elestrin?

Do not apply sunscreen to the area where the gel was applied for at least 25 minutes. Do not apply sunscreen to the area where the gel was applied for 7 or more consecutive days.

Do not allow others to come in contact with the area of skin where you applied the gel for at least two hours after you apply Elestrin.

If you get Elestrin in your eyes, rinse your eyes right away with warm clean water to flush out any Elestrin. Seek medical attention if needed.

Grapefruit and grapefruit juice may interact with estradiol and lead to potentially dangerous effects. Discuss the use of grapefruit products with your doctor.

Avoid fire, flames or smoking until the gel has dried. Elestrin contains alcohol. Alcohol-based gels are flammable.

Never apply Elestrin to the breast or in or around the vagina.

What are possible food and drug interactions associated with Elestrin?

If Elestrin is taken with certain other drugs, the effects of either could be increased, decreased, or altered. It is especially important to check with your doctor before combining Elestrin with the following: carbamazepine; clarithromycin; erythromycin; grapefruit juice; itraconazole; ketoconazole; phenobarbital; rifampin; ritonavir; and St. John's wort preparations.

What are the possible side effects of Elestrin?

Side effects cannot be anticipated. If any develop or change in intensity, tell your doctor as soon as possible. Only your doctor can determine if it is safe for you to continue taking this drug.

Side effects may include: bloating, blood clots, breast cancer, breast pain, cancer of the uterus, dementia, enlargement of benign tumors of the uterus ("fibroids"), fluid retention, gallbladder disease, hair loss, headache, irregular vaginal bleeding or spotting, heart attack, high blood pressure, high blood sugar, liver problems, nausea and vomiting, ovarian cancer, stomach cramps, stroke, vaginal yeast infection

Some of the warning signs of serious side effects include: breast lumps, changes in speech, changes in vision, chest pain, unusual vaginal bleeding, dizziness and faintness, leg pain, severe headaches, shortness of breath, vomiting

Call your healthcare provider right away if you get any of these warning signs, or any other unusual symptom that concerns you.

These are not all the possible side effects of Elestrin. For more information, ask your healthcare provider or pharmacist.

Can I receive Elestrin if I am pregnant or breastfeeding?

Elestrin is intended for post-menopausal women. Tell your doctor if you are pregnant, planning to become pregnant, or are breastfeeding. Estrogen products should not be used during pregnancy. Avoid using Elestrin if you are breastfeeding, since this drug passes into breast milk.

What should I do if I miss a dose of Elestrin?
If you miss a dose, do not double the dose. If your next dose is less than 12 hours away, it is best just to wait and apply your normal dose the next day. If it is more than 12 hours until the next dose, apply the dose you missed and resume your normal dosing the next day.

How should I store Elestrin?
Store at room temperature, 20° to 25°C (68° to 77°F); excursions permitted at 15° to 30°C (59° to 86°F).

Eletriptan hydrobromide See Relpax, page 1129.

ELIDEL
Generic name: Pimecrolimus

What is Elidel?
Elidel cream is a prescription medicine used on the skin to treat eczema (atopic dermatitis), and is in a class of medicines called topical calcineurin inhibitors. This drug is for people ages 2 and older who do not have a weakened immune system. Elidel cream is used on the skin for short periods, and if needed, treatment may be repeated with breaks in between.

What is the most important information I should know about Elidel?
The safety of using Elidel cream for a long period of time is not known. A very small number of people who have used Elidel cream have had skin cancer or lymphoma. However, a link with the use of Elidel cream has not been shown. Do not use Elidel cream continuously for a long period of time; use this cream only on areas of your skin that have eczema; and do not use this on a child under 2 years old.

See "How should I take Elidel?" for proper procedures on how to use this product.

Elidel is for external use only. Do not get it in your eyes, nose, or mouth. If you get it in your eyes, rinse at once with cool tap water.

If your condition worsens, does not improve after 6 weeks of using Elidel, or if a feeling of warmth or a burning sensation at the application site is severe or persists for more than 1 week contact your doctor.

Elidel may cause you to become sunburned more easily. Avoid the sun, sunlamps, or tanning booths until you know how you react to Elidel. Use sunscreen or wear protective clothing if you must be outside for more than a short time.

Elidel may be harmful if swallowed. If you ingest it, contact your poison control center or emergency room right away.

Who should not take Elidel?

Do not take this medication if you are allergic to any of its ingredients. Also, this drug should not be used on children under age 2.

What should I tell my doctor before I take the first dose of Elidel?

Tell your doctor about all prescription, over-the-counter, and herbal medications you are taking before beginning treatment with Elidel. Also, talk to your doctor about your complete medical history, especially if you have a skin disease called Netherton's syndrome (a rare inherited condition), have chicken pox or herpes, have a weak immune system, are receiving any form of light therapy (phototherapy, UVA, or UVB), or if you are pregnant/planning to become pregnant/breastfeeding.

What is the usual dosage?

The information below is based on the dosage guidelines your doctor uses. Depending on your condition and medical history, your doctor may prescribe a different regimen. Do not change the dosage or stop taking your medication without your doctor's approval.

Adults: Elidel cream is usually applied to the affected skin twice daily, until symptoms disappear. This drug should not be used for prolonged periods of time. If signs and symptoms persist beyond 6 weeks, patients should be re-examined by their doctor to confirm the initial diagnosis.

How should I take Elidel?

Wash your hands before using Elidel cream. When applying the cream after a bath or shower, make sure your skin is dry. Apply a thin layer only to the affected skin areas, twice a day, as directed by your doctor. Do not bathe, shower or swim right after applying Elidel Cream. This could wash off the cream.

You can use moisturizers with Elidel Cream. Make sure you check with your doctor first about the products that are right for you. Because the skin of patients with eczema can be very dry, it is important to keep up good skin care practices. If you use moisturizers, apply them after Elidel cream.

What should I avoid while taking Elidel?

Do not bathe, shower, or swim right after applying Elidel cream. This could wash off the cream.

Do not use sun lamps, tanning beds, or get treatment with ultraviolet light therapy during treatment with Elidel cream. Limit sun exposure during treatment, even when the medicine is not on your skin. If you need to be outdoors after applying Elidel cream, wear loose fitting clothing that protects the treated area from the sun. Ask your doctor what other types of protection from the sun you should use.

Do not cover the skin being treated with bandages, dressings or wraps. You can wear normal clothing.

Do not use Elidel cream in the eyes. If Elidel cream gets in your eyes, rinse them with cold water.

Do not swallow Elidel cream. If you do, call your doctor.

What are possible food and drug interactions associated with Elidel?

If Elidel is taken with certain other drugs, the effects of either could be increased, decreased, or altered. It is especially important to check with your doctor before combining Elidel with the following: azole antifungals such as ketoconazole; calcium channel blockers such as diltiazem; and macrolide antibiotics such as erythromycin.

What are the possible side effects of Elidel?

Side effects cannot be anticipated. If any develop or change in intensity, tell your doctor as soon as possible. Only your doctor can determine if it is safe for you to continue taking this drug.

Side effects may include: burning, chicken pox, cold sores, common cold/stuffy nose, cough, fever, flu, headache, shingles, sore throat, swollen glands, warts

The most common side effect at the skin application site is burning or a feeling of warmth. These side effects are usually mild or moderate, happen during the first 5 days of treatment, and usually clear up in a few days. Call your doctor if the burning feeling is severe or lasts for more than 1 week.

Can I receive Elidel if I am pregnant or breastfeeding?

The effects of Elidel during pregnancy and breastfeeding are unknown. Tell your doctor immediately if you are pregnant, plan to become pregnant, or are breastfeeding.

What should I do if I miss a dose of Elidel?

If you miss a dose of Elidel, use it as soon as possible. If it is almost time for your next dose, skip the missed dose and go back to your regular dosing schedule. Do not use 2 doses at once.

How should I store Elidel?

Store Elidel at room temperature, between 59 and 86 degrees F (15 and 30 degrees C). Store away from heat, moisture, and light. Do not freeze. Do not leave Elidel in your car in cold or hot weather. Make sure the cap on the tube is tightly closed. Keep Elidel out of the reach of children.

ELOCON

Generic name: Mometasone furoate

What is Elocon?

Elocon is a cortisone-like steroid available in cream, ointment, and lotion form. It is used to treat certain itchy rashes and other inflammatory skin conditions.

What is the most important information I should know about Elocon?

When you use Elocon, you inevitably absorb some of the medication through your skin and into the bloodstream. Too much absorption of Elocon can lead to unwanted side effects elsewhere in the body. Avoid using large amounts of Elocon over large areas, and do not cover with airtight dressings such as plastic wrap or adhesive bandages unless your doctor directs you to do so.

Elocon is for external use only. Avoid contact with the eyes. Do not use Elocon on the face, underarms, or groin area unless advised to do so by your healthcare provider.

Use Elocon cream only for the skin problem for which it is intended.

Stop using Elocon when the skin area returns to normal. Contact your health care provider if improvement is not seen within 2 weeks.

Ask your health care provider before using other medicine containing steroids. If you are uncertain whether your other medications contain corticosteroids, check with your pharmacist.

Caution is advised when using Elocon in children; they may be more sensitive to its effects. Elocon should not be used in children younger than 2 years old; safety and effectiveness in these children have not been confirmed. Corticosteroids may affect growth rate in children and teenagers in some cases. They may need regular growth checks while they use Elocon.

Look at the "How should I take this medication?" section for proper procedure on how to use Elocon.

Who should not take Elocon?

Do not use Elocon if you have ever had an allergic reaction to it or any other steroid medication.

What should I tell my doctor before I take the first dose of Elocon?

Tell your doctor about all prescription, over-the-counter, and herbal medication you are taking before beginning treatment with this drug. Also, talk to your doctor about your complete medical history, especially if you have acne-like lesions, measles, inflammation around your mouth, chickenpox, have recently had a vaccination, have any kind of skin infection or atrophy (wasting) of your skin.

What is the usual dosage?
The information below is based on the dosage guidelines your doctor uses. Depending on your condition and medical history, your doctor may prescribe a different regimen. Do not change the dosage or stop taking your medication without your doctor's approval.

Adults: Apply a thin film of Elocon to the affected skin areas once daily.

Children 2 years and older: Use should be limited to the least amount necessary. Use of steroids over a long period of time may interfere with growth and development in this age group. Elocon cream and ointment may be used for children aged 2 and older, but not for more than 3 weeks.

How should I take Elocon?
Apply a thin film of the cream or ointment or a few drops of the lotion to the affected skin once a day. Massage gently until it disappears.

Elocon is for use only on the skin. Be careful to keep it out of your eyes.

For the most effective and economical use of Elocon lotion, hold the tip of the bottle very close to (but not touching) the affected skin and squeeze the bottle gently.

Once you have applied Elocon, do not cover the skin with an airtight bandage, a tight diaper, plastic pants, or any other airtight dressing unless your doctor tells you otherwise. This could encourage excessive absorption of the medication into your bloodstream.

Wash your hand after applying Elocon unless your hands are part of the treated area.

What should I avoid while taking Elocon?
Be careful not to use Elocon for a longer time than prescribed. If you do, you may disrupt your ability to make your own natural adrenal corticoid hormones (hormones secreted by the outer layer of the adrenal gland).

Elocon is for external use only. Avoid getting it into your eyes. Do not use it to treat anything other than the condition for which it was prescribed.

Do not use Elocon cream or ointment on your face, underarms, or groin area unless your doctor tells you to.

What are possible food and drug interactions associated with Elocon?
If this medication is used with certain other drugs, the effects of either could be increased, decreased, or altered. Always check with your doctor before combining this drug with any other medication.

What are the possible side effects of Elocon?
Side effects cannot be anticipated. If any develop or change in intensity, notify your doctor as soon as possible. Only your doctor can determine if it is safe for you to continue using Elocon.

Side effects may include: acne-like pimples, allergic skin rash, boils, burning, damaged skin, dryness, excessive hairiness, infected hair follicles, infection of the skin, irritation, itching, light colored patches on skin, prickly heat, rash around the mouth, skin atrophy and wasting, softening of the skin, stretch marks, tingling or stinging

Can I receive Elocon if I am pregnant or breastfeeding?
The effects of taking Elocon during pregnancy are unknown. If you are pregnant or plan to become pregnant, inform your doctor immediately. You should not use Elocon while breastfeeding, since absorbed hormone could make its way into breast milk and harm the nursing infant.

What should I do if I miss a dose of Elocon?
If you miss a dose of Elocon, use it as soon as possible. If it is almost time for your next dose, skip the missed dose and go back to your regular dosing schedule. Do not use 2 doses at once.

How should I store Elocon?
Store Elocon between 59 and 86 degrees F (15 and 30 degrees C). Store away from heat, moisture, and light. Do not store in the bathroom. Keep Elocon out of the reach of children.

EMSAM
Generic name: Selegiline patch

What is Emsam?
Emsam is a skin patch prescribed to treat major depression.

What is the most important information I should know about Emsam?
Emsam is not approved for use in children or adolescents.

Antidepressant medicines may increase suicidal thoughts or actions in some children, teenagers, and young adults when the medicine is first started. Depression and other serious mental illnesses are the most important causes of suicidal thoughts and actions. Some people may have a particularly high risk of having suicidal thoughts or actions. These include people who have (or have a family history of) bipolar disorder (also called manic-depressive illness) or suicidal thoughts or actions.

Pay close attention to any changes, especially sudden changes, in mood, behaviors, thoughts, or feelings. This is very important when an antidepressant medicine is first started or when the dose is changed.

Call the doctor right away to report new or sudden changes in mood, behavior, thoughts, or feelings. Signs to watch for include new or worsening depression, new or worsening anxiety, agitation, insomnia, hostility, panic attacks, restlessness, extreme hyperactivity, and suicidal thinking or behavior.

Keep all follow-up visits as scheduled, and call the doctor between visits as needed, especially if you have concerns about symptoms.

Emsam is a monoamine oxidase inhibitor (MAOI). This class of drugs, including Emsam, can cause a sudden, large increase in blood pressure (hypertensive crisis) if you consume foods and drinks that contain high amounts of tyramine.

Who should not take Emsam?
You should not use Emsam if you are taking another medication that will interact with it, or if you are allergic to any of the ingredients in it. Talk with your doctor to find the best way to treat depression.

Do not take Emsam if you have a condition call pheochromocytoma.

What should I tell my doctor before I take the first dose of Emsam?
Tell your doctor about all prescription, over-the-counter, and herbal medications you are taking before beginning treatment with Emsam. Also, talk to your doctor about your complete medical history, including heart problems, manic episodes, seizures, fainting, and if you are pregnant or planning to become pregnant. Tell your doctor if you are breastfeeding.

What is the usual dosage?
The information below is based on the dosage guidelines your doctor uses. Depending on your condition and medical history, your doctor may prescribe a different regimen. Do not change the dosage or stop taking your medication without your doctor's approval.

Adults: Emsam patches are available in three different dosage strengths: 6 milligrams (mg)/24hours, 9 mg/24 hours, and 12 mg/24hour. Your doctor will adjust the dose to best fit your needs.

How should I take Emsam?
Apply Emsam patch to dry, smooth skin on your upper chest or back (below the neck and above the waist), upper thigh, or to the outer surface of the upper arm. Choose a new site each time you change your patch. Do not use the same site two days in a row.

What should I avoid while taking Emsam?
You must not eat foods or drink beverages that contain high amounts of tyramine while using Emsam 9 mg/24hours and 12 mg/24 hours

patches. (You do not have to make any diet changes with the Emsam 6 mg/24 hours patch.)

Do not take other medicines while using Emsam or for 2 weeks after you remove your last patch unless your doctor has told you to do so.

Do not drive or operate dangerous machinery until you know how Emsam affects you. Emsam may impair your judgment, ability to think, or coordination.

Do not drink alcoholic beverages while using Emsam.

What are possible food and drug interactions associated with Emsam?

If Emsam is taken with certain other drugs, the effects of either could be increased, decreased, or altered. It is especially important to check with your doctor before combining Emsam with the following: amphetamines; antiseizure medication; all other antidepressants; carbamazepine and oxcarbazepine; cold medicines; Demerol; diet/weight loss pills; pain medication; and St. John's wort. Some of these medications need to be stopped for at least a week before you can start using Emsam.

While on Emsam, avoid tyramine-rich foods such as dried or aged meats (sausages/salami), fava beans, aged cheeses, beer on tap, yeast, sauerkraut, and soybean products.

What are the possible side effects of Emsam?

Side effects cannot be anticipated. If any develop or change in intensity, tell your doctor as soon as possible. Only your doctor can determine if it is safe for you to continue taking this drug.

Side effects may include: increase in blood pressure (hypertensive crisis*); increased depression; mania or hypomania in people who have a history of bipolar disorder; low blood pressure

Can I receive Emsam if I am pregnant or breastfeeding?

The effects of Emsam during pregnancy and breastfeeding are unknown. Talk with your doctor before taking this drug if you are pregnant, plan to become pregnant, or are breastfeeding.

What should I do if I miss a dose of Emsam?

If you forget to change your patch after 24 hours, remove the old patch, put on a new patch in a different area and continue to follow your original schedule.

---

* Symptoms of a hypertensive crisis include the sudden onset of severe headache, nausea, stiff neck, a fast heartbeat or a change in the way your heart beats, excessive sweating, and confusion. If you suddenly develop these symptoms, seek emergency medical treatment right away.

How should I store Emsam?

Store at room temperature, in the original pouches that the patches come in.

ENABLEX

Generic name: Darifenacin

What is Enablex?

Enablex is a prescription medicine used for the treatment of overactive bladder (OAB) in adults. Symptoms of OAB are having a strong need to go to the bathroom right away (urgency), leaking or wetting accidents (urinary incontinence), having to go to the bathroom too often (urinary frequency). This medication gives OAB symptom relief by targeting specific receptors on the bladder that cause involuntary muscle spasms. Enablex helps control the bladder muscle and helps restore control of urination.

What is the most important information I should know about Enablex?

Do not drive or perform other possibly unsafe tasks until you know how you react to Enablex; this drug may cause dizziness or blurred vision. These effects may become worse if you take Enablex with alcohol or certain medicines.

Heat exhaustion or heatstroke due to decreased sweating can occur while you are taking Enablex; you may become overheated in a warm environment or during increased physical activity. Seek immediate medical attention if you experience sudden or severe tiredness, weakness, anxiety, dizziness, or fainting.

Enablex may cause urinary retention (difficulty urinating), gastric retention (delayed emptying of the stomach), and narrow angle glaucoma.

Who should not take Enablex?

Do not take Enablex if you are allergic to any of its ingredients.

Also, do not take this drug if you are not able to empty your bladder (urinary retention), have delayed or slow emptying of your stomach (gastric retention), or if you have an eye problem called uncontrolled narrow-angle glaucoma.

What should I tell my doctor before I take the first dose of Enablex?

Tell your doctor about all prescription, over-the-counter, and herbal medications you are taking before beginning treatment with Enablex. Also, talk to your doctor about your complete medical history, especially if you have any stomach or intestinal problems, or problems with constipation; have trouble emptying your bladder or you have a weak urine stream;

have myasthenia gravis (muscle problems); have an eye problem called narrow-angle glaucoma; have liver problems; or if you are pregnant or plan to become pregnant.

What is the usual dosage?
The information below is based on the dosage guidelines your doctor uses. Depending on your condition and medical history, your doctor may prescribe a different regimen. Do not change the dosage or stop taking your medication without your doctor's approval.

Adults: The recommended starting dose of Enablex is 7.5 milligrams (mg) once per day. Based on individual response, the dose may increase to 15mg taken once daily; this may occur as early as 2 weeks after starting therapy.

Special populations: Patients with moderate liver impairment or those who are taking specific drugs should not exceed a daily Enablex dose of 7.5mg. Enablex is not recommended for use in patients with severe liver impairment.

The safety and effectiveness of Enablex in pediatric patients have not been established.

How should I take Enablex?
Enablex should be taken once a day with liquid, with or without food. This drug should be swallowed whole and should not be crushed, split, or chewed.

What should I avoid while taking Enablex?
Avoid potentially hazardous activities (eg, driving) when beginning treatment with Enablex. The drug may cause blurred vision.

Do not become overheated in hot weather or during activity; heatstroke may occur.

Avoid the consumption of alcohol while you are on Enablex.

What are possible food and drug interactions associated with Enablex?
If Enablex is taken with certain other drugs, the effects of either could be increased, decreased, or altered. It is especially important to check with your doctor before combining Enablex with the following: anticholinergic drugs, antifungal medicines, clarithromycin, digoxin, flecainide, itraconazole, ketoconazole, midazolam, nefazodone, nelfinavir, ritonavir, scopolamine, thioridazine, and tricyclic antidepressants such as amitriptyline and imipramine.

What are the possible side effects of Enablex?
Side effects cannot be anticipated. If any develop or change in intensity, tell your doctor as soon as possible. Only your doctor can determine if it is safe for you to continue taking this drug.

Side effects may include: blurred vision, constipation, dry mouth, overheated feeling, diarrhea, dizziness, dry eyes, flu-like symptoms, headache, nausea, stomach pain, stomach upset, weakness, back pain, bloody or cloudy urine, inability to urinate despite an urge to do so

Can I receive Enablex if I am pregnant or breastfeeding?
The effects of Enablex during pregnancy and breastfeeding are unknown. Tell your doctor immediately if you are pregnant, plan to become pregnant, or are breastfeeding.

What should I do if I miss a dose of Enablex?
If you miss a dose of Enablex, take it as soon as possible. If it is almost time for your next dose, skip the missed dose and go back to your regular dosing schedule. Do not take 2 doses at once.

How should I store Enablex?
Store Enablex at 77 degrees F (25 degrees C). Brief storage at temperatures between 59 and 86 degrees F (15 and 30 degrees C) is permitted. Store away from heat, moisture, and light. Do not store in the bathroom. Keep Enablex out of the reach of children.

Enalapril maleate *See Vasotec, page 1376.*

Enalapril maleate and felodipine *See Lexxel, page 740.*

Enalapril maleate and hydrochlorothiazide *See Vaseretic, page 1374.*

Entacapone *See Comtan, page 331.*

Entecavir *See Baraclude, page 197.*

Epinephrine *See EpiPen, below.*

EPIPEN
Generic name: Epinephrine

What is EpiPen?
EpiPen is used in the emergency department for the treatment of severe allergic reactions (anaphylaxis) to insect stings or bites, foods, drugs, and other allergens.

What is the most important information I should know about EpiPen?
EpiPens are pre-filled automatic injection devices for use during allergic emergencies. They are to be injected into your outer thigh and must be carried with you at all times.

Refer to "How should I take EpiPen?" for proper procedures on how to use EpiPen.

Never put your thumb, fingers, or hand over the black tip of the auto-injector. Do NOT remove the gray activation cap until ready to use.

Never inject EpiPen into hands, fingers, feet, or toes. Doing so may cause a loss of blood flow and result in tissue damage to these areas. If you accidentally inject EpiPen into any of these areas, seek immediate emergency medical attention.

EpiPen does not contain latex.

Immediately after using this product, go to the nearest hospital emergency room. You may need further medical attention. Tell the doctor or health care provider that you have received an injection of epinephrine. Show the doctor the thigh where the injection was given. Give your used EpiPen to the doctor for inspection and proper disposal.

Who should not take EpiPen?

There are no absolute reasons why you should not use EpiPen. This drug should be used more cautiously in those who are allergic to any ingredient in EpiPen.

What should I tell my doctor before I take the first dose of EpiPen?

Tell your doctor about all prescription, over-the-counter, and herbal medications you are taking before beginning treatment with EpiPen. Also, talk to your doctor about your complete medical history, especially if you have heart problems, thyroid problems, high blood pressure, angle-closure glaucoma, mental or mood disorders, asthma, depression, an irregular heartbeat, or diabetes. In addition, talk to your doctor if you are pregnant or plan on becoming pregnant.

What is the usual dosage?

The information below is based on the dosage guidelines your doctor uses. Depending on your condition and medical history, your doctor may prescribe a different regimen. Do not change the dosage or stop taking your medication without your doctor's approval.

Adults: The usual EpiPen dose for adults is 0.3 mg.

Children: The usual EpiPen dose for children is 0.15mg or 0.30 mg depending upon the body weight. (A dosage of 0.15mg may be more appropriate for patients weighing less than 30kg.) A dosage of 0.01mg per kilogram of body weight is appropriate.

How should I take EpiPen?

In case of emergency, inject this medication as directed by your doctor or a healthcare professional.

Check EpiPen regularly. Replace the injector unit if it contains particles, is discolored, or is cracked or damaged in any way.

Never put your thumb, fingers, or hand over the black tip of the auto-injector. Do NOT remove the gray activation cap until ready to use.

Directions for Use: Unscrew the yellow or green cap off of the EpiPen carrying case and remove the product from its storage tube. Grasp unit with the black tip pointing downward. Form fist around the unit (black tip down).

With your other hand, pull off the gray safety release. Hold black tip near outer thigh. Swing and jab firmly into outer thigh until it clicks so that the unit is perpendicular (at a 90° angle) to the thigh. (Auto-injector is designed to work through clothing.) Hold firmly against thigh for approximately 10 seconds. (The injection is now complete. Window on auto-injector will show red.)

Remove unit from thigh and massage injection area for 10 seconds. Call 911 and seek immediate medical attention.

Carefully place the used EpiPen (without bending the needle), needle-end first, into the storage tube of the carrying case that provides built-in needle protection after use. Then screw the cap of the storage tube back on completely, and take it with you to the hospital emergency room.

Inject EpiPen only into the outer thigh. Do not inject into the buttocks or into a vein.

Immediately after use, go to the nearest hospital emergency room. You may need further medical attention. Tell the doctor or healthcare provider that you have received an injection of epinephrine. Show the thigh where the injection was given. Give your used EpiPen to the doctor for inspection and proper disposal.

Keep this product, as well as syringes and needles, out of the reach of children and pets. Do not reuse needles, syringes, or other materials. Ask your healthcare provider how to dispose of these materials after use. Follow all local rules for disposal.

What should I avoid while taking EpiPen?
Avoid using solutions that are either discolored or cloudy. Do not inject anywhere else except your outer thigh.

Never put your thumb, fingers, or hand over the black tip of the auto-injector. Do NOT remove the gray activation cap until ready to use.

Do not reuse needles, syringes, or other materials.

What are possible food and drug interactions associated with EpiPen?
If EpiPen is used with certain other drugs, the effects of either could be increased, decreased, or altered. It is especially important to check with your doctor before combining EpiPen with the following: amitriptyline, amoxapine, bucindolol, carteolol, carvedilol, clomipramine, desipramine, dilevalol, dothiepin, doxepin, entacapone, halothane, imipramine,

levobunolol, linezolid, lofepramine, metipranolol, nadolol, nortriptyline, opipramol, oxprenolol, penbutolol, pindolol, propranolol, protriptyline, rocuronium, sotalol, tertatolol, timolol, and trimipramine.

What are the possible side effects of EpiPen?

Side effects cannot be anticipated. If any develop or change in intensity, tell your doctor as soon as possible. Only your doctor can determine if it is safe for you to continue taking this drug.

Side effects may include: sweating, nausea, vomiting, difficulty breathing, dizziness, weakness, tremors, headache, nervousness, anxiety, increased heart rate, palpitations, difficulty sleeping, fearfulness

Can I receive EpiPen if I am pregnant or breastfeeding?

The effects of EpiPen during pregnancy and breastfeeding are unknown. Talk to your healthcare provider if you are pregnant, plan to become pregnant or are breastfeeding due to the potential harm to the baby.

What should I do if I miss a dose of EpiPen?

If you miss a dose of EpiPen, contact your doctor right away.

How should I store EpiPen?

Keep the EpiPen nearby and ready for use at all times. Store at 25°C (77°F); excursions permitted to 15°C-30°C (59°F-86°F). Protect from light. Do NOT store in refrigerator. Do NOT expose to extreme cold or heat. For example, do NOT store in your vehicle's glove box. Keep out of the reach of children.

EPIVIR

Generic name: Lamivudine

What is Epivir?

Epivir is used to treat human immunodeficiency virus (HIV) infection. The drug is taken along with zidovudine, another HIV medication.

What is the most important information I should know about Epivir?

The Epivir/zidovudine combination does not completely eliminate HIV or totally restore the immune system. There is still a danger of serious infections; see your doctor regularly for monitoring and tests.

Epivir does not stop the spread of HIV to others through blood or sexual contact. Use barrier methods of birth control (eg, condoms) if you have HIV infection. Do not share needles, injection supplies, or items like toothbrushes or razors.

Epivir can cause an enlarged liver and the chemical imbalance known as lactic acidosis. This serious and sometimes fatal side effect is more likely in women, people who are overweight, and those who have been taking drugs such as Epivir for an extended period of time. Signs of lactic acidosis include fatigue, nausea, abdominal pain, and a feeling of un-wellness. Contact your doctor if you experience any of these symptoms. Treatment with Epivir may have to be discontinued.

Some people receiving drugs for HIV experience a redistribution of body fat, leading to extra fat around the middle, a hump on the back, and wasting in the arms, legs, and face. Researchers don't know whether this represents a long-term health problem or not.

Do not drive or perform other possibly unsafe tasks until you know how you react to Epivir; this medication may cause drowsiness or dizziness. These effects may be worse if you take it with alcohol or certain medicines.

Do not stop taking Epivir, even for a short period of time. If you do, the virus may grow resistant to the medicine and become harder to treat.

If you have the hepatitis B virus, your doctor will perform lab tests for several months after you stop taking Epivir. Some patients have experienced a worsening of the hepatitis B virus after stopping the use of Epivir. Tell your doctor about any new or unusual symptoms that you notice after stopping treatment with this medication.

Epivir contains sucrose and may affect your blood sugar. Check blood sugar levels closely. Ask your doctor before you change the dose of your diabetes medicine.

Who should not take Epivir?
Do not use Epivir if you are hypersensitive to Epivir or any of its ingredients.

What should I tell my doctor before I take the first dose of Epivir?
Tell your doctor about all prescription, over-the-counter, and herbal medication you are taking before beginning treatment with this drug. Also, talk to your doctor about your complete medical history, especially if you have a history of hepatitis B or liver problems, muscle problems, an abnormal blood cell count, kidney problems, diabetes, lactic acidosis, a nerve disorders, or pancreatitis.

What is the usual dosage?
The information below is based on the dosage guidelines your doctor uses. Depending on your condition and medical history, your doctor may prescribe a different regimen. Do not change the dosage or stop taking your medication without your doctor's approval.

Adults: The usual dose (either tablets or liquid) is 150 milligrams (mg) twice daily or 300 mg once a day. Your doctor may adjust the dosage if you have kidney problems or weigh less than 110 pounds.

Children 3 months to 16 years: The usual dose is 4 milligrams per 2.2 pounds of body weight twice a day, up to a maximum of 150 mg twice daily. The safety of Epivir in combination with antiretroviral drugs other than zidovudine has not been established in children.

DOSE ADJUSTMENT: It is recommended that the dose of Epivir be adjusted in accordance with a patient's kidney function. Tell your doctor if you have a history of kidney disease or problems with your kidneys so that the dose of this medication may be adjusted.

How should I take Epivir?

It's important to keep adequate levels of Epivir in your bloodstream at all times, so you need to keep taking this medication regularly, just as prescribed, even when you're feeling better. Epivir may be taken with or without food. Take Epivir at the same time each day.

What should I avoid while taking Epivir?

Do not drive or perform other possibly unsafe tasks until you know how you react to Epivir; this medication may cause drowsiness or dizziness. These effects may be worse if you take it with alcohol or certain medicines.

Do not stop taking Epivir, even for a short period of time. If you do, the virus may grow resistant to the medicine and become harder to treat.

Do not share needles, injection supplies, or items like toothbrushes or razors. Use barrier methods of birth control (eg, condoms) if you have HIV infection. Epivir does not stop the spread of HIV to others through blood or sexual contact.

What are possible food and drug interactions associated with Epivir?

Combining Epivir with the HIV drug zalcitabine is not recommended. Check with your doctor before combining Epivir with sulfamethoxazole and trimethoprim.

What are the possible side effects of Epivir?

Side effects cannot be anticipated. If any develop or change in intensity, inform your doctor as soon as possible. Only your doctor can determine if it is safe for you to continue taking Epivir.

Side effects may include: abdominal cramps and pains, allergic reaction, anemia, chills, cough, depression, diarrhea, dizziness, enlarged lymph nodes, enlarged spleen, fatigue, fever, general feeling of illness, hair loss, headache, hives, insomnia and other sleep problems, itching, joint pain, liver damage, lost appetite, mouth sores, muscle and bone pain, muscle weakness or wasting, nasal problems, nausea, pancreatitis, prickling or tingling sensation, skin rashes, stomach upset, vomiting, weakness, wheezing

Side effects in children may include: abnormal breathing sounds/wheezing; cough; diarrhea; ear problems; fever; mouth inflammation; nasal discharge; nausea; stuffy nose; swollen lymph nodes; vomiting

Epivir can cause an enlarged liver and the chemical imbalance known as lactic acidosis. This serious and sometimes fatal side effect is more likely in women, people who are overweight, and those who have been taking drugs such as Epivir for an extended period. Signs of lactic acidosis include fatigue, nausea, abdominal pain, and a feeling of unwellness. Contact your doctor if you experience any of these symptoms. Treatment with Epivir may have to be discontinued.

Can I receive Epivir if I am pregnant or breastfeeding?
The effects of Epivir during pregnancy have not been adequately studied, but there is reason to suspect some risk. If you are pregnant, plan to become pregnant, or are breastfeeding notify your doctor immediately. Mothers infected with HIV who are currently on Epivir should not breastfeed due to the risk of passing the HIV infection or the drug to the baby.

What should I do if I miss a dose of Epivir?
If you miss a dose of Epivir, take it as soon as possible. If it is within 2 hours of your next dose, skip the missed dose and go back to your regular dosing schedule. Do not take 2 doses at once.

How should I store Epivir?
Store Epivir at 77 degrees F (25 degrees C). Brief storage at temperatures between 59 and 86 degrees F (15 and 30 degrees C) is permitted. Store away from heat, moisture, and light. Do not store in the bathroom. Keep Epivir out of the reach of children.

Eplerenone *See Inspra, page 659.*

Eprosartan mesylate *See Teveten, page 1294.*

Eprosartan mesylate and hydrochlorothiazide
See Teveten HCT, page 1296.

EQUETRO
Generic name: Carbamazepine for bipolar disorder

What is Equetro?
Equetro is used to treat acute manic and mixed episodes of bipolar I disorder.
A mixed episode is when a manic episode occurs with a major depressive episode (depressed mood, loss of interest or pleasure in nearly all activities).

What is the most important information I should know about Equetro?

Patients with a history of adverse hematologic (blood) reaction to any drug may be particularly at risk of bone marrow depression.

Carbamazepine should not be used in patients with a history of hypersensitivity to the drug, or known sensitivity to any of the tricyclic compounds (such as amitriptyline, desipramine, imipramine, protriptyline, and nortriptyline). In rare cases, serious but fatal dermatological reactions may occur. Call your doctor immediately if you develop a rash after staring Equetro therapy.

Do not take Equetro at the same time as class of antidepressant medications called monoamine oxidase inhibitors (MAOIs). Before administration of carbamazepine, discontinue MAOIs for a minimum of 14 days, or longer if the clinical situation permits.

Do not begin treatment with Equetro if you are already being treated with a drug containing carbamazepine.

If stopped abruptly, Equetro may cause a seizure in epileptic people.

If you experience symptoms such as fever, sore throat, ulcers in the mouth, or easy bruising, contact your doctor immediately, as this may be a sign of a more serious side effect of Equetro.

Do not take Equetro if you are pregnant, plan to become pregnant, or nursing due to serious side effects associated with the drug.

Do not engage in activities that require mental alertness or coordination, such as operating machinery or driving, after taking Equetro until you know how the medication affects you.

Patients with increased intraocular pressure (glaucoma) should be closely observed during therapy.

Who should not take Equetro?

Do not use Equetro if you have had problems with your bone marrow, or if you are allergic to any ingredients.

Carbamazepine should not be used in patients with a history of known sensitivity to any of the tricyclic compounds (such as amitriptyline, desipramine, imipramine, protriptyline, and nortriptyline).

Anyone taking an MAOI should not take Equetro.

Do not take Equetro if you are pregnant, plan to become pregnant, or nursing due to serious side effects associated with the drug.

What should I tell my doctor before I take the first dose of Equetro?

Tell your doctor about all prescription, over-the-counter, and herbal medications you are taking before beginning treatment with Equetro. Also, talk to your doctor about your complete medical history, especially if you have a history of liver problems, seizure disorder, problems with your blood, increased ocular pressure (glaucoma), or if you are currently pregnant, plan on becoming pregnant, or are breastfeeding. In addition, you should tell your doctor if you are currently on or have been on an MAOI within the last 14 days, or if you have a known sensitivity to any of the tricyclic compounds (such as amitriptyline, desipramine, imipramine, protriptyline, and nortriptyline).

What is the usual dosage?

The information below is based on the dosage guidelines your doctor uses. Depending on your condition and medical history, your doctor may prescribe a different regimen. Do not change the dosage or stop taking your medication without your doctor's approval.

Adults: The usual dosage of Equetro is 400 milligrams (mg) per day usually given in divided doses of 200 mg two times a day. The dosage may be adjusted by 200 mg increments. The maximum dosage of this drug is 1600 mg/day.

How should I take Equetro?

Equetro capsules may be swallowed whole, or opened and sprinkled over food such as applesauce. Capsules may be taken with or without food. Do not crush or chew the capsules.

What should I avoid while taking Equetro?

Avoid potentially harmful activities, such as driving and operating machinery, until you see how Equetro affects you, as this drug may cause dizziness and blurred vision.

Equetro contains carbamazepine and should not be used in combination with any other medications containing carbamazepine

What are possible food and drug interactions associated with Equetro?

If Equetro is taken with certain other drugs, the effects of either could be increased, decreased, or altered. It is especially important to check with your doctor before combining Equetro with the following: acetaminophen, alprazolam, amitriptyline, bupropion, buspirone, citalopram, clobazam, clonazepam, clozapine, cyclosporine, delavirdine, desipramine, diazepam, dicumarol, doxycycline, ethosuximide, felbamate, felodipine, glucocorticoids, haloperidol, itraconazole, lamotrigine, levothyroxine, lorazepam, methadone, midazolam, mirtazapine, nortriptyline, olanzapine, oral contraceptives, oxcarbazepine, phenytoin, praziquantel, protease inhibitors, quetiapine, risperidone, theophylline, topiramate, tiagabine, tramadol, triazolam, trazodone, valproate, warfarin, ziprasidone, and zonisamide.

What are the possible side effects of Equetro?

Side effects cannot be anticipated. If any develop or change in intensity, tell your doctor as soon as possible. Only your doctor can determine if it is safe for you to continue taking this drug.

Side effects may include: blurred vision, dizziness, dry mouth, itchiness, muscle problems, nausea, speech problems, vomiting

Can I receive Equetro if I am pregnant or breastfeeding?
Do not take Equetro if you are pregnant, plan to become pregnant, or breastfeeding. This drug may cause severe problems during pregnancy, such as spina bifida (an opening in the fetus's spinal cord). Also, this drug may pass into breast milk and should not be used if you are breastfeeding.

How should I store Equetro?
Store at room temperature and keep away from light and moisture.

ERAXIS
Generic name: Anidulafungin

What is Eraxis?
Eraxis is used to treat fungal infections caused by *Candida,* including infections in the lining of the abdomen (intra-abdominal abscess and peritonitis) and throat infections.

What is the most important information I should know about Eraxis?
Eraxis is not a self-administered antifungal. This drug is most likely given in a hospital setting, by a doctor or nurse.

Do not drive or perform other possibly unsafe tasks until you know how you react to Eraxis; this drug may cause dizziness or blurred vision. These effects may worsen if you take Eraxis with alcohol or certain medicines.

Eraxis only works against fungus; it does not treat viral infections (eg, the common cold).

Who should not take Eraxis?
Do not take Eraxis if you are allergic to anidulafungin, any of its other ingredients, or if you have had sensitivity to other echinocandin antifungals (such as caspofungin) in the past.

What should I tell my doctor before I take the first dose of Eraxis?
Tell your doctor about all prescription, over-the-counter, and herbal medications you are taking to avoid a possible interaction with Eraxis. Also, talk to your doctor about your complete medical history before beginning treatment with Eraxis. In addition, tell your doctor if you are pregnant, plan to become pregnant, or are breastfeeding.

What is the usual dosage?

The information below is based on the dosage guidelines your doctor uses. Depending on your condition and medical history, your doctor may prescribe a different regimen. Do not change the dosage or stop taking your medication without your doctor's approval.

Candidemia and Most Candida Infections (abdominal)

Adults: The recommended dose for candidemia and most *Candida* infections is a single 200 milligram (mg) dose of Eraxis on day 1, followed by 100 mg daily dose thereafter. Duration of treatment should be based on the patient's clinical response. In general, treatment with Eraxis should continue for at least 14 days after the positive fungal test.

Esophageal (throat) Candidiasis

Adults: The recommended dose for throat infections is a single 100 mg loading dose of Eraxis on Day 1, followed by 50 mg daily dose thereafter. Treatment should continue for a minimum of 14 days and for at least 7 days following the last symptom.

How should I take Eraxis?

Eraxis will be administered by your doctor. To clear up your infection completely, use Eraxis for the full course of treatment. Keep using it even if you feel better in a few days.

What should I avoid while taking Eraxis?

Do not drive or perform other possibly unsafe tasks until you know how you react to Eraxis; this drug may cause dizziness or blurred vision. These effects may become worse if you take it with alcohol or certain medicines.

Keep using Eraxis even if you feel better in a few days.

Eraxis will be administered by your doctor, keep your regular doctor appointments.

What are possible food and drug interactions associated with Eraxis?

There have been no drug or food interactions which have been documented that interfere with Eraxis when given at the recommended dosing. However, it is important to discuss with your doctor all prescription and non-prescription medications and supplements that you are currently taking.

What are the possible side effects of Eraxis?

Side effects cannot be anticipated. If any develop or change in intensity, tell your doctor as soon as possible. Only your doctor can determine if it is safe for you to continue taking this drug.

Side effects may include: diarrhea, headache, nausea, rash, upset stomach, vomiting, swelling, redness at the injection site, dark urine, fever, chills, or persistent sore throat, irregular heartbeat, leg redness, pale stools, shortness of breath, unusual bruising or bleeding, yellowing of the skin or eyes, or sever allergic reactions (rash, hives, itching, tightness in the chest, swelling of the face, lips, or tongue)

Can I receive Eraxis if I am pregnant or breastfeeding?
If you are pregnant, planning to become pregnant, or are nursing, talk to your doctor before taking Eraxis. The effects of Eraxis on pregnancy are unknown, and it may pass into breast milk.

What should I do if I miss a dose of Eraxis?
If you miss a dose of Eraxis, use it as soon as possible. If it is almost time for your next dose, skip the missed dose and go back to your regular dosing schedule. Do not use 2 doses at once.

How should I store Eraxis?
Eraxis is usually handled and stored by a healthcare provider.

Ergotamine tartate and caffeine See *Cafergot, page 240*.

Erlotinib hydrochloride See *Tarceva, page 1259*.

Escitalopram oxalate See *Lexapro, page 734*.

Esomeprazole magnesium See *Nexium, page 879*.

Esterified estrogens and methyltestosterone See *Estratest/ Estratest H.S., page 504*.

ESTRACE
Generic name: Estradiol

What is Estrace?
Estrace is a medicine that contains estrogen hormones. It is used to reduce moderate to severe hot flashes associated with menopause. It is also used to treat dryness, itching and burning in the vaginal area. It may also be used to treat certain hormonal imbalances and certain cancers in men and women. Estrace may also be used to prevent the thinning of bones (osteoporosis).

What is the most important information I should know about Estrace?
Estrace may increase the chances of getting cancer of the uterus. Contact your doctor if vaginal bleeding of unknown cause occurs. This could be a sign of a serious condition requiring immediate medical attention.

Using Estrace with progestins may increase risk of dementia.

Do not use estrogens with or without progestins to prevent heart disease, heart attacks, or strokes. The use of Estrace with or without progestins may increase your chances of getting heart attacks, strokes, breast cancer and blood clots.

If you have high blood pressure, high cholesterol (fat in the blood), diabetes, are overweight, or if you use tobacco, you may have a higher chance of getting heart disease. Ask your healthcare provider for ways to lower your chances for getting heart disease.

Do not drive or perform other possibly unsafe tasks until you know how you react to Estrace; this medication may cause dizziness. This effect may be worse if you take it with alcohol or certain medicines.

Limit alcoholic beverages while you are taking Estrace.

Estrace may cause dark skin patches on your face (melasma). Exposure to the sun may make these patches darker and you may need to avoid prolonged sun exposure and sunlamps. Consult your doctor regarding the use of sunscreens and protective clothing.

Estrace may increase the risk of blood clots. The risk may be greater if you smoke (especially in women older than 35 years of age).

Contact your doctor if vaginal discomfort occurs or if you suspect you have developed an infection while taking Estrace.

Additional monitoring of your dose or condition may be necessary if you are presently taking an azole antifungal (eg, itraconazole), carbamazepine, a macrolide antibiotic (eg, erythromycin), ritonavir, cimetidine, or St. John's Wort.

If you wear contact lenses and you develop problems with them, contact your doctor.

If you will be having surgery or will be confined to a chair or bed for a long period of time (such as a long plane flight), notify your doctor beforehand. Special precautions may need to be taken in these circumstances while you are taking Estrace.

Estrace may interfere with certain lab tests. Be sure your doctor and lab personnel know you are taking Estrace

Some of these products may contain the dye tartrazine (FD&C Yellow No. 5), which can cause allergic reactions in certain patients. If you previously had allergic reactions to the dye tartrazine, contact your doctor or pharmacist to determine if the product you are taking contains the dye tartrazine.

Estrace may affect your blood sugar. Check blood sugar levels closely. Ask your doctor before you change the dose of your diabetes medicine.

Nonprescription therapy to help prevent bone loss in menopausal women includes a weight-bearing exercise plan, an adequate daily calcium and vitamin D intake. Consult your doctor or pharmacist for more details.

While you are using estrogens, it is important to visit your doctor at least once a year for a check-up.

Have a breast exam and mammogram (breast X-ray) every year unless your healthcare provider tells you something else. If members of your family have had breast cancer or if you have ever had breast lumps or an abnormal mammogram (breast x-ray), you may need to have more frequent breast examinations.

If you experience any of these warning signals (or any other unusual symptoms), call your doctor immediately: abnormal bleeding from the vagina; pain in the calves or chest, sudden shortness of breath, or coughing blood; sever headache or vomiting, dizziness, faintness, changes in vision or speech, weakness or numbness of an arm or leg; breast lumps; yellowing of the skin or eyes; pain, selling, or tenderness in the abdomen.

Who should not take Estrace?

Do not take Estrace if you have unusual vaginal bleeding that has not been evaluated by your doctor or if you currently have or have had certain cancers.

Do not take Estrace if you had a stroke or heart attack in the past year.

Do not take Estrace if you currently have or have had liver problems or blood clots.

Do not take Estrace if you are allergic to Estrace and its formulation.

Do not take Estrace if you have recently given birth, are breastfeeding, or if you think you are pregnant.

If you are going to have surgery of will be on bed rest you may need to stop taking Estrace.

Contact your doctor if you fit any of the previously mentioned circumstances and are currently taking Estrace.

What should I tell my doctor before I take the first dose of Estrace?

Tell your doctor about all prescription, over-the-counter, and herbal medications you are taking before beginning treatment with Estrace. Also, talk to your doctor about you complete medical history, especially if you have any heart problems, a family history of breast cancer, yellowing of the whites of the eyes or skin during pregnancy or with past estrogen use, have a vaginal infection or womb problems (uterine fibroids, endometriosis, or other uterine problems), asthma, a certain blood disorder (porphyria), cholesterol or lipid problems, depression, diabetes, excessive weight gain, gallbladder disease, high blood pressure, lupus, low thyroid hormone levels, migraine headaches, pancreas disease, seizures, if you smoke, currently have or have had kidney or liver problems in the past, and if you will be having surgery..In addition, tell your doctor if you are pregnant, plan on becoming pregnant, or are breastfeeding.

What is the usual dosage?

The information below is based on the dosage guidelines your doctor uses. Depending on your condition and medical history, your doctor

may prescribe a different regimen. Do not change the dosage or stop taking your medication without your doctor's approval.

When estrogen is prescribed for a postmenopausal woman with a uterus, a progestin should also be initiated to reduce the risk of endometrial cancer. A woman without a uterus does not need progestin. Use of estrogen, alone or in combination with a progestin, should be with the lowest effective dose and for the shortest duration consistent with treatment goals and risks for the individual woman.

Patients should be reevaluated periodically as clinically appropriate (3-month to 6-month intervals) to determine if treatment is still necessary. For women who have a uterus, adequate diagnostic measures, such as endometrial sampling, when indicated, should be undertaken to rule out malignancy in cases of undiagnosed persistent or recurring abnormal vaginal bleeding.

Prevention of Osteoporosis
Adults: Use the lowest dose approved by your doctor.

Treatment of Advanced Androgen-Dependent Carcinoma of the Prostate
Adults: The usual dose is 1 to 2 mg three times daily.

Treatment of Breast Cancer
Adults: The usual dose is 10 mg three times daily for a period of at least three months.

Treatment of Female Decreased Estrogen Due to Hypogonadism, Castration, or Primary Ovarian Failure
Adults: The usual dose is 1 to 2 mg daily, to be adjusted after monitoring.

Treatment of Moderate to Severe Vasomotor Symptoms, Vulval and Vaginal Atrophy Associated with Menopause
Adults: The usual dose is 1 to 2 mg daily of Estrace. Administration should be cyclic (e.g. 3 weeks on and 1 week off). Attempts to discontinue or taper medication should be made after 3 month and 6 month intervals.

How should I take Estrace?

Start at the lowest dose and follow-up with the doctor to see how well that dose is working for you. You should see your doctor every 3 to 6 months to reevaluate dosing.

Take Estrace by mouth with or without food. If stomach upset occurs, take with food to reduce the stomach irritation.

Grapefruit and grapefruit juice may increase the risk of this drug's side effects. Talk to your doctor before including grapefruit or grapefruit juice into you diet while you are taking Estrace.

While you are using estrogens, it is important to visit your doctor at least once a year for a check-up.

What should I avoid while taking Estrace?

Do not miss your doctor appointments as they are important in evaluating your therapy. Also, do not miss or increase dose of Estrace without consulting with your doctor. Avoid giving Estrace to other people.

Do not use estrogens with or without progestins to prevent heart disease, heart attacks, or strokes.

Do not drive or perform other possibly unsafe tasks until you know how you react to Estrace; this medication may cause dizziness.

Limit alcoholic beverages while you are taking Estrace.

Avoid prolonged sun exposure and sunlamps. Estrace may cause dark skin patches on your face (melasma); exposure to the sun may make these patches darker.

What are possible food and drug interactions associated with Estrace?

If Estrace is taken with certain other drugs, the effects of either could be increased, decreased, or altered. It is especially important to check with your doctor before combining Estrace with the following: clarithromycin, ginseng, itraconazole, ketoconazole, levothyroxine, licorice, phenobarbital, phenytoin, prednisone, rifampin, St Johns Wort, succinylcholine, tacrine, tipranavir, and warfarin.

What are the possible side effects of Estrace?

Side effects cannot be anticipated. If any develop or change in intensity, tell your doctor as soon as possible. Only your doctor can determine if it is safe for you to continue taking this drug.

Side effects may include: headache, breast pain, spotting or breakthrough bleeding, abdominal cramps/bloating, nausea, vomiting, hair loss, darkening of skin, fluid retention, high blood pressure, back pain, dark urine, depression, dizziness, fainting, memory problems, mental or mood changes, muscle pain, painful or difficult urination

If you experience any of these warning signals (or any other unusual symptoms), call your doctor immediately: abnormal bleeding from the vagina; pain in the calves or chest, sudden shortness of breath, or coughing blood; sever headache or vomiting, dizziness, faintness, changes in vision or speech, weakness or numbness of an arm or leg; breast lumps; yellowing of the skin or eyes; pain, selling, or tenderness in the abdomen.

Can I receive Estrace if I am pregnant or breastfeeding?

You should not use Estrace if you are pregnant, plan on becoming pregnant or breastfeeding due to potential harm to the baby. If you are or will be breastfeeding while using Estrace, check with your doctor to discuss any possible risks to your baby. (Estrace may be found in breast milk.)

What should I do if I miss a dose of Estrace?

If you miss a dose, take it as soon as you remember with food. If it is close to the time of your next dose, skip it and resume your scheduled dose. Do not double up.

How should I store Estrace?

Store Estrace at room temperature, 59 to 86 degrees F (15 to 30 degrees C), in a tight, light-resistant container. Store away from heat, moisture, and light. Do not store in your bathroom. Keep Estrace out of the reach of children.

Estradiol *See Estrace, page 495; Estrasorb, below; Estring, page 508; EstroGel, page 513; Estrogen patches, page 517; or Vagifem, page 1362.*

Estradiol and levonorgestrel transdermal system *See Climara Pro, page 304.*

Estradiol and norethindrone acetate *See CombiPatch, page 324.*

Estradiol gel *See Elestrin, page 470.*

ESTRASORB
Generic name: Estradiol

What is Estrasorb?

Estrasorb is a medicine that contains the hormone estrogen. It is used to reduce hot flashes associated with menopause.

It is also used to treat dryness, itching and burning in the vaginal area. These symptoms may occur when estrogen levels drop during menopause.

What is the most important information I should know about Estrasorb?

Estrogens increase the chances of getting cancer of the uterus. Report any unusual vaginal bleeding right away while you are using Estrasorb. Vaginal bleeding after menopause may be a warning sign of cancer of the uterus.

When estrogen is prescribed for a postmenopausal woman with a uterus, progestin should also be initiated to reduce the risk of endometrial cancer. A woman without a uterus does not need progestin.

Use of estrogen, alone or in combination with a progestin, should be with the lowest effective dose and for the shortest duration consistent with treatment goals and risks for the individual women. Patients should be re-evaluated periodically as clinically appropriate (at 3 to 6-month intervals) to determine if treatment is still necessary.

For women with a uterus, adequate diagnostic measures, such as endometrial sampling, when indicated, should be undertaken to rule out malignancy in cases of undiagnosed persistent or recurring abnormal vaginal bleeding

Do not use estrogens with or without progestins to prevent heart disease, heart attacks, strokes or dementia. Using estrogens with or without progestins may increase your chances of getting heart attacks, strokes, breast cancer, and blood clots.

Using estrogens with or without progestins may increase your risk of dementia.

If you have high blood pressure, high cholesterol (fat in the blood), diabetes, are overweight, or if you use tobacco, you may have a higher risk of developing heart disease. Ask your healthcare provider for ways to lower your risk for heart disease.

Do not drive or perform other possibly unsafe tasks until you know how you react to Estrasorb; this medication may cause dizziness. This effect may be worse if you take it with alcohol or certain medicines.

Limit alcoholic beverages while you are taking Estrasorb.

Estrasorb may cause dark skin patches on your face (melasma). Exposure to the sun may make these patches darker; you may need to avoid prolonged sun exposure and sunlamps. Consult your doctor regarding the use of sunscreens and protective clothing.

Estrasorb may increase the risk of blood clots. This risk may be greater if you smoke (especially in women older than 35 years of age).

Contact your doctor if vaginal discomfort occurs or if you suspect you have developed an infection while taking Estrasorb.

If you wear contact lenses and you develop problems with them, tell your doctor.

If you will be having surgery or will be confined to a chair or bed for a long period of time (such as a long plane flight), notify your doctor beforehand. Special precautions may need to be taken in these circumstances while you are taking Estrasorb.

Estrasorb may interfere with certain lab tests. Be sure your doctor and lab personnel know you are taking Estrasorb.

Estrasorb may affect your blood sugar. Check blood sugar levels closely and discuss with your doctor before changing the dose of your diabetes medicine.

Have a breast exam and mammogram (breast X-ray) every year unless your healthcare provider directs you to do differently. If members of your family have had breast cancer or if you have ever had breast lumps or an abnormal mammogram (breast x-ray), you may need to have more frequent breast examinations.

Estrasorb is an emulsion that is applied each day to the skin of both thighs and calves. It is not known if Estrasorb will be absorbed as well if applied to other parts of the body.

Estrasorb is packaged in foil pouches. Do not open the pouches until just before you apply Estrasorb.

Who should not take Estrasorb?

Do not take Estrasorb if you are allergic to any of its ingredients.

Hormone therapy should not be started if you have unusual vaginal bleeding and if you currently have or have had certain cancers. If you have had cancer, talk with your healthcare provider about whether you should use Estrasorb.

Also, do not take this drug if you have had a stroke or heart attack in the past year, currently have or have had blood clots, or think you may be pregnant.

What should I tell my doctor before I take the first dose of Estrasorb?

Tell your doctor about all prescription, over-the-counter, and herbal medications you are taking before beginning treatment with Estrasorb. Also, talk to your doctor about your complete medical history, especially if you have a family history of breast cancer; have yellowing of the whites of the eyes or skin during pregnancy or with past estrogen use; have a vaginal infection or uterine problems (fibroids, endometriosis, or other uterine problems); asthma; a certain blood disorder (porphyria); cholesterol or lipid problems; depression; diabetes; excessive weight gain; gallbladder disease; high blood pressure; lupus; low thyroid hormone levels; migraine headaches; pancreas disease; seizures; if you smoke; currently have or have had kidney or liver problems in the past; and if you will be having surgery. In addition, tell your doctor if you are pregnant, plan to become pregnant, or are breastfeeding.

What is the usual dosage?

The information below is based on the dosage guidelines your doctor uses. Depending on your condition and medical history, your doctor may prescribe a different regimen. Do not change the dosage or stop taking your medication without your doctor's approval.

Adults: The usual dosage of Estrasorb is 3.48 grams daily.

If you are switching from oral estrogen to Estrasorb (an emulsion) stop taking the oral estrogen and wait 1 week before using Estrasorb. However, if symptoms return, you may start using Estrasorb sooner.

How should I take Estrasorb?

Apply Estrasorb in the morning. If you shower or take a bath, be sure your skin is dry before applying this medication.

Do not apply Estrasorb to any skin on your thighs and calves that appears to be red or irritated.

Do not apply sunscreen and Estrasorb at the same time because sunscreen may affect the amount of estradiol you absorb.

Allow the cream to be absorbed before putting on any clothing. Do not open the pouches until just before you apply Estrasorb.

Estrasorb should be applied in a comfortable sitting position to clean, dry skin on both legs each morning. Each foil-laminated pouch of Estrasorb should be opened individually. Cut or tear the first foil-laminated pouch at the notches indicated near the top of the pouch.

Apply the emulsion in the pouch to the top of the left thigh, being careful to push the entire contents from the bottom through the neck of the pouch. Using one hand or both hands, rub the emulsion into the entire left thigh and left calf for three minutes until thoroughly absorbed. Rub any excess material remaining on both hands on the buttocks.

Cut or tear the second foil-laminated pouch at the notches indicated near the top of the pouch. Apply the emulsion in the pouch to the top of the right thigh, being careful to push the entire contents from the bottom through the neck of the pouch. Using one hand or both hands rub the emulsion into the entire right thigh and right calf for three minutes until thoroughly absorbed. Rub any excess material remaining on both hands on the buttocks.

Allow the application areas to dry completely before covering with clothing to avoid transfer to other individuals. On completion of Estrasorb application, both hands should be washed with soap and water to remove any residual estradiol.

What should I avoid while taking Estrasorb?

After applying Estrasorb, avoid coming into contact with other people before washing your hands.

Do not open the pouches until just before you apply Estrasorb.

Do not apply Estrasorb to any skin on your thighs and calves that appears to be red or irritated.

Do not apply sunscreen and Estrasorb at the same time because sunscreen may affect the amount of estradiol you absorb.

Grapefruit and grapefruit juice may increase the risk of Estrasorb's side effects. Talk to your doctor before including grapefruit or grapefruit juice in your diet while you are taking Estrasorb.

What are possible food and drug interactions associated with Estrasorb?

If Estrasorb is taken with certain other drugs, the effects of either could be increased, decreased, or altered. It is especially important to check with your doctor before combining Estrasorb with the following: carbamazepine, clarithromycin, ginseng, itraconazole, ketoconazole, levothyroxine, licorice, phenobarbital, phenytoin, prednisone, rifampin, St Johns Wort, succinylcholine, tacrine, tipranavir, and warfarin.

What are the possible side effects of Estrasorb?
Side effects cannot be anticipated. If any develop or change in intensity, tell your doctor as soon as possible. Only your doctor can determine if it is safe for you to continue taking this drug.

Side effects may include: breast pain, hair loss, headache, irregular vaginal bleeding or spotting, nausea and vomiting, skin irritation/redness/rash, stomach/abdominal cramps/bloating

Warning signs of serious side effects: breast lumps, calf or leg swelling, changes in speech, changes in vision, chest pain, depression, dizziness and faintness, fever, memory problems, mental or mood changes, pains in your legs, severe headaches, shortness of breath, unusual vaginal bleeding, vomiting

Can I receive Estrasorb if I am pregnant or breastfeeding?
You should not use Estrasorb if you are pregnant, plan on becoming pregnant, or breastfeeding due to potential harm to the baby. If you are or will be breastfeeding while using Estrasorb, check with your doctor to discuss any possible risks to your baby. (Estrasorb may be found in breast milk.)

What should I do if I miss a dose of Estrasorb?
If you miss a dose of Estrasorb, use it as soon as possible. If it is almost time for your next dose, skip the missed dose and go back to your regular dosing schedule. Do not use 2 doses at once.

How should I store Estrasorb?
Store Estrasorb at room temperature, between 59 and 86 degrees F (15 and 30 degrees C). Store in original packaging until just before use. Store away from heat, moisture, and light. Do not store in the bathroom. Keep Estrasorb out of the reach of children.

ESTRATEST/ESTRATEST H.S.
Generic name: Esterified estrogens and methyltestosterone

What is Estratest/Estratest H.S.?
Estratest/Estratest H.S. is used to ease some symptoms of menopause, such as moderate to severe hot flashes (feelings of warmth in the face, neck, and chest, or sudden strong feelings of heat and sweating) and the burning, itching, and severe dryness in and around the vagina.

**What is the most important information
I should know about Estratest/Estratest H.S.?**

Estrogens increase the chances of getting cancer of the uterus. Tell your doctor about any unusual vaginal bleeding right away while you are taking estrogens. Vaginal bleeding after menopause may be a warning sign of cancer of the uterus. Your doctor should check any unusual vaginal bleeding to find out the cause.

When estrogen is prescribed for a postmenopausal woman with a uterus, a progestin should also be initiated to reduce the risk of endometrial cancer. A woman without a uterus does not need progestin. Use of estrogen, alone or in combination with a progestin, should be with the lowest effective dose and for the shortest duration consistent with treatment goals and risks for the individual woman. Patients should be reevaluated periodically as clinically appropriate (such as every 3 to 6-months) to determine if treatment is still necessary.

For women who have a uterus, adequate diagnostic measures, such as endometrial sampling, when indicated, should be undertaken to rule out malignancy in cases of undiagnosed persistent or recurring abnormal vaginal bleeding.

Do not use estrogens with or without progestins to prevent heart disease, heart attacks, or strokes. Using estrogens with or without progestins may increase your chances of getting heart attacks, high blood pressure, strokes, breast cancer, and blood clots. Using estrogens with progestins may increase your risk of dementia. You and your healthcare provider should talk regularly about whether you still need treatment with Estratest/Estratest H.S.

If you have high blood pressure, high cholesterol (fat in the blood), diabetes, are overweight, or if you use tobacco, you may have a higher risk of developing heart disease. Ask your healthcare provider for ways to lower your risk for heart disease.

Do not drive or perform other possibly unsafe tasks until you know how you react to Estratest; this medication may cause dizziness. This effect may be worse if you take it with alcohol or certain medicines.

Limit alcoholic beverages while you are taking Estratest.

Estratest may cause dark skin patches on your face (melasma). Exposure to the sun may make these patches darker; you may need to avoid prolonged exposure to the sun, sunlamps, and tanning beds. Consult your doctor regarding the use of sunscreens and protective clothing.

If you will be having surgery or will be confined to a chair or bed for a long period of time (such as a long plane flight), notify your doctor 3 to 4 weeks in advance. Special precautions may need to be taken in these circumstances while you are taking Estratest.

Have a breast exam and mammogram (breast X-ray) every year unless your healthcare provider directs you to do differently. If members of your family have had breast cancer or if you have ever had breast lumps or an abnormal mammogram (breast x-ray), you may need to have more frequent breast examinations.

You and your healthcare provider should talk regularly (for example, every 3 to 6 months) about the dose you are taking and whether you still need treatment with Estratest.

Who should not take Estratest/Estratest H.S.?

Do not start taking Estratest/Estratest H.S. if you have unusual vaginal bleeding, or if you currently have or have had certain cancers. Estrogens may increase the risk of developing certain types of cancers, including cancer of the breast or uterus.

Do not take Estratest if you had a stroke or heart attack in the past year.

Do not take Estratest if you currently have or have had blood clots or liver problems.

Do not take Estratest if you think you may be pregnant.

Do not take this drug if you are allergic to any of its ingredients.

What should I tell my doctor before
I take the first dose of Estratest/Estratest H.S.?

Tell your doctor about all prescription, over-the-counter, and herbal medications you are taking before beginning treatment with Estratest/Estratest H.S. Also, talk to your doctor about your complete medical history, especially if you have experienced asthma (wheezing); epilepsy (seizures); migraine; gall bladder disease; inflammation of the pancreas; diabetes; high cholesterol, lipids, or triglycerides; endometriosis; lupus; or problems with your heart, liver, thyroid, or kidneys.

If you are breastfeeding, tell your doctor before beginning treatment with this drug.

What is the usual dosage?

The information below is based on the dosage guidelines your doctor uses. Depending on your condition and medical history, your doctor may prescribe a different regimen. Do not change the dosage or stop taking your medication without your doctor's approval.

Adults: The usual dosage is 1 tablet of Estratest or 1 to 2 tablets of Estratest H.S. daily. Administration should be cyclic, for example, three weeks on and one week off.

How should I take Estratest/Estratest H.S.?

Take Estratest/Estratest H.S. by mouth with or without food.

This medication can be taken alone or in combination with progestin. If you do not have a uterus, there is no need to take progestin with Estratest/Estratest H.S.

Estrogens should be used at the lowest dose possible for your treatment and only as long as needed. You and your healthcare provider should talk regularly (for example, every 3 to 6 months) about the dose you are taking and whether you still need treatment with Estratest/ Estratest H.S.

What should I avoid while taking Estratest/Estratest H.S.?

Do not use estrogens with or without progestins to prevent heart disease, heart attacks, or stroke.

Do not drive or perform other possibly unsafe tasks until you know how you react to Estratest; this medication may cause dizziness.

Limit alcoholic beverages while you are taking Estratest.

Avoid prolonged exposure to sun, sunlamps, and tanning beds. Estratest may cause dark skin patches on your face (melasma); exposure to the sun may make these patches darker.

What are possible food and drug interactions associated with Estratest/Estratest H.S.?

If Estratest/Estratest H.S. is taken with certain other drugs, the effects of either could be increased, decreased, or altered. It is especially important to check with your doctor before combining Estratest with the following: anticoagulants such as warfarin, carbamazepine, cyclosporine, hydrocortisone, insulin, macrolide, oxyphenbutazone, phenobarbital, phenytoin, rifampin, succinylcholine, tacrolimus, and tricyclic antidepressants such as amitriptyline.

What are the possible side effects of Estratest/Estratest H.S.?

Side effects cannot be anticipated. If any develop or change in intensity, tell your doctor as soon as possible. Only your doctor can determine if it is safe for you to continue taking this drug.

Side effects may include: abnormal skin sensation, acne, bloating, breast enlargement, breast pain, changes in sex drive, fluid retention, hair loss, headache, irregular vaginal bleeding/spotting, stomach cramps/ nausea, deepening of voice, spotty dark patches on the face, unusual body hair growth or body movements

Serious side effects may include: breast lumps, changes in speech, changes in vision, chest pain, dizziness, leg pain, severe headaches, shortness of breath, unusual vaginal bleeding, vomiting

Can I receive Estratest/Estratest H.S. if I am pregnant or breastfeeding?

Estratest/Estratest H.S. should not be used during pregnancy. Tell your doctor immediately if you are pregnant or plan to become pregnant.

If you are or will be breastfeeding while using Estratest, check with your doctor to discuss any possible risks to your baby. (Estratest has been found in breast milk.)

What should I do if I miss a dose of Estratest/Estratest H.S.?

If you miss a dose of Estratest, take it as soon as possible that same day. If it is almost time for your next dose or it is the next day, skip the missed dose and go back to your regular dosing schedule. Do not take 2 doses at once.

How should I store Estratest/Estratest H.S.?

Store Estratest/Estratest H.S. at room temperature, between 59 and 86 degrees F (15 and 30 degrees C). Store away from heat, moisture, and light. Do not store in the bathroom. Keep Estratest out of the reach of children.

ESTRING

Generic name: Estradiol

What is Estring?

Estring is a type of estrogen therapy used to relieve vaginal and urinary symptoms that occur when there is no estrogen in a woman's body after menopause.

What is the most important information I should know about Estring?

Estrogens, as those found in Estring, may increase the risk of cancer of the uterus in post-menopausal women. Contact your healthcare provider if you experience vaginal bleeding of unknown cause.

Estrogens should not be used during pregnancy. Estrogens do not prevent miscarriage (spontaneous abortion) and are not needed in the days following childbirth. If you take estrogens during pregnancy, your unborn child has a greater than usual chance of having birth defects. The risk of developing these defects is small, but greater than the risk in children whose mothers did not take estrogens during pregnancy. These birth defects may affect the baby's urinary system and sex organs.

Do not use estrogens with or without progestins to prevent heart disease, heart attacks, stroke or dementia. Using estrogens with or without progestins may increase your chances of getting heart attacks, stroke, breast cancer, and blood clots. Also, using estrogens with or without progestins may increase your risk of dementia.

Toxic shock syndrome (TSS) has been reported in a few patients using vaginal rings. TSS is a rare but serious and sometimes fatal condition. Symptoms of TSS may include fever nausea, vomiting, diarrhea, muscle pain, dizziness or lightheadedness, fainting, or a sunburn-like rash. Tell your doctor right away if you notice these effects.

If you have high blood pressure, high cholesterol (fat in the blood), diabetes, are overweight, or if you use tobacco, you may have a higher chance for developing heart disease. Ask your healthcare provider for ways to lower your risk for heart disease.

It will take about 2 to 3 weeks to restore the tissue of the vagina and urinary tract to a healthier condition and to feel the full effect of Estring in relieving vaginal and urinary symptoms. If your symptoms persist for more than a few weeks after beginning Estring therapy, contact your doctor or healthcare provider.

Do not drive or perform other possibly unsafe tasks until you know how you react to Estring; this drug may cause dizziness. This effect may be worse if you take it with alcohol or certain medicines.

Limit alcoholic beverages while you are using Estring.

Estring may cause dark skin patches on your face (melasma). Exposure to the sun may make these patches darker and you may need to avoid prolonged exposure to sun, sunlamps, and tanning beds. Consult your doctor regarding the use of sunscreens and protective clothing.

Estring may increase the risk of blood clots (especially in women older than 35 years). The risk may be greater if you smoke.

Contact your healthcare provider if vaginal discomfort occurs or if you suspect you have developed an infection while taking Estring.

If you wear contact lenses and you develop problems with them, contact your doctor.

If you will be having surgery or will be confined to a chair or bed for a long period of time (such as a long plane flight), notify your doctor beforehand. Special precautions may need to be taken in these circumstances while you are taking Estring.

Your doctor should reevaluate you every 3 to 6 months to determine whether or not you need to continue taking Estring.

Estring may interfere with certain lab tests. Be sure your doctor and lab personnel know you are using Estring.

Estring may affect your blood sugar. Check blood sugar levels closely and discuss with your doctor before changing the dose of your diabetes medicine.

Have a breast exam and mammogram (breast X-ray) every year unless your healthcare provider tells you something else. If members of your family have had breast cancer or if you have ever had breast lumps or an abnormal mammogram, you may need to have breast examinations more often.

One of the most frequently reported effects associated with the use of Estring is an increase in vaginal secretions. These secretions are like those that occur normally prior to menopause and indicate that Estring is working. However, if the secretions are associated with a bad odor or vaginal itching or discomfort, be sure to contact your doctor or healthcare provider.

Most women and their partners experience no discomfort with Estring in place during intercourse, so it is NOT necessary that the ring be removed before intercourse. If Estring should cause you or your partner any discomfort, you may remove it prior to intercourse. Be sure to reinsert Estring as soon as possible afterwards.

There have been rare reports of Estring falling out in some women following intense straining or coughing. If this should occur, simply wash Estring with lukewarm (NOT hot) water and reinsert it.

Estring may slide down into the lower part of the vagina as a result of the abdominal pressure or straining that sometimes accompanies constipation. If this should happen, gently guide Estring back into place with your finger.

Who should not take Estring?

Estring should not be used if you are pregnant, plan to become pregnant, or breastfeeding. This therapy may cause birth defects in your child. Also, do not use Estring if you have unusual vaginal bleeding, or a history of certain types of cancer (eg, breast or uterine).

Do not use Estring if you currently have or have had blood clots. Do not use Estring if you have had a stroke or heart attack within the past year. Do not use Estring if you have known liver disease. In addition, do not use Estring if you have a known hypersensitivity to any of the ingredients found in this product.

What should I tell my doctor before I take the first dose of Estring?

Tell your doctor about all prescription, over-the-counter, and herbal medications you are taking before beginning therapy with Estring. Also, talk to your doctor about your complete medical history, especially if you have had cancer of the breast(s) or uterus; abnormal vaginal bleeding; yellowing of the eyes or skin during pregnancy or with past estrogen use; have a vaginal infection or womb problems (uterine fibroids, endometriosis, or other uterine problems); asthma; a certain blood disorder (porphyria); cholesterol or lipid problems; depression; diabetes; excessive weight gain; gallbladder disease; high blood pressure; lupus; low thyroid hormone levels; migraine headaches; pancreas disease; seizures; if you smoke; currently have or have had kidney or liver problems in the past; and if you will be having surgery. In addition, tell your doctor if you are pregnant, plan on becoming pregnant, or are breastfeeding.

What is the usual dosage?

The information below is based on the dosage guidelines your doctor uses. Depending on your condition and medical history, your doctor may prescribe a different regimen. Do not change the dosage or stop taking your medication without your doctor's approval.

Estring should be inserted into the vagina and left in place for 90 days. After this time, if it is necessary, Estring should be replaced. Estring can be inserted and removed by you or your doctor or healthcare provider.

Estrogens should be used only as long as needed. You and your health-care provider should talk regularly (for example, every 3 to 6 months) about whether you still need treatment with Estring.

It will take about 2 to 3 weeks to restore the tissue of the vagina and urinary tract to a healthier condition and to feel the full effect of Estring in relieving vaginal and urinary symptoms. If your symptoms persist for more than a few weeks after beginning Estring therapy, contact your doctor or healthcare provider.

How should I take Estring?

To insert Estring, choose the position that is most comfortable for you: standing with one leg up, squatting, or lying down.

After washing and drying your hands, remove Estring from its pouch using the tear-off notch on the side. (Since the ring becomes slippery when wet, be sure your hands are dry before handling it.)

Hold Estring between your thumb and index finger and press the opposite sides of the ring together; the ring should be pressed into an oval. Gently push the compressed ring into your vagina as far as you can. The exact position is not critical as long as it is placed in the upper third of the vagina.

Wash your hands immediately after using Estring.

When Estring is in place, you should not feel anything. If you feel discomfort, Estring is probably not far enough inside. Gently push it further into the vagina. There is no danger of Estring being pushed too far up in the vagina or getting lost. Estring can only be inserted as far as the end of the vagina, where the cervix (the narrow, lower end of the uterus) will block Estring from going any further.

Estring may slide down into the lower part of the vagina as a result of the abdominal pressure or straining that sometimes accompanies constipation. If this should happen, gently guide Estring back into place with your finger.

After 90 days there will no longer be enough estradiol in the ring to maintain its full effect in relieving your vaginal or urinary symptoms. Estring should be removed at that time and replaced with a new Estring, if your doctor determines that you need to continue your therapy.

To remove Estring, wash and dry your hands thoroughly. Assume a comfortable position, either standing with one leg up, squatting, or lying down.

Loop (or hook) your finger through the ring and gently pull it out. Discard the used ring in a waste receptacle. (Do not flush Estring.)

What should I avoid while taking Estring?

Do not miss your doctor appointments as they are important in evaluating your therapy. Avoid giving Estring to other people.

Do not use estrogens with or without progestins to prevent heart disease, heart attacks, or strokes.

Do not drive or perform other possibly unsafe tasks until you know how you react to Estring; this medication may cause dizziness.

Limit alcoholic beverages while you are taking Estring.

Avoid prolonged sun exposure and sunlamps because Estring may cause dark skin patches on your face (melasma); exposure to the sun may make these patches darker.

What are possible food and drug interactions associated with Estring?

If Estring is taken with certain other drugs, the effects of either could be increased, decreased, or altered. It is especially important to check with your doctor before combining Estring with the following: anticoagulants (blood thinning medications) such as warfarin; azole antifungals such as ketoconazole; erythromycin; phenobarbital; phenytoin; prednisone; rifampin; ritonavir; succinylcholine; and tacrine.

What are the possible side effects of Estring?

Side effects cannot be anticipated. If any develop or change in intensity, tell your doctor as soon as possible. Only your doctor can determine if it is safe for you to continue taking this drug.

Side effects may include: bloating (water retention), breast tenderness/ enlargement, hair loss, headache, nausea, spotty darkening of skin on the face, vomiting

Serious side effects may include: abnormal vaginal bleeding, breast lumps, changes in vision or speech, coughing blood, dizziness, faintness, pain in the lower legs or chest, pain/swelling/tenderness of the stomach, severe headache, shortness of breath, vomiting, weakness/numbness of arm(s) or leg(s)

Can I receive Estring if I am pregnant or breastfeeding?

Do not use Estring if you are pregnant, plan to become pregnant, or are breastfeeding.

What should I do if I miss a dose of Estring?

If you forget and have not inserted a new ring after 90 days, contact your doctor to establish a new schedule for Estring.

How should I store Estring?

Store Estring at room temperature, between 59 and 86 degrees F (15 and 30 degrees C). Store in the original packaging until just before use. Store away from heat, moisture, and light. Do not store in the bathroom. Keep Estring out of the reach of children.

ESTROGEL
Generic name: Estradiol

What is EstroGel?
EstroGel is used to ease some symptoms of menopause, such as moderate to severe hot flashes (feelings of warmth in the face, neck, and chest, or sudden strong feelings of heat and sweating) and the burning, dryness, and itching in/around the vagina.

What is the most important information I should know about EstroGel?
Estrogens, such as those found in EstroGel, increase the risk for developing cancer of the uterus. Contact your doctor if vaginal bleeding of unknown cause occurs.

Do not use estrogens with or without progestins to prevent heart disease, heart attacks, stroke, or dementia. Using estrogens with or without progestins may increase your risk for heart attack, strokes, breast cancer, dementia, and blood clots.

When estrogen is prescribed for a postmenopausal woman with an intact uterus, a progestin should also be initiated to reduce the risk of endometrial cancer. A woman without a uterus does not need progestin. Use of estrogen, alone or in combination with a progestin, should be limited to the shortest duration consistent with treatment goals and risks for the individual woman.

Patients should be reevaluated periodically as clinically appropriate (such as at 3 to 6-month intervals) to determine if treatment is still necessary. For women who have an intact uterus, adequate diagnostic measures, such as endometrial sampling, when indicated, should be undertaken to rule out malignancy in cases of undiagnosed persistent or recurring abnormal vaginal bleeding.

If you have high blood pressure, high cholesterol (fat in the blood), diabetes, are overweight, or if you use tobacco, you may have a greater risk of developing heart disease. Ask your healthcare provider for ways to lower your risk for heart disease.

If someone else is exposed to EstroGel by direct contact with the gel, that person should wash the area of contact with soap and water as soon as possible. The longer the gel is in contact with the skin before washing, the greater the chance that the other person will absorb some of the estrogen hormone. (This caution is especially important for men and children.)

EstroGel is for external use only. Do not get it in your eyes, nose, vagina, or mouth. If you get it in any of these areas, rinse right away with warm clean water. Seek medical attention if needed.

Check with your doctor before you apply sunscreen to the application site while using EstroGel. If you will be swimming, wait for as long as possible after applying EstroGel before going into the water.

EstroGel is flammable. Avoid fire, flame, or smoking until the medicine has dried on your skin.

Eating grapefruit or drinking grapefruit juice may increase the risk of EstroGel side effects. Talk to your doctor before including grapefruit or grapefruit juice in your diet while you are taking EstroGel.

Tell your doctor or dentist that you take EstroGel before you receive any medical or dental care, emergency care, or surgery. If possible, EstroGel should be stopped at least 4 to 6 weeks before surgery or any time you might be confined to a bed or chair for a long period of time (such as a long plane flight, car ride, bed-rest, or illness).

EstroGel may cause dark patches of skin on your face. Exposure to the sun may make these patches darker. If patches develop, use sunscreen or wear protective clothing when exposed to the sun, sunlamps, or tanning booths.

If you wear contact lenses and you develop problems with them, tell your doctor.

EstroGel may affect your blood sugar. Check blood sugar levels closely and discuss with your doctor before changing the dose of your diabetes medicine.

EstroGel may interfere with certain lab tests. Be sure your doctor and lab personnel know you are using EstroGel.

Have a breast exam and mammogram (breast X-ray) every year unless your healthcare provider directs you differently. If members of your family have had breast cancer or if you have ever had breast lumps or an abnormal mammogram (breast x-ray), you may need to have more frequent breast examinations.

Have an annual gynecologic exam.

Who should not take EstroGel?

Do not begin therapy with EstroGel if you have unusual vaginal bleeding that has not been evaluated by your doctor.

Do not take EstroGel if you currently have or have had certain cancers (eg, breast or uterine); if you had a stroke or heart attack in the past year; if you currently have or have had liver problems or blood clots.

Do not take EstroGel if you are pregnant or breastfeeding. Also, do not take EstroGel if you are allergic to any of its ingredients.

What should I tell my doctor before I take the first dose of EstroGel?

Tell your doctor about all prescription, over-the-counter, and herbal medications you are taking before beginning treatment with EstroGel. Also, talk to your doctor about your complete medical history, especially if you have asthma (wheezing); epilepsy (seizures); had your uterus removed (hysterectomy); a history of cancer; high blood cholesterol or lipid levels; diabetes; headaches; gallbladder or pancreas problems; a history of yellowing of the eyes or skin during pregnancy or with past estrogen use;

the blood disease porphyria; a family history of blood clots (such as in the legs, lungs, or eyes); migraine; endometriosis; lupus; or problems with your heart, liver, thyroid, or kidneys. Your doctor should know if you are scheduled for surgery or need to be on bed rest.

In addition, tell your doctor if you are currently pregnant, plan to become pregnant, or are breastfeeding.

What is the usual dosage?

The information below is based on the dosage guidelines your doctor uses. Depending on your condition and medical history, your doctor may prescribe a different regimen. Do not change the dosage or stop taking your medication without your doctor's approval.

The usual dosage of EstroGel is 1.25 grams (g), or 1 pump, applied to the arm once per day.

How should I take EstroGel?

EstroGel is for external use only. Do not get it in your eyes, nose, vagina, or mouth. If you get it in any of these areas, rinse right away with warm clean water.

EstroGel's pump must only be primed the first time it is being used. Remove the large pump cover and completely depress the pump. (Fully depress the pump twice for the 93-gram pump or 3 times for the 50-gram pump and the 25-gram pump.) Discard the unused gel by thoroughly rinsing it down the sink or placing it in the household trash in a manner that avoids accidental exposure or ingestion by household members or pets.

After priming, the pump is ready to use. One complete pump depression will dispense the same amount of EstroGel each time.

Apply EstroGel at the same time each day.

Apply your daily dose of gel to clean, dry, unbroken skin. If you take a bath, shower, or use a sauna, apply your EstroGel dose following these activities. If you go swimming, try to leave as much time as possible between applying your EstroGel dose and going swimming.

To apply, collect the gel into the palm of your hand by pressing the pump firmly and fully with one fluid motion without hesitation. Apply the gel to 1 arm using your hand. Spread the gel as thinly as possible over the entire area on the inside and outside of your arm from wrist to shoulder.

Always place the small protective cap back on the tip of the pump and the large pump cover over the top of the pump after each use.

Wash your hands with soap and water after applying the gel to reduce the chance that the medicine will spread from your hands to other people.

It is **not** necessary to massage or rub in EstroGel. Simply allow the gel to dry for up to 5 minutes before dressing.

Do not allow others to apply the gel for you.

What should I avoid while taking EstroGel?

It is important that you do not spread the medicine to others, especially men and children. Be sure to wash your hands after applying EstroGel. Do not allow others to make contact with the area of skin where you applied the gel for at least one hour after application. Alcohol-based gels are flammable. Avoid fire, flame or smoking until the gel has dried.

Do not apply EstroGel to skin that is irritated or broken. Do not apply it to your face, in or around the vagina, or to your breasts. Do not allow others to apply the gel for you.

Avoid prolonged sun exposure and sunlamps because EstroGel may cause dark skin patches on your face (melasma); exposure to the sun may make these patches darker.

Do not use estrogens with or without progestins to prevent heart disease, heart attacks, stroke, or dementia.

What are possible food and drug interactions associated with EstroGel?

If EstroGel is taken with certain other drugs, the effects of either could be increased, decreased, or altered. It is especially important to check with your doctor before combining EstroGel with the following: carbamazepine, erythromycin, grapefruit or grapefruit juice, ketoconazole, levothyroxine, phenobarbital, phenytoin, rifampin, ritonavir, and St. John's wort.

What are the possible side effects of EstroGel?

Side effects cannot be anticipated. If any develop or change in intensity, tell your doctor as soon as possible. Only your doctor can determine if it is safe for you to continue taking this drug.

Side effects may include: bloating, breast pain, hair loss, headache, irregular vaginal bleeding or spotting, nausea, stomach cramps, vomiting

Serious side effects may include: breast lumps, changes in speech and vision, chest pain, dizziness, faintness, leg pain, severe headache, shortness of breath, unusual vaginal bleeding, vomiting

Can I receive EstroGel if I am pregnant or breastfeeding?

You should not use EstroGel if you are pregnant, plan on becoming pregnant or are breastfeeding due to potential harm to the baby.

If you are or will be breastfeeding while using EstroGel, check with your doctor to discuss any possible risks to your baby. (EstroGel is found in breast milk.)

What should I do if I miss a dose of EstroGel?

If you miss a dose, do not double the dose on the next day to catch up. If your next dose is less than 12 hours away, it is best just to wait and apply your normal dose the next day. If it is more than 12 hours until the next dose, apply the dose you missed and resume your normal dosing the next day.

How should I store EstroGel?

Store EstroGel at room temperature, between 68 and 77 degrees F (20 and 25 degrees C) with the cap secured. Brief storage at temperatures between 59 and 86 degrees F (15 and 30 degrees C) is permitted. Store away from heat, moisture, and light. Do not store in the bathroom. Keep EstroGel out of the reach of children.

Estrogen and progestin *See Activella, page 21.*

ESTROGEN PATCHES
Generic name: Estradiol

What are Estrogen patches?

Estrogen patches are used to reduce symptoms of menopause, including feelings of warmth in the face, neck, and chest; the sudden intense episodes of heat and sweating known as hot flashes; dry, itchy external genitals; and vaginal irritation. They are also prescribed for other conditions that cause low levels of estrogen, and some doctors prescribe them for teenagers who fail to mature at the usual rate. Certain estrogen patches are also prescribed to help prevent osteoporosis.

What is the most important information I should know about Estrogen patches?

Because estrogens have been linked with an increased risk of breast, uterine, and endometrial cancer (cancer in the lining of the uterus), it is essential to have regular mammograms and checkups. Report any unusual vaginal bleeding to your doctor immediately.

Hormone replacement therapy using estrogens, with or without progestin, should not be used to prevent heart disease. Recent studies have confirmed an increased rate of heart attack, stroke, and dangerous blood clots among women taking estrogen or estrogen combinations for 5 years. Blood clots can lead to phlebitis, stroke, heart attack, a loss of blood supply to the lungs, a blockage in the blood vessels serving the eye, and other serious disorders. Because of these risks, hormone replacement therapy should be given at the lowest effective dose for the shortest possible time. Your doctor will determine the dosage that is best for you.

Contact your doctor right away if you notice any of the following symptoms: abdominal pain, tenderness, or swelling; abnormal bleeding of the vagina; breast lumps; coughing up blood; difficulty with speech; pain in your chest or calves; severe headache, dizziness, or faintness; skin irritation, redness, or rash; sudden shortness of breath; vision changes; weakness or numbness of an arm or leg; or yellowing of the skin or eyes.

Who should not take Estrogen patches?

Estrogen patches should not be used during pregnancy. You should also avoid this product if you have any of the following: unexplained vaginal bleeding; known or suspected breast cancer; any type of tumor stimulated by estrogen; phlebitis; blood clots in the lung; a clotting disorder; active or recent (within the last year) heart disease, heart attack, or stroke; liver disease or liver problems, or an allergy to any component of the patch.

What should I tell my doctor before I take the first dose of Estrogen patches?

Tell your doctor about all prescription, over-the-counter, and herbal medications you are taking before beginning treatment with this drug. Also talk to your doctor about your complete medical history, especially if you have clot-related disorders, including heart attack and stroke, pulmonary embolism (a clot in the lungs), and thrombophlebitis (a clot in the veins); high blood pressure; high triglycerides; diabetes; thyroid problems; asthma; epilepsy; migraine headaches; heart problems; kidney problems; endometriosis; or gallbladder disease.

What is the usual dosage?

The information below is based on the dosage guidelines your doctor uses. Depending on your condition and medical history, your doctor may prescribe a different regimen. Do not change the dosage or stop taking your medication without your doctor's approval.

Your doctor will determine the dosage that is right for you. Typically, hormone replacement therapy should be started at the lowest possible dose and for the shortest duration needed to relieve your symptoms. You should be evaluated every 3 to 6 months.

How should I take Estrogen patches?

Each patch is individually sealed in a protective pouch and is applied directly to the skin. Apply the adhesive side to a clean, dry area of your skin on the trunk of your body (including the buttocks and abdomen). Do not apply to your breasts or waist. Firmly press the patch in place with the palm of your hand for about 10 seconds, to make sure the edges are flat against your skin.

Contact with water during bathing, swimming, or showering will not affect the patch.

What should I avoid while taking Estrogen patches?

Because the application site must be rotated, avoid using any particular site more than once a week.

What are possible food and drug interactions associated with Estrogen patches?

If you take certain other drugs while using estrogen, the effects of either could be increased, decreased, or altered. It is especially important to check with your doctor before taking the following: alcohol, barbiturates such as phenobarbital and secobarbital, blood thinners such as warfarin, cimetidine, clarithromycin, dantrolene, epilepsy drugs such as carbamazepine and phenytoin, erythromycin, grapefruit juice, itraconazole, ketoconazole, rifampin, ritonavir, St. John's wort, steroids such as prednisone, and tricyclic antidepressants such as amitriptyline and imipramine.

What are the possible side effects of Estrogen patches?

Side effects cannot be anticipated. If any develop or change in intensity, tell your doctor as soon as possible. Only your doctor can determine if it is safe for you to continue taking this drug.

Side effects may include: anxiety, back pain, breakthrough bleeding, breast tenderness, constipation, depression, flu-like symptoms, headache, high blood pressure, hot flushes, insomnia, indigestion, nausea, neck pain, sinus problems, skin redness and irritation at the site of the patch, upper respiratory tract infection, weight gain

Can I receive Estrogen patches if I am pregnant or breastfeeding?

Estrogens should not be used during pregnancy or immediately after childbirth. Use of estrogens during pregnancy has been linked to reproductive tract problems in the children. If you are pregnant or plan to become pregnant, notify your doctor immediately. Estrogens decrease the quantity and quality of breast milk. If this medication is essential to your health, your doctor may advise you to discontinue breastfeeding until your treatment is finished.

What should I do if I miss a dose of Estrogen patches?

If you forget to apply a new patch when you are supposed to, do it as soon as you remember. If it is almost time to change patches anyway, skip the one you missed and go back to your regular schedule. Do not apply more than the prescribed number of patches at a time.

How should I store Estrogen patches?

Store the patches at room temperature, in their sealed pouches.

Estropipate See Ogen, page 933.

ESTROSTEP FE

Generic name: Norethindrone acetate and ethinyl estradiol

What is Estrostep Fe?

Estrostep Fe is an oral contraceptive indicated for the prevention of pregnancy in women who elect to use oral contraceptives as a method of contraception.

Estrostep Fe is also indicated for the treatment of moderate acne in females who are 15 years and older and have a need for oral contraception in addition to having acne. Estrostep Fe is only indicated if the female has begun menstruation, has failed therapy with topical acne treatments, and is able to stay on therapy with Estrostep Fe for at least 6 months.

What is the most important information
I should know about Estrostep Fe?
Cigarette smoking increases the risk of serious cardiovascular side effects (such as blood clots, heart attacks, and stroke) when combined with oral contraceptives such as Estrostep Fe. This risk increases with age and with heavy smoking (15 or more cigarettes per day) and is significantly increased in women over 35 years of age. Women who use oral contraceptives should be strongly advised not to smoke.

Estrostep Fe does not protect against transmission of HIV (AIDS) and other sexually transmitted diseases.

You may need to use back-up birth control, such as condoms or a spermicide when you first start using this medication. Follow your doctor's instructions.

If you experience vomiting or diarrhea for any reason, or if you are taking medication (such as an antibiotic), make sure to use a back-up birth control method (such as condoms or spermicide) until you check with your doctor.

You may have breakthrough bleeding, especially during the first 3 months. Do not stop taking Estrostep Fe if you experience spotting, light bleeding, or you feel sick; the problem will usually go away. Tell your doctor if this bleeding continues or is heavy.

If you wear contact lenses and notice a change in vision or an inability to wear your lenses, tell your doctor.

Oral contraceptives may cause edema (fluid retention), with swelling of the fingers or ankles, and may raise your blood pressure. If you experience fluid retention, contact your doctor.

Estrostep Fe may cause dark skin patches on your face (melasma). Exposure to the sun may make these patches darker; you may need to avoid prolonged exposure to the sun, sunlamps, and tanning beds. Consult your doctor regarding the use of sunscreens and protective clothing.

If you need to have any type of medical tests or surgery, or if you will be on bed rest, you may need to stop using this medication for a short time. Any doctor or surgeon who treats you should know that you are using birth control pills.

Contact your doctor if you notice any unusual symptoms.

Who should not take Estrostep Fe?
Estrostep Fe should not be used by women with blood clots or a history of blood clots, heart disease, breast cancer, endometrial cancer, abnormal genital bleeding, or liver problems.

Estrostep Fe should not be used by pregnant women. Also, do not use Estrostep Fe if you have an allergy to it or any of its ingredients.

What should I tell my doctor before I take the first dose of Estrostep Fe?

Tell your doctor about all prescription, over-the-counter, and herbal medications you are taking before beginning treatment with Estrostep Fe. Also, talk to your doctor about your complete medical history, especially if you have any heart problems, liver problems, diabetes, elevated cholesterol or triglycerides, high blood pressure, migraines, headaches, epilepsy, mental depression, gallbladder disease, kidney disease, history of irregular menstrual periods, circulation problems, a history of stroke, abnormal vaginal bleeding, blood clots or cancer. In addition tell your doctor if you are pregnant, plan on becoming pregnant, you recently gave birth or are breastfeeding.

What is the usual dosage?

The information below is based on the dosage guidelines your doctor uses. Depending on your condition and medical history, your doctor may prescribe a different regimen. Do not change the dosage or stop taking your medication without your doctor's approval.

Adults: Each white tablet (1 mg norethindrone and 20 mcg ethinyl estradiol) dispenser has been preprinted with the days of the week, starting with Sunday. Take the appropriate tablet once daily. The brown tablets (75 mg ferrous fumarate) should be taken the same way after all 21 white tablets have been administered.

For acne treatment, follow the same guidelines for use of Estrostep Fe as an oral contraceptive.

How should I take Estrostep Fe?

Take as directed based on the regimen of your choice. Consult with your doctor to decide upon a proper regimen and make sure you make all follow-up appointments. You have a choice of which day to start taking your first pack of pills. Decide with your doctor or clinic which is the best day for you. Pick a time of day which will be easy to remember. During the first week of initiating therapy, an additional method of contraception is recommended.

Tablets should be taken regularly at the same time each day and can be taken without regard to meals. The chewable tablet may be chewed or swallowed whole. If chewed, drink a full glass of water just after you swallow the pill.

Day 1 start: Pick the day label strip that starts with the first day of your period. (This is the day you start bleeding or spotting, even if it is almost midnight when the bleeding begins.) Place this day label strip on the tablet dispenser over the area that has the days of the week (starting with Sunday) printed on the plastic. Take the first "active" white pill during the first 24 hours of your period. You will not need to use a back-up method of birth control, since you are starting the pill at the beginning of your period.

Sunday start: Take the first "active" white pill on the Sunday after your period starts, even if you are still bleeding. If your period begins on Sunday, start the pack that same day. Use another method of birth control as a back-up method if you have sex anytime from the Sunday you start your first pack until the next Sunday (7 days). Condoms or spermicide are good back-up methods of birth control.

WHEN YOU FINISH A PACK OR SWITCH YOUR BRAND OF PILLS:

21 pills: Wait 7 days to start the next pack. You will probably have your period during that week. Be sure that no more than 7 days pass between 21-day packs.

28 pills: Start the next pack on the day after your last "reminder" pill. Do not wait any days between packs.

Menstruation usually begins in two or three days, but may begin as late as the fourth or fifth day after the brown tablets have been started. In any event, the next course of tablets should be started without interruption. If spotting occurs while you are taking white tablets, continue the medication without interruption.

At times there may be no menstrual period after a cycle of pills. Therefore, if you miss one menstrual period but have taken the pills *exactly as you were supposed to,* continue as usual into the next cycle. If you have not taken the pills correctly and miss a menstrual period, *you may be pregnant* and should stop taking oral contraceptives until your doctor or healthcare provider determines whether or not you are pregnant. Until you can get to your doctor or healthcare provider, use another form of contraception. If two consecutive menstrual periods are missed, you should stop taking pills until it is determined whether or not you are pregnant.

What should I avoid while taking Estrostep Fe?

Do not smoke while using birth control pills, especially if you are older than 35. Smoking can increase your risk of blood clots, stroke, or heart attack caused by birth control pills.

Avoid having unprotected sex because birth control pills will not protect you from sexually transmitted diseases including HIV and AIDS.

Avoid prolonged exposure to sun, sunlamps, and tanning beds because Estrostep Fe may cause dark skin patches on your face (melasma); exposure to the sun may make these patches darker.

What are possible food and drug interactions associated with Estrostep Fe?

If Estrostep Fe is taken with certain other drugs, the effects of either could be increased, decreased, or altered. It is especially important to check with your doctor before combining Estrostep Fe with the following: acetaminophen; barbiturates (eg, phenobarbital, pentobarbital); carbamazepine; clofibric acid; cyclosporine; morphine; phenytoin; prednisolone; rifampin; St John's wort; temazepam; and theophylline.

What are the possible side effects of Estrostep Fe?
Side effects cannot be anticipated. If any develop or change in intensity, tell your doctor as soon as possible. Only your doctor can determine if it is safe for you to continue taking this drug.

Side effects may include: breakthrough bleeding, breast pain or tenderness, change in weight or appetite, edema, decreased sex drive, depression, freckles or darkening of facial skin, headache, increased hair growth, loss of hair, migraine, nausea, problems with contact lenses, nervousness, dizziness, loss of menstrual period, stomach cramps/bloating, vaginal itching, vomiting

Can I receive Estrostep Fe if I am pregnant or breastfeeding?
You should not use Estrostep Fe if you are pregnant, plan on becoming pregnant or breastfeeding due to potential harm to the baby.

What should I do if I miss a dose of Estrostep Fe?
If you miss 1 white pill, take it as soon as you remember. Take the next pill at your regular time. This means you may take 2 pills in 1 day.

If you miss 2 white pills (week 1 or week 2), take 2 pills on the day you remember and 2 pills the next day. Then resume to 1 pill a day until you finish the pack.

If you miss 2 white pills (week 3): Day-1 starter: Throw out the rest of the pill pack and start a new pack that same day. Sunday starter: Continue with 1 pill every day until Sunday. On Sunday, throw out the pack and start a new pack. You may not have your period this month, but this is expected. However, if you miss your period 2 months in a row, call your doctor or clinic because you might be pregnant. You MUST use another birth control method (such as condoms or spermicide) as a back-up method of birth control until you have taken a white "active" pill every day for 7 days.

If you miss 3 or more white pills (during the first 3 weeks): Day-1 starter: Throw out the rest of the pill pack and start a new pack that same day. Sunday starter: Keep taking 1 pill every day until Sunday. On Sunday, throw out the rest of the pack and start a new pack of pills that same day. You MUST use another birth control method (such as condoms or spermicide) as a back-up method of birth control until you have taken a white "active" pill every day for 7 days.

If you are unsure what to do about the pills you have missed, use a back-up method anytime you have sex until the next time you see your doctor. Keep taking the white pills each day until your next doctor's appointment.

How should I store Estrostep Fe?
Store Estrostep Fe at room temperature and away from children. Do not store above 25° C (77° F). Protect from moisture, heat, light, and humidity. Store tablets inside the pouch when not in use.

Eszopiclone *See Lunesta, page 776.*

Ethinyl estradiol and norelgestromin *See Ortho Evra,*
page 956.

Ethinyl estradiol and norethindrone acetate *See femHRT,*
page 543.

Ethotoin *See Peganone, page 987.*

ETODOLAC

What is Etodolac?
Etodolac, a nonsteroidal anti-inflammatory drug, is available in regular and extended-release forms. Both forms are used to relieve the inflammation, swelling, stiffness, and joint pain of osteoarthritis (the most common form of arthritis) and rheumatoid arthritis. Regular etodolac is also used to relieve pain in other situations.

What is the most important information I should know about Etodolac?
You should have frequent checkups with your doctor if you take etodolac regularly. Ulcers or internal bleeding can occur without warning.

Call your doctor if you have any signs or symptoms of stomach or intestinal ulcers or bleeding, blurred vision or other eye problems, skin rash, weight gain, or fluid retention and swelling.

This drug should be used with caution if you have kidney or liver disease; and it can cause liver inflammation in some people.

If you are taking etodolac over an extended period of time, your doctor may check your blood for anemia.

This drug can increase water retention. Use with caution if you have heart disease or high blood pressure.

Who should not take Etodolac?
If you are sensitive to or have ever had an allergic reaction to etodolac, or if you have had asthma attacks, hives, or other allergic reactions caused by aspirin or other nonsteroidal anti-inflammatory drugs, you should not take this medication; it might cause a severe allergic reaction. Make sure your doctor is aware of any drug reactions you have experienced; and be careful about taking this drug if you have asthma—even if you've never

had a drug reaction before. If you do suffer an allergic reaction, call for emergency help immediately.

What should I tell my doctor before I take the first dose of Etodolac?

Tell your doctor about all prescription, over-the-counter, and herbal medications you are taking before beginning treatment with etodolac. Also, talk to your doctor about your complete medical history, especially if you have heart disease, high blood pressure, kidney or liver disease, anemia, ulcers, or gastrointestinal problems.

What is the usual dosage?

The information below is based on the dosage guidelines your doctor uses. Depending on your condition and medical history, your doctor may prescribe a different regimen. Do not change the dosage or stop taking your medication without your doctor's approval.

General Pain Relief

Adults: Take 200 to 400 milligrams (mg) every 6 to 8 hours as needed. Ordinarily, you should not take more than 1,000 mg a day, although your doctor may increase the dose to 1,200 mg a day if absolutely necessary.

Osteoarthritis and Rheumatoid Arthritis

Adults: The starting dose of etodolac is 300 mg 2 or 3 times a day, or 400 or 500 mg twice a day. The usual daily maximum ranges from 600 to 1,000 mg, although your doctor may prescribe as much as 1,200 mg a day if necessary. The usual dose of the extended-release tablets is 400 to 1,200 mg taken once a day.

How should I take Etodolac?

Take this medication exactly as prescribed by your doctor. The doctor may instruct you to take etodolac with food or an antacid, and with a full glass of water. Never take it on an empty stomach.

What should I avoid while taking Etodolac?

Do not take aspirin or any other anti-inflammatory medieations while taking etodolac, unless your doctor tells you to do so.

What are possible food and drug interactions associated with Etodolac?

If etodolac is taken with certain other drugs, the effects of either could be increased, decreased, or altered. It is especially important to check with your doctor before combining etodolac with the following: aspirin, cyclosporine, digoxin, lithium, methotrexate, phenylbutazone, and warfarin.

What are the possible side effects of Etodolac?

Side effects cannot be anticipated. If any develop or change in intensity, inform your doctor as soon as possible. Only your doctor can determine if it is safe for you to continue taking etodolac.

Side effects may include: abdominal pain, black stools, blurred vision, chills, constipation, depression, diarrhea, dizziness, fever, gas, increased frequency of urination, indigestion, itching, nausea, nervousness, rash, ringing in ears, painful or difficult urination, vomiting, weakness

Can I receive Etodolac if I am pregnant or breastfeeding?

The effects of etodolac during pregnancy have not been adequately studied. However, you should definitely not take it in late pregnancy. If you are pregnant or plan to become pregnant, inform your doctor immediately. Etodolac may appear in breast milk and could affect a nursing infant. If this medication is essential to your health, your doctor may advise you to discontinue breastfeeding until your treatment with this medication is finished.

What should I do if I miss a dose of Etodolac?

Take the forgotten dose as soon as you remember. If it is almost time for the next dose, skip the one you missed and go back to your regular schedule. Never double the dose.

How should I store Etodolac?

Store at room temperature. Protect capsules from moisture. Protect the regular tablets from light; protect the extended-release tablets from excessive heat and humidity.

Etonogestrel and ethinyl estradiol *See NuvaRing, page 924.*

Etravirine *See Intelence, page 666.*

EVISTA

Generic name: Raloxifene hydrochloride

What is Evista?

Evista is prescribed to treat and help prevent osteoporosis.

What is the most important information I should know about Evista?

Because of Evista's tendency to promote clots, you should not take it during long periods of immobilization such as recovery from surgery or prolonged bed rest, or for 72 hours beforehand. If you are scheduled for surgery, make sure the doctor is aware that you are taking Evista. For the same reason, if you are going on a trip where your movement will be restricted, make a point of periodically getting up and walking around.

Evista is not needed prior to menopause and shouldn't be taken until menopause has passed. It has not been studied in premenopausal women and its use is not recommended.

If you develop unusual uterine bleeding or breast problems while taking Evista, tell your doctor immediately.

Never combine Evista with estrogen hormones.

Who should not take Evista?

Evista is not for use by women who are—or could become—pregnant. You should also avoid this drug if you have a history of blood clot formation, including deep vein thrombosis (blood clot in the legs), pulmonary embolism (blood clot in the lungs), and retinal vein thrombosis (blood clot in the retina of the eye), since Evista increases the risk of clots. Avoid the drug, too, if it gives you an allergic reaction.

What should I tell my doctor before I take the first dose of Evista?

Tell your doctor about all prescription, over-the-counter, and herbal medications you are taking before beginning treatment with this drug. Also, talk to your doctor about your complete medical history, especially if you have congestive heart failure, liver problems, cancer, or high triglycerides.

What is the usual dosage?

The information below is based on the dosage guidelines your doctor uses. Depending on your condition and medical history, your doctor may prescribe a different regimen. Do not change the dosage or stop taking your medication without your doctor's approval.

Postmenopausal women: The recommended dosage is one 60-milligram tablet once a day.

How should I take Evista?

Take Evista once daily, at any time, with or without food.

What should I avoid while taking Evista?

Due to the risk of blood clots, avoid prolonged bed rest or restricted movement.

What are possible food and drug interactions associated with Evista?

If Evista is taken with certain other drugs, the effects of either could be increased, decreased, or altered. It is especially important to check with your doctor before combining Evista with the following: cholestyramine, clofibrate, diazepam, diazoxide, ibuprofen, indomethacin, naproxen, and warfarin.

What are the possible side effects of Evista?

Side effects cannot be anticipated. If any develop or change in intensity, tell your doctor as soon as possible. Only your doctor can determine if it is safe for you to continue taking this drug.

Side effects may include: abdominal pain, arthritis, breast pain, bronchitis, chest pain, depression, diarrhea, dizziness, fever, flu symptoms, gas, gynecological problems, headache, hot flashes, increased cough, indigestion, infection, insomnia, joint pain, leg cramps, muscle ache, nasal inflammation, nausea, rash, sinusitis, sore throat, stomach and intestinal problems, sweating, swelling, tendon soreness, uterine discharge, urinary tract infection, vomiting, weight gain

Can I receive Evista if I am pregnant or breastfeeding?

Evista can harm a developing baby. Do not use if you are or may become pregnant. Also avoid breastfeeding while taking Evista.

What should I do if I miss a dose of Evista?

Take it as soon as you remember. If it is almost time for your next dose, skip the one you missed and go back to your regular schedule. Never take a double dose.

How should I store Evista?

Store at room temperature.

EXELON

Generic name: Rivastigmine tartrate

What is Exelon?

Exelon is used to treat mild-to-moderate dementia in Alzheimer's disease and Parkinson's disease patients.

What is the most important information I should know about Exelon?

Exelon may cause you to develop significant gastrointestinal adverse reactions such as nausea, vomiting, and decreased appetite. This is more likely to occur if you are taking Exelon capsules or oral solution. It is less likely to occur if you are using the Exelon patch.

Exelon may cause you to experience weight loss which may be attributed to the gastrointestinal effects with which Exelon is associated.

All forms of Exelon (capsules, oral solution, or patches) may cause diarrhea, increase your chances of developing a seizure, and may cause or worsen extrapyramidal symptoms such as tremor.

Who should not take Exelon?
Do not take Exelon if you are allergic to it or to any of its ingredients.

What should I tell my doctor before I take the first dose of Exelon?
Tell your doctor about all prescription, over-the-counter, and herbal medications you are taking before beginning treatment with Exelon. Also, talk to your doctor about your complete medical history before beginning treatment with Exelon, especially if you have a history of stomach ulcers, heart problems, breathing or lung problems, and are taking nonsteroidal anti-inflammatory drugs (NSAIDs).

What is the usual dosage?
The information below is based on the dosage guidelines your doctor uses. Depending on your condition and medical history, your doctor may prescribe a different regimen. Do not change the dosage or stop taking your medication without your doctor's approval.

Dementia in Alzheimer's disease
The usual dosage of Exelon for dementia in Alzheimer's patients is 3-6 milligrams (mg) taken twice a day if given in the oral solution or tablet form. Doses may be increased at a minimum of two-week intervals with a maximum of 12 mg per day.

If Exelon is given as a patch, then initially the 4.6 milligram (mg) patch should be worn for 24 hours. After 4 weeks of treatment, and if you do not experience any significant side effects (nausea, vomiting, diarrhea, loss of appetite), the patch strength may be increased to the 9.5 milligram (mg) patch and it should be worn for 24 hours and then replaced with a new patch.

Dementia in Parkinson's disease
The usual dosage of Exelon for dementia in Parkinson's patients is 1.5-6 mg taken twice a day if given in the oral solution or tablet form. Doses may be increased at a minimum of 4-week intervals with a maximum of 12 mg per day.

If Exelon is given as a patch, then initially the 4.6 milligrams (mg) patch should be worn for 24 hours. After 4 weeks of treatment, and if you do not experience any significant side effects (eg, nausea, vomiting, diarrhea, loss of appetite), the patch strength may be increased to the 9.5 milligram (mg) patch. It should be worn for 24 hours and then replaced with a new patch.

How should I take Exelon?
Exelon capsules and oral solution should be taken with meals in the morning and the evening. Exelon oral solution may be taken straight, or may be mixed with a small glass of water, cold fruit juice, or soda.

The oral solution and capsules may be used interchangeably as long as the dosage remains the same.

If you are using the Exelon patch, it should be applied to the upper or lower back or to the upper arm or chest area.

If you are a caretaker and feel that the patient will pull the patch off before he or she is supposed to, place the Exelon patch on the patient's back. Avoid placing the patch in an area where it can be rubbed off by tight clothing. Before applying the patch, make sure the area where you are applying is clean, dry, and hairless, free of any powder, oil, moisturizer, or lotion, and free of cuts, rashes, or irritations.

The Exelon patch should be worn for 24 hours. After 24 hours, remove the patch and apply a new patch to a different spot of skin. Do not apply a new patch to a previously used spot for at least 14 days.

What should I avoid while taking Exelon?
Exelon may cause you to develop neurological effects (eg, seizures). Therefore, avoid participating in potentially hazardous activities (eg, driving, operating machinery) unless your physician has told you otherwise.

What are possible food and drug interactions associated with Exelon?
If Exelon is taken with certain other drugs, the effects of either could be increased, decreased, or altered. It is especially important to check with your doctor before combining Exelon with anticholinergic medications, succinylcholine, other cholinomimetic drugs, and similar neuromuscular blocking agents or cholinergic agonists (such as bethanechol).

What are the possible side effects of Exelon?
Side effects cannot be anticipated. If any develop or change in intensity, tell your doctor as soon as possible. Only your doctor can determine if it is safe for you to continue taking this drug.

Side effects for Exelon Capsules and Solution may include: anxiety, confusion, constipation, depression, dizziness, diarrhea, fatigue, feeling of uneasiness or out of sorts, hallucinations, headache, flu-like symptoms, increased blood pressure, increased sweating, indigestion, insomnia, intestinal gas, loss of appetite, loss of consciousness or fainting, nausea, stomach pain, tremor, urinary tract infection, vomiting, weight loss, weakness, worsening symptoms if you have Parkinson's disease

Side effects for Exelon Patch may include: anxiety, diarrhea, dizziness, depression, headache, indigestion, insomnia, loss of appetite, nausea, skin irritation at the site of patch application, stomach pain, vomiting, weakness, weight loss

Can I receive Exelon if I am pregnant or breastfeeding?

The effects of Exelon during pregnancy and breastfeeding are unknown. Talk with your doctor before taking this drug if you are pregnant, plan to become pregnant, or are breastfeeding.

What should I do if I miss a dose of Exelon?

If you miss taking a dose of Exelon tablets or oral solution, take it as soon as you remember. If it is almost time for your next dose, skip the missed dose and return to your normal dosing schedule. Do not take a double dose.

If you miss applying the Exelon patch, apply it as soon as you remember. Then apply the next patch at the usual time you take your dose. Do not apply two patches at once to make up for the missed dose.

If you have missed taking Exelon for several days, contact your physician before restarting therapy with Exelon.

How should I store Exelon?

Store the Exelon capsules at room temperature and in a tight container. Exelon oral solution can also be stored at room temperature, in an upright position and protected from freezing. If Exelon oral solution is combined with cold fruit juice or soda, the mixture may be stored at room temperature for four hours.

Store Exelon patches at room temperature. Do not use Exelon patches beyond the expiration date that is listed on the carton and pouch.

Exenatide See Byetta, page 235.

EXFORGE

Generic name: Amlodipine and valsartan

What is Exforge?

Exforge is used to treat high blood pressure. It contains two medicines: amlodipine, a calcium channel blocker; and valsartan, an angiotensin receptor blocker (ARB).

What is the most important information I should know about Exforge?

If you become pregnant, stop taking Exforge immediately. Using this medication during pregnancy can cause fetal injury or death. Talk to your doctor if you plan to become pregnant while taking Exforge.

Who should not take Exforge?

Do not take Exforge if you are pregnant or plan to become pregnant. Exforge should not be used in people less than 18 years old.

What should I tell my doctor before I take the first dose of Exforge?

Tell your doctor about all prescription, over-the-counter, and herbal medications you are taking before beginning treatment with Exforge. Also, talk to your doctor about your complete medical history, especially if you have heart problems, liver problems, or kidney problems, or if you are vomiting and have a lot of diarrhea. Tell your doctor if you are pregnant plan to become pregnant, or are breastfeeding.

What is the usual dosage?

The information below is based on the dosage guidelines your doctor uses. Depending on your condition and medical history, your doctor may prescribe a different regimen. Do not change the dosage or stop taking your medication without your doctor's approval.

Adults: The usual starting dose is 5 milligrams (mg) of amlodipine and 160 mg of valsartan once daily.

How should I take Exforge?

Take Exforge as prescribed by your doctor, once each day, with or without food.

What should I avoid while taking Exforge?

Avoid becoming pregnant while taking Exforge.

What are possible food and drug interactions associated with Exforge?

If Exforge is used with certain other drugs, the effects of either could be increased, decreased, or altered. It is especially important to check with your doctor before combining Exforge with potassium supplements or potassium-sparing diuretics such as spironolactone, triamterene, and amiloride.

What are the possible side effects of Exforge?

Side effects cannot be anticipated. If any develop or change in intensity, tell your doctor as soon as possible. Only your doctor can determine if it is safe for you to continue taking this drug.

Side effects may include: swelling of the hands, ankles, or feet; nasal congestion; upper respiratory infection; dizziness

Can I receive Exforge if I am pregnant or breastfeeding?

Exforge is not recommended during pregnancy or breastfeeding. Talk to your doctor before taking this drug if you are pregnant, plan to become pregnant, or are breastfeeding.

What should I do if I miss a dose of Exforge?

If you miss a dose, take it as soon as you remember. If it is almost time for your next dose, skip the one you missed and return to your regular dosing schedule. Do not double the dose.

How should I store Exforge?

Store at room temperature.

EXTINA
Generic name: Ketoconazole foam

What is Extina?

Extina foam is used on the skin (topically) for a condition called seborrheic dermatitis in adults and children 12 years and older who have normal immune system function. Seborrheic dermatitis is a skin condition that affects the scalp, body, ears and face, and causes red, flaky, greasy looking skin.

What is the most important information I should know about Extina?

Extina foam is for skin use only. Do not use in the eyes, mouth or vagina.

Keep the Extina foam can away from and do not spray it near fire, open flame, or direct heat. Extina foam is flammable. Never throw the Extina foam can into a fire, even if the can is empty.

Tell your doctor if the area of application shows signs of increased irritation.

Who should not take Extina?

Extina should not be used by individuals younger than age 12 or by people whose immune system is not working properly.

What should I tell my doctor before I take the first dose of Extina?

Tell your doctor about all prescription, over-the-counter, and herbal medication you are taking before beginning treatment with Extina. Also, talk to your doctor about your complete medical history.

What is the usual dosage?

The information below is based on the dosage guidelines your doctor uses. Depending on your condition and medical history, your doctor may prescribe a different regimen. Do not change the dosage or stop taking your medication without your doctor's approval.

Adults and children 12 years and older: Extina foam should be applied to the affected area(s) twice daily for 4 weeks.

How should I take Extina?

Hold the container upright, and dispense Extina foam into the cap of the can or other cool surface in an amount sufficient to cover the affected area(s). Dispensing directly onto hands is not recommended, as the foam will begin to melt immediately upon contact with warm skin. Pick up small amounts of Extina foam with the fingertips, and gently massage into the affected area(s) until the foam disappears.

For areas on the body with hair, part the hair so that Extina foam may be applied directly to the skin (rather than on the hair).

Avoid contact with the eyes, mouth, or vagina.

What should I avoid while taking Extina?

Extina foam is flammable. Avoid fire, flame and/or smoking during and immediately following application.

What are possible food and drug interactions associated with Extina?

If Extina is taken with certain other drugs, the effect of either medication could be increased, decreased, or altered. Always check with your doctor before combining Extina with any other medication.

What are the possible side effects of Extina?

Side effects cannot be anticipated. If any develop or change in intensity, tell your doctor as soon as possible. Only your doctor can determine if it is safe for you to continue taking this drug.

Side effects may include: redness, itchiness, rash, burning at the application site

Can I receive Extina if I am pregnant or breastfeeding?

The effect of Extina foam during pregnancy and breastfeeding are unknown. Tell your doctor if you are pregnant, plan to become pregnant, or are breastfeeding.

What should I do if I miss a dose of Extina?

If you miss a dose of Extina, apply it as soon as you remember.

How should I store Extina?

Store the can of Extina foam at room temperature. Do not place the can in the refrigerator or freezer. Keep the can away from all sources of fire and heat. Do not leave the can in direct sunlight.

Ezetimbe and simvastatin *See Vytorin, page 1408.*

Ezetimibe *See Zetia, page 1469.*

FACTIVE
Generic name: Gemifloxacin

What is Factive?
Factive is an antibiotic. It is used to treat adults 18 years or older with bronchitis or pneumonia (lung infections) caused by certain bacteria (germs).

Sometimes, other germs called viruses infect the lungs. The common cold is a virus. Factive, like other antibiotics, does not treat viruses.

What is the most important information I should know about Factive?
Factive should not be given to adolescents or children; the effects of this drug on people less than 18 years old are unknown. Also, do not take Factive if you are breastfeeding.

Who should not take Factive?
Do not take Factive if you are allergic to any of its ingredients or to any antibiotic called a quinolone. If you develop hives, difficulty breathing, or other symptoms of a severe allergic reaction, seek emergency treatment right away. If you develop a skin rash, stop taking Factive and call your doctor.

What should I tell my doctor before I take the first dose of Factive?
Tell your doctor about all prescription, over-the-counter, and herbal medications you are taking before beginning treatment with Factive. Also, talk to your doctor about your complete medical history, especially if you are pregnant/plan to become pregnant or nursing, have a heart problem (such as recent heart attack or slow heart beat), or have kidney problems.

What is the usual dosage?
The information below is based on the dosage guidelines your doctor uses. Depending on your condition and medical history, your doctor may prescribe a different regimen. Do not change the dosage or stop taking your medication without your doctor's approval.

Bronchitis
Adults: The usual dosage is one 320 milligrams (mg) tablet daily, for 5 days.

Pneumonia
Adults: The usual dosage is one 320 mg tablet daily, for 7 days.

How should I take Factive?
Take Factive at the same time each day. This drug can be taken with or without food. Swallow the tablet whole, and drink plenty of fluids with it. Do not chew the Factive tablet.

What are possible food and drug interactions associated with Factive?

If Factive is taken with certain other drugs, the effects of either could be increased, decreased, or altered. It is especially important to check with your doctor before combining Factive with the following: Antacids containing aluminum or magnesium, antiarrhythmics, antipsychotics, corticosteroids, oral or by injection, didanosine, diuretics, such as furosemide and hydrochlorothiazide, erythromycin, iron (ferrous sulfate), mutlivitamins containing zinc, sucralfate, tricyclic antidepressant.

What are the possible side effects of Factive?

Side effects cannot be anticipated. If any develop or change in intensity, tell your doctor as soon as possible. Only your doctor can determine if it is safe for you to continue taking this drug.

Side effects may include: Change in the way things taste in your mouth, diarrhea, dizziness, headache, nausea, rash, stomach pain, vomiting

Can I receive Factive if I am pregnant or breastfeeding?

The effects of Factive during pregnancy and breastfeeding are unknown. Tell your doctor immediately if you are pregnant, plan to become pregnant, or are breastfeeding.

What should I do if I miss a dose of Factive?

If you miss a dose of Factive, take it as soon as you remember. Do not take more than 1 dose in a day.

How should I store Factive?

Store at room temperature.

Famciclovir See *Famvir, below.*

Famotidine See *Pepcid, page 997.*

FAMVIR
Generic name: Famciclovir

What is Famvir?

Famvir is an antiviral medication used to stop/minimize the symptoms of recurrent genital herpes. It is also used to minimize the outbreaks of genital herpes, cold sores, and the rash and pain of shingles (herpes zoster).

What is the most important information I should know about Famvir?

Famvir is not a cure for herpes. This drug may not stop the spread of herpes to others. If you are sexually active, you may still pass herpes to your partner while taking Famvir. Even if you are not currently having an outbreak, herpes may still be spread to your partner.

Who should not take Famvir?
Do not use Famvir if you are allergic to any of its ingredients.

What should I tell my doctor before I take the first dose of Famvir?
Tell your doctor about all prescription, over-the-counter, and herbal medications you are taking before beginning treatment with Famvir. Also, talk to your doctor about your complete medical history, especially if you are over 65, have liver or kidney problems, or you are pregnant/planning to become pregnant or breastfeeding.

What is the usual dosage?
The information below is based on the dosage guidelines your doctor uses. Depending on your condition and medical history, your doctor may prescribe a different regimen. Do not change the dosage or stop taking your medication without your doctor's approval.

Recurrent Genital Herpes
Adults: The usual dosage is two 500 milligram (mg) tablets as soon as you feel the beginning of an outbreak (within 6 hours), and two more tablets about 12 hours later.

Suppression of Recurrent Genital Herpes
Adults: The usual dosage is one 250 mg tablet in the morning and one at night. This treatment may continue for up to a year.

Cold Sores
Adults: The usual dosage is three 500 mg tablets taken all together at the first sign of an outbreak (within 1 hour).

Shingles
Adults: The usual dosage is 500 mg every 8 hours, for 7 days. Take the first tablet as soon as shingles in diagnosed (within 3 days of the first symptoms).

How should I take Famvir?
Famvir can be taken with or without food.

What should I avoid while taking Famvir?
Avoid engaging in unprotected sexual activity. Genital herpes may still be passed to your partner while you are on Famvir and/or you do not have visible sores.

What are possible food and drug interactions associated with Famvir?

If Famvir is taken with certain other drugs, the effects of either could be increased, decreased, or altered. It is especially important to check with your doctor before combining Famvir with the following: Probenecid.

What are the possible side effects of Famvir?

Side effects cannot be anticipated. If any develop or change in intensity, tell your doctor as soon as possible. Only your doctor can determine if it is safe for you to continue taking this drug.

Side effects may include: Diarrhea, fatigue, headache, nausea, stomach pain

Can I receive Famvir if I am pregnant or breastfeeding?

The effects of Famvir during pregnancy and breastfeeding are unknown. Tell your doctor immediately if you are pregnant, plan to become pregnant, or are breastfeeding.

How should I store Famvir?

Store at room temperature.

Felbamate See Felbatol, below.

FELBATOL

Generic name: Felbamate

What is Felbatol?

Felbatol is used alone or with other drugs to treat partial seizures with or without generalization (seizures in which consciousness may be retained or lost). It is also used with other medications to treat seizures associated with Lennox-Gastaut syndrome (a childhood condition characterized by brief loss of awareness and muscle tone).

Felbatol is usually used only when other medications have failed to control severe cases of epilepsy.

What is the most important information I should know about Felbatol?

Felbatol, taken by itself or with other prescription and/or non-prescription drugs, can result in a very rare and potentially fatal blood abnormality in which red blood cell count declines drastically. Warning signs of this abnormality, called aplastic anemia, include weakness, fatigue, and a tendency to easily bruise or bleed.

Taking Felbatol can also result in potentially fatal liver damage. Warning signs of a liver problem include dark urine, loss of appetite, stomach upset, and yellow skin or eyes. Tell your doctor immediately if you develop these symptoms. The sooner Felbatol is discontinued, the better your chances of recovery.

Felbatol should not be used by patients until there has been a complete discussion of the potential risks and benefits and the patient, parent, or guardian has provided written informed consent.

Who should not take Felbatol?

Do not take Felbatol if you are sensitive to or have ever had an allergic reaction to the medication or similar drugs. Also, do not take Felbatol if you have ever had any blood abnormalities or liver problems.

What should I tell my doctor before I take the first dose of Felbatol?

Tell your doctor about all prescription, over-the-counter, and herbal medications you are taking before beginning treatment with Felbatol. Also, talk to your doctor about your complete medical history, especially if you have liver disease, a history of blood abnormalities, or a history of kidney problems.

What is the usual dosage?

The information below is based on the dosage guidelines your doctor uses. Depending on your condition and medical history, your doctor may prescribe a different regimen. Do not change the dosage or stop taking your medication without your doctor's approval.

Adults and children 14 years and older: Whether Felbatol is taken alone or with other antiepileptic drugs, the usual starting dose is 1,200 milligrams (mg) per day divided into smaller doses and taken 3-4 times daily. Your doctor may gradually increase your daily dose to as much as 3,600 mg.

If you are already taking a drug to control your epilepsy, your doctor will reduce your dosage when you add Felbatol.

Children 2 to 14 years old with Lennox-Gastaut Syndrome: The usual dose is 15 mg per 2.2 pounds (lb) of body weight per day divided into smaller doses 3-4 times daily. Your doctor may gradually increase your child's dose to 45 mg per 2.2 lb of body weight per day.

Your doctor will reduce the amount of any other epilepsy drug your child is taking when starting Felbatol.

How should I take Felbatol?

Take Felbatol exactly as prescribed by your doctor. Felbatol should not be stopped suddenly. This could increase the frequency of your seizures.

If you are taking Felbatol liquid, shake well before using. You can take Felbatol tablets with or without food.

What should I avoid while taking Felbatol?

Do not stop taking Felbatol even if you feel better. Continue taking Felbatol to prevent seizures from recurring.

Avoid prolonged exposure to sunlight because Felbatol may increase the sensitivity of the skin to sunlight.

What are possible food and drug interactions associated with Felbatol?

If Felbatol is taken with certain other drugs, the effects of either could be increased, decreased, or altered. It is especially important to check with your doctor before combining Felbatol with any of the following: carbamazepine, phenobarbital, and phenytoin.

What are the possible side effects of Felbatol?

Side effects cannot be anticipated. If any develop or change in intensity, tell your doctor as soon as possible. Only your doctor can determine if it is safe for you to continue taking this drug.

Side effects in adults taking Felbatol alone may include: anxiety, constipation, diarrhea, fatigue, headache, inability to fall or stay asleep, loss of appetite, nausea, sinus inflammation, upper respiratory tract infection, upset stomach, vomiting

Side effects in adults taking Felbatol with other medications may include: abnormal stride, abnormal taste, abnormal vision, anxiety, constipation, depression, dizziness, double vision, fatigue, headache, inability to fall or stay asleep, loss of appetite, nervousness, sleepiness, tremor, upper respiratory tract infection, upset stomach, vomiting

Side effects in children taking Felbatol with other medication may include: abnormally small pupils (pinpoint pupils), abnormal stride, abnormal thoughts, constipation, coughing, fatigue, fever, headache, hiccups, inability to control urination, inability to fall or stay asleep, lack of muscle coordination, loss of appetite, mood changes, nervousness, pain, rash, red or purple spots on the skin, sleepiness, sore throat, unstable emotions, upper respiratory tract infections, upset stomach, vomiting, weight loss

Can I receive Felbatol if I am pregnant or breastfeeding?

The effects of Felbatol during pregnancy and breastfeeding are unknown. Tell your doctor immediately if you are pregnant, plan to become pregnant, or are breastfeeding.

What should I do if I miss a dose of Felbatol?

Take the forgotten dose as soon as you remember. If it is almost time for your next dose, skip the one you missed and go back to your regular schedule. Never take a double dose.

How should I store Felbatol?
Store Felbatol at room temperature in a tightly closed container and away from excessive heat and moisture.

FELDENE

Generic name: Piroxicam

What is Feldene?
Feldene is used to relieve the signs and symptoms of both osteoarthritis and rheumatoid arthritis.

What is the most important information I should know about Feldene?
Nonsteroidal anti-inflammatory drugs (NSAIDs), such as Feldene, may increase the chance of a heart attack or stroke that can lead to death. This chance increases with longer use of NSAID medicines and in people who have heart disease. NSAIDs should never be used right before or after a heart surgery called a coronary artery bypass graft (CABG).

NSAIDs may cause ulcers and bleeding in the stomach and intestines at any time during treatment. This can happen without warning symptoms and may cause death. The chance of a person getting an ulcer or bleeding increases with taking medicines called corticosteroids (anti-inflammatory drugs) and anticoagulants (blood thinners), longer use, smoking, drinking alcohol, older age, or having poor health.

It may take up to 12 days to feel the full benefit of this medication; however, you will notice some relief as soon as you start taking this medication.

Who should not take Feldene?
Do not take Feldene if you are allergic to it or to any of its ingredients. You should also avoid this medication if you have breathing problems such as asthma, allergic reactions to aspirin or to similar medications, or have just had CABG surgery.

What should I tell my doctor before I take the first dose of Feldene?
Tell your doctor about all prescription, over-the-counter, and herbal medications you are taking before beginning treatment with Feldene. Also, talk to your doctor about your complete medical history, especially if you have heart problems, stomach problems, kidney disease, high blood pressure, or you are pregnant or plan to become pregnant.

What is the usual dosage?
The information below is based on the dosage guidelines your doctor uses. Depending on your condition and medical history, your doctor

may prescribe a different regimen. Do not change the dosage or stop taking your medication without your doctor's approval.

Adults: The usual dosage of Feldene is 20 milligrams (mg) once per day. If needed, your doctor may instruct you to divide this dosage into smaller doses.

How should I take Feldene?
Take Feldene exactly as indicated by your doctor. To prevent upset stomach and side effects, take this medication with food. Never take it on an empty stomach.

What should I avoid while taking Feldene?
Never take Feldene on an empty stomach. Avoid the use of other painkillers known as NSAIDs such as Motrin (ibuprofen) and products containing aspirin.

What are possible food and drug interactions associated with Feldene?
If Feldene is taken with certain other drugs, the effects of either could be increased, decreased, or altered. It is especially important to check with your doctor before combining Feldene with the following: ACE inhibitors, aspirin, diuretics, lithium, methotrexate, piroxicam, and warfarin.

What are the possible side effects of Feldene?
Side effects cannot be anticipated. If any develop or change in intensity, tell your doctor as soon as possible. Only your doctor can determine if it is safe for you to continue taking this drug.

Side effects may include: constipation, diarrhea, dizziness, gas, heartburn, nausea, stomach pain, vomiting

Serious side effects may include: blood in stool, chest pain, itchiness, nausea, shortness of breath/trouble breathing, skin rash/blisters, slurred speech, swelling of face or throat, vomiting blood, weakness in one part/side of your body, yellowing of eyes and skin. If you experience any of these symptoms, contact your doctor right away

Can I receive Feldene if I am pregnant or breastfeeding?
The effects of Feldene during pregnancy and breastfeeding are unknown. Tell your doctor immediately if you are pregnant, plan to become pregnant, or are breastfeeding.

What should I do if I miss a dose of Feldene?
Take the forgotten dose as soon as you remember. If it is almost time for your next dose, skip the one you missed and go back to your regular schedule. Never take a double dose.

How should I store Feldene?
Store at room temperature.

Felodipine See Plendil, page 1036.

FEMHRT
Generic name: Ethinyl estradiol and norethindrone acetate

What is femHRT?
femHRT is a hormone replacement therapy for women experiencing un-comfortable symptoms of menopause, such as vaginal itching and hot flashes. Also, femHRT prevents the thinning of bones (osteoporosis) that usually happens when a woman enters menopause.

What is the most important information I should know about femHRT?
femHRT is an estrogen/progestin combination drug. Do not use estrogens and progestins to prevent heart disease, heart attacks, or strokes. Using estrogens and progestins may increase your risk of heart attack, stroke, breast cancer, and blood clots in the legs and lungs. femHRT should be used at the lowest effective dose for the shortest period.

Who should not take femHRT?
You should not take femHRT if you are pregnant, planning to become pregnant or are breastfeeding. If you have abnormal vaginal bleeding, have or had certain cancers, had your uterus removed (hysterectomy), have liver disease or have had a heart attack/stroke, do not take femHRT. Talk with your doctor about other treatment options for your menopausal symptoms.

What should I tell my doctor before I take the first dose of femHRT?
Tell your doctor about all prescription, over-the-counter, and herbal medications you are taking before beginning treatment with femHRT. Also, talk to your doctor about your complete medical history, especially if you are pregnant, plan to become pregnant, or are breastfeeding.

What is the usual dosage?
The information below is based on the dosage guidelines your doctor uses. Depending on your condition and medical history, your doctor may prescribe a different regimen. Do not change the dosage or stop taking your medication without your doctor's approval.
The usual dosage of femHRT is one pill, once per day, every day.

How should I take femHRT?

You can take femHRT any time of day, with or without food. However, it's usually easier to plan to take it at the same time each day; for example, just after brushing your teeth or before you go to bed.

What are possible food and drug interactions associated with femHRT?

If femHRT is taken with certain other drugs, the effects of either could be increased, decreased, or altered. It is especially important to check with your doctor before combining femHRT with the following: acetamino-phen, blood pressure medications, blood thinners, clarithromycin, cyclo-sporin, diabetes medications, erythromycin, estrogens, grapefruit juice, intraconazole, ketoconazole, oral contraceptives, prednisolone, ritonavir, theophylline.

What are the possible side effects of femHRT?

Side effects cannot be anticipated. If any develop or change in intensity, tell your doctor as soon as possible. Only your doctor can determine if it is safe for you to continue taking this drug.

Side effects may include: Abdominal pain, breast tenderness or enlarge-ment, enlargement of uterine fibroids (benign growths in the uterus), headache, nausea and vomiting, retention of extra fluid (edema), spotty darkening of the skin

Can I receive femHRT if I am pregnant or breastfeeding?

Like other estrogen/progestin therapies, it is not recommended to take femHRT if you are pregnant, planning to become pregnant, or are breast-feeding.

What should I do if I miss a dose of femHRT?

If you forget to take your pill at the usual time, take it as soon as you remember. If it is almost time for your next pill, skip the missed pill and take the next one in the pack. Do not take two pills at once.

How should I store femHRT?

Store at room temperature.

Fenofibrate *See Antara, page 110; Tricor, page 1332; or Triglide, page 1334.*

Fentanyl buccal *See Fentora, page 545.*

Fentanyl transdermal system *See Duragesic, page 452.*

FENTORA
Generic name: Fentanyl buccal

What is Fentora?
Fentora is used to manage breakthrough cancer pain (sudden painful episodes) in patients who are opioid-tolerant.

What is the most important information I should know about Fentora?
Fentora has high potential for abuse, and should only be used to treat opioid-tolerant patients who experience persistent cancer pain. Fentora is not recommended for temporary or post-operative pain, such as pain from a medical or dental procedure.

Fentora comes in two different products, tablets and lozenges. Take Fentora exactly as indicated by your doctor and never switch or substitute these products without your doctor's approval.

Keep Fentora out of the reach of children. This drug contains medicine in amounts that could be fatal to children and babies.

Who should not take Fentora?
Fentora should not be taken to control temporary pain from injuries, surgery, and headaches, including migraines.

Do not take Fentora if you are not opioid-tolerant; it may cause life-threatening breathing problems. Also, you should not take Fentora if you are allergic to it or to any of its ingredients.

What should I tell my doctor before I take the first dose of Fentora?
Tell your doctor about all prescription, over-the-counter, and herbal medications you are taking before beginning treatment with Fentora. Also, talk to your doctor about your complete medical history, especially if you are not opioid-tolerant, if you are taking medications knows as monoamine oxidase inhibitors (MAOIs), or if you are pregnant, plan to become pregnant, or are breastfeeding.

What is the usual dosage?
The information below is based on the dosage guidelines your doctor uses. Depending on your condition and medical history, your doctor may prescribe a different regimen. Do not change the dosage or stop taking your medication without your doctor's approval.

Adults: The usual starting dose is 100 micrograms (mcg). Use 1 dose of Fentora for an episode of breakthrough cancer pain. If your breakthrough cancer pain is not relieved after 30 minutes, use only 1 more dose of Fentora at this time. Wait at least 4 more hours before using Fentora again for another episode of breakthrough cancer pain.

How should I take Fentora?

The Fentora tablet should be placed between the cheek and gum and left to disintegrate for 14-25 minutes. After 30 minutes, any remaining pieces of the tablet could be swallowed with a glass of water. Do not split, suck, chew, or swallow whole Fentora tablets; this will result in a lower concentration in the body.

What should I avoid while taking Fentora?

Do not split, suck, chew, or swallow whole Fentora tablets. Also, do not take Fentora if you are pregnant, planning to become pregnant, or are breast-feeding. This drug may cause harm to your unborn child, and my cause breathing problems in your nursing baby. Do not drive, operate heavy machinery, or do other dangerous activities until you know how Fentora affects you. Fentora can make you sleepy. Ask your doctor when it is okay to do these activities. Do not drink alcohol while using Fentora. It can increase your chance of getting dangerous side effects.

What are possible food and drug interactions associated with Fentora?

If Fentora is taken with certain other drugs, the effects of either could be increased, decreased, or altered. It is especially important to check with your doctor before combining Fentora with the following: amprenavir, aprepitant, diltiazem, erythromycin, fluconazole, fosamprenavir, grapefruit juice, or verapamil.

What are the possible side effects of Fentora?

Side effects cannot be anticipated. If any develop or change in intensity, tell your doctor as soon as possible. Only your doctor can determine if it is safe for you to continue taking this drug.

Side effects may include: dizziness, drowsiness, headache, nausea, sleepiness, vomiting

Can I receive Fentora if I am pregnant or breastfeeding?

Do not take Fentora if you are pregnant, planning to become pregnant, or are breastfeeding. This drug may pass into your breast milk causing breathing problems in your baby.

What should I do if I miss a dose of Fentora?

Fentora is not a regularly scheduled medicine. It should only be used for breakthrough cancer pain. Remember to continue taking your regularly used around-the-clock opioid medicine and take Fentora only when you experience an episode of breakthrough pain.

How should I store Fentora?

Store Fentora at room temperature until ready to use. Always keep Fentora out of reach of children and in a secure place to protect from theft. If a child accidentally takes Fentora, get emergency help right away.

Fexofenadine hydrochloride See Allegra, page 64.

FINACEA
Generic name: Azelaic acid

What is Finacea?
Finacea is a gel used to treat mild to moderate rosacea (a skin condition marked by red eruptions, usually on the cheeks and nose).

What is the most important information I should know about Finacea?
Finacea is to be used in only on your affected skin. Never use it orally, in your eyes, or vaginally.

This medicine has been known to occasionally have a bleaching effect on the skin. Report any abnormal changes in skin color to your doctor.

You should keep using Finacea regularly, even if you see no immediate improvement. It may take a few weeks before you see results.

Who should not take Finacea?
Do not use Finacea if you are allergic to it or to any ingredient of the gel or if you have a history of allergies to propylene glycol (an additive in many facial products).

What should I tell my doctor before I take the first dose of Finacea?
Tell your doctor about all prescription, over-the-counter, and herbal medication you are taking before beginning treatment with Finacea. Also, talk to your doctor about your complete medical history.

What is the usual dosage?
The information below is based on the dosage guidelines your doctor uses. Depending on your condition and medical history, your doctor may prescribe a different regimen. Do not change the dosage or stop taking your medication without your doctor's approval.

Adults: The usual dose of Finacea is a thin film applied twice a day, once in the morning and again in the evening.

How should I take Finacea?
Use Finacea once in the morning and again in the evening. Wash the areas to be treated with very mild soap or a soapless cleansing lotion and pat dry with a soft towel. Apply a thin film of the medication and gently, but thoroughly, massage it into the skin. Wash your hands afterwards. You can apply makeup after Finacea has dried.

What should I avoid while taking Finacea?

Finacea should not come into contact with the mouth, eyes, and other mucous membranes.

Avoid any foods and beverages that might provoke redness, flushing, and blushing such as spicy foods, hot foods and drinks, and alcoholic beverages.

Use only very mild soaps or soapless cleansing lotion for facial cleansing. Avoid alcoholic cleansers, tinctures and astringents, abrasives, and peeling agents. Do not use dressings or wrappings that block contact with air.

What are possible food and drug interactions associated with Finacea?

No interactions have been reported.

What are the possible side effects of Finacea?

Side effects cannot be anticipated. If any develop or change in intensity, tell your doctor as soon as possible. Only your doctor can determine if it is safe for you to continue taking this drug.

Side effects may include: burning, itching, itchy spots, scaling or dry skin, stinging, tingling

Can I receive Finacea if I am pregnant or breastfeeding?

The effects of Finacea during pregnancy and breastfeeding are unknown. Tell your doctor immediately if you are pregnant, plan to become pregnant, or are breastfeeding. Use caution if you are nursing while using Finacea.

What should I do if I miss a dose of Finacea?

Apply it as soon as you remember. If it is almost time for your next application, skip the one you missed and go back to your regular schedule.

How should I store Finacea?

Store at room temperature.

Finasteride *See Propecia, page 1086, or Proscar, page 1093.*

FIORICET

Generic name: Butalbital, acetaminophen, and caffeine

What is Fioricet?

Fioricet is used for the relief of tension headache symptoms caused by muscle contractions in the head, neck, and shoulder area.

What is the most important information I should know about Fioricet?

Mental and physical dependence (addiction) can occur with the use of barbiturates such as butalbital when these drugs are taken in higher than recommended doses over long periods of time.

Who should not take Fioricet?

Do not take Fioricet if you are allergic to it or to any of its ingredients.

Do not take this medication if you have an inherited metabolic disorder that affects the liver or bone marrow (porphyria).

What should I tell my doctor before I take the first dose of Fioricet?

Tell your doctor about all prescription, over-the-counter, and herbal medication you are taking before beginning treatment with Fioricet. Also, talk to your doctor about your complete medical history, especially if you have kidney or liver disease, have severe stomach pain, a history of prior substance abuse, or if you drink more than 3 alcoholic beverages per day.

What is the usual dosage?

The information below is based on the dosage guidelines your doctor uses. Depending on your condition and medical history, your doctor may prescribe a different regimen. Do not change the dosage or stop taking your medication without your doctor's approval.

Adults: The usual dose of Fioricet is 1 or 2 tablets taken every 4 hours as needed. Do not take more than 6 tablets per day.

Fioricet may cause excitement, depression, and confusion in older people. Your doctor will prescribe a dose individualized to suit your needs.

Children: The safety and efficacy of Fioricet has not been established in children less than 12 years of age.

How should I take Fioricet?

Take Fioricet exactly as prescribed. Do not increase the amount you take without your doctor's approval. You may take Fioricet with food or milk if it upsets your stomach.

What should I avoid while taking Fioricet?

Fioricet can cause drowsiness or dizziness. Use caution when driving, operating machinery, or performing other hazardous activities.

Avoid taking Fioricet with sleeping pills, anti-allergy medications, sedatives, and tranquilizers. These may also make you drowsy.

Do not drink alcohol while taking Fioricet. Doing so may result in increased drowsiness and dizziness and may also damage your liver.

Avoid taking other medications that contain acetaminophen, such as Tylenol. Avoid taking in too much caffeine.

What are possible food and drug interactions associated with Fioricet?

If Fioricet is taken with certain other drugs, the effects of either could be increased, decreased, or altered. It is especially important to check with your doctor before combining Fioricet with the any of the following: antihistamines such as diphenhydramine, anxiety medicines such as alprazolam or diazepam, monoamine oxidase inhibitors such as phenelzine and tranylcypromine, muscle relaxants such as cyclobenzaprine, narcotic pain relievers such as codeine or propoxyphene, and tranquilizers such as chlordizaepoxide, chlorpromazine, and haloperidol.

What are the possible side effects of Fioricet?

Side effects cannot be anticipated. If any develop or change in intensity, tell your doctor as soon as possible. Only your doctor can determine if it is safe for you to continue taking this drug.

Side effects may include: stomach pain, dizziness, drowsiness, intoxicated feeling, light-headedness, nausea, sedation, shortness of breath, vomiting

Can I receive Fioricet if I am pregnant or breastfeeding?

The effects of Fioricet during pregnancy and breastfeeding are unknown. Tell your doctor immediately if you are pregnant, plan to become pregnant, or are breastfeeding. Do not breastfeed while taking Fioricet.

What should I do if I miss a dose of Fioricet?

Take it as soon as you remember. If it is almost time for your next dose, skip the missed dose and go back to your regular schedule. Never take 2 doses at the same time.

How should I store Fioricet?

Store at room temperature in a tight, light-resistant container.

FIORINAL

Generic name: Butalbital, aspirin, and caffeine

What is Fiorinal?

Fiorinal is used for the relief of tension headache symptoms caused by muscle contractions in the head, neck, and shoulder area.

What is the most important information I should know about Fiorinal?

Mental and physical dependence can occur with the use of barbiturates such as butalbital when these drugs are taken in higher than recommended doses over long periods of time.

Who should not take Fiorinal?
Do not take Fiorinal if you are allergic to or intolerant to aspirin, butalbital, or caffeine.

Do not take this medication if you have an inherited metabolic disorder that affects the liver or bone marrow (porphyria).

When aspirin is given to children and teenagers suffering from flu or chickenpox, it can cause a dangerous neurological disease called Reye's syndrome. Therefore, do not use Fiorinal under these circumstances.

Fiorinal contains aspirin. Do not take Fiorinal if you have a stomach (peptic) ulcer or a disorder that affects the blood clotting process. Aspirin may irritate the stomach lining and may cause bleeding.

**What should I tell my doctor before
I take the first dose of Fiorinal?**
Tell your doctor about all prescription, over-the-counter, and herbal medication you are taking before beginning treatment with Fiorinal. Let you doctor know if you have had a head injury, have a history of substance abuse, or if you are taking blood thinners. Also, talk to your doctor about your complete medical history, especially if you have: a bleeding disorder, Addison's disease (an adrenal gland disorder), an enlarged prostate, asthma, difficulty urinating, stomach (peptic) ulcers, or an underactive thyroid.

What is the usual dosage?
The information below is based on the dosage guidelines your doctor uses. Depending on your condition and medical history, your doctor may prescribe a different regimen. Do not change the dosage or stop taking your medication without your doctor's approval.

The usual dose of Fiorinal is 1 or 2 capsules taken every 4 hours. Do not take more than 6 capsules in a day.

How should I take Fiorinal?
For best relief, take Fiorinal as soon as a headache begins.

Take Fiorinal with a full glass of water or food to reduce stomach irritation

Take Fiorinal exactly as prescribed. Do not increase the amount you take without your doctor's approval, and do not take the drug for longer than prescribed.

What should I avoid while taking Fiorinal?
Avoid taking Fiorinal with alcohol or other medications that can make you feel drowsy. Use caution when driving, operating machinery, or performing other hazardous activities. If you drink alcohol during therapy with Fiorinal, this can increase your risk of stomach bleeding.

Do not take more Fiorinal than prescribed. Fiorinal may be habit-forming.

Avoid other aspirin-containing products.

What are possible food and drug interactions associated with Fiorinal?

If Fiorinal is taken with certain other drugs, the effects of either could be increased, decreased, or altered. It is especially important to check with your doctor before combining Fiorinal with the any of the following: acetazolamide, alcohol; blood-thinning drugs such as warfarin; insulin; MAO inhibitors, such as the antidepressants phenelzine and tranylcypromine; mercaptopurine; methotrexate; narcotic pain relievers such as codeine and morphine; nonsteroidal anti-inflammatory drugs such as ibuprofen or naproxen; oral diabetes drugs such as glyburide; probenecid; sleeping pills; steroid medications such as prednisone; sulfinpyrazone; and tranquilizers such as alprazolam, chlordiazepoxide, and diazepam.

What are the possible side effects of Fiorinal?

Side effects cannot be anticipated. If any develop or change in intensity, tell your doctor as soon as possible. Only your doctor can determine if it is safe for you to continue taking this drug.

Side effects may include: dizziness, drowsiness

Can I receive Fiorinal if I am pregnant or breastfeeding?

The effects of Fiorinal during pregnancy and breastfeeding are unknown. Tell your doctor immediately if you are pregnant, plan to become pregnant, or are breastfeeding. Do not breastfeed while taking Fiorinal.

What should I do if I miss a dose of Fiorinal?

If you take Fiorinal on a regular schedule, take the forgotten dose as soon as you remember. If it is almost time for your next dose, skip the missed dose and go back to your regular schedule. Do not take 2 doses at once.

How should I store Fiorinal?

Store at room temperature. Keep the container tightly closed.

FIORINAL WITH CODEINE

Generic name: Butalbital, codeine phosphate, aspirin, and caffeine

What is Fiorinal with Codeine?

Fiorinal with Codeine is prescribed for the relief of tension headache caused by stress and muscle contraction in the head, neck, and shoulder area. It combines a sedative-barbiturate (butalbital), a narcotic pain reliever and cough suppressant (codeine), a non-narcotic pain and fever reliever (aspirin), and a stimulant (caffeine).

What is the most important information
I should know about Fiorinal with Codeine?

Barbiturates such as butalbital and narcotics such as codeine can be habit-forming (addicting) when taken in higher than recommended doses over long periods of time.

Who should not take Fiorinal with Codeine?

Do not take Fiorinal with Codeine if you have ever had an allergic reaction to butalbital, codeine, aspirin, caffeine, or other pain relievers.

Do not take this medication if you have a tendency to bleed too much; asthma (wheezing) associated with aspirin or other nonsteroidal anti-inflammatory drugs such as ibuprofen; nasal polyps (growths or nodules); peptic (stomach) ulcer; porphyria (an inherited metabolic disorder affecting the liver and bone marrow); severe liver damage; severe vitamin K deficiency; and swelling due to water retention.

When aspirin is given to children and teenagers with chickenpox or flu, it can cause a dangerous neurological disease called Reye's syndrome. Therefore, do not use Fiorinal with Codeine under these circumstances.

What should I tell my doctor before
I take the first dose of Fiorinal with Codeine?

Tell your doctor about all prescription, over-the-counter, and herbal medication you are taking before beginning treatment with Fiorinal with Codeine. Also, talk to your doctor about your complete medical history, especially if you have Addison's disease (an adrenal gland disorder), asthma, a bleeding disorder, difficulty urinating, an enlarged prostate, stomach (peptic) ulcers, or underactive thyroid.

Tell your doctor if you have had a head injury, have a history of substance abuse, or if you are taking blood thinners.

What is the usual dosage?

The information below is based on the dosage guidelines your doctor uses. Depending on your condition and medical history, your doctor may prescribe a different regimen. Do not change the dosage or stop taking your medication without your doctor's approval.

Adults: The usual dose of Fiorinal with Codeine is 1 to 2 capsules taken every 4 hours. Do not take more than 6 capsules per day.

Children: The safety and effectiveness of butalbital has not been established in children less than 12 years of age.

How should I take Fiorinal with Codeine?

Take Fiorinal with Codeine with a full glass of water or food to reduce stomach irritation.

Take Fiorinal with Codeine exactly as prescribed.

What should I avoid while taking Fiorinal with Codeine?

Do not take Fiorinal with Codeine more frequently than prescribed and do not increase the amount you take without your doctor's approval.

Avoid taking this medication with other drugs that can make you feel drowsy. Use caution when driving, operating machinery, or performing other hazardous activities. Alcohol taken during therapy with Fiorinal can increase the risk of stomach bleeding.

Avoid other aspirin-containing products.

What are possible food and drug interactions associated with Fiorinal with Codeine?

If Fiorinal with Codeine is taken with certain other drugs, the effects of either could be increased, decreased, or altered. It is especially important to check with your doctor before combining Fiorinal with Codeine with any of the following: acetazolamide; alcohol; beta-blocking blood pressure drugs such as atenolol and propranolol; blood-thinning drugs such as warfarin; MAO inhibitors, such as the antidepressants phenelzine or tranylcypromine; insulin; mercaptopurine; methotrexate; narcotic pain relievers such as codeine and morphine; nonsteroidal anti-inflammatory drugs such as ibuprofen or naproxen; oral contraceptives; oral diabetes drugs such as glyburide; probenecid; sleeping pills; steroid medications such as prednisone; sulfinpyrazone; and tranquilizers such as alprazolam, chlordiazepoxide, and diazepam.

What are the possible side effects of Fiorinal with Codeine?

Side effects cannot be anticipated. If any develop or change in intensity, tell your doctor as soon as possible. Only your doctor can determine if it is safe for you to continue taking this drug.

Side effects may include: stomach pain, dizziness, drowsiness, nausea

Can I receive Fiorinal with Codeine if I am pregnant or breastfeeding?

The effects of Fiorinal with Codeine during pregnancy and breastfeeding are unknown. Tell your doctor immediately if you are pregnant, plan to become pregnant, or are breastfeeding. Do not breastfeed while taking Fiorinal with Codeine.

What should I do if I miss a dose of Fiorinal with Codeine?

If you take the drug on a regular schedule, take the dose you skipped as soon as you remember. If it is almost time for your next dose, skip the missed dose and go back to your regular schedule. Do not take 2 doses at once.

How should I store Fiorinal with Codeine?

Store at room temperature. Keep the container tightly closed.

FLAGYL

Generic name: Metronidazole

What is Flagyl?

Flagyl is used to treat certain vaginal and urinary tract infections in men and women; amebic dysentery and liver abscess; and infections of the abdomen, blood, bones and joints, brain, lung, heart, and skin caused by certain bacteria.

What is the most important information I should know about Flagyl?

Do not drink alcoholic beverages while taking Flagyl. The combination can cause abdominal cramps, nausea, vomiting, headaches, and flushing. It can also change the taste of the alcoholic beverage. Also, avoid over-the-counter medications containing alcohol, such as certain cough and cold products.

It is important to avoid skipping doses of Flagyl or discontinuing Flagyl before you have completed the full course of therapy that your doctor has prescribed. You may feel better shortly after you begin therapy with Flagyl. However, if you skip doses, or do not complete the full course of therapy, then the effectiveness of Flagyl in treating your condition may be decreased and make the use of Flagyl or other antibiotics less effective if used for any future illnesses.

Who should not take Flagyl?

Do not take Flagyl if you are allergic to it or to drugs which are similar to it. Do not use Flagyl during the first 3 months of pregnancy for the treatment of trichomoniasis.

What should I tell my doctor before I take the first dose of Flagyl?

Tell your doctor about all prescription, over-the-counter, and herbal medication you are taking before beginning treatment with Flagyl. Also, talk to your doctor about your complete medical history, especially if you have central nervous system diseases; epilepsy or another seizure disorder; a fungal infection; or liver disease.

What is the usual dosage?

The information below is based on the dosage guidelines your doctor uses. Depending on your condition and medical history, your doctor may prescribe a different regimen. Do not change the dosage or stop taking your medication without your doctor's approval.

Amebiasis

Adults: **Acute intestinal amebiasis:** 750 milligrams (mg) taken by mouth 3 times daily for 5-10 days. **Amebic liver abscess:** 500 mg or 750 mg taken by mouth 3 times daily for 5-10 days.

Children: The usual dose is 35-50 mg per 2.2 pounds of body weight per day, divided into 3 doses a day and taken by mouth for 10 days.

Anaerobic Bacterial Infections
Adults: The usual oral dosage is 7.5 mg per 2.2 pounds (lb) of body weight taken by mouth every 6 hours. Do not take more than 4 grams (g) during a 24-hour period. The usual duration of therapy is 7 to 10 days; however this may vary depending on where the infection is located in your body. For more serious infections, Flagyl will be given as an I.V. through your vein.

Trichomoniasis
Adults: *Females:* 1-day treatment: 2 grams (g) given either as a single dose or in 2 divided doses of 1 g each taken in the same day; 7-day course of treatment: 250 mg taken 3 times daily for 7 consecutive days.

Males: Your doctor will individualize your dosing regimen based on the severity of your infection and how well you respond to treatment.

How should I take Flagyl?
Flagyl works best when there is a constant amount of drug in the blood. Take your doses at evenly spaced intervals and try to avoid missing any doses.

If you are being treated for the sexually transmitted genital infection called trichomoniasis, your doctor may want to treat your partner at the same time, even if there are no symptoms. Try to avoid sexual intercourse until the infection is cured. If you do have sex, use a condom.

Flagyl can be taken with or without food. It may cause dry mouth. Hard candy, chewing gum, or bits of ice can help to relieve the problem.

What should I avoid while taking Flagyl?
Do not drink alcohol while taking Flagyl. Avoid taking over-the-counter medications containing alcohol. Avoid taking Flagyl if you have taken disulfiram within the last 2 weeks.

Avoid skipping any doses of Flagyl. Skipping doses or not completing the full course of therapy, as your doctor has prescribed, may decrease the effectiveness of Flagyl and make the use of Flagyl or other antibiotics less effective if used for any future illnesses.

What are possible food and drug interactions associated with Flagyl?
If Flagyl is taken with certain other drugs, the effects of either could be increased, decreased, or altered. It is especially important to check with your doctor before combining Flagyl with any of the following: alcoholic beverages, cimetidine, disulfiram, lithium, oral coumarin anticoagulants (eg, warfarin), phenobarbital, and phenytoin.

What are the possible side effects of Flagyl?

Side effects cannot be anticipated. If any develop or change in intensity, tell your doctor as soon as possible. Only your doctor can determine if it is safe for you to continue taking this drug.

Two serious side effects that have occurred with Flagyl are seizures and numbness or tingling in the arms, legs, hands, and feet. If you experience either of these symptoms, stop taking the medication and call your doctor immediately.

Side effects may include: abdominal cramps, constipation, unpleasant metallic taste, diarrhea, headache, loss of appetite, nausea, upset stomach, vomiting

Can I receive Flagyl if I am pregnant or breastfeeding?

The effects of Flagyl during pregnancy and breastfeeding are unknown. Do not use Flagyl during the first 3 months of pregnancy for the treatment of trichomoniasis. Discuss other treatment options with your doctor before beginning Flagyl therapy if you are pregnant. Tell your doctor immediately if you are pregnant, plan to become pregnant, or are breastfeeding. Do not breastfeed while you are taking Flagyl.

What should I do if I miss a dose of Flagyl?

Take it as soon as you remember. If it is almost time for your next dose, skip the missed dose and go back to your regular schedule. Do not take 2 doses at once.

How should I store Flagyl?

Store below 77° F (25°C) and protect it from light.

Flecainide acetate See Tambocor, page 1255.

FLECTOR

Generic name: Diclofenac epolamine

What is Flector?

Flector Patch is a nonsteroidal anti-inflammatory drug used as a last resort to relieve acute pain due to minor strains, sprains, and bruises.

What is the most important information I should know about Flector?

NSAIDs (nonsteroidal anti-inflammatory drugs) may increase the risk of blood clots, heart attack, and stroke, which can be fatal. Patients with heart problems or who are prone to have heart problems may be at greater risk.

NSAIDs also cause an increased risk of serious gastrointestinal adverse events including bleeding, ulceration, and perforation of the stomach, which can be fatal. These events can occur at anytime during use and without warning symptoms. Elderly patients are at a greater risk.

Flector should not be used to treat patients who have recently undergone CABG (coronary artery bypass graft) surgery or patients who are allergic to NSAIDs.

Flector Patch should not be applied to skin that is damaged due to eczema, infection, burns wounds, etc. Flector may also cause serious, skin adverse reactions which may occur without warning, patients should watch for any signs such as a rash, blisters, etc.

Flector should be used with caution in patients with high blood pressure and water retention or heart failure. Flector should not be used by patients who experience wheezing or who have a runny nose after taking aspirin.

Flector should be avoided in late pregnancy.

Taking NSAIDs long-term may result in kidney damage. Patients who have liver dysfunction and are taking Flector should be monitored.

Patients using Flector for extended periods may bleed more easily and should test regularly for anemia.

Patients should report any unexplained weight gain or edema to their doctors.

Patients can tape the patch down if it begins to peel off at the edges. Flector should not be worn while showering or bathing.

Flector should be discarded out of the reach of children and pets.

Who should not take Flector?

Do not use Flector if you are allergic to it or any of its ingredients. Also, you should not take Flector if are allergic to aspirin, other NSAIDs, or if you have recently undergone CABG surgery.

What should I tell my doctor before I take the first dose of Flector?

Tell your doctor about all prescription, over-the-counter, and herbal medications you are taking, before beginning treatment with Flector. Also, talk to your doctor about your complete medical history, especially if you have any ulcers or gastrointestinal problems, high blood pressure, kidney or liver disease, heart problems, wheezing, or allergies to aspirin.

What is the usual dosage?

The information below is based on the dosage guidelines your doctor uses. Depending on your condition and medical history, your doctor may prescribe a different regimen. Do not change the dosage or stop taking your medication without your doctor's approval.

Adults: The recommended dose is one patch to the most painful area twice a day.

How should I take Flector?

Flector patches should be applied to skin that is intact and should not be worn while bathing or showering. After applying the patch, patients or their caregivers should wash their hands.

What should I avoid while taking Flector?

Do not apply Flector Patch to non-intact or damaged skin resulting from injuries (burns, wounds) or other medical conditions (eczema, dermatitis).

Avoid showering or bathing while a Flector Patch is applied.

What are possible food and drug interactions associated with Flector?

If Flector is taken with certain other drugs, the effects of either could be increased, decreased, or altered. It is especially important to check with your doctor before combining Flector with any of the following: ACE-inhibitors (captopril, enalapril, fosinopril, etc.), aspirin, diuretics (furosemide and thiazides such as hydrochlorothiazide, etc.), lithium, methotrexate, and warfarin.

What are the possible side effects of Flector?

Side effects cannot be anticipated. If any develop or change in intensity, tell your doctor as soon as possible. Only your doctor can determine if it is safe for you to continue taking this drug.

Side effects may include: skin reactions at the application site, including rash, burning, dryness, discoloration, blistering, itching and inflammation, nausea, headache, vomiting, diarrhea, drowsiness, dizziness

Can I receive Flector if I am pregnant or breastfeeding?

The effects of Flector during pregnancy and breastfeeding are unknown. Talk with your doctor before taking this drug if you are pregnant, plan to become pregnant, or are breastfeeding.

What should I do if I miss a dose of Flector?

Ask your doctor or pharmacist for advice. Never double the dose.

How should I store Flector?

Store at room temperature.

FLEXERIL

Generic name: Cyclobenzaprine hydrochloride

What is Flexeril?

Flexeril is a muscle relaxant used to relieve muscle spasms due to sprains, strains, or pulls.

What is the most important information I should know about Flexeril?

Flexeril is not a substitute for the physical therapy, rest, or exercise that your doctor orders for proper healing. Although Flexeril relieves the pain of strains and sprains, it is not useful for other types of pain.

Who should not take Flexeril?

Do not take Flexeril if you are taking antidepressant drugs known as monoamine oxidase inhibitors (MAOIs) such as phenelzine or tranylcypromine or if you have taken an MAOI within the last 2 weeks. Avoid Flexeril if you are allergic to it or if you have an overactive thyroid gland.

Do not take Flexeril if you have recently had a heart attack, if you have chronic heart failure, or suffer from an irregular heartbeat.

What should I tell my doctor before I take the first dose of Flexeril?

Tell your doctor about all prescription, over-the-counter, and herbal medication you are taking before beginning treatment with Flexeril. Also, talk to your doctor about your complete medical history, especially if you are elderly, have liver disease, have ever had the eye condition called glaucoma, or if you have ever been unable to urinate. Let your doctor know if you have irregular heartbeats or other heart problems.

What is the usual dosage?

The information below is based on the dosage guidelines your doctor uses. Depending on your condition and medical history, your doctor may prescribe a different regimen. Do not change the dosage or stop taking your medication without your doctor's approval.

Adults: The usual dose of Flexeril is 5 milligrams (mg) taken 3 times a day. The dose may be increased to 10 mg taken 3 times a day.

How should I take Flexeril?

Flexeril may be taken with or without food. Flexeril should be used only for short periods (no more than 3 weeks).

Flexeril may cause dry mouth. Sucking a hard candy, chewing gum, or melting ice chips in your mouth can provide temporary relief.

What should I avoid while taking Flexeril?

Do not take Flexeril for more than 2-3 weeks.

Flexeril can make you feel drowsy or less alert. Use caution when driving or operating dangerous machinery. Avoid participating in any hazardous activity that requires full mental alertness until you know how Flexeril affects you.

Avoid alcoholic beverages while taking Flexeril.

What are possible food and drug interactions associated with Flexeril?

If Flexeril is taken with certain other drugs, the effects of either could be increased, decreased, or altered. It is especially important to check with your doctor before combining Flexeril with the following: antidepressants known as MAOIs, such as phenelzine and tranylcypromine; barbiturates such as phenobarbital; guanethidine and other high blood pressure drugs; drugs that slow the central nervous system, such as alprazolam and triazolam; and tramadol.

What are the possible side effects of Flexeril?

Side effects cannot be anticipated. If any develop or change in intensity, tell your doctor as soon as possible. Only your doctor can determine if it is safe for you to continue taking this drug.

Side effects may include: dizziness, drowsiness, dry mouth

Can I receive Flexeril if I am pregnant or breastfeeding?

The effects of Flexeril during pregnancy and breastfeeding are unknown. Tell your doctor immediately if you are pregnant, plan to become pregnant, or are breastfeeding. Do not breastfeed while taking Flexeril.

What should I do if I miss a dose of Flexeril?

If it is within an hour or so of your scheduled time, take the missed dose as soon as you remember. If you do not remember until later, skip the missed dose and go back to your regular schedule. Do not take 2 doses at once.

How should I store Flexeril?

Store away from heat, light, and moisture.

FLOMAX

Generic name: Tamsulosin hydrochloride

What is Flomax?

Flomax is used for the treatment of benign prostates hyperplasia (BPH). BPH is the swelling of the prostate gland, which may in-turn block the flow of urine. Symptoms of BPH are a weak or interrupted urinary stream, a feeling that you cannot empty your bladder completely, a feeling of delay or hesitation when you start to urinate, a need to urinate often, especially at night, or a feeling that you must urinate right away. Flomax relaxes the muscles of the prostate and increases urine flow.

What is the most important information I should know about Flomax?

Flomax is not indicated for use in women.

Flomax capsules can cause a sudden drop in blood pressure, especially following the first dose or when changing doses of capsules. Such a drop in blood pressure may be cause fainting, dizziness, or lightheadedness. Therefore, get up slowly from a chair or bed at any time until you learn how you react to Flomax capsules. You should not drive or do any hazardous activities until you are used to the side effects of this drug. If you begin to feel dizzy, sit down until you feel better.

Who should not take Flomax?
Do not take Flomax if you are allergic to any of its ingredients.

What should I tell my doctor before I take the first dose of Flomax?
Tell your doctor about all prescription, over-the-counter, and herbal medications you are taking before beginning treatment with Flomax. Also, talk to your doctor about your entire medical history.

What is the usual dosage?
The information below is based on the dosage guidelines your doctor uses. Depending on your condition and medical history, your doctor may prescribe a different regimen. Do not change the dosage or stop taking your medication without your doctor's approval.

Adults: The usual dosage of Flomax is 0.4 milligrams (mg) daily. If there is no response to this strength, it may be increased to 0.8 mg daily.

How should I take Flomax?
Flomax should be taken 30 minutes after the same meal, everyday. Do not crush, chew, or open Flomax capsules.

What should I avoid while taking Flomax?
Avoid any dangerous activities, such as driving or operating heavy machinery, until you know how Flomax affects you.

What are possible food and drug interactions associated with Flomax?
If Flomax is taken with certain other drugs, the effects of either could be increased, decreased, or altered. It is especially important to check with your doctor before combining Flomax with the following: cimetidine, fluoxetine, ketoconazole, warfarin, and other drugs like Flomax.

What are the possible side effects of Flomax?
Side effects cannot be anticipated. If any develop or change in intensity, tell your doctor as soon as possible. Only your doctor can determine if it is safe for you to continue taking this drug.

Side effects may include: back pain, chest pain, cough, diarrhea, dizziness, headache, infection, nausea, sinus infection, sleeplessness, sore throat, weakness

Can I receive Flomax if I am pregnant or breastfeeding?
Flomax is not indicated for use in women.

What should I do if I miss a dose of Flomax?
If you miss a dose, take it as soon as you remember. If it is almost time for your next dose, skip the dose you missed and return to your normal dosing schedule. Do not double your next dose.

How should I store Flomax?
Store at room temperature and keep out of reach of children.

FLONASE
Generic name: Fluticasone propionate

What is Flonase?
Flonase nasal spray is used to treat nasal symptoms (stuffy or runny nose) associated with seasonal and year-round nasal allergies, as well as year-round non-allergic nasal symptoms. Flonase is an anti-inflammatory medication that reduces the inflammation in the nasal passages causing these nasal symptoms.

**What is the most important information
I should know about Flonase?**
Steroids, including Flonase, can suppress your immune system, making it difficult for your body to fight infections. Therefore, it is important to avoid exposure to chickenpox and measles when taking Flonase, especially if you have not had these infections or been properly immunized before.

Because steroids may slow down the rate of growth in children, their growth should be checked regularly.

Once you start using Flonase, a decrease of your nasal symptoms may be seen after 12 hours, but maximal benefit may not be noted until several days after.

Avoid spraying this medication into your eyes.

Do not use more of your medicine or take it more often than your doctor has prescribed. The maximum total daily dose should not exceed 2 sprays in each nostril.

Who should not take Flonase?
Do not use Flonase if you are allergic to it or to any of its ingredients.

Flonase should also be avoided in patients who have experienced recent nasal septal ulcers, nasal surgery, or nasal trauma until healing has occurred.

Flonase Nasal Spray is not recommended for children under 4 years of age.

What should I tell my doctor before I take the first dose of Flonase?

Tell your doctor about all prescription, over-the-counter, and herbal medication you are taking before beginning treatment with Flonase. Also, talk to your doctor about your complete medical history, especially if you experience: weakness, dizziness, fatigue, joint/muscular pain, feeling of decreased energy, depression or any other symptoms you cannot explain; have been exposed to chickenpox or measles; have experienced recent nasal septal (the section of the nose that divides the left and right nostrils) ulcers, nasal surgery, or nasal trauma; have asthma and are receiving long-term corticosteroid treatment.

Tell your doctor if you are taking any medication containing ritonavir (a medication commonly used to treat HIV or AIDS).

What is the usual dosage?

The information below is based on the dosage guidelines your doctor uses. Depending on your condition and medical history, your doctor may prescribe a different regimen. Do not change the dosage or stop taking your medication without your doctor's approval.

Adults: The recommended starting dose is 2 sprays in each nostril once daily or divided into 1 spray in each nostril twice daily. For long-term therapy, the dose may be reduced to 1 spray in each nostril once daily.

Adolescents and children 4 years and older: The recommended starting dose is 1 spray in each nostril once daily. If symptom relief is not obtained, the dose may be increased to 2 sprays in each nostril once daily. Once adequate control is achieved, the dosage should be decreased to 1 spray in each nostril once daily.

The maximum total daily dose should not exceed 2 sprays in each nostril.

For Seasonal Allergic Rhinitis
Adults and children 12 years and older:
May use up to 2 sprays in each nostril once daily as needed for symptom control.

How should I take Flonase?

Prime the pump according to the manufacturer's directions. Blow your nose to clear nostrils. For each spray, close one nostril. Tilt head slightly forward keeping the bottle upright and carefully insert the nasal applicator into the other nostril. Start to breathe in through the nose and while breathing in, press firmly down on the applicator to release the spray holding the bottle as before described. Avoid spraying into eyes and breathe gently inward through the nostril. Breathe out through your mouth.

Once you have administered the required number of sprays, wipe the nasal applicator with a clean tissue and replace the dust cover.

Do not use this bottle for more than the labeled number of sprays, even if the bottle is not completely empty.

What should I avoid while taking Flonase?

Do not exceed the recommended maximum dose of 2 sprays in each nostril per day.

Do not take the drug ritonavir while taking this medication.

What are possible food and drug interactions associated with Flonase?

If Flonase is taken with certain other drugs, the effects of either could be increased, decreased, or altered. It is especially important to check with your doctor before combining Flonase with ketoconazole or ritonavir.

What are the possible side effects of Flonase?

Side effects cannot be anticipated. If any develop or change in intensity, tell your doctor as soon as possible. Only your doctor can determine if it is safe for you to continue taking this drug.

Side effects may include: cataracts, headache, increased eye pressure, nasal burning or irritation, nasal fungal infections, nasal septum perforation, nosebleed, throat inflammation, wheezing

Can I receive Flonase if I am pregnant or breastfeeding?

The effects of Flonase during pregnancy and breastfeeding are unknown. Tell your doctor immediately if you are pregnant, plan to become pregnant, or are breastfeeding.

What should I do if I miss a dose of Flonase?

If you miss a dose, skip the dose you missed and return to your next scheduled dose. Do not double your dose.

How should I store Flonase?

Store at room temperature.

FLOVENT HFA

Generic name: Fluticasone propionate

What is Flovent HFA?

Flovent HFA contains a medicine called fluticasone propionate, which is a synthetic corticosteroid. Corticosteroids are natural substances found in the body that help fight inflammation. Corticosteroids are used to treat asthma because they reduce airway inflammation.

Flovent HFA is used to treat asthma in patients 4 years of age and older.

When inhaled regularly, Flovent HFA also helps to prevent symptoms of asthma.

Flovent HFA comes in 3 strengths. Your doctor has prescribed the one that is best for your condition.

What is the most important information I should know about Flovent HFA?

It may take 1 to 2 weeks or longer for this medicine to work. It's very important to keep taking Flovent HFA regularly—every day—even if you do not feel any symptoms.

Do not use Flovent HFA as a fast-acting inhaler for sudden relief of symptoms.

Flovent HFA is intended for patients 4 years of age and older. You should supervise your child when he or she uses Flovent HFA, following the instructions provided by your child's doctor.

People taking medications that suppress the immune system are more susceptible to infections than healthy individuals. For example, chickenpox and measles can have a more serious or even fatal course in children or adults using corticosteroids.

Fluticasone will not stop an asthma attack that has already started. It is used to prevent attacks. Therefore, you should always have a short-acting, "rescue" inhaler, such as an albuterol inhaler.

Who should not take Flovent HFA?

Do not take this medication if you are allergic to Flovent HFA or any of its ingredients, or any other orally inhaled corticosteroids.

Also, you should not take Flovent HFA if you have an acute asthma attack or status asthmaticus.

What should I tell my doctor before I take the first dose of Flovent HFA?

Tell your doctor about all prescription, over-the-counter, and herbal medication you are taking before beginning treatment with Flovent HFA. Also, talk to your doctor about your complete medical history, especially if you are exposed to chickenpox or measles, or if you are pregnant, plan to become pregnant, or are breastfeeding.

What is the usual dosage?

The information below is based on the dosage guidelines your doctor uses. Depending on your condition and medical history, your doctor may prescribe a different regimen. Do not change the dosage or stop taking your medication without your doctor's approval.

Adults and adolescents 12 years and older: If you are currently using an inhaled bronchodilator, the recommended starting dose is 88 micrograms (mcg) twice a day. The maximum dose is 440 mcg twice a day.

If you are currently using another steroid inhaler, the starting dose ranges from 88 to 220 mcg twice daily. The maximum dose is 440 mcg twice a day.

If you are taking oral steroid tablets, the recommended starting dose is 440 mcg twice a day. The maximum dose is 880 mcg twice a day. Your doctor will slowly decrease your dose of steroid tablets, and then lower your dose of Flovent.

Children 4 to 11 years: The recommended starting dose is 88 mcg twice a day, regardless of prior therapy. The maximum daily dose is 88 mcg twice a day.

How should I take Flovent HFA?

Shake the inhaler well for 5 seconds immediately before each use. Prime the inhaler before using it for the first time by releasing 4 test sprays into the air away from your face, shaking well for 5 seconds before each spray. In cases where the inhaler has not been used for more than 7 days or when it has been dropped, prime the inhaler again by shaking well for 5 seconds and releasing 1 test spray into the air away from your face. Remove the cap from the mouthpiece. Breathe out fully through your mouth. While breathing in deeply and slowly through your mouth, fully depress the top of the metal canister with your index finger. Hold your breath as long as possible or up to 10 seconds, and then breathe normally. Wait about 30 seconds and shake the inhaler again. Repeat the steps. After you finish taking your dose, rinse your mouth with water and spit it out. Do not swallow.

Clean the inhaler at least once a week after the evening dose.

When the counter on the inhaler reads 020, you should refill your Flovent HFA or ask your doctor if you need another refill. When the counter reads 000, throw it out because you will not receive the right amount of medicine if you keep using it.

If you are using other inhaled medicines, ask your doctor for instructions on when to use it while using Flovent HFA.

What should I avoid while taking Flovent HFA?

Do not inhale more doses or use your Flovent HFA more often than your doctor has prescribed.

Avoid activities or environments where you are exposed to allergens. Clean areas where dust or pet fur may make your asthma or allergies worse.

Avoid exposure to known sources of infection. Stay away from people with chicken pox, measles, or any other type of infection. Your immune system may not be strong enough to fight off an infection while you are using Flovent HFA.

Avoid spraying the medication into your eyes. Never breathe into the inhalers. Avoid using expired medication because you will not receive the right amount of medicine if you keep using it.

What are possible food and drug interactions associated with Flovent HFA?

If Flovent HFA is taken with certain other drugs, the effects of either could be increased, decreased, or altered. It is especially important to check with your doctor before combining Flovent HFA with other corticosteroids, ketoconazole, or ritonavir.

What are the possible side effects of Flovent HFA?

Side effects cannot be anticipated. If any develop or change in intensity, tell your doctor as soon as possible. Only your doctor can determine if it is safe for you to continue taking this drug.

Side effects may include: cold, headache, throat irritation, thrush (fungal infection) in the mouth and throat, upper respiratory tract infection

Side effects more common in children may include: bronchitis, diarrhea, ear infection, fever, inflammation of the nose and throat, viral infection, vomiting

Can I receive Flovent HFA if I am pregnant or breastfeeding?

The effects of Flovent HFA during pregnancy and breastfeeding are unknown. Tell your doctor immediately if you are pregnant, plan to become pregnant, or are breastfeeding.

What should I do if I miss a dose of Flovent HFA?

If you miss a dose, just take your next scheduled dose when it is due. Do not double the dose.

How should I store Flovent HFA?

Store at room temperature.

FLOXIN

Generic name: Ofloxacin

What is Floxin?

Floxin tablets are used in adults to treat various infections. This includes chronic bronchitis, pneumonia, skin infections, vaginal and urinary tract infections, pelvic inflammatory disease that is caused by certain sexually transmitted diseases, and prostate infections.

What is the most important information I should know about Floxin?

The use of Floxin may cause you to develop a serious allergic reaction. It is important to immediately notify your physician if you develop any type of rash, difficulty breathing, hives, swelling of the lips, tongue, or face, or throat tightening.

Floxin may increase your risk of developing tendonitis (inflammation of the tendons) or tendon rupture. This risk is increased in patients who are older (over 60 years old), patients who are taking corticosteroids, and in patients who have undergone kidney, heart, or lung transplants. It is therefore important to immediately notify your physician if you experience tendon pain, swelling or inflammation.

Floxin may also increase the risk of developing seizures. It is important to notify your physician if you have any type of seizure disorder.

In addition, Floxin may cause you to develop peripheral neuropathy (changes in sensation and possible nerve damage). It is important to notify your physician immediately if you develop any type of pain, burning, tingling, numbness, or weakness in your arms, hands, legs, or feet.

The use of Floxin may cause you to develop sensitivity to the sun (photosensitivity) and to sunlamps and tanning beds. It is important to limit your time in the sun as well as avoid sunlamps, and tanning beds while taking Floxin tablets. It is important to immediately notify your physician if you develop any type of sunburn, blisters, or swelling of your skin.

Floxin may cause you to develop serious heart rhythm changes. Notify your physician immediately if you have a change in heart beat or if you feel faint.

You may develop diarrhea. It is important to contact your physician if you develop watery or bloody stools while on therapy or after discontinuing therapy.

Who should not take Floxin?

Do not take Floxin if you have had any type of previous allergic reaction to it or have ever had an allergic reaction to similar drugs in its class (quinolones).

What should I tell my doctor before I take the first dose of Floxin?

Tell your doctor about all prescription, over-the-counter, and herbal medication you are taking before beginning treatment with Floxin. Also, talk to your doctor about your complete medical history, especially if you are elderly, have kidney or liver disease, diabetes, have a history of cardiac arrhythmias, or a seizure disorder.

What is the usual dosage?

The information below is based on the dosage guidelines your doctor uses. Depending on your condition and medical history, your doctor may prescribe a different regimen. Do not change the dosage or stop taking your medication without your doctor's approval.

Adults: The usual dosage is 200 milligrams (mg) to 400 milligrams (mg) given every 12 hours. Your dose will vary depending on the type of infection you have and how well your kidneys function.

How should I take Floxin?

Take Floxin exactly as prescribed by your doctor. Complete the full course of therapy for best results. Take Floxin with or without food. Be sure to drink plenty of fluids while taking Floxin tablets.

While taking Floxin tablets, it is important to avoid taking antacids containing calcium, magnesium, or aluminum; sucralfate; iron; multivitamins containing zinc; and didanosine within two hours before or after taking Floxin tablets.

What should I avoid while taking Floxin?

Avoid sunlamps and tanning beds. It is important to limit your exposure to sun. Floxin tablets can make your skin sensitive to sun, sunlamps, and tanning beds. Consequently, this may cause you to develop a severe sunburn, blisters or swelling of your skin. Notify your physician immediately if any of these symptoms occur and wear protective clothing and sunscreen when you are exposed to sunlight.

Floxin may cause dizziness or lightheadedness. It is important to avoid performing potentially hazardous tasks (eg, driving, operating machinery, engaging in activities that require mental alertness) until you are use to the effects of Floxin tablets.

What are possible food and drug interactions associated with Floxin?

If Floxin is taken with certain other drugs, the effects of either could be increased, decreased, or altered. It is especially important to check with your doctor before combining Floxin tablets with the following: antacids containing aluminum, calcium, or magnesium; antidiabetic agents (eg, insulin, glyburide), cimetidine, cyclosporine, didanosine, iron, multivitamins containing zinc, non-steroidal anti-inflammatory drugs, probenecid, sucralfate, theophylline, and warfarin.

What are the possible side effects of Floxin?

Side effects cannot be anticipated. If any develop or change in intensity, tell your doctor as soon as possible. Only your doctor can determine if it is safe for you to continue taking this drug.

Side effects of Floxin tablets may include: diarrhea, difficulty sleeping, dizziness, headache, itching of genital area in women, nausea, vaginal inflammation, vomiting

Tendon rupture can occur during or after therapy with Floxin. Stop taking Floxin and contact your doctor if you feel pain, inflammation, or rupture of a tendon.

Can I receive Floxin if I am pregnant or breastfeeding?

The effects of Floxin during pregnancy are unknown. Inform your doctor if you are pregnant or planning to become pregnant.

The effects of Floxin tablets are found in breast milk. Do not breastfeed while using Floxin tablets.

What should I do if I miss a dose of Floxin?
If you miss a dose of Floxin, take it as soon as you remember. If it is almost time for your next dose, skip the missed dose and go back to your regular dosing schedule. Do not take a double dose.

How should I store Floxin?
Store Floxin tablets at room temperature in a tightly closed container.

Fluconazole See Diflucan, page 417.

FLULAVAL
Generic name: Influenza virus vaccine

What is FluLaval?
FluLaval is an influenza virus vaccine indicated for active immunization of adults 18 year and older against influenza disease caused by influenza virus subtypes A and type B contained in the vaccine.

What is the most important information I should know about FluLaval?
If Guillain-Barre syndrome (an uncommon inflammatory disorder in which your body's immune system attacks your nerves, typically causing severe weakness and numbness) has occurred within 6 weeks of receipt of a prior influenza vaccine, the decision to give FluLaval should be based on careful consideration of the potential benefits and risks.

Individuals with bleeding disorders or receiving anticoagulants are at risk of hematoma (internal bleeding) formation following a FluLaval injection.

Patients lacking an adequate immune response may have a reduced immune response to FluLaval.

Who should not take FluLaval?
FluLaval is not indicated for use in children.

FluLaval is contraindicated in patients who are known to have allergic reactions to egg proteins (eggs or egg products), chicken proteins, or any ingredient of FluLaval. Also, it is contraindicated if the patient had any life-threatening reaction to previous influenza vaccination.

Immunization should be delayed in a patient with an acute neurologic disorder but should be considered when the disease process has been stabilized.

What should I tell my doctor before I take the first dose of FluLaval?

Tell your doctor about all prescription, over-the-counter, and herbal medication you are taking before beginning treatment with FluLaval. Also, talk to your doctor about your complete medical history, especially if you have allergic reactions to egg or chicken proteins, are pregnant or planning to become pregnant, or if you have a history of any neurologic disorder.

What is the usual dosage?

The information below is based on the dosage guidelines your doctor uses. Depending on your condition and medical history, your doctor may prescribe a different regimen. Do not change the dosage or stop taking your medication without your doctor's approval.

A single 0.5 mL intramuscular injection preferably in the region of the deltoid muscle of the upper arm.

How should I take FluLaval?

Inspect FluLaval for any particular matter or discoloration prior to administration. Shake the vial vigorously each time before withdrawing a dose of vaccine. A separate sterile syringe and needle should be used for each injection to prevent transmission of infectious agents. A needle length of greater than 1 inch is preferred because needles less than 1 inch might be of insufficient length to penetrate muscle tissue in certain adults.

What should I avoid while taking FluLaval?

Avoid exposing yourself to known sources of infection.

What are possible food and drug interactions associated with FluLaval?

If FluLaval is taken with certain other drugs, the effects of either could be increased, decreased, or altered. It is especially important to check with your doctor before combining FluLaval with any of the following: phenytoin, theophylline, and warfarin.

What are the possible side effects of FluLaval?

Side effects cannot be anticipated. If any develop or change in intensity, tell your doctor as soon as possible. Only your doctor can determine if it is safe for you to continue taking this drug.

Side effects may include: pain, redness, swelling at the injection site, headache, fatigue, low grade fever

Can I receive FluLaval if I am pregnant or breastfeeding?

The effects of FluLaval during pregnancy and breastfeeding are unknown. Tell your doctor immediately if you are pregnant, plan to become pregnant, or are breastfeeding.

What should I do if I miss a dose of FluLaval?
Most people need only one dose of this medicine.

How should I store FluLaval?
Store the vial in refrigerator at 2° and 8°C (36° and 46°F). Do not freeze. Discard if the vaccine has been frozen. Once entered, a multi-dose vial, and any residual contents, should be discarded after 28 days.

FLUMADINE
Generic name: Rimantadine

What is Flumadine?
Flumadine is used to prevent and treat influenza A, a viral infection.

**What is the most important information
I should know about Flumadine?**
Be sure to use Flumadine for the full course of treatment. Your symptoms may start to improve before the infection is completely treated. The virus could also become less sensitive to this or other medicines. This could make the infection harder to treat in the future.

Do not drive or perform other possibly unsafe tasks until you know how you react to Flumadine; this medicaiton may cause dizziness or drowsiness. These effects may be worse if you take it with alcohol or certain medicines.

Check with your doctor if you will be receiving a live nasal flu vaccine or have received one within the past 14 days. You should usually not start taking Flumadine until 2 weeks after you receive a live nasal flu vaccine. You should usually not receive a live nasal flu vaccine within 48 hours after you stop taking Flumadine.

Use Flumadine with caution if you have a history of epilepsy or had a seizure episode in the past. There have been some reports of seizure-like activity in patients with a history of seizures that were not on an anticonvulsant medication while taking Flumadine.

Who should not take Flumadine?
Do not take Flumadine if you are sensitive to the drug or to amantadine.

**What should I tell my doctor before
I take the first dose of Flumadine?**
Tell your doctor about all prescription, over-the-counter, and herbal medication you are taking before beginning treatment with Flumadine. Also, talk to your doctor about your complete medical history, especially if you have epilepsy or any other seizure disorder, or if you have kidney or liver disease. In addition, tell your doctor if you have received a live nasal flu vaccine within the past 14 days.

What is the usual dosage?
The information below is based on the dosage guidelines your doctor uses. Depending on your condition and medical history, your doctor may prescribe a different regimen. Do not change the dosage or stop taking your medication without your doctor's approval.

Prevention of Influenza A
Adults and children 10 years and older: The recommended dose is 100 milligrams (mg) taken 2 times a day.

Children younger than 10 years old: The daily recommended dose is 5 mg per 2.2 pounds (lb) of body weight. The daily dose should not exceed 150mg.

Treatment of Influenza A
Adults and children 10 years and older: The recommended dose is 100 mg taken 2 times a day, continued for 7 days after you start feeling ill. Flumadine therapy should be initiated as soon as possible, preferably within 48 hours after onset of signs and symptoms of influenza A infection.

In patients with severe liver dysfunction, kidney failure, and those who are elderly a dose reduction to 100mg daily is recommended.

How should I take Flumadine?
Take Flumadine exactly as directed by your doctor. Flumadine may be taken with or without food.

If you are taking Flumadine to treat the flu, start taking it as soon as possible. It works best if you begin taking it within 48 hours after you start having flu symptoms.

Take Flumadine for the full course of treatment. Do not miss any doses.

What should I avoid while taking Flumadine?
Use caution when driving, operating machinery, or performing other hazardous activities. Flumadine may cause dizziness.

Be sure to use Flumadine for the full course of treatment. Your symptoms may start to improve before the infection is completely treated.

What are possible food and drug interactions associated with Flumadine?
If Flumadine is taken with certain other drugs, the effects of either could be increased, decreased, or altered. It is especially important to check with your doctor before combining Flumadine with acetaminophen, aspirin, cimetidine, and live influenza virus vaccine.

What are the possible side effects of Flumadine?

Side effects cannot be anticipated. If any develop or change in intensity, tell your doctor as soon as possible. Only your doctor can determine if it is safe for you to continue taking this drug.

Side effects may include: abdominal pain, difficulty falling or staying asleep, dizziness, dry mouth, feeling tired or weak, headache, loss of appetite, nausea, nervousness, vomiting

Can I receive Flumadine if I am pregnant or breastfeeding?

The effects of Flumadine during pregnancy and breastfeeding are unknown. Tell your doctor immediately if you are pregnant, plan to become pregnant, or are breastfeeding. Do not breastfeed while taking Flumadine.

What should I do if I miss a dose of Flumadine?

Take the missed dose as soon as you remember. If it is almost time for your next dose, skip the missed dose and take your next regularly scheduled dose. Do not take 2 doses at once.

How should I store Flumadine?

Store Flumadine at 77 degrees F (25 degrees C). Brief storage at temperatures between 59 and 86 degrees F (15 and 30 degrees C) is permitted. Store away from heat, moisture, and light. Do not store in the bathroom. Keep Flumadine out of the reach of children..

Flunisolide See AeroBid, page 48.

Fluocinonide 0.1% See Vanos, page 1373.

Fluorometholone See FML, page 581.

Fluoxetine hydrochloride See Prozac, page 1103.

Flurazepam hydrochloride See Dalmane, page 373.

Flurbiprofen See Ansaid, page 107.

Fluticasone furoate See Veramyst, page 1380.

Fluticasone propionate See Cutivate, page 361; Flonase, page 563; or Flovent HFA, page 565.

Fluticasone propionate and salmeterol See Advair Diskus, page 41, or Advair HFA, page 44.

Fluvastatin sodium See Lescol/Lescol XL, page 712.

FLUVOXAMINE MALEATE

What is Fluvoxamine maleate?

Fluvoxamine is used to treat obsessive-compulsive disorder.

What is the most important information I should know about Fluvoxamine maleate?

Antidepressants can increase the risk of suicidal thinking and behavior in children and teenagers. Adult and pediatric patients taking antidepressants should be watched closely for changes in moods or actions, especially when they first start therapy or when their dose is increased or decreased. Patients and their families should contact the doctor immediately if new symptoms develop or seem to get worse. Signs to watch for include anxiety, hostility, insomnia, restlessness, impulsive or dangerous behavior, and thoughts about suicide or dying.

Never take fluvoxamine if you are taking another class of antidepressant drugs called monoamine oxidase inhibitors (MAOIs) or if you have stopped taking an MAOI in the last 14 days. MAOI drugs include phenelzine, tranylcypromine, and isocarboxazid. Taking fluvoxamine in close proximity or concurrently with an MAOI can result in serious—sometimes fatal—reactions, including high body temperature, coma, and seizures.

A life-threatening condition called serotonin syndrome (serious changes in how your brain, muscles, and digestive system work) can occur when you take fluvoxamine with medicines known as triptans, which are used to treat migraine headaches. Signs and symptoms of serotonin syndrome include restlessness, diarrhea, hallucinations, coma, loss of coordination, nausea, fast heartbeat, vomiting, increased body temperature, rapid changes in blood pressure, and overactive reflexes. Serotonin syndrome may be more likely to occur when starting or increasing the dose of fluvoxamine or a triptan.

Who should not take Fluvoxamine maleate?

Do not take fluvoxamine if you are sensitive to the drug. Never take fluvoxamine if you are taking alosetron, astemizole, cisapride, MAOIs, terfenadine, thioridazine, or tizanidine.

What should I tell my doctor before I take the first dose of Fluvoxamine maleate?

Tell your doctor about all prescription, over-the-counter, and herbal medications you are taking before beginning treatment with fluvoxamine. Also, talk to your doctor about your complete medical history, especially if you have liver disease, a history of seizure disorders, suffer from mania, or experience worsening symptoms of depression and/or suicidal thoughts.

What is the usual dosage?

The information below is based on the dosage guidelines your doctor uses. Depending on your condition and medical history, your doctor may prescribe a different regimen. Do not change the dosage or stop taking your medication without your doctor's approval.

Adults: The usual starting dose is 50 milligrams (mg) taken daily at bedtime. The dose may be increased depending upon your response. The maximum daily dose is 300 mg. If you take more than 100 mg a day, your doctor will divide the total amount into 2 doses. If the doses are not equal, you should take the larger dose at bedtime.

Elderly patients, or patients with impaired liver function, might require a lower starting dose.

Children 8 to 17 years old: The recommended starting dose is 25 mg taken at bedtime. The dose may be increased to a maximum of 200 mg daily for children under 11 years, and 300 mg for children 11 to 17 years. Larger daily dosages are divided in two, as for adults.

How should I take Fluvoxamine maleate?

Take fluvoxamine with or without food, exactly as prescribed by your doctor.

What should I avoid while taking Fluvoxamine maleate?

Do not stop taking fluvoxamine without first talking to your doctor. An abrupt decrease in dose could cause withdrawal symptoms such as mood problems, tiredness, insomnia, and tingling sensations.

Use caution when driving, operating machinery, or performing hazardous activities. Fluvoxamine can cause dizziness or drowsiness.

Use alcohol cautiously. Alcohol may increase drowsiness and dizziness while taking fluvoxamine or affect your condition.

What are possible food and drug interactions associated with Fluvoxamine maleate?

If fluvoxamine is taken with certain other drugs, the effects of either could be increased, decreased, or altered. It is especially important to check with your doctor before combining fluvoxamine with the following: antidepressants such as amitriptyline, clomipramine, or imipramine; blood pressure medications known as beta-blockers, including metoprolol and propranolol; blood thinners such as aspirin and aspirin-related products, or warfarin; carbamazepine; clozapine; diltiazem; lithium; methadone; mexiletine; migraine headache drugs such as almotriptan and sumatriptan; nonsteroidal anti-inflammatory drugs such as ibuprofen or naproxen; phenytoin; pimozide; quinidine; tacrine; theophylline; thioridazine; tranquilizers and sedatives such as alprazolam, diazepam, midazolam, and triazolam; and tryptophan.

What are the possible side effects of Fluvoxamine maleate?

Side effects cannot be anticipated. If any develop or change in intensity, tell your doctor as soon as possible. Only your doctor can determine if it is safe for you to continue taking this drug.

Side effects may include: abnormal ejaculation, agitation, anxiety, diarrhea, difficulty falling or staying asleep, dizziness, dry mouth, headache, indigestion, nausea, nervousness, sleepiness, sweating, tremor, vomiting, weakness, weight loss

Can I receive Fluvoxamine maleate if I am pregnant or breastfeeding?

The effects of fluvoxamine during pregnancy and breastfeeding are unknown. Tell your doctor immediately if you are pregnant, plan to become pregnant, or are breastfeeding. Do not breastfeed while taking fluvoxamine.

What should I do if I miss a dose of Fluvoxamine maleate?

If you are taking 1 dose a day, skip the missed dose and go back to your regular schedule. If you are taking 2 doses a day, take the missed dose as soon as possible, then go back to your regular schedule. Never take 2 doses at the same time.

How should I store Fluvoxamine maleate?

Store at room temperature and protect from moisture.

Fluvoxamine maleate, extended-release See Luvox CR, page 778.

FLUZONE

Generic name: Influenza virus vaccine

What is Fluzone?

Fluzone is an inactivated influenza virus vaccine indicated for active immunization against influenza disease caused by influenza virus subtypes A and type B.

What is the most important information I should know about Fluzone?

Recurrence of Guillain-Barre syndrome has been associated with the administration of influenza virus vaccine. If Guillain-Barre syndrome has occurred within 6 weeks of receiving prior influenza virus vaccine, the decision to give Fluzone should be based on careful consideration of the potential benefits and risks.

Patients lacking an adequate immune response may have a reduced immune response to Fluzone.

In case you experience a severe allergic reaction to Fluzone, appropriate medical treatment and supervision must be available to manage the possible allergic response.

The immune response to Fluzone may be lower in patients 65 years of age and older when compared to the immune response in younger patients.

Fluzone contains killed viruses and cannot cause influenza virus. Fluzone stimulates the immune system to produce antibodies that protect against the influenza virus.

Fluzone may not protect everyone against the influenza virus. It is recommended to get an influenza virus vaccine once a year because immunity during the year after receiving vaccination declines, and circulating strains of the influenza virus change each year.

Who should not take Fluzone?

You should not be given Fluzone if you are allergic to egg proteins or any ingredient of Fluzone. Also, you should not be given Fluzone if you have had a previous severe reaction to any influenza virus vaccine.

The safety and effectiveness of Fluzone have not been established in children younger than 6 months old.

What should I tell my doctor before I take the first dose of Fluzone?

Tell your doctor about all prescription, over-the-counter, and herbal medication you are taking before beginning treatment with Fluzone. Also, talk to your doctor about your complete medical history, especially if you have Guillain-Barre syndrome, lack an adequate immune response, or you are pregnant or planning to become pregnant, or breastfeeding.

What is the usual dosage?

The information below is based on the dosage guidelines your doctor uses. Depending on your condition and medical history, your doctor may prescribe a different regimen. Do not change the dosage or stop taking your medication without your doctor's approval.

Adults: One 0.5mL dose, intramuscular injection

Children 6 through 35 months old: Previously unvaccinated: Two 0.25 mL doses, intramuscular injection, one on day 1 followed by another 0.25 mL dose at least 1 month later. *Previously vaccinated (ie, received two doses within the same season):* One 0.25 mL dose, intramuscular injection

Children 36 months through 8 years old: Previously unvaccinated: Two 0.5 mL doses, one on day 1 followed by another 0.5 mL dose at least one month later. *Previously vaccinated (ie, received two doses within the same season):* One 0.5mL dose, intramuscular injection

Children 9 years old and older: One 0.5mL dose, intramuscular injection

How should I take Fluzone?

Inspect Fluzone vaccine syringes and vials for any particular matter or discoloration prior to administration. If any of this is present, Fluzone should not be given.

Shake the syringe and single-dose vials well before administering Fluzone. Shake the multi-dose vial each time before withdrawing a dose.

Fluzone is given as an intramuscular (directly into the muscle) injection only. It is preferred to give Fluzone in the deltoid muscle (rounded outline part of your shoulder) in adults and children over 36 months of age. Fluzone should not be injected into the gluteal region or into areas where there may be a major nerve trunk.

In children 36 months and younger, the anterolateral aspect of the thigh should be used.

If Fluzone is to be given at the same time as another injectable vaccine(s), the vaccine(s) should be given at different injection sites.

What should I avoid while taking Fluzone?

Fluzone should not be injected into the gluteal region or into areas where there may be a major nerve trunk. Fluzone should not be given at the same injection site if being administered at the same time as another vaccine(s).

What are possible food and drug interactions associated with Fluzone?

If Fluzone is taken with certain other drugs, the effects of either could be increased, decreased, or altered. It is especially important to check with your doctor before combining Fluzone with other vaccines (Fluzone should not be mixed with another vaccine in the same syringe or vial) or immunosuppressive drugs (the immune response to Fluzone may be reduced).

What are the possible side effects of Fluzone?

Side effects cannot be anticipated. If any develop or change in intensity, tell your doctor as soon as possible. Only your doctor can determine if it is safe for you to continue taking this drug.

Side effects may include: soreness at injection site, tenderness, pain, swelling, malaise, headache, muscle pain

Can I receive Fluzone if I am pregnant or breastfeeding?

The effects of Fluzone during pregnancy and breastfeeding are unknown. Tell your doctor immediately if you are pregnant, plan to become pregnant, or are breastfeeding.

What should I do if I miss a dose of Fluzone?
Most people need only one dose of Fluzone. If your child needs a second dose of Fluzone, it is very important for your child to receive the second dose on schedule. If you must cancel the appointment for the second dose, make another appointment as close to that date as possible.

How should I store Fluzone?
Store in the refrigerator at 2° to 8°C (35° to 46°F). Do not freeze. Between uses, return the multi-dose vial to the refrigerator. Throw out if frozen or if it is after the expiration date shown on the label.

FML
Generic name: Fluorometholone

What is FML?
FML is available as an eye ointment or suspension that is used to treat steroid-responsive inflammation of the eyelid and the eye itself.

What is the most important information I should know about FML?
Do not use FML more often or for a longer period of time than your doctor instructs. Overuse can increase the risk of side effects and lead to eye damage. If your eye problems return, do not use any leftover FML without first asking your doctor.

If inflammation or pain lasts longer than 48 hours or becomes worse, discontinue FML and call your doctor.

FML is packaged as a sterile medicine. Avoid touching the tip of the bottle to any surfaces, including your eye, to decrease the spread of possible infections to your eye.

Benzalkonium chloride, which is the preservative in FML, may be absorbed by soft contact lenses. If you wear soft contact lenses, you should wait at least 15 minutes after instilling FML suspension to insert your soft contact lenses.

Who should not take FML?
Do not use FML if you have ever had an allergic reaction or are sensitive to it or to any of its ingredients. You should not use FML if you are allergic to other steroid medications. .

FML is not prescribed for patients with certain viral, fungal, and bacterial infections of the eye.

What should I tell my doctor before I take the first dose of FML?
Tell your doctor about all prescription, over-the-counter, and herbal medication you are taking before beginning treatment with FML. Also, talk to your doctor about your complete medical history, especially if you

have cataracts or other eye diseases; glaucoma (elevated pressure in the eye causing optic nerve damage and loss of vision); a history of herpes simplex; or if you are pregnant, planning to become pregnant, or breast-feeding.

What is the usual dosage?
The information below is based on the dosage guidelines your doctor uses. Depending on your condition and medical history, your doctor may prescribe a different regimen. Do not change the dosage or stop taking your medication without your doctor's approval.

Adults: FML Ointment: Apply a small amount of ointment (about ½-inch ribbon) between the lower eyelid and eyeball 1-3 times a day. During the first 24-48 hours, the frequency of dosing may be increased to one application every 4 hours. Do not discontinue therapy prematurely. *FML Liquifilm:* Place 1 drop of suspension between the lower eyelid and eyeball 2-4 times a day. During the first 24-48 hours, the frequency of dosing may be increased to one instillation every 4 hours. Do not discontinue therapy prematurely.

How should I take FML?
FML may increase the chance of infection from contact lenses. Your doctor may advise you to stop wearing your contacts while using FML.

Use FML exactly as prescribed. Do not stop until your doctor advises you to do so. To avoid spreading infection, do not let anyone else use your prescription.

To administer FML eye drops, wash your hands thoroughly. Shake well before using. Gently pull your lower eyelid down to form a pocket between your eye and eyelid. Hold the eye drop bottle on the bridge of your nose or on your forehead.

Do not touch the applicator tip to any surface, including your eye. Tilt your head back and squeeze FML into your eye. Close your eyes gently. Keep them closed for 1-2 minutes. Do not rinse the dropper. Wait 5-10 minutes before using a second eye medication.

To administer FML ointment, wash your hands thoroughly. Hold the tube in your hand for a few minutes to warm it up so that the ointment comes out easily. Tilt your head back slightly and pull down gently on your lower eyelid. Apply a thin film of ointment into your lower eyelid. Close your eye and roll your eyeball around in all directions for 1-2 minutes.

If you are applying another eye medication, allow at least 10 minutes before your next application.

What should I avoid while taking FML?
Do not touch the dropper or tube opening to any surface, including your eyes or hands. If it becomes dirty it could cause an infection in your eye.

FML may cause blurred vision. Use caution when driving, operating machinery, or performing other potentially hazardous activities.

If you wear contact lenses, ask your doctor if you can wear them while you are using FML.

What are possible food and drug interactions associated with FML?

No significant interactions with food or other drugs have been reported at this time. However, always tell your doctor about any medicines you take, including over-the-counter drugs, vitamins, and herbal supplements.

What are the possible side effects of FML?

Side effects cannot be anticipated. If any develop or change in intensity, tell your doctor as soon as possible. Only your doctor can determine if it is safe for you to continue taking this drug.

Side effects may include: allergic reactions, blurred vision, burning or stinging, cataract formation, corneal ulcers, dilation of the pupil, drooping eyelids, eye inflammation and infection including pinkeye, eye irritation, increased eye pressure, slow wound healing, taste alterations, secondary eye infections

Can I receive FML if I am pregnant or breastfeeding?

The effects of FML during pregnancy and breastfeeding are unknown. Tell your doctor immediately if you are pregnant, plan to become pregnant, or are breastfeeding. Do not use FML if you are breastfeeding.

What should I do if I miss a dose of FML?

Apply the ointment or instill the suspension as soon as you remember. If it is almost time for your next dose, skip the missed dose and return to your regular schedule. Do not apply/instill a double dose.

How should I store FML?

Store at room temperature and protect from heat.

FOCALIN

Generic name: Dexmethylphenidate hydrochloride

What is Focalin?

Focalin is a central nervous stimulant used to treat attention deficit hyperactivity disorder (ADHD) in children.

What is the most important information I should know about Focalin?

Excessive doses of Focalin over a long period of time can produce addiction. It is also possible to develop tolerance to the drug, so that larger doses are needed to produce the original effect. Because of these dangers, be sure to check with your doctor before making any change in dosage. Do not stop the drug without your doctor's supervision.

Who should not take Focalin?

Do not take Focalin if you are sensitive to the drug, or have marked anxiety, tension, and agitation. Focalin can make your symptoms worse.

Do not take Focalin if you have motor tics (repeated, uncontrollable twitches) or a family history or diagnosis of Tourette's syndrome (severe and multiple tics).

Do not take Focalin if you are taking monoamine oxidase inhibitors (MAOIs) such as phenelzine or tranylcypromine or within 14 days after stopping this type of medication.

Do not take this drug if you have glaucoma (elevated pressure in the eye).

Focalin should not be used in children less than 6 years of age because it has not been studied in this age group.

What should I tell my doctor before I take the first dose of Focalin?

Tell your doctor about all prescription, over-the-counter, and herbal medications you are taking before beginning treatment with Focalin. Also, talk to your doctor about your complete medical history, especially if you have any mental or physical problems. Also, inform your doctor of any drug or alcohol abuse, depression, psychosis, epilepsy/seizures, high blood pressure, heart conditions, glaucoma, or if you or any of your family has a history of tics/Tourette's syndrome.

Also tell your doctor if you or your child is pregnant, planning to become pregnant, or is breastfeeding.

What is the usual dosage?

The information below is based on the dosage guidelines your doctor uses. Depending on your condition and medical history, your doctor may prescribe a different regimen. Do not change the dosage or stop taking your medication without your doctor's approval.

Focalin has not been studied in children under 6 years of age.

If you have never taken Focalin before, the usual starting dose is 5 milligrams (mg) a day. For those who are switching from Ritalin, the starting Focalin dose is half the amount of the Ritalin dose. In either case, the total daily dose of Focalin should be divided into 2 doses taken at least 4 hours apart.

Depending on your response, your doctor may increase the dose by 2.5-5 mg a day, up to a maximum of 20 mg (10 mg 2 times a day). Increases are usually made at weekly intervals.

How should I take Focalin?

Focalin can be taken with or without food. The drug is usually taken 2 times a day, at least 4 hours apart, but your doctor may adjust the schedule depending on your child's response. Take Focalin exactly as prescribed.

What should I avoid while taking Focalin?

Use caution when driving, operating machinery, or performing other hazardous activities. Focalin may cause dizziness, drowsiness, or blurred vision. This drug may interfere with your ability to concentrate.

Do not share Focalin with anyone else. Focalin should not be used to prevent or treat normal fatigue.

What are possible food and drug interactions associated with Focalin?

If Focalin is taken with certain other drugs, the effects of either could be increased, decreased, or altered. It is especially important to check with your doctor before combining Focalin with the following: antiseizure drugs such as phenobarbital, phenytoin, primidone; antidepressant drugs, including MAOIs (phenelzine, tranylcypromine), serotonin reuptake inhibitors (fluoxetine, paroxetine), and tricyclics (amitriptyline, imipramine); blood pressure drugs such as clonidine; cold or allergy medicines that contain decongestants; blood thinners such as warfarin or aspirin; ephedra; and St. John's wort.

What are the possible side effects of Focalin?

Side effects cannot be anticipated. If any develop or change in intensity, tell your doctor as soon as possible. Only your doctor can determine if it is safe for you to continue taking this drug.

Side effects may include: decreased appetite, fever, nausea, stomach pain, increased blood pressure and heart rate, new or worsening behavior and thought problems, aggressive behavior, new psychotic symptoms, slowing of growth

Can I receive Focalin if I am pregnant or breastfeeding?

The effects of Focalin during pregnancy and breastfeeding are unknown. Tell your doctor immediately if you are pregnant, plan to become pregnant, or are breastfeeding.

What should I do if I miss a dose of Focalin?

Take it as soon as you remember. If it is almost time for your next dose, skip the missed dose and return to your regular schedule. Never take 2 doses at the same time.

How should I store Focalin?
Store in a cool, dry place in a tightly closed, light-resistant container.

FOCALIN XR
*Generic name: Dexmethylphenidate hydrochloride,
    extended-release*

What is Focalin XR?
Focalin XR is a once-daily treatment for attention deficit hyperactivity disorder (ADHD).

What is the most important information I should know about Focalin XR?
Dexmethylphenidate, the active ingredient in Focalin XR, helps increase attention and decrease impulsiveness and hyperactivity in patients with ADHD.

Who should not take Focalin XR?
You should not take Focalin XR if you have significant anxiety, tension or agitation. This drug may make these symptoms worse. Also, do not take Focalin XR if you have glaucoma, tics from Tourette's syndrome (or a family history of Tourette's syndrome), if you are taking MAOIs, or if you are allergic to any of the ingredients in this drug.

What should I tell my doctor before I take the first dose of Focalin XR?
Tell your doctor about all prescription, over-the-counter, and herbal medications you are taking before beginning treatment with Focalin XR. Also, talk to your doctor about your complete medical history, especially if you have any mental or physical problems. Also, inform your doctor of any drug or alcohol abuse, depression, psychosis, epilepsy/seizures, high blood pressure, heart conditions, glaucoma, or if you or any of your family has a history of tics/Tourette's syndrome.

What is the usual dosage?
The information below is based on the dosage guidelines your doctor uses. Depending on your condition and medical history, your doctor may prescribe a different regimen. Do not change the dosage or stop taking your medication without your doctor's approval.

Focalin XR is available in 5, 10 and 20 milligram (mg) extended-release capsules, and should be taken once each morning.

How should I take Focalin XR?
Focalin XR capsules may be taken at the same time each day, with or without food. The capsules may be swallowed whole, or opened and sprinkled

over a spoon of applesauce. The capsule should not be crushed, chewed, nor have its contents divided.

What should I avoid while taking Focalin XR?

Use caution when driving, operating heavy machinery, or performing other activities that require alertness. Focalin may cause dizziness, drowsiness, or blurred vision. This drug may interfere with your ability to concentrate.

What are possible food and drug interactions associated with Focalin XR?

If Focalin XR is taken with certain other drugs, the effects of either could be increased, decreased, or altered. It is especially important to check with your doctor before combining Focalin XR with the following: antidepressants (such as MAOIs or SSRIs), antiseizure medications, blood thinners, clomipramine, desipramine, imipramine, phenobarbital, phenytoin, primidone, and cold or allergy preparations containing decongestants.

What are the possible side effects of Focalin XR?

Side effects cannot be anticipated. If any develop or change in intensity, tell your doctor as soon as possible. Only your doctor can determine if it is safe for you to continue taking this drug.

Side effects may include: anxiety, dependence, dizziness, dry mouth, jitteriness, slowed growth (in both weight and height) in children, throat pain, upset stomach

Also, if you have blurred vision see your doctor immediately—this may be a sign of a more serious problem.

Can I receive Focalin XR if I am pregnant or breastfeeding?

The effects of Focalin XR during pregnancy and breastfeeding are unknown. Talk with your doctor before taking this drug if you are pregnant, plan to become pregnant, or are breastfeeding.

How should I store Focalin XR?

Store at room temperature in a clean, dry place.

FORADIL AEROLIZER

Generic name: Formoterol fumarate

What is Foradil Aerolizer?

Foradil Aerolizer consists of Foradil capsules and an Aerolizer inhaler. Foradil Aerolizer is a long-acting beta2-agonist (LABA) used for asthma, exercise-induced bronchospasm, and chronic obstructive pulmonary disease (COPD). Foradil Aerolizer helps control asthma in people who need regular treatment with short-acting inhalers. Foradil Aerolizer is also used to relieve tightening of the airways in people with chronic obstructive pulmonary disease (COPD), including chronic bronchitis and emphysema. Taken on an as-needed basis, Foradil Aerolizer can also be used to prevent exercise-induced tightening of the airways.

What is the most important information I should know about Foradil Aerolizer?

Foradil Aerolizer is used to prevent asthma attacks. Do not use Foradil Aerolizer for the relief of acute asthma symptoms. Your doctor will prescribe a short-acting inhaler such as albuterol to use for acute asthma attacks.

Foradil Aerolizer may increase the risk of asthma-related death. It should only be used as additional therapy if you are not adequately controlled on other asthma-controlling medications or if your disease is severe enough to require treatment with two medications.

You should never swallow Foradil capsules. Foradil capsules are only to be used with the Aerolizer inhaler that comes with Foradil Aerolizer. Never place a capsule in the mouthpiece of the Aerolizer inhaler.

Foradil Aerolizer should not be used as a substitute for oral or inhaled corticosteroids.

Who should not take Foradil Aerolizer?

Do not take Foradil Aerolizer if you are sensitive to any component of the medication, including lactose (milk sugar) or milk protein.

What should I tell my doctor before I take the first dose of Foradil Aerolizer?

Tell your doctor about all prescription, over-the-counter, and herbal medications you are taking before beginning treatment with Foradil. Also, talk to your doctor about your complete medical history, especially if your asthma is significantly worsening, or if you have high blood pressure, heart disease, an abnormal heart rhythm, a seizure disorder, thyroid disease, diabetes, kidney or liver disease, pregnant or planning to become pregnant, or breastfeeding.

What is the usual dosage?

The information below is based on the dosage guidelines your doctor uses. Depending on your condition and medical history, your doctor may prescribe a different regimen. Do not change the dosage or stop taking your medication without your doctor's approval.

Adults: Foradil Aerolizer comes as a powder-filled capsule to inhale by mouth using a special inhaler. See "How Should I Take Foradil Aerolizer?" below.

Asthma
Adults and children 5 years of age and older: For the long-term control of asthma, the recommended dosage is 1 capsule every 12 hours. Do not use more than 2 capsules per day.

Prevention of Exercise-Induced Asthma
Adults and children 5 years of age and older: The recommended dosage is 1 capsule at least 15 minutes before exercise. If a second dose is needed the same day, take it at least 12 hours after the first dose. Do not use more than 2 capsules per day. If you are already taking Foradil Aerolizer on a regular twice-daily basis, do not take an extra dose before exercise.

Chronic Obstructive Pulmonary Disease
Adults: The usual dosage is 1 capsule every 12 hours. Do not use more than 2 capsules a day. If your usual dosage does not provide relief, check with your doctor. Other treatments may have to be added to your regimen.

How should I take Foradil Aerolizer?

Foradil capsules are intended for use only with the Aerolizer inhaler. They should not be swallowed.

To use the system, place a capsule in the well of the Aerolizer, then press and release the buttons on the side of the device. This will pierce the capsule. The medication is released into the air stream when you breathe in rapidly and deeply through the mouthpiece. Do not exhale into the device or use a spacer with this medication. Detailed instructions are supplied with your prescription. If you have any questions, ask your doctor or pharmacist.

On rare occasions, the capsule may break into small pieces that can reach the throat or mouth during inhalation. A screen built into the inhaler should prevent any capsule pieces from being inhaled. To reduce the chance of the capsules breaking, store them in a dry place and keep them in their blister pack until just before use. Pierce the capsule only once.

Be sure your hands are dry before handling the capsules and be careful to keep the Aerolizer dry. Do not wash any part of the device. Throw away the Aerolizer when your prescription is finished and replace it with the new one provided with each refill.

After use, open the inhaler and remove and throw away the empty capsule.

What should I avoid while taking Foradil Aerolizer?

Do not use Foradil Aerolizer with a spacer and never exhale into the Foradil Aerolizer device.

Never take the Aerolizer inhaler apart.

Never place a Foradil capsule directly into the mouthpiece of the Aerolizer inhaler. Never leave a used Foradil capsule in the Aerolizer inhaler chamber.

Always use the new Aerolizer inhaler that comes with your next refill. Do not use the Aerolizer inhaler from your last refill.

Avoid exposing Foradil capsules to moisture.

Avoid situations that may trigger an asthma attack.

Do not use Foradil Aerolizer more often than prescribed. Excessive use can cause heart irregularities. Tell your doctor immediately if you experience chest pain, palpitations, rapid heart rate, or tremor.

Do not use Foradil with other long-acting beta-agonists such as salmeterol.

What are possible food and drug interactions associated with Foradil Aerolizer?

If Foradil Aerolizer is taken with certain other drugs, the effects of either could be increased, decreased, or altered. It is especially important to check with your doctor before combining Foradil Aerolizer with the following: antibiotics such as clarithromycin and erythromycin, antidepressants categorized as tricyclics (such as amitriptyline and imipramine), antidepressants categorized as monoamine oxidase inhibitors (such as phenelzine and tranylcypromine), antifungals (such as fluconazole, itraconazole, and ketoconazole), beta-blockers used to control high blood pressure (such as atenolol and metoprolol), xanthine derivatives (such as theophylline), steroids (such as hydrocortisone and prednisone), and water pills (diuretics) such as furosemide and hydrochlorothiazide.

What are the possible side effects of Foradil Aerolizer?

Side effects cannot be anticipated. If any develop or change in intensity, tell your doctor as soon as possible. Only your doctor can determine if it is safe for you to continue taking this drug.

Side effects may include: anxiety, bronchitis, chest infection, chest pain, difficulty breathing, difficulty falling or staying asleep, difficulty speaking, dizziness, dry mouth, fever, inflammation of the tonsils or sinuses, itchiness, rash, tremor, upper respiratory tract infection, viral infection, worsening of asthma, fast and irregular heart beat, headache, nervousness, muscle cramps, nausea, tiredness, low blood potassium, high blood acid

Can I receive Foradil Aerolizer if I am pregnant or breastfeeding?

The effects of Foradil Aerolizer during pregnancy and breastfeeding are unknown. Tell your doctor immediately if you are pregnant, plan to become pregnant, or are breastfeeding. Foradil Aerolizer is recommended only if the potential benefit outweighs the potential risk. Use Foradil Aerolizer with caution if you are nursing. It is not known whether Foradil Aerolizer appears in breast milk.

What should I do if I miss a dose of Foradil Aerolizer?

Take it as soon as you remember. If it is almost time for your next dose, skip the one you missed and go back to your regular schedule. Never take 2 doses at once.

How should I store Foradil Aerolizer?

Store at room temperature, away from heat and moisture. Leave the capsules in the blister pack until needed for use. Always throw out the Aerolizer by the "Use by" date.

FORADIL CERTIHALER

Generic name: Formoterol fumarate

What is Foradil Certihaler?

Foradil Certihaler is a long-acting beta2-agonist (LABA). It is used long-term, twice a day, to control symptoms of asthma and prevent symptoms such as wheezing in adults and children ages 5 and older.

What is the most important information I should know about Foradil Certihaler?

LABA medicines such as Foradil Certihaler may increase the chance of death from asthma problems in patients with asthma.

Foradil Certihaler should not be used to treat sudden symptoms of asthma. Always have a short-acting beta2-agonist medicine with you to treat asthma attacks. If you are not sure that you have an inhaled short-acting beta2 agonist, contact your healthcare provider to have one prescribed for you.

Foradil Certihaler is not a substitute for oral or inhaled corticosteroids.

Foradil Certihaler should not be the only medicine being used for your asthma. Foradil Certihaler should be used as additional therapy if you are not adequately controlled on other asthma-controlling medications or if your disease is severe enough to require treatment with two medications.

Call your healthcare provider if breathing problems worsen over time while using Foradil Certihaler. You may need different treatment.

Who should not take Foradil Certihaler?

LABA medicines such as Foradil Certihaler may increase the chance of death from asthma problems; therefore, this medicine is not for adults and children with asthma who are well-controlled with another asthma-controller medicine, such as a low-to-medium dose of an inhaled corticosteroid, or patients who only need short-acting beta2-agonist medicines once in awhile.

Foradil Certihaler should not be used in patients with a history of hypersensitivity to formoterol fumarate or to any components of this product, including lactose (milk sugar) or milk protein.

What should I tell my doctor before I take the first dose of Foradil Certihaler?

Tell your doctor about all prescription, over-the-counter, and herbal medications you are taking before beginning treatment with Foradil Certihaler. Also, talk to your doctor about your complete medical history, especially if you have heart problems, high blood pressure, seizures, thyroid problems, diabetes, or if you are pregnant, plan to become pregnant, or are breastfeeding.

Tell your doctor if you allergic to Foradil Certihaler, any other medicines, or food products. Foradil Certihaler contains lactose (milk sugar) and a small amount of milk proteins. Individuals who have a severe milk protein allergy may have an allergic reaction to Foradil Certihaler.

What is the usual dosage?

The information below is based on the dosage guidelines your doctor uses. Depending on your condition and medical history, your doctor may prescribe a different regimen. Do not change the dosage or stop taking your medication without your doctor's approval.

Adults and children 5 years of age and older: The usual dosage is one 10-microgram (mcg) inhalation from the Foradil Certihaler every 12 hours. You must not exhale into the device. The total daily dose of Foradil Certihaler should not exceed one inhalation twice daily (20 mcg total daily dose).

Do not stop using Foradil Certihaler or reduce doses of other asthma medication taken along with Foradil Certihaler unless told to do so by your healthcare provider because your symptoms might get worse. Foradil Certihaler should not be the only medicine prescribed for your asthma. It should not be used if your healthcare provider decides that another asthma-controller medicine alone does not control your asthma or that you need 2 asthma-controller medicines.

How should I take Foradil Certihaler?

Use Foradil Certihaler exactly as prescribed. Foradil Certihaler should be administered only by the oral inhalation route. You must not exhale into the device. The total daily dose of Foradil Certihaler should not exceed one inhalation twice daily (20 mcg total daily dose). More frequent administration or administration of a larger number of inhalations is not recommended. Do not change or stop any of your medicines to control or treat your breathing problems. Your healthcare provider will adjust your medicines as needed. Make sure you always have a short-acting beta2-agonist medicine with you. Use your short-acting beta2-agonist medicine if you have breathing problems between doses of Foradil Certihaler. Do not use a spacer device with Foradil Certihaler. Do not breathe into Foradil Certihaler. Children should use Foradil Certihaler with an adult's help, as instructed by the child's healthcare provider.

To use the inhaler: While holding the inhaler level, breathe out (exhale) away from the inhaler, then close your lips firmly over mouthpiece. Breathe in (inhale) quickly with one fast, deep breath. Hold your breath for at least 5 seconds. Exhale away from the inhaler. Double-check air holes to see if they opened completely. After you have received the dose, close the cap all the way until it clicks shut. The counter will now show you have one less dose left in the inhaler. If the display number did not decrease by one after this step, but you still received your dose of medicine, stop using the inhaler and contact your pharmacist.

You should never use Foradil Certihaler with a spacer and never exhale into the device. The inhaler should never be washed and should be kept dry.

What should I avoid while taking Foradil Certihaler?

Avoid exposing the Foradil Certihaler to moisture.

Never use a spacer with Foradil Certihaler and never exhale into the device.

Do not use other LABA medicines while you are using Foradil Certihaler. Other LABA medicines include Foradil Aerolizer (formoterol fumarate inhalation powder), Serevent Diskus (salmeterol xinofoate inhalation powder), or Advair Diskus (fluticasone propionate and salmeterol inhalation powder), Brovana (arformoterol tartrate inhalation solution), or Symbicort (budesonide and formoterol fumarate dehydrate solution aerosol).

What are possible food and drug interactions associated with Foradil Certihaler?

If Foradil Certihaler is taken with certain other drugs, the effects of either could be increased, decreased, or altered. It is especially important to check with your doctor before combining Foradil Certihaler with the following: beta-blockers such as metoprolol, diuretics such as hydrochlorothiazide or furosemide, monoamine oxides inhibitors such as tranylcypromine, steroids such as prednisone, xanthine derivatives such as theophylline, and tricyclic antidepressants such as amitriptyline.

What are the possible side effects of Foradil Certihaler?

Side effects cannot be anticipated. If any develop or change in intensity, tell your doctor as soon as possible. Only your doctor can determine if it is safe for you to continue taking this drug.

Side effects may include: Chest pain, fast, irregular heartbeat, increased blood pressure; headache; tremor; nervousness; dry mouth; muscle cramps; nausea; dizziness; tiredness; trouble sleeping, low blood potassium, high blood sugar, high blood acid

Signs of a serious allergic reactions include: rash, hives, swelling of the face, mouth, and tongue, and breathing problems, increased blood pressure, rapid heart rate, chest pain, and nervousness.

Tell your healthcare provider about any side effect that bothers you or that does not go away. These are not all the side effects associated with Foradil Certihaler.

Can I receive Foradil Certihaler if I am pregnant or breastfeeding?

The effects of Foradil during pregnancy and breastfeeding are unknown. Tell your doctor immediately if you are pregnant, plan to become pregnant, or are breastfeeding.

What should I do if I miss a dose of Foradil Certihaler?

If you miss a dose of Foradil Certihaler, just skip that dose. Take your next dose at your usual time. Never take 2 doses at one time.

How should I store Foradil Certihaler?

Store Foradil Certihaler at room temperature. Protect Foradil Certihaler from heat and moisture. Use Foradil Certihaler before the expiration date which is marked on the label on the underside of the inhaler. Keep Foradil Certihaler out of the reach of children. Keep your Foradil Certihaler inhaler dry. Handle with dry hands.

Formoterol *See Perforomist, page 1007.*

Formoterol fumarate *See Foradil Aerolizer, page 587, or Foradil Certihaler, page 591.*

FORTICAL NASAL SPRAY

Generic name: Calcitonin-salmon (rDNA origin)

What is Fortical Nasal Spray?

Fortical Nasal Spray is similar to calcitonin, a natural protein found in the body. It reduces the rate of calcium loss from bones. Fortical Nasal Spray is indicated to treat bone weakening (osteoporosis) in women going through menopause for more than 5 years who have very weak bones. Fortical Nasal Spray not only stops osteoporosis, but may reverse the disease and increase bone strength.

Fortical Nasal Spray helps make bones stronger and less likely to break. Fortical Nasal Spray is recommended for use in conjunction with adequate calcium and vitamin D intake for maximum benefit.

What is the most important information I should know about Fortical Nasal Spray?

Although no allergic reactions have been reported with Fortical Nasal Spray, calcitonin-salmon has been reported to cause serious allergic reactions such as shock, difficulty breathing, wheezing, and swelling of the throat or tongue. If you have a suspected allergy to Fortical Nasal Spray, a skin test should be considered prior to beginning therapy.

Periodic nose exams are recommended due to possible changes in nasal conditions. Nose exams should be done before you start using Fortical Nasal Spray and when you experience nasal discomfort while you are using it.

Fortical Nasal Spray is not a substitute for calcium supplements. Fortical Nasal Spray will help you gain the maximum benefit from your calcium replacement therapy. It is important to take all the calcium and vitamin D supplements as instructed by your doctor.

Who should not take Fortical Nasal Spray?
You should not take Fortical Nasal Spray if you are allergic to calcitonin-salmon.

What should I tell my doctor before I take the first dose of Fortical Nasal Spray?
Tell your doctor about all prescription, over-the-counter, and herbal medications you are taking, as well as your complete medical history before beginning treatment with Fortical Nasal Spray. Also, tell your doctor if you are pregnant or planning to become pregnant, nursing, have any nasal conditions, or if you are going to have surgery.

What is the usual dosage?
The information below is based on the dosage guidelines your doctor uses. Depending on your condition and medical history, your doctor may prescribe a different regimen. Do not change the dosage or stop taking your medication without your doctor's approval.

Adults: The usual dose of Fortical Nasal Spray is 1 spray per day into your nostril, alternating nostrils daily.

How should I take Fortical Nasal Spray?
Before administration of the first dose, allow the bottle to reach room temperature. Remove the protective cap and clip from the bottle of Fortical Nasal Spray. Hold the bottle upright and depress the two white side arms of the pump toward the bottle at least 5 times until a full spray is produced. Once the nasal spray has been primed for the first time, it is not necessary to re-prime it before each use. To use the spray, the nozzle should be carefully placed into the nostril with the head in the upright position and the pump firmly depressed toward the bottle. You do not need to inhale. It is important to hold the nasal spray in an upright position to be able to deliver an accurate dose.

You may not feel the mist from the nasal spray because it is so fine. It is all right if some of the spray drips. One spray will give you the amount of medication needed.

Use Fortical Nasal Spray every day, alternating nostrils each time. If you use your right nostril one day, use the left nostril the next day.

Replace the lock tab and cap after using Fortical Nasal Spray. Do not return the medication to the refrigerator. It should be kept at room temperature and thrown out 30 days after its first use.

What should I avoid while taking Fortical Nasal Spray?

Avoid spraying Fortical Nasal Spray into the same nostril every day. If you use the right nostril one day, use the left nostril the next day.

Avoid wasting the medication by testing the sprayer.

What are possible food and drug interactions associated with Fortical Nasal Spray?

No formal studies have been done to evaluate drug interactions with Fortical Nasal Spray. Currently, no drug interactions have been observed. Prior use of diphosphonates in postmenopausal women with osteoporosis have not been assessed, but its use in patients with Paget's disease of the bone appears to reduce the anti-resorptive response to Fortical Nasal Spray.

What are the possible side effects of Fortical Nasal Spray?

Side effects cannot be anticipated. If any develop or change in intensity, tell your doctor as soon as possible. Only your doctor can determine if it is safe for you to continue taking this drug.

Side effects may include: back pain, dizziness, nasal symptoms (including dryness, crusting, redness, irritation, itching, tenderness, soreness, irritation, thick feeling, paleness, infection, nasal cavity narrowing, infection, bleeding, runny nose), headache, joint pain

Can I receive Fortical Nasal Spray if I am pregnant or breastfeeding?

The effects of Fortical Nasal Spray on pregnancy and nursing are unknown. Tell your doctor if you are pregnant, planning to become pregnant, or are nursing.

What should I do if I miss a dose of Fortical Nasal Spray?

If you missed a dose of Fortical Nasal Spray, take it as soon as you remember. Never take 2 doses at once.

How should I store Fortical Nasal Spray?

Store the unopened medication in the refrigerator. Do not freeze. After opening the package, keep the bottle at room temperature for 30 days. Make sure it stands upright. Throw out 30 days after first use.

FOSAMAX
Generic name: Alendronate sodium

What is Fosamax?
Fosamax is used to treat or prevent osteoporosis (thinning of bone) in women after menopause. It lowers the risk of having a hip or spinal fracture. In men with osteoporosis, it is used to increase bone mass. Fosamax is also used to treat osteoporosis in men or women who are taking corticosteroids such as prednisone. This drug is also used to treat Paget's disease, a painful condition that weakens and deforms the bones, in men and women. Fosamax tablets are used to prevent and treat osteoporosis, whereas Fosamax oral solution is only used for the treatment of osteoporosis.

What is the most important information I should know about Fosamax?
Improvements in bone density may be seen as early as 3 months after you start therapy with Fosamax, even though you may not be able to see or feel any differences. You must take Fosamax exactly as directed to help make sure it works and to help lower the chance of problems in your esophagus.

If you have chest pain, new or worsening heartburn, or have trouble or pain when you swallow, stop taking Fosamax and call your doctor.

Fosamax is not a hormone.

Who should not take Fosamax?
Do not take Fosamax if you have certain problems with your esophagus, cannot stand or sit upright for at least 30 minutes, have low levels of calcium in your blood, or are allergic to Fosamax or any of its ingredients. You should not take Fosamax oral solution if you have trouble swallowing liquids.

What should I tell my doctor before I take the first dose of Fosamax?
Tell your doctor about all prescription, over-the-counter, and herbal medications you are taking before beginning treatment with Fosamax. Also, talk to your doctor about your complete medical history, especially if you have problems with swallowing, are on hormone replacement therapy, have stomach or digestive problems, kidney problems, are unable to stand or sit upright for at least 30 minutes, pregnant or planning to become pregnant, or breastfeeding.

What is the usual dosage?
The information below is based on the dosage guidelines your doctor uses. Depending on your condition and medical history, your doctor

may prescribe a different regimen. Do not change the dosage or stop taking your medication without your doctor's approval.

Paget's Disease
Adults: The usual dose is 40 milligrams (mg) taken once a day for 6 months.

Prevention of Postmenopausal Osteoporosis
Adults: The usual dose is one 35-mg tablet taken once weekly or one 5-mg tablet taken once daily.

Steroid-Induced Osteoporosis
Adults: The usual dose is one 5-mg tablet taken once daily. In postmenopausal women not receiving estrogen, the usual dose is one 10-mg tablet taken once daily.

Treatment of Osteoporosis in Men
Adults: The usual dose is one 70-mg tablet taken once weekly, or one bottle of 70-mg oral solution taken once weekly, or one 10-mg tablet taken once daily.

Treatment of Postmenopausal Osteoporosis
Adults: The usual dose is one 70 mg tablet once weekly or one bottle of 70 mg oral solution once weekly or one 10 mg tablet once daily.

How should I take Fosamax?

Take Fosamax exactly as prescribed. Fosamax works only if it is taken on an empty stomach. Take Fosamax after you get up for the day and before your first meal, drink, medicine or supplement. Take it while you are sitting or standing. Swallow the Fosamax tablet with a full glass (6-8 oz) of plain water only. Do not take Fosamax with mineral water, coffee, tea, or juice.

Some forms of Fosamax are taken once a day. Others are taken only once a week. If you take Fosamax once a week, take it on the same day each week.

To ensure that you get a correct dose, measure the Fosamax oral solution with a dose-measuring spoon, dropper, or cup and not a regular tablespoon. Drink an additional 2 oz of water after you take your dose.

Do not chew or suck on the tablet. After you swallow your Fosamax dose, wait at least 30 minutes before you lie down, before you eat or drink except for plain water, and before you take other medicines, including antacids, calcium, and other supplements and vitamins.

Do not lie down after taking Fosamax until at least 30 minutes have passed and you have had your first meal of the day.

What should I avoid while taking Fosamax?

Do not eat, drink, or take other medicines or supplements before taking Fosamax. Do not take Fosamax at bedtime or before getting up for the day. Do not eat, drink or take other medicines or supplements until after at least 30 minutes of taking Fosamax. Do not lie down for at least 30 minutes after taking Fosamax, and do not lie down until after your first meal of the day.

What are possible food and drug interactions associated with Fosamax?

If Fosamax is taken with certain other drugs, the effects of either could be increased, decreased, or altered. It is especially important to check with your doctor before combining Fosamax with the following: antacids, aspirin, calcium supplements, and nonsteroidal anti-inflammatory drugs such as ibuprofen or naproxen.

What are the possible side effects of Fosamax?

Side effects cannot be anticipated. If any develop or change in intensity, tell your doctor as soon as possible. Only your doctor can determine if it is safe for you to continue taking this drug.

Side effects may include: abdominal pain; acid regurgitation; bone and joint pain; constipation; diarrhea; gas; indigestion; muscle pain; nausea; vomiting; full or bloated feeling; black or bloody stools; eye pain; rash that may get worse in sunlight; hair loss; headache; dizziness; change in sense of taste; and swelling in the joints, hands or legs, and bone

Stop taking Fosamax and call your doctor right away if you experience chest pain, new or worsening heartburn, or trouble or pain when swallowing. Tell your doctor if you develop severe bone, muscle, or joint pain.

Can I receive Fosamax if I am pregnant or breastfeeding?

The effects of Fosamax during pregnancy and breastfeeding are unknown. Tell your doctor immediately if you are pregnant, plan to become pregnant, or are breastfeeding. Use caution if you breastfeed while taking Fosamax.

What should I do if I miss a dose of Fosamax?

If you are taking Fosamax on a daily basis, do not take a missed dose later in the day. Instead, skip it and go back to your regular schedule the next morning.

If you miss a dose of once weekly Fosamax, take the missed dose the morning after you remember. Then return to taking one dose once a week as originally scheduled on their chosen day. Do not take 2 doses at once.

How should I store Fosamax?

Keep the container tightly closed and store at room temperature. Do not freeze the oral solution.

FOSAMAX PLUS D
Generic name: Alendrónate sodium and cholecalciferol

What is Fosamax Plus D?
Fosamax Plus D contains alendronate sodium and vitamin D3 (chole-calciferol) Fosamax Plus D provides a week's worth of vitamin D3, but some patients may need more vitamin D than what is in Fosamax Plus D. Your doctor may recommend additional vitamin D supplements. Fosamax Plus D is used for the treatment of osteoporosis (thinning bones) in women after menopause. It reduces the chance of having a hip or spinal break. It is also used to increase bone mass in men with osteoporosis.

What is the most important information I should know about Fosamax Plus D?
Improvement in bone density may be seen as early as 3 months after you start therapy with Fosamax Plus D even though you may not be able to see or feel and differences. You should take Fosamax Plus D exactly as directed to help make sure it works and to help lower the chance of problems in your esophagus.

If you have chest pain, new or worsening heartburn, or have trouble or pain when you swallow, stop taking Fosamax Plus D and call your doctor.

Fosamax Plus D should not be used to treat vitamin D deficiency. Fosamax Plus D is not a hormone.

Who should not take Fosamax Plus D?
Do not take Fosamax Plus D if you have certain problems with your esophagus, cannot stand or sit upright for at least 30 minutes, have low levels of calcium in your blood, severe kidney disease, or if you are allergic to Fosamax Plus D or any of its ingredients. This medication should not be used in women before menopause.

What should I tell my doctor before I take the first dose of Fosamax Plus D?
Tell your doctor about all prescription, over-the-counter, and herbal medications you are taking before beginning treatment with Fosamax Plus D. Also, talk to your doctor about your complete medical history, especially if you have or have had problems with swallowing, stomach or digestive problems, kidney problems, sarcoidosis, leukemia, lymphoma, are pregnant or planning to become pregnant, breastfeeding, or about other medical problems you have or have had in the past.

What is the usual dosage?
The information below is based on the dosage guidelines your doctor uses. Depending on your condition and medical history, your doctor

may prescribe a different regimen. Do not change the dosage or stop taking your medication without your doctor's approval.

Adults: The recommended dosage for osteoporosis in both men and women is one 70-milligram (mg)/2800 IU or one 70-mg/5800 IU tablet once weekly.

How should I take Fosamax Plus D?

Take 1 tablet of Fosamax Plus D on the same day once a week. You should take the tablet after you get up for the day and before your first meal, drink, or other medicines or supplements. Fosamax Plus D only works on an empty stomach. Take Fosamax Plus D while you are sitting or standing up. Swallow the tablet with a full glass (6-8 oz) of plain water only. Do not take Fosamax Plus D with coffee or tea, juice, or any other beverage. Do not chew or suck on the tablet. After swallowing the tablet, wait at least 30 minutes before you lie down, your first meal or drink (except plain water), or before taking other medicines or supplements. You may sit, stand, or walk and do normal activities. You should not lie down until after your first meal of the day. For Fosamax Plus D to work, you must keep taking it as long as is instructed by your doctor.

What should I avoid while taking Fosamax Plus D?

Do not eat, drink, or take other medicines or supplements before taking Fosamax Plus D. Wait for at least 30 minutes after taking Fosamax Plus D to eat, drink, or take other medicines or supplements. Do not lie down for at least 30 minutes after taking Fosamax Plus D. Do not lie down until after your first meal of the day.

What are possible food and drug interactions associated with Fosamax Plus D?

If Fosamax Plus D is taken with certain other drugs, the effects of either could be increased, decreased, or altered. It is especially important to check with your doctor before combining Fosamax Plus D with the following: antacids, aspirin, anticonvulsants, bile acid sequestrants (such as cholestyramine, colestipol), calcium supplements, cimetidine, mineral oils, olestra, orlistat, and thiazide diuretics.

What are the possible side effects of Fosamax Plus D?

Side effects cannot be anticipated. If any develop or change in intensity, tell your doctor as soon as possible. Only your doctor can determine if it is safe for you to continue taking this drug.

Side effects may include: black or bloody bowel movements, bloating, bone, muscle, or joint pain, change in taste, constipation, diarrhea, gas, headache, nausea, stomach pain, vomiting, eye pain, rash that may be worse to sunlight, hair loss, dizziness, swelling in the joints, hands or legs

Stop taking Fosamax Plus D and call your doctor right away if you experience chest pain, new or worsening heartburn, or trouble or pain when swallowing. Also call your doctor if you develop severe bone, muscle, or joint pain.

Reaction symptoms may include: inflammation, irritation, ulcers of the esophagus (which may sometimes bleed)

Can I receive Fosamax Plus D if I am pregnant or breastfeeding?
The effects of Fosamax Plus D during pregnancy and breastfeeding are unknown. Talk with your doctor before taking this drug if you are pregnant, plan to become pregnant, or are breastfeeding.

What should I do if I miss a dose of Fosamax Plus D?
If you miss a dose, take only 1 Fosamax Plus D tablet on the morning after you remember. Do not take 2 tablets on the same day. Continue your usual schedule of 1 Fosamax Plus D tablet once a week on your chosen day.

How should I store Fosamax Plus D?
Store at room temperature, away from moisture and light. You should keep the tablets in the original blister package until use.

Fosamprenavir calcium See Lexiva, page 736.

Fosfomycin tromethamine See Monurol, page 849.

Fosinopril sodium See Monopril, page 844.

Fosinopril sodium and hydrochlorothiazide See Monopril HCT, page 846.

FROVA
Generic name: Frovatriptan succinate

What is Frova?
Frova is used to treat migraine attacks in adults. This drug should only be taken for a migraine headache. Do not use Frova to treat headaches that might be caused by other conditions.

What is the most important information I should know about Frova?
Frova may cause heart problems. If there is already a heart condition, such as coronary artery disease (CAD), this drug should not be used. This drug should not be given to anyone who would have symptoms of CAD,

such as high blood pressure, high cholesterol, smoking, obesity, diabetes, a family history of CAD, menopause, or men over 40 years of age.

Who should not take Frova?
Do not take Frova if you are allergic to any of its ingredients. You should not use this drug if you have high blood pressure, heart problems, migraines, have had a stroke, or circulation/blood flow problems.

What should I tell my doctor before I take the first dose of Frova?
Tell your doctor about all prescription, over-the-counter, and herbal medications you are taking before beginning treatment with Frova. Also, talk to your doctor about your complete medical history, especially if you have heart problems, a history of chest pain, diabetes.

What is the usual dosage?
The information below is based on the dosage guidelines your doctor uses. Depending on your condition and medical history, your doctor may prescribe a different regimen. Do not change the dosage or stop taking your medication without your doctor's approval.

Adults: The usual dosage of Frova is one tablet taken by mouth with liquid. If the headache recurs after initial relief, a second tablet may be taken, as long as you have waited 2 hours between doses. The maximum daily dose of Frova is 3 tablets.

How should I take Frova?
Take the Frova tablet with liquids.

What are possible food and drug interactions associated with Frova?
If Frova is taken with certain other drugs, the effects of either could be increased, decreased, or altered. It is especially important to check with your doctor before combining Frova with the following: almotriptan, eletriptan hydrobromide, ergotamine medications, naratriptan, rizatriptan, selective serotonin reuptake inhibitor (ssri), such as fluoxetine, fluvoxamine, paroxetine, and sertraline, sumatriptan, zolmitriptan.

What are the possible side effects of Frova?
Side effects cannot be anticipated. If any develop or change in intensity, tell your doctor as soon as possible. Only your doctor can determine if it is safe for you to continue taking this drug.

Side effects may include: Chest pain, dizziness, dry mouth, feeling hot or cold, headache, hot flashes, indigestion, pain in joints or bones, tingling, tiredness

Can I receive Frova if I am pregnant or breastfeeding?
The effects of Frova during pregnancy and breastfeeding are unknown. Tell your doctor immediately if you are pregnant, plan to become pregnant, or are breastfeeding.

How should I store Frova?
Store at room temperature.

Frovatriptan succinate *See Frova, page 602.*

Furosemide *See Lasix, page 709.*

Gabapentin *See Neurontin, page 872.*

GABITRIL
Generic name: Tiagabine hydrochloride

What is Gabitril?
Gabatril is indicated as add-on therapy in adults and children 12 years and older for the treatment of partial seizures.

What is the most important information I should know about Gabitril?
Gabitril is approved as add-on therapy for the management of partial seizure disorders. In patients not diagnosed with epilepsy, seizures have occurred in patients taking Gabitril.

Most seizures in patients without epilepsy occurred soon after starting Gabitril, after a dose increase, or after several months of treatment. Seizures have occurred at very low doses of Gabitril.

Safety and effectivenss of Gabitril have not been established for any indications other than as add-on therapy for partial seizures in adults and children 12 years and older.

Do not abruptly stop taking Gabitril because of the possibility of increasing seizure frequency. If you are having problems, talk to your doctor before stopping any medications.

Although rare, a very serious and possibly fatal rash may occur with the use of Gabitril.

Who should not take Gabitril?
Gabitril is contraindicated in patients who have demonstrated an allergic reaction to this drug or any of its ingredients.

What should I tell my doctor before I take the first dose of Gabitril?
Tell your doctor about all prescription, over-the-counter, and herbal medications you are taking before beginning treatment with Gabitril. Also, talk to your doctor about your complete medical history, especially if you have

liver problems, are pregnant or plan to become pregnant, breastfeeding or plan to breastfeed, have a mental condition, or status epilepticus.

What is the usual dosage?
The information below is based on the dosage guidelines your doctor uses. Depending on your condition and medical history, your doctor may prescribe a different regimen. Do not change the dosage or stop taking your medication without your doctor's approval.

Patients Who Are Taking Enzyme-inducing Antiepilepsy Drugs (carbamazapine, phenytoin, primidone, and phenobarbital)
Adolescents 12 to 18 years old: Gabitril should be initiated at 4 mg once daily. Modification of concomitant antiepilepsy drugs is not necessary, unless clinically indicated. The total daily dose of Gabitril may be increased by 4 mg at the beginning of Week 2. Thereafter, the total daily dose may be increased by 4 to 8 mg at weekly intervals until clinical response is achieved, or up to 32 mg/day. The total daily dose should be given in divided doses two to four times daily.

Adults: Gabitril should be initiated at 4 mg once daily. Modification of concomitant antiepilepsy drugs is not necessary, unless clinically indicated. The total daily dose of Gabitril may be increased by 4 to 8 mg at weekly intervals until clinical response is achieved, or up to 56 mg/day. The total daily dose should be given in divided doses two to four times daily. Doses above 56 mg/day have not been systematically evaluated in adequate and well-controlled clinical trials.

Patients who are only taking non-enzyme-inducing AEDS require lower doses of Gabitril than the patients receiving enzyme-inducing agents.

How should I take Gabitril?
Gabitril should be taken after a meal or snack.

What should I avoid while taking Gabitril?
This drug may make you dizzy or drowsy; use caution when engaging in activities requiring alertness such as driving or using machinery. Avoid alcoholic beverages.

What are possible food and drug interactions associated with Gabitril?
If Gabitril is taken with certain other drugs, the effects of either could be increased, decreased, or altered. It is especially important to check with your doctor before combining Gabitril with the following: carbamazepine, phenobarbital, phenytoin, and valproate.

What are the possible side effects of Gabitril?
Side effects cannot be anticipated. If any develop or change in intensity, tell your doctor as soon as possible. Only your doctor can determine if it is safe for you to continue taking this drug.

Side effects may include: dizziness, lack of energy, drowsiness, nausea, nervousness, tremor, abdominal pain, difficulty concentrating

Can I receive Gabitril if I am pregnant or breastfeeding?
If you are a woman of childbearing age, be sure to notify your doctor if you become pregnant or intend to become pregnant while taking Gabitril. Also tell your doctor if you are breastfeeding or plan to breastfeed. Gabitril should be used in women who are pregnant or nursing only if the benefits clearly outweigh the risks.

What should I do if I miss a dose of Gabitril?
If you forget to take Gabitril at your scheduled time, take it as soon as you remember. However, if it is almost time for your next dose, skip the missed dose. Do not take a double dose of Gabitril. Do not attempt to make up a missed dose by increasing the next dose.

How should I store Gabitril?
Store Gabitril at room temperature. Protect from light and moisture.

Galantamine hydrobromide *See Razadyne ER/Razadyne, page 1122.*

GANTRISIN
Generic name: Acetyl sulfisoxazole

What is Gantrisin?
Gantrisin is a children's medication used to treat severe, repeated, or long-lasting urinary tract infections including pyelonephritis (bacterial kidney inflammation), pyelitis (inflammation of the part of the kidney that drains urine into the ureter), and cystitis (inflammation of the bladder).

This drug is also used in combination with another drug to treat bacterial meningitis. It is also prescribed as a preventive measure for children who have been exposed to meningitis.

Middle ear infections can be treated with Gantrisin in combination with penicillin or erythromycin.

Gantrisin is also used in combination with pyrimethamine in the treatment of infections such as chancroid (venereal disease causing enlargement and ulceration of lymph nodes in the groin), trachoma and inclusion conjunctivitis (eye infections), nocardiosis (bacterial disease affecting the lungs, skin, and brain), and toxoplasmosis (parasitic disease transmitted by infected cats, their feces, or litter boxes, and by undercooked meat).

Malaria that does not respond to the drug chloroquine can also be treated with Gantrisin in combination with other drugs.

What is the most important information I should know about Gantrisin?

Notify your doctor at the first sign of a reaction such as skin rash, sore throat, fever, joint pain, cough, shortness of breath or other breathing difficulties, abnormal skin paleness, reddish or purplish skin spots, or yellowing of the skin or whites of the eyes.

Rare but severe reactions—sometimes fatal—have occurred with the use of sulfa drugs like as Gantrisin. These reactions include sudden and severe liver damage, agranulocytosis (a severe blood disorder), and Stevens-Johnson syndrome (severe blistering of the skin).

Children taking sulfa drugs such as Gantrisin should have their blood counts checked frequently.

Who should not take Gantrisin?

Your child should not use Gantrisin if they are sensitive to sulfonamides. Also, do not use this drug to treat infants less than 2 months of age except in rare cases, pregnant women at the end of pregnancy, and mothers nursing infants less than 2 months of age.

What should I tell my doctor before I take the first dose of Gantrisin?

Tell your doctor about all prescription, over-the-counter, and herbal medications you are taking before beginning treatment with Gantrisin. Also, talk to your doctor about your complete medical history, especially if your child has liver or kidney disease, severe allergies or asthma, glucose-6-phosphate dehydrogenase deficiency (an inherited disorder), diabetes, decreased bone marrow function, or any blood disorders.

What is the usual dosage?

The information below is based on the dosage guidelines your doctor uses. Depending on your condition and medical history, your doctor may prescribe a different regimen. Do not change the dosage or stop taking your medication without your doctor's approval.

Adults: This medication should not be given to infants under 2 months of age except in the treatment of congenital toxoplasmosis (a parasitic infection contracted by pregnant women and passed along to the fetus).

Children 2 months and older: The usual starting dose is half the regular dose, or 75 milligrams (mg) per 2.2 pounds of body weight divided into 4-6 doses taken over 24 hours. Do not give more than 6 grams (g) over 24 hours.

The usual dose for children 2 months of age or older is 150 milligrams (mg) per 2.2 pounds (lb) of body weight divided into 4-6 doses taken over 24 hours. The maximum dose should not exceed more than 6 grams per 24 hours.

Gantrisin pediatric suspension supplies 500 mg in each teaspoonful (5 milliliters).

How should I take Gantrisin?

Be sure your child takes Gantrisin exactly as prescribed. It is important that the child drink plenty of fluids while taking this medication in order to prevent formation of crystals or stones in the urine.

Gantrisin is available as a suspension and should be shaken well before each dose. To make sure you are giving an accurate dose, ask your pharmacist for a specially marked measuring spoon.

What should I avoid while taking Gantrisin?

Gantrisin works best when there is a constant amount of the drug in the blood and urine. To help keep a constant level, try to make sure your child does not miss any doses and takes them at evenly spaced intervals, around the clock.

Avoid prolonged sun exposure, tanning beds, or sunlamps. Use sunscreen and protective clothing when outdoors.

What are possible food and drug interactions associated with Gantrisin?

If Gantrisin is taken with certain other drugs, the effects of either could be increased, decreased, or altered. It is especially important to check with your doctor before combining Gantrisin with the following: blood-thinners such as warfarin, diabetes drugs such as glyburide, methotrexate, and thiopental.

What are the possible side effects of Gantrisin?

Side effects cannot be anticipated. If any develop or change in intensity, tell your doctor as soon as possible. Only your doctor can determine if it is safe for your child to continue taking this drug.

Side effects may include: allergic reactions, anemia and other blood disorders, angioedema (swelling of the face, lips, tongue, and throat), bluish discoloration of the skin, cough, dizziness, hallucinations, hepatitis, inflammation of the mouth or tongue, kidney failure, lack or loss of appetite, nausea, palpitations, presence of blood or crystals in urine, rapid heartbeat, reddish or purplish skin spots, severe skin welts or swelling, skin eruptions, skin rash, vomiting

Can I receive Gantrisin if I am pregnant or breastfeeding?

Do not use Gantrisin during pregnancy. Do not breastfeed while taking Gantrisin.

What should I do if I miss a dose of Gantrisin?
Give Gantrisin to your child as soon as you remember. If it is almost time for the next dose, skip the missed dose and go back to the regular schedule. Never give 2 doses at the same time.

How should I store Gantrisin?
Keep Gantrisin in the container it came in. Keep it tightly closed, store it at room temperature, and away from moist places and direct light.

GARDASIL
Generic name: Human papillomavirus vaccine

What is Gardasil?
Gardasil is a vaccine used in girls and women 9-26 years of age for the prevention of cervical cancer and genital warts caused by human papillomavirus (HPV) types 6, 11, 16, and 18.

What is the most important information I should know about Gardasil?
This vaccine is not intended to be used for treatment of active genital warts and cervical caner. This vaccine will not protect against diseases that are not caused by HPV.

Patients with impaired immune responsiveness may have reduced antibody response to active immunization.

The safety and efficacy of Gardasil have not been evaluated in children younger than 9 years and adults above the age of 26 years.

Gardasil should not be given to individuals with bleeding disorders unless the potential benefits clearly outweigh the risk of administration.

Who should not take Gardasil?
Gardasil is contraindicated in patients who are allergic to the active substances or to any of the ingredients of the vaccine.

What should I tell my doctor before I take the first dose of Gardasil?
Tell your doctor about all prescription, over-the-counter, and herbal medication you are taking before beginning treatment with Gardasil. Also, talk to your doctor about your complete medical history, especially if you are pregnant or planning to become pregnant, and a bleeding disorder such as hemophilia.

What is the usual dosage?
The information below is based on the dosage guidelines your doctor uses. Depending on your condition and medical history, your doctor

may prescribe a different regimen. Do not change the dosage or stop taking your medication without your doctor's approval.

Gardasil should be administered intramuscularly as 3 separate 0.5mL doses according to the following schedule: First dose at elected date, Second dose at 2 months after the first dose, and Third dose at 6 months after the first dose.

How should I take Gardasil?

Gardasil should be administered intramuscularly in the deltoid region of the upper arm or in the higher anterolateral area of the thigh. Gardasil must not be injected intravascularly. Fainting may follow any vaccination, so patients should be observed approximately 15 minutes after administration. The prefilled syringe is for single use only and should not be used for more than 1 individual. For single-use vials a separate sterile syringe and needle must be used for each individual. Do not use the product if particulates are present or if it appears discolored. The vaccine should be used as supplied; no dilution or reconstitution is necessary. The full recommended dose of the vaccine should be used. Shake well before use. Withdraw the 0.5mL dose of vaccine from the single dose vial using a sterile needle and syringe. Once the single dose vial has been penetrated, the withdrawn vaccine should be used promptly. For prefilled syringe use, inject the entire contents of the syringe.

What should I avoid while taking Gardasil?

Do not drive or engage in activities that require alertness and coordination.

What are possible food and drug interactions associated with Gardasil?

If Gardasil is taken with certain other drugs, the effects of either could be increased, decreased, or altered. It is especially important to check with your doctor before combining Gardasil with immunosuppressant medications.

What are the possible side effects of Gardasil?

Side effects cannot be anticipated. If any develop or change in intensity, tell your doctor as soon as possible. Only your doctor can determine if it is safe for you to continue taking this drug.

Side effects may include: Injection site pain/swelling, fever, nausea, dizziness

Can I receive Gardasil if I am pregnant or breastfeeding?

The effects of Gardasil during pregnancy and breastfeeding are unknown. Tell your doctor immediately if you are pregnant, plan to become pregnant, or are breastfeeding.

What should I do if I miss a dose of Gardasil?

Contact your doctor if you miss a Gardasil dose or if you get behind schedule. The next dose should be given as soon as possible. There is no need to start over.

How should I store Gardasil?

Store at room temperature. Do not freeze. Protect from light.

Gatifloxacin See Zymar, page 1506.

Gemfibrozil See Lopid, page 756.

Gemifloxacin See Factive, page 535.

GEODON

Generic name: Ziprasidone hydrochloride

What is Geodon?

Geodon is a psychotropic medicine used in the treatment of both schizophrenia and bipolar mania (both manic and mixed episodes). A manic episode is a period of abnormally and persistently elevated, unreserved, or irritable mood. A mixed episode is a manic episode with a major depressive episode (depressed mood, loss of interest or pleasure in nearly all activities).

What is the most important information I should know about Geodon?

Geodon should not be used in patients who have psychosis due to dementia (such as Alzheimer's disease). Using this drug in a person with dementia may lead to an increased risk of death.

It may take a few weeks for Geodon to work; do not stop taking the drug if you do not see results right away.

Call your doctor immediately if you feel faint or feel a change in the way that your heart beats as this may be a sign of an abnormal heart rhythm.

Avoid potentially hazardous activities, such as driving or operating machinery, until you know the affect Geodon has on you. This drug has been shown to cause sleepiness.

Geodon may cause a drop in your blood pressure, especially when you first start taking this medication or if the dose is increased. If this happens, try not to stand up too quickly and contact your doctor concerning this problem.

It is unknown if Geodon directly causes high blood glucose levels or diabetes, but when taking this drug you should monitor for symptoms of hyperglycemia (such as frequent thirst, urination, and/or hunger, fatigue, weight loss, blurred vision, dry mouth, or poor wound healing).

Who should not take Geodon?

Do not take Geodon if you are allergic to any of its ingredients. This drug should not be taken if you have heart problems (such as a recent heart attack, severe heart failure or heart rhythm irregularities), even if you are taking anti-arrhythmic medication.

What should I tell my doctor before I take the first dose of Geodon?

Tell your doctor about all prescription, over-the-counter, and herbal medications you are taking before beginning treatment with Geodon. Also, talk to your doctor about your complete medical history, especially if you have diabetes, a history of heart disease in your family, any problems with your heart beat, fainting or dizziness, or if are pregnant, expecting to become pregnant, or breastfeeding. Also, inform your doctor if you have previously been allergic to Geodon or any of its ingredients and if you have a known history of low potassium or magnesium levels in your blood.

What is the usual dosage?

The information below is based on the dosage guidelines your doctor uses. Depending on your condition and medical history, your doctor may prescribe a different regimen. Do not change the dosage or stop taking your medication without your doctor's approval.

Bipolar Mania
Adults: The usual dose of Geodon capsules is 40 milligrams (mg) twice per day on the first day of treatment. On the second day, the dose should be increased to 60-80 mg twice per day. Dose adjustments should be within the range of 40-80 mg twice daily, based on tolerability and the how well the drug is working for you.

If taken through injection, the maximum dosage allowed is 40 mg per day, in 10-20 mg injections (10 mg injections can be given every 2 hours while 20 mg injections may be given every 4 hours.)

Schizophrenia
Adults: The usual dosage of Geodon capsules is 20 mg twice per day. This daily dose may be adjusted in certain individuals based on clinical status to up to 80 mg twice a day. The dosing adjustment, if indicated, should occur at intervals of no less than 2 days.

Geodon has not been shown to be safe or effective in the treatment of those under the age of 18 years old.

How should I take Geodon?

Take Geodon only as directed by your doctor. Geodon capsules should be swallowed whole with food. It is best to take Geodon at the same time every day. It may take a few weeks for Geodon to work; do not stop taking the drug or change the dose if you do not see results right away.

What should I avoid while taking Geodon?

Avoid potentially hazardous activities, such as driving or operating machinery, until you know the affect Geodon has on you. This drug has been shown to cause sleepiness.

Since medications of the same drug class as Geodon may interfere with the ability of the body to adjust to heat, it is best to avoid situations involving high temperature or humidity.

Avoid consuming alcoholic beverages while taking Geodon.

What are possible food and drug interactions associated with Geodon?

If Geodon is taken with certain other drugs, the effects of either could be increased, decreased, or altered. It is especially important to check with your doctor before combining Geodon with the following: arsenic, carbamazepine, chlorpromazine, dofetilide, dolasetron, droperidol, gatifloxacin, halofantrine, ketoconazole, levomethadyl, mefloquine, mesoridazine, moxifloxacin, pentamidine, pimozide, probucol, quinidine, sotalol, sparfloxacin, tacrolimus, and thioridazine.

What are the possible side effects of Geodon?

Side effects cannot be anticipated. If any develop or change in intensity, tell your doctor as soon as possible. Only your doctor can determine if it is safe for you to continue taking this drug.

Side effects may include: anxiety, back pain, diarrhea, dizziness, dry mouth, flu, headache, injection site pain, nausea, sleepiness, stomach pain/upset stomach, vomiting, weakness

A rare but serious condition known as neuroleptic malignant syndrome can occur with Geodon. If you experience a very high fever, rigidity in your muscles, shaking, confusion, sweating, or increased heart rate and blood pressure, contact your doctor immediately for this may be fatal.

Can I receive Geodon if I am pregnant or breastfeeding?

The effects of Geodon during pregnancy and breastfeeding are unknown. Tell your doctor immediately if you are pregnant, plan to become pregnant, or are breastfeeding. Geodon should only be used during pregnancy if the potential benefit justifies the risk to the fetus.

How should I store Geodon?

Store at room temperature. If Geodon is mixed into injection solution, it will last for 24 hours at room temperature, or 7 days if kept refrigerated.

GLEEVEC
Generic name: Imatinib mesylate

What is Gleevec?
Gleevec is used to treat Philadelphia chromosome positive chronic myeloid leukemia (Ph+ CML), a cancer of white blood cells, and also for the treatment of a rare form of stomach cancer called gastrointestinal stromal tumor (GIST). It is also used to treat certain tumors of the stomach and digestive system. Gleevec works by turning off specific proteins in cancer cells that cause cancer to replicate.

What is the most important information I should know about Gleevec?
Women of childbearing potential should be advised to avoid becoming pregnant.

Gleevec is often associated with edema (swelling caused by fluid in your body's tissues) and occasionally serious fluid retention. Patient should be weighed and monitored regularly for signs and symptoms of fluid retention.

Treatment with Gleevec is also associated with low levels of certain blood cells. Complete blood counts should be performed weekly for the first month, biweekly for the second, and periodically thereafter.

Severe congestive heart failure and left ventricular dysfunction have occasionally been reported in patients taking Gleevec. Liver problems, muscle or bone pain (including gastrointestinal bleeding), and skin blistering have also been reported with Gleevec. Your doctor should check you closely for any serious complications periodically throughout treatment.

Gleevec is sometimes associated with gastrointestinal irritation. It is important to take Gleevec with food and a large glass of water to minimize this problem.

Who should not take Gleevec?
Patients who are allergic to imatinib or to any other component of Gleevec should not use this drug.

What should I tell my doctor before I take the first dose of Gleevec?
Tell your doctor about all prescription, over-the-counter, and herbal medications you are taking before beginning treatment with Gleevec. Also, talk to your doctor about your complete medical history, especially if you are experiencing swelling or weight gain from water retention, have a history of liver, kidney, or heart disease, are pregnant or could be pregnant, or are breastfeeding.

What is the usual dosage?
The information below is based on the dosage guidelines your doctor uses. Depending on your condition and medical history, your doctor may prescribe a different regimen. Do not change the dosage or stop taking your medication without your doctor's approval.

Ph+ CML, Chronic Phase
Adults: 400 milligrams (mg) per day; a dose increase from 400 to 600 mg may be considered in the absence of severe adverse reactions and failure to achieve adequate response.

Children: The recommended dose of Gleevec for children with newly diagnosed Ph+ CML is 340 mg/m^2/day (not to exceed 600 mg). The recommended dose for children with Ph+ chronic phase CML recurrent after stem cell transplant or who are resistant to interferon-alpha therapy is 260 mg/m^2/day.

Ph+ CML, Accelerated Phase and Blast Crisis
Adults: 600 mg/day; a dose increase from 600 to 800 mg may be considered in the absence of adverse reactions and failure to achieve adequate responses

Ph+ Acute Lymphoblastic Leukemia (ALL), Relapsed/Refractory
Adults: 600 mg/day

Myelodysplastic/Myeloproliferative Diseases (MDS/MPD)
Adults: 400 mg/day

Aggressive Systemic Mastocytosis (ASM) Without D816V C-Kit Mutation or C-Kit Mutational Status Unknown Not Responding to Other Therapies
Adults: 400 mg/day

ASM Associated with Eosinophilia
Adults: 100 mg/day starting dose, a dose increase from 100 to 400 mg may be considered in the absence of adverse reactions if assessments demonstrate insufficient response to therapy.

Hypereosinophilic Syndrome/Chronic Eosinophilic Leukemia (HES/CEL)
Adults: 400 mg/day; for patients with HES/CEL with FIP1L1-PDGFR$_{alpha}$ fusion kinase, a starting dose of 100 mg/day is recommended; a dose increase from 100 to 400 mg may be considered in the absence of adverse reactions

Dermatofibrosarcoma Protuberans (DFSP)
Adults: 800 mg/day

Unresectable and/or Metastatic, Malignant GIST:
Adults: 400 to 600 mg/day

How should I take Gleevec?

Gleevec should be taken with food and a large glass of water. For patients unable to swallow the film-coated tablets, the tablets may be dispersed in a glass of water or apple juice.

What should I avoid while taking Gleevec?

Gleevec should not be taken with grapefruit juice. Females of childbearing age should avoid becoming pregnant. Sexually active females should use adequate contraception.

What are possible food and drug interactions associated with Gleevec?

If Gleevec is taken with certain other drugs, the effects of either could be increased, decreased, or altered. It is especially important to check with your doctor before combining Gleevec with the following: acetaminophen, alfentanil, atanazavir, carbamazepine, clarithromycin, cyclosporine, dexamethasone, diergotamine, dihydropyridine calcium channel blockers, erythromycin, ergotamine, fentanyl, grapefruit juice, HMG-CoA reductase inhibitors or "statins," indinavir, itraconazole, ketoconazole, nefazadone, nelfinavir, phenobarbital, phenytoin, pimozide, quinidine, rifampicin, ritonavir, saquinavir, sirolimus, St. John's wort, tacrolimus, telithromycin, triazolobenzodiazepines, voriconazole, warfarin

What are the possible side effects of Gleevec?

Side effects cannot be anticipated. If any develop or change in intensity, tell your doctor as soon as possible. Only your doctor can determine if it is safe for you to continue taking this drug.

Side effects may include: nausea, vomiting, fluid retention, muscle cramps, rash, diarrhea, heartburn, headache

Can I receive Gleevec if I am pregnant or breastfeeding?

Tell your doctor immediately if you are pregnant, plan to become pregnant, or are breastfeeding. Women of childbearing age should avoid becoming pregnant while being treated with Gleevec.

What should I do if I miss a dose of Gleevec?

If you miss a dose, take the medicine as soon as you remember, making sure you also eat a meal and drink a large glass of water. If it is almost time for your next meal, skip the missed dose and take the medicine when you eat your next meal. Do not take extra medicine to make up the missed dose.

How should I store Gleevec?

Store at room temperature in a tightly closed container. Protect from moisture.

Glimepiride *See Amaryl, page 75.*

Glipizide *See Glucotrol/Glucotrol XL, page 620.*

Glipizide and metformin hydrochloride *See Metaglip, page 802.*

GLUCOPHAGE/GLUCOPHAGE XR
Generic name: Metformin hydrochloride

What is Glucophage/Glucophage XR?
Glucophage and Glucophage XR are used to treat type 2 diabetes. Regular Glucophage tablets are taken two or three times daily. The extended-release form, Glucophage XR, is available for once-daily dosing.

What is the most important information I should know about Glucophage/Glucophage XR?
Glucophage/Glucophage XR could cause a very rare—but potentially fatal—side effect known as lactic acidosis. It is caused by a buildup of lactic acid in the blood. The problem is most likely to occur in people whose liver or kidneys are not working well, and in those who have multiple medical problems, take several medications, or have congestive heart failure. The risk also is higher if you are an older adult or drink alcohol. Lactic acidosis is a medical emergency that must be treated in a hospital. Notify your doctor immediately if you experience any of the following: dizziness, extreme weakness or tiredness, light-headedness, low body temperature, rapid breathing or trouble breathing, sleepiness, slow or irregular heartbeat, unexpected or unusual stomach discomfort, or unusual muscle pain.

You should not take Glucophage/Glucophage XR for 2 days before and after having an X-ray procedure (such as an angiogram) that uses an injectable dye. Also, if you are going to have surgery, except minor surgery, you should stop taking Glucophage/Glucophage XR. Once you have resumed normal food and fluid intake, your doctor will tell you when you can start drug therapy again.

If you are taking Glucophage/Glucophage XR, you should check your blood or urine periodically for abnormal sugar (glucose) levels.

Glucophage/Glucophage XR does not usually cause hypoglycemia (low blood sugar). However, it remains a possibility, especially in older, weak, and undernourished people and those with kidney, liver, adrenal, or pituitary gland problems. The risk of low blood sugar increases when Glucophage is combined with other diabetes medications. The risk is also boosted by missed meals, alcohol, and excessive exercise. To avoid low blood sugar, you should closely follow the diet and exercise plan suggested by your doctor.

If your blood sugar becomes unstable due to the stress of a fever, injury, infection, or surgery, your doctor may temporarily take you off Glucophage/Glucophage XR and ask you to take insulin instead.

You should stop taking Glucophage/Glucophage XR if you become seriously dehydrated, since this increases the likelihood of developing lactic acidosis. Tell your doctor if you lose a significant amount of fluid due to vomiting, diarrhea, fever, or some other condition.

The effectiveness of any oral antidiabetic, including Glucophage/Glucophage XR, may decrease with time. This may occur because of either a diminished responsiveness to the medication or a worsening of the diabetes.

Who should not take Glucophage/Glucophage XR?

Glucophage/Glucophage XR is processed primarily by the kidneys, and can build up to excessive levels in the body if the kidneys aren't working properly. It should be avoided if you have kidney disease or your kidney function has been impaired by a condition such as shock, blood poisoning, or a heart attack.

You should not use Glucophage/Glucophage XR if you need to take medicine for congestive heart failure.

Do not take Glucophage/Glucophage XR if you have ever had an allergic reaction to metformin.

Do not take Glucophage/Glucophage XR if you have metabolic or diabetic ketoacidosis (a life-threatening medical emergency caused by insufficient insulin and marked by excessive thirst, nausea, fatigue, pain below the breastbone, and fruity breath). Diabetic ketoacidosis should be treated with insulin.

What should I tell my doctor before I take the first dose of Glucophage/Glucophage XR?

Tell your doctor about all prescription, over-the-counter, and herbal medications you are taking before beginning treatment with this drug. Also, talk to your doctor about your complete medical history, especially if you have kidney or liver problems.

What is the usual dosage?

The information below is based on the dosage guidelines your doctor uses. Depending on your condition and medical history, your doctor may prescribe a different regimen. Do not change the dosage or stop taking your medication without your doctor's approval.

Your doctor will tailor your dosage to your individual needs.

Glucophage

Adults: The usual starting dose is one 500-milligram tablet twice a day, taken with morning and evening meals. Your doctor may increase your daily dose by 500 milligrams at weekly intervals, based on your response up to a total of 2,000 milligrams. An alternative starting dose is one

850-milligram tablet a day, taken with the morning meal. Your doctor may increase this by 850 milligrams at 14-day intervals, to a maximum of 2,550 milligrams a day. The usual maintenance dose ranges from 1,500 to 2,550 milligrams daily. If you take more than 2,000 milligrams a day, your doctor may recommend that the medication be divided into three doses, taken with each meal.

Children 10 to 16 years old: The usual starting dose is one 500-milligram tablet twice a day with meals. The dosage may be increased by 500 milligrams at weekly intervals up to a maximum of 2,000 milligrams daily.

Glucophage XR
Adults: The usual starting dose is one 500-milligram tablet once daily with the evening meal. Your doctor may increase your dose by 500 milligrams at weekly intervals, up to a maximum dosage of 2,000 milligrams a day. If a single 2,000-milligram dose fails to control your blood sugar, you may be asked to take 1,000-milligram doses twice a day. If you need more than 2,000 milligrams a day, the doctor will switch you to regular Glucophage.

The safety and effectiveness of Glucohpage XR in children have not been established.

How should I take Glucophage/Glucophage XR?
Do not take more or less of this medication than directed by your doctor. The drug should be taken with food to reduce the possibility of nausea or diarrhea, especially during the first few weeks of therapy.

If taking Glucophage XR, be sure to swallow the tablet whole; do not crush it or chew it. The inactive ingredients in the tablet may occasionally appear in the stool. This is not a cause for concern.

What should I avoid while taking Glucophage/Glucophage XR?
Avoid drinking too much alcohol while taking this drug. Heavy drinking increases the danger of lactic acidosis and can also trigger an attack of low blood sugar.

What are possible food and drug interactions associated with Glucophage/Glucophage XR?
If Glucophage/Glucophage XR is taken with certain other drugs, the effects of either could be increased, decreased, or altered. It is especially important to check with your doctor before combining this medication with the following: alcohol, amiloride, calcium channel blockers (heart medications) such as nifedipine and verapamil, cimetidine, decongestants or airway-opening drugs such as albuterol and pseudoephedrine, digoxin, estrogens, furosemide, glyburide, isoniazid, major tranquilizers such as chlorpromazine, morphine, niacin, nifedipine, oral contraceptives, phenytoin, procainamide, quinidine, quinine, ranitidine, steroids such as prednisone, thyroid hormones such as levothyroxine, triam-

terene, trimethoprim, vancomycin, and diuretics such as hydrochloro-thiazide.

What are the possible side effects of Glucophage/Glucophage XR?

Side effects cannot be anticipated. If any develop or change in intensity, tell your doctor as soon as possible. Only your doctor can determine if it is safe for you to continue taking this drug.

Side effects may include: abdominal discomfort, diarrhea, gas, headache, indigestion, nausea, vomiting, weakness

Can I receive Glucophage/Glucophage XR if I am pregnant or breastfeeding?

If you are pregnant or plan to become pregnant, tell your doctor immediately. Glucophage/Glucophage XR have not been studied during pregnancy. It is not known whether Glucophage/Glucophage XR appears in breast milk. Therefore, women should discuss with their doctors whether to discontinue the medication or to stop breastfeeding. If the medication is discontinued and if diet alone does not control glucose levels, then your doctor may consider insulin injections.

What should I do if I miss a dose of Glucophage/Glucophage XR?

Take it as soon as you remember. If it is almost time for your next dose, skip the one you missed and go back to your regular schedule. Never take 2 doses at the same time.

How should I store Glucophage/Glucophage XR?

Store it at room temperature.

GLUCOTROL/GLUCOTROL XL

Generic name: Glipizide

What is Glucotrol/Glucotrol XL?

Glucotrol is used to treat high blood sugar in type 2 (non-insulin-dependent) diabetes in combination with diet and exercise. Glucotrol helps the body release more of its own insulin and respond better to it; it also lowers the amount of sugar (glucose) made by the body. Glucotrol also comes in an extended-release form called Glucotrol XL, which allows the medicine to be released slowly over 24 hours.

What is the most important information I should know about Glucotrol/Glucotrol XL?

Treatment with Glucotrol may increase the risk of death from heart disease compared with treatment of diabetes with diet alone or diet plus insulin.

Glucotrol may cause severe hypoglycemia (very low levels of sugar in your blood). This can happen if you do not follow your diet, exercise too much, drink alcohol, are under stress, or get sick. It can also happen if your dose of Glucotrol is higher than you need or if you're taking other glucose-lowering drugs. Your doctor will decide how to adjust your medication. Never adjust the dose yourself. Elderly, debilitated, and malnourished patients and those with adrenal or pituitary insufficiency are more susceptible to hypoglycemia. It may be difficult to recognize the signs and symptoms of hypoglycemia in the elderly and patients taking "beta-blockers" (a type of drug used to treat high blood pressure).

Glucotrol is an aid to, not a substitute for, good diet and exercise. Failure to follow a sound diet and exercise plan can lead to serious complications, such as dangerously high or low blood sugar levels. Glucotrol cannot be used in place of insulin. It is not an oral form of insulin.

Who should not take Glucotrol/Glucotrol XL?
Do not take Glucotrol if you are sensitive to the drug or any of its components.

Do not use Glucotrol if you are suffering from diabetic ketoacidosis (a life-threatening medical emergency caused by low insulin levels and marked by excessive thirst, nausea, fatigue, pain below the breastbone, and fruity-smelling breath). Diabetic ketoacidosis should be treated with insulin.

What should I tell my doctor before I take the first dose of Glucotrol/Glucotrol XL?
Tell your doctor about all prescription, over-the-counter, and herbal medications you are taking before beginning treatment with Glucotrol. Also, talk to your doctor about your complete medical history, especially if you ever had diabetic ketoacidosis, have a history of kidney or liver disease, thyroid disease, chronic (continuing) diarrhea or type 1 diabetes, if you have a serious infection, illness, or injury, need surgery, have narrowing of the stomach or intestines, or are pregnant or might be pregnant, or are breastfeeding.

What is the usual dosage?
The information below is based on the dosage guidelines your doctor uses. Depending on your condition and medical history, your doctor may prescribe a different regimen. Do not change the dosage or stop taking your medication without your doctor's approval.

Glucotrol
Adults: The usual starting dose is 5 milligrams (mg) taken before breakfast. Depending upon your blood sugar response, your doctor may increase the initial dose in increments of 2.5 to 5 mg. The maximum recommended daily dose is 40 mg. Total daily dosages above 15 mg are usually divided into 2 equal doses that are taken before meals.

Elderly or liver impairment: The usually starting dose is 2.5 mg.

For patients whose daily insulin intake is 20 units or less, insulin may be discontinued and Glucotrol therapy may be began at usual dosages.

For patients whose daily insulin intake is more than 20 units, the insulin dose should be reduced by 50% and Glucotrol therapy may be started at the usual dosages.

Glucotrol XL
Adults: The usual starting dose is 5 mg each day at breakfast. After 3 months, your doctor may increase the dose to 10 mg daily. The maximum recommended dose is 20 mg.

Elderly or liver impairment: The usually starting dose is 5 mg.

For patients whose daily insulin intake is 20 units or less, insulin may be discontinued and Glucotrol XL therapy may be started at the usual dosages.

For patients whose daily insulin intake is more than 20 units, the insulin dose should be reduced by 50% and Glucotrol XL therapy may begin at usual dosages.

How should I take Glucotrol/Glucotrol XL?

Take Glucotrol exactly as prescribed. To achieve the best control over blood sugar levels, Glucotrol should be taken 30 minutes before a meal. However, the exact dosing schedule as well as the dosage amount must be determined by your doctor.

Glucotrol XL should be taken with breakfast. Swallow the tablets whole. Do not chew, crush, or divide them. This damages the tablet and will release too much medicine into your body. Do not be alarmed if you notice something that looks like a tablet in your stool; it is only the empty shell that has been eliminated.

What should I avoid while taking Glucotrol/Glucotrol XL?

Follow diet, medication, and exercise routines closely. Changing any of these things can affect blood sugar levels.

Avoid alcohol as it can interfere with your blood sugar levels and your diabetes treatment.

What are possible food and drug interactions associated with Glucotrol/Glucotrol XL?

If Glucotrol is taken with certain other drugs, the effects of either could be increased, decreased, or altered. it is especially important to check with your doctor before combining Glucotrol with the following: alcohol, aspirin, beta-blockers (eg, atenolol and metoprolol), calcium-blockers (eg diltiazem, nifedipine, verapamil), chloramphenicol, cimetidine, clofibrate, corticosteroids (eg, dexamethasone and prednisone), diuretics (eg, water pills such as hydrochlorothiazide or furosemide), epinephrine, estrogens, fluconazole, gemfibrozil, isoniazid, mao inhibitors (eg, phenelzine and tranylcypromine), miconazole, nicotinic acid, nonsteroidal anti-inflammatory drugs (eg, ibuprofen or naproxen), norepinephrine, oral contraceptives, phenothiazines, phenytoin, probenecid, pseudoephedrine, rifampin, sulfa drugs (eg, sulfamethoxazole), thyroid drugs, warfarin

What are the possible side effects of Glucotrol/Glucotrol XL?

Side effects cannot be anticipated. If any develop or change in intensity, tell your doctor as soon as possible. Only your doctor can determine if it is safe for you to continue taking this drug.

Side effects may include: constipation, diarrhea, dizziness, drowsiness, gas, headache, hives, itching, low blood sugar, nervousness, sensitivity to light, skin rash and eruptions, stomach pain, tremors

Glucotrol and Glucotrol XL can cause low blood sugar. This risk is increased by missed meals, alcohol, other diabetes medications, and excessive exercise. Low blood sugar is also more likely in older people, those with kidney or liver problems, and those with adrenal or pituitary gland diseases. To avoid low blood sugar, follow the dietary and exercise regimen suggested by your doctor.

Symptoms of mild low blood sugar may include: blurred vision, cold sweats, dizziness, fast heartbeat, fatigue, headache, hunger, light-headedness, nausea, nervousness, weakness, trembling, tingling in the lips or hands

Symptoms of more severe low blood sugar may include: coma, disorientation, pale skin, seizures, shallow breathing

If you experience any of these signs and symptoms of hypoglycemia, eat or drink something with sugar in it right away, such as a regular (not diet) soft drink, orange juice, honey, sugar candy, or glucose tablets. If you do not feel better or if your blood sugar does not go up, call your doctor immediately. If your doctor is unavailable in an emergency, call 911 or have someone drive you the nearest emergency room.

Can I receive Glucotrol/Glucotrol XL if I am pregnant or breastfeeding?

The effects of Glucotrol during pregnancy and breastfeeding are unknown. Tell your doctor immediately if you are pregnant, plan to become pregnant, or are breastfeeding.

What should I do if I miss a dose of Glucotrol/Glucotrol XL?

Take it as soon as you remember. If it is almost time for your next dose, skip the one you missed and go back to your regular schedule. Never take 2 doses at the same time.

How should I store Glucotrol/Glucotrol XL?

Store Glucotrol at room temperature away from heat and moisture.

GLUCOVANCE
Generic name: Glyburide and metformin hydrochloride

What is Glucovance?
Glucovance, as an adjunct with diet and exercise, is used to treat type 2 diabetes. This drug combines two glucose-lowering drugs, glyburide and metformin. Glyburide lowers blood sugar primarily by causing more of the body's own insulin to be released, and metformin lowers blood sugar, in part, by helping your body use your own insulin more effectively.

What is the most important information I should know about Glucovance?
Glucovance can cause a rare, but serious condition called lactic acidosis (a build up of an acid in the blood) that can be potentially fatal. Lactic acidosis is a medical emergency and must be treated in the hospital. Stop taking Glucovance and call your doctor right away if you: feel very weak or tired, have muscle pain, have trouble breathing, have stomach pain with nausea, vomiting, and diarrhea, feel cold, especially in your arms and legs, feel dizzy or lightheaded, have a slow or irregular heartbeat, or if a medical condition suddenly changes.

You have a higher chance for getting lactic acidosis with if you have kidney or liver problems, have congestive heart failure that requires treatments with medicines, drink a lot of alcohol, get dehydrated (lose a large amount of body fluids). Dehydration can happen if you are sick with a fever, have diarrhea, or from vomiting. Dehydration can also happen when you sweat a lot with activity or exercise and don't drink enough fluids. You also have a higher chance of getting lactic acidosis if you have certain x-ray tests with injectable dyes used, have surgery, have a heart attack, severe infection, or stroke, or are 80 years of age or older and not had your kidney function tested.

Glucovance may cause hypoglycemia (very low levels of blood sugar). This can happen if you do not follow your diet, exercise too much, drink alcohol, under stress, or get sick. It can also happen if you take other glucose-lowering drugs. Elderly, debilitated, and malnourished patients and those with adrenal or pituitary insufficiency are more susceptible to hypoglycemia. It may be difficult to recognize signs and symptoms of hypoglycemia in the elderly and patients taking "beta-blockers" (type of drug used to treat high blood pressure).

If you experience signs and symptoms of hypoglycemia, eat or drink something with sugar in it right away, such as regular (not diet) soft drink, orange juice, honey, sugar candy, or glucose tablets. If you do not feel better or your blood glucose does not go up, call your doctor immediately. If your doctor is unavailable for an emergency, call 911 or have someone drive you to the nearest emergency room.

Glucovance is an aid to, not a substitute for, good diet and exercise.

Failure to follow a sound diet and exercise plan can lead to serious complications, such as dangerously high or low blood sugar levels.

Who should not take Glucovance?

Do not begin treatment with Glucovance if you have kidney disease, congestive heart failure treated with medications, drink alcohol excessively, are dehydrated, or have high blood ketone or acid levels (including diabetic ketoacidosis).

Do not use Glucovance if you are scheduled to undergo surgery or an x-ray procedure involving special dye or contrast agents.

Do not use Glucovance if you have a serious infection, a history or heart attack or stroke, are 80 years of age or older and have not had your kidney function tested, or are allergic to any of its ingredients.

What should I tell my doctor before I take the first dose of Glucovance?

Tell your doctor about all prescription, over-the-counter, and herbal medications you are taking before beginning treatment with Glucovance. Also, talk to your doctor about your complete medical history, especially if you have an illness that causes severe diarrhea, vomiting, or fever; or you have heart, kidney or liver problems, or if you have low levels of vitamin B_{12}, are pregnant or planning to become pregnant, or are breastfeeding. Your doctor should also know if you are going to have surgery or an x-ray procedure that requires special dye or contrast agents.

What is the usual dosage?

The information below is based on the dosage guidelines your doctor uses. Depending on your condition and medical history, your doctor may prescribe a different regimen. Do not change the dosage or stop taking your medication without your doctor's approval.

Patients with Inadequate Glycemic Control on Diet and Exercise
Adults: 1.25 milligrams (mg)/250 mg once or twice daily is the recommended starting dose; dosage increases should be made in increments of 1.25 mg/250 mg per day every 2 weeks

Patients with Inadequate Glycemic Control on a Sulfonylurea and/or Metformin
2.5 mg/500 mg or 5 mg/500 mg twice daily is the recommended starting dose; daily dose should be titrated in increments of no more than 5 mg/500 mg

Do not exceed the maximum daily dose of 20 mg/2000 mg.

How should I take Glucovance?

Glucovance should be taken with meals.

What should I avoid while taking Glucovance?

Do not change your diet, medication, and exercise routines. Changing any of these could affect blood sugar levels.

Avoid alcohol. It can interfere with your blood sugar levels and your diabetes treatment.

What are possible food and drug interactions associated with Glucovance?

If Glucovance is taken with certain other drugs, the effects of either could be increased, decreased, or altered. it is especially important to check you're your doctor before combining Glucovance with the following: amiloride, beta-adrenergic blocking agents, calcium channel blockers, chloramphenicol, coumarins, ciprofloxacin, corticosteroids, digoxin, estrogens, furosemide, isoniazid, miconazole, morphine, monoamine oxidase inhibitors, nicotinic acid, nifedipine, nonsteroidal anti-inflammatory drugs (eg, ibuprofen), oral contraceptives, phenothiazines, phenytoin, procainamide, probenacid, quinidine, quinine, ranitidine, salicylates, sulfonamides, sympathomimetics, thiazide diuretics, thyroid products, trimethoprim, vancomycin.

What are the possible side effects of Glucovance?

Side effects cannot be anticipated. If any develop or change in intensity, tell your doctor as soon as possible. Only your doctor can determine if it is safe for you to continue taking this drug.

Side effects may include: diarrhea, nausea, upset stomach, upper respiratory infection, headache, vomiting, dizziness, abdominal pain

Symptoms of hypoglycemia (low blood sugar): dizziness, hunger, lightheadedness, shakiness

If you experience signs and symptoms of hypoglycemia, eat or drink something with sugar in it right away, such as regular (not diet) soft drink, orange juice, honey, sugar candy, or glucose tablets. If you do not feel better or your blood glucose does not go up, call your doctor immediately. If your doctor is unavailable for an emergency, call 911 or have someone drive you to the nearest emergency room.

Symptoms of lactic acidosis: dizziness, feeling cold, irregular/slow heartbeat, lightheadedness, muscle pain, stomach problems, tired or uncomfortable, trouble breathing

Lactic acidosis is a medical emergency and must be treated in the hospital.

Can I receive Glucovance if I am pregnant or breastfeeding?

The effects of Glucovance during pregnancy are unknown. Tell your doctor immediately if you are pregnant, plan to become pregnant, or are breastfeeding.

What should I do if I miss a dose of Glucovance?

If you miss a dose of Glucovance, take it as soon as possible. Of it is almost time for your next dose, skip the missed dose and go back to your regular dosing schedule. Do not take 2 doses at once.

How should I store Glucovance?

Store at room temperature.

GLUMETZA

Generic name: Metformin hydrochloride extended release

What is Glumetza?

Glumetza is used along with diet and exercise to improve blood sugar control in adults with type 2 diabetes. Glumetza may also be used with another anti-diabetes medicine called a sulfonylurea or with insulin. Glumetza helps control your blood sugar levels by helping your body respond better to the insulin it makes naturally.

What is the most important information I should know about Glumetza?

Glumetza can cause a rare, but serious condition called lactic acidosis (a build up of an acid in the blood) that can be potentially fatal. Lactic acidosis is a medical emergency and must be treated in the hospital. Stop taking Glumetza and call your doctor right away if you: feel very weak or tired, have muscle pain, have trouble breathing, have stomach pain with nausea, vomiting, and diarrhea, feel cold, especially in your arms and legs, feel dizzy or lightheaded, have a slow or irregular heartbeat, or if a medical condition suddenly changes.

You have a higher chance for getting lactic acidosis with Glumetza if you have kidney or liver problems, have congestive heart failure that requires treatments with medicines, drink a lot of alcohol, get dehydrated (lose a large amount of body fluids). Dehydration can happen if you are sick with a fever, have diarrhea, or from vomiting. Dehydration can also happen when you sweat a lot with activity or exercise and don't drink enough fluids. You also have a higher chance of getting lactic acidosis if you have certain x-ray tests with injectable dyes used, have surgery, have a heart attack, severe infection, or stroke, or are 80 years of age or older and not had your kidney function tested.

Who should not take Glumetza?

Do not take Glumetza if you have kidney problems, heart failure that is treated with medicines, are allergic to Glumetza or to any of its ingredients, or have a condition called metabolic acidosis, including diabetic ketoacidosis. Diabetic ketoacidosis should be treated with insulin.

What should I tell my doctor before I take the first dose of Glumetza?

Tell your doctor about all prescription, over-the-counter, and herbal medications you are taking before beginning treatment with Glumetza. Also, talk to your doctor about your complete medical history, especially if you have kidney, liver or heart problems, drink a lot of alcohol, or if you are pregnant, planning to become pregnant or are breastfeeding.

What is the usual dosage?

The information below is based on the dosage guidelines your doctor uses. Depending on your condition and medical history, your doctor may prescribe a different regimen. Do not change the dosage or stop taking your medication without your doctor's approval.

Adults: The usual starting dose of Glumetza is 1000 milligrams (mg) a day, taken with food in the evening. Dosage increases should be made in increments of 500 mg a week, up to a maximum of 2000 mg once-a-day with the evening meal. If glycemic control is not achieved with 2000 mg once daily, a trial of 1000 mg twice daily should be considered.

Glumetza plus Insulin Therapy
Adults: Continue your current insulin dose upon starting Glumetza. Glumetza should be started at 500 mg once daily in patients also receiving insulin therapy. For patients not responding adequately, Glumetza should be increased by 500 mg after approximately 1 week and by 500 mg every week thereafter until adequate glycemic control is achieved without exceeding the maximum daily dose. The insulin dose should be decreased by 10-25% when plasma fasting glucose concentrations decrease to >120 mg/dL. Further adjustments should be individualized.

How should I take Glumetza?

Take Glumetza once a day in the evening with food. Swallow tablets whole. Never crush, split, or chew Glumetza tablets.

Take Glumetza exactly as prescribed. Your doctor will usually start you on a low dose and increase your dose slowly. Do not change your dose unless your doctor tells you to.

It is normal to see the tablet shell and a soft mass of the inactive ingredients in your stool.

While you are on Glumetza therapy, stay on your diet and exercise program, and test your blood sugar regularly as directed by your doctor.

What should I avoid while taking Glumetza?

Avoid excessive alcohol use while taking Glumetza. This means you should not binge drink for short periods or drink a lot of alcohol on a regular basis. Alcohol can increase the chance of getting lactic acidosis.

What are possible food and drug interactions associated with Glumetza?

If Glumetza is taken with certain other drugs, the effects of either could be increased, decreased, or altered. It is especially important to check with your doctor before combining Glumetza with the following: amiloride, calcium channel blockers, corticosteroids, digoxin, diuretics (eg, furosemide); estrogens, isoniazid; morphine, nicotinic acid, nifedipine, oral contraceptives, phenothiazines, phenytoin, procainamide, quinidine, quinine, ranitidine, sympathomimetics, thyroid medications, triamterene, trimethoprim, vancomycin

What are the possible side effects of Glumetza?

Side effects cannot be anticipated. If any develop or change in intensity, tell your doctor as soon as possible. Only your doctor can determine if it is safe for you to continue taking this drug.

Side effects may include: diarrhea, nausea, and upset stomach.

Symptoms of lactic acidosis: dizziness, feeling cold, irregular/slow heartbeat, lightheadedness, muscle pain, stomach problems, tired or uncomfortable, trouble breathing

Lactic acidosis is a medical emergency and must be treated in the hospital.

Can I receive Glumetza if I am pregnant or breastfeeding?

Treatment with Glumetza is not recommended during pregnancy or breastfeeding. If you are pregnant, planning to become pregnant, or are nursing, talk to your doctor about your therapy options.

What should I do if I miss a dose of Glumetza?

If you miss a dose of Glumetza, resume dosing according to schedule.

How should I store Glumetza?

Store at room temperature.

Glyburide See Diabeta, page 410, or Micronase, page 826.

Glyburide and metformin hydrochloride See Glucovance, page 624.

GLYSET
Generic name: Miglitol

What is Glyset?
Glyset is used as an add-on treatment to diet to improve high blood sugar levels caused by type 2 diabetes mellitus. Glyset may also be used in combination with a sulfonylurea (such as Glipizide, Glimepiride, or Glyburide) when diet plus either Glyset or a sulfonylurea alone do not result in adequate blood sugar control.

What is the most important information I should know about Glyset?
Glyset itself does not cause low blood sugar even when administered to patients in the fasted state. However, when Glyset is given in combination with a sulfonylurea or insulin, it will cause a further lowering of blood sugar.

It is important to continue to adhere to dietary instructions, a regular exercise program, and regular testing of urine or blood glucose.

Glyset when administered alone should not cause hypoglycemia (very low levels of blood sugar that could be life-threatening). However, sulfonylureas and insulin may cause hypoglycemia. When Glyset is administered with a sulfonylurea drug or insulin, the combination will further lower your blood glucose and has the potential of causing hypoglycemia.

When diabetic patients are exposed to stress such as fever, infection, trauma, or surgery, a temporary loss of blood glucose may occur. When this happens, temporary insulin therapy may be necessary.

Who should not take Glyset?
Do not use Glyset if you have diabetic ketoacidosis (inadequate insulin levels resulting in high blood sugar and accumulation of organic acids and ketones in the blood.), inflammatory bowel disease, colonic ulceration, partial intestinal obstruction, or chronic intestinal disease.

Glyset should not be used by anyone allergic to the drug or any of its components.

What should I tell my doctor before I take the first dose of Glyset?
Tell your doctor about all prescription, over-the-counter, and herbal medications you are taking before beginning treatment with Glyset. Also, talk to your doctor about your complete medical history, especially if you are pregnant or planning to become pregnant, or have intestinal or kidney disease.

What is the usual dosage?
The information below is based on the dosage guidelines your doctor uses. Depending on your condition and medical history, your doctor

may prescribe a different regimen. Do not change the dosage or stop taking your medication without your doctor's approval.

Adults: The recommended starting dosage of Glyset is 25 milligrams (mg), given orally 3 times a day. However, some patients may benefit by starting at 25 mg once daily to minimize side effects, then gradually increase the frequency of administration to 3 times a day.

The usual maintenance dose of Glyset is 50 mg 3 times a day, although some patients may benefit from increasing the dose to 100 mg 3 times a day.

The maximum recommended dosage of Glyset is 100 mg 3 times a day.

How should I take Glyset?
Glyset should be taken orally 3 times a day with the first bite of each main meal.

What should I avoid while taking Glyset?
Avoid drinking alcohol while taking this medication because it may increase your risk of developing hypoglycemia.

Use caution when engaging in activities that require alertness such as driving or operating machinery because you may experience blurred vision, dizziness, or drowsiness from very high or low blood sugar levels.

What are possible food and drug interactions associated with Glyset?
If Glyset is taken with certain other drugs, the effects of either could be increased, decreased, or altered. It is especially important to check with your doctor before combining Glyset with the following: amylase, digoxin, glyburide, intestinal absorbents (eg, charcoal), metformin, propranolol, ranitidine

What are the possible side effects of Glyset?
Side effects cannot be anticipated. If any develop or change in intensity, tell your doctor as soon as possible. Only your doctor can determine if it is safe for you to continue taking this drug.

Side effects may include: abdominal pain, diarrhea, excess gas in stomach, skin rash

Symptoms of hypoglycemia (low blood sugar): dizziness, hunger, lightheadedness, shakiness

If you experience signs and symptoms of hypoglycemia, eat or drink something with sugar in it right away, such as regular (not diet) soft drink, orange juice, honey, sugar candy, or glucose tablets. If you do not feel better or your blood glucose does not go up, call your doctor immediately. If your doctor is unavailable for an emergency, call 911 or have someone drive you to the nearest emergency room.

Can I receive Glyset if I am pregnant or breastfeeding?

The effects of Glyset during pregnancy and breastfeeding are unknown. Tell your doctor immediately if you are pregnant, plan to become pregnant, or are breastfeeding.

What should I do if I miss a dose of Glyset?

If you miss a dose and have completed your meal, skip the missed dose. Take the next dose with the next meal. Do not take 2 doses at once.

How should I store Glyset?

Store at room temperature.

Goserelin acetate *See Zoladex, page 1487.*

Guaifenesin and codeine phosphate *See Tussi-Organidin NR, page 1343.*

GUANFACINE HYDROCHLORIDE

What is Guanfacine hydrochloride?

Guanfacine is given alone or in combination with other drugs, especially thiazide diuretics, for the treatment of high blood pressure.

What is the most important information I should know about Guanfacine hydrochloride?

You must take guanfacine regularly for it to be effective. Since blood pressure declines gradually, it may be several weeks before you get the full benefit of guanfacine. You must continue taking it even if you are feeling well. Guanfacine does not cure high blood pressure; it only keeps it under control.

Do not abruptly stop taking guanfacine. It may cause rebound or "overshoot" hypertension (sudden increase in blood pressure) and also cause nervousness and anxiety. This is very dangerous and could result in a medical emergency.

Who should not take Guanfacine hydrochloride?

Do not take guanfacine if you are allergic or sensitive to the drug.

What should I tell my doctor before I take the first dose of Guanfacine hydrochloride?

Tell your doctor about all prescription, over-the-counter, and herbal medications you are taking before beginning treatment with guanfacine. Also, talk to your doctor about your complete medical history, especially if you have atherosclerosis (hardening and narrowing of the arteries); heart disease; kidney or liver disease; or have suffered a recent heart attack or stroke.

What is the usual dosage?

The information below is based on the dosage guidelines your doctor uses. Depending on your condition and medical history, your doctor may prescribe a different regimen. Do not change the dosage or stop taking your medication without your doctor's approval.

Adults: The recommended initial dose of guanfacine when given alone or in combination with another drug is 1 milligram (mg) taken daily at bedtime. If after 3-4 weeks of therapy, 1 mg does not give a satisfactory result, a dose of 2 mg may be given. Higher daily doses have been used, but side effects increase significantly with doses of 3 mg/day.

Children: The safety and effectiveness of guanfacine have not been established in children <12 years of age.

How should I take Guanfacine hydrochloride?

Take guanfacine exactly as prescribed by your doctor. Guanfacine should be taken at bedtime, since it will probably cause drowsiness.

In some cases, you may take 2 evenly spaced doses per day rather than a single dose at bedtime.

What should I avoid while taking Guanfacine hydrochloride?

Since guanfacine causes drowsiness and may also make you dizzy, do not drive, climb, or perform hazardous tasks until you find out exactly how guanfacine affects you.

While taking guanfacine, drink alcoholic beverages with care. You may feel intoxicated after drinking only a small amount of alcohol.

If you have been taking guanfacine for a while, do not stop taking it without speaking to your doctor. Stopping abruptly may result in nervousness, rapid pulse, anxiety, heartbeat irregularities, and so-called rebound high blood pressure (higher than before you started taking guanfacine). If you do have rebound high blood pressure, it will probably develop 2-4 days after your last dose of guanfacine. Rebound high blood pressure, if it occurs, will usually decrease and then disappear over a period of 2-4 days.

What are possible food and drug interactions associated with Guanfacine hydrochloride?

If guanfacine is taken with certain other drugs, the effects of either could be increased, decreased, or altered. It is especially important to check with your doctor before combining guanfacine with the following: barbiturates (eg, amobarbital, secobarbital, phenobarbital), benzodiazepines (eg, alprazolam or diazepam), phenothiazines (eg, chlorpromazine or thioridazine), phenytoin

What are the possible side effects of Guanfacine hydrochloride?
Side effects cannot be anticipated. If any develop or change in intensity, tell your doctor as soon as possible. Only your doctor can determine if it is safe for you to continue taking this drug.

Side effects may include: constipation, dizziness, dry mouth, feeling tired, headache, impotence, sleepiness, weakness, insomnia, fainting, involuntary leakage of urine (urinary incontinence), pink eye (conjunctivitis), tingling or numbness, depression, skin reactions/rash

**Can I receive Guanfacine hydrochloride if I am
pregnant or breastfeeding?**
The effects of guanfacine during pregnancy and breastfeeding are unknown. Tell your doctor immediately if you are pregnant, plan to become pregnant, or are breastfeeding. Use caution when taking guanfacine while breastfeeding.

What should I do if I miss a dose of Guanfacine hydrochloride?
Take the missed dose as soon as you remember. If it is almost time for your next dose, skip the missed dose and go back to your regular schedule. Never take 2 doses at once. If you miss taking guanfacine for 2 or more days in a row, check with your doctor.

How should I store Guanfacine hydrochloride?
Store at room temperature in a tight, light-resistant container.

HALCION
Generic name: Triazolam

What is Halcion?
Halcion is used in adults for the short-term treatment of insomnia.

**What is the most important information
I should know about Halcion?**
Halcion is not indicated for use in children.

After taking Halcion, you may get out of bed without being fully awake and perform an activity that you do not know you are doing (such as sleep-driving a car, making or eating food, talking on the phone, having sex, or sleep-walking). The next morning you may not have any recollection of this. Drinking alcohol or taking other medications that make you sleepy increases the chances of doing these activities.

You may have withdrawal symptoms for 1 to 2 days if you stop taking Halcion suddenly. These symptoms may include trouble sleeping, unpleasant feelings, stomach and muscle cramps, vomiting, sweating, shakiness and seizures.

Who should not take Halcion?

Do not take Halcion if you are allergic to it or any of its components, if you drink alcohol, cannot guarantee a full night's sleep, or are pregnant or considering becoming pregnant.

What should I tell my doctor before I take the first dose of Halcion?

Tell your doctor about all prescription, over-the-counter, and herbal medications you are taking before beginning treatment with Halcion. Also, talk to your doctor about your complete medical history, especially if you have a history of depression, mental illness, suicidal thoughts, drug or alcohol abuse or addiction, kidney or liver disease, lung disease or breathing problems, and if you are pregnant, plan to become pregnant, or are breastfeeding.

What is the usual dosage?

The information below is based on the dosage guidelines your doctor uses. Depending on your condition and medical history, your doctor may prescribe a different regimen. Do not change the dosage or stop taking your medication without your doctor's approval.

Adults: The recommended dose for most adults is 0.25 milligrams (mg). In some patients, a lower dose may be prescribed and the maximum daily dose should not exceed 0.5 mg.

How should I take Halcion?

Halcion should be taken right before you go to bed or after you have gone to bed and have had trouble falling asleep. Do not take Halcion with or right after a meal. Try to get a full night's sleep before you must be active again.

What should I avoid while taking Halcion?

You should never stop taking this medication without consulting your doctor first. Driving or operating dangerous machinery or participating in any hazardous activity is not recommended after taking Halcion until you are fully awake.

What are possible food and drug interactions associated with Halcion?

If Halcion is taken with certain other drugs, the effects of either could be increased, decreased, or altered. It is especially important to check with your doctor before combining this medication with any the following: flumazenil, grapefruit juice, itraconazole, isoniazid, ketoconazole, macrolide antibiotics, nefazodone, other sleep medications, oral contraceptives, and ranitidine.

What are the possible side effects of Halcion?

Side effects cannot be anticipated. If any develop or change in intensity, inform your doctor as soon as possible. Only your doctor can determine if it is safe for you to continue taking this drug.

Side effects may include: coordination difficulties, drowsiness, dizziness, headache, pins and needles sensations

Serious side effects may include: severe allergic reactions, getting out of bed while not being fully awake and performing an activity that you do not know you are doing, memory loss, anxiety, and abnormal thoughts or behavior. If you experience any of these serious side effects, contact your doctor immediately.

Can I receive Halcion if I am pregnant or breastfeeding?

There is a risk of potential fetal harm and an increased risk of congenital malformations; therefore, Halcion should not be used during pregnancy. Since the effects of Halcion during breastfeeding are unknown, its use should be avoided. If you are pregnant or planning to become pregnant, tell your doctor immediately.

What should I do if I miss a dose of Halcion?

If you missed a dose, skip it. Never take an extra dose to make up for a missed dose. Keep in mind that this medication is used just to help you sleep.

How should I store Halcion?

Store at room temperature and protect from light.

Halobetasol propionate *See Ultravate, page 1352.*

HALOPERIDOL

What is Haloperidol?

Haloperidol is an antipsychotic drug used to treat schizophrenia. It is also used to control tics and vocal utterances of Tourette's disorder in adults and children. Additionally, it is used to treat children with severe aggressive behavior or hyperactive children with aggression when other treatments are ineffective.

What is the most important information I should know about Haloperidol?

Haloperidol has caused death in elderly people taking it for psychological problems.

Patients with a condition known as severe toxic central nervous system depression or those who have Parkinson's disease should not take haloperidol. Since haloperidol may cause heart-related side effects, your doctor will monitor heart function while on this medication.

If you experience muscle stiffness, high body temperature, or irregular heartbeat, contact your doctor immediately as these may be signs of a serious side effect.

Caution should be used in patients with heart problems, receiving antiseizure medications, or receiving blood thinners, since haloperidol has the potential to interfere with the effect of these drugs.

Patients receiving haloperidol and lithium should be monitored closely, since the combined use of these medications may affect the brain.

Who should not take Haloperidol?

You should not take haloperidol if you have psychological problems, as determined by your doctor.

Patients with Parkinson's disease or a condition known as severe toxic central nervous system depression should not take haloperidol.

Haloperidol should not be given to anyone in a comatose state.

What should I tell my doctor before I take the first dose of Haloperidol?

Tell your doctor about all prescription, over-the-counter, and herbal medications you are taking before beginning treatment with haloperidol. Also, talk to your doctor about your complete medical history, especially if you have heart problems, are receiving antiseizure medications, blood thinners, or any other agent that affects the brain.

What is the usual dosage?

The information below is based on the dosage guidelines your doctor uses. Depending on your condition and medical history, your doctor may prescribe a different regimen. Do not change the dosage or stop taking your medication without your doctor's approval.

Adults: Usual dosages for adults with moderate symptoms are from 0.5 milligrams (mg) to 2 mg twice daily or three times daily. For severe symptoms, the usual dosage is 3-5 mg twice or three times daily.

Children 3 to 12 years: Haloperidol is given according to the child's weight and may start at 0.5 mg daily. Depending on the response, the dosage may be increased by the doctor. Doses may be given twice or three times daily.

How should I take Haloperidol?

Take this medication exactly as directed by your physician.

What should I avoid while taking Haloperidol?

Avoid alcohol use, as well as other agents that affect the brain, since they may cause more sedative effects.

Haloperidol may impair the mental and/or physical abilities required for the performance of hazardous tasks such as operating machinery or driving a motor vehicle. Use caution when performing such tasks.

What are possible food and drug interactions associated with Haloperidol?

If haloperidol is used with certain other drugs, the effects of either could be increased, decreased, or altered. It is especially important to check with your doctor before combining haloperidol with the following: alcohol, antiseizure drugs, blood thinners, and heart medications.

What are the possible side effects of Haloperidol?

Side effects cannot be anticipated. If any develop or change in intensity, tell your doctor as soon as possible. Only your doctor can determine if it is safe for you to continue taking this drug.

Side effects may include: fast heartbeat, Parkinson's-like symptoms, neck spasms/involuntary muscle spasms, insomnia, restlessness, agitation, headache, confusion

Can I receive Haloperidol if I am pregnant or breastfeeding?

The effects of haloperidol during pregnancy and breastfeeding are unknown. Tell your doctor immediately if you are pregnant, plan to become pregnant, or are breastfeeding.

What should I do if I miss a dose of Haloperidol?

Skip the dose and continue with your normal dosing schedule.

How should I store Haloperidol?

Store at room temperature.

HELIDAC THERAPY

*Generic name: Bismuth subsalicylate, metronidazole,
  and tetracycline hydrochloride*

What is Helidac Therapy?

Helidac is used to treat *Helicobacter pylori,* a bacterium that can cause stomach ulcers.

What is the most important information I should know about Helidac Therapy?

Follow the medication regimen exactly as directed in order to cure the infection.

Who should not take Helidac Therapy?

Helidac should not be used in children, if you are pregnant or nursing, if you have kidney or liver disease, or if you are sensitive to any component of the drug. Do not take Helidac if you are allergic to aspirin.

What should I tell my doctor before I take the first dose of Helidac Therapy?

Tell your doctor about all prescription, over-the-counter, and herbal medications you are taking before beginning treatment with Helidac. Also, talk to your doctor about your complete medical history, especially if you have any blood disorders, suffer from seizures or epilepsy, or have kidney or liver disease.

What is the usual dosage?

The information below is based on the dosage guidelines your doctor uses. Depending on your condition and medical history, your doctor may prescribe a different regimen. Do not change the dosage or stop taking your medication without your doctor's approval.

Adults: The recommended dosage (taken 4 times daily for 14 days at mealtimes and at bedtime) is bismuth subsalicylate: 525 milligrams (mg) in two 262.4-mg chewable tablets; metronidazole: 250-mg in one 250 mg tablet; and tetracycline hydrochloride: 500 mg in one 500-mg capsule.

Your doctor may also prescribe an H2 antagonist (a class of drug used to treat ulcers) to take along with your Helidac therapy.

How should I take Helidac Therapy?

There are 4 pills in each dose of Helidac. The 2 pink tablets (bismuth subsalicylate) should be chewed and swallowed. The white tablet (metronidazole) and the orange and white capsule (tetracycline) should be swallowed whole. Be sure to drink at least 8 ounces of fluid with each dose to prevent stomach upset, especially at bedtime.

What should I avoid while taking Helidac Therapy?

Do not drink alcohol during therapy and for at least 1 day after completing treatment.

Avoid prolonged exposure to sunlight or artificial sunlight. Helidac increases sensitivity to sunlight and severe burning may result. Wear sunscreen or protective clothing when you are outside.

Avoid taking antacids, dairy products, iron supplements, laxatives, or multivitamins within 2 hours of taking Helidac.

What are possible food and drug interactions associated with Helidac Therapy?

If Helidac is taken with certain other drugs, the effects of either could be increased, decreased, or altered. it is especially important to check with your doctor before combining Helidac with the following: antacids containing aluminum, calcium, or magnesium, aspirin, blood thinners such as warfarin, cimetidine, diabetes medications such as glyburide or insulin, iron, lithium, methoxyflurane, penicillin, phenobarbital, phenytoin, probenecid, sodium bicarbonate, sulfinpyrazone, zinc

Helidac can interfere with birth control. Use an additional form of birth control, such as condoms, during Helidac Therapy.

For 1 hour before and 2 hours after each dose of Helidac, avoid eating dairy products. They can interfere with Helidac therapy's absorption.

Do not start Helidac therapy if you have taken the anti-alcohol drug disulfiram within the past 2 weeks.

What are the possible side effects of Helidac Therapy?
Side effects cannot be anticipated. If any develop or change in intensity, tell your doctor as soon as possible. Only your doctor can determine if it is safe for you to continue taking this drug.

Side effects may include: abdominal pain, darkening of the stool, discoloration of the tongue, diarrhea, nausea, vomiting

Can I receive Helidac Therapy if I am pregnant or breastfeeding?
Helidac therapy should not be used if you are pregnant or breastfeeding. Talk to your doctor if you are pregnant, plan to become pregnant, or are breastfeeding. If pregnancy is detected, immediately stop taking Helidac.

What should I do if I miss a dose of Helidac Therapy?
Take the next dose at the appointed time and continue with your regular schedule until Helidac therapy is completed. Do not take 2 doses at once. If you miss more than 4 doses, contact your doctor.

How should I store Helidac Therapy?
Store at room temperature.

HEPAGAM B
Generic name: Hepatitis B immune globulin

What is HepaGam B?
HepaGam B is used to treat patients who have had a brief encounter (ingestion or sexual contact) with blood contaminated by the hepatitis B virus. The injection can also be used for babies born to HBV-infected mothers.

What is the most important information I should know about HepaGam B?
HepaGam B is made from human plasma and therefore may contain viruses or other pathogens. The plasma is screened and cleaned of viruses

such as HIV, HBV, and hepatitis C virus (HCV), but may contain infections such as Creutzfeldt-Jacob ("mad cow") disease.

HepaGam B contains a type of sugar (maltose) that may interfere with antidiabetes treatments.

Who should not take HepaGam B?
Do not take HepaGam B if you are allergic to any of its ingredients.

What should I tell my doctor before I take the first dose of HepaGam B?
Tell your doctor about all prescription, over-the-counter, and herbal medications you are taking before beginning treatment with HepaGam B. Also, talk to your doctor about your complete medical history, especially if you are diabetic, pregnant, or are breastfeeding.

What is the usual dosage?
The information below is based on the dosage guidelines your doctor uses. Depending on your condition and medical history, your doctor may prescribe a different regimen. Do not change the dosage or stop taking your medication without your doctor's approval.

Adults: The usual dosage for exposure to HBV blood/plasma is an injection of 0.06 milliliters (mL)/kilogram (kg) of body weight as soon as possible after exposure (within 24 hours if possible).

Infants: The usual dosage for a baby born to an infected mother is 0.5 mL after the baby is stable, but within 12 hours of birth.

How should I take HepaGam B?
HepaGam B should be injected by your nurse or doctor in the upper leg (thigh), upper arm, or buttocks. If it is injected in the buttocks, it should only be given in the upper or outer regions, not in the center.

What should I avoid while taking HepaGam B?
Avoid receiving any other types of vaccinations within 3 months of treatment with HepaGam B.

What are possible food and drug interactions associated with HepaGam B?
If HepaGam B is taken with certain other drugs, the effects of either could be increased, decreased, or altered. It is especially important to check with your doctor before combining HepaGam B with any other vaccination. All other vaccinations should be avoided for at least 3 months; you may have to be revaccinated with HepaGam B after receiving a different type of live vaccination.

What are the possible side effects of HepaGam B?
Side effects cannot be anticipated. If any develop or change in intensity, tell your doctor as soon as possible. Only your doctor can determine if it is safe for you to continue taking this drug.

Side effects may include: injection-site pain, aching joints, muscle pain, allergic reaction, chills, cold/flu symptoms, fainting, fever, headache, lightheadedness, nausea, vomiting

Can I receive HepaGam B if I am pregnant or breastfeeding?
The effects of HepaGam B during pregnancy and breastfeeding are unknown. Talk with your doctor before taking this drug if you are pregnant, plan to become pregnant, or are breastfeeding.

What should I do if I miss a dose of HepaGam B?
HepaGam B is only administered under very specific circumstances in a hospital or office setting.

How should I store HepaGam B?
HepaGam B is only administered under very specific circumstances in a hospital or office setting.

Hepatitis B immune globulin See *HepaGam B, page 640.*

Human papillomavirus vaccine See *Gardasil, page 609.*

Hydralazine hydrochloride and *isosorbide dinitrate*
  See *BiDil, page 221.*

Hydrochlorothiazide and *triamterene* See *Dyazide, page 456.*

HYDROCHLOROTHIAZIDE

What is Hydrochlorothiazide?
Hydrochlorothiazide is a diuretic used to treat high blood pressure and other conditions that require the elimination of excess fluid from the body. These conditions include congestive heart failure, cirrhosis of the liver, corticosteroid and estrogen therapy, and kidney disorders. When used for high blood pressure, hydrochlorothiazide can be used alone or with other high blood pressure medications.

What is the most important information I should know about Hydrochlorothiazide?
If you have high blood pressure, you must take hydrochlorothiazide regularly for it to be effective. Since blood pressure declines gradually, it may

be several weeks before you get the full benefit of hydrochlorothiazide. You must continue taking it even if you are feeling well. Hydrochlorothiazide does not cure high blood pressure; it only keeps it under control.

Who should not take Hydrochlorothiazide?
Do not take hydrochlorothiazide if you are unable to urinate or if you are sensitive to or have ever had an allergic reaction to this drug or similar drugs. If you are sensitive to sulfa or other sulfonamide-derived drugs, you should not take this drug.

What should I tell my doctor before I take the first dose of Hydrochlorothiazide?
Tell your doctor about all prescription, over-the-counter, and herbal medications you are taking before beginning treatment with hydrochlorothiazide. Also, talk to your doctor about your complete medical history, especially if you have a history of allergy or asthma, diabetes, gout, kidney or liver disease, or if you have systemic lupus erythematosus (a form of rheumatism).

What is the usual dosage?
The information below is based on the dosage guidelines your doctor uses. Depending on your condition and medical history, your doctor may prescribe a different regimen. Do not change the dosage or stop taking your medication without your doctor's approval.

High Blood Pressure
Adults: The usual starting dose is 25 milligrams (mg) daily. The dose may be increased to 50 mg daily, given as a single dose or 2 divided doses. Dosages should be adjusted when this medication is used with other high blood pressure drugs.

Water Retention
Adults: The usual dosage is 25 to 100 mg daily as a single or divided dose. Your doctor may put you on a day on/day off schedule or some other alternate day schedule to suit your needs.

Children: The usual dosage is 0.5 to 1 mg per pound per day in a single dose or 2 divided doses. Do not exceed 37.5 mg per day in infants up to 2 years of age or 100 mg per day in children 2-12 years of age.

Infants less than 6 months of age may require doses up to 1.5 mg per pound per day in 2 divided doses.

How should I take Hydrochlorothiazide?
Take hydrochlorothiazide exactly as prescribed by your doctor.

To reduce nighttime urination, take hydrochlorothiazide early in the day unless otherwise directed by your doctor.

What should I avoid while taking Hydrochlorothiazide?

Do not stop taking hydrochlorothiazide suddenly even if you feel better.

Use caution when driving, operating machinery, or performing other hazardous activities as hydrochlorothiazide may cause dizziness.

Avoid using alcohol because it may increase the side effects of hydrochlorothiazide.

Avoid a diet high in salt. Too much salt may cause the body to retain water and may decrease the effects of hydrochlorothiazide.

Dehydration, excessive sweating, severe diarrhea or vomiting could deplete your body's fluids and may cause low blood pressure. Avoid becoming overheated in hot weather and during exercise.

What are possible food and drug interactions associated with Hydrochlorothiazide?

If hydrochlorothiazide is taken with certain other drugs, the effects of either could be increased, decreased, or altered. It is especially important to check with your doctor before combining hydrochlorothiazide with the following: alcohol, barbiturates such as phenobarbital, blood pressure drugs such as methyldopa, cholestyramine, colestipol, corticosteroids such as prednisone, diabetes drugs such as glyburide or insulin, digoxin, lithium, narcotics such as morphine or methadone, NSAIDs such as ibuprofen or naproxen, norepinephrine, skeletal muscle relaxants such as tubocurarine

What are the possible side effects of Hydrochlorothiazide?

Side effects cannot be anticipated. If any develop or change in intensity, tell your doctor as soon as possible. Only your doctor can determine if it is safe for you to continue taking this drug.

Side effects may include: abdominal cramping, diarrhea, dizziness upon standing up, headache, loss of appetite, low blood pressure, low potassium (leading to symptoms such as dry mouth, excessive thirst, weak or irregular heartbeat, muscle pain or cramps), stomach irritation, stomach upset, weakness

Can I receive Hydrochlorothiazide if I am pregnant or breastfeeding?

The effects of hydrochlorothiazide during pregnancy and breastfeeding are unknown. Tell your doctor immediately if you are pregnant, plan to become pregnant, or are breastfeeding. Do not breastfeed while taking hydrochlorothiazide.

What should I do if I miss a dose of Hydrochlorothiazide?

If you forget a dose, take it as soon as you remember. If it is almost time for your next dose, skip the missed dose and go back to your regular schedule. Do not take 2 doses at the same time.

How should I store Hydrochlorothiazide?
Keep container tightly closed. Protect from light, moisture, and freezing cold. Store at room temperature.

Hydrocodone bitartrate and acetaminophen See Vicodin, page 1388.

Hydrocodone bitartrate and ibuprofen See Vicoprofen, page 1390.

Hydrocodone polistirex, chlorpheniramine polistirex See Tussionex, page 1341.

Hydrocortisone acetate and iodoquinol See Alcortin A gel, page 56.

HYDROCORTISONE SKIN PREPARATIONS

What is Hydrocortisone skin preparations?
Hydrocortisone creams, lotions, and ointments are used to relieve a variety of inflammatory skin conditions and itchy rashes.

What is the most important information I should know about Hydrocortisone skin preparations?
When you apply a hydrocortisone cream, lotion, or ointment, some of the drug will be absorbed through your skin and into the bloodstream. Avoid using large amounts of hydrocortisone over large areas of your body. Do not cover areas of your body on which you have applied hydrocortisone with airtight dressings such as plastic wrap or adhesive bandages, unless directed to do so by your doctor. Doing so may lead to unwanted side effects.

Who should not take Hydrocortisone skin preparations?
Do not use hydrocortisone if you sensitive to any component of the drug.

What should I tell my doctor before I take the first dose of Hydrocortisone skin preparations?
Tell your doctor about all prescription, over-the-counter, and herbal medications you are taking before beginning treatment with hydrocortisone. Also, talk to your doctor about your complete medical history, especially if you have a bacterial, fungal, or viral infection.

What is the usual dosage?
The information below is based on the dosage guidelines your doctor uses. Depending on your condition and medical history, your doctor

may prescribe a different regimen. Do not change the dosage or stop taking your medication without your doctor's approval.

Adults: Apply hydrocortisone cream or lotion to the affected area 2 to 4 times a day, depending on the severity of the condition.

Children: Limit use to the least amount necessary, as directed by your doctor.

How should I take Hydrocortisone skin preparations?

Use hydrocortisone exactly as directed, and only to treat the condition for which your doctor prescribed it.

Apply hydrocortisone skin preparations directly to the affected area.

If you are using hydrocortisone for psoriasis or a condition that has been difficult to cure, your doctor may advise you to use a bandage or covering over the affected area. If an infection develops, remove the bandage and contact your doctor.

What should I avoid while taking Hydrocortisone skin preparations?

Hydrocortisone skin preparations are for external use only. Avoid contact with the eyes.

Do not use plastic bandages, dressings, or diapers that do not allow air to circulate to the area unless your doctor tells you to do so.

Avoid using other topical medications, harsh or abrasive soaps, or cosmetics on the affected area without first talking to your doctor.

What are possible food and drug interactions associated with Hydrocortisone skin preparations?

If hydrocortisone skin preparations are used with certain other drugs, the effects of either could be increased, decreased, or altered. It is especially important to check with your doctor before combining them with other drugs.

What are the possible side effects of Hydrocortisone skin preparations?

Side effects cannot be anticipated. If any develop or change in intensity, tell your doctor as soon as possible. Only your doctor can determine if it is safe for you to continue taking this drug.

Side effects may include: acne-like skin eruptions; burning; dryness; growth of excessive hair; inflammation around the mouth, hair follicles, and skin; irritation; itching, peeling skin; prickly heat; secondary infection; skin softening; stretch marks; unusual lack of skin color

Can I receive Hydrocortisone skin preparations if I am pregnant or breastfeeding?
The effects of hydrocortisone during pregnancy and breastfeeding are unknown. Tell your doctor immediately if you are pregnant, plan to become pregnant, or are breastfeeding. Use hydrocortisone sparingly, and only with your doctor's permission, when breastfeeding.

What should I do if I miss a dose of Hydrocortisone skin preparations?
Apply it as soon as you remember. If it is almost time for the next dose, skip the missed dose and go back to your regular schedule.

How should I store Hydrocortisone skin preparations?
Keep the container tightly closed, and store it at room temperature, away from heat. Protect from freezing.

Hydroxychloroquine sulfate See *Plaquenil, page 1030.*

Hydroxyzine pamoate See *Vistaril, page 1400.*

Hyoscyamine sulfate See *Levsin, page 730.*

HYTRIN
Generic name: Terazosin hydrochloride

What is Hytrin?
Hytrin is used alone or in combination with other drugs to treat high blood pressure. Hytrin is also used to relieve the symptoms of benign prostatic hyperplasia or BPH (an enlargement of the prostate gland surrounding the urinary canal).

What is the most important information I should know about Hytrin?
If you have high blood pressure, you must take Hytrin regularly for it to be effective. Since blood pressure declines gradually, it may be several weeks before you get the full benefit of Hytrin. You must continue taking it even if you are feeling well. Hytrin does not cure high blood pressure; it only keeps it under control.

Who should not take Hytrin?
Do not take Hytrin if you are sensitive to it or have ever had an allergic reaction to it.

What should I tell my doctor before I take the first dose of Hytrin?
Tell your doctor about all prescription, over-the-counter, and herbal medications you are taking before beginning treatment with Hytrin. Also, talk to your doctor about your complete medical history, especially if you have kidney or liver disease.

What is the usual dosage?
The information below is based on the dosage guidelines your doctor uses. Depending on your condition and medical history, your doctor may prescribe a different regimen. Do not change the dosage or stop taking your medication without your doctor's approval.

Benign Prostatic Hyperplasia
Adults: The usual starting dose is 1 milligram (mg) taken at bedtime. Your doctor will gradually increase the dose to 10 mg, taken once a day for at least 4 to 6 weeks.

If you stop taking Hytrin for several days or longer, your doctor will restart your treatment with 1 mg at bedtime.

High Blood Pressure
Adults: The usual starting dose is 1 mg at bedtime. Your doctor may slowly increase the dose until your blood pressure has been lowered sufficiently. The usual recommended dosage range is 1-5 mg taken once or twice a day. Some people may require doses as high as 20-40mg per day.

How should I take Hytrin?
Take Hytrin with or without food. Take your first dose at bedtime.

What should I avoid while taking Hytrin?
Hytrin can cause fainting or low blood pressure, especially at the start of therapy. Avoid driving and performing hazardous tasks for 12 hours after the first dose, after a dosage increase, or if your therapy is interrupted then resumed.

Avoid becoming overheated in hot weather and during exercise. Low blood pressure, dizziness, and fainting could result.

What are possible food and drug interactions associated with Hytrin?
If Hytrin is taken with certain other drugs, the effects of either could be increased, decreased, or altered. It is especially important to check with your doctor before combining Hytrin with: nonsteroidal anti-inflammatory painkillers such as ibuprofen and naproxen, and other blood pressure medications such as enalapril, hydrochlorothiazide, or verapamil.

What are the possible side effects of Hytrin?

Side effects cannot be anticipated. If any develop or change in intensity, tell your doctor as soon as possible. Only your doctor can determine if it is safe for you to continue taking this drug.

Side effects may include: difficult or labored breathing, dizziness, headache, heart palpitations, light-headedness upon standing, nausea, pain in the arms and legs, sleepiness, stuffy nose, weakness

Hytrin has been associated with rare cases of priapism (painful penile erection lasting for hours). Seek medical attention right away because priapism can lead to permanent impotence if it is not treated.

Can I receive Hytrin if I am pregnant or breastfeeding?

The effects of Hytrin during pregnancy and breastfeeding are unknown. Tell your doctor immediately if you are pregnant, plan to become pregnant, or are breastfeeding. Do not breastfeed while you are taking Hytrin.

What should I do if I miss a dose of Hytrin?

Take it as soon as you remember. If it is almost time for the next dose, skip the missed dose and go back to your regular schedule. Do not take 2 doses at the same time.

How should I store Hytrin?

Store at room temperature in a cool, dry place. Protect from light.

HYZAAR

Generic name: Losartan potassium and hydrochlorothiazide

What is Hyzaar?

Hyzaar is a combination drug used to treat high blood pressure. It consists of losartan, which belongs to the class of angiotensin II receptor blockers, and hydrochlorothiozide, which is a diuretic. Hyzaar is also used to reduce the risk of stroke in patients with high blood pressure and left ventricular hypertrophy (thickening of the heart muscle).

What is the most important information I should know about Hyzaar?

Do not use Hyzaar during the second or third trimesters of pregnancy. This drug can cause injury and even death to the developing fetus. Tell your doctor immediately if you think you might be pregnant.

You must take Hyzaar regularly for it to be effective. Since blood pressure declines gradually, it may take several weeks for you to get the full benefit of Hyzaar. You must continue taking it even if you are feeling well. Hyzaar does not cure blood pressure. It only keeps it under control.

Who should not take Hyzaar?
Do not take Hyzaar if you are sensitive to any component of this drug, if you are sensitive to sulfa drugs, or if you are unable to urinate.

What should I tell my doctor before I take the first dose of Hyzaar?
Tell your doctor about all prescription, over-the-counter, and herbal medications you are taking before beginning treatment with Hyzaar. Also, talk to your doctor about your complete medical history, especially if you have kidney or liver disease, gout, diabetes, high cholesterol, a history of allergy or asthma, or systemic lupus erythematosus.

What is the usual dosage?
The information below is based on the dosage guidelines your doctor uses. Depending on your condition and medical history, your doctor may prescribe a different regimen. Do not change the dosage or stop taking your medication without your doctor's approval.

High Blood Pressure
Adults: Hyzaar comes in 3 strengths: 50/12.5 mg (50 milligrams of losartan and 12.5 mg of hydrochlorothiazide), 100/12.5mg, and 100/25mg. The usual starting dose is one 50/12.5mg tablet per day.

   If your blood pressure does not respond to this dose after about 3 weeks, the doctor may increase the dose to two 50/12.5 mg tablets taken once daily or one 100/25mg tablet taken once daily.

High Blood Pressure with Left Ventricular Hypertrophy
The usual starting dose is one 50/12.5 mg tablet taken once daily. The dose may be increased to one 100/12.5mg or 100/25mg tablet taken once daily.

How should I take Hyzaar?
Take Hyzaar exactly as prescribed. It can be taken with or without food. Try to take it at the same time each day so that it is easier to remember.

What should I avoid while taking Hyzaar?
Hyzaar may cause dizziness or drowsiness. Use caution when driving, operating machinery, or performing other hazardous activities. Use alcohol cautiously. Alcohol may increase drowsiness and dizziness while you are taking Hyzaar.

   Use caution when rising from a sitting or lying position. Hyzaar may cause low blood pressure and you may feel lightheaded or faint. Excessive sweating, severe diarrhea, or vomiting can deplete your body fluids and cause your blood pressure to drop too low. Be careful when exercising and in hot weather.

   Avoid a diet high in salt. Too much salt may cause your body to retain water and may decrease the effects of hydrochlorothiazide. Avoid using salt substitutes without first talking to your doctor.

Avoid spending too much time in natural or artificial sunlight. Hyzaar may make your skin more sensitive to sunlight. Wear sunscreen and protective clothing.

What are possible food and drug interactions associated with Hyzaar?

If Hyzaar is taken with certain other drugs, the effects of either could be increased, decreased, or altered. It is especially important to check with your doctor before combining Hyzaar with the following: barbiturates, blood pressure drugs such as atenolol or nifedipine, cholestyramine, colestipol, corticosteroids such as prednisone, diabetes drugs such as insulin or glyburide, diuretics that increase the level of potassium in your body (eg, spironolactone, triamterene and amiloride), fluconazole, lithium, narcotics such as morphine or methadone, NSAIDs such as ibuprofen or naproxen, norepinephrine, potassium supplements, rifampin, salt substitutes containing potassium, skeletal muscle relaxants such as tubocurarine

What are the possible side effects of Hyzaar?

Side effects cannot be anticipated. If any develop or change in intensity, tell your doctor as soon as possible. Only your doctor can determine if it is safe for you to continue taking this drug.

Side effects may include: dizziness, upper respiratory tract infection

Can I receive Hyzaar if I am pregnant or breastfeeding?

When used in the second or third trimester of pregnancy, Hyzaar can cause injury or even death to the unborn child. Stop taking Hyzaar as soon as you know you are pregnant. If you are pregnant or plan to become pregnant, tell your doctor immediately. Do not breastfeed while taking Hyzaar.

What should I do if I miss a dose of Hyzaar?

Take the missed dose as soon as you remember. If it is almost time for your next dose, skip the missed dose and go back to your regular schedule. Do not take 2 doses at once.

How should I store Hyzaar?

Keep in a tightly closed container at room temperature. Protect from light.

Ibandronate sodium See Boniva, page 223.

Ibuprofen See Motrin, page 850.

Ibuprofen lysine See NeoProfen, page 870.

Imatinib mesylate See Gleevec, page 614.

Imipramine See Tofranil/Tofranil-PM, page 1312.

IMITREX
Generic name: Sumatriptan succinate

What is Imitrex?
Imitrex is used to treat migraine headaches. It does not prevent or reduce the number of migraines you have. Imitrex should only be used to ease the pain of the actual migraine attack.

Imitrex is available as tablets, injection and nasal spray.

What is the most important information I should know about Imitrex?
Imitrex should not be used in people who have heart problems such as coronary artery disease (CAD). Also, this drug should not be taken by those who have symptoms or risk factors for CAD but are as yet undiagnosed (eg, high blood pressure, high cholesterol, smoker, overweight or obese, diabetes, family history of CAD, menopause, men over 40 years).

Imitrex may increase your blood pressure and should therefore not be taken by people who have uncontrolled blood pressure.

Who should not take Imitrex?
Do not begin treatment with Imitrex if you are allergic to any of its ingredients. Also, do not take this drug if you have liver problems, high blood pressure, heart problems, or you are taking any other medications with ergotamine or within 2 weeks of taking an MAOI.

What should I tell my doctor before I take the first dose of Imitrex?
Tell your doctor about all prescription, over-the-counter, and herbal medications you are taking before beginning treatment with Imitrex. Also, talk to your doctor about your complete medical history, especially if you have heart problems, high blood pressure, liver or kidney problems, seizures (epilepsy), or you are taking other medications for migraines.

What is the usual dosage?
The information below is based on the dosage guidelines your doctor uses. Depending on your condition and medical history, your doctor may prescribe a different regimen. Do not change the dosage or stop taking your medication without your doctor's approval.

Tablets
Adults: The usual dosage of Imitrex tablets is 25 milligrams (mg), 50 mg, or 100 mg taken at the first sign of a migraine. If the pain is not relieved,

another dose may be taken 2 hours after the first; the maximum daily dosage of Imitrex is 200 mg.

Nasal Spray
Adults: Imitrex nasal spray is available as 5 mg or 20 mg. A 10-mg dose may be achieved by the administration of a single 5-mg dose in each nostril. The usual dose is a single nasal spray in 1 nostril. If your headache comes back, you can take a second nasal spray anytime after 2 hours after you took the first spray.

For any attack where you have no response to the first nasal spray, do not take a second nasal spray without first talking with your healthcare provider. Do not take more than a total of 40 mg of Imitrex nasal spray in any 24-hour period. The safety of treating an average of more than 4 headaches in a 30-day period has not been established.

Injection
Adults: The maximum single recommended adult dose of Imitrex injection is 6 mg given subcutaneously (under the skin). The maximum recommended dose that may be given in 24 hours is two 6-mg injections separated by at least 1 hour.

How should I take Imitrex?
Imitrex tablet should be swallowed whole with water or fluids at the first sign of a migraine attack.

Imitrex Injection should only be administered subcutaneously, under the skin.

What are possible food and drug interactions associated with Imitrex?
If Imitrex is taken with certain other drugs, the effects of either could be increased, decreased, or altered. It is especially important to check with your doctor before combining Imitrex with the following: ergotamine, monoamine oxidase (MAO) inhibitors, and selective serotonin reuptake inhibitors (SSRIs).

What are the possible side effects of Imitrex?
Side effects cannot be anticipated. If any develop or change in intensity, tell your doctor as soon as possible. Only your doctor can determine if it is safe for you to continue taking this drug.

Side effects may include: burning/tingling/prickly sensation on the skin, chest pain or tightness, cold/warm sensation, dizziness, dry mouth, nausea, neck/throat/jaw pain, sleepiness/tiredness, vomiting

Can I receive Imitrex if I am pregnant or breastfeeding?
The effects of Imitrex during pregnancy and breastfeeding are unknown. Tell your doctor immediately if you are pregnant, plan to become pregnant, or are breastfeeding.

What should I do if I miss a dose of Imitrex?
Take the missed dose as soon as you remember. If it is almost time for your next dose, skip the missed dose and go back to your regular schedule. Do not take 2 doses at once.

How should I store Imitrex?
Store at room temperature, away from light and heat. Keep the injection in the carrying case that comes with it.

Immune globulin intravenous (human) *See Privigen, page 1072.*

IMODIUM
Generic name: Loperamide hydrochloride

What is Imodium?
Imodium is used to treat diarrhea. Imodium is also available in several over-the-counter forms.

What is the most important information I should know about Imodium?
If you are taking Imodium for acute diarrhea, tell your doctor if you develop a fever, if you notice blood or mucus in your stools, if you develop abdominal swelling or bulging, or if your symptoms do not improve within 2 days. For chronic diarrhea, tell your doctor if there is no improvement after 10 days.

It is important to maintain adequate hydration during treatment.

Who should not take Imodium?
Do not take Imodium if you are sensitive to any component of the drug, if you have abdominal pain without diarrhea, or if you have blood in your stools and a fever higher than 101 degrees.

What should I tell my doctor before I take the first dose of Imodium?
Tell your doctor about all prescription, over-the-counter, and herbal medications you are taking before beginning treatment with Imodium. Also, talk to your doctor about your complete medical history, especially if you have a condition that could be complicated by constipation, inflammation or irritation of the intestines or colon, liver disease, blood or mucus in the stool, or if you have a fever of 101°F or higher.

What is the usual dosage?
The information below is based on the dosage guidelines your doctor uses. Depending on your condition and medical history, your doctor

may prescribe a different regimen. **Do not change the dosage or stop taking your medication without your doctor's approval.**

Adults and children 12 years and older: The usual dosage is 2 capsules after your first loose bowel movement and 1 capsule after each loose movement thereafter. Do not take more than 8 capsules in 24 hours.

Children 8-12 years who weigh more than 66 pounds: The usual dosage is 1 capsule taken 3 times a day after the first loose stool. Do not give more than 3 capsules in 24 hours.

Children 6-8 years who weigh 44-66 pounds: The usual dosage is 1 capsule taken 2 times a day after the first loose stool. Do not give more than 2 capsules in 24 hours.

Children 2-5 years who weigh 28-44 pounds: The nonprescription liquid formulation (Imodium A-D 1 milligram/5 milliliters) should be used.
Imodium is not recommended in children under 2 years of age.

How should I take Imodium?
Take Imodium exactly as directed. Take the capsules with 4 to 8 ounces of water.
Diarrhea can quickly lead to dehydration. Drink plenty of water or other clear liquids until your diarrhea stops.

What should I avoid while taking Imodium?
Imodium may cause tiredness, drowsiness, or dizziness. Be careful when driving or operating machinery.

What are possible food and drug interactions associated with Imodium?
If Imodium is taken with certain other drugs, the effects of either could be increased, decreased, or altered. It is especially important to check with your doctor before combining Imodium with quinidine, ritonavir, or saquinavir.

What are the possible side effects of Imodium?
Side effects cannot be anticipated. If any develop or change in intensity, tell your doctor as soon as possible. Only your doctor can determine if it is safe for you to continue taking this drug.

Side effects may include: abdominal pain, constipation, dry mouth, gas, nausea, vomiting, increased blood sugar, dizziness

Can I receive Imodium if I am pregnant or breastfeeding?
The effects of Imodium during pregnancy and breastfeeding are unknown. Tell your doctor immediately if you are pregnant, plan to become pregnant, or are breastfeeding. Small amounts of Imodium may appear in breast milk. Avoid using Imodium if you are breastfeeding.

What should I do if I miss a dose of Imodium?

If Imodium is taken on a regular schedule and a dose is missed, skip the missed dose and take only the next regularly scheduled dose. Do not take 2 doses at once.

How should I store Imodium?

Store at room temperature, away from moisture and heat.

Indinavir sulfate *See Crixivan, page 357.*

INDOCIN
Generic name: Indomethacin

What is Indocin?

Indocin is used to relieve the inflammation, swelling, stiffness, and joint pain associated with moderate or severe rheumatoid arthritis and osteoarthritis (the most common form of arthritis), and ankylosing spondylitis (arthritis of the spine). It is also used to treat bursitis (inflammation and pain around joints), tendinitis (acute painful shoulder), acute gouty arthritis, and other kinds of pain.

What is the most important information I should know about Indocin?

Indocin may increase the chance of a heart attack or stroke that can lead to death. This chance increases with longer use of Indocin or if you have heart disease. Symptoms include chest pain, shortness of breath, weakness, and slurred speech.

Indocin can cause ulcers and bleeding in the stomach and intestines at any time during treatment. Ulcers and bleeding can happen without warning symptoms and may cause death. Symptoms include abdominal pain or blood in the stool. The risk of getting an ulcer or bleeding increases the longer you use the medication; if you smoke or drink alcohol; are older, or in poor health; or if you take corticosteroids such as prednisone or blood thinners such as warfarin.

Who should not take Indocin?

Do not take Indocin if you are sensitive to any component of the drug. Also, do not take Indocin if you have asthma, hives, or allergic reactions after taking aspirin or other nonsteroidal anti-inflammatory drugs (NSAIDs), or right before or after a heart surgery called a coronary artery bypass graft.

Do not use Indocin suppositories if you have a history of rectal inflammation or recent rectal bleeding.

What should I tell my doctor before I take the first dose of Indocin?

Tell your doctor about all prescription, over-the-counter, and herbal medication you are taking before beginning treatment with Indocin. Also, talk to your doctor about your complete medical history, especially if you drink more than 3 alcoholic beverages a day or if you have: a bleeding disorder, an allergy to aspirin or any other NSAIDs, an ulcer or bleeding in the stomach, chronic heart failure, fluid retention, heart disease, high blood pressure, kidney or liver disease.

What is the usual dosage?

The information below is based on the dosage guidelines your doctor uses. Depending on your condition and medical history, your doctor may prescribe a different regimen. Do not change the dosage or stop taking your medication without your doctor's approval.

Adults: This medication is available in capsule, liquid, and suppository form. The following dosages are for the capsule form. If you prefer the liquid form ask your doctor to make the proper substitution. Do not try to convert Indocin or dosage yourself.

Acute Gouty Arthritis
The usual dose is 50 milligrams (mg) taken 3 times a day until pain is reduced to a tolerable level (usually 3-5 days). Your doctor will advise you when to stop taking Indocin for this condit

Bursitis or Tendinitis
The usual dose is 75-150 mg daily divided into 3-4 small doses for 1-2 weeks, until symptoms disappear.

Moderate to Severe Rheumatoid Arthritis, Osteoarthritis, Ankylosing Spondylitis
The usual dose is 25 mg taken 2-3 times a day, increasing to a total daily dose of 150-200 mg.

Your doctor may prescribe a single daily 75-mg capsule of Indocin SR in place of regular Indocin.

Children: Safety and effectiveness in children 14 years of age and younger have not been established.

How should I take Indocin?

Take Indocin exactly as prescribed by your doctor. You should take Indocin with food or an antacid, and with a full glass of water. Never take Indocin on an empty stomach.

If you are using Indocin for arthritis, it should be taken regularly. If you are taking the liquid form of this medicine, shake the bottle well before each use.

Indocin SR capsules should be swallowed whole, not crushed or broken.

Do not lie down for about 20-30 minutes after taking Indocin. This helps prevent irritation that could lead to trouble in swallowing.

If you are using the suppository form of this medicine:

If the suppository is too soft to insert, hold it under cool water or chill it before removing the wrapper.

Remove the foil wrapper and moisten your rectal area with cool tap water.

Lie down on your side and use your finger to push the suppository well up into the rectum. Hold your buttocks together for a few seconds.

Indocin suppositories should be kept inside the rectum for at least 1 hour so that your body can absorb all the medicine.

What should I avoid while taking Indocin?

Indocin may increase the sensitivity of the skin to sunlight. Avoid prolonged exposure to natural and artificial sunlight. Use a sunscreen and wear protective clothing when exposed to the sun.

Avoid alcohol or use it with moderation. If you drink more than 3 alcoholic beverages a day, Indocin may increase the risk of dangerous stomach bleeding.

Many over-the-counter cough, cold, allergy, and pain medications contain aspirin or other NSAIDs such as ibuprofen or naproxen. These medications may interact with Indocin.

What are possible food and drug interactions associated with Indocin?

If Indocin is taken with certain other drugs, the effects of either could be increased, decreased, or altered. It is especially important to check with your doctor before combining Indocin with the following: aspirin, blood pressure medications, including beta-blockers (atenolol, propranol), ACE inhibitors (enalapril, monopril), and angiotensin II receptor antagonists (losartan, valsartan), blood-thinners such as warfarin, captopril, cyclosporine, diflunisal, digoxin, lithium, loop diuretics such as furosemide, methotrexate, other NSAIDs such as ibuprofen or naproxen, potassium-sparing water pills such as spironolactone, probenecid, thiazide-type water pills such as hydrochlorothiazide, triamterene.

What are the possible side effects of Indocin?

Side effects cannot be anticipated. If any develop or change in intensity, tell your doctor as soon as possible. Only your doctor can determine if it is safe for you to continue taking this drug.

Side effects may include: Abdominal pain, constipation, depression, diarrhea, dizziness, fatigue, headache, heartburn, indigestion, nausea, ringing in the ears, sleepiness or excessive drowsiness, stomach pain, stomach upset, vertigo, vomiting

Can I receive Indocin if I am pregnant or breastfeeding?

The effects of Indocin during pregnancy and breastfeeding are unknown. Tell your doctor immediately if you are pregnant, plan to become pregnant, or are breastfeeding.

If taken late in pregnancy, Indocin may cause prenatal heart problems. It may also slow contractions and lead to a delayed delivery.

Do not breastfeed while you are taking Indocin.

What should I do if I miss a dose of Indocin?

Take the forgotten dose as soon as you remember. If it is time for your next dose, skip the missed dose and return to your regular schedule. Never take 2 doses at once.

How should I store Indocin?

The liquid and suppository forms of Indocin may be stored at room temperature. Keep both forms from extreme heat, and protect the liquid from freezing.

Indomethacin *See Indocin, page 656.*

Influenza virus vaccine *See Afluria, page 51; FluLaval, page 571; or Fluzone, page 578.*

INSPRA

Generic name: Eplerenone

What is Inspra?

Inspra is used to treat people who develop congestive heart failure after a heart attack. Inspra is also used to treat high blood pressure, whether taken alone or with other medicines.

What is the most important information I should know about Inspra?

Inspra may increase potassium in the blood (hyperkalemia), which may lead to serious and life-threatening heart problems such as an irregular heartbeat (arrhythmia).

Who should not take Inspra?

Do not take Inspra if you are allergic to any of its ingredients, have kidney problems, high blood potassium levels, diabetes, or if you are taking certain kinds of medicines for fungal infections, depression, or HIV/AIDS.

What should I tell my doctor before I take the first dose of Inspra?

Tell your doctor about all prescription, over-the-counter, and herbal medications you are taking before beginning treatment with Inspra. Also, talk to your doctor about your complete medical history, especially if you have kidney problems or if you are pregnant, plan to become pregnant, or are breastfeeding.

What is the usual dosage?

The information below is based on the dosage guidelines your doctor uses. Depending on your condition and medical history, your doctor may prescribe a different regimen. Do not change the dosage or stop taking your medication without your doctor's approval.

Adults: The usual starting dosage of Inspra is 25 mg daily. Over 4 weeks, the dosage should be increased to a maximum of 50 mg daily.

How should I take Inspra?

Take Inspra at the same time everyday, with or without food.

What should I avoid while taking Inspra?

Avoid taking potassium pills or diuretics (water pills).

What are possible food and drug interactions associated with Inspra?

If Inspra is taken with certain other drugs, the effects of either could be increased, decreased, or altered. It is especially important to check with your doctor before combining Inspra with the following: clarithromycin, itraconazole, ketoconazole, nefazodone, nelfinavir, ritonavir, and troleandomycin.

What are the possible side effects of Inspra?

Side effects cannot be anticipated. If any develop or change in intensity, tell your doctor as soon as possible. Only your doctor can determine if it is safe for you to continue taking this drug.

Side effects may include: cough, diarrhea, dizziness, flulike symptoms, drowsiness

Can I receive Inspra if I am pregnant or breastfeeding?

The effects of Inspra during pregnancy and breastfeeding are unknown. Tell your doctor immediately if you are pregnant, plan to become pregnant, or are breastfeeding.

What should I do if I miss a dose of Inspra?

If you miss a dose, take it as soon as you remember. If it is close to your next dose, skip it and continue on your normal medication schedule. Do not take 2 doses at once.

How should I store Inspra?
Store at room temperature.

Insulin See Novolin, page 919.

INSULIN

What is Insulin?
Insulin is prescribed for diabetes when diet modifications and oral medications fail to correct the condition. Insulin is a hormone produced by the pancreas, a large gland that lies near the stomach. This hormone is necessary for the body's correct use of food, especially sugar. Insulin apparently works by helping sugar penetrate the cell wall, where it is then utilized by the cell. In people with diabetes, the body either does not make enough insulin, or the insulin that is produced cannot be used properly.

What is the most important information I should know about Insulin?
Regardless of the type of insulin you use, you should follow carefully the dietary and exercise guidelines prescribed by your doctor. Failure to follow these guidelines or to take your insulin as prescribed may result in serious and potentially life-threatening complications such as hypoglycemia (lowered blood sugar levels).

If you are ill, you should check your urine for ketones (acetone), and notify your doctor if the test is positive. This condition can be life-threatening.

Wear personal identification that states clearly that you are diabetic. Carry a sugar-containing product such as hard candy to offset any symptoms of low blood sugar.

Do not change the type of insulin or even the model and brand of syringe or needle you use without your physician's instruction. Failure to use the proper syringe may lead to improper dosage levels of insulin.

If you become ill from any cause, especially with nausea and vomiting or fever, your insulin requirements may change. It is important to eat as normally as possible. If you have trouble eating, drink fruit juices, soda, or clear soups, or eat small amounts of bland foods. Test your urine and/or blood sugar and tell your doctor at once. If you have severe and prolonged vomiting, seek emergency medical care.

If you are taking insulin, you should check your glucose levels with home blood and urine testing devices. If your blood tests consistently show above-normal sugar levels or your urine tests consistently show the presence of sugar, your diabetes is not properly controlled, and you should tell your doctor.

Who should not take Insulin?
Insulin should be used only to correct diabetic conditions.

What should I tell my doctor before
I take the first dose of Insulin?
Tell your doctor about all prescription, over-the-counter, and herbal medications you are taking before beginning treatment with this drug. Also, talk to your doctor about your complete medical history, especially about recent episodes of nausea, vomiting, or any other illness.

What is the usual dosage?
The information below is based on the dosage guidelines your doctor uses. Depending on your condition and medical history, your doctor may prescribe a different regimen. Do not change the dosage or stop taking your medication without your doctor's approval.

Your doctor will specify which insulin to use, how much, when, and how often to inject it. Your dosage may be affected by changes in food, activity, illness, medication, pregnancy, exercise, travel, or your work schedule. Proper control of your diabetes requires close and constant cooperation with your doctor. Failure to use your insulin as prescribed may result in serious and potentially fatal complications.

How should I take Insulin?
Take your insulin exactly as prescribed, being careful to follow your doctor's dietary and exercise recommendations. Before taking your injection, carefully read and follow the manufacturer's instructions on how to prepare your pre-filled pen or syringe. Clean the injection area with alcohol first; typical areas of injection are the abdomen, thighs, and arms. Insert the needle and push the plunger as far as it will go. Do not rub the injection area. To avoid skin damage, the next injection should be made at least half an inch from the previous site.

Some insulins should be clear, and some have a cloudy precipitate. Find out what your insulin should look like and check it carefully before using.

What should I avoid while taking Insulin?
To avoid infection or contamination, use disposable needles and syringes or sterilize your reusable syringe and needle carefully. Always keep handy an extra supply of insulin as well as a spare syringe and needle.

Use alcohol carefully, since excessive alcohol consumption can cause low blood sugar. Don't drink unless your doctor has approved it.

What are possible food and drug interactions
associated with Insulin?
Follow your physician's dietary guidelines as closely as you can and inform your physician of any medication, either prescription or non-pre-

scription, that you are taking. Specific medications, depending on the amount present, that affect insulin levels or its effectiveness include: alcohol, ACE inhibitors such as the blood pressure medications benazepril and quinapril, anabolic steroids, appetite suppressants such as diethylpropion, aspirin, beta-blocking blood pressure medicines such as atenolol and metoprolol, diuretics such as furosemide and hydrochlorothiazide, epinephrine, estrogens, isoniazid, major tranquilizers such as chlorpromazine and thioridazine, MAO inhibitors (drugs such as the antidepressants phenelzine and tranylcypromine), niacin, octreotide, oral contraceptives, oral diabetes drugs, phenytoin, steroid medications such as prednisone, sulfa antibiotics such as sulfamethoxazole, and thyroid medications such as levothyroxine.

What are the possible side effects of Insulin?

Side effects cannot be anticipated. If any develop or change in intensity, tell your doctor as soon as possible. Only your doctor can determine if it is safe for you to continue taking this drug.

While side effects from insulin use are rare, allergic reactions or low blood sugar may pose significant health risks. Your doctor should be notified if any of the following occur:

Mild allergic reactions: swelling, itching or redness at the injection site (usually disappears within a few days or weeks)

More serious allergic reactions: fast pulse, low blood pressure, perspiration, rash over the entire body, shortness of breath, shallow breathing, or wheezing

Low blood sugar may develop in poorly controlled or unstable diabetes. Consuming sugar or a sugar-containing product will usually correct the condition, which can be brought about by taking too much insulin, missing or delaying meals, exercising or working more than usual, an infection or illness, a change in the body's need for insulin, drug interactions, or consuming alcohol.

Symptoms of low blood sugar include: abnormal behavior, anxiety, blurred vision, cold sweat, confusion, depressed mood, dizziness, drowsiness, fatigue, headache, hunger, inability to concentrate, light-headedness, nausea, nervousness, personality changes, rapid heartbeat, restlessness, sleep disturbances, slurred speech, sweating, tingling in the hands, feet, lips, or tongue, tremor, unsteady movement

Symptoms of insufficient insulin include: drowsiness, flushing, fruity breath, heavy breathing, loss of appetite, rapid pulse, thirst

An overdose of insulin can cause low blood sugar (hypoglycemia). Symptoms include: depressed mood, dizziness, drowsiness, fatigue, headache, hunger, inability to concentrate, irritability, nausea, nervousness, personality changes, rapid heartbeat, restlessness, sleep disturbances, slurred speech, sweating, tingling, tremor, and unsteady movements. Your doctor should be contacted immediately if these symptoms of severe low blood sugar occur. Eating sugar or a sugar-based product will often correct the condition. If you suspect an overdose, seek medical attention immediately.

Can I receive Insulin if I am pregnant or breastfeeding?

Insulin is considered safe for pregnant women, but pregnancy may make managing your diabetes more difficult. Properly controlled diabetes is essential for the health of the mother and the developing baby; therefore, it is extremely important that pregnant women follow closely their physician's dietary and exercise guidelines and prescribing instructions. Since insulin does not pass into breast milk, it is safe for nursing mothers. It is not known whether genetically engineered insulin lispro appears in breast milk.

What should I do if I miss a dose of Insulin?

Your doctor should tell you what to do if you miss an insulin injection or meal.

How should I store Insulin?

Store insulin in a refrigerator (but not in the freezer) or in another cool, dark place. Do not expose insulin to heat or direct sunlight.

Some brands of pre-filled syringes can be kept at room temperature for a week or a month. The vial or cartridge of genetically engineered insulin lispro can be kept unrefrigerated for up to 28 days. Check your product's label. Never use insulin after the expiration date that is printed on the label and carton.

Insulin detemir See Levemir, page 722.

Insulin glulisine See Apidra, page 114.

INTAL
Generic name: Cromolyn sodium

What is Intal?

Intal is used to manage asthma, to prevent asthma attacks, and to prevent and treat seasonal and chronic allergies. It is available in different forms.

What is the most important information I should know about Intal?

Intal does not stop an asthma attack that has already started—it is used to prevent attacks.

When taken to prevent severe bronchial asthma, it can take up to 4 weeks before you feel its maximum benefit. Do not stop using Intal suddenly without the advice of your doctor.

Who should not take Intal?
Do not use Intal if you are sensitive to any component of this drug.

What should I tell my doctor before I take the first dose of Intal?
Tell your doctor about all prescription, over-the-counter, and herbal medications you are taking before beginning treatment with Intal. Also, talk to your doctor about your complete medical history, especially if you have kidney or liver disease.

What is the usual dosage?
The information below is based on the dosage guidelines your doctor uses. Depending on your condition and medical history, your doctor may prescribe a different regimen. Do not change the dosage or stop taking your medication without your doctor's approval.

Management of Bronchial Asthma
Adults and children 5 years and older: The usual starting dose of the Intal Inhaler Aerosol Spray is 2 metered sprays taken at regular intervals, 4 times daily. This is the maximum dose that should be taken, and lower dosages may be effective in children. This drug should be used only after an asthma attack has been controlled and you can inhale adequately.

Prevention of an Acute Asthma Attack Following Exercise or Exposure to Cold Air or Environmental Agents
Adults and Children 5 years and older: The usual dose of the Intal Inhaler Aerosol Spray is 2 metered sprays shortly before exposure to the irritant (10 to 15 minutes but no more than 60 minutes).

How should I take Intal?
Make sure the canister is properly inserted into the inhaler unit. Take the cover off the mouthpiece. Shake the inhaler gently. If the mouthpiece cover is not present, inspect the inhaler for the presence of foreign objects.

Hold Inhaler and exhale slowly and fully, expelling as much air as possible. Do not breathe into the inhaler— it could clog the inhaler valve. Place the mouthpiece into your mouth, close your lips around it, and tilt your head back. Keep your tongue below the opening of the inhaler. While breathing in deeply and slowly through the mouth, fully depress the top of the metal canister with your index finger. Remove the inhaler from your mouth. Hold your breath for several seconds, then breathe out slowly. This step is very important. It allows the drug to spread throughout your lungs. Repeat steps 2-5, then replace the mouthpiece cover.

What should I avoid while taking Intal?

Avoid spraying in the eyes. Do not stop taking Intal until your doctor tells you to. It may be some time before you begin to notice effects from this medication.

What are possible food and drug interactions associated with Intal?

If Intal is taken with certain other drugs, the effects of either could be increased, decreased, or altered. Always check with your doctor before combining Intal with other drugs.

What are the possible side effects of Intal?

Side effects cannot be anticipated. If any develop or change in intensity, tell your doctor as soon as possible. Only your doctor can determine if it is safe for you to continue taking this drug.

Side effects may include: cough, throat irritation or dryness, nausea, wheezing. bad taste

Can I receive Intal if I am pregnant or breastfeeding?

The effects of Intal during pregnancy and breastfeeding are unknown. Tell your doctor immediately if you are pregnant, plan to become pregnant, or are breastfeeding.

What should I do if I miss a dose of Intal?

If you miss a dose, take it as soon as you remember. Then take the rest of that day's doses at equally spaced intervals. Do not take 2 doses at once.

How should I store Intal?

Store at room temperature, away from light and heat.

INTELENCE

Generic name: Etravirine

What is Intelence?

Intelence is used to treat HIV infection in adults. It must be used in combination with other HIV medications.

What is the most important information I should know about Intelence?

Intelence is not a cure for HIV infection. It does not reduce the risk of passing HIV to others through sexual contact, sharing needles, or being exposed to blood. The long-term effects of Intelence are not known.

Who should not take Intelence?

At this time there are no known reasons to avoid using Intelence.

What should I tell my doctor before I take the first dose of Intelence?

Tell your doctor about all prescription, over-the-counter, and herbal medications you are taking before beginning treatment with Intelence. Also tell your doctor about your complete medical history, especially if you have liver problems (including hepatitis B or C), or if you are pregnant, plan to become pregnant, or are breastfeeding.

What is the usual dosage?

The information below is based on the dosage guidelines your doctor uses. Depending on your condition and medical history, your doctor may prescribe a different regimen. Do not change the dosage or stop taking your medication without your doctor's approval.

Adults: The usual dosage is 200 milligrams taken twice a day.

How should I take Intelence?

You should take Intelence every day exactly as prescribed by your doctor. The usual dosage is 2 tablets twice a day (for a total of 4 tablets a day) following a meal. The tablets should be swallowed whole with liquids such as water.

What should I avoid while taking Intelence?

You should not chew or crush the tablets. Never take Intelence on an empty stomach. Do not change your dose or stop taking Intelence without talking to your doctor.

What are possible food and drug interactions associated with Intelence?

If Intelence is taken with certain drugs, the effects of either could be increased, decreased, or altered. It is especially important to check with your doctor before combining Intelence with the following: other HIV medicines, drugs used to treat abnormal heart rhythms, blood thinners, anticonvulsants, antifungals, antibiotics such as clarithromycin, antimycobacterials such as rifampin and rifabutin, drugs used to treat tuberculosis, sleeping medications such as diazepam, corticosteroids, cholesterol-lowering drugs known as statins, immunosuppressants, narcotic painkillers, drugs used to treat erectile dysfunction, and the herb St. John's wort.

What are the possible side effects of Intelence?

Side effects cannot be anticipated. If any develop or change in intensity, tell your doctor as soon as possible. Only your doctor can determine if it is safe for you to continue taking this drug.

Side effects may include: skin rash, diarrhea, nausea, abdominal pain, vomiting, headache, changes in body shape or fat, immune reconstitution syndrome (signs of inflammation from opportunistic infections that may occur as the medicine works to control the HIV infection and strengthen the immune system)

Can I receive Intelence if I am pregnant or breastfeeding?
Intelence should be avoided during pregnancy and breastfeeding. Talk with your doctor before taking this drug if you are pregnant, plan to become pregnant, or are breastfeeding.

What should I do if I miss a dose of Intelence?
If it is within 6 hours of the time you usually take Intelence, take the missed dose as soon as possible following a meal. Then take your next dose at the regularly scheduled time. If you miss a dose of Intelence by more than 6 hours of the time you usually take it, wait and take the next dose at the regularly scheduled time. Do not double the next dose to make up for the missed dose.

How should I store Intelence?
Store at room temperature.

INVEGA
Generic name: Paliperidone

What is Invega?
Invega is used to treat schizophrenia and is known as an "atypical antipsychotic" medicine.

What is the most important information I should know about Invega?
Elderly patients with dementia (such as that seen in Alzheimer's disease) who are treated with atypical antipsychotics have a higher chance for death; Invega is not approved to treat dementia.

In rare cases, Invega may cause neuroleptic malignant syndrome (NMS), a life-threatening nervous system condition that causes a high fever, stiff muscles, sweating, a fast or irregular heart beat, change in blood pressure, and confusion. NMS can also affect your kidneys. NMS is a medical emergency. Call your doctor right away if you experience any of these symptoms.

Invega may also cause tardive dyskinesia, a movement disorder characterized by slow or jerky facial or body movements. Call your doctor right away if you experience uncontrollable muscle movements.

Antipsychotic therapy has induced hyperglycemia (high blood sugar) and diabetes that has progressed to coma or death in extreme cases. Patients with diabetes or those at risk for diabetes should have their blood sugar monitored often.

Overheating and dehydration may occur due to Invega therapy. Take precautions when exercising or doing activities in the heat and stay hydrated.

Take care when driving or using machinery until you know how Invega affects you as you may experience impaired judgment, thinking, and motor skills.

Dizziness and fainting caused by a drop in blood pressure may occur during Invega therapy, especially when you first start taking Invega or when the dose is increased. Get up slowly after sitting or lying down.

Who should not take Invega?

You should not take Invega if you are allergic to paliperidone, risperidone, or to any of the ingredients in Invega.

You should not take Invega if you have pre-existing severe gastrointestinal narrowing (trouble swallowing, inflammation of the small bowel, "short gut syndrome," peritonitis, cystic fibrosis, chronic intestinal pseudo-obstruction, or Meckel's diverticulum).

Invega tablets should only be used in patients who are able to swallow the tablet whole.

What should I tell my doctor before I take the first dose of Invega?

Tell your doctor about all prescription, over-the-counter, and herbal medications you are taking before beginning treatment with Invega. Also, talk to your doctor about your complete medical history, especially past or current heart problems, seizures, diabetes or elevated blood sugar, liver disease, and if you regularly drink alcohol. Tell your doctor if you have or have had problems with your esophagus, stomach or small or large intestine. Inform your doctor if you are pregnant, trying to become pregnant, or are breastfeeding.

What is the usual dosage?

The information below is based on the dosage guidelines your doctor uses. Depending on your condition and medical history, your doctor may prescribe a different regimen. Do not change the dosage or stop taking your medication without your doctor's approval.

Adults: The usual dose is 6 milligrams (mg) daily. Some patients may benefit from either higher doses up to 12 mg/day or a lower dose of 3 mg/day. If needed, the dose can be increased in increments of 3 mg/day at intervals of at least 5 days.

The maximum recommended daily dose is 12 mg/day.

Adults with moderate to severe kidney disease: The maximum recommended dose is 3 mg once daily.

How should I take Invega?

Take Invega once a day in the morning. Swallow Invega tablets whole with water or another liquid. Do not chew, divide, or crush Invega tablets. Invega can be taken with or without food.

What should I avoid while taking Invega?

Avoid drinking alcohol while taking Invega. Be careful not to overexert yourself; be cautious of excessive sweating and keep yourself fully hydrated.

What are possible food and drug interactions associated with Invega?

If Invega is taken with certain other drugs, the effects of either could be increased, decreased, or altered. It is especially important to check with your doctor before combining Invega with the following: alcohol and other central nervous system drugs, amiodarone, chlorpromazine, gatifloxacin, levodopa and other dopamine agonists, moxifloxacin, procainamide, quinidine, sotalol, and thioridazine.

What are the possible side effects of Invega?

Side effects cannot be anticipated. If any develop or change in intensity, tell your doctor as soon as possible. Only your doctor can determine if it is safe for you to continue taking this drug.

Side effects may include: abdominal pain, anxiety, back pain, visual disturbances, cough, disturbed digestion, excessive salivary secretions, fainting, fast heart beat, fatigue, pain in the extremities, headache, high blood pressure, high blood sugar and diabetes, impaired judgment or thinking, involuntary movements, dizziness upon standing, muscle stiffness, nausea, overheating and dehydration, restlessness, seizures, drowsiness, suicidal thoughts, trouble swallowing, upset stomach, weakness

Can I receive Invega if I am pregnant or breastfeeding?

The effects of Invega during pregnancy and breastfeeding are unknown. Tell your doctor immediately if you are pregnant, plan to become pregnant, or are breastfeeding. Taking Invega while breastfeeding is not recommended.

What should I do if I miss a dose of Invega?

If you miss a dose, take it as soon as you remember. If it is almost time for your next dose (less than 12 hours away), skip that dose and resume your normal dosing schedule. Do not take two doses together.

How should I store Invega?

Store at room temperature away from moisture.

Ipratropium bromide *See Atrovent, page 150.*

Ipratropium bromide and albuterol sulfate *See Combivent, page 327, or DuoNeb, page 450.*

Irbesartan *See Avapro, page 164.*

Irbesartan and hydrochlorothiazide *See Avalide, page 155.*

ISENTRESS
Generic name: Raltegravir

What is Isentress?
Isentress is used to treat HIV infection. It must be taken in combination with other HIV medications.

What is the most important information I should know about Isentress?
Isentress is not a cure for HIV infection. It does not reduce the risk of passing HIV to others through sexual contact, sharing needles, or being exposed to blood.

The long-term effects of using Isentress are not known.

Who should not take Isentress?
At this time, there are no known reasons to avoid taking Isentress.

What should I tell my doctor before I take the first dose of Isentress?
Tell your doctor about all prescription, over-the-counter, and herbal medications you are taking before beginning treatment with Isentress.

Also tell your doctor about your complete medical history, especially if you have any allergies or you are pregnant, plan to become pregnant, or are breastfeeding.

What is the usual dosage?
The information below is based on the dosage guidelines your doctor uses. Depending on your condition and medical history, your doctor may prescribe a different regimen. Do not change the dosage or stop taking your medication without your doctor's approval.

Adults: The usual dose is 400 milligrams twice a day.

How should I take Isentress?
Take Isentress exactly as prescribed by your doctor. Take the tablet twice a day by mouth. It can be taken with or without food.

What should I avoid while taking Isentress?

Do not change your dose or stop taking Isentress without talking to your doctor.

What are possible food and drug interactions associated with Isentress?

If Isentress is used with certain other drugs, the effects of either could be increased, decreased, or altered. Always check with your doctor before combining Isentress with other medications, especially rifampin or other medicines used to treat HIV.

What are the possible side effects of Isentress?

Side effects cannot be anticipated. If any develop or change in intensity, tell your doctor as soon as possible. Only your doctor can determine if it is safe for you to continue taking this drug.

Side effects may include: diarrhea, headache, nausea, rash, skin reactions

Can I receive Isentress if I am pregnant or breastfeeding?

Isentress should be avoided during pregnancy and breastfeeding. Talk with your doctor before taking this drug if you are pregnant, plan to become pregnant, or are breastfeeding.

What should I do if I miss a dose of Isentress?

If you miss a dose, take it as soon as you remember. If you do not remember until it is time for your next dose, skip the missed dose and go back to your regular schedule. Do not double the dose to make up for the missed dose.

How should I store Isentress?

Store at room temperature.

Isometheptene mucate, dichloralphenazone, and acetaminophen See Midrin, page 828.

ISORDIL

Generic name: Isosorbide dinitrate

What is Isordil?

Isordil is prescribed to prevent angina pectoris (suffocating chest pain), which occurs when the heart arteries become constricted and sufficient oxygen does not reach the heart tissues. Isordil dilates the blood vessels by relaxing the muscles in their walls. Oxygen flow improves as the vessels relax, and chest pain is prevented.

What is the most important information I should know about Isordil?

Isordil may cause severe low blood pressure (possibly marked by dizziness or fainting), especially when you stand or sit up quickly. Alcohol may worsen this condition. People taking diuretics (water pills) or those who have low blood pressure should use Isordil with caution.

Who should not take Isordil?

Do not take Isordil if you are allergic to any of its ingredients, or to other nitrates or nitrites.

What should I tell my doctor before I take the first dose of Isordil?

Tell your doctor about all prescription, over-the-counter, and herbal medications you are taking before beginning treatment with Isordil. Also, talk to your doctor about your complete medical history, especially if you have anemia, glaucoma, a previous head injury or heart attack, heart disease, low blood pressure, or thyroid disease.

What is the usual dosage?

The information below is based on the dosage guidelines your doctor uses. Depending on your condition and medical history, your doctor may prescribe a different regimen. Do not change the dosage or stop taking your medication without your doctor's approval.

Adults: The usual starting dose of Isordil is 5 milligrams (mg) to 20 mg, 2 or 3 times daily. For maintenance therapy, between 10 mg to 40 mg, 2 or 3 times daily is recommended.

How should I take Isordil?

Take exactly as prescribed by your doctor.

What should I avoid while taking Isordil?

Avoid abruptly stopping this medication because it could result in additional chest pain. You should follow your doctor's plan for a gradual withdrawal schedule.

What are possible food and drug interactions associated with Isordil?

If Isordil is taken with certain other drugs, the effects of either could be increased, decreased, or altered. It is especially important to check with your doctor before combining Isordil with the following: alcohol, dilitiazem hydrochloride, nifedipine, and sildenafil citrate (Viagra).

What are the possible side effects of Isordil?

Side effects cannot be anticipated. If any develop or change in intensity, tell your doctor as soon as possible. Only your doctor can determine if it is safe for you to continue taking this drug.

Side effects may include: dizziness, headache, lightheadedness, low blood pressure, weakness

Can I receive Isordil if I am pregnant or breastfeeding?

The effects of Isordil during pregnancy and breastfeeding are unknown. Tell your doctor immediately if you are pregnant, plan to become pregnant, or are breastfeeding.

What should I do if I miss a dose of Isordil?

Take it as soon as you remember. If the next dose is within 6 hours, skip the missed dose and go back to your regular schedule. Do not take 2 doses at the same time.

How should I store Isordil?

Store at room temperature, in a tightly closed container. Protect from light and excessive heat.

Isosorbide dinitrate See Isordil, page 672.

ISOSORBIDE MONONITRATE

What is Isosorbide mononitrate?

Isosorbide is used to prevent angina pectoris—crushing chest pains that result when partially clogged arteries restrict the flow of oxygen-rich blood to the heart muscle. Isosorbide does not relieve angina attacks already underway.

What is the most important information I should know about Isosorbide mononitrate?

Isosorbide may cause severe low blood pressure (possibly marked by dizziness or fainting), especially when you are standing or if you sit up quickly. People taking blood pressure medication, those who have low blood pressure should use isosorbide with caution.

Who should not take Isosorbide mononitrate?

Do not use isosorbide if you are allergic to it or to other heart medications containing nitrates or nitrites.

What should I tell my doctor before I take the first dose of Isosorbide mononitrate?

Tell your doctor about all prescription, over-the-counter, and herbal medications you are taking before beginning treatment with isosorbide. Also, talk to your doctor about your complete medical history, especially if you have had a heart attack, have congestive heart failure, a form of heart disease known as hypertrophic cardiomyopathy (thickening of the heart muscle), low blood pressure, suffer from migraines, or have kidney or liver disease.

What is the usual dosage?

The information below is based on the dosage guidelines your doctor uses. Depending on your condition and medical history, your doctor may prescribe a different regimen. Do not change the dosage or stop taking your medication without your doctor's approval.

Adults: The usual starting dose is 30 milligrams (mg) or 60 mg once daily. After several days the dosage may be increased to 120 mg once daily. In rare cases, a dosage of 240 mg may be required.

How should I take Isosorbide mononitrate?

The daily dose of isosorbide should be taken when you wake up in the morning. Do not chew or crush the tablets, swallow them whole with a half-glassful of water.

What should I avoid while taking Isosorbide mononitrate?

Do not abruptly stop taking isosorbide. This can worsen your condition.

Isosorbide may cause dizziness. Avoid driving, operating machinery, or performing other tasks that require concentration until you know how this drug affects you.

Avoid drinking alcohol while taking isosorbide. Alcohol combined with isosorbide can result in very low blood pressure possibly resulting in fainting or falling.

Isosorbide may cause headaches. Do not try to avoid the headaches by changing your dose. If your headache stops, it may mean the drug has lost its effectiveness. Aspirin or acetaminophen may relieve the pain.

Avoid the concurrent use of Viagra, Cialis or Levitra as these may increase the risk of a severe drop in blood pressure.

What are possible food and drug interactions associated with Isosorbide mononitrate?

If isosorbide is taken with certain other drugs, the effects of either could be increased, decreased, or altered. It is especially important to check with your doctor before combining isosorbide with the following: calcium-blocking blood pressure medications such as diltiazem, nifedipine, and verapamil; erectile dysfunction drugs such as Viagra, Cialis and Levitra

What are the possible side effects of Isosorbide mononitrate?
Side effects cannot be anticipated. If any develop or change in intensity, tell your doctor as soon as possible. Only your doctor can determine if it is safe for you to continue taking this drug.

Side effects may include: dizziness, headache, restlessness, constipation, diarrhea, nausea, vomiting, lightheadedness, low blood pressure.

Can I receive Isosorbide mononitrate if I am pregnant or breastfeeding?
The effects of isosorbide during pregnancy and breastfeeding are unknown. Tell your doctor immediately if you are pregnant, plan to become pregnant, or are breastfeeding.

What should I do if I miss a dose of Isosorbide mononitrate?
Take your dose of isosorbide as soon as you remember. If the next dose is in less than 2 hours, skip the one you missed and go back to your regular schedule. Do not take 2 doses at the same time.

How should I store Isosorbide mononitrate?
Keep isosorbide in the container it came in, tightly closed. Store it at room temperature and away from excess heat and moisture.

Isotretinoin See Accutane, page 9.

Isradipine See DynaCirc CR, page 461.

Itraconazole See Sporanox, page 1216.

JANUMET
Generic name: Sitagliptin and metformin

What is Janumet?
Janumet contains 2 prescription medicines: sitagliptin and metformin. Janumet can be used along with diet and exercise to lower blood sugar in adult patients with type 2 diabetes.

What is the most important information I should know about Janumet?
Janumet can cause a rare but serious condition called lactic acidosis. Tell your doctor if you experience any of the following symptoms: feeling very weak, tired, or uncomfortable (malaise), unusual muscle pain, unusual sleepiness, rapid breathing that you can't explain, unusual or unexpected stomach problems (such as nausea or vomiting), low body temperature, feeling dizzy or lightheaded, suddenly having a slow or uneven heartbeat

Tell your doctor if you are undergoing an x-ray procedure. Janumet should be temporarily discontinued during this time.

Avoid drinking excessive alcohol while taking Janumet. Do not binge drink for short periods or drink a lot of alcohol on a regular basis.

Who should not take Janumet?

Do not take Janumet if you are allergic to Janumet, metformin, or sitagliptin or any of the ingredients of Janumet. You should also not take Janumet if you have: type 1 diabetes, metabolic acidosis or diabetic ketoacidosis, kidney disease, or if you are going to receive an injection of a dye or contrast agents for an x-ray procedure.

What should I tell my doctor before I take the first dose of Janumet?

Tell your doctor about all prescription, over-the-counter, and herbal medications you are taking before beginning treatment with Janumet. Also, talk to your doctor about your complete medical history, especially if you have ever had a history of liver, kidney, or heart problems. Tell your doctor if you drink alcohol frequently or are a binge drinker. Tell your doctor if you are pregnant, plan to become pregnant, or are breastfeeding.

What is the usual dosage?

The information below is based on the dosage guidelines your doctor uses. Depending on your condition and medical history, your doctor may prescribe a different regimen. Do not change the dosage or stop taking your medication without your doctor's approval.

Adults: The starting dose of Janumet should be based on the patient's current regimen. Janumet should be given twice daily with meals. The following doses are available: 50 milligrams (mg) sitagliptin/500 mg metformin HCl and 50 mg sitagliptin/1000 mg metformin HCl.

How should I take Janumet?

You should take Janumet with food to decrease your chances getting an upset stomach.

What should I avoid while taking Janumet?

Avoid excessive alcohol while taking Janumet. You should not binge drink for short periods, and you should not drink a lot of alcohol on a regular basis.

What are possible food and drug interactions associated with Janumet?

If Janumet is taken with certain other drugs, the effect of either medication could be increased, decreased, or altered. It is especially important to check with your doctor before combining with the following medications:

calcium channel blockers, cimetidine, corticosteroids, digoxin, diuretics, estrogen, furosemide, isoniazid, nicotinic acid, nifedipine, oral contraceptives, phenytoin, and thyroid medications.

What are the possible side effects of Janumet?
Side effects cannot be anticipated. If any develop or change in intensity, tell your doctor as soon as possible. Only your doctor can determine if it is safe for you to continue taking this drug.

Side effects may include: stuffy or runny nose, sore throat, upper respiratory infection, diarrhea, nausea and vomiting, gas, stomach discomfort, indigestion, weakness, headache

Can I receive Janumet if I am pregnant or breastfeeding?
The effects of Janumet during pregnancy and breastfeeding are unknown. Tell your doctor immediately if you are pregnant, or plan to become pregnant, or are breastfeeding.

What should I do if I miss a dose of Janumet?
If you miss a dose, take it with food as soon as you remember. If you do not remember until it is time for your next dose, skip the missed dose and go back to your regular schedule. Do not take 2 doses of Janumet at once.

How should I store Janumet?
Store at room temperature in a tightly closed container.

JANUVIA
Generic name: Sitagliptin phosphate

What is Januvia?
Januvia is used along with diet and exercise to lower blood sugar in patients with type 2 diabetes. Januvia can be taken alone or with certain other medications used for diabetes if they do not provide enough control.

What is the most important information I should know about Januvia?
Talk to your doctor if you experience excess thirst or urination, or fruity-scented breath. These may be signs of high blood sugar (glucose) and improper blood glucose control.

Who should not take Januvia?
Do not take Januvia if you have type 1 diabetes or diabetic ketoacidosis (increased ketones in the blood or urine).

What should I tell my doctor before I take the first dose of Januvia?

Tell your doctor about all prescription, over-the-counter, and herbal medications you are taking before beginning treatment with Januvia. Also, talk to your doctor about your complete medical history, especially if you are pregnant, plan to become pregnant, or are breastfeeding, if you have kidney problems, any allergies; or if you are taking digoxin. During periods of stress on the body, such as fever, trauma, infection or surgery, your medication needs may change; contact your doctor right away.

What is the usual dosage?

The information below is based on the dosage guidelines your doctor uses. Depending on your condition and medical history, your doctor may prescribe a different regimen. Do not change the dosage or stop taking your medication without your doctor's approval.

Adults: The recommended dose for adults is 100 milligrams (mg) taken once daily with or without food. If you have kidney problems, your doctor may prescribe lower doses of Januvia.

How should I take Januvia?

You should take Januvia once a day with or without food. Your doctor may prescribe Januvia along with other medications that lower blood sugar. It is important to follow any dietary, exercise, and glucose monitoring instructions from your doctor while taking this medication.

What are possible food and drug interactions associated with Januvia?

It is especially important to check with your doctor before combining Januvia with Digoxin. Talk with your doctor or pharmacist about any other medications you are taking in order to make sure the effects of the medications will not be altered.

What are the possible side effects of Januvia?

Side effects cannot be anticipated. If any develop or change in intensity, tell your doctor as soon as possible. Only your doctor can determine if it is safe for you to continue taking this drug.

Side effects may include: headache, stomach discomfort and diarrhea, sore throat, stuffy or runny nose, upper respiratory infection

Symptoms of a serious allergic reaction include: rash, hives, and swelling of the face, lips, tongue, and throat that may cause difficulty in breathing or swallowing. If you have an allergic reaction, stop taking Januvia and call your doctor right away. Your doctor may prescribe a medication to treat your allergic reaction and a different medication for your diabetes.

Can I receive Januvia if I am pregnant or breastfeeding?

The effects of Januvia during pregnancy and breastfeeding are unknown. Tell your doctor immediately if you are pregnant, plan to become pregnant, or are breastfeeding.

What should I do if I miss a dose of Januvia?

If you miss a dose, take it as soon as you remember. If you do not remember until it is time for your next dose, skip the missed dose and go back to your regular schedule. Do not take 2 doses at once.

How should I store Januvia?

Store at room temperature.

KALETRA

Generic name: Lopinavir and ritonavir

What is Kaletra?

Kaletra is a combination of two medicines, lopinavir and ritonavir, used to treat HIV-infected people. Kaletra is always used with other anti-HIV medicines. Kaletra is a protease inhibitor, which blocks a chemical that HIV needs to multiply itself. HIV infection destroys CDr, or T cells, which are important to the immune system. Kaletra may increase the number of T cells and reduce the amount of HIV in the blood, which reduces the chance of death or infections that happen when your immune system is weak.

What is the most important information I should know about Kaletra?

Kaletra does not cure human immunodeficiency virus (HIV) infection or acquired immune deficiency syndrome (AIDS), nor does it reduce the risk of passing HIV to others through sexual contact or blood contamination.

Combining Kaletra with certain other medications can cause serious, even life-threatening, reactions. See "What are possible food and drug interactions associated with this medication?" below before taking Kaletra with any other medication.

There have been reports of inflammation of the pancreas (sometimes fatal) in people taking Kaletra. Tell your doctor if you experience abdominal pain, nausea, or vomiting while taking Kaletra.

Who should not take Kaletra?

Do not take Kaletra if you are allergic to the medication or any of its ingredients, including ritonavir or lopinavir. Do not take Kaletra if you are taking certain medicines. (See "What are possible food and drug interactions associated with Kaletra?")

What should I tell my doctor before I take the first dose of Kaletra?

Tell your doctor about all prescription, over-the-counter, and herbal medications you are taking before beginning treatment with Kaletra. Also, talk to your doctor about your complete medical history, especially if you have diabetes; hemophilia; or liver problems, including infection with hepatitis B or hepatitis C.

What is the usual dosage?

The information below is based on the dosage guidelines your doctor uses. Depending on your condition and medical history, your doctor may prescribe a different regimen. Do not change the dosage or stop taking your medication without your doctor's approval.

Tablets

Adults and children 12 years and older: Each Kaletra tablet contains 200 milligrams (mg) of lopinavir and 50 mg of ritonavir. For patients who have not taken any anti-HIV medications in the past, your doctor may prescribe 2 tablets (400/100 mg) taken 2 times each day or 4 tablets (800/200 mg) taken once daily. For patients with experience with anti-HIV medications, the usual dose is 2 tablets (400/100mg) taken 2 times each day.

Oral Suspension

Adults and children 12 years and older: For patients who have not taken any anti-HIV medications in the past, your doctor may prescribe either 5 milliliters (mL) taken 2 times each day or 10mL to be taken 1 time each day. For patients with experience with anti-HIV medications, the usual dose is 5 mL taken 2 times each day.

Capsules

Adults and children 12 years and older: For patients who have not taken any anti-HIV medications in the past, your doctor may prescribe either 3 capsules taken 2 times each day or 6 capsules taken once daily. For patients with experience with anti-HIV medications, the usual dose is 3 capsules taken 2 times each day.

Dosage adjustments may be made depending on the other medicines you are taking.

Children 6 months to 12 years: The usual dose is calculated based on weight.

How should I take Kaletra?

Take Kaletra oral solution with food to help it work most effectively.

Kaletra tablets can be taken with or without food. Kaletra tablets and capsules should be swallowed whole and not chewed, broken, or crushed. Let your doctor know when your Kaletra supply starts to run low.

What should I avoid while taking Kaletra?

Avoid doing things that can spread HIV infection, since Kaletra doesn't stop you from passing HIV to others. Practice safe sex and do not share needles or personal items that can have blood or bodily fluids on them.

Avoid taking any new medications without first talking to your doctor (see "What are possible food and drug interactions associated with this medication?" below).

Do not stop taking Kaletra unless your doctor tells you to do so. If the medicine is stopped for even a short time, the amount of HIV in your blood may increase, or the virus may develop resistance to Kaletra and become harder to treat.

What are possible food and drug interactions associated with Kaletra?

If Kaletra is taken with certain other drugs, the effects of either could be increased, decreased, or altered. If you use birth control pills or a contraceptive patch, you should use an additional or different kind of contraception, because Kaletra can affect the effectiveness of contraceptives.

Combining Kaletra with certain medications can cause serious, even life-threatening, reactions. It is important to check with your doctor before combining Kaletra with the following: astemizole, cholesterol-lowering medicines (such as lovastatin, simvastatin, and atorvastatin), cisapride, ergot-based medications that are often used for migraines (such as dihydroergotamine, ergonovine, ergotamine, and methylergonovine), midazolam, pimozide, rifampin, St. John's wort, terfenadine, triazolam.

It is also very important to check with your doctor before combining Kaletra with the following medications: amprenavir, carbamazepine, didanosine, disulfiram, efavirenz, fluticasone propionate, metronidazole, nelfinavir, nevirapine, phenobarbital, phenytoin, rifabutin, sildenafil, tadalafil, vardenafil.

What are the possible side effects of Kaletra?

Side effects cannot be anticipated. If any develop or change in intensity, tell your doctor as soon as possible. Only your doctor can determine if it is safe for you to continue taking this drug.

Side effects may include: abdominal pain, abnormal bowel movements, diarrhea, feeling weak/tired, headache, nausea, skin rash (in children)

Can I receive Kaletra if I am pregnant or breastfeeding?

The effects of Kaletra during pregnancy and breastfeeding are unknown. Tell your doctor immediately if you are pregnant, plan to become pregnant, or are breastfeeding. Do not breastfeed if you have HIV, as there is a chance that the virus can be transmitted via breastfeeding.

What should I do if I miss a dose of Kaletra?
It is important that you do not miss any doses. If you miss a dose of Kaletra, take it as soon as possible. If it is almost time for your next dose, wait and take the next dose at the regular time. Do not take 2 doses at once.

How should I store Kaletra?
Store Kaletra tablets at room temperature; avoid excessive heat and do not expose Kaletra tablets to high humidity outside the pharmacy container for longer than 2 weeks.

Kaletra oral solution and capsules can be used within 2 months if stored at room temperature. If you refrigerate your Kaletra oral solution and capsules, you will be able to use it until the printed expiration date. Avoid exposing Kaletra oral solution and capsules to excessive heat.

KEFLEX
Generic name: Cephalexin hydrochloride

What is Keflex?
Keflex is an antibiotic used to treat infections of the respiratory tract, the middle ear, the bones, the skin, and the reproductive and urinary systems.

**What is the most important information
I should know about Keflex?**
If you are allergic to either penicillin or cephalosporin antibiotics in any form, consult your doctor before taking Keflex. If there is a possibility that you are allergic to both types of medication and if a reaction occurs, it could be extremely severe. If you take the drug and feel signs of a reaction, seek medical attention immediately.

Your doctor will only prescribe Keflex to treat a bacterial infection. Keflex will not cure a viral infection such as the common cold. It is important to take the full dosage schedule of Keflex, even if you're feeling better in a few days. Not completing the full dosage schedule may decrease the drug's effectiveness and increase the chances that the bacteria may become resistant to Keflex and similar antibiotics.

Who should not take Keflex?
Do not take Keflex if you are allergic to this drug or any cephalosporins.

**What should I tell my doctor before
I take the first dose of Keflex?**
Tell your doctor about all prescription, over-the-counter, and herbal medications you are taking before beginning treatment with Keflex. Also, talk to your doctor about your complete medical history, especially if you have kidney or liver disease, are taking a blood thinner, or have a history of stomach or intestinal disease such as inflammation of the large intestine.

What is the usual dosage?
The information below is based on the dosage guidelines your doctor uses. Depending on your condition and medical history, your doctor may prescribe a different regimen. Do not change the dosage or stop taking your medication without your doctor's approval.

Throat, Skin, and Urinary Tract Infections
Adults: The usual dose is 500 milligrams (mg) every 12 hours. Urinary tract infections should be treated for 7 to 14 days. If the infection is more severe, you may need larger doses.

Other Infections
Adults: The usual dose is 250 mg every 6 hours.

The usual dose for children under 15 years of age is 25 to 50 mg per 2.2 pounds of body weight, divided into smaller doses.

Middle Ear Infections
Children: For middle ear infections, the dose is 75 to 100 mg per 2.2 pounds per day, divided into 4 doses.

Strep Throat and Skin Infections
Children: For strep throat in children over 1 year of age and for skin infections, the dose may be divided into 2 doses taken every 12 hours. For strep throat infections, Keflex should be taken for at least 10 days. Your doctor may double the dose if your child has a severe infection.

How should I take Keflex?
Keflex can be taken with or without food. However, if the drug upsets your stomach, you may want to take it after you have eaten.

Take Keflex at even intervals around the clock as prescribed by your doctor.

If you are taking the liquid form of Keflex, use the specially marked spoon to measure each dose accurately.

What should I avoid while taking Keflex?
Do not give Keflex to other people and do not use it for other infections.

What are possible food and drug interactions associated with Keflex?
If Keflex is taken with certain other drugs, the effects of either could be increased, decreased, or altered. It is especially important to check with your doctor before combining Keflex with the following: antidiarrhea medications such as Imodium, metformin, oral contraceptives, and probenecid.

What are the possible side effects of Keflex?

Side effects cannot be anticipated. If any develop or change in intensity, tell your doctor as soon as possible. Only your doctor can determine if it is safe for you to continue taking this drug.

Side effects may include: diarrhea, allergic reactions, abdominal pain

Can I receive Keflex if I am pregnant or breastfeeding?

The effects of Keflex during pregnancy and breastfeeding are unknown. Tell your doctor immediately if you are pregnant, plan to become pregnant, or are breastfeeding. Use caution when taking Keflex while breastfeeding.

What should I do if I miss a dose of Keflex?

If you take this medication twice a day and it is within 6 hours of your next dose, skip the missed dose and take the next dose as scheduled. However, if you have more than 6 hours until your next dose, take the missed dose as soon as you remember and continue with your normal dosing schedule. If you take 3 or more doses a day, take the missed dose only if there are greater than 4 hours until your next dose. If not, skip the missed dose and continue with your normal dosing schedule. If you miss or skip a dose, do not take 2 doses at once.

How should I store Keflex?

Store the capsules and tablets at room temperature. Store the liquid suspension in a refrigerator and throw out any unused medication after 14 days.

KEPPRA/KEPPRA XR

Generic name: Levetiracetam

What is Keppra/Keppra XR?

Keppra is used to treat several types of seizures in both adults and children with epilepsy: partial onset seizures in adults and children (4 years and older), myoclonic seizures in adults, and juvenile myoclonic epilepsy in children 12 years and older. Keppra is used to treat primary generalized tonic-clonic seizures in adults and idiopathic generalized epilepsy in children >6 years.

Keppra XR (an extended-release form) is used to treat partial onset seizures in patients 16 years and older.

What is the most important information I should know about Keppra/Keppra XR?

Keppra may cause sleepiness, coordination problems, and behavior problems when being taken for adult partial onset seizures. In children, Keppra may cause sleepiness and behavior problems when it is taken for partial onset seizures.

Who should not take Keppra/Keppra XR?

Do not take Keppra if you are allergic to any of the ingredients in either the tablets or oral solution.

What should I tell my doctor before I take the first dose of Keppra/Keppra XR?

Tell your doctor about all prescription, over-the-counter, and herbal medications you are taking before beginning therapy with Keppra. Also, talk to your doctor about your complete medical history, including if you have kidney disease, are pregnant or plan on becoming pregnant while on this medication, or are breastfeeding.

What is the usual dosage?

The information below is based on the dosage guidelines your doctor uses. Depending on your condition and medical history, your doctor may prescribe a different regimen. Do not change the dosage or stop taking your medication without your doctor's approval.

Adults and children 16 years and older: The usual dose is 1000 milligrams (mg)/day (given as 500 mg 2 times a day).

Children 4 to 16 years: The usual starting dose is 20 mg/kilogram (kg) per day (taken as 10 mg/kg 2 times a day). The daily dose should be increased every 2 weeks by increments of 20 mg/kg to the recommended daily dose of 60 mg/kg (30 mg/kg twice per day).

Keppra XR may be dosed at 1000 to 3000 mg per day. Your doctor may adjust your dose if you have kidney problems.

How should I take Keppra/Keppra XR?

Keppra is taken orally with or without food. If you are taking Keppra twice a day, then take it once in the morning and once at night. Take Keppra at the same times each day. Swallow the tablets whole; do not chew or crush the tablets.

What should I avoid while taking Keppra/Keppra XR?

Avoid driving, operating machinery, or performing other activities that need your complete focus until you know how this drug affects you. Keppra may make you sleepy or dizzy.

Avoid becoming pregnant while being treated with Keppra.

What are possible food and drug interactions associated with Keppra/Keppra XR?

If Keppra is taken with certain other drugs, the effects of either could be increased, decreased, or altered. Always check with your doctor before combining any other medication with Keppra.

What are the possible side effects of Keppra/Keppra XR?
Side effects cannot be anticipated. If any develop or change in intensity, tell your doctor as soon as possible. Only your doctor can determine if it is safe for you to continue taking this drug.

Side effects may include: depression, dizziness, headache, loss of appetite, nasal infection, nervousness, pain, sleepiness, sore throat, weakness, behavior changes

Can I receive Keppra/Keppra XR if I am pregnant or breastfeeding?
If you are pregnant, planning to become pregnant, or are breastfeeding, talk to your doctor before beginning treatment with Keppra. It is not recommended to be pregnant while receiving this type of epileptic therapy.

How should I store Keppra/Keppra XR?
Store at room temperature away from heat and light.

KETEK
Generic name: Telithromycin

What is Ketek?
Ketek is an antibiotic used to treat adults over 18 years of age who have a lung infection called community-acquired pneumonia. This type of pneumonia is caused by certain bacterial germs. Ketek is not for other types of infections caused by bacteria, and like other antibiotics, Ketek does not kill viruses.

What is the most important information I should know about Ketek?
Do not take Ketek if you have myasthenia gravis. Myasthenia gravis is a rare disease that causes muscle weakness. Patients with myasthenia gravis who have taken Ketek have sometimes experienced life-threatening breathing problems.

Ketek can also cause other serious side effects, including severe liver damage. Do not take Ketek if you have ever had side effects of the liver while taking Ketek, or any of the group of antibiotics known as macrolides, such as erythromycin, azithromycin, clarithromycin, and dirithromycin. Stop Ketek and call your doctor right away if you have signs of liver problems. Do not take another dose unless your doctor tells you to. Signs of liver problems include: dark urine, increased tiredness, itchy skin, light-colored stools, loss of appetite, right upper belly pain, yellowing of the skin and/or eyes.

Who should not take Ketek?

Do not take Ketek if you have myasthenia gravis. Also, do not take Ketek if you have had an allergic reaction to, or have had side effects on the liver to Ketek, or to any of the group of antibiotics known as macrolides (see "What is the most important information I should know about Ketek?"). Do not take Ketek if you are taking cisapride or pimozide.

What should I tell my doctor before I take the first dose of Ketek?

Tell your doctor about all prescription, over-the-counter, and herbal medications you are taking before beginning treatment with Ketek. Also, talk to your doctor about your complete medical history, especially if you have myasthenia gravis. Tell your doctor if you or someone in your family has a rare heart condition known as QTc prolongation, or any other heart problems. Tell your doctor if you are being treated for heart rhythm disturbances with certain medicines knows as antiarrhythmics. Be sure to let your doctor know if you have low blood potassium or magnesium; or heart, liver, or kidney disease.

What is the usual dosage?

The information below is based on the dosage guidelines your doctor uses. Depending on your condition and medical history, your doctor may prescribe a different regimen. Do not change the dosage or stop taking your medication without your doctor's approval.

Adults: The usual dosage is 800 milligrams (mg), or 2 tablets, taken 1 time each day for 7-10 days, depending on the type of infection being treated.

How should I take Ketek?

Ketek tablets should be swallowed whole and may be taken with or without food. To make sure that all bacteria are killed, take all of the medication that was prescribed for you, even if you begin to feel better. You should contact your doctor if your condition is not improving while taking Ketek or if you took too much of the medication.

What should I avoid while taking Ketek?

Ketek may cause problems with vision, particularly when looking quickly between objects close by and objects far away. Most vision problems are mild to moderate and occur following the first or second dose. However, severe cases have been reported and vision problems may occur after any dose during treatment. These problems may last several hours and sometimes come back with the next dose. Ketek may also cause you to faint, especially if you are also experiencing nausea, vomiting, and lightheadedness.

If visual difficulties or fainting occur, you should avoid driving a motor vehicle, operating heavy machinery, or engaging in otherwise hazardous activities.

Taking Ketek with certain other medications may lead to serious side effects, therefore, you should talk to your doctor before taking these medications (see "What are possible food and drug interactions associated with this medication?").

What are possible food and drug interactions associated with Ketek?

If Ketek is taken with certain other drugs, the effects of either could be increased, decreased, or altered. It is especially important to check with your doctor before combining Ketek with the following: atorvastatin, carbamazepine, cisapride, cyclosporine, digoxin, dofetilide, ergot alkaloid derivatives, hexobarbital, itraconazole, ketoconazole, lovastatin, metoprolol, midazolam, phenobarbital, phenytoin, pimozide, procainamide, rifampin, quinidine, simvastatin, sirolimus, tacrolimus, theophylline.

What are the possible side effects of Ketek?

Side effects cannot be anticipated. If any develop or change in intensity, tell your doctor as soon as possible. Only your doctor can determine if it is safe for you to continue taking this drug.

Side effects may include: Diarrhea, dizziness, headache, nausea, vomiting

Ketek has the potential to affect the heart. In rare cases, this may result in an abnormal heartbeat, which may result in a fainting spell. Contact your doctor if you have a fainting spell and stop taking Ketek immediately.

An intestinal infection is another serious side effect of taking Ketek. Call your doctor if you get watery diarrhea; diarrhea that does not go away; or bloody stools, which may be accompanied by stomach cramps and a fever, up to 2 months after you have finished your antibiotic.

Can I receive Ketek if I am pregnant or breastfeeding?

The effects of Ketek during pregnancy and breastfeeding are unknown. Tell your doctor immediately if you are pregnant, plan to become pregnant, or are breastfeeding.

What should I do if I miss a dose of Ketek?

If you miss a dose, take it as soon as you remember. If it is almost time for your next dose, wait and take the next dose at the regular time. Do not take more than 1 dose of Ketek in a 24-hour period.

How should I store Ketek?

Store Ketek tablets at room temperature.

Ketoconazole *See Nizoral, page 900.*

Ketoconazole foam *See Extina, page 533.*

KETOROLAC TROMETHAMINE

What is Ketorolac tromethamine?
Ketorolac, a nonsteroidal anti-inflammatory drug, is used to relieve moderately severe, acute pain. It is prescribed for a limited amount of time (no more than 5 days for adults and as a single dose for children), not for long-term therapy.

What is the most important information
I should know about Ketorolac tromethamine?
Ketorolac can cause serious side effects, including ulcers and internal bleeding. Never take it for more than 5 days.

This drug should be used with caution if you have kidney or liver disease. It may cause liver inflammation or kidney problems in some people.

If you are an older adult or are taking blood thinners, use this drug cautiously.

Ketorolac is not recommended for long-term use, since side effects increase over time. This medication should be taken for no more than 5 days.

Who should not take Ketorolac tromethamine?
Do not take ketorolac if it has ever given you an allergic reaction. Also avoid this medication if you have ever had an allergic reaction—such as nasal polyps (tumors), swelling of the face, limbs, and throat, hives, wheezing, light-headedness—to aspirin or other nonsteroidal anti-inflammatory drugs (NSAIDs).

Do not take ketorolac if you have ever had a peptic ulcer or stomach or intestinal bleeding. Avoid it if you have severe kidney disease or bleeding problems.

Never combine this drug with aspirin, NSAIDs, or probenecid. Make sure your doctor is aware of any drug reactions you have experienced.

What should I tell my doctor before
I take the first dose of Ketorolac tromethamine?
Tell your doctor about all prescription, over-the-counter, and herbal medications you are taking before beginning treatment with ketorolac. Also talk to your doctor about your complete medical history, especially if you have ever had kidney or liver problems, ulcers, intestinal bleeding, heart disease, high blood pressure, or if you are taking blood thinners.

What is the usual dosage?

The information below is based on the dosage guidelines your doctor uses. Depending on your condition and medical history, your doctor may prescribe a different regimen. Do not change the dosage or stop taking your medication without your doctor's approval.

Adults: Your doctor may give you ketorolac intravenously or intramuscularly to start, then have you switch to the tablets. Most patients take 2 tablets for the first dose (20 milligrams) and then 1 tablet (10 milligrams) every 4 to 6 hours. You should not take more than 40 milligrams per day and should not take ketorolac for more than 5 days in all.

Children: For children under 16, the doctor may prescribe a single dose of ketorolac, by intravenous or intramuscular injection, after an operation. Ketorolac is not recommended for children under 2 years.

How should I take Ketorolac tromethamine?

Take ketorolac exactly as prescribed. Take it with a full glass of water. Ketorolac works fastest when taken on an empty stomach, but an antacid can be taken if it causes upset.

What should I avoid while taking Ketorolac tromethamine?

Avoid lying down for about 20 minutes after taking ketorolac. This will help to prevent irritation of your upper digestive tract.

What are possible food and drug interactions associated with Ketorolac tromethamine?

If ketorolac is taken with certain other drugs, the effects of either could be increased, decreased, or altered. It is especially important to check with your doctor before combining ketorolac with the following: blood pressure medication such as ACE inhibitors, antidepressants, antiepileptic drugs, aspirin and other NSAIDs, blood thinners such as warfarin, lithium, antianxiety medication, methotrexate, probenecid, alprazolam, and diuretics.

What are the possible side effects of Ketorolac tromethamine?

Side effects cannot be anticipated. If any develop or change in intensity, inform your doctor as soon as possible. Only your doctor can determine if it is safe for you to continue using ketorolac.

Side effects may include: diarrhea, dizziness, drowsiness, headache, indigestion, nausea, stomach and intestinal pain, swelling due to fluid retention

Can I receive Ketorolac tromethamine if I am pregnant or breastfeeding?

Ketorolac should not be taken late in pregnancy; during this period, it can harm the developing baby. If you are pregnant or plan to become pregnant, inform your doctor immediately. Ketorolac appears in breast milk and could affect a nursing infant. This medication should not be used while you are breastfeeding.

What should I do if I miss a dose of Ketorolac tromethamine?
If you take ketorolac on a regular schedule, take it as soon as you remember. If it is almost time for your next dose, skip the one you missed and go back to your regular schedule. Never take 2 doses at the same time.

How should I store Ketorolac tromethamine?
Store at room temperature, away from light.

Ketotifen fumarate See Zaditor, page 1441.

KINRIX
Generic name: Diphtheria, tetanus, pertussis,
poliovirus vaccine

What is Kinrix?
Kinrix is a vaccine given by injection to children 4 to 6 years old to prevent diphtheria, tetanus, pertussis (whooping cough), and polio.

What is the most important information I should know about Kinrix?
As with other vaccines, there is a risk of allergic reactions. Signs of severe allergic reactions may include hives, difficulty breathing, and swelling of the throat. If any of these events occur, seek immediate medical attention. Such rare events usually occur before leaving the doctor's office. Kinrix should be avoided in children less than 4 years old and more than 7 years old.

Who should not take Kinrix?
Kinrix should not be used in children less than 4 years old and more than 7 years old. In addition, it should also not be used in children who are allergic to any ingredient in Kinrix, have an allergy to latex, or have a history of allergic reactions to any vaccine that protects against diphtheria, tetanus, pertussis or polio.

Kinrix should not be given to children who have experienced a brain or nervous system disorder within 7 days after receiving a pertussis-containing vaccine, have had Guillain-Barre syndrome after a tetanus-containing vaccine, or have had any of the following problems within 48 hours after a dose of a pertussis-containing vaccine: high fever (105 degrees or more), a shock-like state, persistent crying lasting 3 hours or more, or seizures with or without fever within 3 days of vaccination.

What should I tell my doctor before I take the first dose of Kinrix?

Tell the doctor about all prescription and over-the-counter medications your child is taking, as well as any vaccines your child has received, before beginning treatment with Kinrix. Also tell the doctor about your child's complete medical history, including a tendency to have seizures, history of a weakened immune system, or a history of allergic reactions to vaccines.

What is the usual dosage?

The information below is based on the dosage guidelines your doctor uses. Depending on your condition and medical history, your doctor may prescribe a different regimen. Do not change the dosage or stop taking your medication without your doctor's approval.

Children 4 to 6 years: The usual dosage is 0.5 milliliter (mL) as a single intramuscular injection.

How should I take Kinrix?

Kinrix will be injected by a nurse or doctor in the upper leg (thigh), upper arm, or buttocks.

What should I avoid while taking Kinrix?

Vaccination is the best way to protect against diphtheria, tetanus, pertussis, and polio. Avoid missing any regularly scheduled vaccines the doctor has recommended for your child.

What are possible food and drug interactions associated with Kinrix?

If Kinrix is taken with certain other drugs, the effects of either could be increased, decreased, or altered. It is especially important to check with your doctor before combining Kinrix with the following: corticosteroids, cytotoxic drugs, and immunosuppressive therapies including chemotherapy and radiation.

What are the possible side effects of Kinrix?

As with any other vaccine, there is a risk of allergic reactions. Signs of severe allergic reactions may include hives, difficulty breathing, and swelling of the throat. If any of these events occur, seek immediate medical attention.

Side effects cannot be anticipated. If any develop or change in intensity, tell your doctor as soon as possible. Only your doctor can determine if it is safe for your child to receive this vaccine.

Side effects may include: pain, redness, or swelling at the injection site; fever; loss of appetite

Can I receive Kinrix if I am pregnant or breastfeeding?
The effects of Kinrix during pregnancy and breastfeeding are unknown.

What should I do if I miss a dose of Kinrix?
Ask your doctor for advice.

How should I store Kinrix?
Your doctor will store Kinrix in the refrigerator.

KLONOPIN
Generic name: Clonazepam

What is Klonopin?
Klonopin is used alone or with other drugs to treat seizure disorders. It is also used to treat panic disorder, which is characterized by unexpected attacks of overwhelming panic along with fear of having additional future attacks.

What is the most important information I should know about Klonopin?
Physical and/or psychological dependence can occur with Klonopin.

Withdrawal effects are possible if the medication is stopped suddenly after long-term use or after high-dose treatment. Do not stop taking Klonopin suddenly without first talking to your doctor. Your doctor may want to gradually reduce the dose.

When you start Klonopin, you may experience impaired judgment, thinking, or motor skills. You should not drive or operate dangerous machinery until you know how this medication will affect you. Consuming alcohol, a CNS depressant, may intensify or worsen the side effects of Klonopin.

When on Klonopin, your doctor should monitor your blood liver function during long-term therapy due to possible side effects.

When used in patients with several different types of seizure disorders, Klonopin may increase the incidence or onset of generalized tonic-clonic seizures. These patients may require the addition of appropriate anticonvulsants or an increase in their dosage.

When Klonopin is used in conjunction with valproic acid, there is a risk of absence status (a continual series of seizures).

Who should not take Klonopin?
Do not use Klonopin if you are sensitive to or have ever had an allergic reaction to it or similar drugs, such as chlordiazepoxide and diazepam.

Do not take Klonopin if you have severe liver disease or the eye condition known as acute narrow-angle glaucoma (increased pressure in the eye). Patients with open-angle glaucoma who are receiving appropriate treatment may use Klonopin.

What should I tell my doctor before I take the first dose of Klonopin?

Tell your doctor about all prescription, over-the-counter, and herbal medication you are taking before beginning treatment with Klonopin. Also, talk to your doctor about your complete medical history, especially if you have kidney or liver disease, seizures, are depressed or have suicidal thoughts, are on valproic acid or any other anticonvulsants, have several different types of coexisting seizure disorders, have a history of sensitivity to Klonopin or other benzodiazepines, or have a history of substance abuse. In addition, tell your doctor if you are pregnant, planning on becoming pregnant, or breastfeeding.

What is the usual dosage?

The information below is based on the dosage guidelines your doctor uses. Depending on your condition and medical history, your doctor may prescribe a different regimen. Do not change the dosage or stop taking your medication without your doctor's approval.

Panic Disorder

Adults: The usual starting dose is 0.25 milligrams (mg) taken twice a day. The dose may be increased by 1 mg per day after 3 days. Some people may need as much as 4 mg per day; for these patients the dose should be incrementally increased by 0.125 to 0.25 mg twice a day every 3 days until the panic disorder is controlled or until the side effects become too bothersome.

Klonopin therapy should be stopped slowly, with a decrease of 0.125 mg twice a day every 3 days, until the drug is completely withdrawn.

Elderly: There is no clinical trial experience with the use of Klonopin in patients 65 years and older. In general, elderly patients should be started on a low dose of Klonopin and observed closely.

Children: The safety and effectiveness of Klonopin to treat panic disorder have not been established in children under age 18.

Seizure Disorders

Adults: The usual starting dose is 1.5 mg per day divided into 3 doses. The dose may be increased by 0.5-1 mg every 3 days until seizures are controlled or the side effects become too bothersome. The maximum daily dose is 20 mg.

Elderly: There is no clinical trial experience with the use of Klonopin is patients 65 years and older. In general, elderly patients should be started on a low dose of Klonopin and observed closely.

Children: The starting dose for infants and children up to 10 years old or up to 66 pounds should be 0.01-0.03 mg per 2.2 pounds of body weight per day. Do not give more than 0.05 mg per 2.2 pounds of body weight per day. The dose may be increased by 0.25-0.5 mg every 3 days, up to 0.1-0.2 mg per 2.2 pounds of body weight a day, until seizures are controlled or the side effects become too bothersome.

How should I take Klonopin?

Take Klonopin exactly as prescribed. Klonopin is available as a tablet or as a wafer that melts in your mouth. Take Klonopin tablets with water and swallow the tablet whole. The wafers can be taken with or without water. With dry hands, peel back the foil on the blister pack. Do not push the wafer through the foil. Immediately after opening the blister, remove the wafer and place it on your tongue. You must take the wafer right after opening the blister. It will melt rapidly in your mouth.

What should I avoid while taking Klonopin?

Klonopin will cause drowsiness and may cause dizziness. Use caution when driving, operating machinery, or performing other hazardous activities. Avoid using Klonopin with other drugs that may cause drowsiness or dizziness. Use alcohol cautiously. Alcohol may increase drowsiness and dizziness while taking Klonopin. Alcohol may also increase the risk of having a seizure.

Klonopin can be habit-forming and can lose its effectiveness as you build up a tolerance to it. You may experience withdrawal symptoms, such as convulsions, hallucinations, tremor, and abdominal and muscle cramps, if you stop using Klonopin suddenly. You should only stop or change your dose only after first talking to your doctor.

What are possible food and drug interactions associated with Klonopin?

If Klonopin is taken with certain other drugs, the effects of either could be increased, decreased, or altered. It is especially important to check with your doctor before combining Klonopin with the following: amphotericin, antidepressants (imipramine, phenelzine, and tranylcypromine), barbiturates, carbamazepine, chlorpromazine, diazepam, haloperidol, narcotic pain relievers (meperidine and morphine), nystatin, other anticonvulsants (phenytoin and divalproex), and sedatives (triazolam).

What are the possible side effects of Klonopin?

Side effects cannot be anticipated. If any develop or change in intensity, tell your doctor as soon as possible. Only your doctor can determine if it is safe for you to continue taking this drug.

Side effects may include: depression, dizziness, fatigue, flu, inflamed sinuses or nasal passages, lack of coordination, memory problems, menstrual problems, nervousness, sleepiness, upper respiratory tract infection

Klonopin can also cause aggressive behavior, agitation, anxiety, excitability, hostility, irritability, nervousness, nightmares, sleep disturbances, and vivid dreams.

Can I receive Klonopin if I am pregnant or breastfeeding?
Do not take Klonopin if you are pregnant or planning on becoming pregnant. Talk to your doctor first. Do not take Klonopin while breastfeeding. There have been suggested associations between the use of anticonvulsants by women with epilepsy and an elevated incidence of birth defects in children born to these women. The use of Klonopin in women of childbearing potential should be weighed carefully by the patient and her doctor.

What should I do if I miss a dose of Klonopin?
If it is within an hour after the missed time, take the dose as soon as you remember. If you do not remember until later, skip the missed dose and go back to your regular schedule. Never take two doses at the same time.

How should I store Klonopin?
Store at room temperature. Keep away from heat, light, and moisture.

LABETALOL HYDROCHLORIDE

What is Labetalol hydrochloride?
Labetalol is used to treat high blood pressure. It can be used alone or in combination with other high blood pressure medications, especially thiazide diuretics such as hydrochlorothiazide and loop diuretics such as furosemide.

What is the most important information I should know about Labetalol hydrochloride?
Labetalol has caused severe liver damage in some people. Although this is a rare occurrence, if you develop any symptoms of abnormal liver function—itching, dark urine, continuing loss of appetite, yellow eyes and skin, or unexplained flu-like symptoms—contact your doctor immediately.

This medication may mask the symptoms of low blood sugar or alter blood sugar levels. If you are diabetic, discuss this with your doctor.

Notify your doctor or dentist that you are taking labetalol if you have a medical emergency, and before you have surgery or dental treatment.

Who should not take Labetalol hydrochloride?

You should not take labetalol if you suffer from an obstructive airway disease such as bronchial asthma, congestive heart failure, heart block (a heart irregularity), inadequate blood supply to the circulatory system (cardiogenic shock), a severely slow heartbeat, or any other condition that causes severe and continued low blood pressure. Also, do not take this medication if you are sensitive to or have ever had an allergic reaction to labetalol or any of the product's ingredients.

What should I tell my doctor before I take the first dose of Labetalol hydrochloride?

Tell your doctor about all prescription, over-the-counter, and herbal medications you are taking before beginning treatment with this drug. Also, talk to your doctor about all your medical conditions, especially if you have a history of congestive heart failure, kidney or liver disease, asthma, chronic bronchitis, emphysema, or other bronchial diseases.

What is the usual dosage?

The information below is based on the dosage guidelines your doctor uses. Depending on your condition and medical history, your doctor may prescribe a different regimen. Do not change the dosage or stop taking your medication without your doctor's approval.

Adults: Your doctor will adjust the dosages to fit your needs. The usual starting dose is 100 milligrams, 2 times per day, alone or with a diuretic drug. After 2 to 3 days of checking your blood pressure, your doctor may begin increasing your dose by 100 milligrams, 2 times per day, at intervals of 2 to 3 days. The regular dose ranges from 200 to 400 milligrams, 2 times per day. Some people may require total daily dosage of as much as 1,200 to 2,400 milligrams, either alone or with a thiazide diuretic. In these cases, your doctor will observe the drug's effect and adjust your dose accordingly.

How should I take Labetalol hydrochloride?

Labetalol can be taken with or without food. The amount of labetalol absorbed into your bloodstream is actually increased by food.

What should I avoid while taking Labetalol hydrochloride?

Labetalol should not be stopped suddenly. This can cause chest pain and heart attack. Dosage should be gradually reduced.

What are possible food and drug interactions associated with Labetalol hydrochloride?

If labetalol is taken with certain other drugs, the effects of either could be increased, decreased, or altered. It is especially important to check with your doctor before taking labetalol with the following: airway opening drugs such as albuterol, antidepressant medications such as amitripty-line, cimetidine, diabetes drugs such as glyburide, epinephrine, insulin, nitroglycerin, nonsteroidal anti-inflammatory drugs such as ibuprofen, ritodrine, and verapamil.

What are the possible side effects of Labetalol hydrochloride?
Side effects cannot be anticipated. If any develop or change in intensity, tell your doctor as soon as possible. Only your doctor can determine if it is safe for you to continue taking this drug.

Side effects may include: dizziness, fatigue, indigestion, nausea, stuffy nose

Can I receive Labetalol hydrochloride if I am pregnant or breastfeeding?
The effects of labetalol during pregnancy have not been adequately stud-ied. If you are pregnant or plan to become pregnant, inform your doctor immediately. Labetalol appears in breast milk and could affect a nurs-ing infant. If this medication is essential to your health, your doctor may advise you to discontinue breastfeeding until your treatment is finished.

What should I do if I miss a dose of Labetalol hydrochloride?
Take it as soon as you remember. If it is almost time for your next dose, skip the one you missed and go back to your regular schedule. Never take 2 doses at the same time.

How should I store Labetalol hydrochloride?
Store at room temperature.

LAMICTAL
Generic name: Lamotrigine

What is Lamictal?
Lamictal is used either alone or in combination with other medicines to treat seizures in adults and children 2 years and older.

Lamictal is also used for maintenance treatment of bipolar disorder to help prevent mood swings in adults 18 years and older.

What is the most important information I should know about Lamictal?
All patients who are currently taking or are about to start drugs for epi-lepsy should be closely monitored for changes in behavior that indicate the emergence or worsening of suicidal thoughts or behavior or depres-sion.

Rarely, serious and possibly fatal rashes have been reported with the use of Lamictal. Although most patients who develop rash while receiving Lamictal have mild to moderate symptoms, some individuals may develop a serious skin reaction that requires hospitalization. Because of this risk, it's important to contact your doctor immediately if you develop any of the following: fever, hives, painful sores in your mouth or around your eyes, skin rash, swelling of your lips or tongue, swollen lymph glands.

These serious skin reactions are most likely to happen within the first 8 weeks of treatment and occur more often in children than adults. They are also more likely to happen if you take Lamictal with the anticonvulsant valproate (Depakene or Depakote); if you take a higher starting dose of Lamictal than your doctor prescribed; or if you increase your dose of Lamictal faster than prescribed.

Who should not take Lamictal?
Do not take Lamictal if you are allergic to the medication or any of its ingredients.

Lamictal is not approved for treating children or teenagers with mood disorders such as bipolar disorder or depression.

What should I tell my doctor before I take the first dose of Lamictal?
Tell your doctor about all prescription, over-the-counter, and herbal medications you are taking before beginning treatment with Lamictal. Also, talk to your doctor about your complete medical history, especially if you have kidney, liver, or heart problems; or if you have thoughts of harming yourself or committing suicide.

What is the usual dosage?
The information below is based on the dosage guidelines your doctor uses. Depending on your condition and medical history, your doctor may prescribe a different regimen. Do not change the dosage or stop taking your medication without your doctor's approval.

There are very specific calculations for your starting dose and dosage increase schedule based on your age, weight, medical condition, and other medications you're taking. The dose of Lamictal must be increased slowly, generally every 1 to 2 weeks. It may take several weeks or months before your final dosage can be determined by your doctor.

How should I take Lamictal?
Lamictal tablets should be swallowed whole; chewing them may leave a bitter taste.

Lamictal CD is a form that comes as Chewable Dispersible tablets that may be swallowed whole, chewed, or mixed in water or diluted fruit juice. If chewing them, drink some water to aid in swallowing. To mix in liquid, add the tablets to a small amount of water or juice (1 teaspoon or enough to cover the tablets) in a glass. Approximately 1 minute later, mix the solution and take the entire amount at once.

What should I avoid while taking Lamictal?

Do not abruptly stop taking Lamictal without consulting your doctor first. Do not start or stop estrogen-containing birth control pills while taking Lamictal unless you have discussed with your doctor any dosage adjustments that might be necessary. Use caution before driving a car or operating complex, hazardous machinery until you know if Lamictal affects your ability to perform these tasks.

What are possible food and drug interactions associated with Lamictal?

If Lamictal is taken with certain other drugs, the effects of either could be increased, decreased, or altered. It is especially important to check with your doctor before combining Lamictal with the following: carbamazepine, estrogen-containing birth control pills, medicines that inhibit folic acid metabolism, oxcarbazepine, phenobarbital, phenytoin, primidone, rifampin, topiramate, and valproate.

What are the possible side effects of Lamictal?

Side effects cannot be anticipated. If any develop or change in intensity, tell your doctor as soon as possible. Only your doctor can determine if it is safe for you to continue taking this drug.

Side effects may include: blurred or double vision, coordination problems, dizziness, headache, insomnia, nausea, rash, sleepiness, vomiting

The most serious side effect of Lamictal is a rash that can be life-threatening. See "What is the most important information I should know about Lamictal?"

Can I receive Lamictal if I am pregnant or breastfeeding?

The effects of Lamictal during pregnancy are not known. Lamictal can pass into breast milk, and the effects on the infant are unknown. Tell your doctor immediately if you are pregnant, plan to become pregnant, or are breastfeeding.

What should I do if I miss a dose of Lamictal?

Never double your dose of Lamictal if you miss a dose. Skip the missed dose and return to your regular schedule.

How should I store Lamictal?

Store at room temperature away from heat and light.

LAMISIL

Generic name: Terbinafine hydrochloride

What is Lamisil?

Lamisil is used to treat fungal infections. The tablets are used for fungus of the toenail or fingernail. The cream and solution are used for other fungal infections such as athlete's foot, jock itch, and ringworm. The solution is also used to treat tinea versicolor, a fungal infection that produces brown, tan, or white spots on the trunk of the body. Lamisil oral granules are used for the treatment of tinea capitis (a fungal infection of the scalp hair follicles) in adults and children 4 years and older.

What is the most important information I should know about Lamisil?

Lamisil works gradually. It usually takes a week for results to start becoming apparent. Toenail infections require 12 weeks of treatment; fingernail infections require 6 weeks. The condition can continue to improve for 2-6 weeks after completing treatment, though it may take more time for nails to grow in. It may take about 10-12 months for toenails and about 4-6 months for fingernails to grow in completely.

If you see no change at all after a full week of applying the cream or solution, notify your doctor; the problem may not be fungal.

Changes in the lens and retina of the eye have been reported in people taking Lamisil. If you notice any changes in your vision while taking the tablets, notify your doctor.

Lamisil has been known to cause rare cases of liver damage. If you develop warning signs such as nausea, loss of appetite, or fatigue, alert your doctor. Lamisil is not recommended if you have liver disease or kidney problems.

If you suffer from the autoimmune disorder lupus erythematosus, you will not be able to take Lamisil.

Isolated cases of decreases in white blood cell count have been reported. In all of the reported cases to date, these have been reversible. If you have problems with your immune system, your doctor may need to monitor your white blood cell count carefully if you take Lamisil for more than 6 weeks. In some cases, Lamisil therapy may need to be discontinued.

Lamisil has, in rare instances, caused very severe skin reactions. If you develop a steadily worsening rash, stop taking the tablets and call your doctor immediately.

If you develop another kind of infection while taking Lamisil, tell your doctor. Lamisil may decrease your ability to fight infection.

Do not use Lamisil cream or solution in the eye, mouth, nose, or vagina. In case of accidental contact with the eyes, rinse them thoroughly with running water and call your doctor if symptoms continue.

If you develop skin irritation, redness, itching, burning, blistering, swelling, or oozing while using the cream or solution, notify your doctor.

Who should not take Lamisil?
Do not take Lamisil if you are sensitive to any component of the drug or if you have lupus erythematosus.

What should I tell my doctor before I take the first dose of Lamisil?
Tell your doctor about all prescription, over-the-counter, and herbal medications you are taking before beginning treatment with Lamisil. Also, talk to your doctor about your complete medical history, especially if you have diabetes, kidney or liver disease, a weak immune system, or lupus erythematosus.

What is the usual dosage?
The information below is based on the dosage guidelines your doctor uses. Depending on your condition and medical history, your doctor may prescribe a different regimen. Do not change the dosage or stop taking your medication without your doctor's approval.

CREAM AND GEL

Athlete's Foot
Adults: For athlete's foot found only on the soles of the feet and not between the toes, use the cream twice a day for 2 weeks. For athlete's foot found between the toes, use the cream twice a day for 1 week. Do not use for more than 4 weeks.

Jock Itch and Ringworm
Adults: Apply to the affected and closely surrounding areas once a day for at least 1 week. Do not use for more than 4 weeks.

SOLUTION

Athlete's Foot and Tinea Versicolor
Adults: Apply to the affected and closely surrounding areas twice a day for 1 week.

Jock Itch and Ringworm
Adults: Apply to the affected and closely surrounding areas once a day for 1 week.

TABLETS

Fungal Infection of the Fingernails
Adults: The usual dose is 250 milligrams (mg) once a day for 6 weeks.

Fungal Infection of the Toenails
Adults: The usual dose is 250 mg once a day for 12 weeks.

The safety and efficacy of Lamisil tablets and cream have not been established in children under 12.

ORAL GRANULES

Tinea Capitis
Adults and children 4 years and older: Dosing is based upon body weight, but typically 1 to 2 packets should be taken each day. Treatment should last 6 weeks.

How should I take Lamisil?
Take Lamisil tablets exactly as directed. Lamisil can be taken with or without food. For best results, be sure to take the complete course of your medicine. Continue using Lamisil for the full amount of time your doctor prescribes, even if your symptoms being to improve.

Before applying the cream, gel, or solution, wash the affected area with soap and water and dry completely before applying. Use enough solution to wet the entire area, and to cover the affected skin and surrounding area. Do not cover the treated area with dressings unless directed by your doctor.

Take Lamisil oral granules with a soft nonacidic food such as mashed potatoes (do not use applesauce or a fruit-based food). Swallow the combination of food and granules without chewing.

What should I avoid while taking Lamisil?
Avoid alcohol while taking Lamisil. Alcohol and Lamisil can both affect the liver.

Do not apply Lamisil cream, gel, or solution to the breast. Avoid getting Lamisil cream, gel, or solution in your eyes, nose, mouth, or vagina. Do not use the spray form on your face. In case of accidental contact with the eyes, rinse your eyes thoroughly with running water and call your doctor if the symptoms persist.

Avoid using bandages or wraps on areas of your body on which you have applied Lamisil cream or solution.

What are possible food and drug interactions associated with Lamisil?
If Lamisil is taken with certain other drugs, the effects of either could be increased, decreased, or altered. It is especially important to check with your doctor before combining Lamisil with the following: antidepressants (such as fluoxetine, imipramine, paroxetine, phenelzine, sertraline, and tranylcypromine), cimetidine, cyclosporine, beta-blockers (such as atenolol and propranolol), flecainide, propafenone, rasagiline, rifampin, and selegiline.

What are the possible side effects of Lamisil?

Side effects cannot be anticipated. If any develop or change in intensity, tell your doctor as soon as possible. Only your doctor can determine if it is safe for you to continue taking this drug.

Side effects may include: (Tablets) diarrhea, headache, rash, upset stomach; (cream and solution) burning or irritation, itching, dryness, peeling, rash

Lamisil tablets have been known to cause rare cases of liver damage. If you develop warning signs such as nausea, loss of appetite, or fatigue, tell your doctor immediately.

Changes in the lens and retina of the eye have been reported in people taking Lamisil. If you notice any vision changes while taking Lamisil, tell your doctor.

Can I receive Lamisil if I am pregnant or breastfeeding?

The effects of during pregnancy and breastfeeding are unknown. Tell your doctor immediately if you are pregnant, plan to become pregnant, or are breastfeeding. It is not recommended to take Lamisil while breastfeeding.

What should I do if I miss a dose of Lamisil?

Take it as soon as you remember. If it is almost time for your next dose, skip the missed dose and return to your regular schedule. Do not take 2 doses at once.

How should I store Lamisil?

Lamisil tablets should be stored in a tight container, away from direct light, at or below room temperature. Store Lamisil oral granules at room temperature.

Lamivudine *See Epivir, page 487.*

Lamivudine and zidovudine *See Combivir, page 329.*

Lamotrigine *See Lamictal, page 699.*

LANOXIN

Generic name: Digoxin

What is Lanoxin?

Lanoxin is used to treat mild to moderate chronic heart failure and atrial fibrillation (irregular, fast heartbeat).

What is the most important information I should know about Lanoxin?

You should not stop taking Lanoxin without first speaking to your doctor. Suddenly withdrawing the drug could cause a serious change in your heart function. Even if you feel better, you need to keep taking this medication to help the heart work properly.

Do not drive or perform other possibly unsafe tasks until you know how you react to Lanoxin; this drug may cause dizziness or blurred vision. These effects may be worse if you take it with alcohol or certain medicines.

Tell your doctor or dentist that you take Lanoxin before you receive any medical or dental care, emergency care, or surgery. Your doctor may schedule lab tests, including electrocardiogram (ECG), electrolytes, and blood digoxin levels, periodically while you use Lanoxin. These tests will monitor your condition or check for side effects. Be sure to keep all doctor and lab appointments.

Who should not take Lanoxin?

Do not take Lanoxin if you are sensitive to the drug or if you have an abnormal heart rhythm known as ventricular fibrillation.

What should I tell my doctor before I take the first dose of Lanoxin?

Tell your doctor about all prescription, over-the-counter, and herbal medications you are taking before beginning treatment with Lanoxin. Also, talk to your doctor about your complete medical history, especially if you have calcium, potassium, or magnesium imbalances; certain heart problems, including sinus node disease, AV block, a disorder of the left ventricle, or Wolff-Parkinson-White syndrome, abnormal heart rhythms or extra heartbeats; a history of heart attack, kidney disease, underactive or overactive thyroid, fainting due to heart problems, or liver or lung problems.

What is the usual dosage?

The information below is based on the dosage guidelines your doctor uses. Depending on your condition and medical history, your doctor may prescribe a different regimen. Do not change the dosage or stop taking your medication without your doctor's approval.

If you are receiving Lanoxin for the first time, you may be rapidly "digitalized" (a larger first dose may be given, followed by smaller maintenance doses), or gradually "digitalized" (maintenance doses only), depending on your doctor's recommendation. If your doctor feels you need rapid digitalization, your first few doses may be given through your veins. You will then be switched to tablets or capsules for long-term maintenance.

Adults: A single initial dose of 500 micrograms (mcg) to 750 mcg usually produces a minimal affect within half an hour to 2 hours; the maximal affect occurs in 2 to 6 hours. Additional doses of 125 mcg to 375 mcg may be given cautiously at 6- to 8-hour intervals.

A typical maintenance dose might be 0.125 milligrams (mg) or 0.25 mg taken once daily, but individual requirements vary widely. Your doctor will determine the exact dose based on your needs. Therapy is generally initiated at a dose of 250 mcg once daily in patients >70 years with good kidney function; at 125 mcg once daily in patients >70 years or those with impaired kidney function, and at 62.5 mcg in patients with marked kidney impairment.

Doses may be increased every 2 weeks according to response.

Children: Infants and young children usually have their daily dose divided into smaller doses. Children >10 years take adult dosages in proportion to body weight. The dosage will be determined by your doctor.

How should I take Lanoxin?

Take Lanoxin exactly as prescribed. It is usually taken once daily. Take Lanoxin on an empty stomach. However, if the drug upsets your stomach, you can take it with food.

Do not stop taking Lanoxin without first speaking to your doctor. A sudden absence of the drug could cause a serious change in your heart function. Even if you feel better, you need to keep taking this medication to help the heart work properly.

Lanoxin is available in tablet, capsule, liquid, and injectable forms. If you are taking the liquid form, use the specially marked dropper that comes with it.

Do not use Lanoxin injection if it contains particles, is cloudy or discolored, or if the vial is cracked or damaged. Keep this product, as well as syringes and needles, out of the reach of children and pets. Do not reuse needles, syringes, or other materials. Ask your healthcare provider how to dispose of these materials after use. Follow all local rules for disposal.

What should I avoid while taking Lanoxin?

Avoid taking Lanoxin with high-bran/high-fiber foods, such as certain breakfast cereals.

Do not change from one form of Lanoxin to another without first talking to your doctor or pharmacist.

Do not drive or perform other possibly hazardous tasks until you know how you react to Lanoxin; this drug may cause dizziness or blurred vision. These effects may be worse if you take it with alcohol or certain medicines.

Do not miss any doctor or lab appointments. Lab tests, including electrocardiogram (ECG), electrolytes, and blood digoxin levels, may be performed while you use Lanoxin.

What are possible food and drug interactions associated with Lanoxin?

If Lanoxin is taken with certain other drugs, the effects of either could be increased, decreased, or altered. It is especially important to check with your doctor before combining Lanoxin with the following: alprazolam, amiodarone, antacids, anticancer drugs such as cyclophosphamide, beta-blockers (such as atenolol and propranolol), calcium channel blockers (such as diltiazem or verapamil), cholestyramine, clarithromycin, cough, cold, and allergy remedies, diphenoxylate, erythromycin, indomethacin, itraconazole, kaolin-pectin, metoclopramide, neomycin, propafenone, propantheline, quinidine, rifampin, spironolactone, succinylcholine, sulfasalazine, tetracycline, thyroid hormones.

What are the possible side effects of Lanoxin?

Side effects cannot be anticipated. If any develop or change in intensity, tell your doctor as soon as possible. Only your doctor can determine if it is safe for you to continue taking this drug.

Side effects may include: breast development in males, change in heartbeat, confusion, diarrhea, dizziness, headache, loss of appetite, lower stomach pain, nausea, rash, vomiting, weakness

Digoxin can produce visual disturbances (blurred or yellow vision), apathy, and mental disturbances (such as anxiety, depression, delirium, and hallucinations). If you experience any of these symptoms, contact your doctor.

Can I receive Lanoxin if I am pregnant or breastfeeding?

The effects of Lanoxin during pregnancy and breastfeeding are unknown. Tell your doctor immediately if you are pregnant, plan to become pregnant, or are breastfeeding. Use caution when taking Lanoxin while breastfeeding because this drug is found in breast milk.

What should I do if I miss a dose of Lanoxin?

If you remember within 12 hours, take it immediately. If you remember later, skip the missed dose and go back to your regular schedule. Never take 2 doses at the same time. If you miss doses 2 or more days in a row, talk to your doctor.

How should I store Lanoxin?

Store Lanoxin at room temperature in the container it came in, tightly closed, and away from moist places and direct light.

Lansoprazole See Prevacid, page 1057.

LASIX

Generic name: Furosemide

What is Lasix?

Furosemide is a diuretic (water pill) used to treat high blood pressure. It is also used to treat swelling due to fluid retention associated with heart failure or kidney or liver disease.

What is the most important information I should know about Lasix?

Lasix acts quickly, usually within 1 hour. However, since blood pressure declines gradually, it may be several weeks before you get the full benefit of Lasix. You must continue taking it even if you are feeling well. Lasix does not cure high blood pressure; it only keeps it under control.

Do not drive or perform other possibly unsafe tasks until you know how you react to Lasix; this drug may cause dizziness or blurred vision. These effects may be worse if you take it with alcohol or certain medicines.

Lasix may cause dizziness, lightheadedness, or fainting; alcohol, hot weather, exercise, or fever may increase these effects. To prevent these side effects, sit up or stand slowly, especially in the morning. Sit or lie down at the first sign of any of these effects.

Lasix is a strong diuretic. Using too much of this drug can lead to serious water and mineral loss. Therefore, it is important that you be monitored by your doctor. Promptly notify your doctor if you become very thirsty, have a dry mouth, become confused, or develop muscle cramps/weakness.

Lasix may affect your blood sugar. Check blood sugar levels closely. Ask your doctor before you change the dose of your diabetes medicine.

Your doctor may also prescribe a potassium supplement while you take Lasix. Check with your doctor before you use a salt substitute or other product that has potassium in it.

If you have high blood pressure, do not use nonprescription products that contain stimulants, such as diet pills or cold medicines.

Lasix may cause you to become sunburned more easily. Avoid the sun, sunlamps, or tanning booths until you know how you react to Lasix. Use sunscreen or wear protective clothing if you must be outside for more than a short time.

Tell your doctor or dentist that you take Lasix before you receive any medical or dental care, emergency care, or surgery.

Who should not take Lasix?

Do not use Lasix if you cannot urinate or if you are sensitive to the drug.

What should I tell my doctor before I take the first dose of Lasix?

Tell your doctor about all prescription, over-the-counter, and herbal medications you are taking before beginning treatment with Lasix. Also, talk to your doctor about your complete medical history, especially if you have abnormal electrolyte levels, an allergy to sulfa medicines, diabetes, fluid in your abdomen (ascites), gout, a history of heart attack, hearing problems, kidney or liver disease. Also tell your doctor if you have low urine output, lupus erythematosus, porphyria (a blood disorder), or if you are dehydrated or on a low-salt diet.

What is the usual dosage?

The information below is based on the dosage guidelines your doctor uses. Depending on your condition and medical history, your doctor may prescribe a different regimen. Do not change the dosage or stop taking your medication without your doctor's approval.

Fluid Retention

Adults: The usual starting dose is 20 to 80 milligrams (mg). If needed, the same dose can be taken 6 to 8 hours later, or the dose may be increased. Your doctor may raise the dosage by 20 to 40 mg with successive administration 6 to 8 hours after the previous dose, until the desired effect is achieved. This dosage is then taken 1 to 2 times a day thereafter. The maximum daily dose is 600 mg.

High Blood Pressure

Adults: The usual starting dose is 80 mg, divided into 2 smaller doses. Your doctor will adjust the dosages and may add other high blood pressure medications if Lasix is not enough. To prevent an excessive drop in blood pressure, the dosage of other agents or Lasix should be reduced when new blood pressure medicines are being added.

In general, dose selection as well as dose adjustments in elderly patients should be made with caution; therapy is usually initiated at the low end of the dosing range.

Children: The usual starting dose is 2 mg per 2.2 pounds of body weight given as a single oral dose. If the response is not satisfactory, the dosage may be increased by 1 to 2 mg per 2.2 pounds of body weight 6 to 8 hours after the previous dose. The dose should not exceed 6 mg per 2.2 pounds of body weight.

How should I take Lasix?

Take Lasix exactly as prescribed by your doctor. To reduce nighttime urination, take Lasix early in the day unless otherwise directed by your doctor. Lasix is taken with or without food.

What should I avoid while taking Lasix?

Avoid using cough and cold products while taking Lasix. They contain ingredients that may increase your blood pressure.

Use alcohol with caution. Alcohol may increase the side effects of Lasix.

Do not drive or perform other possibly unsafe tasks until you know how you react to Lasix; this drug may cause dizziness or blurred vision.

Do not sit or stand up quickly when you begin treatment with Lasix, especially in the morning. Sit or lie down at the first sign of dizziness, and lightheadedness.

Avoid the sun, sunlamps, or tanning booths until you know how you react to Lasix. Use sunscreen or wear protective clothing if you must be outside for more than a short time.

What are possible food and drug interactions associated with Lasix?

If Lasix is taken with certain other drugs, the effects of either could be increased, decreased, or altered. It is especially important to check with your doctor before combining Lasix with the following: aminoglycoside antibiotics such as amikacin and gentamicin, ACE inhibitors such as captopril, aspirin and other salicylates, barbiturates, blood pressure drugs such as doxazosin and terazosin, chloral hydrate, corticosteroids, digoxin, ethacrynic acid, ibuprofen, indomethacin, lithium, narcotics such as codeine, norepinephrine, succinylcholine, sucralfate, tubocurarine

What are the possible side effects of Lasix?

Side effects cannot be anticipated. If any develop or change in intensity, tell your doctor as soon as possible. Only your doctor can determine if it is safe for you to continue taking this drug.

Side effects may include: blood disorders, dizziness, loss of appetite, muscle spasms, reddish or purplish spots on the skin, restlessness, ringing in the ears, sensitivity to sunlight, yellow eyes and skin, lightheadedness, calf pain or tenderness, confusion, dry mouth, fast or irregular heartbeat

Can I receive Lasix if I am pregnant or breastfeeding?

The effects of Lasix during pregnancy and breastfeeding are unknown. Tell your doctor immediately if you are pregnant, plan to become pregnant, or are breastfeeding. Use caution when taking Lasix while breastfeeding because this drug is found in breast milk.

What should I do if I miss a dose of Lasix?

Take the forgotten dose as soon as you remember. If it is almost time for your next dose, skip the missed dose and go back to your regular schedule. Never take 2 doses at the same time.

How should I store Lasix?

Store at room temperature away from heat and moisture in a tight, light-resistant container. Do not store in the bathroom. Exposure to light may cause Lasix to develop a slight discoloration. Do not take discolored tablets.

Latanoprost *See Xalatan, page 1423.*

Leflunomide *See Arava, page 121.*

LESCOL/LESCOL XL

Generic name: Fluvastatin sodium

What is Lescol/Lescol XL?

Lescol and Lescol XL (an extended-release form) are medications called statins that are used to lower cholesterol. They lower the LDL (bad) cholesterol and triglycerides in your blood. They can raise your HDL (good) cholesterol as well. Lescol and Lescol XL are for people whose cholesterol has not come down enough with exercise and a low-fat diet alone.

Lescol and Lescol XL may also be used in people with heart disease (coronary artery disease) to slow the buildup of too much cholesterol in the arteries of the heart, and therefore lower the chances of needing procedures to help restore blood flow to the heart.

Lescol and Lescol XL are also prescribed for adolescents who have a hereditary form of high cholesterol and have not been able to lower it with exercise and a low-fat diet alone.

What is the most important information I should know about Lescol/Lescol XL?

Treatment with Lescol or Lescol XL has not been shown to prevent heart attacks or stroke.

Taking Lescol or Lescol XL is not a substitute for following a healthy low-fat and low-cholesterol diet and exercising to lower your cholesterol. Follow the diet and exercise program given to you by your health care provider.

Do not take this drug if you are pregnant, think you may be pregnant, or planning to become pregnant. Women who may become pregnant should use effective birth control while taking Lescol or Lescol XR. Check with your doctor if you have questions about using birth control.

Do not drive or perform other possibly unsafe tasks until you know how you react to this drug, as it may cause dizziness. This effect may be worse if you take it with alcohol or certain medicines.

Drinking alcohol daily or in large amounts may increase the risk of liver problems with Lescol. Check with your doctor before drinking alcohol while you are taking Lescol.

Tell your doctor or dentist that you take Lescol before you receive any medical or dental care, emergency care, or surgery.

Do not take more than the recommended dose without checking with your doctor.

Report any unexplained muscle pain, tenderness, or weakness to your doctor right away, especially if you also have a fever or general body discomfort.

Who should not take Lescol/Lescol XL?

Do not take Lescol or Lescol XL if you are pregnant, think you may be pregnant, or are planning to become pregnant, since this medication may harm an unborn baby. Likewise, do not take Lescol or Lescol XL if you are breastfeeding, as it can pass into your breast milk and may harm your baby.

Do not take Lescol or Lescol XL if you have liver problems or if you are allergic to the medication or any of its ingredients.

What should I tell my doctor before I take the first dose of Lescol/Lescol XL?

Tell your doctor about all prescription, over-the-counter, and herbal medications you are taking before beginning treatment with Lescol or Lescol XL. Also, talk to your doctor about your complete medical history, especially if you have low blood pressure, a serious infection, have recently undergone major surgery or had a serious injury, a history of seizures, chronic muscle aches or weakness; diabetes; or problems with your thyroid, kidneys, or liver. Also let the doctor know if you drink more than 2 glasses of alcohol daily.

Let your doctor know if you cannot swallow tablets whole. You may need Lescol capsules or a different medicine instead of Lescol XL tablets.

What is the usual dosage?

The information below is based on the dosage guidelines your doctor uses. Depending on your condition and medical history, your doctor may prescribe a different regimen. Do not change the dosage or stop taking your medication without your doctor's approval.

Lescol and Lescol XL have the same active ingredient. However, Lescol is a capsule that is taken 1 or 2 times a day and Lescol XL is an extended-release tablet that is taken once a day.

Adults: The recommended starting dose is dependent on your individual LDL cholesterol goal. If your goal requires more than a 25% reduction, the recommended starting dose is 40 milligrams (mg) once or twice daily (Lescol) and 80 mg once daily (Lescol XL). If your LDL goal requires less than a 25% reduction, a starting dose of 20 mg daily may be used.

Kidney impairment: Fluvastatin has not been studied at doses greater than 40 mg in patients with severe kidney impairment; therefore caution should be exercised when treating such patients at higher doses.

Adolescents 10 to 16 years: The recommended starting dose is one 20-mg Lescol capsule. The doctor will adjust the dose as needed, usually every 6 weeks, up to a maximum of 80 mg a day. The maximum dose can be taken either as one 40-mg Lescol capsule twice a day (morning and evening), or as a single 80-mg Lescol XL tablet taken in the evening.

Adolescent girls must have been menstruating for at least 1 year before taking Lescol or Lescol XL.

How should I take Lescol/Lescol XL?

Your doctor will likely start you on a low-fat and low-cholesterol diet and exercise plan before giving you Lescol or Lescol XL. Stay on this diet and exercise plan while taking the medication. Your doctor may do blood tests to check your cholesterol levels during treatment with Lescol or Lescol XL. Your dose may be changed based on these blood test results.

Take Lescol capsules or Lescol XL tablets at the same time every evening. Sometimes Lescol capsules are also taken every morning. Both medications should be swallowed whole with liquid, and they can be taken with or without food. Do not break, crush, or chew Lescol XL tablets or open Lescol capsules.

If you are taking a Lescol in addition to a bile acid resin (such as cholestyramine), Lescol should be administered at bedtime, at least 2 hours following the resin to avoid a significant interaction due to drug binding to resin.

Continue to take Lescol even if you feel well. Do not miss any doses.

What should I avoid while taking Lescol/Lescol XL?

Avoid getting pregnant or taking the medication while breastfeeding. If you do get pregnant, stop taking Lescol or Lescol XL right away and call your doctor.

Avoid missing any doses. Keep taking the medicine even if you feel well.

Do not drive or perform other possibly unsafe tasks until you know how you react to Lescol; this drug may cause dizziness. This effect may be worse if you take it with alcohol or certain medicines.

Avoid excessive alcohol use. Drinking daily or in large amounts may increase the risk of liver problems with Lescol. Check with your doctor before drinking alcohol while you are taking Lescol.

What are possible food and drug interactions associated with Lescol/Lescol XL?

If Lescol or Lescol XL is taken with certain other drugs, the effects of either could be increased, decreased, or altered. It is especially important to check with your doctor before combining either of these drugs with the following: blood thinners such as warfarin, cholestyramine, cimetidine, cyclosporine, diclofenac, digoxin, erythromycin, fibrates, fluconazole, gemfibrozil, glyburide, niacin, omeprazole, phenytoin, ranitidine, and rifampin.

In addition, tell your doctor if you take medicines for any of the following: your immune system, cholesterol, infections, heart failure, seizures, diabetes, and heartburn or stomach ulcers.

What are the possible side effects of Lescol/Lescol XL?

Side effects cannot be anticipated. If any develop or change in intensity, tell your doctor as soon as possible. Only your doctor can determine if it is safe for you to continue taking this drug.

Side effects may include: diarrhea, flu-like symptoms, headaches, muscle pain, sinus infection, stomach pain, stomach upset, tiredness, trouble sleeping

When taking Lescol or Lescol XL, some people may develop more serious side effects, such as severe muscle problems that can sometimes lead to kidney problems, including kidney failure. You have a higher chance for developing muscle problems if you are taking certain other medicines with Lescol or Lescol XL. Another serious side effect is liver problems. Your doctor may do blood tests to check your liver before you start taking Lescol or Lescol XL, and periodically during treatment.

Call your doctor right away if you have any of the following symptoms: muscle problems like weakness, tenderness, or pain that happen without a good reason; especially if you also have a fever or feel more tired than usual; nausea and vomiting; passing brown or dark-colored urine; feeling more tired than usual; your skin and the whites of your eyes are yellow; stomach pain

Can I receive Lescol/Lescol XL if I am pregnant or breastfeeding?

Do not use Lescol if you are pregnant, it may cause harm to the fetus. Avoid becoming pregnant while you are taking it. If you think you may be pregnant, contact your doctor right away. Do not breastfeed while you are taking Lescol; this drug is found in breast milk.

What should I do if I miss a dose of Lescol/Lescol XL?

If you miss a dose of Lescol or Lescol XL, take it as soon as you remember. If it has been more than 12 hours since your last dose, wait and take the next dose at your regular time. Do not take 2 doses of Lescol or Lescol XL at the same time.

How should I store Lescol/Lescol XL?

Store at room temperature and protect from light.

LETAIRIS
Generic name: Ambrisentan

What is Letairis?
Letairis is used to treat high blood pressure in the arteries of your lungs (pulmonary arterial hypertension, or PAH). It can help improve your ability to exercise and help slow down the worsening of your physical condition.

What is the most important information I should know about Letairis?
Letairis can cause liver injury. Your doctor will have your blood tested before you start Letairis and once a month after that to check your liver function.

Letairis can cause serious birth defects if taken during pregnancy. Women must not be pregnant when they start taking Letairis or become pregnant while on this medication. Women who are able to get pregnant must have a negative pregnancy test before beginning treatment and each month during treatment. Women who are able to get pregnant must use two different methods of birth control at the same time during treatment with Letairis and for 1 month after stopping Letairis. If you miss your period or think you may be pregnant, tell your doctor right away.

Letairis is only available through a restricted program called the Letairis Education and Access Program (LEAP). In order to receive this medication, you must talk to your doctor, understand the risks and benefits of taking this medication, and agree to all of the instructions in the LEAP program.

Who should not take Letairis?
Do not take Letairis if you are pregnant or become pregnant during treatment with Letairis. You also should not take Letairis if your blood tests show possible liver injury.

What should I tell my doctor before I take the first dose of Letairis?
Tell your doctor about all prescription, over-the-counter, and herbal medications you are taking before beginning treatment with Letairis. Also, talk to your doctor about your complete medical history, especially if you are pregnant, plan to become pregnant, or have liver problems.

What is the usual dosage?
The information below is based on the dosage guidelines your doctor uses. Depending on your condition and medical history, your doctor may prescribe a different regimen. Do not change the dosage or stop taking your medication without your doctor's approval.

Adults: The usual initial dosage is 5 milligrams (mg) once daily with or without food. Your doctor may increase your dose to 10 mg once daily if the lower dose is well tolerated.

How should I take Letairis?
You may take Letairis with or without food. The tablets should be swallowed whole and not split, crushed, or chewed.

What should I avoid while taking Letairis?
Avoid becoming pregnant while on this medication. Also, avoid breastfeeding your baby while on this medication unless your doctor instructs otherwise.

What are possible food and drug interactions associated with Letairis?
If Letairis is taken with certain other drugs, the effects of either could be increased, decreased, or altered. It is especially important to check with your doctor before combining Letairis with cyclosporine A, ketoconazole, or omeprazole.

What are the possible side effects of Letairis?
Side effects cannot be anticipated. If any develop or change in intensity, tell your doctor as soon as possible. Only your doctor can determine if it is safe for you to continue taking this drug.

Side effects may include: fluid retention; swelling of hands, legs, ankles, and feet; stuffy nose; flushing; stomach pain; constipation; headache; shortness of breath; sinus inflammation; palpitations; red and sore throat and nose

Can I receive Letairis if I am pregnant or breastfeeding?
You cannot take Letairis if you are pregnant or plan to become pregnant due to the potential harm to the baby. Breastfeeding is not recommended while on this medication.

What should I do if I miss a dose of Letairis?
If you miss a dose, take it as soon as you remember that day. Then, take your next dose at the regular time the next day. Do not take two doses at the same time to make up for a missed dose.

How should I store Letairis?
Store Letairis at room temperature in the package it comes in.

Levalbuterol *See Xopenex, page 1432, or Xopenex HFA, page 1435.*

LEVAQUIN
Generic name: Levofloxacin

What is Levaquin?
Levaquin is a quinolone antibiotic used to treat many types of bacteria that can infect the lungs, sinuses, skin, and urinary tract in adults.

What is the most important information I should know about Levaquin?
Serious and sometimes fatal allergic reactions have been reported in people taking Levaquin. If you know that you are allergic to some antibiotics, you may also be allergic to Levaquin. Talk to your doctor about all of the antibiotics to which you are allergic. Contact your doctor if your condition is not improving while taking Levaquin.

You may begin to feel better quickly; however, in order to make sure that all bacteria are killed, you should complete the full course of medication. Do not take more than the prescribed dose of Levaquin even if you missed a dose by mistake. You should not take a double dose.

Sometimes viruses rather than bacteria may infect the lungs and sinuses (for example, the common cold). Levaquin like other antibiotics does not kill viruses.

Long-term or repeated use of Levaquin may cause a second infection. Tell your doctor if signs of a second infection occur. Your medicine may need to be changed to treat this.

Liver damage has been reported in patients receiving Levaquin. Call your doctor right away if you have unexplained symptoms such as nausea or vomiting, stomach pain, fever, weakness, abdominal pain or tenderness, itching, unusual or unexplained tiredness, loss of appetite, light colored bowel movements, dark colored urine or yellowing of your skin or the whites of your eyes.

Pain, swelling, and tears of the Achilles, shoulder, or hand tendons have been reported in patients receiving Levaquin. The risk for tendon tears is higher if you are over 65 years old and if you are taking corticosteroids. If you develop pain, swelling, or rupture of a tendon, you should stop taking Levaquin, avoid exercise and strenuous use of the affected area, and contact your healthcare professional.

Sun sensitivity (photosensitivity), which can appear as skin eruptions or severe sunburn, can occur in some patients taking quinolone antibiotics after exposure to sunlight or artificial ultraviolet (UV) light (eg, tanning beds). Avoid excessive exposure to sunlight or artificial UV light while taking Levaquin. Use sunscreen and wear protective clothing if out in the sun. If photosensitivity develops, contact your physician.

Do not drive or perform other possibly unsafe tasks until you know how you react to Levaquin; this drug may cause dizziness or lightheadedness. These effects may be worse if you take it with alcohol or certain medicines.

If you have diabetes and you develop a hypoglycemic (low sugar in the blood) reaction while on Levaquin; you should stop taking Levaquin and call your healthcare professional.

Convulsions have been reported in patients receiving quinolone antibiotics, including Levaquin. If you have experienced convulsions in the past, be sure to let your physician know that you have a history of convulsions.

Quinolones, including Levaquin, may also cause central nervous system stimulation, which may lead to tremors, restlessness, anxiety, lightheadedness, confusion, hallucinations, paranoia, depression, nightmares, insomnia, and rarely, suicidal thoughts or acts.

Diarrhea that usually ends after treatment is a common problem caused by antibiotics. A more serious form of diarrhea can occur during or up to 2 months after the use of antibiotics. If you develop a watery and bloody stool with or without stomach cramps and fever, contact your physician as soon as possible.

In a few people, Levaquin like some other antibiotics may produce a small effect on the heart that is seen on an electrocardiogram test. The rare heart problem is called QT prolongation and can cause an abnormal heartbeat and can be very dangerous. The chances of this event are increased in those with a family history of prolonged QT interval, low potassium, and who are taking drugs to control heart rhythm, called class IA (quinidine, procainamide) or class III (amiodarone, sotalol) antiarrhythmic agents. You should call your healthcare professional right away if you have any prolonged heart palpitations (a change in the way your heart beats) or a loss of consciousness (fainting spells).

Levaquin may produce false-positive urine screening results for opiates using commercially available immunoassay kits. Confirmation of positive opiate screens by more specific methods may be necessary.

Who should not take Levaquin?

Do not take Levaquin if you are allergic to the medication; any of its ingredients; or to any other quinolones, such as ciprofloxacin. Levaquin is not recommended for children. Levaquin is also not recommended for use by pregnant or nursing women.

What should I tell my doctor before I take the first dose of Levaquin?

Tell your doctor about all prescription, over-the-counter, and herbal medications you are taking before beginning treatment with Levaquin. Also, talk to your doctor about your complete medical history, especially if you have diabetes, liver problems, tendon problems (inflammation), Alzheimer's disease, irregular heartbeat, history of chest pain or heart attack, kidney disease, or a history of convulsions.

What is the usual dosage?

The information below is based on the dosage guidelines your doctor uses. Depending on your condition and medical history, your doctor may prescribe a different regimen. Do not change the dosage or stop taking your medication without your doctor's approval.

Adults >18 years: Levaquin tablets or oral solution may be prescribed at 250, 500, or 750 milligrams (mg) daily. Levaquin oral solution comes in a dose of 25 mg per milliliter (mL).

The usual dose of Levaquin Injection is 250 mg or 500 mg administered by slow infusion over 60 minutes every 24 hours or 750 mg administered by slow infusion over 90 minutes every 24 hours.

Anthrax Inhalation Infection

Adults and children >50 kg and >6 years: The usual dose is 500 mg taken 1 time each day for 60 days.

If the child weighs >50kg, the preferred dose is 8 mg per kilogram (not exceeding 250 mg per dose) 2 times a day for 60 days.

The safety of Levaquin use in adults for more than 28 days or in pediatric use for more than 14 days has not been studied. Therefore, prolonged Levaquin treatment should only be used when the benefit outweighs the risk.

Respiratory Tract Infection

Adults: The usual dose for bronchitis and pneumonia is 500 mg taken 1 time each day for 7 to 14 days, or 750 mg taken 1 time each day for 5 to 14 days. The usual dose for sinus infections is 500 mg taken daily for 10 to 14 days, or 750 mg taken daily for 5 days.

Skin Infection

Adults: The usual dose is 500, or 750 mg taken daily for 7 to 14 days.

Urinary Tract Infection, and Prostate and Kidney Inflammation

Adults: The usual dose for urinary tract infections is 250 mg taken daily for 3 to 10 days. Chronic prostate inflammation is treated with 500 mg taken daily for 28 days; kidney inflammation is treated with 250 mg taken daily for 10 days.

How should I take Levaquin?

Levaquin should be taken once a day for the full number of days it has been prescribed. Levaquin tablets should be swallowed and may be taken with or without food. Levaquin oral solution should be taken 1 hour before or 2 hours after eating. Try to take Levaquin at the same time each day, and make sure to drink a lot of fluids while you are taking Levaquin. Many antacids and multivitamins may interfere with the absorption of Levaquin. Therefore, you should take Levaquin either 2 hours before or 2 hours after taking these products.

Do not use Levaquin injection if it contains particles, is cloudy or discolored, or if the vial is cracked or damaged. Keep this product, as well as syringes and needles, out of the reach of children and pets. Do not reuse needles, syringes, or other materials. Ask your health care provider how to dispose of these materials after use. Follow all local rules for disposal.

You may begin to feel better quickly; however, in order to make sure that all bacteria are killed, you should complete the full course of medication. Do not take more than the prescribed dose of Levaquin even if you missed a dose by mistake. You should not take a double dose.

What should I avoid while taking Levaquin?

You should be careful about driving or operating machinery until you are sure Levaquin does not make you dizzy. Some quinolone antibiotics have been associated with a higher sensitivity to the sun or other sources of ultraviolet light, such as the artificial ultraviolet light used in tanning salons. You should avoid excessive exposure to sunlight or artificial ultraviolet light while you are taking Levaquin. Use sunscreen and wear protective clothing if out in the sun.

Do not stop taking Levaquin or alter the dose of this medication without first contacting your doctor.

Do not use Levaquin injection if it contains particles, is cloudy or discolored, or if the vial is cracked or damaged. Do not reuse needles, syringes, or other materials.

What are possible food and drug interactions associated with Levaquin?

If Levaquin is taken with certain other drugs, the effects of either could be increased, decreased, or altered. It is especially important to check with your doctor before combining Levaquin with the following medications: amiodarone, antacids, antidepressants astemizole, cisapride, corticosteroids such as prednisone, didanosine, dofetilide, droperidol, haloperidol, ketoconazole, insulin or oral diabetes medicines, iron, macrolide antibiotics such as erythromycin, methadone, multivitamins, NSAIDs, paliperidone, phenothiazines such as chlorpromazine, pimozide, procainamide, quinidine, ranolazine, sotalol, sucralfate, telithromycin, theophylline, warfarin

What are the possible side effects of Levaquin?

Side effects cannot be anticipated. If any develop or change in intensity, tell your doctor as soon as possible. Only your doctor can determine if it is safe for you to continue taking this drug.

Side effects may include: abdominal pain, diarrhea, dizziness, gas, itching, nausea, rash, vaginal irritation in women

If you develop other serious side effects, you should let your doctor know as soon as they occur. You should stop taking Levaquin and call your doctor right away if you develop any of the following: hives, skin rash, or other symptoms of an allergic reaction, low blood sugar reaction, pain, swelling, or rupture of a tendon, pain, tingling, numbness, and/or weakness in general.

You may get diarrhea that ends after your treatment with Levaquin stops. However, Levaquin may also lead to a more serious type of diarrhea that can occur up to 2 months after you stop taking the medication. If you have watery or bloody stools, which may or may not be accompanied by stomach cramps and fever, call your doctor right away.

Can I receive Levaquin if I am pregnant or breastfeeding?
The effects of Levaquin during pregnancy and breastfeeding are unknown. Tell your doctor immediately if you are pregnant, plan to become pregnant, or are breastfeeding.

What should I do if I miss a dose of Levaquin?
If you miss a dose of Levaquin, take it as soon as your remember. But, do not take more than the prescribed dose of Levaquin. You should not take 2 doses at once.

How should I store Levaquin?
Store Levaquin at room temperature, in a tightly closed container.

LEVEMIR
Generic name: Insulin detemir [rDNA origin]

What is Levemir?
Levemir is used once or twice daily for the treatment of adults or children with diabetes mellitus type 1, or adults with diabetes mellitus type 2 who require long-acting insulin to control their high blood sugar levels.

What is the most important information I should know about Levemir?
Do not make any changes with your insulin dose unless you have talked to your doctor. Your insulin needs may change because of illness, stress, other medicines, or changes in diet or activity level. Talk to your doctor about adjusting your insulin dose and before engaging in any new activity (such as a new exercise regimen or diet plan). Illness, especially with nausea and vomiting, may cause your insulin requirements to change. Even if you are not eating, you still require insulin. You and your doctor should establish a sick day plan to use in case of illness. When you are sick, test your blood/urine frequently and call your doctor as instructed.

Take Levemir exactly as prescribed. Do not miss any doses. Contact your doctor if you missed a dose.

Do not use Levemir with an insulin infusion pump. Do NOT dilute Levemir Cartridges or mix it with other insulin.

Consuming alcohol, including beer and wine, may increase and lengthen the risk of hypoglycemia (overly low blood sugar) when you take Levemir. Do not drink alcohol without discussing it first with your doctor.

Be careful when you drive a car or operate machinery until you know how you respond to Levemir. Your ability to concentrate or react may be reduced if you have hypoglycemia. Ask your doctor if you should drive if you have frequent hypoglycemia or reduced or absent warning signs of hypoglycemia.

Tell your doctor or dentist that you take Levemir before you receive any medical or dental care, emergency care, or surgery. Carry an ID card at all times that says you have diabetes.

An insulin reaction resulting from low blood sugar levels (hypoglycemia) may occur if you take too much insulin, skip a meal, or exercise too much. It is a good idea to carry a reliable source of glucose (eg, tablets or gel) to treat low blood sugar. If this is not available, you should eat or drink a quick source of sugar like table sugar, honey, candy, orange juice, or non-diet soda. This will raise your blood sugar level quickly. Tell your doctor right away if this happens. To prevent low blood sugar, eat meals at the same time each day and do not skip meals.

Developing a fever or infection, eating significantly more than prescribed, or missing your dose of insulin may cause high blood sugar (hyperglycemia). High blood sugar may make you feel confused, drowsy, or thirsty. It can also make you flush, breathe faster, or have a fruit-like breath odor. If these symptoms occur, tell your doctor right away.

Lab tests, including fasting blood glucose levels or hemoglobin A_{1c}, may be performed while you use Levemir. Be sure to keep all doctor and lab appointments.

Who should not take Levemir?
Do not take Levemir if you are allergic to any of its ingredients.

What should I tell my doctor before I take the first dose of Levemir?
Tell your doctor about all prescription, over-the-counter, and herbal medications you are taking to avoid a possible interaction with Levemir. Also talk with your doctor about your complete medical history, especially if you have nerve problems, thyroid problems, adrenal gland problems, pituitary problems, diabetic ketoacidosis, use 3 or more injections daily, are fasting, have high blood sodium levels, are on a low-salt diet, or have kidney or liver problems.

What is the usual dosage?
The information below is based on the dosage guidelines your doctor uses. Depending on your condition and medical history, your doctor may prescribe a different regimen. Do not change the dosage or stop taking your medication without your doctor's approval.

Doses of insulin are measured in units. Levemir is available as a U-100 insulin. One milliliter (mL) of U-100 contains 100 units of insulin detemir. (1 mL = 1 cc). Only U-100 type syringes should be used for injection to ensure proper dosing.

Adults and children 6 to 17 years: The usual dosage of Levemir is taken once or twice a day. If it is prescribed once daily, it should be taken with either your morning or evening meal. If Levemir is prescribed twice-daily, then take a morning dose, and then an evening dose may be taken either 12 hours after the morning dose, with your evening meal, or at bedtime. The dose of Levemir should be adjusted according to measurements of sugar in your blood.

How should I take Levemir?
Inspect Levemir visually prior to administration and only use if the solution appears clear, odorless, and colorless.

Use the proper injection technique taught to you by your doctor. Refer to the package insert that accompanies Levemir for detailed instructions.

Inject Levemir deep under the skin, NOT into a vein or muscle. Injection sites within an injection area (abdomen, thigh, upper arm) must be rotated from one injection to the next. Check with your doctor if you notice a depression in the skin or skin thickening at the injection site. You may need to change your injection technique.

Levemir should not be mixed or diluted with any other insulin preparations.

Follow your doctor's instructions about monitoring your blood sugar. Do not make any changes with your insulin unless you have talked to your doctor. Your insulin needs may change because of illness, stress, other medicines, or changes in diet or activity level. Talk to your doctor about how to adjust your insulin dose. If you will be traveling across time zones, consult your doctor concerning adjustments in your insulin schedule.

It is important that you use a new needle for each injection. After each injection, remove the needle without recapping and dispose of it in a puncture-resistant container.

What should I avoid while taking Levemir?
Do not inject Levemir in the same place twice; rotate injection sites. Do not mix this insulin with any other insulin, and should only be used if the solution is clear and colorless.

Do NOT take more than the recommended dose, use more often than prescribed, or change the type or dose of insulin you are using without checking with your doctor. Do not miss a Levemir dose.

Consuming alcohol, including beer and wine, may increase and lengthen the risk of hypoglycemia (too low blood sugar) when you take Levemir. Be careful when you drive a car or operate machinery until you know how you react to Levemir. Your ability to concentrate or react may be reduced if you have hypoglycemia. Ask your doctor if you should drive if you have frequent hypoglycemia or reduced or absent warning signs of hypoglycemia. Exercise or activity level may change the way your body uses insulin. Check with your doctor before you start an exercise program because your dose may need to be changed.

What are possible food and drug interactions associated with Levemir?

If Levemir is taken with certain other drugs, the effects of either could be increased, decreased, or altered. It is especially important to check with your doctor before combining Levemir with the following: ACE inhibitors, antidiabetic drugs (oral), beta-blockers, clonidine, corticosteroids, danazol, disopyramide, diuretics, estrogens, fibrates, fluoxetine, guanethidine, isoniazid, MAO inhibitors, phenothiazine derivatives, progestogens (eg, in oral contraceptives), propoxyphene, reserpine, salicylates, somatostatin analog (eg, octreotide), somatropin, sulfonamide antibiotics, sympathomimetic agents (eg, epinephrine, albuterol, terbutaline), thyroid hormones

What are the possible side effects of Levemir?

Side effects cannot be anticipated. If any develop or change in intensity, tell your doctor as soon as possible. Only your doctor can determine if it is safe for you to continue taking this drug.

Side effects may include: allergic reactions/injection site reactions, low blood sugar (hypoglycemia), rash, weight gain

Hyperglycemia (high blood sugar) is a common side effect. It also occurs when there is a conflict between the amount of carbohydrates (source of glucose) from your food, the amount of glucose used by your body, and the amount and timing of insulin dosing. Speak to your doctor about the warning signs of hypoglycemia.

Developing a fever or infection, eating significantly more than prescribed, or missing your dose of insulin may cause high blood sugar (hyperglycemia). High blood sugar may make you feel confused, drowsy, or thirsty. It can also make you flush, breathe faster, or have a fruit-like breath odor. If these symptoms occur, tell your doctor right away.

In patients with type 1 or insulin-dependent diabetes, long-lasting hyperglycemia can cause diabetic ketoacidosis (DKA). The first symptoms of DKA usually come on slowly, over a period of hours or days, and include feeling drowsy, flushed face, thirst, loss of appetite, and fruity odor on the breath. With DKA, urine tests show large amounts of glucose and ketones. Heavy breathing and a rapid pulse are more severe symptoms.

If uncorrected, long-lasting hyperglycemia or DKA can lead to nausea, vomiting, stomach pains, dehydration, loss of consciousness, or even death. Therefore, it is important that you obtain medical help right away.

What should I do if I miss a dose of Levemir?

It is very important to follow your insulin regimen exactly. Do NOT miss any doses. Ask your doctor for specific instructions to follow in case you ever miss a dose of insulin.

Can I receive Levemir if I am pregnant or breastfeeding?

Before taking Levemir, talk to your doctor if you are pregnant, planning to become pregnant, or are breastfeeding. There is a risk of Levemir causing harm to your unborn baby, or passing through your breast milk.

How should I store Levemir?

Unopened vials and PenFill cartridges: Store unopened vials and Pen-Fill cartridges in a refrigerator (36°F to 46°F; 2°C to 8°C) but not in the freezer. Do not use Levemir if it has been frozen. Keep unopened Levemir vials and PenFill cartridges in the carton so they will stay clean and protected from light because the product is light sensitive.

Punctured vials: After initial use, the punctured vials should be stored in a refrigerator but not in a freezer. If refrigeration is not possible, the vial that you are currently using can be kept at room temperature up to 42 days, as long as it is kept below 30°C [86°F]. Throw away un-refrigerated vials after 42 days from the first use, even if they still contain insulin.

Punctured cartridges: After initial use (the rubber membrane has been punctured), do not refrigerate the punctured Levemir PenFill cartridges. However, keep them as cool as possible (below 30°C [86°F]). The PenFill cartridge that you are currently using can be kept at room temperature up to 42 days, as long as they are kept below 30°C [86°F]. Throw away unrefrigerated disposable Levemir PenFill cartridges after 42 days from the cartridges first use, even if it still contains Levemir.

Keep all disposable PenFill cartridges and vials away from direct heat and sunlight.

***Levetiracetam** See Keppra/Keppra XR, page 685.*

LEVITRA
Generic name: Vardenafil hydrochloride

What is Levitra?

Levitra is used to treat erectile dysfunction (ED) in men. Levitra helps increase blood flow to the penis during sexual stimulation, helping to achieve and sustain an erection.

What is the most important information I should know about Levitra?

Levitra can cause your blood pressure to drop suddenly to an unsafe level if it is taken with certain other medicines. A sudden drop in blood pressure could cause you to get dizzy, faint, or have a heart attack or stroke. Sit up or stand slowly, especially in the morning. Alcohol, hot weather, exercise, or fever may increase these effects. Sit or lie down at the first sign of any of these effects.

Do not take Levitra if you take any medicines called nitrates, or if you use any recreational drugs called poppers. Tell all your healthcare providers that you take Levitra. If you need emergency medical care for a heart problem, it will be important for your healthcare provider to know when you last took Levitra.

Levitra does not increase a man's sexual desire; protect a man or his partner against sexually transmitted diseases; serve as a male form of birth control; or cure erectile dysfunction (ED).

Do not drive or perform other possibly unsafe tasks until you know how you react to Levitra; this drug may cause dizziness, drowsiness, fainting, or blurred vision. These effects may be worse if you take it with alcohol or certain medicines.

Patients with heart problems who take Levitra may be at increased risk for heart-related side effects, including heart attack or stroke. Symptoms of a heart attack may include chest, shoulder, neck, or jaw pain; numbness of an arm or leg; severe dizziness, headache, nausea, stomach pain, or vomiting; fainting; or vision changes. Symptoms of a stroke may include confusion; vision or speech changes; one-sided weakness; or fainting. Contact your doctor or seek medical attention right away if you experience these symptoms.

Levitra may rarely cause a prolonged, painful erection. This could happen even when you are not having sex. If this is not treated right away, it could lead to permanent sexual problems such as impotence. Contact your doctor right away if this happens.

Levitra may uncommonly cause mild, temporary vision changes (such as blurred vision, sensitivity to light, blue/green color tint to vision). Contact your doctor if vision changes persist or are severe.

Who should not take Levitra?

Levitra is not for women or for children under the age of 18. Do not take Levitra if you have been told by your doctor not to have sexual activity because of health problems. Sexual activity can put an extra strain on your heart, especially if your heart is already weak from a heart attack (within the past 6 months) or heart disease. Do not take Levitra if you are allergic to it or any of its ingredients.

Do not take Levitra if you are taking medicines called nitrates. Nitrates are commonly used to treat angina—a symptom of heart disease that causes pain in your chest, jaw, or down your arm. Nitrates include nitroglycerin, which is found in tablets, sprays, ointments, pastes, or patches. Nitrates can also be found in other medicines, such as isosorbide dinitrate or isosorbide mononitrate. Some recreational drugs called poppers, such as amyl nitrate and butyl nitrate, also contain nitrates. Do not use Levitra if you are using these drugs. Ask your doctor or pharmacist if you are not sure if any of your medicines are nitrates.

Do not take Levitra if you have low blood pressure, uncontrolled high blood pressure, certain hereditary degenerative eye problems (retinitis pigmentosa), and severe liver or kidney problems (that require dialysis). Talk to your doctor to see if you can use Levitra.

What should I tell my doctor before I take the first dose of Levitra?

Tell your doctor about all prescription, over-the-counter, and herbal medications you are taking before beginning treatment with Levitra. Also, talk to your doctor about your complete medical history, especially if you have heart problems such as angina, heart failure, irregular heartbeat, or have had a heart attack or stroke. Ask your doctor if it is safe for you to have sexual activity. Tell your doctor if you or any family members have a rare heart condition known as prolongation of the QT interval. Let your doctor know if you have a deformed penis shape; Peyronie's disease; or if you have had an erection that lasted more than 4 hours. Also, tell your doctor if you have eye problems, such as retinitis pigmentosa; severe vision loss; macular degeneration; or nonarteritic anterior ischemic optic neuropathy (NAION). Other conditions that you should discuss with your doctor include: bleeding problems, blood cell problems (such as sickle cell anemia, cancer of the plasma cells, or leukemia), kidney problems, liver problems, low blood pressure, stomach ulcers, uncontrolled high blood pressure.

What is the usual dosage?

The information below is based on the dosage guidelines your doctor uses. Depending on your condition and medical history, your doctor may prescribe a different regimen. Do not change the dosage or stop taking your medication without your doctor's approval.

Adults >18 years: The usual dose of Levitra is 10 milligrams (mg) taken no more than 1 time each day, 1 hour before sexual activity. The dose may be increased to a maximum recommended dose of 20 mg or decreased to 5 mg based on efficacy and side effects, The maximum recommended dosing frequency is once per day.

Elderly: Older patients, 65 years and older, should start with a daily dose of 5 mg.

Liver impairment: Should start with a daily dose of 5mg. No dosage adjustment is required in these patients. Those with moderate liver impairment should not exceed a daily dose of 10mg.

Levitra may be altered by other medications. Talk to your doctor about all of the medication that you are currently taking and how they may potentially affect Levitra dosage.

How should I take Levitra?

Take 1 Levitra tablet about 1 hour before sexual activity. Some form of sexual stimulation is needed for an erection to happen with Levitra. Levitra may be taken with or without food. Do not take Levitra more often than once daily, or as directed by your doctor.

What should I avoid while taking Levitra?

Do not use Levitra with medicines or drugs containing nitrates. Also, medicines called alpha-blockers, which are sometimes prescribed for prostate problems or high blood pressure, can cause problems when they are taken with Levitra. Taking both drugs can lower blood pressure significantly and lead to fainting. You should contact your doctor if alpha-blockers or other drugs that lower blood pressure are prescribed to you by another physician.

Do not drive or perform other possibly unsafe tasks until you know how you react to Levitra; this drug may cause dizziness, drowsiness, fainting, or blurred vision. These effects may be worse if you take it with alcohol or certain medicines.

Do not take Levitra more than once in a 24-hour period.

Do not sit or stand up too quickly when you start taking Levitra, especially in the morning. Sit or lie down at the first sign of dizziness.

What are possible food and drug interactions associated with Levitra?

If Levitra is taken with certain other drugs, the effects of either could be increased, decreased, or altered. It is especially important to check with your doctor before combining Levitra with the following: alfuzosin, doxazosin, erythromycin, indinavir, itraconazole, ketoconazole, medicines that treat abnormal heartbeat, including quinidine, procainamide, amiodarone, and sotalol, nitrates, other medicines or treatments for ED, prazosin, ritonavir, tamsulosin, terazosin

What are the possible side effects of Levitra?

Side effects cannot be anticipated. If any develop or change in intensity, tell your doctor as soon as possible. Only your doctor can determine if it is safe for you to continue taking this drug.

Side effects may include: dizziness, flushing, headache, indigestion, runny or stuffy nose, upset stomach

Levitra may also lead to some other less common side effects. Priapism, or an erection that won't go away, is an uncommon but serious side effect of Levitra. If you get an erection that lasts more than 4 hours, you should get medical help right away. Levitra may also lead to color vision changes, such as seeing a blue tinge to objects or having difficulty telling the difference between the colors blue and green. If you experience a sudden decrease or loss of vision in one or both eyes, seek medical attention immediately.

What should I do if I miss a dose of Levitra?
If you miss a dose of Levitra and you still intend to engage in sexual activity, take it as soon as you remember. Continue to take it as directed by your doctor.

Can I receive Levitra if I am pregnant or breastfeeding?
Levitra is not for women and children.

How should I store Levitra?
Store Levitra at 77 degrees F (25 degrees C). Brief storage at temperatures between 59 and 86 degrees F (15 and 30 degrees C) is permitted.
   Store away from heat, moisture, and light. Do not store in the bathroom.

Levocetirizine See Xyzal, page 1437.

Levofloxacin See Levaquin, page 718.

Levonorgestrel See Plan B, page 1028.

Levonorgestrel and ethinyl estradiol See Lybrel, page 780, or Seasonique, page 1177.

Levothyroxine sodium See Synthroid, page 1247.

LEVSIN
Generic name: Hyoscyamine sulfate

What is Levsin?
Levsin is used to treat stomach, intestinal, and urinary tract disorders that involve cramps, colic, bladder spasms, peptic ulcer disease, diverticulitis, irritable bowel syndrome, cystitis, pancreatitis, or other painful muscle contractions. It also helps to reduce the rigidity, tremors, and runny nose commonly associated with Parkinson's disease.
   Levsin also reduces secretions and can help control conditions such as excessive sweating and drooling. In addition, Levsin is used before surgery to reduce secretions of the nose, lungs, salivary glands, and stomach.

What is the most important information I should know about Levsin?

Levsin may make you sweat less, causing your body temperature to increase and putting you at risk of heat stroke. Avoid becoming overheated in hot weather or while you are being active.

Do not drive or perform other possibly unsafe tasks until you know how you react to Levsin; this drug may cause drowsiness, dizziness, blurred vision, or lightheadedness. These effects may be worse if you take it with alcohol or certain medicines.

Levsin will add to the effects of alcohol and other medicines that may cause drowsiness (such as sleep aids and muscle relaxants). Ask your pharmacist if you have any questions about which medicines may cause drowsiness.

Caution is advised when using Levsin in children; they may be more sensitive to its effects. Safety and effectiveness in children >2 years have not been confirmed.

Who should not take Levsin?

Do not take Levsin if you have bowel or digestive tract obstruction or paralysis, glaucoma, myasthenia gravis, severe ulcerative colitis, or urinary tract disorders.

People who must avoid phenylalanine should not take NuLev tablets (one available form of Levsin).

What should I tell my doctor before I take the first dose of Levsin?

Tell your doctor about all prescription, over-the-counter, and herbal medications you are taking before beginning treatment with Levsin. Also, talk to your doctor about your complete medical history, especially if you have: heart or blood vessel problems such as an irregular heartbeat, heart disease, prostate problems, nerve problems, diarrhea, fever, have been very ill or are in poor health, if you are at risk of glaucoma, have hiatal hernia associated with inflammation of the lower part of the esophagus, high blood pressure, kidney disease, numbness or tingling in your hands or feet, thyroid problems.

What is the usual dosage?

The information below is based on the dosage guidelines your doctor uses. Depending on your condition and medical history, your doctor may prescribe a different regimen. Do not change the dosage or stop taking your medication without your doctor's approval.

Levsin comes in several forms, including tablets, sublingual (dissolved under the tongue) tablets, tablets that dissolve on the tongue (NuLev), sustained-release capsules (Levsinex Timecaps), sustained-release tablets (Levbid), liquid, drops, and an injectable solution.

Levsin, Levsin/SL, and NuLev Tablets
Adults and children ≥12 years: The usual dose is 1 to 2 tablets every 4 hours or as needed. Do not take more than 12 tablets in 24 hours.

Children 2 to <12 years: The usual dose is ½ to 1 tablet every 4 hours or as needed. Do not give your child more than 6 tablets in 24 hours.

Levsin Elixir
Adults and children ≥12 years: The recommended dosage is 1 to 2 teaspoonfuls every 4 hours or as needed. Do not take more than 12 teaspoonfuls in 24 hours.

Children 2 to <12 years: Dosage is by body weight and will be determined by your doctor. Doses may be given every 4 hours or as needed. Do not give your child more than 6 teaspoonfuls in 24 hours.

Levbid Extended-Release Tablets
Adults and children ≥12 years: The dosage is 1 to 2 tablets every 12 hours. The tablets are scored so that you can break them in half if your doctor wants you to. Do not crush or chew them. You should not take more than 4 tablets in 24 hours.

Levsin Drops
Adults and children ≥12 years: The recommended dosage is 1 to 2 milliliters (mL) every 4 hours or as needed, but no more than 12 mL in 24 hours.

Children 2 to <12 years: The usual dosage is ¼ to 1 mL every 4 hours or as needed. Do not give your child more than 6 mL in 24 hours.

Children <2 years: Your doctor will determine the dosage based on body weight. The doses may be repeated every 4 hours or as needed.

Levsinex Timecaps
Adults and children ≥12 years: The recommended dosage is 1 to 2 capsules every 12 hours. Your doctor may adjust the dosage to 1 capsule every 8 hours as needed. Do not take more than 4 capsules in 24 hours.

How should I take Levsin?

Take Levsin exactly as prescribed. Although the sublingual tablets (Levsin/SL) are designed to be dissolved under the tongue, they may also be chewed or swallowed. The regular tablets should be swallowed. Do not crush or chew Levbid extended-release tablets. NuLev tablets should be placed on the tongue, allowed to melt, and then swallowed. They can be taken with or without water.

Levsin is usually taken 30 to 60 minutes before a meal. Follow your doctor's specific instructions for taking Levsin.

Make sure to measure the liquid form of Levsin with a special dose-measuring spoon or cup, not with a regular tablespoon.

If you are taking antacids, take Levsin before meals and the antacids after meals.

Levsin can cause dry mouth. For temporary relief, suck on a hard candy or chew gum.

Proper dental care is important while you are taking Levsin. Brush and floss your teeth and visit the dentist regularly.

Levsin may make your eyes more sensitive to sunlight. It may help to wear sunglasses.

What should I avoid while taking Levsin?

Levsin may cause dizziness, drowsiness, or blurred vision. Use caution when driving, operating machinery, or performing other hazardous activities. Avoid using alcohol. It may increase drowsiness and dizziness while you are taking Levsin.

Avoid becoming overheated. Levsin may make you sweat less and you may be at greater risk of heat stroke.

What are possible food and drug interactions associated with Levsin?

If Levsin is taken with certain other drugs, the effects of either could be increased, decreased, or altered. It is especially important to check with your doctor before combining Levsin with the following: antimuscarinics such as dicyclomine, amantadine, antacids, antidepressants (including MAOIs and tricyclics), antihistamines, haloperidol, tranquilizers such as chlorpromazine and prochlorperazine

What are the possible side effects of Levsin?

Side effects cannot be anticipated. If any develop or change in intensity, tell your doctor as soon as possible. Only your doctor can determine if it is safe for you to continue taking this drug.

Side effects may include: allergic reactions, bloating, blurred vision, confusion, constipation, decreased sweating, dilated pupils, dizziness, drowsiness, dry mouth, excitement, headache, heart palpitations, hives, impotence, inability to urinate, insomnia, itching, lack of coordination, loss of sense of taste, nausea, nervousness, rapid heartbeat, skin reactions, speech problems, vomiting, weakness

Can I receive Levsin if I am pregnant or breastfeeding?

The effects of Levsin during pregnancy and breastfeeding are unknown. Tell your doctor immediately if you are pregnant, plan to become pregnant, or are breastfeeding. Use caution when breastfeeding because Levsin is found in breast milk.

What should I do if I miss a dose of Levsin?

Take it as soon as you remember. If it is almost time for your next dose, skip the missed dose and go back to your regular schedule. Do not take 2 doses at once.

How should I store Levsin?

Store Levsin at room temperature. Store away from heat, moisture, and light. Do not store in the bathroom.

LEXAPRO

Generic name: Escitalopram oxalate

What is Lexapro?

Lexapro is used to treat major depression in adults and adolescents 12 to 17 years old. Lexapro is also used to treat generalized anxiety disorder in adults.

What is the most important information I should know about Lexapro?

Lexapro is not approved for use in children less than 12 years old.

Antidepressant medicines may increase suicidal thoughts or actions in some children, teenagers, and young adults when the medicine is first started. Depression and other serious mental illnesses are the most important causes of suicidal thoughts and actions. Some people may have a particularly high risk of having suicidal thoughts or actions. These include people who have (or have a family history of) bipolar disorder (also called manic-depressive illness) or suicidal thoughts or actions.

Pay close attention to any changes, especially sudden ones, in mood, behaviors, thoughts, or feelings. This is very important when an antidepressant medicine is first started or when the dose is changed.

Call your doctor right away to report new or sudden changes in mood, behavior, thoughts, or feelings. Signs to watch for include new or worsening depression, new or worsening anxiety, agitation, insomnia, hostility, panic attacks, restlessness, extreme hyperactivity, and suicidal thinking or behavior.

Keep all follow-up visits as scheduled, and call the doctor between visits as needed, especially if you have concerns about symptoms.

Abrupt discontinuation of this drug or any antidepressant could cause side effects such as irritability, agitation, dizziness, headache, insomnia, and many others. Do not stop taking this medication without first consulting your physician.

Taking Lexapro at the same time you are taking aspirin, aspirin-related products, or any other blood thinner or anticoagulant increases the risk of bleeding.

Who should not take Lexapro?

Do not use Lexapro if you are taking pimozide or a monoamine oxidase inhibitor (MAOI), if you are allergic to Lexapro, or if you are sensitive to any component of the drug.

What should I tell my doctor before I take the first dose of Lexapro?

Tell your doctor about all medications you are taking before beginning treatment with Lexapro. Also, talk to your doctor about your complete medical history, especially if you have a bleeding disorder, kidney or liver disease, a history of seizures or mania, or experience worsening symptoms of depression and/or suicidal thoughts.

What is the usual dosage?

The information below is based on the dosage guidelines your doctor uses. Depending on your condition and medical history, your doctor may prescribe a different regimen. Do not change the dosage or stop taking your medication without your doctor's approval.

Adults: The recommended starting dose is 10 milligrams (mg) once daily. If necessary, your doctor may increase the dose to 20 mg after a minimum of 1 week. The higher dose is not recommended for most older adults and people with liver problems.

Adolescents 12 to 17 years old: For treating major depression, the recommended starting dose is 10 mg once daily. If necessary, the doctor may increase the dose to 20 mg after a minimum of 3 weeks.

How should I take Lexapro?

Lexapro is available in tablet and liquid forms and can be taken with or without food in the morning or evening. Although improvement usually begins within 1-4 weeks, treatment may continue for several months.

What should I avoid while taking Lexapro?

Do not stop taking Lexapro without first talking to your doctor. An abrupt decrease in dose could cause withdrawal symptoms such as mood problems, fatigue, insomnia, and tingling sensations.

Because Lexapro can cause dizziness or drowsiness, use caution when driving, operating machinery, or performing hazardous activities until you know how the drug affects you. It's also best to avoid alcohol while taking Lexapro.

Do not take Celexa (citalopram) while you are taking Lexapro, since the two drugs are related.

What are possible food and drug interactions associated with Lexapro?

If Lexapro is taken with certain other drugs, the effects of either could be increased, decreased, or altered. It is especially important to check with your doctor before combining Lexapro with the following: antidepressants, painkillers, sedatives, and tranquilizers and other drugs that act on the brain; aspirin and other blood thinners such as warfarin; carbamazepine; cimetidine; citalopram; ketoconazole; lithium; metoprolol; migraine drugs known as triptans, such as sumatriptan and zolmitriptan; nonsteroidal anti-inflammatory drugs such as ibuprofen and naproxen; narcotic painkillers such as oxycodone; and tryptophan.

Never combine Lexapro with any drug classified as an MAOI. Drugs in this category include the antidepressants phenelzine and tranylcypromine. Lexapro and MAOIs should not be taken together or within 14 days of each other. Combining these drugs with Lexapro can cause serious and even fatal reactions such as high body temperature, muscle rigidity, twitching, and agitation leading to delirium and coma.

What are the possible side effects of Lexapro?
Side effects cannot be anticipated. If any develop or change in intensity, tell your doctor as soon as possible. Only your doctor can determine if it is safe for you to continue taking this drug.

Side effects may include: decreased sex drive and inability to have an orgasm, difficulty falling or staying asleep, ejaculation problems, fatigue, increased sweating, nausea, sleepiness

Can I receive Lexapro if I am pregnant or breastfeeding?
The effects of Lexapro during pregnancy and breastfeeding are unknown. Tell your doctor immediately if you are pregnant, plan to become pregnant, or are breastfeeding. If you decide to breastfeed, Lexapro is not recommended.

What should I do if I miss a dose of Lexapro?
Take it as soon as you remember. If it is almost time for your next dose, skip the missed dose and go back to your regular schedule. Never take two doses at the same time.

How should I store Lexapro?
Store at room temperature away from moisture and heat.

LEXIVA
Generic name: Fosamprenavir calcium

What is Lexiva?
Lexiva is used to treat people with HIV infection, always in combination with other anti-HIV medicines. Lexiva belongs to a class of anti-HIV medicines called protease inhibitors. When used in combination therapy, Lexiva may help lower the amount of HIV found in your blood; raise certain cell counts; and keep your immune system as healthy as possible, so it can fight infection.

What is the most important information I should know about Lexiva?

Lexiva does not cure human immunodeficiency virus (HIV) infection or acquired immune deficiency syndrome (AIDS), nor does it reduce the risk of passing HIV to others through sexual contact or blood exposure. It is not known if Lexiva will help you live longer or experience fewer of the medical problems, such as opportunistic infections, associated with HIV or AIDS.

Lexiva can cause dangerous and life-threatening interactions if taken with certain other medicines (see "What are possible food and drug interactions associated with this medication?"). You should know all of the medicines you take, including vitamins and herbal supplements; and keep a list that you can show to your healthcare providers and pharmacists. Do not start any new medicines while you are taking Lexiva without talking with your healthcare provider or pharmacist.

Women who use birth control pills should choose a different kind of contraception. The use of Lexiva and Norvir (ritonavir) in combination with birth control pills may be harmful to your liver. The use of Lexiva may decrease the effectiveness of birth control pills. Talk to your healthcare provider about choosing an effective contraceptive.

Use barrier forms of contraception (eg, condoms) if you have HIV infection. Do not share needles, injection supplies, or items like toothbrushes or razors.

When your medicine supply is low, get more from your doctor or pharmacist as soon as you can. Do not stop taking Lexiva, even for a short period of time. If you do, the virus may grow resistant to the medicine and become harder to treat.

Lexiva may improve immune system function. This may reveal hidden infections in some patients. Tell your doctor right away if you notice signs or symptoms of an infection (such as: fever, sore throat, weakness, cough, shortness of breath) after you start Lexiva.

Changes in body fat (such as an increased amount of fat in the upper back, neck, breast, and trunk, and loss of fat from the legs, arms, and face) may occur in some patients taking Lexiva. The cause and long-term effects of these changes are unknown. Discuss any concerns with your doctor.

Lexiva may raise your blood sugar. Check blood sugar levels closely. High blood sugar may make you feel confused, drowsy, or thirsty. It can also make you flush, breathe faster, or have a fruit-like breath odor. If these symptoms occur, tell your doctor right away.

Eating grapefruit or drinking grapefruit juice while you are taking Lexiva may increase the amount of Lexiva in your blood. This may increase your risk for serious side effects. Talk with your doctor before including grapefruit juice in your diet.

If you take an aluminum- or magnesium-containing antacid, ask your doctor or pharmacist how to take it with Lexiva.

Lab tests, including liver function, cholesterol or triglyceride levels, white blood cell count, and blood sugar levels, may be performed while you use Lexiva. These tests may be used to monitor your condition or check for side effects. Be sure to keep all doctor and lab appointments.

Who should not take Lexiva?

Do not take Lexiva if you are allergic to it or any of its ingredients. Do not take Lexiva if you are allergic to, or are taking amprenavir or sulfa medicines. Do not take Lexiva if you are also taking amprenavir. See "What are possible food and drug interactions associated with this medication?" below for a list of drugs you should not take in combination with Lexiva.

What should I tell my doctor before I take the first dose of Lexiva?

Tell your doctor about all prescription, over-the-counter, and herbal medications you are taking before beginning treatment with Lexiva. Lexiva can cause serious interactions if taken with certain other medications. Also, talk to your doctor about your complete medical history, especially if you have diabetes; hemophilia; kidney or liver problems; or are allergic to sulfa medicines. Before you take Lexiva, talk to your doctor if you are pregnant, planning to become pregnant, or are breastfeeding. Women who use birth control pills should use an additional or different kind of contraception, since Lexiva may decrease the effectiveness of birth control pills. Talk to your doctor about choosing an effective contraceptive. If you take Lexiva, birth control pills, and other drugs in combination, you may be harming your liver.

What is the usual dosage?

The information below is based on the dosage guidelines your doctor uses. Depending on your condition and medical history, your doctor may prescribe a different regimen. Do not change the dosage or stop taking your medication without your doctor's approval.

Adults: The usual dose is 700 milligrams (mg) taken twice daily, in combination with ritonavir. The maximum dosage is 2 tablets or 1400 mg taken twice daily when Lexiva is used alone.

Children 2 to 18 years: The recommended dosage of Lexiva in patients 2 years of age and older should be calculated based on body weight (kg) and should not exceed 1400mg twice daily. When Lexiva is given alone to children, 1400mg twice daily may be used in patients weighing at least 47kg.

Children between 2 and 5 years old can take Lexiva suspension at a dose of 30 mg per kilogram twice daily without exceeding a dose of 1,400 mg twice daily. Children 6 years and older can receive either Lexiva suspension at a dose of 30 mg per kilogram twice daily without exceeding a dose of 1400 mg twice daily or they can receive 18 mg per kilogram of the oral suspension without exceeding a dose of 700 mg twice daily(in combination ritonavir).

Liver impairment: Lexiva should be used with caution in patients with liver impairment. A reduced dose of 700 mg twice daily should be used in these patients. If the liver impairment is moderate in severity, the daily Lexiva dose should be reduced to 700 mg twice daily (without ritonavir) or 450 mg twice daily if used in combination with ritonavir. If the liver impairment is severe, the dose should be reduced to 350 mg twice daily (alone). There is not data on the use of Lexiva in combination with ritonavir in patients with severe liver impairment.

How should I take Lexiva?

Lexiva tablets may be taken with or without food. Do not take more or less than your prescribed dose at any one time. Do not change your dose or stop taking Lexiva unless your doctor tells you to do so. If the medicine is stopped for even a short time, the amount of HIV virus in your blood may increase. When your supply of Lexiva or other anti-HIV medicine starts to run low, get more from your doctor or pharmacy.

Continue taking Lexiva even if you start to feel better. Do not miss any doses.

If you take an aluminum- or magnesium-containing antacid, ask your doctor or pharmacist how to take it with Lexiva

Adults should take Lexiva oral suspension without food. Children should take Lexiva suspension with food. If vomiting occurs within 30 minutes after dosing, the dose should be repeated. Shake Lexiva Oral Suspension vigorously before each use.

What should I avoid while taking Lexiva?

Do not use certain medicines while you are taking Lexiva (see "What are possible food and drug interactions associated with this medication?"). Do not breastfeed while taking Lexiva.

Avoid doing things that can spread HIV infection, since Lexiva doesn't stop you from passing HIV to others. Do not have any kind of sex without protection. Practice safe sex by using a latex or polyurethane condom to lower the chance of sexual contact with semen, vaginal secretions, or blood. You should never use or share dirty needles. Also, do not share personal items that can have blood or body fluids on them, like toothbrushes and razor blades.

What are possible food and drug interactions associated with Lexiva?

If Lexiva is taken with certain other drugs, the effects of either could be increased, decreased, or altered. It is especially important to check with your doctor before combining Lexiva with the following: amprenavir, cisapride, ergot medicines, such as dihydroergotamine, ergonovine, ergotamine, and methylergonovine, flecainide, grapefruit (whole fruit or juice), midazolam, pimozide, propafenone, triazolam.

What are the possible side effects of Lexiva?
Side effects cannot be anticipated. If any develop or change in intensity, tell your doctor as soon as possible. Only your doctor can determine if it is safe for you to continue taking this drug.

Side effects may include: diarrhea, nausea, vomiting, headache, fatigue

Sometimes, Lexiva can cause diabetes or affect blood sugar in people who are already diabetic. Lexiva may also increase the risk of bleeding problems in some patients with hemophilia. Lexiva may cause skin rashes, changes in blood tests, or changes in body fat. In some patients, Lexiva may worsen liver disease if you already have liver problems.

Can I receive Lexiva if I am pregnant or breastfeeding?
The effects of Lexiva during pregnancy and breastfeeding are unknown. Tell your doctor immediately if you are pregnant, plan to become pregnant, or are breastfeeding. You should not breastfeed if you are HIV-positive because of the chance of passing the HIV virus to your baby through your milk.

What should I do if I miss a dose of Lexiva?
It is important that you not miss any doses. If you miss a dose of Lexiva by more than 4 hours, wait and take the next dose at the regular time. However, if you miss a dose by fewer than 4 hours, take your missed dose right away then take your next dose at the regular time.

How should I store Lexiva?
Store Lexiva at 77°F (25°C). Brief storage at temperatures between 59° and 86°F (15° and 30°C) is permitted. Store away from heat, moisture, and light. Do not store in the bathroom. Keep the container tightly closed. Do not use after the expiration date.

LEXXEL
Generic name: Enalapril maleate and felodipine

What is Lexxel?
Lexxel is used alone or in combination with other blood pressure medications to treat high blood pressure. It combines 2 blood pressure drugs: an ACE inhibitor and a calcium channel blocker. Lexxel is not usually the first drug that should be used when starting to treat hypertension.

What is the most important information I should know about Lexxel?

When used in pregnancy during the second and third trimesters, Lexxel can cause injury and even death to the developing fetus. Notify your doctor immediately if you think you might be pregnant.

During the first few days of Lexxel therapy you may experience some lightheadedness, especially in the morning. Be careful when sitting or standing up. Excessive perspiration and dehydration may lead to an excessive fall in blood pressure because of reduction in fluid in your body. Vomiting or diarrhea may also lead to a fall in blood pressure. If you feel faint when taking Lexxel, contact your doctor immediately.

Do not drive or perform other possibly unsafe tasks until you know how you react to Lexxel; this drug may cause dizziness or lightheadedness. These effects may be worse if you take it with alcohol or certain medicines.

Check with your doctor before you use a salt substitute or a product that has potassium in it.

Proper dental care is important while you are taking Lexxel. Brush and floss your teeth and visit the dentist regularly. Good dental hygiene decreases the incidence and severity of side effects such as gum swelling.

Patients who take medicine for high blood pressure often feel tired or run down for a few weeks after starting treatment. Be sure to take your medicine even if you may not feel "normal." Tell your doctor if you develop any new symptoms.

Lexxel may not work as well in black patients. They may also be at greater risk of side effects. Contact your doctor if your symptoms do not improve or if they become worse.

Lexxel may cause you to become sunburned more easily. Avoid the sun, sunlamps, or tanning booths until you know how you react to Lexxel. Use sunscreen or wear protective clothing if you must be outside for more than a short time.

Tell your doctor or dentist that you take Lexxel before you receive any medical or dental care, emergency care, or surgery.

Lab tests, including liver function, kidney function, complete blood cell counts, and blood pressure, may be performed while you use Lexxel. These tests may be used to monitor your condition or check for side effects. Be sure to keep all doctor and lab appointments.

If you notice any sign of an infection (such as sore throat and fever) contact your doctor for this may be due to a side effect of Lexxel.

Who should not take Lexxel?

Do not take Lexxel if you are sensitive to any component of the drug or if you have ever developed a swollen throat and difficulty swallowing (angioedema) while taking drugs that are similar to Lexxel, such as captopril or enalapril.

What should I tell my doctor before I take the first dose of Lexxel?

Tell your doctor about all prescription, over-the-counter, and herbal medications you are taking before beginning treatment with Lexxel. Also, talk to your doctor about your complete medical history, especially if you have a history of drug induced angioedema, have collagen vascular disease (a connective tissue disorder), kidney or liver disease, are receiving dialysis, have bone marrow suppression, low blood counts, low blood sodium, high blood potassium, the blood disease porphyria, lupus, slow heart beat, heart disease, or heart failure.

What is the usual dosage?

The information below is based on the dosage guidelines your doctor uses. Depending on your condition and medical history, your doctor may prescribe a different regimen. Do not change the dosage or stop taking your medication without your doctor's approval.

Adults: Lexxel is available in 2 strengths: Lexxel 5-2.5 contains 5 milligrams (mg) of enalapril and 2.5 mg of felodipine; Lexxel 5-5 contains 5 mg of each.

The usual starting dose is 1 tablet of Lexxel 5-5 once a day. If there is no change in your blood pressure after 1 to 2 weeks, the doctor may increase your dose to 2 tablets once a day. If your blood pressure still remains too high, the dose may be increased to 4 tablets of Lexxel 5-2.5 once a day. The doctor may also add a diuretic (water pill) containing a thiazide to your regimen.

If you have kidney disease, your doctor may start you at a lower dose.

How should I take Lexxel?

Take Lexxel exactly as prescribed. Lexxel can be taken with a light meal or without food; take with food if stomach upset occurs. However, a high-fat meal can reduce its effectiveness. Also, be careful when drinking grapefruit juice, as it can increase Lexxel's impact. Swallow Lexxel tablets whole. Do not divide, crush, or chew the tablet.

Continue to take Lexxel even if you do not see results right away. You may feel worse before you feel better.

What should I avoid while taking Lexxel?

Lexxel may cause dizziness or drowsiness. Use caution when driving, operating machinery, or performing other hazardous activities.

Lexxel sometimes causes a severe drop in blood pressure. The danger is especially great if you have been taking diuretics (water pills), or if you have heart disease, kidney disease, or a potassium or salt imbalance. Excessive sweating, severe diarrhea, and vomiting are also dangerous because they can rob the body of water. This can cause a dangerous drop in blood pressure. If you feel light-headed or faint, have chest pain, or feel your heart racing, contact your doctor immediately.

Do not use salt substitutes or potassium supplements while taking Lexxel.

Avoid the sun, sunlamps, or tanning booths until you know how you react to Lexxel. Use sunscreen or wear protective clothing if you must be outside for more than a short time.

Do not sit of stand up too quickly when beginning Lexxel therapy, especially in the morning. Lay down at the first sign of dizziness and lightheadedness.

What are possible food and drug interactions associated with Lexxel?

If Lexxel is taken with certain other drugs, the effects of either could be increased, decreased, or altered. It is especially important to check with your doctor before combining Lexxel with the following: cimetidine, diuretics such as furosemide or hydrochlorothiazide or those that leave potassium in the body such as amiloride, spironolactone, and triamterene, epilepsy medications such as carbamazepine, phenobarbital, and phenytoin, erythromycin, glyburide, grapefruit juice, high-fat meals, itraconazole, ketoconazole, lithium, nonsteroidal anti-inflammatory drugs such as ibuprofen or naproxen, potassium supplements, tacrolimus.

What are the possible side effects of Lexxel?

Side effects cannot be anticipated. If any develop or change in intensity, tell your doctor as soon as possible. Only your doctor can determine if it is safe for you to continue taking this drug.

Side effects may include: dizziness, headache, swelling, lightheadedness when sitting or standing up, drowsiness, nausea, persistent dry cough, fatigue, vomiting

If you experience swelling of the face, extremities, eyes, lips, tongue, difficulty in swallowing or breathing, immediately report them to your doctor. Do not take any more doses of Lexxel without first consulting with your doctor.

Can I receive Lexxel if I am pregnant or breastfeeding?

Do not take Lexxel while you are pregnant. When taken during the final 6 months, the ACE inhibitor in Lexxel can cause birth defects, prematurity, and even death in the developing fetus or newborn baby. If you are pregnant, tell your doctor immediately. Do not breastfeed while you are taking Lexxel because the drug is found in breast milk.

What should I do if I miss a dose of Lexxel?

Take it as soon as you remember. If it is almost time for your next dose, skip the missed dose and go back to your regular schedule. Never take 2 doses at the same time.

How should I store Lexxel?
Store Lexxel at room temperature, below 86°F. Store away from heat, moisture, and light. Do not store in the bathroom.

LIALDA
Generic name: Mesalamine

What is Lialda?
Lialda is a medicine that is taken to cause remission of active, mild-to-moderate ulcerative colitis.

What is the most important information I should know about Lialda?
Lialda has been associated with a syndrome that may be difficult to distinguish from an ulcerative colitis flare-up. If you experience cramping, abdominal pain, bloody diarrhea, fever, headache or rash, talk to your doctor immediately.

Some patients taking mesalamine have reported heart-related reactions, such as inflammation of the heart muscle and inflammation of the lining of the heart. Tell your doctor if you have any heart conditions.

Tell your doctor if you are allergic to any over the counter or prescription medications.

Who should not take Lialda?
You should not take Lialda if you are allergic to salicylates (including mesalamine or aspirin) or to any of the ingredients of Lialda.

What should I tell my doctor before I take the first dose of Lialda?
Tell your doctor about all prescription, over-the-counter, and herbal medication you are taking before beginning treatment with Lialda. Also, talk to your doctor about your complete medical history, especially if you have ever had a history of kidney, liver, or heart disease. Tell your doctor if you have a condition called pyloric stenosis. Also, tell your doctor about any medication allergies that you may have.

What is the usual dosage?
The information below is based on the dosage guidelines your doctor uses. Depending on your condition and medical history, your doctor may prescribe a different regimen. Do not change the dosage or stop taking your medication without your doctor's approval.

Adults: The recommended dose is two to four 1.2-gram tablets taken once daily with a meal for a total daily dose of 2.4 grams or 4.8 grams. Treatment duration is up to 8 weeks.

How should I take Lialda?
Swallow Lialda tablets whole. Do not crush or chew tablets.

What should I avoid while taking Lialda?
You should avoid crushing or chewing Lialda tablets.

What are possible food and drug interactions associated with Lialda?
If Lialda is taken with certain other drugs, the effect of either medication could be increased, decreased, or altered. It is especially important to check with your doctor before combining Lialda with the following medications: azathioprine, nonsteroidal anti-inflammatory drugs (NSAIDs), 6-mercaptopurine.

What are the possible side effects of Lialda?
Side effects cannot be anticipated. If any develop or change in intensity, tell your doctor as soon as possible. Only your doctor can determine if it is safe for you to continue taking this drug.

Side effects may include: headache, gas, loss of hair, itching

Can I receive Lialda if I am pregnant or breastfeeding?
The effects of Lialda during pregnancy and breastfeeding are unknown. Tell your doctor immediately if you are pregnant, or plan to become pregnant, or are breastfeeding.

What should I do if I miss a dose of Lialda?
If you miss a dose of Lialda, take it as soon as you remember. However, if it is almost time for your next dose, skip the missed dose and take only your next regularly scheduled dose. Do not take two doses at the same time.

How should I store Lialda?
Store Lialda at room temperature. Protect the medicine from moisture by keeping the bottle closed tightly.

LIBRAX
Generic name: Chlordiazepoxide hydrochloride and clidinium bromide

What is Librax?
Librax is used with other medications for the treatment of peptic ulcers, irritable bowel syndrome (spastic colon), and acute enterocolitis (inflammation of the colon and small intestine). It combines a benzodiazepine—chlordiazepoxide—and clidinium, which is an antispasmodic medication.

What is the most important information I should know about Librax?

Because of its sedative effects, you should not operate heavy machinery, drive, or engage in other hazardous tasks that require you to be mentally alert while you are taking Librax.

Who should not take Librax?

Do not take Librax if you have glaucoma (elevated pressure in the eye), an enlarged prostate, or a bladder obstruction. If you are sensitive to or have ever had an allergic reaction to any component of this drug, you should not take Librax.

What should I tell my doctor before I take the first dose of Librax?

Tell your doctor about all prescription, over-the-counter, and herbal medications you are taking before beginning treatment with Librax. Also, talk to your doctor about your complete medical history, especially if you have glaucoma, difficulty urinating or a bladder obstruction, or an enlarged prostate.

What is the usual dosage?

The information below is based on the dosage guidelines your doctor uses. Depending on your condition and medical history, your doctor may prescribe a different regimen. Do not change the dosage or stop taking your medication without your doctor's approval.

Adults: The usual dose is 1 to 2 capsules, 3 to 4 times a day before meals and at bedtime.

How should I take Librax?

Take Librax before meals and at bedtime. Librax can make your mouth dry. For temporary relief, suck a hard candy or chew gum.

What should I avoid while taking Librax?

Avoid drinking alcohol while taking Librax; as it may increase its drowsiness and dizziness side effects.

Because of its sedative effects, you should not operate heavy machinery, drive, or engage in other hazardous tasks that require you to be mentally alert while you are taking Librax.

Librax can be habit-forming and has been associated with drug dependence and addiction. Be very careful taking Librax if you have ever had problems with alcohol or drug abuse. Never take more than the prescribed amount.

In addition, you should not stop taking Librax suddenly, because of the risk of withdrawal symptoms (convulsions, cramps, tremors, vomiting, sweating, depression, and sleeplessness). If you have been taking Librax over a long period of time, your doctor will decrease your dose gradually.

Avoid becoming overheated; Librax decreases sweating and therefore may increase the risk of heat stroke.

What are possible food and drug interactions associated with Librax?

If Librax is taken with certain other drugs, the effects of either could be increased, decreased, or altered. It is especially important to check with your doctor before combining Librax with any of the following: alcohol, antidepressants known as monoamine oxidase inhibitors MAOIs, such as phenelzine or tranylcypromine, belladonna, benzodiazepines such as alprazolam and diazepam, blood-thinners such as warfarin, diphenhydramine, ketoconazole, major tranquilizers such as chlorpromazine and trifluoperazine, potassium supplements.

What are the possible side effects of Librax?

Side effects cannot be anticipated. If any develop or change in intensity, tell your doctor as soon as possible. Only your doctor can determine if it is safe for you to continue taking this drug.

Side effects may include: blurred vision, changes in sex drive, confusion, constipation, drowsiness, dry mouth, fainting, lack of coordination, liver problems, minor menstrual irregularities, nausea, skin eruptions, swelling due to fluid retention, urinary difficulties, yellowing of skin and eyes

Can I receive Librax if I am pregnant or breastfeeding?

Several studies have found an increased risk of birth defects if Librax is taken during the first 3 months of pregnancy. Therefore, Librax is rarely recommended for use by pregnant women. If you are pregnant, plan to become pregnant, or are breastfeeding, inform your doctor immediately.

What should I do if I miss a dose of Librax?

Take it as soon as you remember. If it is almost time for your next dose, skip the one you missed and go back to your regular schedule. Do not take 2 doses at once.

How should I store Librax?

Store away from heat, light, and moisture.

LIBRIUM

Generic name: Chlordiazepoxide hydrochloride

What is Librium?

Librium is used to treat anxiety disorders. It is also prescribed for short-term relief of the symptoms of anxiety, symptoms of withdrawal in acute alcoholism, and anxiety and apprehension before surgery.

What is the most important information I should know about Librium?

Librium has the potential to cause dependence.

You could experience withdrawal symptoms if you stop taking Librium abruptly. Do not discontinue the drug or change your dose without your doctor's approval.

Who should not take Librium?

Do not use Librium if you are allergic to any of its ingredients.

What should I tell my doctor before I take the first dose of Librium?

Tell your doctor about all prescription, over-the-counter, and herbal medications you are taking before beginning treatment with Librium. Also, talk to your doctor about your complete medical history, especially if you have kidney or liver disease, porphyria (a rare metabolic disorder), or suffer from depression or have suicidal thoughts.

What is the usual dosage?

The information below is based on the dosage guidelines your doctor uses. Depending on your condition and medical history, your doctor may prescribe a different regimen. Do not change the dosage or stop taking your medication without your doctor's approval.

Mild to Moderate Anxiety
Adults: The usual dose is 5 or 10 milligrams (mg) taken 3-4 times a day.

Children 6 years and older: The usual dose is 5 mg taken 2-4 times a day. Some children may need to take 10 mg, 2-3 times a day.

The drug is not recommended for children under 6 years of age.

Severe Anxiety
Adults: The usual dose is 20 or 25 mg taken 3-4 times a day.

Apprehension and Anxiety before Surgery
Adults: On days before surgery, the usual dose is 5-10 mg taken 3-4 times a day.

Withdrawal Symptoms of Acute Alcoholism
Adults: The injectable form is usually used initially. Following this is the oral medication starting at doses from 50-100 mg, to be followed by repeated doses as needed up to 300 mg per day. The doctor will repeat this dose, up to a maximum of 300 mg per day, until agitation is controlled. The dose will then be reduced as much as possible.

In elderly patients, your doctor may limit the dose to the smallest effective amount in order to avoid over-sedation or lack of coordination. The usual dose is 5 mg taken 2-4 times per day.

How should I take Librium?
Take Librium exactly as prescribed.

What should I avoid while taking Librium?
Librium may cause you to become drowsy or less alert. Do not drive or operate dangerous machinery or participate in any hazardous activity that requires full mental alertness until you know how you react to Librium.

Avoid alcohol while taking Librium as it may increase drowsiness and dizziness caused by Librium.

What are possible food and drug interactions associated with Librium?
If Librium is taken with certain other drugs, the effects of either could be increased, decreased, or altered. It is especially important to check with your doctor before combining Librium with the following: antacids, antidepressant drugs known as MAO inhibitors, including phenelzine and tranylcypromine, antihistamines, antipsychotic drugs such as chlorpromazine and trifluoperazine, antiseizure drugs such as carbamazepine and phenytoin, barbiturates, blood-thinners, cimetidine, disulfiram, levodopa, muscle relaxants such as cyclobenzaprine, narcotic pain relievers, tranquilizers and sedatives such as alprazolam, diazepam, midazolam, and triazolam.

What are the possible side effects of Librium?
Side effects cannot be anticipated. If any develop or change in intensity, tell your doctor as soon as possible. Only your doctor can determine if it is safe for you to continue taking this drug.

Side effects may include: confusion, constipation, drowsiness, fainting, increased or decreased sex drive, liver problems, lack of muscle coordination, minor menstrual irregularities, nausea, skin rash or eruptions, swelling due to fluid retention, yellow eyes and skin

Side effects due to rapid decrease or abrupt withdrawal from Librium may include: abdominal and muscle cramps, convulsions, exaggerated feeling of depression, sleeplessness, sweating, tremors, vomiting

Can I receive Librium if I am pregnant or breastfeeding?
Do not take Librium if you are pregnant or planning to become pregnant. There may be an increased risk of birth defects. Do not breastfeed while you are taking Librium.

What should I do if I miss a dose of Librium?
Take it as soon as you remember if it is within an hour or of your scheduled time. If you do not remember until later, skip the dose you missed and go back to your regular schedule. Do not take two doses at once.

How should I store Librium?
Store at room temperature away from heat, light, and moisture.

Linezolid See Zyvox, page 1514.

LIPITOR
Generic name: Atorvastatin calcium

What is Lipitor?
Lipitor is a type of medication called a statin. It lowers cholesterol in your blood. Lipitor lowers the "bad" LDL cholesterol and triglycerides in your blood. It can raise the "good" HDL cholesterol as well. Lipitor is for adults and children over 10 years old whose cholesterol does not come down enough with exercise and a low-fat diet alone. Lipitor can lower the risk for heart attack or stroke in patients who have risk factors for heart disease such as age, smoking, high blood pressure, low HDL cholesterol levels, heart disease in the family; or high blood sugar with risk factors such as eye problems, kidney problems, smoking, or high blood pressure.

**What is the most important information
I should know about Lipitor?**
Taking Lipitor is not a substitute for following a healthy low-fat and low-cholesterol diet and exercising to lower your cholesterol.

Do not take Lipitor if you are pregnant or think you may be pregnant, or if you are planning to become pregnant.

Lipitor can cause serious side effects, especially if taken with certain other medicines (see "What are possible food and drug interactions associated with this medication?" below).

Who should not take Lipitor?
If you are pregnant or plan to become pregnant, you should not take Lipitor, since this medication may harm an unborn baby. Likewise, do not take Lipitor if you are breastfeeding, as it can pass into your breast milk. Do not take Lipitor if you have liver problems; or if you are allergic to the medication, or any of its ingredients.

**What should I tell my doctor before
I take the first dose of Lipitor?**
Tell your doctor about all prescription, over-the-counter, and herbal medication you are taking before beginning treatment with Lipitor. Be sure to tell your doctor if you take medicines for any of the following: birth control, cholesterol, heart failure, HIV or AIDS, infections, or the immune system. Also, talk to your doctor about your complete medical history,

especially if you drink more than 2 glasses of alcohol daily, or if you have diabetes. Tell your doctor if you have muscle aches or weakness, or problems with your kidney, liver, or thyroid.

What is the usual dosage?
The information below is based on the dosage guidelines your doctor uses. Depending on your condition and medical history, your doctor may prescribe a different regimen. Do not change the dosage or stop taking your medication without your doctor's approval.

Adults >17 years: The usual starting dose of Lipitor is 10 or 20 milligrams (mg) taken 1 time each day, with a maximum dose of 80 mg daily.

Lipitor starts to work in about 2 weeks. Your cholesterol levels will be checked during treatment with Lipitor, and your dosage may be changed based on the results.

Children and adolescents 10 to 17 years: The usual dose is 10 mg daily, with a maximum dose of 20 mg daily.

Adolescent girls must be having periods before taking Lipitor.

How should I take Lipitor?
Your doctor will likely start you on a low-fat and low-cholesterol diet before giving you Lipitor. Stay on this diet while taking the medication.

Do not break Lipitor tablets before you take them. Take Lipitor every day at about the same time each day. Lipitor can be taken with or without food.

What should I avoid while taking Lipitor?
Do not get pregnant or take the medication while breastfeeding. If you do get pregnant, stop taking Lipitor right away and call your doctor.

Avoid drinking grapefruit juice while taking Lipitor.

What are possible food and drug interactions associated with Lipitor?
If Lipitor is taken with certain other drugs, the effects of either could be increased, decreased, or altered. It is especially important to check with your doctor before combining Lipitor with any of the following: cimetidine, clarithromycin, colestipol, cyclosporine, digoxin, erythromycin, grapefruit juice, itraconazole, ketoconazole, oral contraceptives, spironolactone.

What are the possible side effects of Lipitor?
Side effects cannot be anticipated. If any develop or change in intensity, tell your doctor as soon as possible. Only your doctor can determine if it is safe for you to continue taking this drug.

Side effects may include: constipation, diarrhea, gas, headache, muscle and joint pain, rash, stomach pain, upset stomach

Some people may develop more serious side effects while taking Lipitor. These side effects may include severe muscle problems that can sometimes lead to kidney problems, including kidney failure. You have a higher chance for developing muscle problems if you are taking certain other medicines with Lipitor. Another serious side effect is liver problems.

Call your doctor right away if you have any of the following symptoms: muscle problems like weakness, tenderness, or pain that happen without a good reason, especially if you also have a fever or feel more tired than usual; nausea and vomiting; passing brown or dark-colored urine; stomach pain; your skin and whites of your eyes become yellow

Can I receive Lipitor if I am pregnant or breastfeeding?
No. Lipitor may cause harm to an unborn or newborn baby, and should not be taken during pregnancy or breastfeeding.

What should I do if I miss a dose of Lipitor?
If you miss a dose of Lipitor, take it as soon as you remember. If it has been more than 12 hours since your last dose, wait and take the next dose at your regular time. Do not take 2 doses of Lipitor at the same time.

How should I store Lipitor?
Store Lipitor at room temperature.

Lisdexamfetamine dimesylate See Vyvanse, page 1411.

Lisinopril See Zestril, page 1465.

Lisinopril and hydrochlorothiazide See Zestoretic, page 1462.

LOESTRIN 24 FE
Generic name: Norethindrone acetate and ethinyl estradiol

What is Loestrin 24 FE?
Loestrin 24 FE is an oral contraceptive pill for the prevention of pregnancy.

What is the most important information I should know about Loestrin 24 FE?
This product (like all oral contraceptives) is intended to prevent pregnancy. It does not protect against HIV infection (AIDS) and other sexually transmitted diseases. Cigarette smoking increases the risk of serious problems with your heart and blood vessels from oral contraceptive use. This risk increases with age and with the amount of smoking (>15 ciga-

rettes per day) and is apparent in women >35 years of age. Women who use oral contraceptives should not smoke.

If you miss pills, you could get pregnant. This includes starting the pack late. The more pills you miss, the more likely you are to get pregnant.

Who should not take Loestrin 24 FE?

If you have a history of heart attack or stroke, history of blood clots in the legs, lungs or eyes, chest pain, severe high blood pressure, headaches with neurological symptoms, high blood sugar with complications involving the kidneys, eyes, nerves or blood vessels, abnormal vaginal bleeding, known or suspected breast/uterine/ovarian cancer, you should not take Loestrin 24 FE.

Also, if you plan to have surgery that will leave you immobile for a period of time, you should not use this type of birth control. Loestrin 24 FE should not be used if you are allergic to it or any of its ingredients, are pregnant or planning to become pregnant, or if you have kidney or liver disease.

What should I tell my doctor before I take the first dose of Loestrin 24 FE?

Tell your doctor about all prescription, over-the-counter, and herbal medications you are taking before beginning treatment with Loestrin 24 FE. Also, talk to your doctor about your complete medical history, especially if you have high blood pressure, diabetes, heart problems, liver or kidney problems, or if you have had any type of cancer (especially breast), a heart attack, or a stroke. Your doctor should know if you have unexplained vaginal bleeding, recently had an abortion or miscarriage, recently had a baby, or if you are pregnant.

What is the usual dosage?

The information below is based on the dosage guidelines your doctor uses. Depending on your condition and medical history, your doctor may prescribe a different regimen. Do not change the dosage or stop taking your medication without your doctor's approval.

Adults: Loestrin 24 FE should be taken in the dosage prescribed by your doctor, every 24 hours.

How should I take Loestrin 24 FE?

Take one pill of Loestrin 24 FE everyday at the same time, with or without food.

What are possible food and drug interactions associated with Loestrin 24 FE?

If Loestrin 24 FE is taken with certain other drugs, the effects of either could be increased, decreased, or altered. It is especially important to check with your doctor before combining Loestrin 24 FE with any of the following: antibiotics, anticonvulsants, HIV medicines, St. John's wort.

What are the possible side effects of Loestrin 24 FE?
Side effects cannot be anticipated. If any develop or change in intensity, tell your doctor as soon as possible. Only your doctor can determine if it is safe for you to continue taking this drug.

Side effects may include: bleeding or spotting between menstrual periods, breast tenderness, difficulty wearing contact lenses, nausea, vomiting, weight gain

These side effects, especially nausea and vomiting, may decrease or subside within the first three months of use.

Can I receive Loestrin 24 FE if I am pregnant or breastfeeding?
You should not use Loestrin 24 FE if you are pregnant, planning to become pregnant, or are breastfeeding.

What should I do if I miss a dose of Loestrin 24 FE?
If you forget to take your pill, take it as soon as you remember. It is okay to take 2 pills in one day, though it may cause you to be slightly nauseous.

How should I store Loestrin 24 FE?
Store at room temperature, in a dry area.

LOMOTIL
Generic name: Diphenoxylate hydrochloride and atropine sulfate

What is Lomotil?
Lomotil is a combination product used to treat diarrhea.

What is the most important information I should know about Lomotil?
Follow Lomotil dosing instructions strictly. Taking too much Lomotil may result in a suppression of your breathing and coma, possibly leading to brain damage, and even death.

When taking Lomotil, drink adequate fluids as directed by your doctor.

Lomotil is not recommended for use in children under age 2. Keep Lomotil in a child-resistant container and away from children.

Who should not take Lomotil?
You should not take Lomotil if you have a known sensitivity or allergy to Lomotil, have a liver disorder known as obstructive jaundice, or have

been diagnosed by your doctor as having diarrhea due to bacteria called pseudomembranous enterocolitis or enterotoxin-producing bacteria.

What should I tell my doctor before I take the first dose of Lomotil?

Tell your doctor about all prescription, over-the-counter, and herbal medications you are taking before beginning treatment with Lomotil. Also, talk to your doctor about your complete medical history, especially if you have been diagnosed with a condition called ulcerative colitis, have liver and kidney disease or impairment, or you are taking a medication known as a monoamine oxidase inhibitor (MAOI).

What is the usual dosage?

The information below is based on the dosage guidelines your doctor uses. Depending on your condition and medical history, your doctor may prescribe a different *regimen*. Do not change the dosage or stop taking your medication without your doctor's approval.

Adults and adolescents over 12 years: The usual starting dose of Lomotil is 2 tablets taken 4 times a day or 10 mL (2 teaspoonfuls) of Lomotil liquid 4 times per day. Based on your body's response to Lomotil, your doctor may reduce your dose to 2 tablets daily or 10 mL daily.

Children 2 to 12 years: In children under 13 years old, only give Lomotil liquid, do not give Lomotil tablets. The usual starting dose for children is based on age and weight and is given 4 times daily:

2 years/24-31 lbs: 1.5-3 mL; 3 years/26-35 lbs: 2-3 mL; 4 years/31-44 lbs: 2-4 mL; 5 years/35-51 lbs: 2.5-4.5 mL; 6-8 years/38-71 lbs: 2.5-5 mL; 8-12 years: 51-121 lbs: 3.5-5 mL

Your child's doctor may prescribe a lower dose based on your child's symptoms.

How should I take Lomotil?

Take Lomotil exactly as prescribed by your doctor. Space out the dosing times evenly throughout the day and take Lomotil at the same times every day. If using Lomotil liquid for a child, use the plastic dropper provided for measuring and giving doses.

What should I avoid while taking Lomotil?

Until you know how Lomotil affects you, be careful doing activities that require alertness, such as driving a car or operating machinery. Also, avoid drinking alcohol while taking this drug.

What are possible food and drug interactions associated with Lomotil?

If Lomotil is taken with certain other drugs, the effects of either could be increased, decreased, or altered. It is especially important to check with your doctor before combining Lomotil with any of the following: alcohol, barbiturates (medications such as phenobarbital), monoamine oxidase inhibitors (MAOIs), tranquilizers

What are the possible side effects of Lomotil?
Side effects cannot be anticipated. If any develop or change in intensity, tell your doctor as soon as possible. Only your doctor can determine if it is safe for you to continue taking this drug.

Side effects may include: numbness of arms and legs, euphoria, depression, overall sick feeling/lethargy, confusion, tiredness/drowsiness, dizziness, restlessness, headache, urinary retention, flushing (redness of the skin), dryness of the mucous membranes or skin, increase in body temperature, rapid beating of the heart

Can I receive Lomotil if I am pregnant or breastfeeding?
The effects of Lomotil during pregnancy are unknown. Tell your doctor immediately if you are pregnant or plan to become pregnant. You should tell your doctor if you are breastfeeding; Lomotil is excreted in breast milk and may affect your baby.

What should I do if I miss a dose of Lomotil?
If you miss a dose of Lomotil do not double your next dose. Skip the dose and return to your normal dosing schedule.

How should I store Lomotil?
Store at room temperature.

Loperamide hydrochloride See Imodium, page 654.

LOPID
Generic name: Gemfibrozil

What is Lopid?
Lopid is a cholesterol-regulating medication. It is used to lower the levels of triglycerides in your blood when diet and exercise alone have not lowered them enough and when you are at risk for pancreatitis (inflammation of the pancreas). Lopid is also used to reduce the chances of developing coronary artery disease if you are at risk and have not responded to diet and exercise, or to other medications. Lopid can also be used to decrease your very low density lipoprotein (VLDL) cholesterol ("bad" cholesterol), while increasing your high density lipoprotein (HDL) cholesterol ("good" cholesterol).

What is the most important information I should know about Lopid?

Taking Lopid is not a substitute for following a healthy, low-fat and low-cholesterol diet and exercising to lower your cholesterol.

If you experience any muscle pain, tenderness, or weakness while taking Lopid, contact you doctor immediately. These can be signs of a rare but serious muscle disease known as myositis.

Lopid may increase the risk of developing gallbladder disease, including gallstones.

Lopid can increase your risk of developing cancer; discuss your individual risk with your doctor.

If you are taking a blood-thinning medication (anticoagulant), Lopid may affect the drug's levels in your blood. Your doctor may monitor you by performing blood tests and may decrease the dose of the anticoagulant.

Because Lopid can cause changes in the levels of important cells in your blood, your doctor may take blood samples from you periodically during your first 12 weeks taking Lopid.

Liver injury can occur from taking Lopid. Your doctor may want to check your liver function during your treatment with Lopid.

Use caution taking Lopid if you have kidney disease; Lopid can worsen kidney function.

Who should not take Lopid?

You should not take Lopid if you are currently taking cerivastatin, another medication for cholesterol. You should also not take Lopid if you have liver or severe kidney dysfunction, including primary biliary cirrhosis, pre-existing gallbladder disease, or are hypersensitive to Lopid.

What should I tell my doctor before I take the first dose of Lopid?

Tell your doctor about all prescription, over-the-counter, and herbal medication you are taking before beginning treatment with Lopid. Also, talk to your doctor about your complete medical history, especially if you have a history of gallstones, cancer, muscle aches or weakness, problems with your liver or kidneys, or you are taking blood-thinning medications.

What is the usual dosage?

The information below is based on the dosage guidelines your doctor uses. Depending on your condition and medical history, your doctor may prescribe a different regimen. Do not change the dosage or stop taking your medication without your doctor's approval.

Adults: The usual dose is 1200mg a day split into two doses; one taken in the morning and the other in the evening.

How should I take Lopid?

You should take Lopid 30 minutes before a meal, preferably in the morning and evening.

What are possible food and drug interactions associated with Lopid?

If Lopid is taken with certain other drugs, the effects of either could be increased, decreased, or altered. It is especially important to check with your doctor before combining Lopid with the following: bood-thinning medications (anticoagulants), cholesterol-lowering medications called HMG-CoA reductase inhibitors, repaglinide.

What are the possible side effects of Lopid?

Side effects cannot be anticipated. If any develop or change in intensity, tell your doctor as soon as possible. Only your doctor can determine if it is safe for you to continue taking this drug.

Side effects may include: Abdominal pain, acute appendicitis, diarrhea, fatigue, headache, indigestion, nausea/vomiting

Can I receive Lopid if I am pregnant or breastfeeding?

Tell your doctor immediately if you are pregnant, plan to become pregnant, or are nursing. Lopid should be used in pregnancy only if the potential benefit justifies the potential risk to the fetus. It is not known whether Lopid is excreted in breast milk. A decision should be made whether to discontinue nursing or to discontinue the drug, taking into account the importance of the drug to the mother.

What should I do if I miss a dose of Lopid?

If you miss a dose of Lopid, do not double your next dose. Skip the missed dose and return to your normal dosing schedule.

How should I store Lopid?

Store Lopid at room temperature and away from light and moisture.

Lopinavir and ritonavir See Kaletra, page 680.

LOPRESSOR

Generic name: Metoprolol tartrate

What is Lopressor?

Lopressor is a medication known as beta-blocker that is used to treat high blood pressure, chest pain (angina), and heart attack.

What is the most important information I should know about Lopressor?

Do not abruptly stop taking Lopressor without first consulting your doctor. Suddenly stopping Lopressor therapy may lead to worsening angina or even a heart attack.

Lopressor may mask the signs and symptoms of low blood sugar, especially in people with high blood sugar (diabetes). If you have diabetes, monitor your blood sugar frequently, especially when you first start taking Lopressor.

If you have a disease that can make it hard to breathe such as wheezing (asthma) or chronic obstructive pulmonary disease (COPD), or thyroid problems, Lopressor can worsen your condition. Tell your doctor immediately if you experience shortness of breath.

If you have a tumor of the adrenal gland, which causes high blood pressure (pheochromocytoma), your doctor will prescribe you another type of blood pressure medication before you start taking Lopressor.

Inform your physician or dentist before undergoing any type of surgery that you are taking Lopressor.

Who should not take Lopressor?

You should not take Lopressor if you have been diagnosed with heart conditions called sinus bradycardia (a type of slow heartbeat), heart block >1st degree, cardiogenic shock, severe heart failure or sick-sinus syndrome. You should not take Lopressor if your heart beats >45 times per minute or if your systolic blood pressure (the top number) is >100mmHg. Also, you should not take Lopressor if you have been diagnosed with a severe peripheral circulatory disorder (in which blood flow to the legs and arms is reduced), pheochromocytoma or if are allergic to it or any of its ingredients.

What should I tell my doctor before I take the first dose of Lopressor?

Tell your doctor about all prescription, over-the-counter, and herbal medications you are taking before beginning treatment with Lopressor. Also, talk to your doctor about your complete medical history, especially if you have high blood sugar, wheezing, shortness of breath, or any other disease that can make it hard for you to breathe, overactive thyroid, or if you have suffered a heart attack before. Tell your doctor if you have a history of severe allergic reactions to allergens, because Lopressor may decrease the effectiveness of epinephrine.

What is the usual dosage?

The information below is based on the dosage guidelines your doctor uses. Depending on your condition and medical history, your doctor may prescribe a different regimen. Do not change the dosage or stop taking your medication without your doctor's approval.

Angina Pectoris
Adults: The usual starting dose is 100 milligrams (mg) a day, split into 2 doses. If necessary, your doctor may increase your individual dose up to 400 mg per day.

High Blood Pressure
Adults: The usual starting dose is 100 mg a day, split into 2 doses. If necessary, your doctor may increase your individual dose up to 450 mg per day.

Heart Attack
If your doctor suspects that you are having a heart attack, he/she may give you Lopressor at a dose of 5 mg intravenously every 2 minutes for a total of 3 doses. Depending on your response, your doctor may give you additional intravenous doses, and after 2 days may start you on 100 mg per day in divided doses.

How should I take Lopressor?
You should take Lopressor with or immediately following meals, and should take it at the same time every day.

What should I avoid while taking Lopressor?
You should avoid operating an automobile or heavy machinery as well as engaging in other tasks that require mental alertness until you know how Lopressor will affect you.

What are possible food and drug interactions associated with Lopressor?
If Lopressor is taken with certain other drugs, the effects of either could be increased, decreased, or altered. It is especially important to check with your doctor before combining Lopressor with the following: bupronion, cimetidine, diphenhydramine, hydroxychloroquine, paroxetine, propafenone, quinidine, quinine, reserpine (or any other catecholamine-depleting medications), ritonavir, terbinafine, thioridazine.

If you have a history of severe allergic reactions to common allergens, Lopressor may cause you to have a more severe reaction if you come in contact with these allergens.

What are the possible side effects of Lopressor?
Side effects cannot be anticipated. If any develop or change in intensity, tell your doctor as soon as possible. Only your doctor can determine if it is safe for you to continue taking this drug.

Side effects may include: low blood pressure, tiredness, dizziness, depression, confusion, short-term memory loss, headache, nightmares, sleeplessness, shortness of breath, slow heart-rate, vomiting, diarrhea, itching, rash, heart block, heart failure

Can I receive Lopressor if I am pregnant or breastfeeding?

The effects of Lopressor during pregnancy and breastfeeding are unknown. Lopressor is excreted in breast milk. Tell your doctor immediately if you are pregnant, plan to become pregnant, or are breastfeeding.

What should I do if I miss a dose of Lopressor?

If you miss a dose of Lopressor, do not double your next dose. Skip the missed dose and return to your normal dosing schedule.

How should I store Lopressor?

Store at room temperature and away from heat, light, and moisture.

LOPROX

Generic name: Ciclopriox

What is Loprox?

Loprox is a medication applied to the outer layer of the skin or scalp that is used to treat common fungal infections.

**What is the most important information
I should know about Loprox?**

Loprox is only meant to be applied to the outer surface of the skin, and should not be used near the eyes. Stop using Loprox and contact your doctor immediately if you experience any allergic reaction such as itching, burning, blistering, or swelling in the areas to which you apply Loprox.

Apply Loprox for the entire amount of time your doctor tells you to, even if your symptoms improve early on. Tell your doctor if your symptoms do not improve within 4 weeks of using Loprox. While using Loprox, make sure not to apply tight bandages or dressings over the treated skin.

Who should not take Loprox?

You should not use Loprox if you have a known allergy or sensitivity to Loprox.

**What should I tell my doctor before
I take the first dose of Loprox?**

Tell your doctor about all prescription, over-the-counter, and herbal medications you are taking before beginning treatment with Loprox. Also, talk to your doctor about your complete medical history, especially if you have an allergy or sensitivity to Loprox.

What is the usual dosage?

The information below is based on the dosage guidelines your doctor uses. Depending on your condition and medical history, your doctor may prescribe a different regimen. Do not change the dosage or stop taking your medication without your doctor's approval.

Cream, Gel, Suspension
Adults and children >10 years: Gently massage Loprox into the affected and surrounding skin twice daily, in the morning and evening. You may see an improvement of your symptoms within the first week. If you don't see an improvement after 4 weeks, contact your doctor.

Shampoo
Adults and children >10 years: Wet hair and apply approximately 1 teaspoon (5 mL) of Loprox shampoo to the scalp; 2 teaspoons (10 mL) may be used for long hair. Lather and leave on hair and scalp for 3 minutes. Avoid contact with eyes. Rinse off. Treatment should be repeated twice per week for 4 weeks, with a minimum of 3 days between applications.

How should I take Loprox?
If using Loprox lotion, make sure to shake the bottle well before each use.
   Gently massage Loprox onto the affected areas, including the immediate surrounding skin to ensure the Loprox is effective. It should be applied around the same times each day.

What should I avoid while taking Loprox?
Avoid applying tight bandages or wound dressings to the same area to which you apply Loprox.

What are possible food and drug interactions associated with Loprox?
If Loprox is taken with certain other drugs, the effects of either could be increased, decreased, or altered. It is especially important to check with your doctor before combining Loprox with any other product also applied to the skin.

What are the possible side effects of Loprox?
Side effects cannot be anticipated. If any develop or change in intensity, tell your doctor as soon as possible. Only your doctor can determine if it is safe for you to continue taking this drug.

Side effects may include: itching or burning of the area to which Loprox is applied.

Can I receive Loprox if I am pregnant or breastfeeding?
The effects of Loprox during pregnancy and breastfeeding are unknown. Tell your doctor immediately if you are pregnant, plan to become pregnant, or are breastfeeding.

What should I do if I miss a dose of Loprox?
If you forget to apply Loprox, do not apply double the amount next time you use Loprox. Skip the missed application and return to your normal dosing schedule.

How should I store Loprox?
Loprox should be stored at room temperature.

Lorazepam *See Ativan, page 143.*

Losartan potassium *See Cozaar, page 352.*

Losartan potassium and hydrochlorothiazide *See Hyzaar, page 649.*

LOTENSIN
Generic name: Benazepril hydrochloride

What is Lotensin?
Lotensin is a type of blood pressure lowering medication known as an angiotensin converting enzyme (ACE) inhibitor. Lotensin is used to lower your blood pressure when taken alone or in combination with other medications.

**What is the most important information
I should know about Lotensin?**
When taken during pregnancy, ACE inhibitors such as Lotensin can cause injury and even death to the developing baby. If you are pregnant or plan on becoming pregnant, stop taking Lotensin and contact your doctor immediately.

Lotensin can cause a rare but serious allergic reaction leading to extreme swelling of the face, lips, tongue, throat, or gut (causing severe abdominal pain). If you experience any of these symptoms, seek emergency medical attention right away.

Lotensin may rarely cause a yellowing of the skin or eyes (jaundice), which can be a sign of liver injury. If this occurs tell your doctor immediately.

Lotensin may cause lightheadedness or fainting, especially upon standing from a lying or sitting position.

Lotensin may decrease your levels of infection-fighting white blood cells, especially if you have lupus erythematosus or kidney disease. If you have these diseases your doctor will most likely monitor you closely by taking regular blood samples. If you get any type of infection (sore throat/fever) while taking Lotensin, promptly report it to your doctor.

Lotensin should be taken with caution in patients who have congestive heart failure.

Who should not take Lotensin?
You should not take Lotensin if you have had a previous allergic reaction or are sensitive to Lotensin or any other ACE inhibitor.

What should I tell my doctor before I take the first dose of Lotensin?

Tell your doctor about all prescription, over-the-counter, and herbal medications you are taking before beginning treatment with Lotensin. Also, talk to your doctor about your complete medical history, especially if you are pregnant or plan on becoming pregnant, if you have lupus, heart failure or kidney disease, or if you have ever had an allergy or sensitivity to an ACE inhibitor such as Lotensin.

What is the usual dosage?

The information below is based on the dosage guidelines your doctor uses. Depending on your condition and medical history, your doctor may prescribe a different regimen. Do not change the dosage or stop taking your medication without your doctor's approval.

Adults: The usual starting dose is 10 milligrams (mg) once a day. Your doctor may increase your daily dose to 20 to 40 mg per day as one dose or split into multiple doses.

Children ages >6 years: In children, usual doses of Lotensin range from 0.1 to 0.6 mg per 2.2 pounds of body weight per day.

How should I take Lotensin?

Lotensin can be taken with or without food, at the same time every day.

What should I avoid while taking Lotensin?

Avoid driving or operating heavy machinery until you know how Lotensin will affect you. Also avoid becoming dehydrated while taking Lotensin; this could cause your blood pressure to drop too low.

What are possible food and drug interactions associated with Lotensin?

If Lotensin is taken with certain other drugs, the effects of either could be increased, decreased, or altered. It is especially important to check with your doctor before combining Lotensin with any of the following: antidiabetes medications, diuretics (hydrochlorothiazide, spironolactone, amiloride, triamterene), lithium, potassium supplements, salt substitutes containing potassium

What are the possible side effects of Lotensin?

Side effects cannot be anticipated. If any develop or change in intensity, tell your doctor as soon as possible. Only your doctor can determine if it is safe for you to continue taking this drug.

Side effects may include: headache, dizziness, cough, fatigue, nausea

Can I receive Lotensin if I am pregnant or breastfeeding?

Taking Lotensin while you are pregnant could cause serious harm or even death to your unborn baby. Tell your doctor immediately if you are pregnant, plan to become pregnant, or are breastfeeding.

What should I do if I miss a dose of Lotensin?

If you forget to take Lotensin, skip the dose you missed and then return to your normal dosing schedule. Do not take 2 doses at once.

How should I store Lotensin?

Store Lotensin at room temperature in a tightly closed container protected from light.

LOTENSIN HCT

Generic name: Benazepril hydrochloride and hydrochlorothiazide

What is Lotensin HCT?

Lotensin is a combination product that contains two medicines: Benazepril, an ACE inhibitor, and hydrochlorothiazide, a diuretic. These two medications work together to lower blood pressure in patients who may not have had adequate blood pressure lowering from other medications.

What is the most important information I should know about Lotensin HCT?

When taken during pregnancy, angiotensin converting enzyme (ACE) inhibitors such as Lotensin HCT can cause injury and even death to the developing baby. If you are pregnant or plan on becoming pregnant, stop taking Lotensin HCT and contact your doctor immediately.

Lotensin HCT can cause a rare but serious allergic reaction leading to extreme swelling of the face, lips, tongue, throat, or gut (causing severe abdominal pain). If you experience any of these symptoms seek emergency medical attention.

Lotensin HCT may rarely cause a yellowing of the skin or eyes (jaundice), which can be a sign of liver injury. If this occurs tell your doctor immediately.

Lotensin HCT may cause lightheadedness or fainting, especially upon standing from a lying or sitting position.

Lotensin HCT may decrease your blood levels of infection-fighting white blood cells, especially if you have lupus erythematosus or kidney disease. If you have these diseases, your doctor will most likely monitor you closely by taking regular blood samples. If you get any type of infection (sore throat/fever) while taking Lotensin HCT, promptly report it to your doctor.

Lotensin HCT may activate lupus or gout (severe and painful inflammation of joints) in certain susceptible patients.

If you have diabetes, Lotensin HCT may increase your blood sugar levels; check your blood sugar frequently.

Lotensin HCT should be taken with caution in patients who have congestive heart failure.

Who should not take Lotensin HCT?

You should not take Lotensin HCT if you do not produce urine, you have a history of sensitivity or allergic reaction to an ACE inhibitor, or you are allergic to sulfonamide-derived medications.

What should I tell my doctor before I take the first dose of Lotensin HCT?

Tell your doctor about all prescription, over-the-counter, and herbal medications you are taking before beginning treatment with Lotensin HCT. Also, talk to your doctor about your complete medical history, especially if you are pregnant or plan on becoming pregnant. Tell your doctor if you have diabetes, heart failure, lupus, liver or kidney disease, or if you have ever had an allergy or sensitivity to an ACE inhibitor or sulfonamide-derived medications.

What is the usual dosage?

The information below is based on the dosage guidelines your doctor uses. Depending on your condition and medical history, your doctor may prescribe a different regimen. Do not change the dosage or stop taking your medication without your doctor's approval.

Adults: Usual doses range from 10/12.5 milligrams (mg), 10 mg of benazepril and 12.5 mg of hydrochlorothiazide) to 20/25 mg taken once daily. Your doctor may increase your dose based on your individual condition and blood pressure.

How should I take Lotensin HCT?

You should take Lotensin HCT with or without food at the same time every day.

What should I avoid while taking Lotensin HCT?

Avoid driving or operating heavy machinery until you know how Lotensin HCT will affect you. Also avoid becoming dehydrated while taking Lotensin HCT; this could cause your blood pressure to drop too low.

What are possible food and drug interactions associated with Lotensin HCT?

If Lotensin HCT is taken with certain other drugs, the effects of either could be increased, decreased, or altered. It is especially important to check with your doctor before combining Lotensin HCT with any of the following: diuretics (such as hydrochlorothiazide, spironolactone, amiloride, triamterene), cholestyramine, colestipol, lithium, norepineph-rine, NSAIDs such as ibuprofen or naproxen, insulin, potassium supple-ments, salt substitutes containing potassium

What are the possible side effects of Lotensin HCT?

Side effects cannot be anticipated. If any develop or change in intensity, tell your doctor as soon as possible. Only your doctor can determine if it is safe for you to continue taking this drug.

Side effects may include: headache, dizziness, cough, fatigue, nausea, impotence, muscle rigidity

Can I receive Lotensin HCT if I am pregnant or breastfeeding?

Taking Lotensin HCT while you are pregnant could cause serious harm or even death to your unborn baby. Tell your doctor immediately if you are pregnant, plan to become pregnant, or are breastfeeding. Lotensin HCT is excreted in breast milk; talk to your doctor before breastfeeding and taking Lotensin HCT.

What should I do if I miss a dose of Lotensin HCT?

If you forget to take Lotensin HCT, skip the dose you missed and then return to your normal dosing schedule. Do not take 2 doses at once.

How should I store Lotensin HCT?

Store Lotensin HCT at room temperature in a tightly closed container protected from light.

Loteprednol etabonate ophthalmic suspension See Alrex, *page 70.*

LOTREL

Generic name: Amlodipine besylate and benazepril hydrochloride

What is Lotrel?

Lotrel contains 2 prescription medicines that work together to lower blood pressure: amlodipine besylate, a calcium channel blocker, and benazepril hydrochloride, an ACE inhibitor. Your doctor will prescribe Lotrel only after other medicines haven't worked.

What is the most important information I should know about Lotrel?

When taken during pregnancy, ACE inhibitors such as Lotrel can cause injury and even death to the developing baby. If you are pregnant or plan on becoming pregnant, stop taking Lotrel and contact your doctor immediately.

Lotrel can cause a rare but serious allergic reaction leading to extreme swelling of the face, lips, tongue, throat, or gut (causing severe abdominal pain). If you experience any of these symptoms, seek emergency medical attention right away.

Lotrel may rarely cause a yellowing of the skin or eyes (jaundice), which can be a sign of liver injury. If this occurs, tell your doctor immediately.

Lotrel may cause lightheadedness or fainting, especially upon standing from a lying or sitting position.

If you get any type of infection (sore throat/fever) while taking Lotrel, promptly report it to your doctor. Lotrel may decrease your blood levels of infection-fighting white blood cells, especially if you have lupus erythematosus or kidney disease. If you have these diseases your doctor will most likely monitor you closely by taking regular blood samples.

Lotrel should be taken with caution in patients who have congestive heart failure.

Lotrel is not for the initial treatment of high blood pressure, and is usually given to patients who have not had adequate blood pressure lowering effects from other medications.

Who should not take Lotrel?

You should not take Lotrel if you have had a previous allergic reaction or are sensitive to Lotrel or any other ACE inhibitor or calcium channel blocker medications.

What should I tell my doctor before I take the first dose of Lotrel?

Tell your doctor about all prescription, over-the-counter, and herbal medications you are taking before beginning treatment with Lotrel, especially medications for high blood pressure or heart failure, diuretics (water pills), or lithium. Also, talk to your doctor about your complete medical history, especially if you are pregnant or plan on becoming pregnant, if you are breastfeeding, if you have a heart condition, liver or kidney problems, diabetes (high blood sugar), lupus, or if you have ever had an allergy or sensitivity to an ACE inhibitor or calcium channel blocker. Tell your doctor or dentist you are taking Lotrel if you are going to have surgery, allergy shots for bee stings, or kidney dialysis.

What is the usual dosage?

The information below is based on the dosage guidelines your doctor uses. Depending on your condition and medical history, your doctor may prescribe a different regimen. Do not change the dosage or stop taking your medication without your doctor's approval.

Adults: Usual doses of Lotrel are 2.5/10 milligrams (mg), 2.5 mg of amlodipine and 10 mg of benazepril to 10/40 mg taken once daily. Your doctor may increase or decrease your individual dose based on your condition and blood pressure.

How should I take Lotrel?
Lotrel can be taken with or without food and should be taken at the same time every day.

What should I avoid while taking Lotrel?
Avoid driving or operating heavy machinery until you know how Lotrel will affect you. Avoid becoming dehydrated and drink adequate fluids while taking Lotrel, to prevent your blood pressure from dropping too low.

What are possible food and drug interactions associated with Lotrel?
If Lotrel is taken with certain other drugs, the effects of either could be increased, decreased, or altered. It is especially important to check with your doctor before combining Lotrel with any of the following: blood pressure drugs, diuretics (such as hydrochlorothiazide, spironolactone, amiloride, triamterene), heart failure drugs, lithium, potassium supplements, salt substitutes containing potassium.

What are the possible side effects of Lotrel?
Side effects cannot be anticipated. If any develop or change in intensity, tell your doctor as soon as possible. Only your doctor can determine if it is safe for you to continue taking this drug.

Side effects may include: headache, cough, dizziness, swelling, fluid retention

Rare, but more serious side effects include: allergic reactions (swelling of your face, eyelids, tongue or throat), difficulty swallowing, asthma (wheezing) or other breathing problems; low blood pressure

Can I receive Lotrel if I am pregnant or breastfeeding?
When used in pregnancy, ACE inhibitors can cause injury and even death to the developing fetus. When pregnancy is detected, Lotrel should be discontinued as soon as possible. It is not known whether Lotrel is excreted into breast milk. It is recommended that nursing be discontinued while Lotrel is administered.

What should I do if I miss a dose of Lotrel?
If you forget to take Lotrel, take it as soon as you remember. If it is more than 12 hours, just take your next dose at the regular time. Do not take 2 doses at once.

How should I store Lotrel?
Store Lotrel at room temperature, away from moisture.

LOTRISONE
Generic name: Clotrimazole and betamethasone dipropionate

What is Lotrisone?
Lotrisone cream and lotion are used on the skin to treat fungal infections of the feet, groin, and body, especially if those fungal infections are inflamed and have symptoms of redness and/or itching. Lotrisone contains clotrimazole and betamethasone dipropionate. Clotrimazole works against fungus, and betamethasone dipropionate is a corticosteroid used to help relieve redness, swelling, itching, and other discomforts of fungal infections.

What is the most important information I should know about Lotrisone?
Lotrisone is for external, topical use on the skin only. Lotrisone is not to be used in children, or to treat diaper rash. Also, do not use Lotrisone near the eyes, mouth, or in the vagina.

Do not use Lotrisone cream or lotion for longer than 4 weeks. Prolonged use may lead to unwanted side effects. Notify your doctor if your condition persists beyond the recommended treatment time.

Who should not take Lotrisone?
Lotrisone cream and lotion are not recommended for use in children under the age of 17 because topical corticosteroids, such as Lotrisone, may be absorbed through the skin, possibly leading to hormone imbalances that can be serious and can slow a child's growth.

Do not use Lotrisone for diaper rash. Do not use if you are allergic or sensitive to clotrimazole and betamethasone dipropionate; other corticosteroids or imidazoles; or any ingredients in Lotrisone.

What should I tell my doctor before I take the first dose of Lotrisone?
Tell your doctor about all prescription, over-the-counter, and herbal medications you are taking before beginning treatment with Lotrisone. Also, talk to your doctor about your complete medical history, especially if you are using other corticosteroid-containing products.

What is the usual dosage?
The information below is based on the dosage guidelines your doctor uses. Depending on your condition and medical history, your doctor may prescribe a different regimen. Do not change the dosage or stop taking your medication without your doctor's approval.

Foot Fungal Infections
Adults and adolescents over 17 years: The usual treatment is to apply sufficient cream or lotion into the affected and surrounding skin areas 2 times a day, in the morning and evening, for 4 weeks. Notify your doctor if there is no improvement after 2 weeks of treatment on the feet.

Groin and Body Fungal Infections
Adults and adolescents over 17 years: The usual treatment is to apply sufficient cream or lotion into the affected and surrounding skin areas 2 times a day, in the morning and evening, for 2 weeks. Notify your doctor if there is no improvement after 1 week of treatment on the groin or body.

How should I take Lotrisone?

Lotrisone lotion should be well shaken before each use. Gently massage sufficient Lotrisone cream or lotion into the affected and surrounding areas 2 times a day, in the morning and evening.

Do not use more than 45 grams of Lotrisone cream per week or more than 45 milliliters of Lotrisone lotion per week. Even if your symptoms improve, you should continue to take Lotrisone for the full prescribed treatment time.

What should I avoid while taking Lotrisone?

Do not use Lotrisone cream or lotion for longer than 4 weeks for any condition. Prolonged use of Lotrisone cream or lotion may lead to unwanted side effects.

Do not use any bandage, cover, or wrap over the area where you have applied Lotrisone. If you are using Lotrisone cream or lotion in the groin area, it is especially important to use the medication for 2 weeks only, and to apply the cream or lotion sparingly. Do not use Lotrisone cream or lotion near the eyes, mouth, or vagina.

What are possible food and drug interactions associated with Lotrisone?

If Lotrisone is taken with certain other drugs, the effects of either could be increased, decreased, or altered. It is especially important to check with your doctor before combining Lotrisone with other corticosteroids.

What are the possible side effects of Lotrisone?

Side effects cannot be anticipated. If any develop or change in intensity, tell your doctor as soon as possible. Only your doctor can determine if it is safe for you to continue taking this drug.

Side effects may include: acne, allergic skin reactions, change in skin color, dryness, increased hair, infection of the hair follicles, irritation, itching, skin thinning, stretch marks

Can I receive Lotrisone if I am pregnant or breastfeeding?

The effects of Lotrisone during pregnancy and breastfeeding are unknown. Tell your doctor immediately if you are pregnant, plan to become pregnant, or are breastfeeding.

What should I do if I miss a dose of Lotrisone?

If you miss a dose of Lotrisone, apply it as soon as you remember. If it is almost time for your next dose, skip the dose you missed and go back to your regular schedule.

How should I store Lotrisone?

Lotrisone cream or lotion should be stored at room temperature. The Lotrisone lotion bottle should be stored upright.

Lovastatin See Mevacor, page 814.

Lovastatin and niacin See Advicor, page 46.

LOVAZA
Generic name: Omega-3-acid ethyl esters

What is Lovaza?

Lovaza is used together with diet and exercise to help lower triglyceride levels in the blood. Lovaza works by lowering the body's production of triglycerides. High levels of triglycerides can lead to coronary artery disease, heart disease, and stroke.

What is the most important information I should know about Lovaza?

This medication is only part of a complete program of treatment that also includes diet, exercise, and weight control. Follow your diet, medication, and exercise routines very closely.

Who should not take Lovaza?

Do not use this medication if you are allergic to fish or soybeans. Do not take Lovaza if you are allergic to the medication or any or its ingredients.

What should I tell my doctor before I take the first dose of Lovaza?

Tell your doctor about all prescription, over-the-counter, and herbal medications you are taking before beginning treatment with Lovaza. Also, talk to your doctor about your complete medical history, especially if you have diabetes (high blood sugar), or an underactive thyroid.

What is the usual dosage?
The information below is based on the dosage guidelines your doctor uses. Depending on your condition and medical history, your doctor may prescribe a different regimen. Do not change the dosage or stop taking your medication without your doctor's approval.

Adults: The usual starting dose of Lovaza is 4 grams (g) once daily, and it may be taken as a single 4-g dose (4 capsules) or as 2-g doses (2 capsules taken twice a day).

How should I take Lovaza?
Take Lovaza with food. Do not take it in larger amounts, or longer than recommended by your doctor. Follow the directions on your prescription label.

What should I avoid while taking Lovaza?
Avoid eating foods that are high in fat or cholesterol. This medication will not be as effective in lowering your triglycerides if you do not follow the diet plan recommended by your doctor. Avoid drinking alcohol. It can increase your triglycerides and may make your condition worse.

What are possible food and drug interactions associated with Lovaza?
If Lovaza is taken with certain other drugs, the effects of either could be increased, decreased, or altered. It is especially important to check with your doctor before combining Lovaza with any of the following: blood thinners, estrogens, heart medications known as beta blockers, and thiazides (water pills).

What are the possible side effects of Lovaza?
Side effects cannot be anticipated. If any develop or change in intensity, tell your doctor as soon as possible. Only your doctor can determine if it is safe for you to continue taking this drug.

Side effects may include: back pain, belching, body aches, chest pain, chills, fever, flu-like symptoms, mild skin rash, uneven heartbeats, unusual or unpleasant taste in your mouth, upset stomach

Side effects other than those listed here may also occur. Talk to your doctor about any side effect that seems unusual or that is especially bothersome.

Can I receive Lovaza if I am pregnant or breastfeeding?
The effects of Lovaza during pregnancy and breastfeeding are unknown. Tell your doctor immediately if you are pregnant, plan to become pregnant, or are breastfeeding.

What should I do if I miss a dose of Lovaza?

Take the missed dose as soon as you remember. If it is almost time for your next dose, skip the missed dose and take the medicine at the next regularly scheduled time. Do not take extra medicine to make up the missed dose.

How should I store Lovaza?

Store this medication at room temperature away from moisture and heat. Do not freeze.

Lubiprostone See Amitiza, page 84.

LUMIGAN

Generic name: Bimatoprost solution

What is Lumigan?

Lumigan is for high eye pressure, also called intraocular pressure (IOP), in people with the eye conditions open-angle glaucoma or ocular hypertension.

What is the most important information I should know about Lumigan?

Lumigan may darken the color of your iris (colored part of the eye), eyelid, and eyelashes. Lumigan may also cause permanent brown pigmentation of the iris. Lumigan may also increase the growth or change the direction of growth of your eyelashes and small hairs around your eye. If you stop using Lumigan, the discoloration of your eyelids or eyelashes is reversible; however the discoloration of the iris is most likely permanent. If you notice any discoloration or changes in these areas of the eye, inform your doctor so that you can be appropriately monitored.

When using Lumigan, do not allow the tip of the bottle to touch your eye, fingers, or any other surface, as serious eye infections may occur if your bottle becomes contaminated. You should contact your doctor immediately if you experience any eye injury, infection, or eyelid reactions before continuing to use Lumigan.

Soft contact lenses should be removed before putting Lumigan drops in your eye, and then reinserted after at least 15 minutes. If you also use other eye drops, wait at least 5 minutes before instilling Lumigan after applying other products.

Who should not take Lumigan?

Do not use Lumigan if you have a known sensitivity or allergy to this product.

What should I tell my doctor before I take the first dose of Lumigan?

Mention all prescription, over-the-counter, and herbal medications you are taking before beginning treatment with Lumigan. Also, talk to your doctor about your complete medical history, especially if you have macular edema, inflammation, infection, or any other eye injury; have scheduled eye surgery; or you wear contact lenses.

What is the usual dosage?

The information below is based on the dosage guidelines your doctor uses. Depending on your condition and medical history, your doctor may prescribe a different regimen. Do not change the dosage or stop taking your medication without your doctor's approval.

Adults: The usual dosage of Lumigan is 1 drop in the affected eye(s) once daily in the evening. Do not exceed more than the once-daily dosage because frequent administration may decrease the intraocular-pressure lowering effect.

How should I take Lumigan?

You should instill the drop of solution into your eye(s) in the evening, taking extra care not to allow the tip of the bottle to touch any surface, including your eye or fingers. If you wear contact lenses, make sure to take them off before instilling Lumigan, and wait at least 15 minutes before putting them back in. You should wait at least 5 minutes in between using different eye products, including Lumigan.

What should I avoid while taking Lumigan?

You should avoid allowing the tip of your Lumigan bottle to touch other surfaces. You should also avoid inserting contact lenses until at least 15 minutes has elapsed from the time you applied Lumigan to your eye(s).

What are possible food and drug interactions associated with Lumigan?

If Lumigan is taken with certain other drugs, the effects of either could be increased, decreased, or altered. It is especially important to check with your doctor before combining Lumigan with any other product(s) applied to the eye.

What are the possible side effects of Lumigan?

Side effects cannot be anticipated. If any develop or change in intensity, tell your doctor as soon as possible. Only your doctor can determine if it is safe for you to continue taking this drug.

Side effects may include: eye or eyelid redness, growth of eyelashes, visual disturbances, dry eyes, burning or foreign body sensation in the eyes, eye pain, darkening of the eyelashes or skin around the eyes, cataracts, inflammation of the eye or eyelid, an inflammatory condition of the eye known as superficial punctate keratitis, itching of the eyes, eye discharge, tearing, eye sensitivity to light, swelling of the eye

Can I receive Lumigan if I am pregnant or breastfeeding?
The effects of Lumigan during pregnancy and breastfeeding are unknown. Tell your doctor immediately if you are pregnant, plan to become pregnant, or are breastfeeding.

What should I do if I miss a dose of Lumigan?
If you forget to use Lumigan, do not double your next dose. Skip the dose you missed and then return to your normal dosing schedule.

How should I store Lumigan?
Lumigan should be stored in the original container, in the refrigerator or at room temperature.

LUNESTA
Generic name: Eszopiclone

What is Lunesta?
Lunesta is a sleep medication known as a hypnotic. It is used to help if you have trouble falling asleep or staying asleep.

What is the most important information I should know about Lunesta?
If you do not experience an improvement after 7-10 days, contact your doctor to rule out other causes for your sleeping problems.

Inform your doctor immediately if you experience any changes in your behavior or mood, including aggression, agitation, hallucinations, depression, or suicidal thinking.

Lunesta works quickly, and can affect your ability to drive or operate heavy machinery, including the day after you take Lunesta. Do not engage in any activities that require mental alertness right after you take Lunesta or the next day until you know how Lunesta will affect you.

Rarely, Lunesta can cause short-term memory loss, which may be avoided if you are able to devote an entire night to sleep after taking Lunesta.

If you take Lunesta for more than several weeks, you may experience a dependence on Lunesta in order to fall asleep, or a decrease in Lunesta's ability to help you fall asleep.

Withdrawal symptoms may occur if you suddenly stop taking Lunesta, even after taking it for 1 week, but it is more likely to occur with long-term Lunesta therapy.

What should I tell my doctor before I take the first dose of Lunesta?

Tell your doctor about all prescription, over-the-counter, and herbal medications you are taking before beginning treatment with Lunesta. Also, talk to your doctor about your complete medical history, especially if you are over 65 years old, you are depressed or have a history of depression, or you have liver impairment or any disease that makes it difficult to breathe.

What is the usual dosage?

The information below is based on the dosage guidelines your doctor uses. Depending on your condition and medical history, your doctor may prescribe a different regimen. Do not change the dosage or stop taking your medication without your doctor's approval.

Adults: The usual starting dose of Lunesta is 2 milligrams (mg) taken once daily. Your doctor may increase your individual dose to 3 mg daily depending on how Lunesta affects you.

If you are over 65, you have liver impairment, or you are taking certain medications that interact with Lunesta, the usual starting dose is 1 mg daily, and may be increased by your doctor to 2 mg daily.

How should I take Lunesta?

Lunesta should be taken immediately before going to bed. Do not take Lunesta with or right after a meal, and do not take Lunesta unless you are able to get a full night's sleep (7 to 8 hours) before returning to your normal activities.

What should I avoid while taking Lunesta?

Avoid drinking alcohol while taking Lunesta. Also avoid operating an automobile or heavy machinery until you know how Lunesta will affect you.

What are possible food and drug interactions associated with Lunesta?

If Lunesta is taken with certain other drugs, the effects of either could be increased, decreased, or altered. It is especially important to check with your doctor before combining Lunesta with the following: alcohol, clarithromycin, itraconazole, ketoconazole, nefazodone, nelfinavir, olanzapine, other sleep-inducing drugs, ritonavir, rifampicin, and troleandomycin.

What are the possible side effects of Lunesta?

Side effects cannot be anticipated. If any develop or change in intensity, tell your doctor as soon as possible. Only your doctor can determine if it is safe for you to continue taking this drug.

Side effects may include: lightheadedness, dizziness, headache, unpleasant taste, drowsiness, difficulty with coordination

Can I receive Lunesta if I am pregnant or breastfeeding?

Sleep medicines may cause sedation or other potential effects in the unborn baby when used during the last weeks of pregnancy. Be sure to tell your doctor if you are pregnant, if you are planning to become pregnant, or if you become pregnant while taking Lunesta. A very small amount of Lunesta may be present in breast milk after use of the medication. The effects of very small amounts of Lunesta on an infant are not known. Therefore, as with all other prescription sleep medicines, it is recommended that you not take Lunesta if you are breastfeeding a baby.

What should I do if I miss a dose of Lunesta?

If you forget to take a dose of Lunesta, do not double your next dose when you do remember. Take Lunesta as soon as you remember before you go to bed, as long as you can devote a full night to sleep.

How should I store Lunesta?

Store at room temperature.

LUVOX CR

Generic name: Fluvoxamine maleate, extended-release

What is Luvox CR?

Luvox CR is used to treat social anxiety disorder, also known as social phobia. It is also used to treat obsessions and compulsions in patients with obsessive compulsive disorder (OCD).

What is the most important information I should know about Luvox CR?

Luvox CR is not approved for use in children.

Antidepressant medicines may increase suicidal thoughts or actions in some children, teenagers, and young adults when the medicine is first started. Depression and other serious mental illnesses are the most important causes of suicidal thoughts and actions. Some people may have a particularly high risk of having suicidal thoughts or actions. These include people who have (or have a family history of) bipolar disorder (also called manic-depressive illness) or suicidal thoughts or actions.

Pay close attention to any changes, especially sudden changes, in mood, behaviors, thoughts, or feelings. This is very important when an antidepressant medicine is first started or when the dose is changed.

Call the doctor right away to report new or sudden changes in mood, behavior, thoughts, or feelings. Signs to watch for include new or worsening depression, new or worsening anxiety, agitation, insomnia, hostility, panic attacks, restlessness, extreme hyperactivity, and suicidal thinking or behavior.

DRUG IDENTIFICATION GUIDE

Use this section to quickly verify the identity of a capsule, tablet, or other solid oral medication. More than 200 leading tablets and capsules are shown in actual size and color, organized alphabetically by brand name. Each is labeled with its generic name, as well as its strength and the name of its supplier.

Note: While every effort has been made to ensure the faithful reproduction of the product photos in this section, changes in medication size, color, and design are always a possibility. Likewise, all available dosage forms and strengths may not be pictured. When in doubt, it's best to confirm a product's identity with your doctor or pharmacist.

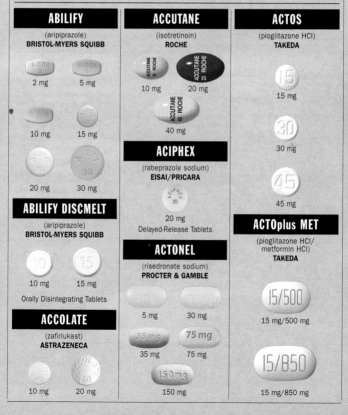

ABILIFY
(aripiprazole)
BRISTOL-MYERS SQUIBB

2 mg | 5 mg
10 mg | 15 mg
20 mg | 30 mg

ABILIFY DISCMELT
(aripiprazole)
BRISTOL-MYERS SQUIBB

10 mg | 15 mg

Orally Disintegrating Tablets

ACCOLATE
(zafirlukast)
ASTRAZENECA

10 mg | 20 mg

ACCUTANE
(isotretinoin)
ROCHE

10 mg | 20 mg
40 mg

ACIPHEX
(rabeprazole sodium)
EISAI/PRICARA

20 mg
Delayed-Release Tablets

ACTONEL
(risedronate sodium)
PROCTER & GAMBLE

5 mg | 30 mg
35 mg | 75 mg
150 mg

ACTOS
(pioglitazone HCl)
TAKEDA

15 mg
30 mg
45 mg

ACTOplus MET
(pioglitazone HCl/
metformin HCl)
TAKEDA

15 mg/500 mg
15 mg/850 mg

ADDERALL

(mixed salts of a single-entity
amphetamine product)
(dextroamphetamine
saccharate/
dextroamphetamine sulfate/
amphetamine aspartate/
amphetamine sulfate)
SHIRE

5 mg

7.5 mg   10 mg

12.5 mg   15 mg

20 mg   30 mg

ADDERALL XR

(mixed salts of a single-entity
amphetamine product)
(dextroamphetamine
saccharate/
dextroamphetamine sulfate/
amphetamine aspartate/
amphetamine sulfate)
SHIRE

5 mg

10 mg

15 mg

20 mg

25 mg

30 mg

Extended-Release Capsules

ADVICOR

(niacin/lovastatin)
ABBOTT

500 mg/20 mg

750 mg/20 mg

1000 mg/20 mg

1000 mg/40 mg

Extended-Release Tablets

AGGRENOX

(aspirin/extended-release
dipyridamole)
BOEHRINGER INGELHEIM

25 mg/200 mg

ALLEGRA

(fexofenadine HCl)
sanofi-aventis, U.S.

30 mg   60 mg

180 mg

ALLEGRA-D 12 HOUR

(fexofenadine HCl/
pseudoephedrine HCl)
sanofi-aventis, U.S.

60 mg/120 mg

Extended-Release Tablets

ALLEGRA-D 24 HOUR

(fexofenadine HCl/
pseudoephedrine HCl)
sanofi-aventis, U.S.

308
AV

180 mg/240 mg

Extended-Release Tablets

ALTACE

(ramipril)
KING

1.25 mg

2.5 mg

5 mg

10 mg

AMBIEN

(zolpidem tartrate)
sanofi-aventis, U.S.

5 mg   10 mg

AMERGE

(naratriptan HCl)
GLAXOSMITHKLINE

1 mg

2.5 mg

AMOXIL

(amoxicillin)
GLAXOSMITHKLINE

500 mg

200 mg
Chewable

400 mg
Chewable

500 mg

875 mg

ANAPROX

(naproxen sodium)
ROCHE

275 mg

ANAPROX DS

(naproxen sodium)
ROCHE

550 mg

ARICEPT

(donepezil HCl)
EISAI/PFIZER

5 mg

10 mg

ARICEPT ODT

(donepezil HCl)
EISAI/PFIZER

5 mg

10 mg

Orally Disintegrating Tablets

ARIMIDEX

(anastrozole)
ASTRAZENECA

1 mg

ARMOUR THYROID

(thyroid, USP)
FOREST

1/4 gr.   1/2 gr.

1 gr.   1 1/2 gr.

2 gr.   3 gr.

4 gr.

5 gr.

ASACOL

(mesalamine)
P&G PHARMACEUTICALS

400 mg

Delayed-Release Tablets

ATACAND

(candesartan cilexetil)
ASTRAZENECA

4 mg   8 mg

16 mg   32 mg

ATACAND HCT

(candesartan cilexetil/
hydrochlorothiazide)
ASTRAZENECA

16 mg/12.5 mg

32 mg/12.5 mg

ATRIPLA

(efavirenz/emtricitabine/
tenofovir disoproxil fumarate)
**BRISTOL-MYERS SQUIBB/
GILEAD SCIENCES, LLC**

600 mg/200 mg/300 mg

AUGMENTIN

(amoxicillin/
clavulanate potassium)
GLAXOSMITHKLINE

125 mg/31.25 mg
Chewable

200 mg/28.5 mg
Chewable

250 mg/62.5 mg
Chewable

400 mg/57 mg
Chewable

AUGMENTIN

(amoxicillin/
clavulanate potassium)
GLAXOSMITHKLINE

250 mg/125 mg

500 mg/125 mg

875 mg/125 mg

AUGMENTIN XR

(amoxicillin/
clavulanate potassium)
GLAXOSMITHKLINE

1000 mg/62.5 mg

AVALIDE

(irbesartan/hydrochlorothiazide)
BRISTOL-MYERS SQUIBB

150 mg/12.5 mg

300 mg/12.5 mg

300 mg/25 mg
Extended-Release Tablets

AVANDAMET

(rosiglitazone maleate/
metformin HCl)
GLAXOSMITHKLINE

1 mg/500 mg

2 mg/500 mg

2 mg/1000 mg

4 mg/500 mg

4 mg/1000 mg

AVANDARYL

(rosiglitazone maleate/
glimepiride)
GLAXOSMITHKLINE

4 mg/1 mg

4 mg/2 mg

4 mg/4 mg

AVANDIA

(rosiglitazone maleate)
GLAXOSMITHKLINE

2 mg   4 mg

8 mg

AVAPRO

(irbesartan)
BRISTOL-MYERS SQUIBB

75 mg   150 mg

300 mg

AVELOX

(moxifloxacin HCl)
SCHERING

400 mg

AVODART

(dutasteride)
GLAXOSMITHKLINE

0.5 mg

AXERT

(almotriptan malate)
ORTHO-MCNEIL

6.25 mg   12.5 mg

AZOR

(amlodipine/olmesartan
medoxomil)
DAIICHI SANKYO

5 mg/20 mg   5 mg/40 mg

10 mg/20 mg   10 mg/40 mg

BARACLUDE

(entecavir)
BRISTOL-MYERS SQUIBB

0.5 mg

1.0 mg

BENICAR

(olmesartan medoxomil)
DAIICHI-SANKYO

5 mg

20 mg

40 mg

BIAXIN

(clarithromycin)
ABBOTT

250 mg

500 mg

BIAXIN XL

(clarithromycin)
ABBOTT

500 mg

Extended-Release Tablets

BONIVA

(ibandronate sodium)
ROCHE

150 mg

CADUET

(amlodipine besylate/
atorvastatin calcium)
PFIZER

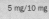

5 mg/10 mg

5 mg/20 mg

5 mg/40 mg

5 mg/80 mg

10 mg/10 mg

10 mg/20 mg

10 mg/40 mg

10 mg/80 mg

CARBATROL
(carbamazepine)
SHIRE

100 mg

200 mg

300 mg

Extended-Release Capsules

CATAPRES
(clonidine HCl)
BOEHRINGER INGELHEIM

0.1 mg   0.2 mg

0.3 mg

CEFTIN
(cefuroxime axetil)
GLAXOSMITHKLINE

250 mg

500 mg

CELEBREX
(celecoxib)
G. D. SEARLE

100 mg

200 mg

CELEXA
(citalopram hydrobromide)
FOREST

10 mg

20 mg

40 mg

CIALIS
(tadalafil)
LILLY

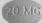
2.5 mg

5 mg

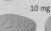
10 mg

 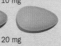
20 mg

CIPRO
(ciprofloxacin HCl)
SCHERING

100 mg

250 mg

500 mg

750 mg

COMBIVIR
(lamivudine/zidovudine)
GLAXOSMITHKLINE

150 mg/300 mg

COMTAN
(entacapone)
NOVARTIS

200 mg

CONCERTA
(methylphenidate HCl)
MCNEIL PEDIATRICS

18 mg

alza27
27 mg

36 mg

54 mg

Extended-Release Tablets

COREG
(carvedilol)
GLAXOSMITHKLINE

3.125 mg   6.25 mg

12.5 mg   25 mg

COUMADIN

(warfarin sodium)
BRISTOL-MYERS SQUIBB

1 mg   2 mg

2.5 mg

3 mg

4 mg   5 mg

6 mg

7.5 mg

10 mg

COZAAR

(losartan potassium)
MERCK

25 mg

50 mg

100 mg

Registered trademark of
E.I. du Pont de Nemours
and Company.

CRESTOR

(rosuvastatin calcium)
ASTRAZENECA

5 mg

10 mg

20 mg

40 mg

CRIXIVAN

(indinavir sulfate)
MERCK

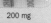

100 mg

200 mg

333 mg

400 mg

CYMBALTA

(duloxetine HCl)
LILLY

20 mg

30 mg

60 mg

Delayed-Release Capsules

DEPAKENE

(valproic acid)
ABBOTT

250 mg

DEPAKOTE

(divalproex sodium)
ABBOTT

125 mg
Sprinkle Capsules

125 mg

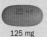

250 mg

500 mg

Delayed-Release Tablets

DEPAKOTE ER

(divalproex sodium)
ABBOTT

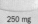

250 mg

500 mg

Extended-Release Tablets

DETROL

(tolterodine tartrate)
PHARMACIA & UPJOHN

1 mg

2 mg

DETROL LA

(tolterodine tartrate)
PHARMACIA & UPJOHN

2 mg

4 mg

Extended-Release Capsules

DIOVAN

(valsartan)
NOVARTIS

40 mg

80 mg

160 mg

320 mg

DUETACT

(pioglitazone HCl/glimepiride)
TAKEDA

30 mg/2 mg

30 mg/4 mg

DYAZIDE

(hydrochlorothiazide/
triamterene)
GLAXOSMITHKLINE

25 mg/37.5 mg

DYNACIRC CR

(isradipine)
RELIANT

5 mg

10 mg

Controlled-Release Tablets

DYNACIRC IR

(isradipine)
RELIANT

2.5 mg

5 mg

EFFEXOR

(venlafaxine HCl)
WYETH

25 mg

37.5 mg

50 mg

75 mg

100 mg

EFFEXOR XR

(venlafaxine HCl)
WYETH

37.5 mg

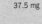

75 mg

150 mg

Extended-Release Capsules

ELDEPRYL

(selegiline HCl)
SOMERSET

5 mg

ENABLEX

(darifenacin)
NOVARTIS

7.5 mg

15 mg

Extended-Release Tablets

EPIVIR

(lamivudine)
GLAXOSMITHKLINE

150 mg

300 mg

EQUETRO

(carbamazepine)
SHIRE

100 mg

200 mg

300 mg

Extended-Release Capsules

ESTRATEST

(esterified estrogens/
methyltestosterone)
SOLVAY

SOLVAY
1026

1.25 mg/2.5 mg

ESTRATEST H.S.

(esterified estrogens/
methyltestosterone)
SOLVAY

SOLVAY
1023

0.625 mg/1.25 mg

EVISTA

(raloxifene HCl)
LILLY

LILLY
4165

60 mg

EXELON

(rivastigmine tartrate)
NOVARTIS

EXELON
1.5 mg

1.5 mg

EXELON
3 mg

3 mg

EXELON
4.5 mg

4.5 mg

EXELON
6 mg

6 mg

EXFORGE

(amlodipine/valsartan)
NOVARTIS

ECE

5 mg/160 mg

UIC

10 mg/160 mg

CSF

5 mg/320 mg

LUF

10 mg/320 mg

FENTORA

(fentanyl buccal tablet)
CEPHALON, INC.

1

100 mcg

2

200 mcg

3

300 mcg

4

400 mcg

6

600 mcg

8

800 mcg

FLOMAX

(tamsulosin HCl)
BOEHRINGER INGELHEIM

Flomax
0.4 mg   BI 58

0.4 mg

FOCALIN

(dexmethylphenidate HCl)
NOVARTIS

D

2.5 mg

D

5 mg

D

10 mg

FOCALIN XR

(dexmethylphenidate HCl)
NOVARTIS

5 mg

NVR   D10

10 mg

NVR   D15

15 mg

NVR   D20

20 mg

Extended-Release Capsules

FOSAMAX

(alendronate sodium)
MERCK

5 mg

10 mg

35 mg

40 mg

70 mg

FOSAMAX PLUS D

(alendronate sodium/
cholecalciferol)
MERCK

70 mg/2800 IU

70 mg/5600 IU

FROVA

(frovatriptan succinate)
ENDO

2.5 mg

GEODON

(ziprasidone HCl)
PFIZER

20 mg

40 mg

60 mg

80 mg

HYTRIN

(terazosin HCl)
ABBOTT

1 mg

2 mg

5 mg

10 mg

HYZAAR

(losartan potassium/
hydrochlorothiazide)
MERCK

50 mg/12.5 mg

100 mg/12.5 mg

100 mg/25 mg

IMITREX

(sumatriptan succinate)
GLAXOSMITHKLINE

25 mg

50 mg

100 mg

INSPRA

(eplerenone)
PFIZER

25 mg   50 mg

INVEGA

(paliperidone)
JANSSEN, L.P.

3 mg

6 mg

9 mg

Extended-Release Tablets

JANUMET

(sitagliptin/metformin HCl)
MERCK

50 mg/500 mg

50 mg/1000 mg

JANUVIA

(sitagliptin)
MERCK

25 mg   50 mg   100 mg

KALETRA

(lopinavir/ritonavir)
ABBOTT

133.3 mg/33.3 mg

Capsules

200 mg/50 mg

Tablets

KEPPRA

(levetiracetam)
UCB

250 mg

500 mg

750 mg

1000 mg

KETEK

(telithromycin)
sanofi-aventis, U.S.

400 mg

KLONOPIN

(clonazepam)
ROCHE

0.5 mg

1 mg   2 mg

KLONOPIN WAFERS

(clonazepam)
ROCHE

0.125 mg

0.25 mg

0.5 mg   1 mg

2 mg

Orally Disintegrating Tablets

LAMICTAL

(lamotrigine)
GLAXOSMITHKLINE

25 mg   100 mg

150 mg   200 mg

LAMISIL

(terbinafine HCl)
NOVARTIS

250 mg

LANOXIN

(digoxin)
GLAXOSMITHKLINE

0.125 mg   0.25 mg

LESCOL

(fluvastatin sodium)
NOVARTIS

20 mg

40 mg

LEVAQUIN

(levofloxacin)
ORTHO-MCNEIL

250 mg

500 mg

750 mg

LEVITRA

(vardenafil HCl)
SCHERING

5 mg   10 mg   20 mg

LEXAPRO

(escitalopram oxalate)
FOREST

5 mg

10 mg

20 mg

LEXIVA

(fosamprenavir calcium)
GLAXOSMITHKLINE

GX LL7

700 mg

LIPITOR

(atorvastatin calcium)
PARKE-DAVIS

10 mg

20 mg

40 mg

80 mg

LOPRESSOR

(metoprolol tartrate)
NOVARTIS

50 mg

100 mg

LOTENSIN

(benazepril HCl)
NOVARTIS

5 mg

10 mg

20 mg

40 mg

LOTENSIN HCT

(benazepril HCl/
hydrochlorothiazide)
NOVARTIS

LOTENSIN HCT

5 mg/6.25 mg

LOTENSIN HCT

10 mg/12.5 mg

LOTENSIN HCT

20 mg/12.5 mg

LOTENSIN HCT

20 mg/25 mg

LOTREL

(amlodipine/benazepril HCl)
NOVARTIS

LOTREL 2255

2.5 mg/10 mg

LOTREL 2260

5 mg/10 mg

LOTREL 2265

5 mg/20 mg

10 mg/20 mg

LUNESTA

(eszopiclone)
SEPRACOR

S190
1 mg

S191
2 mg

S193
3 mg

LYRICA

(pregabalin)
PFIZER

Pfizer   PGN
25

25 mg

Pfizer   PGN
50

50 mg

Pfizer   PGN
75

75 mg

Pfizer   PGN
100

100 mg

Pfizer   PGN
150

150 mg

Pfizer   PGN
200

200 mg

Pfizer   PGN
225

225 mg

Pfizer   PGN
300

300 mg

MAVIK
(trandolapril)
ABBOTT

1 mg

2 mg

4 mg

MAXALT
(rizatriptan benzoate)
MERCK

5 mg   10 mg

MAXALT-MLT
(rizatriptan benzoate)
MERCK

5 mg   10 mg

Orally Disintegrating Tablets

MERIDIA
(sibutramine HCl monohydrate)
ABBOTT

5 mg

10 mg

15 mg

MEVACOR
(lovastatin)
MERCK

20 mg

40 mg

MICARDIS
(telmisartan)
BOEHRINGER INGELHEIM

40 mg

80 mg

MICARDIS HCT
(telmisartan/
hydrochlorothiazide)
BOEHRINGER INGELHEIM

40 mg/12.5 mg

80 mg/12.5 mg

80 mg/25 mg

MIRAPEX.
(pramipexole dihydrochloride)
BOEHRINGER INGELHEIM

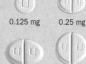

0.125 mg   0.25 mg

0.5 mg   1 mg

1.5 mg

MOBIC
(meloxicam)
BOEHRINGER INGELHEIM

7.5 mg   15 mg

MS CONTIN
(morphine sulfate)
PURDUE FREDERICK

15 mg

30 mg

60 mg

100 mg

200 mg

Controlled-Release Tablets

NAMENDA

(memantine HCl)
FOREST

5 mg

10 mg

NAPROSYN

(naproxen)
ROCHE

250 mg

375 mg

500 mg

NEURONTIN

(gabapentin)
PARKE-DAVIS

100 mg

300 mg

400 mg

600 mg

800 mg

NEXIUM

(esomeprazole magnesium)
ASTRAZENECA

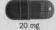
20 mg

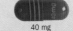
40 mg
Delayed-Release Capsules

NIASPAN

(niacin)
ABBOTT

500 mg

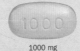
750 mg

1000 mg
Extended-Release Tablets

NOROXIN

(norfloxacin)
MERCK

400 mg

NORVASC

(amlodipine besylate)
PFIZER

2.5 mg   5 mg

10 mg

NORVIR

(ritonavir)
ABBOTT

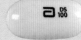
100 mg
Soft Gelatin

OMNICEF

(cefdinir)
ABBOTT

300 mg

OPANA

(oxymorphone HCl)
ENDO

5 mg   10 mg

OPANA ER

(oxymorphone HCl)
ENDO

5 mg   7.5 mg

10 mg   15 mg

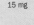
20 mg   30 mg

40 mg
Extended-Release Tablets

OXYCONTIN

(oxycodone HCl)
PURDUE

 10 mg   15 mg

 20 mg   30 mg

40 mg   60 mg

80 mg
Controlled-Release Tablets

PARNATE

(tranylcypromine sulfate)
GLAXOSMITHKLINE

 10 mg

PAXIL

(paroxetine HCl)
GLAXOSMITHKLINE

 10 mg   20 mg

30 mg   40 mg

PAXIL CR

(paroxetine HCl)
GLAXOSMITHKLINE

 12.5 mg   25 mg   37.5 mg
Controlled-Release Tablets

PEPCID

(famotidine)
MERCK

20 mg

 40 mg

PERCOCET

(oxycodone HCl/
acetaminophen)
ENDO

 2.5 mg/325 mg

 5 mg/325 mg

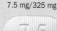 7.5 mg/325 mg

7.5 mg/500 mg

 10 mg/325 mg

 10 mg/650 mg

PERCODAN

(oxycodone HCl/aspirin)
ENDO

 4.8355 mg/325 mg

PERSANTINE

(dipyridamole)
BOEHRINGER INGELHEIM

 25 mg

 50 mg

 75 mg

PLAN B

(levonorgestrel)
DURAMED

 0.75 mg

PLAVIX

(clopidogrel bisulfate)
**BRISTOL-MYERS SQUIBB/
sanofi-aventis, U.S.**

 75 mg

PRANDIN

(repaglinide)
NOVO NORDISK

 0.5 mg

 1 mg

 2 mg

PREMARIN	**PROPECIA**	**PROZAC WEEKLY**

PREMARIN

(conjugated estrogens)
WYETH

0.3 mg

0.45 mg

0.625 mg

0.9 mg

1.25 mg

PREVACID

(lansoprazole)
TAP

15 mg

30 mg

Delayed-Release Capsules

PRISTIQ

(desvenlafaxine)
WYETH

50 mg   100 mg

Extended-Release Tablets

PROPECIA

(finasteride)
MERCK

1 mg

PROSCAR

(finasteride)
MERCK

5 mg

PROTONIX

(pantoprazole sodium)
WYETH

20 mg

40 mg

PROVIGIL

(modafinil)
CEPHALON

100 mg

200 mg

PROZAC

(fluoxetine HCl)
LILLY

10 mg

20 mg

PROZAC WEEKLY

(fluoxetine HCl)
LILLY

90 mg

RAZADYNE

(galantamine HBr)
ORTHO-MCNEIL

4 mg

8 mg

12 mg

RAZADYNE ER

(galantamine HBr)
ORTHO-MCNEIL

8 mg

16 mg

24 mg

Extended-Release Capsules

RELPAX

(eletriptan HBr)
PFIZER

20 mg   40 mg

REQUIP

(ropinirole HCl)
GLAXOSMITHKLINE

0.25-mg Tiltab*

0.5-mg Tiltab*

1-mg Tiltab*

2-mg Tiltab*

3-mg Tiltab*

4-mg Tiltab*

5-mg Tiltab*

RESTORIL

(temazepam)
MALLINCKRODT

7.5 mg

15 mg

22.5 mg

30 mg

RETROVIR

(zidovudine)
GLAXOSMITHKLINE

100 mg   300 mg

REVATIO

(sildenafil citrate)
PFIZER

20 mg

RISPERDAL

(risperidone)
JANSSEN

0.25 mg   0.5 mg

1 mg   2 mg

3 mg

4 mg

RISPERDAL M-TAB

(risperidone)
JANSSEN, L.P.

0.5 mg   1 mg

2 mg

3 mg

4 mg
Orally Disintegrating Tablets

RITALIN

(methylphenidate HCl)
NOVARTIS

5 mg   10 mg   20 mg

RITALIN-LA

(methylphenidate HCl)
NOVARTIS

20 mg

30 mg

40 mg

Extended-Release Capsules

RITALIN-SR

(methylphenidate HCl)
NOVARTIS

20 mg
Sustained-Release Tablets

ROZEREM

(ramelteon)
TAKEDA

8 mg

RYTHMOL

(propafenone HCl)
RELIANT

150 mg   225 mg

300 mg

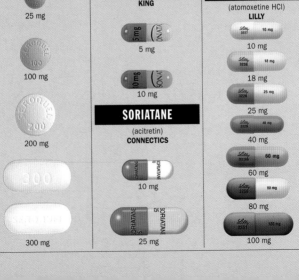

RYTHMOL SR

(propafenone HCl)
RELIANT

225 mg

325 mg

425 mg

Extended-Release Capsules

SANCTURA

(trospium chloride)
ESPRIT

20 mg

SEROQUEL

(quetiapine fumarate)
ASTRAZENECA

25 mg

100 mg

200 mg

300 mg

SINGULAIR

(montelukast sodium)
MERCK

4 mg
Chewable

5 mg
Chewable

10 mg

SKELAXIN

(metaxalone)
KING

800 mg

SONATA

(zaleplon)
KING

5 mg

10 mg

SORIATANE

(acitretin)
CONNECTICS

10 mg

25 mg

STALEVO

(carbidopa/levodopa/entacapone)
NOVARTIS

12.5 mg/50 mg/200 mg

25 mg/100 mg/200 mg

37.5 mg/150 mg/200 mg

50 mg/200 mg/200 mg

STARLIX

(nateglinide)
NOVARTIS

60 mg

120 mg

STRATTERA

(atomoxetine HCl)
LILLY

10 mg

18 mg

25 mg

40 mg

60 mg

80 mg

100 mg

SULAR

(nisoldipine)
SCIELE

 SCI 500

SCI 501

8.5 mg   17 mg

 SCI502

25.5 mg

SCI503

34 mg
Extended-Release Tablets

SUSTIVA

(efavirenz)
BRISTOL-MYERS SQUIBB

 SUSTIVA 50 mg

50 mg

 STIVA 100 mg

100 mg

 SUSTIVA 200 mg

200 mg

 SUSTIVA

600 mg

SYMBYAX

(olanzapine/fluoxetine HCl)
LILLY

 Lilly 3/25

3 mg/25 mg

 Lilly 6/25

6 mg/25 mg

 Lilly 6/50

6 mg/50 mg

 Lilly 12/25

12 mg/25 mg

 Lilly 12/50

12 mg/50 mg

SYNTHROID

(levothyroxine sodium, USP)
ABBOTT

 25   50   75

25 mcg   50 mcg   75 mcg

 88   100   112

88 mcg   100 mcg   112 mcg

 125   137   150

125 mcg   137 mcg   150 mcg

 175   200   300

175 mcg   200 mcg   300 mcg

TAMBOCOR

(flecainide acetate)
3M

 50

50 mg

 100

100 mg

 TR 150

150 mg

TAMIFLU

(oseltamivir phosphate)
ROCHE

 ROCHE 30 mg

30 mg

 ROCHE 45 mg

45 mg

 ROCHE 75 mg

75 mg

TARKA

(trandolapril/verapamil HCl)
ABBOTT

 182

2 mg/180 mg

 241

1 mg/240 mg

 242

2 mg/240 mg

 244

4 mg/240 mg
Extended-Release Tablets

TEGRETOL

(carbamazepine)
NOVARTIS

 TEGRETOL

100 mg chewable

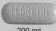 TEGRETOL

200 mg

TEGRETOL XR

(carbamazepine)
NOVARTIS

 T

100 mg

 T

200 mg

 T

400 mg
Extended-Release Tablets

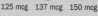
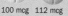

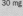
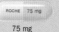

TEKTURNA

(aliskiren)
NOVARTIS

150 mg

300 mg

TEKTURNA HCT

(aliskiren/hydrochlorothiazide)
NOVARTIS

300/12.5 mg

300/25 mg

150/12.5 mg

150/25 mg

TEVETEN

(eprosartan mesylate)
ABBOTT

400 mg

600 mg

TEVETEN HCT

(eprosartan mesy-
late/hydrochlorthiazide)
ABBOTT

600 mg/12.5 mg

600 mg/25 mg

TOPAMAX

(topiramate)
ORTHO-MCNEIL

25 mg

50 mg

100 mg

200 mg

TOPAMAX SPRINKLE

(topiramate)
ORTHO-MCNEIL

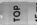

15 mg

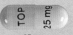

25 mg

TRICOR

(fenofibrate)
ABBOTT

48 mg

145 mg

TRIGLIDE

(fenofibrate)
SCIELE

50 mg

160 mg

TRIZIVIR

(abacavir sulfate/lamivudine/
zidovudine)
GLAXOSMITHKLINE

300 mg/150 mg/300 mg

ULTRACET

(tramadol HCl/acetaminophen)
ORTHO-MCNEIL

37.5mg/325 mg

ULTRAM

(tramadol HCl)
ORTHO-MCNEIL

50 mg

ULTRAM ER
(tramadol HCl)
ORTHO-MCNEIL

100 mg   200 mg   300 mg

Extended-Release Tablets

UNIRETIC
(moexipril HCl/
hydrochlorothiazide)
SCHWARZ PHARMA

7.5 mg/12.5 mg

15 mg/12.5 mg

15 mg/25 mg

VALCYTE
(valganciclovir HCl)
ROCHE

450 mg

VALIUM
(diazepam)
ROCHE

2 mg

5 mg

10 mg

VALTREX
(valacyclovir HCl)
GLAXOSMITHKLINE

500 mg

1 g

VIAGRA
(sildenafil citrate)
PFIZER

25 mg

50 mg

100 mg

VICODIN
(hydrocodone bitartrate/
acetaminophen)
ABBOTT

5 mg/500 mg

VICODIN ES
(hydrocodone bitartrate/
acetaminophen)
ABBOTT

7.5 mg/750 mg

VICODIN HP
(hydrocodone bitartrate/
acetaminophen)
ABBOTT

10 mg/660 mg

VICOPROFEN
(hydrocodone bitartrate/
ibuprofen)
ABBOTT

7.5 mg/200 mg

VIRACEPT
(nelfinavir mesylate)
PFIZER

250 mg

625 mg

VIRAMUNE

(nevirapine)
BOEHRINGER INGELHEIM

200 mg

VIREAD

(tenofovir disoproxil fumarate)
GILEAD SCIENCES

300 mg

VOLTAREN

(diclofenac sodium)
NOVARTIS

25 mg   50 mg

75 mg

VOLTAREN-XR

(diclofenac sodium)
NOVARTIS

100 mg

VYTORIN

(ezetimibe/simvastatin)
MERCK/SCHERING-PLOUGH

10 mg/10 mg   10 mg/20 mg

10 mg/40 mg

10 mg/80 mg

VYVANSE

(lisdexamfetamine dimesylate)
SHIRE US INC.

NRP104 20 mg

20 mg

NRP104 30 mg

30 mg

NRP104 40 mg

40 mg

NRP104 50 mg

50 mg

NRP104 60 mg

60 mg

NRP104 70 mg

70 mg

WELCHOL

(colesevelam HCl)
DAIICHI SANKYO

SANKYO
C01

625 mg

WELLBUTRIN

(bupropion HCl)
GLAXOSMITHKLINE

100 mg   75 mg

WELLBUTRIN SR

(bupropion HCl)
GLAXOSMITHKLINE

WELLBUTRIN SR 100   WELLBUTRIN SR 150

100 mg   150 mg

WELLBUTRIN SR 200

200 mg

Sustained-Release Tablets

WELLBUTRIN XL

(bupropion HCl)
GLAXOSMITHKLINE

WELLBUTRIN XL 150

150 mg

WELLBUTRIN XL 300

300 mg

Extended-Release Tablets

XENICAL

(orlistat)
ROCHE

XENICAL 120   Roche

120 mg

XIFAXAN

(rifaximin)
SALIX

200 mg

XYZAL

(levocetirizine dihydrochloride)
sanofi-aventis

Y   Y

5 mg

ZANTAC

(ranitidine HCl)
GLAXOSMITHKLINE

ZANTAC 150

150 mg

ZANTAC 300

300 mg

ZANTAC EFFERDOSE

(ranitidine HCl)
GLAXOSMITHKLINE

25 mg

150 mg

ZETIA

(ezetimibe)
MERCK/SCHERING-PLOUGH

10 mg

ZIAGEN

(abacavir sulfate)
GLAXOSMITHKLINE

300 mg

ZOCOR

(simvastatin)
MERCK

5 mg

10 mg

20 mg

40 mg

80 mg

ZOLOFT

(sertraline HCl)
PFIZER

25 mg

50 mg

100 mg

ZONEGRAN

(zonisamide)
EISAI

100 mg

ZOVIRAX

(acyclovir)
GLAXOSMITHKLINE

200 mg

400 mg

800 mg

ZYBAN

(bupropion HCl)
GLAXOSMITHKLINE

150 mg

Sustained-Release Tablets

ZYPREXA

(olanzapine)
LILLY

2.5 mg   5 mg

7.5 mg   10 mg

15 mg

20 mg

ZYPREXA ZYDIS

(olanzapine)
LILLY

5 mg   10 mg

15 mg

20 mg

Orally Disintegrating Tablets

Zydis® is a registered trademark
of R.P Scherer Corp.

ZYRTEC

(cetirizine HCl)
PFIZER

5 mg

10 mg

ZYRTEC CHEWABLE

(cetirizine HCl)
PFIZER

5 mg   10 mg

ZYRTEC-D 12 HOUR

(cetirizine HCl/
pseudoephedrine HCl)
PFIZER

5 mg/120 mg

Extended-Release Tablet

ZYVOX

(linezolid)
PFIZER

600 mg

Keep all follow-up visits as scheduled, and call the doctor between visits as needed, especially if you have concerns about symptoms.

Who should not take Luvox CR?
Luvox CR should not be taken if you have an allergy to fluvoxamine or any of the drug's ingredients.

What should I tell my doctor before I take the first dose of Luvox CR?
Tell your doctor about all prescription, over-the-counter, and herbal medications you are taking before beginning treatment with Luvox CR. Also, talk to your doctor about your complete medical history, especially if you have a history of mental health problems. You need to inform your doctor if you are pregnant or planning to become pregnant or are breastfeeding.

What is the usual dosage?
The information below is based on the dosage guidelines your doctor uses. Depending on your condition and medical history, your doctor may prescribe a different regimen. Do not change the dosage or stop taking your medication without you're doctor's approval.

Adults: The recommended starting dose for Luvox CR is 100 milligrams (mg) once daily.

How should I take Luvox CR?
Luvox CR can be taken with or without food as a single daily dose at bedtime. Do not crush or chew capsules

What should I avoid while taking Luvox CR?
Avoid driving or operating machinery until you are certain how this medication affects you.

Avoid drugs that affect the brain as they may impair judgment, thinking, or motor skills when taken with Luvox CR.

What are possible food and drug interactions associated with Luvox CR?
If Luvox CR is taken with certain drugs, the effects of either could be increased, decreased, or altered. It is important to check with your doctor before combining Luvox CR with the following: alcohol, antidepressants (such as amitriptyline, clomipramine, or imipramine), antipsychotics (such as clozapine and thioridazine), aspirin, beta-blockers, carbamazepine, clozapine, diltiazem, lithium, lorazepam, MAOIs, methadone, NSAIDs (such as such as ibuprofen or naproxen), propranolol, ramelteon, serotonergic drugs, sumatriptan, tacrine, thioridazine, tizanidine, tranquilizers and sedatives (such as alprazolam, diazepam, midazolam, and triazolam), triptans, tryptophan, and warfarin.

You should also not take Luvox CR with drugs that are metabolized by a certain liver enzyme (CYP450). Your doctor will check for this interaction.

What are the possible side effects of Luvox CR?
Side effects cannot be anticipated. If any develop or change in intensity, tell your doctor as soon as possible. Only your doctor can determine if it is safe for you to continue taking this drug.

Side effects may include: sleepiness, sweating, tremor, abnormal ejaculation, loss of appetite, weakness, diarrhea, nausea, stomach upset, dizziness, sleeplessness, yawning, anxiety, decreased libido, vomiting, muscle pain

Can I receive Luvox CR if I am pregnant or breastfeeding?
Notify your doctor if you become pregnant or intend to become pregnant during therapy with Luvox CR. Fluvoxamine is secreted in human breast milk. Because of the potential for serious adverse reactions in nursing infants from Luvox CR, a decision should be made whether to discontinue nursing or discontinue the drug, taking into account the importance of the drug to the mother.

How should I store Luvox CR?
Store at room temperature and protect from high humidity.

LYBREL
Generic name: Levonorgestrel and ethinyl estradiol

What is Lybrel?
Lybrel is a birth control pill that contains both levonorgestrel and ethinyl estradiol.

What is the most important information I should know about Lybrel?
Lybrel does not protect against transmission of HIV and other sexually transmitted diseases. Cigarette smoking increases the risk of serious adverse effects on the heart and blood vessels that can be caused by oral contraceptive use.

Who should not take Lybrel?
Do not use Lybrel if you: have unusual vaginal bleeding; have a history of certain cancers, including breast or uterine; had a stroke or heart attack in the past year; have a history of blood clots; have a history of liver problems; are allergic to Lybrel or any of its ingredients; think you may be pregnant; have diabetes complications that affect your circulation; have headaches with aura; have chest pain; or have high blood pressure.

What should I tell my doctor before I take the first dose of Lybrel?

Tell your doctor about all prescription, over-the-counter, and herbal medications you are taking before beginning treatment with Lybrel. Also, talk to your doctor about your complete medical history, especially about any preexisting conditions such as a history of blood clots, high cholesterol, heart problems, diabetes, migraines or seizures, depression, gallbladder disease, irregular periods, or if you have any known or suspected cancers.

What is the usual dosage?

The information below is based on the dosage guidelines your doctor uses. Depending on your condition and medical history, your doctor may prescribe a different regimen. Do not change the dosage or stop taking your medication without your doctor's approval.

Adults: The daily dosage is 1 tablet, which contains 90 micrograms (mcg) of levonorgestrel and 20 mcg of ethinyl estradiol.

How should I take Lybrel?

Take 1 tablet of Lybrel at the same time every day at intervals not exceeding 24 hours. Take the first pill during the first 24 hours of your period. When you finish a pack, start the next pack on the day after your last pill.

What should I avoid while taking Lybrel?

Do not skip days between packs.
   Avoid smoking cigarettes while taking Lybrel.

What are possible food and drug interactions associated with Lybrel?

Certain drugs may interact with birth control pills and make them less effective in preventing pregnancy or may cause unscheduled bleeding. If Lybrel is taken with certain other drugs, the effects of either could be increased, decreased, or altered. It is especially important to check with your doctor before combining Lybrel with rifampin, antiseizure drugs, barbiturates, phenytoin, antibiotics, and herbal products containing St. John's wort.

What are the possible side effects of Lybrel?

Side effects cannot be anticipated. If any develop or change in intensity, tell your doctor as soon as possible. Only your doctor can determine if it is safe for you to continue taking this drug.

Side effects may include: breast lumps, unusual or irregular vaginal bleeding, dizziness, chest pain, shortness of breath, headache, breast pain, hair loss, high blood pressure, increased blood sugar, vaginal yeast infections, fluid retention, liver problems, enlargement of benign tumors of the uterus.

Can I receive Lybrel if I am pregnant or breastfeeding?

Lybrel should not be taken during pregnancy or while breastfeeding. Contact your doctor if you suspect you may be pregnant.

What should I do if I miss a dose of Lybrel?

Take the pill as soon as you remember, then take the next pill at the regular time. This means you take 2 pills the same day. If you missed 2 pills, take 2 pills on the day you remember.

How should I store Lybrel?

Store at room temperature.

LYRICA
Generic name: Pregabalin

What is Lyrica?

Lyrica binds to certain receptors in the brain thought to reduce your ability to feel pain or reduce the occurrence of seizures. It is used in patients 18 years of age and older with nerve pain called diabetic neuropathy, postherpetic infection nerve pain, fibromyalgia (a condition in which there is widespread pain in the muscles and soft tissues surrounding the joints throughout the body), and in combination with other medications to reduce the incidence of seizures.

What is the most important information I should know about Lyrica?

Once you have started to take Lyrica, you should not suddenly stop. If your doctor wants you to discontinue it, he or she will gradually reduce your dose over a minimum of one week.

Lyrica may cause serious allergic reactions. Call your doctor if you experience any of the following symptoms after taking Lyrica: swelling of the face, mouth, lips, tongue, gums, or neck; or if you have trouble breathing.

Lyrica can cause dizziness or sleepiness/tiredness. You should not drive or operate machinery until you know how Lyrica will affect you. You should not drink alcohol or use drugs that may cause you to feel sleepy or tired.

Lyrica may cause changes in your vision, including your ability to focus, leading to blurred vision. If this occurs, tell your doctor immediately. Also contact your doctor immediately if you experience any unexplained muscle pain, tenderness, or weakness, especially if accompanied by fever.

Who should not take Lyrica?
You should not take Lyrica if you have a known sensitivity or allergy to it.

What should I tell my doctor before I take the first dose of Lyrica?
Mention all prescription, over-the-counter, and herbal medications you are taking before beginning treatment with Lyrica. Also, talk to your doctor about your complete medical history, especially if you have a history of developing a tumor(s), have kidney or heart problems, have a bleeding problem or a low blood platelet count, have diabetes, are pregnant or plan to become pregnant, or are breastfeeding. Additionally, if you are a male planning on fathering a child, inform your doctor, as the active ingredient in Lyrica was shown in animal studies to make male animals less fertile and caused sperm abnormalities.

What is the usual dosage?
The information below is based on the dosage guidelines your doctor uses. Depending on your condition and medical history, your doctor may prescribe a different regimen. Do not change the dosage or stop taking your medication without your doctor's approval.

Epilepsy
Adults: The recommended total daily dosage of Lyrica is 150 milligrams (mg) to 600 mg, given in divided doses taken 2-3 times a day in combination with other medications.

Neuropathic Pain Associated with
Diabetic Peripheral Neuropathy
Adults: The usual starting dose is 50 mg taken 3 times daily (150 mg per day). After 1 week, your doctor may increase your total daily dose to 300 mg per day, taken in divided doses.

Management of Fibromyalgia
Adults: The recommended starting dose is 75 mg 2 times a day (150 mg/day) and may be increased to 150 mg 2 times a day (300 mg/day) within 1 week. If you do not benefit from 300 mg/day, your doctor may increase the dose to 225 mg 2 times a day (450 mg/day). Doses above 450 mg/day are not recommended.

Postherpetic Neuralgia
Adults: The usual starting dose is 75 mg 2 times a day, or 50 mg 3 times a day (150 mg per day). Your doctor may increase your dose to 300 mg/day within 1 week based on your individual response.

   If you have significant kidney impairment or disease, your doctor may decrease your dose based on your individual condition.

How should I take Lyrica?
Lyrica should be taken at the same time every day, with or without food.

What should I avoid while taking Lyrica?
You should avoid drinking alcohol, as Lyrica can increase sedation and impair motor skills. You should also avoid driving automobiles or operating heavy machinery until you know how Lyrica will affect you. Do not stop taking Lyrica suddenly, because you may get headaches, nausea, diarrhea, or have trouble sleeping. Also, you may experience more frequent seizures if you already have a seizure disorder. If you need to stop taking Lyrica, your doctor will tell you how to slowly stop taking it.

What are possible food and drug interactions associated with Lyrica?
If Lyrica is taken with certain other drugs, the effects of either could be increased, decreased, or altered. It is especially important to check with your doctor before combining Lyrica with the following: angiotensin converting enzyme (ACE) inhibitors (ie, enalapril, lisinopril, ramipril), antidiabetic medications known as "thiazolidinediones" (ie, rosiglitazone, pioglitazone), CNS depressants such as opiates (ie, oxycodone), or benzodiazepines (ie, lorazepam).

What are the possible side effects of Lyrica?
Side effects cannot be anticipated. If any develop or change in intensity, tell your doctor as soon as possible. Only your doctor can determine if it is safe for you to continue taking this drug.

Side effects may include: dizziness, tiredness, sleepiness, accidental injury, dry mouth, edema (fluid retention), blurred vision, incoordination, lack of concentration, weight gain

Can I receive Lyrica if I am pregnant or breastfeeding?
Lyrica is a pregnancy category C medication, which means that in animal studies adverse effects were observed in the fetuses. Lyrica has not been adequately studied in pregnant women. Tell your doctor immediately if you are pregnant, plan to become pregnant, or are breastfeeding. It is not known whether Lyrica is excreted in breast milk, so your doctor will decide if you should take Lyrica while breastfeeding.

What should I do if I miss a dose of Lyrica?
If you miss a dose by a few hours, take it as soon as you remember. If it is close to your next dose, skip the missed dose and continue with your regular dosing schedule. Do not double your next dose.

How should I store Lyrica?
Store at room temperature.

MACRODANTIN
Generic name: Nitrofurantoin macrocrystals

What is Macrodantin?
Macrodantin is an antibiotic used to treat urinary tract infections caused by bacteria known as *Escherichia coli*, enterococci, *Staphylococcus aureus*, and certain susceptible strains of *Klebsiella* and *Enterobacter* species.

What is the most important information I should know about Macrodantin?
After taking Macrodantin, immediate or delayed chronic lung reactions can occur that could lead to pneumonia, fibrosis of the lung, or death. These serious side effects are rare and are more likely to occur in patients taking Macrodantin 6 months or longer and who are over 65 years old. If you are on long-term Macrodantin therapy, your doctor will monitor your lung function. If you experience any shortness of breath or difficulty breathing, fever, chills, cough, or chest pain, you should notify your doctor immediately.

Macrodantin can cause severe liver reactions that may result in liver damage and even death. If you notice the whites of your eyes or your skin turning yellow, or have severe abdominal pain, inform your doctor immediately.

Macrodantin can cause severe or irreversible peripheral neuropathy (impairment of nerve function in the arms, legs, hands, feet, etc. that causes nerve pain), especially in patients with diabetes, vitamin B deficiency, anemia, electrolyte imbalances, kidney disease, or debilitating diseases.

Macrodantin can deplete the natural bacteria in your gut, allowing overgrowth of bacteria-associated diarrhea. This can occur as much as 2 months after you stop taking Macrodantin and is usually associated with severe abdominal pain, bloody stools, and diarrhea. If you have any of these symptoms, tell your doctor immediately and seek treatment.

Rarely, Macrodantin can cause a severe deficiency of red blood cells in certain patients, including black patients and patients of Mediterranean or Near Eastern descent. This anemia can be reversed upon discontinuing Macrodantin.

Macrodantin should only be used to treat bacterial infections only. It does not treat viral infections like the common cold.

It is important to finish the full course of therapy with Macrodantin even if you start to feel better when you begin taking it. Skipping doses or not finishing the full course of therapy may decrease the effectiveness of the immediate treatment and will also increase the chance that bacteria will develop resistance and cannot be treated by Macrodantin or other antibiotics in the future.

Who should not take Macrodantin?

You should not take Macrodantin if you do not produce urine or a small amount of urine, or if you have significant kidney impairment. Macrodantin should not be taken if you are pregnant at full term (38-42 weeks), during labor and delivery, or if the onset of labor is imminent. Macrodantin should not be given to neonates under 1 month of age. Also, you should not take it if you are known to be allergic or sensitive to it.

What should I tell my doctor before I take the first dose of Macrodantin?

Mention all prescription, over-the-counter, and herbal medications you are taking before beginning treatment with Macrodantin. Also, talk to your doctor about your complete medical history, especially if you are pregnant and at full term (38-42 weeks), if you have liver or kidney disease or impairment, or are over 65.

What is the usual dosage?

The information below is based on the dosage guidelines your doctor uses. Depending on your condition and medical history, your doctor may prescribe a different regimen. Do not change the dosage or stop taking your medication without your doctor's approval.

Adults: The usual dosage is 50-100 milligrams (mg) taken 4 times a day. (If you have an uncomplicated urinary tract infection, your dosage may be lower.) For long-term suppressive therapy, 50-100 mg at bedtime may be adequate.

Children 1 month and older: The usual dosage is 5-7 mg per 2.2 pounds of bodyweight, per day, given in 4 divided doses. For long-term suppressive therapy, doses as low as 1 mg per 2.2 pounds of bodyweight—per 24 hours, given in a single dose or in two divided doses—may be adequate.

Therapy should be continued for one week or for at least 3 days after sterility of the urine is obtained.

How should I take Macrodantin?

Macrodantin should be taken with food to increase its absorption and decrease the occurrence of upset stomach. You should complete the full course of therapy even if you start feeling better.

What should I avoid while taking Macrodantin?

You should avoid taking antacids containing magnesium trisilicate.

What are possible food and drug interactions associated with Macrodantin?

If Macrodantin is taken with certain other drugs, the effects of either could be increased, decreased, or altered. It is especially important to check with your doctor before combining Macrodantin with antacids containing magnesium trisilicate, probenecid, or sulfinpyrazone.

What are the possible side effects of Macrodantin?
Side effects cannot be anticipated. If any develop or change in intensity, tell your doctor as soon as possible. Only your doctor can determine if it is safe for you to continue taking this drug.

Side effects may include: loss of appetite, vomiting, nausea, anorexia, anaphylactic allergic reactions involving the lungs and skin, dizziness, headache, weakness, drowsiness

Can I receive Macrodantin if I am pregnant or breastfeeding?
Macrodantin is a pregnancy category B medication, which means that while some studies have been done in pregnant animals, it has not been studied in pregnant humans. Tell your doctor if you are pregnant or plan to become pregnant, or if you are breastfeeding. Macrodantin is excreted in breast milk. Tell your doctor immediately if you are breastfeeding, so he or she can decide whether you should take Macrodantin.

What should I do if I miss a dose of Macrodantin?
If you forget to take a dose of Macrodantin, do not double your next dose. Skip the dose you missed and return to your normal dosing schedule.

How should I store Macrodantin?
Store at room temperature.

MAVIK
Generic name: Trandolapril

What is Mavik?
Mavik is a type of blood-pressure lowering medication known as an ACE inhibitor. It can be used alone or in combination with other medications. Mavik is also used to help reduce the risk of death from heart failure or left ventricular dysfunction following a heart attack.

What is the most important information I should know about Mavik?
Mavik can cause a rare but serious allergic reaction leading to extreme swelling of the face, lips, tongue, throat, or gut (causing severe abdominal pain). If you experience any of these symptoms, seek emergency medical attention right away.

Mavik may rarely cause a yellowing of the skin or eyes, which can be a sign of liver dysfunction. Notify your doctor immediately if this occurs.

Mavik may cause lightheadedness or fainting caused by very low blood pressure, especially upon standing from a lying or sitting position.

A very low blood pressure can also be caused by not drinking enough fluids, if you sweat too much, or have excessive diarrhea or vomiting. Mavik should be taken with caution in patients who have congestive heart failure.

You should not take any potassium supplements or salt substitutes without talking to your doctor first because Mavik could cause an increase in potassium levels in your blood (hyperkalemia), which can be dangerous. You are at risk of developing hyperkalemia if you have diabetes or kidney problems, or are taking potassium-sparing diuretics or anything with potassium in it.

If you get any type of infection (sore throat/fever) while taking Mavik, promptly report it to your doctor. Mavik may decrease your levels of infection-fighting white blood cells, especially if you have systemic lupus erythematosus or kidney disease. If you have one of these conditions, your doctor will monitor you closely by taking regular blood samples.

When taken during pregnancy, ACE inhibitors such as Mavik can cause injury and even death to the developing baby. If you are pregnant or plan on becoming pregnant, stop taking Mavik and contact your doctor immediately.

Who should not take Mavik?
You should not take Mavik if you have had a previous allergic reaction or are sensitive to Mavik or any other ACE inhibitor.

What should I tell my doctor before I take the first dose of Mavik?
Mention all prescription, over-the-counter, and herbal medications you are taking before beginning treatment with Mavik. Also, talk to your doctor about your complete medical history, especially if you are pregnant or plan on becoming pregnant, planning to undergo any surgery and/or anesthesia, or if you have ever had an allergy or sensitivity to an ACE inhibitor such as Mavik.

What is the usual dosage?
The information below is based on the dosage guidelines your doctor uses. Depending on your condition and medical history, your doctor may prescribe a different regimen. Do not change the dosage or stop taking your medication without your doctor's approval.

Hypertension
Adults: The usual starting dose is 1 milligram (mg) once a day in non-black patients and patients not taking a diuretic. The usual starting dose in black patients is 2 mg once daily. Your doctor may increase your individual dose to 2-4 mg daily. Dose adjustments should be made at intervals of at least 1 week.

Patients treated with 4 mg once daily dosing may be treated with twice daily dosing if they are not adequately responding. If their blood pressure is not controlled with just Mavik, a diuretic may be added.

To reduce the chance of hypotension in patients who are currently being treated with a diuretic, the diuretic should be stopped 2-3 days before starting Mavik, if possible. If blood pressure is not controlled with Mavik alone, the diuretic should be started again. If the diuretic cannot be stopped, an initial dose of Mavik 0.5 mg should be used with careful medical supervision for several hours until blood pressure has been stabilized. The dosage should be subsequently titrated to the optimal response.

Heart Failure Post Myocardial Infarction or Left-Ventricular Dysfunction Post Myocardial Infarction
Adults: The usual starting dose is 1 mg once daily. Your doctor may increase your individual dose up to 4 mg daily.

Renal Impairment (CrCl less than 30 mL/min) or Hepatic Cirrhosis
Adults: The usual starting dose is 0.5 mg daily. Your doctor may or may not increase your dose based on your individual condition.

How should I take Mavik?
Mavik can be taken with or without food and should be taken at the same time every day.

What should I avoid while taking Mavik?
Avoid operating automobiles or heavy machinery until you know how Mavik will affect you. Avoid becoming very dehydrated and drink adequate fluids while taking Mavik, because this could cause your blood pressure to drop too low. Avoid taking potassium supplements or salt substitutes without talking to your doctor first.

What are possible food and drug interactions associated with Mavik?
If Mavik is taken with certain other drugs, the effects of either could be increased, decreased, or altered. It is especially important to check with your doctor before combining Mavik with the following: certain inhalation anesthetics; potassium supplements; salt substitutes containing potassium; thiazide-type diuretics such as hydrochlorothiazide; "potassium sparing" diuretics such as spironolactone, amiloride, triamterene; lithium; or NSAIDs.

What are the possible side effects of Mavik?
Side effects cannot be anticipated. If any develop or change in intensity, tell your doctor as soon as possible. Only your doctor can determine if it is safe for you to continue taking this drug.

Side effects may include: headache, dizziness, diarrhea, cough, low blood pressure, fainting, increased uric acid blood levels, increased nitrogen blood levels, coronary artery bypass graft (CABG) surgery, acid reflux, increased potassium blood levels, slow heart rate, low blood calcium levels, muscle weakness, elevated blood creatinine levels, inflammation of the stomach, cardiogenic shock, intermittent pain and/or weakness of the body, stroke, numbness/weakness

Can I receive Mavik if I am pregnant or breastfeeding?
Mavik is considered a Category D medication. This means that taking it while you are pregnant could cause serious harm or even death to your unborn baby. Tell your doctor immediately if you are pregnant, plan to become pregnant, or are breastfeeding. Mavik is excreted in breast milk, and should not be taken if you are breastfeeding.

What should I do if I miss a dose of Mavik?
If you forget to take Mavik, do not double your next dose. Skip the dose you missed and then return to your normal dosing schedule.

How should I store Mavik?
Store at room temperature in a tightly closed container and protect from light.

MAXALT
Generic name: Rizatriptan benzoate

What is Maxalt?
Maxalt is used for the acute treatment of migraine attacks in adults. It is available as a traditional tablet (Maxalt) or an orally disintegrating tablet (Maxalt-MLT).

Maxalt works to relieve migraines by reducing the swelling of blood vessels surrounding the brain, blocking the release of substances from nerve endings that cause pain, and interrupting the transmission of specific pain signals to the brain.

What is the most important information I should know about Maxalt?
Maxalt should be used only for migraines and not to treat headaches that might be caused by other conditions. Maxalt should only be used when a clear diagnosis of migraine has been established.

Maxalt has the potential of causing coronary vasospasms (a condition in which blood vessels spasm and lead to narrowing). Because of this, it should not be given to patients with heart disease or to those who have risk factors for heart disease. Risk factors for heart disease are high blood pressure, high cholesterol, smoking, obesity, diabetes, a strong family history of heart disease, of if you are a postmenopausal woman or a man older than 40. Your doctor will evaluate you to make sure Maxalt is right for you.

Who should not take Maxalt?

Do not take Maxalt if you are allergic to it or any of its ingredients; if you have uncontrolled high blood pressure, heart disease, or a history of heart disease; or if you have a hemiplegic or basilar migraine. Do not take Maxalt if you have taken monoamine oxidase inhibitors (MAOIs) within the last 2 weeks. Do not take Maxalt within 24 hours of using certain migraine drugs, including triptans and ergotamines.

What should I tell my doctor before I take the first dose of Maxalt?

Mention all prescription, over-the-counter, and herbal medications you are taking before beginning treatment with Maxalt, including those you normally take for a migraine. Also, talk to your doctor about your complete medical history, especially if you have had high blood pressure, chest pain, shortness of breath, heart disease, stroke, or allergies. Discuss any risk factors for heart or blood vessel disease, such as diabetes, high cholesterol, obesity, smoking, and a family history of heart or blood vessel disease, or if you are postmenopausal or a man over 40.

What is the usual dosage?

The information below is based on the dosage guidelines your doctor uses. Depending on your condition and medical history, your doctor may prescribe a different regimen. Do not change the dosage or stop taking your medication without your doctor's approval.

Your doctor will prescribe either a 5 milligram (mg) or 10 mg dose. If your headache comes back, a second dose may be taken anytime after 2 hours of the initial dose. Do not take more than 30 mg of Maxalt in a 24-hour period. If you have no response to the initial dose, call your doctor before taking another tablet.

If you are receiving propranolol, the dose is 5 mg, with a maximum of three doses in a 24-hour period.

How should I take Maxalt?

When you have a migraine headache, take your medication as directed by your doctor. For tablets, swallow the tablet whole with liquid. For orally disintegrating tablets (Maxalt-MLT), open the blister pack with dry hands and place the tablet on your tongue; it will dissolve rapidly and be swallowed with your saliva.

What should I avoid while taking Maxalt?

If you experience side effects such as dizziness, sleepiness, tiredness, or fatigue, do not drive or operate heavy machinery.

What are possible food and drug interactions associated with Maxalt?

If Maxalt is taken with certain other drugs, the effects of either could be increased, decreased, or altered. It is especially important to check with your doctor before combining Maxalt with the following: antidepressants that boost serotonin; monoamine oxidase inhibitors (MAOIs), such as phenelzine and tranylcypromine;triptans and ergotamines; or propranolol.

What are the possible side effects of Maxalt?

Side effects cannot be anticipated. If any develop or change in intensity, tell your doctor as soon as possible. Only your doctor can determine if it is safe for you to continue taking this drug.

Side effects may include: dizziness, fatigue, pain or pressure in the chest or throat, dry mouth, nausea, headache, warm/cold sensations, palpitations, diarrhea, vomiting, tremor, difficulty breathing, flushing, hot flashes

Can I receive Maxalt if I am pregnant or breastfeeding?

Do not use Maxalt if you are pregnant, think you might be pregnant, or are trying to become pregnant, unless you have discussed this with your doctor. The effects of Maxalt while breastfeeding are unknown; talk to your doctor.

What should I do if I miss a dose of Maxalt?

Maxalt should only be taken when needed. It should not be taken on a regular basis, unless otherwise prescribed by your doctor.

How should I store Maxalt?

Store at room temperature and away from heat, light, and moisture. With Maxalt-MLT, do not remove the blister from the outer aluminum pouch until you are ready to take the medication inside.

Meclizine hydrochloride *See Antivert, page 112.*

MEDROL

Generic name: Methylprednisolone

What is Medrol?

Medrol is a steroid medication called a "glucocorticoid" that mimics the action of hormones that naturally occur in your body. These hormones have a variety of effects, including a reduction of inflammation and suppression of the immune system.

Medrol is used to treat certain glandular disorders, rheumatic diseases, collagen diseases, skin conditions, allergic states, diseases of the eye, lung diseases, blood disorders, certain types of cancer, fluid disorders in certain types of kidney dysfunction, certain intestinal diseases, multiple sclerosis, specific parasitic diseases, and tuberculous meningitis.

What is the most important information I should know about Medrol?

You should not receive any live vaccines while taking Medrol.

Medrol can mask the signs and symptoms of mild to severe infections in your body. Inform your doctor if you develop any type of infection before, during, or after taking Medrol.

When taking Medrol you should avoid exposure to chickenpox or measles. If you think you were exposed while taking Medrol, you should contact your doctor immediately.

Taking Medrol for a prolonged period of time may increase your risk of developing cataracts, glaucoma, or optic nerve damage.

Medrol may increase your body's ability to retain salt and water, which can increase your blood pressure.

Medrol may increase the rate at which potassium and calcium are eliminated from your body, which your doctor may want to monitor.

Use Medrol with caution if you have active or latent tuberculosis, a herpes simplex infection of the eye, ulcerative colitis, diverticulitis, stomach ulcers, kidney disease, high blood pressure, osteoporosis, or myasthenia gravis.

You should not abruptly stop taking Medrol. Discontinuation requires a dosage reduction over time to avoid potentially serious side effects, especially in patients who have been taking it for a long time.

Medrol can worsen or initiate mental instabilities such as depression, euphoria, mood swings, insomnia, and personality changes.

Who should not take Medrol?

You should not take Medrol if you have a systemic infection caused by a fungus or you are allergic or sensitive to Medrol.

What should I tell my doctor before I take the first dose of Medrol?

Mention all prescription, over-the-counter, and herbal medications you are taking before beginning treatment with Medrol. Also, talk to your doctor about your complete medical history, especially if you have an infection, liver disease, tuberculosis, glaucoma, cataracts, stomach ulcers, osteoporosis, high blood pressure, ulcerative colitis, diverticulitis, diabetes, or hypothyroidism.

What is the usual dosage?

The information below is based on the dosage guidelines your doctor uses. Depending on your condition and medical history, your doctor may prescribe a different regimen. Do not change the dosage or stop taking your medication without your doctor's approval.

Adults: The initial dosage can range from 4 to 48 milligrams (mg) daily depending on the condition for which you are being treated. Your doctor may also tell you to take a certain dosage of Medrol in the morning every other day to avoid potential side effects.

How should I take Medrol?

Medrol can be taken with or without food, and should be taken at the same time every day, preferably in the morning. Do not abruptly stop taking Medrol. Your doctor will tell you how to slowly stop taking it if you need to.

What should I avoid while taking Medrol?

You should not receive any live vaccines while taking Medrol. Avoid exposure to chickenpox or measles.

What are possible food and drug interactions associated with Medrol?

If Medrol is taken with certain other drugs, the effects of either could be increased, decreased, or altered. It is especially important to check with your doctor before combining Medrol with the following: anticoagulant medications, aspirin, cyclosporine, ketoconazole, phenobarbital, rifampin, phenytoin, or toleandomycin.

What are the possible side effects of Medrol?

Side effects cannot be anticipated. If any develop or change in intensity, tell your doctor as soon as possible. Only your doctor can determine if it is safe for you to continue taking this drug.

Side effects may include: salt retention, congestive heart failure in certain patients, high blood pressure, water retention, potassium loss, muscle weakness, loss of muscle mass, osteoporosis, tendon rupture (particularly of the Achilles tendon), vertebral compression fractures, stomach ulcers, inflammation of the pancreas, bloating, ulcers of the throat, liver injury, impaired wound healing, bruising, thin fragile skin, facial redness, increased sweating, convulsions, dizziness, headache, development of a hormonal disorder called a "Cushingoid state," suppression of growth in children, menstrual irregularities, decreased carbohydrate tolerance, manifestations of diabetes mellitus, increased requirements of insulin or oral hypoglycemic agents in diabetics, cataracts, glaucoma, increased intraocular pressure, bulging of the eyes, itching and other allergic, anaphylactic, or hypersensitivity reactions

Can I receive Medrol if I am pregnant or breastfeeding?

The effects of Medrol during pregnancy and breastfeeding are unknown. Tell your doctor immediately if you are pregnant, plan to become pregnant, or are breastfeeding.

What should I do if I miss a dose of Medrol?
If you miss a dose, do not double your next one. Skip the dose you missed and return to your normal dosing schedule.

How should I store Medrol?
Store at room temperature.

Medroxyprogesterone acetate *See Provera, page 1099.*

Mefenamic acid *See Ponstel, page 1039.*

MEGACE ES
Generic name: Megestrol acetate

What is Megace ES?
Megace ES is used for the treatment of anorexia (loss of appetite), cachexia (malnutrition), or unexplained, significant weight loss in patients with a diagnosis of AIDS.

What is the most important information I should know about Megace ES?
Megace ES may cause severe problems during pregnancy. It is recommended that women of child-bearing age avoid becoming pregnant.

Who should not take Megace ES?
This medication should not be taken if you have a history of being too sensitive to megestrol acetate or any component of the formulation. Do not take this medication if you are or think you may be pregnant.

What should I tell my doctor before I take the first dose of Megace ES?
Mention any prescription, over-the-counter, or herbal medications you are taking before beginning treatment with Megace ES. Also, talk to your doctor about your complete medical history, especially if you are pregnant, planning to become pregnant, or are nursing.

What is the usual dosage?
The information below is based on the dosage guidelines your doctor uses. Depending on your condition and medical history, your doctor may prescribe a different regimen. Do not change your dosage or stop taking your medication without your doctor's approval.

Adults: The recommended initial dosage of Megace ES oral suspension is 625 mg/day (5 mL or one teaspoon daily).

How should I take Megace ES?

Shake contents of the bottle well before pouring into a teaspoon/measuring spoon and swallowing.

What should I avoid while taking Megace ES?

Pregnancy should be avoided while taking this medication.

What are possible food and drug interactions associated with Megace ES?

If Megace ES is taken with certain other drugs, the effects of either could be increased, decreased, or altered. It is especially important to check with your doctor before combining with rifabutin or zidovudine.

What are the possible side effects of Megace ES?

Side effects cannot be anticipated. If any develop or change in intensity, tell your doctor as soon as possible. Only your doctor can determine if it is safe for you to continue taking this drug.

Side effects may include: decreased sex drive, diarrhea, fever, gas, headache, increased blood pressure, impotence, nausea, rash, sleeplessness, upset stomach, vomiting

Can I receive Megace ES if I am pregnant or breastfeeding?

Do not begin therapy with Megace ES if you are pregnant, planning to become pregnant, or are breastfeeding. This drug may cause severe problems during pregnancy. Megace ES may pass into breast milk.

What should I do if I miss a dose of Megace ES?

Take your dose of Megace ES as soon as you remember. If it is almost time for your next dose, skip the one you missed and go back to your regular schedule. Do not double up on doses.

How should I store Megace ES?

Store at room temperature.

Megestrol acetate *See Megace ES, page 795.*

Meloxicam *See Mobic, page 841.*

Memantine hydrochloride *See Namenda, page 858.*

Meperidine hydrochloride *See Demerol, page 389.*

MERIDIA

Generic name: Sibutramine hydrochloride monohydrate

What is Meridia?

Meridia is used to help individuals who are obese to lose weight and keep weight off. Used in conjunction with a low-calorie diet, Meridia may help with weight loss because it affects areas of the brain that control hunger.

What is the most important information I should know about Meridia?

Meridia increases blood pressure or heart rate in some individuals. Do not take Meridia if your blood pressure is not well controlled. Contact your doctor if you experience an increase in blood pressure while taking Meridia.

Your doctor should check your blood pressure and heart rate before you start taking Meridia and continue checking it regularly while you are using it.

Who should not take Meridia?

Do not take Meridia if you have uncontrolled or poorly controlled blood pressure or if you are taking or have taken a medicine called a monoamine oxidase inhibitor (MAOI). Do not take Meridia if you have an eating disorder called anorexia nervosa or bulimia nervosa, or if you are taking weight loss medicines to control your appetite. Do not take Meridia if you are allergic to sibutramine hydrochloride monohydrate or any of Meridia's inactive ingredients.

What should I tell my doctor before I take the first dose of Meridia?

Mention all prescription, over-the-counter, and herbal medications you are taking before beginning treatment with Meridia. Also, talk to your doctor about your complete medical history, especially if you have or have had high blood pressure; heart problems such as a heart attack, heart failure, chest pain, or an irregular heartbeat; stroke or stroke symptoms; liver or kidney problems; glaucoma; thyroid problems; seizures; bleeding problems; gallstones; or depression. Tell your doctor if you are under age 16 or over 65, if you are pregnant, planning to become pregnant, or are nursing.

What is the usual dosage?

The information below is based on the dosage guidelines your doctor uses. Depending on your condition and medical history, your doctor may prescribe a different regimen. Do not change the dosage or stop taking your medication without your doctor's approval.

Adults and adolescents 16 years and older: The recommended initial dose of Meridia is 10 milligrams (mg) once daily; your doctor may increase the dose after 4 weeks to 15 mg daily.

How should I take Meridia?

Take Meridia exactly as prescribed; do not change your dose unless your doctor tells you to do so. You can take Meridia with or without food.

What should I avoid while taking Meridia?

Do not drive, operate heavy machinery, or do other dangerous activities until you know how Meridia affects you.

What are possible food and drug interactions associated with Meridia?

If Meridia is taken with certain other drugs, the effects of either could be increased, decreased, or altered. It is especially important to check with your doctor before combining Meridia with the following: antibiotics, antidepressants, cough and cold medicines, lithium, MAOIs, medicines that increase bleeding, migraine drugs, narcotic painkillers, tryptophan, or other weight-loss medicines.

What are the possible side effects of Meridia?

Side effects cannot be anticipated. If any develop or change in intensity, tell your doctor as soon as possible. Only your doctor can determine if it is safe for you to continue taking this drug.

Common side effects may include: dry mouth, headache, loss of appetite, trouble sleeping, constipation

More serious side effects may include: a large increase in blood pressure or heart rate, seizures, bleeding, and serotonin syndrome, a rare but life-threatening problem which may result in feelings of weakness, restlessness, confusion, or anxiety; a loss of consciousness; rapid heartbeat; fever, vomiting, sweating, shivering, or shaking

Contact your doctor immediately if you experience shortness of breath, rash or hives, or any other effects that bother you or do not go away.

Can I receive Meridia if I am pregnant or breastfeeding?

The effects of Meridia during pregnancy and breastfeeding are unknown.
Using Meridia during pregnancy or while breastfeeding is not recommended. Tell your doctor if you become pregnant or plan to become pregnant while taking Meridia. Do not breastfeed while taking Meridia.

What should I do if I miss a dose of Meridia?

If you miss a dose of Meridia, skip it. Do not take an extra dose to make up for missed doses.

How should I store Meridia?

Store at room temperature. Never leave it in a hot or damp place. Throw away capsules that are out of date or no longer needed.

Mesalamine See Asacol, page 131; Lialda, page 744; or Rowasa, page 1169.

METADATE CD/METADATE ER

Generic name: Methylphenidate hydrochloride

What is Metadate CD/Metadate ER?

Metadate and other brands of methylphenidate are medications known as stimulants and are used in the treatment of attention-deficit/hyperactivity disorder (ADHD).

What is the most important information I should know about Metadate CD/Metadate ER?

Metadate should be an integral part of a total treatment program for ADHD that includes psychological, educational, and social measures. Symptoms of ADHD include continual problems with moderate to severe distractibility, short attention span, hyperactivity, emotional changeability, and impulsiveness.

There are reports of heart problems in patients taking Metadate or other related stimulants. Some of the problems are sudden death in patients with previous heart problems, heart attacks in adults, and increased blood pressure and heart rate. Call your doctor right away if you or your child develops signs of heart problems such as chest pain, shortness of breath, or fainting while taking Metadate.

Metadate can also cause new or worsening symptoms of behavior problems, bipolar illness, and aggressive or hostile behavior. Call your doctor right away if you or your child develops mood or behavior problems.

Excessive doses of Metadate over a long period of time may cause addiction. It is also possible to develop tolerance to the drug, so that larger doses are needed to produce the original effect. Be sure to check with your doctor before making any change in dosage; and stop the drug only under your doctor's supervision.

There is no information regarding the safety and effectiveness of long-term treatment in children. However, slowing of growth has been seen with the long-term use of stimulants, so your doctor will monitor your child carefully while he or she is taking Metadate.

The use of Metadate in children less than 6 years old is not recommended.

Who should not take Metadate CD/Metadate ER?

Metadate should not be taken if you or your child are very anxious, tense, or agitated, have glaucoma, experience tics or have Tourette's syndrome.

Do not take Metadate within 14 days of taking antidepressants called monoamine oxidase inhibitors (MAOIs), or if you are allergic to anything in Metadate.

What should I tell my doctor before I take the first dose of Metadate CD/Metadate ER?

Tell your doctor about all prescription, over-the-counter, and herbal medications you are taking before beginning treatment with Metadate, especially if you are currently taking or have recently taken MAOIs. Also, talk to your doctor about your complete medical history, especially if you have a history of heart problems such as congenital heart defects, heart failure, heart rhythm disorder or recent heart attack, high blood pressure, a personal or family history of mental illness, psychotic disorder, bipolar disorder, depression, suicide attempt, seizures or other convulsion disorders, a history of drug or alcohol addiction, glaucoma, a personal or family history of tics (muscle twitches) or Tourette's syndrome, severe anxiety, tension, or agitation.

What is the usual dosage?

The information below is based on the dosage guidelines your doctor uses. Depending on your condition and medical history, your doctor may prescribe a different regimen. Do not change the dosage or stop taking your medication without your doctor's approval.

Metadate CD

Adults: The recommended starting dose is 20 milligrams (mg) once daily. Your doctor may increase your dose in 10- to 20-mg increments at weekly intervals up to a maximum daily dose of 60 mg.

Children 6 years and older: The recommended starting dose is 20 mg once daily. At weekly intervals, your doctor may increase your child's dose in 10 to 20 mg increments up to a maximum daily dose of 60 mg.

Metadate ER

Adults: These are extended-release tablets that keep working for 8 hours. Your doctor will determine your exact dose.

Children 6 years and older: These tablets keep working for 8 hours, and your doctor will determine the exact dose for your child.

Metadate should not be given to children under 6 years of age.

How should I take Metadate CD/Metadate ER?

Follow your doctor's directions carefully. Metadate CD may also be given by sprinkling the contents of the capsule on a tablespoon of cool applesauce and administering immediately, followed by a drink of water. Do not crush or chew the capsule contents.

Metadate ER tablets must be swallowed whole and never chewed or crushed.

What should I avoid while taking Metadate CD/Metadate ER?

Some people have had visual disturbances such as blurred vision while being treated with Metadate. Be careful if you drive or do anything that requires you to be awake and alert until you know how this medication affects you.

What are possible food and drug interactions associated with Metadate CD/Metadate ER?

If Metadate is taken with certain other drugs, the effects of either could be increased, decreased, or altered. It is especially important to check with your doctor before combining Metadate with any of the following: antidepressants, antiseizure drugs, blood pressure drugs, blood thinners such as warfarin, clonidine, guanethidine, MAOIs, and phenylbutazone.

What are the possible side effects of Metadate CD/Metadate ER?

Side effects cannot be anticipated. If any develop or change in intensity, tell your doctor as soon as possible. Only your doctor can determine if it is safe for you to continue taking this drug.

Side effects may include: inability to fall or stay asleep, nervousness
These side effects can usually be controlled by reducing the dosage and omitting the drug in the afternoon or evening.

More common side effects in children may include: loss of appetite, abdominal pain, weight loss during long-term therapy, inability to fall or stay asleep, abnormally fast heartbeat

Can I receive Metadate CD/Metadate ER if I am pregnant or breastfeeding?

The effects of Metadate during pregnancy and breastfeeding are unknown. Tell your doctor immediately if you are pregnant, plan to become pregnant, or are breastfeeding.

What should I do if I miss a dose of Metadate CD/Metadate ER?

Take the missed dose as soon as you remember. If it is almost time for your next dose, skip the missed dose and take the medicine at your next regularly scheduled time. Do not take a double dose to make up for the missed dose.

How should I store Metadate CD/Metadate ER?

Store at room temperature in a tightly closed, light-resistant container, and protect from moisture.

METAGLIP
Generic name: Glipizide and metformin hydrochloride

What is Metaglip?
Metaglip helps lower blood sugar in people with type 2 diabetes if diet, exercise, or other medications have not. Metaglip contains two different medications that work together to lower blood sugar in part by helping the body use insulin more effectively and prevent it from making too much sugar.

What is the most important information I should know about Metaglip?
A small number of patients who have taken Metaglip have developed a rare but serious side effect known as lactic acidosis. Your chances of developing lactic acidosis increase if you do not have properly functioning kidneys, have kidney disease, heart disease, or liver impairment. Signs and symptoms of lactic acidosis include muscle weakness and pain, difficulty breathing, flulike symptoms, and abdominal pain.

You should not take Metaglip if you have kidney or liver disease, acute or chronic metabolic acidosis, or chronic heart failure. Metaglip can cause your blood sugar to decrease, especially if taken with certain medications or if you have liver, kidney, or heart disease. The signs and symptoms of low blood sugar include lightheadedness, dizziness, shakiness, and hunger.

You should not drink excessively for short or long periods of time while taking Metaglip. Once you have taken Metaglip consistently and have gotten used to its effects, you should inform your doctor immediately if you develop any sudden abdominal pain.

Who should not take Metaglip?
You should not take Metaglip if you have kidney dysfunction or disease, congestive heart failure requiring medication, a known sensitivity or allergy to glipizide or metformin, or acute and chronic metabolic acidosis including diabetic ketoacidosis.

What should I tell my doctor before I take the first dose of Metaglip?
You should tell your doctor that you are taking Metaglip before undergoing any imaging procedure such as an MRI or are scheduled for surgery.

Mention all prescription, over-the-counter, and herbal medications you are taking before beginning treatment with Metaglip. Also, talk to your doctor about your complete medical history, especially if you drink alcohol excessively, are dehydrated, have liver or kidney problems, are taking medications like furosemide or digoxin for chronic heart failure, or are over 80 and have not had your kidney function checked.

What is the usual dosage?

The information below is based on the dosage guidelines your doctor uses. Depending on your condition and medical history, your doctor may prescribe a different regimen. Do not change the dosage or stop taking your medication without your doctor's approval.

The dosage of Metaglip must be individualized on the basis of both effectiveness and tolerance while not exceeding the maximum recommended daily dose of 20 mg glipizide/2,000 mg metformin.

Adults: The usual starting dose is 2.5/250 milligrams (mg) taken once daily with a meal. Depending on your individual fasting blood glucose level, your doctor may increase your dose to 2.5/500 mg taken twice daily, or up to a maximum daily dose of 10/2,000 mg.

How should I take Metaglip?

Metaglip should be taken at the same time every day with food.

What should I avoid while taking Metaglip?

You should avoid drinking alcohol excessively, becoming dehydrated, and allowing your blood sugar to drop by not eating at regular intervals throughout the day.

What are possible food and drug interactions associated with Metaglip?

If Metaglip is taken with certain other drugs, the effects of either could be increased, decreased, or altered. It is especially important to check with your doctor before combining Metaglip with the following: amiloride, antibiotics (sulfonamide-type), antifungal medications, beta blockers, calcium channel blockers (such as nifedipine), chloramphenicol, corticosteroids, coumadin, digoxin, estrogens, phenothiazines (types of antipsychotics), isoniazid, nicotinic acid, oral contraceptives, phenytoin, probenecid, monoamine oxidase inhibitors, morphine, nonsteroidal anti-inflammatory medications (such as acetaminophen), procainamide, quinidine, quinine, ranitidine, sympathomimetic medications, thiazide-type diuretics (as well as other diuretics such as furosemide), thyroid medications, triamterene, trimethoprim, or vancomycin.

What are the possible side effects of Metaglip?

Side effects cannot be anticipated. If any develop or change in intensity, tell your doctor as soon as possible. Only your doctor can determine if it is safe for you to continue taking this drug.

Side effects may include: diarrhea, nausea, upset stomach, low blood sugar

Can I receive Metaglip if I am pregnant or breastfeeding?

You should not take Metaglip during pregnancy without first consulting your doctor. It is not known whether Metaglip is excreted in breast milk.

Tell your doctor immediately if you are pregnant, plan to become pregnant, or are breastfeeding.

What should I do if I miss a dose of Metaglip?
If you forget to take a dose of Metaglip, do not double your next dose. Skip the dose you missed and return to your normal dosing schedule.

How should I store Metaglip?
Store at room temperature.

Metaxalone See Skelaxin, page 1202.

Metformin hydrochloride See Glucophage/Glucophage XR, page 617.

Metformin hydrochloride, extended-release See Glumetza, page 627.

Methamphetamine hydrochloride See Desoxyn, page 403.

Methocarbamol See Robaxin, page 1167.

METHOTREXATE

What is Methotrexate?
Methotrexate is a medicine that inhibits the metabolism of certain types of cells. It is used to treat certain cancers, rheumatoid arthritis (including polyarticular juvenile arthritis), and severe psoriasis.

What is the most important information I should know about Methotrexate?
Methotrexate can cause serious and life-threatening side effects. These side effects can be monitored by your doctor using simple medical tests before they become serious. Your doctor will monitor you when you are taking Methotrexate to check how it affects your body. Inform your doctor immediately of any side effects you experience while taking Methotrexate.

Methotrexate can cause birth defects or fetal death. If you are pregnant, or your partner is pregnant or plans to become pregnant, you should not take Methotrexate. Women should wait at least 1 menstrual cycle after stopping Methotrexate therapy before getting pregnant, and men should wait at least 3 months after stopping Methotrexate therapy before getting their partner pregnant. If you can become pregnant, you should have a pregnancy test before taking Methotrexate. Both men and women should use effective methods of birth control while taking Methotrexate.

You should stop taking Methotrexate and call your doctor right away if you experience diarrhea, mouth sores, a fever, dehydration, cough, bleeding, shortness of breath, any signs of an infection, or a skin rash. Your doctor may also prescribe a folate-containing medication to take in addition to Methotrexate to help reduce possible side effects.

Who should not take Methotrexate?

You should not take Methotrexate if you are pregnant or plan to become pregnant, are breastfeeding, have conditions that weaken your immune system, your bone marrow doesn't make enough blood cells, you have low platelet or white blood cell counts, serious anemia, drink alcohol, have chronic liver disease, or if you are allergic or have a hypersensitivity to Methotrexate.

What should I tell my doctor before I take the first dose of Methotrexate?

Tell your doctor if you are pregnant or your sexual partner is pregnant or plans to become pregnant.

Tell your doctor about all prescription, over-the-counter, and herbal medications you are taking before beginning treatment with Methotrexate. Also, talk to your doctor about your complete medical history, especially if you have kidney problems or are getting dialysis, liver problems, fluid in your stomach area, or if you have lung problems including fluid in your lungs.

What is the usual dosage?

The information below is based on the dosage guidelines your doctor uses. Depending on your condition and medical history, your doctor may prescribe a different regimen. Do not change the dosage or stop taking your medication without your doctor's approval.

Choriocarcinoma and Similar Trophoblastic Diseases
Adults: The usual starting dose is 15-30 milligrams (mg) daily for 3 to 5 days. This is usually repeated 3-5 times with rest periods in between of 1 to several weeks.

Cutaneous T Cell Lymphoma
Adults: The usual dosage is 5-50 mg taken once weekly

Leukemia
Adults: The usual dose is 3.3 mg per square meter of body mass given once daily in combination with other medicines.

Lymphomas
Adults: The usual dose is 10-25 mg daily for 4 to 8 days, but may vary depending on the type or stage of lymphoma being treated.

Psoriasis, Rheumatoid Arthritis, and Juvenile Rheumatoid Arthritis

Adults: The usual starting dose includes a single dose of 7.5 mg taken once a week, or 2.5 mg taken every 12 hours for 3 doses once a week.

Polyarticular-Course Juvenile Rheumatoid Arthritis

Children: The usual starting dose is 10 mg per square meter of body mass taken once a week. Based on the response to this dosage, the doctor may increase the dose to 20-30 mg per square body meter taken once weekly.

How should I take Methotrexate?

Methotrexate should be taken exactly as prescribed by your doctor. You should not take more Methotrexate than prescribed.

For severe psoriasis, rheumatoid arthritis, and juvenile rheumatoid arthritis Methotrexate should be taken weekly, not every day. If you take too much Methotrexate, call your doctor immediately or go to the nearest emergency room.

What should I avoid while taking Methotrexate?

You should avoid getting pregnant or trying to become pregnant, breast-feeding, drinking alcohol, or receiving certain live vaccines.

What are possible food and drug interactions associated with Methotrexate?

If Methotrexate is taken with certain other drugs, the effects of either could be increased, decreased, or altered. It is especially important to check with your doctor before combining Methotrexate with the following: chloramphenicol, nonabsorbable broad-spectrum antibiotics, nonsteroidal anti-inflammatory drugs, phenylbutazone, phenytoin, probenecid, salicylates, sulfonamides, tetracycline, penicillin-type antibiotics, theophylline, trimethoprim/sulfamethoxazole, and vitamins containing folic acid or its derivatives.

What are the possible side effects of Methotrexate?

Side effects cannot be anticipated. If any develop or change in intensity, tell your doctor as soon as possible. Only your doctor can determine if it is safe for you to continue taking this drug.

Side effects may include: birth defects and fetal death; cancer of the lymphatic system (lymphoma); kidney damage; lower white cells, red cells, and platelets in your blood; liver damage; lung disease; opportunistic infections such as *Pneumocystis carinii* pneumonia; severe anemia; severe skin reactions and rashes; soft tissue and bone damage if you are getting radiation therapy at the same time you are taking Methotrexate

Can I receive Methotrexate if I am pregnant or breastfeeding?
Methotrexate should NOT be taken if you are pregnant, plan to become pregnant, or are breastfeeding. Men who are taking Methotrexate should not get their partners pregnant for at least 3 months after last taking Methotrexate.

What should I do if I miss a dose of Methotrexate?
If you forget to take a dose of Methotrexate, ask your doctor if and when you should take your next dose.

How should I store Methotrexate?
Methotrexate should be stored at room temperature.

METHYLDOPA

What is Methyldopa?
Methyldopa is used to treat high blood pressure. It is effective when used alone or with other high blood pressure medications.

**What is the most important information
I should know about Methyldopa?**
Before you begin taking methyldopa, your doctor should perform a complete study of your liver function, and it should be monitored periodically thereafter. If you have a history of liver disease, this medication should be used with caution.

Methyldopa can cause liver disorders. You may develop a fever, jaundice (yellow eyes and skin), or both, usually within the first 2 to 3 months of therapy. If either of these symptoms occurs, stop taking methyldopa and contact your doctor immediately. If the fever and/or jaundice were caused by the medication, your liver function should gradually return to normal.

Hemolytic anemia, a blood disorder in which red blood cells are destroyed, can develop with long-term use of methyldopa; your doctor may do periodic blood counts to check for this problem.

Methyldopa can cause water retention or weight gain in some people.

If you are on dialysis and are taking methyldopa for high blood pressure, your blood pressure may rise after your dialysis treatments.

Notify your doctor or dentist that you are taking methyldopa if you have a medical emergency and before you have surgery or dental treatment.

Who should not take Methyldopa?
If you have liver disease or cirrhosis, or if you have taken methyldopa before and developed liver disease, do not take this medication.

If you are sensitive to or have ever had an allergic reaction to methyldopa, or if you have been prescribed the oral suspension form of methyldopa and have ever had an allergic reaction to sulfites, you should not take this medication.

If you are taking drugs known as monoamine oxidase (MAO) inhibitors, you should not take methyldopa.

What should I tell my doctor before I take the first dose of Methyldopa?
Tell your doctor about all prescription, over-the-counter, and herbal medication you are taking before beginning treatment with indapamide. Also, talk to your doctor about your complete medical history, especially if you have liver problems or blood disorders such as anemia.

What is the usual dosage?
The information below is based on the dosage guidelines your doctor uses. Depending on your condition and medical history, your doctor may prescribe a different regimen. Do not change the dosage or stop taking your medication without your doctor's approval.

Adults: The usual starting dose is 250 milligrams, 2 or 3 times per day in the first 48 hours of treatment. Your doctor may increase or decrease your dose over the next few days to achieve the correct blood pressure. To reduce the effect of any sedation the medication may cause, dosage increases will usually be given in the evening.

The usual maintenance dosage is 500 milligrams to 2 grams per day divided into 2 to 4 doses. The maximum dose is usually 3 grams.

Your doctor will also adjust your dosage of methyldopa when it is taken in combination with certain other high blood pressure drugs.

If you take methyldopa with a non-thiazide high blood pressure medicine, your doctor will limit the initial dosage to 500 milligrams daily divided into small doses.

Dosages will be adjusted, and other high blood pressure drugs may be added, during the first few months of treatment with methyldopa. Those with reduced kidney function may require smaller doses. Older people who are prone to fainting spells due to arterial disease may also require smaller doses.

Children: The usual starting dose is 10 milligrams per 2.2 pounds of body weight daily, divided into 2 to 4 doses. Doses will be adjusted until blood pressure is normal. The maximum daily dose is usually 65 milligrams per 2.2 pounds of body weight or 3 grams, whichever is less.

How should I take Methyldopa?
Take this medication exactly as prescribed. Try not to miss any doses. Do not stop taking the drug without your doctor's knowledge.

What should I avoid while taking Methyldopa?

Methyldopa can cause you to become drowsy or less alert, especially during the first few weeks of therapy or when dosage levels are increased. Avoid driving or participating in any hazardous activity until you know how this drug affects you.

What are possible food and drug interactions associated with Methyldopa?

If methyldopa is taken with certain other drugs, the effects of either could be increased, decreased, or altered. It is especially important to check with your doctor before combining methyldopa with the following: anti-depressants known as MAO inhibitors, dextroamphetamine, imipramine, iron-containing products, lithium, other blood pressure medications, phenylpropanolamine, propranolol, and tolbutamide.

What are the possible side effects of Methyldopa?

Side effects cannot be anticipated. If any develop or change in intensity, inform your doctor as soon as possible. Only your doctor can determine if it is safe for you to continue taking methyldopa.

Side effects may include: drowsiness during the first few weeks of therapy, fluid retention or weight gain, headache, weakness

Can I receive Methyldopa if I am pregnant or breastfeeding?

The use of methyldopa during pregnancy appears to be relatively safe. However, if you are pregnant or plan to become pregnant, inform your doctor immediately. Methyldopa appears in breast milk and could affect a nursing infant. If this medication is essential to your health, your doctor may advise you to discontinue breastfeeding until your treatment is finished.

What should I do if I miss a dose of Methyldopa?

Take it as soon as you remember. If it is almost time for your next dose, skip the one you missed and go back to your regular schedule. Never take 2 doses at the same time.

How should I store Methyldopa?

Keep methyldopa in the container it came in, tightly closed. Store methyldopa tablets at room temperature. Protect from light.

METHYLIN/METHYLIN ER

Generic name: Methylphenidate hydrochloride

What is Methylin/Methylin ER?

Methylin and other brands of methylphenidate are medications known as stimulants and are used in the treatment of attention-deficit/hyperactivity disorder (ADHD). Methylin may help increase attention and decrease impulsiveness and hyperactivity in ADHD patients.

Methylin is also prescribed for the treatment of narcolepsy.

What is the most important information I should know about Methylin/Methylin ER?

Methylin should be an integral part of a total treatment program for ADHD that includes psychological, educational, and social measures. Symptoms of ADHD include continual problems with moderate to severe distractibility, short attention span, hyperactivity, emotional changeability, and impulsiveness.

There are reports of heart and mental problems in patients taking Methylin or other related stimulants. Some of the problems are sudden death in patients with previous heart problems, heart attacks in adults, increased blood pressure and heart rate. Methylin can also cause new or worsening symptoms of behavior problems, bipolar disorder, and aggressive or hostile behavior. Call your doctor right away if you or child develops signs of heart problems such as chest pain, shortness of breath, or fainting while taking Methylin.

Excessive doses of Methylin over a long period of time may cause addiction. It is also possible to develop tolerance to the drug, so that larger doses are needed to produce the original effect. Be sure to check with your doctor before making any change in dosage; and stop the drug only under your doctor's supervision.

There is no information regarding the safety and effectiveness of long-term treatment in children. However, slowing of growth has been seen with the long-term use of stimulants, so your doctor will monitor your child carefully while he or she is taking Methylin.

The use of Methylin in children less than 6 years old is not recommended.

Who should not take Methylin/Methylin ER?

Methylin should not be taken if you or your child are very anxious, tense, or agitated, have glaucoma, thyroid problems, heart problems or recent heart attack, or experience tics or have Tourette's syndrome.

Do not take Methylin within 14 days of taking antidepressants called monoamine oxidase inhibitors (MAOIs), or if you are allergic to anything in Methylin.

What should I tell my doctor before I take the first dose of Methylin/Methylin ER?

Tell your doctor about all prescription, over-the-counter, and herbal medications you are taking before beginning treatment with Methylin, especially if you are currently taking or have recently taken MAOIs. Also, talk to your doctor about your complete medical history, especially if you have a history of heart problems such as congenital heart defects, heart failure, heart rhythm disorder or recent heart attack, high blood pressure, a personal or family history of mental illness, psychotic disorder, bipolar disorder, depression, suicide attempt, epilepsy or other seizure disorders, a history of drug or alcohol addiction, glaucoma, a personal or family history of tics (muscle twitches) or Tourette's syndrome, severe anxiety, tension, or agitation.

What is the usual dosage?
The information below is based on the dosage guidelines your doctor uses. Depending on your condition and medical history, your doctor may prescribe a different regimen. Do not change the dosage or stop taking your medication without your doctor's approval.

Methylin
Adults: The average dosage is 20 to 30 milligrams (mg) a day, divided into 2 or 3 doses, preferably taken 30 to 45 minutes before meals. Some people may need 40 to 60 mg daily, others only 10 to 15 mg. Your doctor will determine the best dose.

Children 6 years and older: The usual starting dose is 5 mg taken twice a day, before breakfast and lunch; your doctor may increase the dose by 5 to 10 mg a week. Your child should not take more than 60 mg in a day. If you do not see any improvement over a period of one month, check with your doctor.

Methylin ER
Adults: These are extended-release tablets that keep working for 8 hours. They may be used in place of Methylin tablets and your doctor will determine the best dose.

Children 6 years and older: Your child's doctor will decide if these extended-release tablets should be used in place of the regular tablets.
Methylin should not be given to children under 6 years of age.

How should I take Methylin/Methylin ER?
Follow your doctor's directions carefully. Methylin tablets should be taken 30 to 45 minutes before meals. Methylin ER tablets must be swallowed whole and never chewed or crushed.

What should I avoid while taking Methylin/Methylin ER?
Some people have had visual disturbances such as blurred vision while being treated with Methylin. Be careful if you drive or do anything that requires you to be awake and alert.

What are possible food and drug interactions associated with Methylin/Methylin ER?
If Methylin is taken with certain other drugs, the effects of either could be increased, decreased, or altered. It is especially important to check

with your doctor before combining Methylin with any of the following: antidepressants, antiseizure drugs, blood pressure drugs, blood thinners such as warfarin, clonidine, guanethidine, MAOIs, and phenylbutazone.

What are the possible side effects of Methylin/Methylin ER?
Side effects cannot be anticipated. If any develop or change in intensity, tell your doctor as soon as possible. Only your doctor can determine if it is safe for you to continue taking this drug.

Side effects may include: inability to fall or stay asleep, nervousness
These side effects can usually be controlled by reducing the dosage and omitting the drug in the afternoon or evening.

More common side effects in children may include: loss of appetite, abdominal pain, weight loss during long-term therapy, inability to fall or stay asleep, abnormally fast heartbeat

Can I receive Methylin/Methylin ER if I am pregnant or breastfeeding?
The effects of Methylin during pregnancy and breastfeeding are unknown. Tell your doctor immediately if you are pregnant, plan to become pregnant, or are breastfeeding.

What should I do if I miss a dose of Methylin/Methylin ER?
Take the missed dose as soon as you remember. If it is almost time for your next dose, skip the missed dose and take the medicine at your next regularly scheduled time. Do not take a double dose to make up for the missed dose.

How should I store Methylin/Methylin ER?
Store at room temperature in a tightly closed, light-resistant container, and protect from moisture.

Methylphenidate hydrochloride *See Concerta, page 333; Metadate CD/Metadate ER, page 799; Methylin/ Methylin ER, page 809; or Ritalin/Ritalin-SR/ Ritalin LA, page 1162.*

Methylphenidate patch *See Daytrana, page 380.*

Methylprednisolone *See Medrol, page 792.*

Metoclopramide hydrochloride *See Reglan, page 1124.*

Metolazone See Zaroxolyn, page 1447.

Metoprolol tartrate See Lopressor, page 758.

METROGEL
Generic name: Metronidazole

What is MetroGel?
MetroGel is a preparation of the drug metronidazole used for the treatment of a skin condition called rosacea. The cream and lotion forms of metronidazole are used for the same problem. All are for external (topical) use only.

What is the most important information I should know about MetroGel?
Metronidazole may irritate the skin. If local irritation occurs, consult your doctor. You may need to use the medication less frequently or to discontinue use.

Who should not take MetroGel?
Do not use topical metronidazole if you have ever had an allergic reaction to metronidazole, or if you have been told that you are sensitive to chemicals called parabens.

What should I tell my doctor before I take the first dose of MetroGel?
Tell your doctor about all prescription, over-the-counter, and herbal medications you are taking before beginning treatment with this drug. Also, talk to your doctor about your complete medical history, especially if you have ever had any abnormalities of the blood.

What is the usual dosage?
The information below is based on the dosage guidelines your doctor uses. Depending on your condition and medical history, your doctor may prescribe a different regimen. Do not change the dosage or stop taking your medication without your doctor's approval.

Adults: Apply a thin layer to the affected area twice a day.

How should I take MetroGel?
After washing the affected area, apply a thin film of the preparation and rub in. Topical metronidazole should be applied twice daily, in the morning and evening. Cosmetics may be used after the drug is applied. (If using the lotion, wait 5 minutes for it to dry.)

What should I avoid while taking MetroGel?

Since this medication may cause tearing of the eye, avoid contact with the eyes. Be sure to wash your hands after applying the medication so as not to irritate the eyes.

What are possible food and drug interactions associated with MetroGel?

Oral metronidazole strengthens the activity of blood thinners such as warfarin. It's not known whether topical preparations have the same effect.

What are the possible side effects of MetroGel?

Side effects cannot be anticipated. If any develop or change in intensity, tell your doctor as soon as possible. Only your doctor can determine if it is safe for you to continue taking this drug.

Side effects may include: burning or stinging, dryness, itching, metallic taste, nausea, redness, skin irritation, tingling or numbness of hands and feet, worsening of rosacea

Can I receive MetroGel if I am pregnant or breastfeeding?

There is no evidence that metronidazole can harm a developing baby. Nevertheless, it should be used during pregnancy only if clearly needed. If you are pregnant or plan to become pregnant, tell your doctor immediately.

Topical metronidazole appears in breast milk. You'll need to choose between nursing your baby or continuing treatment with the drug.

What should I do if I miss a dose of MetroGel?

Apply it as soon as you remember. If it is almost time for your next dose, skip the one you missed and go back to your regular schedule.

How should I store MetroGel?

Store at room temperature. Protect the lotion from freezing.

Metronidazole *See Flagyl, page 555; MetroGel, page 813; or Vandazole, page 1371.*

MEVACOR

Generic name: Lovastatin

What is Mevacor?

Mevacor is a medication called a "statin" that lowers cholesterol in your blood. It can lower the "bad" LDL cholesterol and triglycerides in your blood. Mevacor can raise your "good" HDL cholesterol as well. Mevacor is for people who have not been able to adequately lower their cholesterol with exercise and a low-fat diet alone.

Mevacor may be used in people with heart disease (coronary artery disease) to slow the buildup of too much cholesterol in the arteries of the heart, therefore lowering the chances of needing procedures to help restore blood flow to the heart. Over time, it reduces your chances of experiencing a heart attack or angina.

Mevacor is also prescribed for adolescents who have a hereditary form of high cholesterol and have not been able to adequately lower it with exercise and a low-fat diet alone.

What is the most important information I should know about Mevacor?

Rarely, Mevacor can cause a side effect that can lead to the breakdown of your muscles, and is characterized by sudden muscle pain, weakness, or tenderness. Tell your doctor immediately if you experience these symptoms while taking Mevacor. The chances of this rare side effect increase if you are taking certain other drugs, so tell your doctor about all medications and supplements you are taking before starting Mevacor.

Do not take Mevacor if you are pregnant, think you may be pregnant, or are planning to become pregnant.

Over time, Mevacor may cause liver damage in some patients. When you are taking Mevacor, your doctor may perform simple blood tests to check your liver's health periodically.

Who should not take Mevacor?

You should not take Mevacor if you are pregnant or plan to become pregnant or if you are breastfeeding. You should also not take Mevacor if you have active liver disease or persistent liver damage. Do not take Mevacor if you are allergic to the medication or any of its ingredients.

What should I tell my doctor before I take the first dose of Mevacor?

Tell your doctor about all prescription, over-the-counter, and herbal medications you are taking before beginning treatment with Mevacor. Also, talk to your doctor about your complete medical history, especially if you have ever had chronic muscle aches or weakness, problems with your liver, or kidney disease. Also let the doctor know if you drink more than 2 glasses of alcohol daily.

What is the usual dosage?

The information below is based on the dosage guidelines your doctor uses. Depending on your condition and medical history, your doctor may prescribe a different regimen. Do not change the dosage or stop taking your medication without your doctor's approval.

Adults: The usual starting dose is 20 milligrams (mg) taken once daily, preferably with an evening meal. Your doctor may increase your individual dose up to a maximum of 80 mg taken as one or two doses daily.

Children 10 to 17 years old: The usual daily dose is 10-40 mg taken once or twice daily.

How should I take Mevacor?

Mevacor should be taken with food preferably in the evening. It should be taken at the same time every day.

What should I avoid while taking Mevacor?

Do not get pregnant or take the medication while breastfeeding. If you do get pregnant, stop taking Mevacor right away and call your doctor.

Avoid drinking more than 1 quart of grapefruit juice daily, as this may impair your body's ability to metabolize Mevacor. Avoid alcohol during drug therapy.

What are possible food and drug interactions associated with Mevacor?

If Mevacor is taken with certain other drugs, the effects of either could be increased, decreased, or altered. It is especially important to check with your doctor before combining Mevacor with the following: amiodarone, clarithromycin, cyclosporine, danazol, erythromycin, gemfibrozil, grapefruit juice (>1 quart daily), HIV medications called "protease inhibitors," itraconazole, ketoconazole, nefazodone, niacin, other lipid-lowering drugs, telithromycin, and verapamil.

What are the possible side effects of Mevacor?

Side effects cannot be anticipated. If any develop or change in intensity, tell your doctor as soon as possible. Only your doctor can determine if it is safe for you to continue taking this drug.

Side effects may include: Upset stomach, flatulence, headache, diarrhea, constipation, or stomach pain.

More serious side effects may include: muscle problems, including muscle pain, tenderness or weakness; kidney problems, including kidney failure; and liver problems

You have a greater chance for developing muscle problems if you are taking certain other medicines with Mevacor.

Your doctor may do blood tests to check your liver before you start taking Mevacor, and periodically during treatment.

Call your doctor right away if you have any of the following symptoms: muscle problems such as weakness, tenderness, or pain without apparent cause, especially if you also have a fever or feel more tired than usual;

nausea and vomiting; passing brown or dark-colored urine; unusual fatigue; yellowing of your skin and the whites of your eyes; stomach pain.

Can I receive Mevacor if I am pregnant or breastfeeding?
No. Mevacor may cause fetal harm and should not be taken during pregnancy or while breastfeeding.

What should I do if I miss a dose of Mevacor?
If you miss a dose of this medicine, take it as soon as possible. However, if it is almost time for your next dose, skip the missed dose and go back to your regular dosing schedule. Do not double doses.

How should I store Mevacor?
Mevacor should be stored at room temperature away from light.

MIACALCIN
Generic name: Calcitonin-salmon

What is Miacalcin?
Miacalcin is a protein-like medication that is used to help your bones retain and store calcium. Miacalcin is used to treat osteoporosis in women who are more than 5 years into menopause and who have a low bone mass (compared to healthy pre-menopausal women).

What is the most important information I should know about Miacalcin?
Rarely, Miacalcin can cause serious allergic reactions that require emergency medical attention. If your doctor suspects that you may have an allergy to Miacalcin, he or she will likely test your sensitivity to Miacalcin before prescribing it. If you are using the nasal spray form of Miacalcin, your doctor may periodically examine your nostrils and sinuses to check for any possible side effects of the Miacalcin nasal spray.

Who should not take Miacalcin?
You should not take Miacalcin if you have an allergy to Miacalcin or any of its ingredients.

What should I tell my doctor before I take the first dose of Miacalcin?
Tell your doctor about all prescription, over-the-counter, and herbal medications you are taking before beginning treatment with Miacalcin. Also, talk to your doctor about your complete medical history, especially if you have any ulcerations inside your nostrils or if you have ever had an allergic reaction to Miacalcin.

What is the usual dosage?
The information below is based on the dosage guidelines your doctor uses. Depending on your condition and medical history, your doctor may prescribe a different regimen. Do not change the dosage or stop taking your medication without your doctor's approval.

Adults: The usual dose is 1 spray in one nostril once daily, alternating nostrils every other day.

How should I take Miacalcin?
Miacalcin should be kept in the refrigerator until you are ready to use it. Once you start to use the nasal spray, you should store it at room temperature and in an upright position for up to 35 days.

Before using a new bottle, let the bottle reach room temperature and then "prime" the bottle by pressing down on the pump until a full spray of solution is released.

The nasal spray should only be sprayed in one nostril daily, not both, unless you are otherwise directed by your doctor.

After 30 doses, the nasal spray bottle may not deliver the correct amount of solution even if there is still some in the bottle. Keep track of the number of doses used from the bottle. After 30 sprays, you should start using a new bottle.

What should I avoid while taking Miacalcin?
The use of Miacalcin nasal spray may cause you to develop nasal conditions such as runny nose, sinusitis, or a nosebleed. Therefore, you should avoid using any other nasal agents that may cause irritation to your nose unless you have been directed to do otherwise by your physician.

What are possible food and drug interactions associated with Miacalcin?
There are no reports of food or drug interactions with Micalcin. However, speak to your doctor about any other medications or supplements you are taking.

What are the possible side effects of Miacalcin?
Side effects cannot be anticipated. If any develop or change in intensity, tell your doctor as soon as possible. Only your doctor can determine if it is safe for you to continue taking this drug.

Side effects of the nostrils or nose as a whole may include: bloody nose, dryness, nasal crusts, infection, irritation, itching, redness, runniness or congestion, soreness across bridge of nose, sores, tenderness, thick feeling, uncomfortable feeling

Side effects of the body as a whole may include: back pain, arthritic pain, headache

Can I receive Miacalcin if I am pregnant or breastfeeding?
You should not take Miacalcin during pregnancy unless otherwise prescribed by your physician.

It is not known whether Miacalcin is excreted in breast milk. Tell your doctor immediately if you are pregnant, plan to become pregnant, or are breastfeeding.

What should I do if I miss a dose of Miacalcin?
If you miss a dose of Miacalcin, take it as soon as you remember. If it is almost time for your next dose, skip the dose you missed and return to your normal dosing schedule. Do not double your next dose.

How should I store Miacalcin?
Refrigerate Miacalcin until you are ready to use it. Protect it from freezing.

Once you have opened a bottle, keep it in an upright position and at room temperature for up to 35 days. You should only use 30 sprays per bottle; after 30 sprays, the bottle may not deliver the correct dose.

MICARDIS
Generic name: Telmisartan

What is Micardis?
Micardis is a type of medication called an "angiotensin II receptor antagonist" that blocks certain receptors in your body to help lower your blood pressure.

**What is the most important information
I should know about Micardis?**
If Micardis is taken during your second or third trimester of pregnancy, Micardis can cause serious injury and even death to your unborn baby. If you become pregnant while taking Micardis, stop taking Micardis and tell your doctor immediately.

You should take Micardis cautiously if you have been diagnosed with liver impairment or disease, severe heart failure, kidney disease, or a type of condition called a "biliary obstructive disorder."

If you become dehydrated while taking Micardis, your blood pressure may drop too low and you may feel lightheaded or dizzy. You should stay sufficiently hydrated while taking Micardis to prevent this from occurring.

Who should not take Micardis?
You should not take Micardis if you have ever had an allergic reaction or hypersensitivity to Micardis or any of its ingredients.

Do not take Micardis if you are pregnant. If you get pregnant, stop taking Micardis and call your doctor right away.

What should I tell my doctor before I take the first dose of Micardis?

Tell your doctor about all prescription, over-the-counter, and herbal medications you are taking before beginning treatment with Micardis. Also, talk to your doctor about your complete medical history, especially if you have liver or kidney impairment or disease, biliary obstructive disorders, severe heart failure, are pregnant or plan to become pregnant, or if you are breastfeeding.

What is the usual dosage?

The information below is based on the dosage guidelines your doctor uses. Depending on your condition and medical history, your doctor may prescribe a different regimen. Do not change the dosage or stop taking your medication without your doctor's approval.

Adults: The usual starting dose is 40 milligrams (mg) taken once daily. Your doctor may increase or decrease your individual dose from 20-80 mg based on your condition.

How should I take Micardis?

Micardis should be taken at the same time every day and can be taken with or without food.

What should I avoid while taking Micardis?

You should avoid becoming excessively dehydrated while taking Micardis, as this may cause low blood pressure and lead to lightheadedness or dizziness.

What are possible food and drug interactions associated with Micardis?

If Micardis is taken with certain other drugs, the effects of either could be increased, decreased, or altered. It is especially important to check with your doctor before combining Micardis with digoxin.

What are the possible side effects of Micardis?

Side effects cannot be anticipated. If any develop or change in intensity, tell your doctor as soon as possible. Only your doctor can determine if it is safe for you to continue taking this drug.

Side effects may include: upper respiratory tract infection, back pain, sinus inflammation, diarrhea

Can I receive Micardis if I am pregnant or breastfeeding?

You should not take Micardis if you are pregnant or plan to become pregnant. If taken during your second or third trimester of pregnancy, Micardis can cause serious injury and even death to your unborn baby.

If you become pregnant while taking Micardis, you should stop taking Micardis and tell your doctor immediately.

The effects of Micardis during breastfeeding are unknown. Tell your doctor immediately if you are breastfeeding or plan to breastfeed while taking Micardis.

What should I do if I miss a dose of Micardis?

If you miss a dose of Micardis, take it as soon as you remember. If it is almost time for your next dose, skip the dose you missed and return to your normal dosing schedule. Do not double your next dose.

How should I store Micardis?

Micardis should be stored at room temperature.

MICARDIS HCT

Generic name: Telmisartan and hydrochlorothiazide

What is Micardis HCT?

Micardis HCT contains two different types of medications that work together to help lower your blood pressure. Telmisartan is a type of medication called an "angiotensin II receptor antagonist" that blocks certain receptors in your body to help lower your blood pressure. Hydrochlorothiazide is a medication called a "diuretic" that helps your body get rid of excess fluids, which also lowers your blood pressure.

What is the most important information I should know about Micardis HCT?

If Micardis HCT is taken during your second or third trimester of pregnancy, it can cause serious injury and even death to your unborn baby. If you become pregnant while taking Micardis HCT, you should stop taking Micardis HCT and tell your doctor immediately.

You should take Micardis HCT cautiously if you have been diagnosed with liver impairment or disease, severe heart failure, kidney disease, or a type of condition called a "biliary obstructive disorder."

If you become dehydrated while taking Micardis HCT, your blood pressure may drop too low and you may feel lightheaded or dizzy. You should stay sufficiently hydrated while taking Micardis HCT to prevent this from occurring.

Rarely, Micardis HCT can cause an allergic or hypersensitivity reaction. The chances of this occurring after taking Micardis HCT are increased if you have a history of allergies or bronchial asthma.

Micardis HCT can cause an exacerbation of systemic lupus erythematosus if you have been previously diagnosed with this condition.

Micardis HCT can alter the normal levels of electrolytes (important minerals) in your blood. Your doctor may monitor your electrolyte levels by periodically performing blood tests. Micardis HCT can raise your blood levels of uric acid, therefore increasing your risk of developing gout.

Micardis HCT can also increase your blood sugar levels. If you use insulin your requirements may change, as well as if you take oral medications for diabetes. Even if you do not have diabetes, you may develop diabetes while taking Micardis HCT. During your therapy it is very important that you regularly monitor your blood sugar levels, and report any changes to your doctor.

Who should not take Micardis HCT?
You should not take Micardis HCT if you have ever had an allergic reaction or hypersensitivity to Micardis HCT or any of its ingredients; if you do not produce urine; or if you are allergic to sulfonamide-type medications.

Do not take Micardis HCT if you are pregnant. If you get pregnant, stop taking Micardis HCT and call your doctor right away. Micardis HCT can harm an unborn baby causing injury and even death.

What should I tell my doctor before I take the first dose of Micardis HCT?
Tell your doctor about all prescription, over-the-counter, and herbal medications you are taking before beginning treatment with Micardis HCT. Also, talk to your doctor about your complete medical history, especially if you have liver or kidney impairment or disease, biliary obstructive disorders, lupus, gout, diabetes, severe heart failure, are pregnant or plan to become pregnant, or if you are breastfeeding.

What is the usual dosage?
The information below is based on the dosage guidelines your doctor uses. Depending on your condition and medical history, your doctor may prescribe a different regimen. Do not change the dosage or stop taking your medication without your doctor's approval.

Adults: The usual starting dose is 40/12.5 milligrams (mg) (40mg of telmisartan and 12.5mg of hydrochlorothiazide) taken once daily. Your doctor may increase your individual dose up to 80/25 mg or higher based on your individual response.

How should I take Micardis HCT?
Micardis HCT should be taken at the same time every day and can be taken with or without food.

What should I avoid while taking Micardis HCT?
You should avoid becoming excessively dehydrated while taking Micardis HCT; this may cause low blood pressure and lead to lightheadedness or dizziness.

What are possible food and drug interactions associated with Micardis HCT?

If Micardis HCT is taken with certain other drugs, the effects of either could be increased, decreased, or altered. It is especially important to check with your doctor before combining Micardis HCT with the following: alcohol; barbiturates; cholestyramine and colestipol resins; corticosteroids; diabetes medications, including insulin; digoxin; lithium; narcotics; other medications for high blood pressure; and nonsteroidal anti-inflammatory drugs.

What are the possible side effects of Micardis HCT?

Side effects cannot be anticipated. If any develop or change in intensity, tell your doctor as soon as possible. Only your doctor can determine if it is safe for you to continue taking this drug.

Side effects may include: upper respiratory tract infection, back pain, sinus inflammation, diarrhea, fatigue, or dizziness.

Can I receive Micardis HCT if I am pregnant or breastfeeding?

You should not take Micardis HCT if you are pregnant or plan to become pregnant. If taken during your second or third trimester of pregnancy, Micardis HCT can cause serious injury and even death to your unborn baby. If you become pregnant while taking Micardis HCT, you should stop taking Micardis HCT and tell your doctor immediately.

The effects of Micardis HCT during breastfeeding are unknown. Tell your doctor immediately if you are breastfeeding or plan to breastfeed while taking Micardis HCT.

What should I do if I miss a dose of Micardis HCT?

If you miss a dose of Micardis HCT, take it as soon as you remember. If it is almost time for your next dose, skip the dose you missed and return to your normal dosing schedule. Do not double your next dose.

How should I store Micardis HCT?

Micardis HCT should be stored at room temperature.

MICRO-K

Generic name: Potassium chloride

What is Micro-K?

Micro-K is a specially formulated medication that contains potassium chloride in tiny, coated capsules that release the potassium slowly throughout your gastrointestinal tract. Micro-K is used to treat patients with low potassium levels due to many disease states, toxicity due to digitalis, or those with a condition called hypokalemic familial periodic paralysis.

What is the most important information I should know about Micro-K?

Micro-K may increase your risk of stomach and intestinal bleeding and ulceration. Therefore, you should only take Micro-K if you cannot tolerate liquid or effervescent potassium preparations.

If your body has an impaired ability to excrete potassium, taking Micro-K can cause an increase in your body's potassium level that can result in a heart attack.

If you have chronic kidney disease or any other condition that could potentially result in increased potassium levels, your doctor may perform blood tests regularly to monitor your potassium levels.

Who should not take Micro-K?

You should not take Micro-K if you have high levels of potassium in your blood.

What should I tell my doctor before I take the first dose of Micro-K?

Tell your doctor about all prescription, over-the-counter, and herbal medications you are taking before beginning treatment with Micro-K. Also, talk to your doctor about your complete medical history, especially if you have chronic kidney failure, a systemic acidosis condition such as diabetic acidosis, acute dehydration, extensive tissue breakdown such as with severe burns, or adrenal insufficiency.

What is the usual dosage?

The information below is based on the dosage guidelines your doctor uses. Depending on your condition and medical history, your doctor may prescribe a different regimen. Do not change the dosage or stop taking your medication without your doctor's approval.

Adults: The usual dose for prevention of low potassium is 20 milliequivalents (meq) taken daily (equal to two 750-milligram [mg] capsules taken daily). The usual dose for potassium depletion is 40-100 meq (or 4-10 of the 750 mg capsule) taken daily.

Note: you should never take more than 20 meq (the equivalent of two 750-mg capsules) at the same time.

How should I take Micro-K?

Micro-K should be taken with food and a full glass of water or similar liquid at the same time every day.

Do not suck, chew, or crush the capsules before slowing them. If you have difficulty swallowing capsules, you may open the capsules and sprinkle the contents on soft food such as applesauce or pudding. The food used should not be hot and should be soft enough to be swallowed without chewing. It is important not to chew the contents of the capsules.

What should I avoid while taking Micro-K?

You should avoid taking more Micro-K than your doctor has prescribed unless he or she instructs you otherwise.

Limit the intake of high potassium foods (bananas, fresh fruits/vegetables, fresh meats) as directed by your healthcare professional.

Avoid concomitant use of potassium-containing salt substitutes, and potassium-sparing diuretics.

What are possible food and drug interactions associated with Micro-K?

If Micro-K is taken with certain other drugs, the effects of either could be increased, decreased, or altered. It is especially important to check with your doctor before combining Micro-K with angiotensin-converting enzyme (ACE) inhibitors such as captopril or enalapril and potassium-sparing diuretics such as spironolactone, triamterene, or amiloride.

What are the possible side effects of Micro-K?

Side effects cannot be anticipated. If any develop or change in intensity, tell your doctor as soon as possible. Only your doctor can determine if it is safe for you to continue taking this drug.

Side effects may include: nausea, vomiting, gas, abdominal discomfort, diarrhea, stomach and intestinal ulceration and bleeding

Can I receive Micro-K if I am pregnant or breastfeeding?

The effects of Micro-K during pregnancy are unknown. Tell your doctor immediately if you are pregnant or plan to become pregnant.

If taken during breastfeeding to correct a low potassium level, Micro-K should have little to no effect on the natural potassium level in breast milk.

What should I do if I miss a dose of Micro-K?

If you miss a dose of Micro-K, take it as soon as you remember. If it is almost time for your next dose, skip the dose you missed and return to your normal dosing schedule. Do not double your next dose.

How should I store Micro-K?

Micro-K should be stored at room temperature.

MICRONASE
Generic name: Glyburide

What is Micronase?

Micronase is an oral antidiabetic medication used to treat type 2 diabetes, which occurs when the body either does not make enough insulin or fails to use insulin properly. Insulin transfers sugar from the bloodstream to the body's cells, where it is then used for energy.

There are two forms of diabetes: type 1 and type 2. Type 1 diabetes results from a complete shutdown of normal insulin production and usually requires insulin injections for life, while type 2 diabetes can usually be treated by dietary changes, exercise, and/or oral antidiabetic medications such as Micronase. This medication controls diabetes by stimulating the pancreas to produce more insulin and by helping insulin to work better.

Micronase can be used alone or along with a drug called metformin, if diet plus either drug alone fails to control sugar levels.

What is the most important information I should know about Micronase?

Always remember that Micronase is an aid to, not a substitute for, good diet and exercise. Failure to follow a sound diet and exercise plan can lead to serious complications, such as dangerously high or low blood sugar levels. It is very important for you to monitor your blood sugar regularly and inform your doctor of any changes. Remember, too, that Micronase is *not* an oral form of insulin, and cannot be used in place of insulin.

A recent study showed that treatment with Micronase may increase the risk of heart-related death in patients treated with blood sugar-lowering medications over an extended period of time.

Who should not take Micronase?

You should not take Micronase if you have had an allergic reaction to it or to similar drugs. Also, do not take Micronase if you have type 1 diabetes mellitus and are taking Micronase as your only means of sugar control.

Micronase should not be taken if you are suffering from diabetic ketoacidosis (a life-threatening medical emergency caused by insufficient insulin and marked by excessive thirst, nausea, fatigue, pain below the breastbone, and fruity breath).

What should I tell my doctor before I take the first dose of Micronase?

Tell your doctor about all prescription, over-the-counter, and herbal medication you are taking before beginning treatment with Micronase. Also, talk to your doctor about your complete medical history, especially if you have liver or kidney impairment or disease, don't eat a sufficient amount of calories, exercise excessively, have impaired adrenal or pituitary gland function, or drink alcohol.

What is the usual dosage?

The information below is based on the dosage guidelines your doctor uses. Depending on your condition and medical history, your doctor may prescribe a different regimen. Do not change the dosage or stop taking your medication without your doctor's approval.

Adults: The usual starting dose is 2.5-5 milligrams (mg) taken once daily with breakfast or the first eaten meal. If you are sensitive to drugs that lower blood sugar your doctor may start you on 1.25mg once daily therapy.

Your doctor may increase your individual dose depending on if you are also using insulin or you have taken other oral blood sugar lowering medications. Daily doses greater than 20 milligrams are not recommended.

How should I take Micronase?

Micronase should be taken at the same time every day in the morning with breakfast or with the first meal eaten.

What should I avoid while taking Micronase?

You should avoid drinking alcohol, not eating enough, and exercising excessively.

What are possible food and drug interactions associated with Micronase?

If Micronase is taken with certain other drugs, the effects of either could be increased, decreased, or altered. It is especially important to check with your doctor before combining Micronase with the following: beta-blockers such as the blood pressure medications atenolol and propranolol; blood thinners such as warfarin; calcium channel blockers such as the blood pressure medications diltiazem and nifedipine; certain antibiotics such as ciprofloxacin; chloramphenicol; corticosteroids; estrogens; isoniazid; MAO inhibitors such as the antidepressants phenelzine and tranylcypromine; miconazole; nicotinic acid; nonsteroidal anti-inflammatory drugs such as ibuprofen and naproxen; oral contraceptives; phenothiazines; phenytoin; probenecid; salicylates; sulfonamides; sympathomimetics; thiazide-type diuretics and other diuretics; and thyroid medications.

What are the possible side effects of Micronase?

Side effects cannot be anticipated. If any develop or change in intensity, tell your doctor as soon as possible. Only your doctor can determine if it is safe for you to continue taking this drug.

Side effects may include: allergic reactions, arthritic pain, blistering and irritation of the skin, bloating, heartburn, increased sensitivity to sunlight, itchy skin, low blood sodium levels, low blood sugar, lowering of the number of cells in your blood, nausea, rash

Micronase, like all oral antidiabetics, may cause hypoglycemia (low blood sugar). Signs and symptoms of low blood sugar include dizziness, shakiness, tremor, or light-headedness. The signs of low blood sugar may be hard to recognize if you are elderly or you are taking a medication known as a beta-adrenergic antagonist. Eating sugar or a sugar-based product will often correct mild hypoglycemia. Severe hypoglycemia should be considered a medical emergency, and prompt medical attention is essential.

Can I receive Micronase if I am pregnant or breastfeeding?
The effects of Micronase during pregnancy are unknown. If you remain on Micronase during your pregnancy, you should stop taking Micronase at least 2 weeks before your expected date of delivery.

Tell your doctor immediately if you are pregnant, plan to become pregnant, or are breastfeeding. Drugs similar to Micronase are excreted in breast milk, therefore, discuss with your doctor whether to discontinue breastfeeding or Micronase therapy.

What should I do if I miss a dose of Micronase?
If you miss a dose of Micronase, skip the missed dose and return to your normal dosing schedule. Do not double your next dose.

How should I store Micronase?
Micronase should be stored at room temperature, in a tightly closed container.

MIDRIN
Generic name: Isometheptene mucate, dichloralphenazone, and acetaminophen

What is Midrin?
Midrin is prescribed for the treatment of tension headaches. It is also used to treat vascular headaches such as migraine.

What is the most important information I should know about Midrin?
Midrin can be used only after the headache starts. It does not prevent headaches.

Take Midrin cautiously if you have high blood pressure or any abnormal condition of the blood vessels outside of the heart, or have recently had a cardiovascular attack such as a heart attack or stroke.

Who should not take Midrin?

Unless directed to do so by your doctor, do not take Midrin if you have the eye condition called glaucoma or severe kidney disease, high blood pressure, a physical defect of the heart, or liver disease, or if you are currently taking antidepressant drugs known as MAO inhibitors, including phenelzine and tranylcypromine.

What should I tell my doctor before I take the first dose of Midrin?

Tell your doctor about all prescription, over-the-counter, and herbal medications you are taking before beginning treatment with this drug. Also, talk to your doctor about your complete medical history, especially if you have heart disease, high blood pressure, or have ever had a stroke or heart attack.

What is the usual dosage?

The information below is based on the dosage guidelines your doctor uses. Depending on your condition and medical history, your doctor may prescribe a different regimen. Do not change the dosage or stop taking your medication without your doctor's approval.

Relief of Migraine Headache
Adults: The usual dosage is 2 capsules at once, followed by 1 capsule every hour until the headache is relieved; do not take more than 5 capsules within a 12-hour period.

Relief of Tension Headache
Adults: The usual dosage is 1 or 2 capsules every 4 hours up to a maximum of 8 capsules a day.

How should I take Midrin?

Take this medication exactly as prescribed by your doctor. You should start taking Midrin at the first sign of a migraine attack. Do not take more than the maximum dose of Midrin.

What should I avoid while taking Midrin?

Avoid alcoholic beverages.

What are possible food and drug interactions associated with Midrin?

If Midrin is taken with certain other drugs, the effects of either drug could be increased, decreased, or altered. It is especially important to check with your doctor before combining Midrin with the following: acetaminophen-containing pain relievers, antidepressants classified as MAO inhibitors including phenelzine and tranylcypromine, antihistamines such as diphenhydramine, and central nervous system depressants such as alprazolam, diazepam, and triazolam.

What are the possible side effects of Midrin?

Side effects cannot be anticipated. If any develop or change in intensity, tell your doctor as soon as possible. Only your doctor can determine if it is safe for you to continue taking this drug.

Side effects may include: short periods of dizziness, skin rash

Can I receive Midrin if I am pregnant or breastfeeding?

If you are pregnant, plan to become pregnant, or are breastfeeding, check with your doctor before taking Midrin.

What should I do if I miss a dose of Midrin?

Take this medication only as needed.

How should I store Midrin?

Store at room temperature in a dry place.

Miglitol See Glyset, page 630.

MINIPRESS

Generic name: Prazosin hydrochloride

What is Minipress?

Minipress is a prescription medication that lowers blood pressure in patients with high blood pressure. Minipress can be taken alone or along with other blood pressure-lowering medications.

What is the most important information I should know about Minipress?

If you have high blood pressure, you must take Minipress regularly for it to be effective. Since blood pressure declines gradually, it may be several weeks before you get the full benefit of Minipress; and you must continue taking it even if you are feeling well. Minipress does not cure high blood pressure; it merely keeps it under control.

Minipress may cause fainting and/or rapid heart rate with a sudden loss of consciousness. Your chances of experiencing loss of consciousness are increased if you are also taking other medications for high blood pressure. This side effect can be minimized by taking a low initial dose and slowly increasing your dose to allow your body to become accustomed to Minipress. Commonly, dizziness, drowsiness, or fainting can occur after taking the first dose, especially when rising from a lying or sitting position. If you drink alcohol, are exposed to a hot environment, or are standing for a long time, your chances of experiencing these side effects with the first dose are increased.

Who should not take Minipress?

You should not take Minipress if you are allergic or sensitive to Minipress or any of its ingredients. You should also not take Minipress if you are allergic to a type of medication known as a quinazoline.

What should I tell my doctor before I take the first dose of Minipress?

Tell your doctor about all prescription, over-the-counter, and herbal medication you are taking before beginning treatment with Minipress. Also, talk to your doctor about your complete medical history, especially if you are taking other medications used to treat high blood pressure.

What is the usual dosage?

The information below is based on the dosage guidelines your doctor uses. Depending on your condition and medical history, your doctor may prescribe a different regimen. Do not change the dosage or stop taking your medication without your doctor's approval.

Adults: The usual starting dose is 1 milligram (mg) taken 2 or 3 times daily. Your doctor may slowly increase your individual dose up to 20mg, taken in divided doses, based on your condition.

How should I take Minipress?

Minipress should be taken at the same time every day and may be taken with or without food.

What should I avoid while taking Minipress?

You should avoid excessive exposure to hot environments, standing for prolonged periods of time, becoming dehydrated, and drinking alcohol.

What are possible food and drug interactions associated with Minipress?

If Minipress is taken with certain other drugs, the effects of either could be increased, decreased, or altered. It is especially important to check with your doctor before combining Minipress with the following: diuretics ("water pills") or other medications used to treat high blood pressure such as propranolol.

What are the possible side effects of Minipress?

Side effects cannot be anticipated. If any develop or change in intensity, tell your doctor as soon as possible. Only your doctor can determine if it is safe for you to continue taking this drug.

Side effects may include: Dizziness, drowsiness, headache, irregular heartbeats, lack of energy, nausea, weakness

Can I receive Minipress if I am pregnant or breastfeeding?

The effects of Minipress during pregnancy are unknown. Tell your doctor immediately if you are pregnant, plan to become pregnant, or are breastfeeding. Minipress has been shown to be excreted in breast milk, so you should talk to your doctor about taking this medication if you are breastfeeding.

What should I do if I miss a dose of Minipress?

Take it as soon as you remember. If it is almost time for your next dose, then skip the dose you missed and take your next regular dose. Do not double your dose.

How should I store Minipress?

Minipress should be stored at room temperature away from light.

MINOCIN
Generic name: Minocycline hydrochloride

What is Minocin?

Minocin is a tetracycline-class antibiotic medicine. It is used to treat many kinds of bacterial infections, including: acne; amebic dysentery; anthrax (when penicillin cannot be used); cholera; gonorrhea (when penicillin cannot be used); plague; respiratory infections such as pneumonia; Rocky Mountain spotted fever; syphilis (when penicillin cannot be used); and urinary tract infections, rectal infections, and infections of the cervix caused by certain microbes.

What is the most important information I should know about Minocin?

Minocin may lead to permanent discoloration of the teeth if it is taken during early tooth development. Minocin should not be given to children under 8 years of age.

Minocin should not be taken by women who are pregnant or breastfeeding.

Unless otherwise directed by your doctor, you should take the entire prescribed therapy of Minocin. Do not stop taking Minocin even if you feel better or the signs/symptoms of your infection are clearing.

Who should not take Minocin?

You should not take Minocin if you are allergic to Minocin or other tetracycline antibiotics.

Do not take Minocin if you are pregnant or breastfeeding.

What should I tell my doctor before I take the first dose of Minocin?

Tell your doctor about all prescription, over-the-counter, and herbal medication you are taking before beginning treatment with Minocin. Also, talk to your doctor about your complete medical history, especially if you have kidney or liver problems, are pregnant, plan to become pregnant, or are breastfeeding.

What is the usual dosage?

The information below is based on the dosage guidelines your doctor uses. Depending on your condition and medical history, your doctor may prescribe a different regimen. Do not change the dosage or stop taking your medication without your doctor's approval.

Adults: The usual dosage of Minocin is 200 milligrams (mg) to start with, followed by 100 mg every 12 hours. If more frequent doses are necessary, two or four 50-mg capsules may be taken initially, followed by one 50 mg capsule 4 times daily.

The dosage and the length of time you take the drug can vary according to your condition and the specific infection.

Children over 8 years old: The usual dose is 4 mg per 2.2 pounds of body weight, followed by 2 mg per 2.2 pounds of body weight every 12 hours, not to exceed the usual adult dose.

How should I take Minocin?

You should take Minocin at least 1 hour before meals or 2 hours after meals. The extended-release form should be taken with food. To reduce throat irritation, take Minocin with plenty of fluids.

Take Minocin exactly as your doctor tells you to take it. Skipping doses or not taking all your Minocin may decrease the effectiveness of Minocin or increase the chance that bacteria will develop resistance to Minocin.

What should I avoid while taking Minocin?

You should avoid becoming pregnant or breastfeeding; taking antacids that contain aluminum, calcium, or magnesium; iron-containing products; and excessive exposure to sunlight.

What are possible food and drug interactions associated with Minocin?

If Minocin is taken with certain other drugs, the effects of either could be increased, decreased, or altered. It is especially important to check with your doctor before combining Minocin with the following: an acne medicine called isotretinoin; antacids that contain aluminum, calcium, or magnesium; blood-thinning medications; iron-containing products such as ferrous sulfate; methoxyflurane; migraine medicines called ergot alkaloids; oral birth control pills; and penicillin antibiotic medicines.

What are the possible side effects of Minocin?

Side effects cannot be anticipated. If any develop or change in intensity, tell your doctor as soon as possible. Only your doctor can determine if it is safe for you to continue taking this drug.

Side effects may include: bloody stools, blurred vision, diarrhea, dizziness, headaches, joint pain, light-headedness, rash, stomach cramps, sun sensitivity, tiredness

Can I receive Minocin if I am pregnant or breastfeeding?

Minocin should not be taken if you are pregnant, plan to become pregnant, or if you are breastfeeding. Minocin may cause harm to an unborn infant or developing child under the age of 8.

Tetracycline drugs, like Minocin, are excreted in breast milk. Your doctor may tell you to stop breastfeeding if Minocin is essential to your health.

What should I do if I miss a dose of Minocin?

Take it as soon as you remember, then evenly space out any remaining doses for that day. Never take 2 doses at the same time.

How should I store Minocin?

Minocin should be kept at room temperature, away from excessive heat, light, and moisture.

Minocycline hydrochloride *See Dynacin, page 458, or Minocin, page 832.*

MIRALAX

Generic name: Polyethylene glycol

What is MiraLax?

MiraLax is used to relieve constipation. It works by retaining water in the stool, softening it and increasing the frequency of bowel movements. It may take up to 2 to 4 days to work.

What is the most important information I should know about MiraLax?

Unless your doctor directs otherwise, do not use MiraLax for more than 2 weeks.

Who should not take MiraLax?

Do not take MiraLax if there's any chance that you have a bowel obstruction. Symptoms suggesting an obstruction include abdominal pain or distention, nausea, and vomiting.

Also avoid MiraLax if you are allergic to the active ingredient, polyethylene glycol.

What should I tell my doctor before I take the first dose of MiraLax?
Tell your doctor about all prescription, over-the-counter, and herbal medications you are taking before beginning treatment with this drug. Also talk to your doctor about your complete medical history, especially if you have kidney problems, abdominal pain, or nausea and vomiting.

What is the usual dosage?
The information below is based on the dosage guidelines your doctor uses. Depending on your condition and medical history, your doctor may prescribe a different regimen. Do not change the dosage or stop taking your medication without your doctor's approval.

Adults and adolescents 17 years and older: The usual dose is 17 grams daily.

How should I take MiraLax?
Dissolve 1 capful or packet of MiraLax powder (17 grams) in 8 ounces of water, juice, soda, coffee, or tea. To promote regularity, make sure your diet includes plenty of fiber and fluids, and get regular exercise.

What should I avoid while taking MiraLax?
Remember that MiraLax is not for prolonged use.

What are possible food and drug interactions associated with MiraLax?
No interactions have been reported.

What are the possible side effects of MiraLax?
Side effects cannot be anticipated. If any develop or change in intensity, tell your doctor as soon as possible. Only your doctor can determine if it is safe for you to continue taking this drug.

Side effects may include: bloating, cramps, gas, nausea; diarrhea and excessive frequency with high doses

Can I receive MiraLax if I am pregnant or breastfeeding?
Nothing is known about the effects of MiraLax during pregnancy. If you are pregnant or plan to become pregnant, inform your doctor immediately. MiraLax should be used only if clearly needed. There is no information on the use of MiraLax while nursing. Check with your doctor if you plan to breastfeed.

What should I do if I miss a dose of MiraLax?
Take the forgotten dose as soon as you remember. However, if it is almost time for your next dose, skip the one you missed and return to your regular schedule. Do not take two doses at once.

How should I store MiraLax?
Store at room temperature.

MIRAPEX
Generic name: Pramipexole dihydrochloride

What is Mirapex?
Mirapex is used to treat the signs and symptoms of Parkinson's disease—a progressive disorder marked by muscle rigidity, weakness, shaking, tremor, and eventually difficulty walking and talking.

Mirapex is also used for moderate-to-severe primary Restless Leg Syndrome (RLS). RLS is an urge to move the legs usually accompanied or caused by uncomfortable and unpleasant leg sensations; symptoms begin or worsen during periods of rest or inactivity such as lying or sitting; symptoms are partially or totally relieved by movement such as walking or stretching at least as long as the activity continues; and symptoms are worse or occur only in the evening or night. Difficulty falling asleep may frequently be associated with symptoms of RLS.

What is the most important information I should know about Mirapex?
Mirapex may cause severe drowsiness or tiredness, which may cause you to fall asleep during your daily activities. Some people who have taken Mirapex have had car accidents because they fell asleep while driving. Although many of these patients reported drowsiness while on Mirapex tablets, some perceived that they had no warning signs such as excessive drowsiness, and believed that they were alert immediately prior to the event. Some of these events had been reported as late as one year after the initiation of treatment. You should not drive a car or engage in activities that require mental alertness until you know how Mirapex will affect you.

Certain medications that may also cause drowsiness or that increase the Mirapex levels in your body greatly increase your chances of experiencing sedation or spontaneously falling asleep. Report any new onset or worsening of the symptoms to your doctor immediately.

Who should not take Mirapex?
You should not take Mirapex if you are allergic or sensitive to pramipexole or any other ingredient in the medication.

What should I tell my doctor before I take the first dose of Mirapex?

Tell your doctor about all prescription, over-the-counter, and herbal medication you are taking before beginning treatment with Mirapex. Also, talk to your doctor about your complete medical history, especially if you have low blood pressure, kidney problems, or trouble controlling your muscles. Let your doctor know if you feel sleepy during the day due to any other problem aside from RLS or if you feel dizzy or faint, especially after standing from a sitting or lying down position. You should also talk be sure to tell your doctor if you are pregnant or plan to become pregnant, are breastfeeding, or if you drink alcohol.

What is the usual dosage?

The information below is based on the dosage guidelines your doctor uses. Depending on your condition and medical history, your doctor may prescribe a different regimen. Do not change the dosage or stop taking your medication without your doctor's approval.

Parkinson's Disease

Adults: For the initial treatment of Parkinson's disease, Dosages should be increased gradually from a starting dose of 0.375 milligrams (mg) per day given in three divided doses and should not be increased more frequently than every 5 to 7 days. The typical ascending dosage schedule is: week 1, 0.375 mg/day; week 2, 0.75 mg/day; week 3, 1.5 mg/day; week 4, 2.25 mg/day; week 5, 3 mg/day; week 6, 3.75 mg/day; week 7, 4.5 mg/day.

The maintenance dose of Mirapex for Parkinson's disease is 0.5-1.5 mg, 3 times per day.

Restless Leg Syndrome

Adults: The usual starting dose of Mirapex for RLS is 0.125 milligrams (mg) taken once daily 2-3 hours before bedtime. Your doctor may increase your individual dose every 4-7 days up to a maximum of 0.5 mg per day based on your individual condition.

How should I take Mirapex?

Mirapex should be taken exactly as prescribed and should be taken at the same time every day. Mirapex can be taken with or without food, however taking it with food may lower your chances of experiencing nausea. You should not suddenly stop taking Mirapex without first talking to your doctor. If you have Parkinson's disease and are stopping Mirapex you should slowly decrease your dose over 7 days before stopping all together.

What should I avoid while taking Mirapex?

You should not drive a car, operate machinery, or do anything that requires mental alertness until you know how Mirapex affects you. You should not drink alcohol while taking Mirapex.

What are possible food and drug interactions associated with Mirapex?

If Mirapex is taken with certain other drugs, the effects of either could be increased, decreased, or altered. It is especially important to check with your doctor before combining Mirapex with the following: amantadine; carbidopa/levodopa; cimetidine; tranquilizers or sedatives that belong to classes of medications known as phenothiazines, butyrophenones, or thioxanthenes; diltiazem; metoclopramide; quinidine; quinine; ranitidine; triamterene; and verapamil.

What are the possible side effects of Mirapex?

Side effects cannot be anticipated. If any develop or change in intensity, tell your doctor as soon as possible. Only your doctor can determine if it is safe for you to continue taking this drug.

Side effects may include: arthritis, body discomfort or fatigue, chest pain, constipation, dizziness, drowsiness or sleepiness, dry mouth, hallucinations (your chances are greater of experiencing hallucinations if you are over 65 years old), insomnia, low blood pressure when you sit or stand, nausea, swelling of the lower limbs, vision abnormalities, weakness

Can I receive Mirapex if I am pregnant or breastfeeding?

The effects of Mirapex during pregnancy and breastfeeding are unknown. Tell your doctor immediately if you are pregnant, plan to become pregnant, or are breastfeeding.

What should I do if I miss a dose of Mirapex?

If you miss a dose of Mirapex, take it as soon as you remember. If it is almost time for your next dose, skip the dose you missed and take your next regular dose. Do not double your next dose.

How should I store Mirapex?

Store Mirapex at room temperature, away from light and heat. Keep away from children.

Mirtazapine See Remeron, page 1132.

Misoprostol See Cytotec, page 371.

MOBAN

Generic name: Molindone hydrochloride

What is Moban?

Moban is used to treat the symptoms of schizophrenia.

What is the most important information I should know about Moban?

Moban can cause tardive dyskinesia, a serious sometimes irreversible movement disorder that causes involuntary movements of muscles. The risk for tardive dyskinesia is higher in the elderly and for women. Tell your doctor immediately if you experience any involuntary muscle movements while taking Moban.

Moban can also cause another serious, sometime fatal, disorder known as neuroleptic malignant syndrome, characterized by muscle stiffness, increased body temperature, sweating, changes in mood or consciousness, and a rapid or irregular heartbeat. If you experience any of these symptoms while taking Moban, seek emergency medical attention immediately.

Moban is not to be used with other agents that cause central nervous system depression, such as alcohol, barbiturates, or narcotic pain killers.

Moban should not be used in elderly patients with dementia-related psychosis, since this puts them at an increased risk of serious side effects, including death.

Who should not take Moban?

Do not take Moban if you are allergic to molindone or any other ingredient in Moban.

Moban should not be administered to anyone in a comatose state.

Elderly patients with dementia-related psychosis should not receive Moban due to an increased risk of death.

What should I tell my doctor before I take the first dose of Moban?

Tell your doctor about all prescription, over-the-counter, and herbal medication you are taking before beginning treatment with Moban. Also, talk to your doctor about your complete medical history, especially if you have a history of tardive dyskinesia, neuroleptic malignant syndrome, or have been previously diagnosed with breast cancer.

What is the usual dosage?

The information below is based on the dosage guidelines your doctor uses. Depending on your condition and medical history, your doctor may prescribe a different regimen. Do not change the dosage or stop taking your medication without your doctor's approval.

Adults and children 12 years and older: The usual starting dose is 50 milligrams (mg) to 75 mg per day. Your doctor may increase your dose to 100 mg after 3-4 days of treatment. Based on your individual condition, your dose may be further increased up to 225 mg per day. The dose is usually divided in three to four intervals.

How should I take Moban?
Moban can be taken with or without food. It should be taken at the same time every day.

What should I avoid while taking Moban?
You should not drink alcohol while taking Moban. Moban may cause you to feel drowsy, so you should not operate an automobile or heavy machinery until you know how this medication will affect you. Exercise caution when participating in activities that require alertness.

What are possible food and drug interactions associated with Moban?
If Moban is taken with certain other drugs, the effects of either could be increased, decreased, or altered. It is especially important to check with your doctor before combining Moban with alcohol, barbiturates, and narcotic medications.

Also, be aware that Moban tablets contain calcium, which may interfere with the absorption of tetracycline medications and phenytoin.

What are the possible side effects of Moban?
Side effects cannot be anticipated. If any develop or change in intensity, tell your doctor as soon as possible. Only your doctor can determine if it is safe for you to continue taking this drug.

Side effects may include: dizziness, drowsiness, immobility, involuntary muscle contractions, involuntary muscle movements, muscle restlessness, muscle stiffness, muscle tremors

Can I receive Moban if I am pregnant or breastfeeding?
The effects of Moban during pregnancy and breastfeeding are unknown. Tell your doctor immediately if you are pregnant, plan to become pregnant, or are breastfeeding.

What should I do if I miss a dose of Moban?
If you miss a dose, take it as soon as you remember. If it is almost time for your next dose, skip the dose you missed and take your next regular dose. Do not double your dose to make up for a missed dose.

How should I store Moban?
Store at room temperature in a tightly closed container and away from light.

MOBIC

Generic name: Meloxicam

What is Mobic?

Mobic is a nonsteroidal anti-inflammatory drug, or NSAID, and can reduce inflammation, redness, and pain associated with conditions such as osteoarthritis, rheumatoid arthritis, or Juvenile Rheumatoid Arthritis. Mobic may also be used to treat other types of short-term pain.

What is the most important information I should know about Mobic?

NSAIDs such as Mobic may increase the risk of a heart attack or stroke, which can lead to death. This chance increases if you have taken an NSAID for a long time or if you have heart disease. NSAIDs should never be taken right before or after a heart surgery called a "coronary artery bypass graft" or CABG.

NSAIDs can cause ulcers and bleeding in the stomach and intestines at any time during treatment. The ulcers and bleeding can happen without warning and may cause death. The chance of you getting an ulcer or bleeding increases if you are taking other medications called corticosteroids, anticoagulants (blood thinners), or aspirin; taking NSAIDS for a long time; are a smoker, drink alcohol, are older in age, or in poor health. Signs and symptoms of an ulcer or bleeding include black tarry stools, gnawing or sharp stomach pains, or vomiting. If you experience any of these symptoms, stop taking Mobic and tell your doctor immediately.

Mobic may potentially cause damage to your liver. Some of the warning signs of liver damage can be nausea, vomiting, fatigue, loss of appetite, itching, yellow coloring of skin or eyes, flu-like symptoms, and dark urine. If you experience any of these symptoms, call your doctor right away.

Rarely, Mobic can cause serious and even fatal skin reactions. If you develop any type of rash, fever, blisters, or skin itchiness, you should tell your doctor right away.

Mobic may cause your body to retain water, so you should use caution if you have heart failure, any type of kidney disease, or if you already retain too much water. You should only take NSAIDs exactly as your doctor tells you, at the lowest dose possible for your treatment, and for the shortest time needed. Your blood pressure may increase at any time while taking Mobic, so your doctor may want to monitor it.

Who should not take Mobic?

Do not take Mobic if you've had an asthma attack, hives, or other allergic reaction with aspirin or any other NSAID. You should not take Mobic to treat pain right before or after heart bypass surgery (CABG).

What should I tell my doctor before I take the first dose of Mobic?

Tell your doctor about all prescription, over-the-counter, and herbal medications you are taking before beginning treatment with Mobic. Also, talk to your doctor about your complete medical history, especially if you are pregnant or breastfeeding. NSAIDs such as Mobic should not be taken by pregnant women late in their pregnancy.

What is the usual dosage?

The information below is based on the dosage guidelines your doctor uses. Depending on your condition and medical history, your doctor may prescribe a different regimen. Do not change the dosage or stop taking your medication without your doctor's approval.

Osteoarthritis and Rheumatoid Arthritis

Adults: The recommended starting and maintenance dose taken for the relief of the signs and symptoms of osteoarthritis and rheumatoid arthritis is 7.5 milligrams (mg) once daily. Your doctor may prescribe 15 mg per day depending on your individual condition.

Pauciarticular and Polyarticular Course Juvenile Rheumatoid Arthritis

Children: The usual dose is given using the Mobic oral suspension (liquid) and ranges from 1.5-7.5 mg per day, based on the child's weight.

How should I take Mobic?

Mobic should be taken as directed at the same time every day, and can be taken with or without food. Shake the liquid well before using.

What should I avoid while taking Mobic?

You should not take any other NSAID medicine while taking Mobic. Common over-the-counter NSAIDS include Motrin (ibuprofen) and Aleve (naproxen), as well as many combination products that may contain these medicines.

What are possible food and drug interactions associated with Mobic?

If Mobic is taken with certain other drugs, the effects of either could be increased, decreased, or altered. It is especially important to check with your doctor before combining Mobic with the following: angiotensin converting enzyme (ACE) inhibitors, aspirin, cholestyramine, furosemide, lithium, methotrexate, warfarin, and other prescription NSAIDs such as celecoxib, diclofenac, and diflunisal.

What are the possible side effects of Mobic?

Side effects cannot be anticipated. If any develop or change in intensity, tell your doctor as soon as possible. Only your doctor can determine if it is safe for you to continue taking this drug.

Serious side effects may include: heart attack, stroke, high blood pressure, heart failure from body swelling (fluid retention), kidney problems including kidney failure, bleeding and ulcers in the stomach and intestine, low red blood cells (anemia), life-threatening skin reactions, life-threatening allergic reactions, liver problems including liver failure, asthma attacks in people who have asthma

Other side effects include: stomach pain, acid reflux, diarrhea, nausea, gas, flu like symptoms, dizziness, rash, upper respiratory tract infection

Can I receive Mobic if I am pregnant or breastfeeding?

Mobic is a pregnancy category C medication. This means Mobic has not been adequately tested on pregnant women. You should not take Mobic during pregnancy unless your doctor instructs you to and is aware that you are pregnant. It is not known whether Mobic is excreted in breast milk. Tell your doctor immediately if you are pregnant, plan to become pregnant, or are breastfeeding.

What should I do if I miss a dose of Mobic?

You can take your missed dose as soon as you remember if there are more than 12 hours remaining until your next scheduled dose. If you are within 12 hours of your next dose, skip the missed dose and return to your normal dosing schedule.

You should not double your dose of Mobic.

How should I store Mobic?

Store at room temperature away from heat and light.

Modafinil See *Provigil, page 1101.*

Moexipril hydrochloride See *Univasc, page 1357.*

Moexipril hydrochloride and hydrochlorothiazide
See *Uniretic, page 1354.*

Molindone hydrochloride See *Moban, page 838.*

Mometasone furoate See *Elocon, page 477.*

Mometasone furoate inhalation powder See *Asmanex Twisthaler, page 132.*

Mometasone furoate monohydrate See *Nasonex, page 865.*

MONOPRIL
Generic name: Fosinopril sodium

What is Monopril?
Monopril is a type of blood pressure-lowering medication known as an ACE inhibitor. It stops a chemical in your blood called angiotensin I from becoming a more powerful chemical that raises your blood pressure by making your blood vessels narrower and causing your body to retain salt and water. Monopril is used to lower your blood pressure when taken alone or in combination with other medications.

Monopril is also prescribed to help manage heart failure in combination with conventional therapy, including diuretics with or without digitalis.

What is the most important information I should know about Monopril?
If taken during the second or third trimester of pregnancy, Monopril can cause serious harm or even death to an unborn baby. If you become pregnant while taking Monopril, you should stop taking Monopril immediately and tell your doctor right away.

Monopril can cause a rare but serious allergic reaction leading to extreme swelling of the face, lips, tongue, throat, or gut (causing severe abdominal pain). If you experience any of these symptoms you should seek emergency medical attention right away.

Make sure your doctor knows if you have any type of liver impairment or injury. Monopril may rarely cause a yellowing of the skin or eyes, which can be a sign of liver injury. If this occurs tell your doctor immediately.

Monopril may cause lightheadedness or fainting, especially upon standing from a lying or sitting position. If you get any type of infection (sore throat/fever) while taking Monopril you should promptly report it to your doctor. Monopril may decrease your blood levels of infection fighting white blood cells, especially if you have systemic lupus erythematosus or kidney disease. If you have these diseases your doctor will most likely monitor you closely by taking regular blood samples.

Monopril should be taken with caution in patients who have congestive heart failure or kidney disease.

Who should not take Monopril?
You should not take Monopril if you have had a previous allergic reaction or are sensitive to Monopril or any other ACE inhibitor.

What should I tell my doctor before I take the first dose of Monopril?
Tell your doctor about all prescription, over-the-counter, and herbal medications you are taking before beginning treatment with Monopril. Also,

talk to your doctor about your complete medical history, especially if you are pregnant or plan on becoming pregnant, have congestive heart failure, liver or kidney disease, or if you have ever had an allergy or sensitivity to an ACE inhibitor such as Monopril.

What is the usual dosage?
The information below is based on the dosage guidelines your doctor uses. Depending on your condition and medical history, your doctor may prescribe a different regimen. Do not change the dosage or stop taking your medication without your doctor's approval.

Hypertension
Adults: The usual initial dose is 10 milligrams (mg) taken once daily. The usual maintenance dose is 20-40mg taken once daily, however your doctor may increase your individual dosage up to 80mg taken once daily based on your condition.

Children: The usual dosage for children weighing more than 110 pounds (50kg) is 5 to 10mg taken once daily. An appropriate dosage strength is not available for children weighing less than 110 pounds.

Heart Failure
Adults: The usual initial dose is 10 milligrams (mg) taken once daily. Your doctor will likely observe you at this dose and may increase your daily dose over several weeks up to 20-40mg taken once daily.

How should I take Monopril?
Monopril can be taken with or without food and should be taken at the same time every day.

What should I avoid while taking Monopril?
You should avoid operating automobiles or heavy machinery until you know how Monopril will affect you. You should avoid becoming dehydrated and drink adequate fluids while taking Monopril, because dehydration could cause your blood pressure to drop too low. You should not take salt substitutes or supplements containing potassium unless otherwise directed by your doctor. Separate taking an antacid with Monopril by at least 2 hours.

What are possible food and drug interactions associated with Monopril?
If Monopril is taken with certain other drugs, the effects of either could be increased, decreased, or altered. It is especially important to check with your doctor before combining Monopril with the following: antacids; diuretics; injectable gold products; lithium; potassium-sparing diuretics such as spironolactone, amiloride and triamterene; potassium supplements; salt substitutes containing potassium.

What are the possible side effects of Monopril?

Side effects cannot be anticipated. If any develop or change in intensity, tell your doctor as soon as possible. Only your doctor can determine if it is safe for you to continue taking this drug.

Side effects may include: dizziness, cough, low blood pressure, muscle pain, nausea or vomiting, diarrhea, chest pain, or upper airway infection.

Can I receive Monopril if I am pregnant or breastfeeding?

Monopril should not be taken during pregnancy. Taking Monopril while you are pregnant could cause serious harm or even death to your unborn baby. Tell your doctor immediately if you are pregnant, plan to become pregnant, or are breastfeeding. Monopril is excreted in breast milk, and should not be taken if you are breastfeeding.

What should I do if I miss a dose of Monopril?

If you forget to take Monopril, do not double your next dose. Skip the dose you missed and then return to your normal dosing schedule.

How should I store Monopril?

Store Monopril at room temperature in a tightly closed container and protect from moisture.

MONOPRIL HCT

Generic name: Fosinopril sodium and hydrochlorothiazide

What is Monopril HCT?

Monopril HCT is a combination of two blood pressure-lowering medication classes known as ACE inhibitors and diuretics. ACE inhibitors stop a chemical in your blood called angiotensin I from becoming a more powerful chemical that raises your blood pressure by making your blood vessels narrower and causing your body to retain salt and water. Diuretics help remove excess fluids from your body.

What is the most important information I should know about Monopril HCT?

If taken during the second or third trimester of pregnancy, Monopril HCT can cause serious harm or even death to an unborn baby. If you become pregnant while taking Monopril HCT, you should stop taking Monopril HCT immediately and tell your doctor right away.

Monopril HCT should not be used as the initial blood pressure lowering therapy; it should be used after another blood pressure lowering medication has been tried.

Monopril HCT can cause a rare but serious allergic reaction leading to extreme swelling of the face, lips, tongue, throat, or gut (causing severe abdominal pain). If you experience any of these symptoms you should seek emergency medical attention right away.

Make sure your doctor knows if you have any type of liver impairment or injury. Monopril HCT may rarely cause a yellowing of the skin or eyes, which can be a sign of liver injury. If this occurs tell your doctor immediately.

Monopril HCT may cause lightheadedness or fainting, especially upon standing from a lying or sitting position. If you get any type of infection (sore throat/fever) while taking Monopril HCT you should promptly report it to your doctor. Monopril HCT may decrease your blood levels of infection fighting white blood cells, especially if you have systemic lupus erythematosus or kidney disease. If you have these diseases your doctor will most likely monitor you closely by taking regular blood samples.

Monopril HCT should be taken with caution in patients who have congestive heart failure or kidney disease.

Who should not take Monopril HCT?
You should not take Monopril HCT if you have had a previous allergic reaction or are sensitive to Monopril, any other ACE inhibitor, hydrochlorothiazide, any sulfonamide derived drugs, or any other ingredient in this medication.

You should also not take Monopril HCT if you are having problems urinating.

What should I tell my doctor before I take the first dose of Monopril HCT?
Tell your doctor about all prescription, over-the-counter, and herbal medications you are taking before beginning treatment with Monopril HCT. Also, talk to your doctor about your complete medical history, especially if you are pregnant or plan on becoming pregnant, have congestive heart failure, liver or kidney disease, or if you have ever had an allergy or sensitivity to an ACE inhibitor such as Monopril or a diuretic such as hydrochlorothiazide.

What is the usual dosage?
The information below is based on the dosage guidelines your doctor uses. Depending on your condition and medical history, your doctor may prescribe a different regimen. Do not change the dosage or stop taking your medication without your doctor's approval.

Hypertension
Adults: The usual initial dose is one 10/12.5 mg or 20/12.5 mg tablet taken once daily

How should I take Monopril HCT?
Monopril HCT can be taken with or without food and should be taken at the same time every day.

What should I avoid while taking Monopril HCT?

While taking Monopril HCT, avoid becoming pregnant or breastfeeding. In addition, maintain proper fluid intake and avoid dehydration. If dehydration occurs, lightheadedness and a feeling of faintness may occur.

It is also important that during therapy with Monopril HCT, potassium supplements and salt substitutes containing potassium are avoided unless otherwise directed by your physician. Avoid taking antacids and Monopril HCT simultaneously; separate taking an antacid and Monopril HCT by 2 hours.

What are possible food and drug interactions associated with Monopril HCT?

If Monopril HCT is taken with certain other drugs, the effects of either could be increased, decreased, or altered. It is especially important to check with your doctor before combining Monopril HCT with the following: antacids; cholestyramine; colestipol resins; injectable gold; insulin, lithium; methenamine; nonsteroidal anti-inflammatory drugs (NSAIDs); norepinephrine; potassium-sparing diuretics such as spironolactone, amiloride and triamterene; potassium supplements; salt substitutes containing potassium; tubocurarine.

What are the possible side effects of Monopril HCT?

Side effects cannot be anticipated. If any develop or change in intensity, tell your doctor as soon as possible. Only your doctor can determine if it is safe for you to continue taking this drug.

Side effects may include: Dizziness, chest pain, cough, diarrhea, fatigue, headache, low blood pressure, muscle pain, nausea or vomiting, upper airway infection

Can I receive Monopril HCT if I am pregnant or breastfeeding?

Monopril HCT should not be taken during pregnancy. Taking Monopril HCT while you are pregnant could cause serious harm or even death to your unborn baby. Tell your doctor immediately if you are pregnant, plan to become pregnant, or are breastfeeding. Monopril HCT is excreted in breast milk, and should not be taken if you are breastfeeding.

What should I do if I miss a dose of Monopril HCT?

If you miss a dose of Monopril HCT, take the missed dose as soon as you remember it. If it is almost time for your next dose, skip the missed dose and return to your normal dosing schedule. Do not take a double dose.

How should I store Monopril HCT?

Store Monopril HCT at room temperature in a tightly closed container and protect from moisture.

Montelukast sodium See Singulair, page 1199.

MONUROL
Generic name: Fosfomycin tromethamine

What is Monurol?
Monurol is an antibiotic that treats urinary tract infections in women caused by certain types of bacteria.

What is the most important information I should know about Monurol?
You should not take more than one dose of Monurol for a bladder infection unless otherwise instructed by your doctor. If you do not experience an improvement in your symptoms within 2-3 days after starting Monurol, tell your doctor right away.

Who should not take Monurol?
You should not take Monurol if you are allergic or sensitive to fosfomycin or any other ingredient in Monurol.

What should I tell my doctor before I take the first dose of Monurol?
Tell your doctor about all prescription, over-the-counter, and herbal medications you are taking before beginning treatment with Monurol. Also, talk to your doctor about your complete medical history, especially if you have kidney disease or if you have recurrent bladder infections.

What is the usual dosage?
The information below is based on the dosage guidelines your doctor uses. Depending on your condition and medical history, your doctor may prescribe a different regimen. Do not change the dosage or stop taking your medication without your doctor's approval.

Adults: The usual dosage is one packet of Monurol (equivalent to 3 grams of fosfomycin) taken as a single dose.

How should I take Monurol?
Monurol can be taken with or without food and it should only be taken orally. Dissolve the packet of Monurol granules into approximately one-half cup of water and drink the entire contents immediately after dissolving. Do not use hot water.

What should I avoid while taking Monurol?
Avoid taking more than one dose of Monurol. If your symptoms have not improved after two or three days, contact your physician.

What are possible food and drug interactions associated with Monurol?

If Monurol is taken with certain other drugs, the effects of either could be increased, decreased, or altered. It is especially important to check with your doctor before combining Monurol with medications that increase gastrointestinal motility (stomach and intestinal movement) and metoclopramide.

What are the possible side effects of Monurol?

Side effects cannot be anticipated. If any develop or change in intensity, tell your doctor as soon as possible. Only your doctor can determine if it is safe for you to continue taking this drug.

Side effects may include: diarrhea, headache, vaginal inflammation or infection, nausea, runny nose, back pain, acid reflux, dizziness, weakness, rash

Can I receive Monurol if I am pregnant or breastfeeding?

Tell your doctor immediately if you are pregnant or plan on becoming pregnant in order for you and your doctor to discuss the risks and benefits of Monurol therapy. The effects of Monurol during breastfeeding are unknown. Tell your doctor immediately if you are breastfeeding or plan to breastfeed.

What should I do if I miss a dose of Monurol?

If you miss a dose of Monurol, take it as soon as you remember.

How should I store Monurol?

Monurol should be stored at room temperature.

Morphine sulfate See MS Contin, page 853.

Morphine sulfate, extended-release See Avinza, page 169.

MOTRIN

Generic name: Ibuprofen

What is Motrin?

Motrin is a nonsteroidal anti-inflammatory drug available in both prescription and nonprescription forms. Prescription Motrin is used in adults for relief of the symptoms of rheumatoid arthritis and osteoarthritis, treatment of menstrual pain, and relief of mild to moderate pain. In children aged 6 months and older it can be given to reduce fever and relieve mild to moderate pain. It is also used to relieve the symptoms of juvenile arthritis.

Motrin IB, Children's Motrin, Infants' Motrin, and Motrin Junior are available without a prescription. Check the packages for uses, dosage, and other information on these over-the-counter products.

What is the most important information I should know about Motrin?

You should have frequent checkups with your doctor if you take Motrin regularly. Ulcers or internal bleeding can occur without warning.

This drug should be used with caution if you have kidney or liver disease, or are severely dehydrated; it can cause liver or kidney inflammation or other problems in some people.

Do not take aspirin or any other anti-inflammatory medications while taking Motrin unless your doctor tells you to do so.

If you have a severe allergic reaction, seek medical help immediately.

Motrin may cause vision problems. If you experience any changes in your vision, inform your doctor.

Motrin may prolong bleeding time. If you are taking blood-thinning medication, this drug should be taken with caution.

This drug can cause water retention. It should be used with caution if you have high blood pressure or poor heart function.

Motrin chewable tablets contain phenylalanine. If you have a hereditary disease called phenylketonuria, you should be aware of this.

Who should not take Motrin?

If you are sensitive to or have ever had an allergic reaction to ibuprofen, aspirin, or similar drugs, such as naproxen, or if you have had asthma attacks caused by aspirin or other drugs of this type, or if you have angioedema, a condition whose symptoms are skin eruptions, you should not take this medication. Make sure that your doctor is aware of any drug reactions that you have experienced.

What should I tell my doctor before I take the first dose of Motrin?

Tell your doctor about all prescription, over-the-counter, and herbal medications you are taking before beginning treatment with this drug. Also, talk to your doctor about your complete medical history, especially if you have ever had peptic ulcers or internal bleeding or if you have diabetes, kidney or liver disease, or an infection.

What is the usual dosage?

The information below is based on the dosage guidelines your doctor uses. Depending on your condition and medical history, your doctor may prescribe a different regimen. Do not change the dosage or stop taking your medication without your doctor's approval.

Rheumatoid Arthritis and Osteoarthritis
Adults: The usual dosage is 1,200 to 3,200 milligrams per day divided into 3 or 4 doses. Your doctor will tailor the dose to your individual needs. Symptoms should be reduced within 2 weeks. Daily dosage should not be greater than 3,200 milligrams.

Mild to Moderate Pain
Adults: The usual dose is 400 milligrams every 4 to 6 hours as necessary.

Children 6 months to 12 years: The usual dose is 10 milligrams per 2.2 pounds of body weight every 6 to 8 hours. Do not give the child more than 4 such doses per day.

Menstrual Pain
Adults: The usual dose is 400 milligrams every 4 hours as necessary. Begin treatment when symptoms first appear.

Fever Reduction
Children 6 months to 12 years: The recommended dose is 5 milligrams per 2.2 pounds of body weight if temperature is less than 102.5°F or 10 milligrams per 2.2 pounds of body weight if temperature is 102.5°F or greater. The fever should go down for 6 to 8 hours. Do not give the child more than 40 milligrams per 2.2 pounds of body weight in one day.

Juvenile Arthritis
Children 6 months to 12 years: The usual dose is 30 to 40 milligrams daily per 2.2 pounds of body weight, divided into 3 or 4 doses. Some children may need only 20 milligrams daily per 2.2 pounds.

How should I take Motrin?
Your doctor may ask you to take Motrin with food or an antacid to avoid stomach upset. The suspension can be given with meals or milk if it upsets the stomach. A drink of water or other fluid after taking a chewable tablet can help your body absorb the drug.

What should I avoid while taking Motrin?
Avoid the use of alcohol while taking this medication.

What are possible food and drug interactions associated with Motrin?
If Motrin is taken with certain other drugs, the effects of either could be increased, decreased, or altered. It is especially important to check with your doctor before combining Motrin with the following: aspirin, blood pressure medications known as ACE inhibitors, blood-thinning drugs such as warfarin, diuretics such as furosemide and hydrochlorothiazide, lithium, and methotrexate.

What are the possible side effects of Motrin?

Side effects cannot be anticipated. If any develop or change in intensity, tell your doctor as soon as possible. Only your doctor can determine if it is safe for you to continue taking this drug.

Side effects may include: abdominal cramps or pain, abdominal discomfort, bloating and gas, constipation, diarrhea, dizziness, fluid retention and swelling, headache, heartburn, indigestion, itching, loss of appetite, nausea, nervousness, rash, ringing in ears, stomach pain, vomiting

Can I receive Motrin if I am pregnant or breastfeeding?

The effects of ibuprofen during pregnancy have not been adequately studied. If you are pregnant or plan to become pregnant, inform your doctor immediately. Ibuprofen may appear in breast milk and could affect a nursing infant. If this medication is essential to your health, your doctor may advise you to discontinue breastfeeding until your treatment with this medication is finished.

What should I do if I miss a dose of Motrin?

Take it as soon as you remember. If it is almost time for your next dose, skip the one you missed and go back to your regular schedule. Never take 2 doses at the same time.

How should I store Motrin?

Store at room temperature.

Moxifloxacin hydrochloride See Avelox, page 166.

MS CONTIN
Generic name: Morphine sulfate

What is MS Contin?

MS Contin is a narcotic pain medication that releases its active ingredient (morphine) slowly over time. It is used to treat patients in severe pain who need a painkiller for more than a few days.

What is the most important information I should know about MS Contin?

MS Contin may depress your breathing rate, especially if you are elderly or debilitated, or have conditions that can cause you to become oxygen depleted. You should use caution when taking MS Contin if you have chronic obstructive pulmonary disease (COPD) or any other disease of the lungs that may reduce your breathing rate.

If you have a pre-existing head injury, elevated intracranial pressure (pressure inside the skull), or other injuries to your brain, MS Contin may hide signs of worsening head injuries or may further increase the pressure in your skull.

MS Contin may cause extremely low blood pressure, especially when you rise from laying down or a sitting position.

Taking MS Contin on a regular basis may lead to physical or psychological dependence, potentially leading to drug abuse. If you have taken MS Contin for an extended period of time, you should not suddenly stop taking it. If you discontinue therapy your doctor will gradually reduce your daily dose over time to prevent withdrawal side effects.

Rarely, MS Contin can cause a severe allergic reaction known as anaphylaxis; if you experience any difficulty breathing after taking MS Contin, seek emergency medical attention right away. MS Contin may impair your ability to perform daily tasks that require mental alertness such as driving an automobile.

Who should not take MS Contin?

Do not take MS Contin if you are allergic or sensitive to morphine or any ingredient in MS Contin; if you have a decreased breathing capacity and are not in the presence of emergency medical caregivers; acute or severe asthma; or if you have an intestinal disorder known as "paralytic ileus."

What should I tell my doctor before I take the first dose of MS Contin?

Tell your doctor about all prescription, over-the-counter, and herbal medications you are taking before beginning treatment with MS Contin. Also, talk to your doctor about your complete medical history, especially if you are elderly or debilitated; have severe liver, lung, or kidney impairment; thyroid disease; adrenocortical insufficiency (eg, Addison's Disease); brain depression or coma; psychosis; prostate enlargement, or urethral stricture; acute alcoholism; a spinal condition called kyphoscoliosis; or an inability to swallow.

What is the usual dosage?

The information below is based on the dosage guidelines your doctor uses. Depending on your condition and medical history, your doctor may prescribe a different regimen. Do not change the dosage or stop taking your medication without your doctor's approval.

Adults: MS Contin is usually taken every 12 hours at doses that range from 15 milligrams (mg) to 200 mg per dose. Your individual dose depends on if you have taken another narcotic pain medication in the past or are switching from another pain medication to MS Contin. Your dose is also determined by your doctor based on the type of pain medication you have taken in the past and its dose.

MS Contin 100 and 200 mg tablets are only to be taken by patients who are tolerant of daily doses of morphine of 200 mg and greater for the 100 mg tablet or 400 mg and greater for the 200 mg tablet.

How should I take MS Contin?

MS Contin tablets should be swallowed whole and never chewed or crushed. If a tablet is broken in any way and then taken, this may result in the release of a large enough dose of morphine to be toxic and cause serious side effects.

What should I avoid while taking MS Contin?

You should not drink alcohol or take sleeping aids while taking MS Contin.

What are possible food and drug interactions associated with MS Contin?

If MS Contin is taken with certain other drugs, the effects of either could be increased, decreased, or altered. It is especially important to check with your doctor before combining MS Contin with the following: alcohol; agonist/antagonist pain relievers such as pentazocine, nalbuphine, butorphanol, or buprenorphine; general anesthetics; phenothiazine-type medications; sedatives; and tranquilizers.

What are the possible side effects of MS Contin?

Side effects cannot be anticipated. If any develop or change in intensity, tell your doctor as soon as possible. Only your doctor can determine if it is safe for you to continue taking this drug.

Side effects may include: constipation, lightheadedness, dizziness, lethargy, nausea, vomiting, sweating, euphoria, negative mood changes

Can I receive MS Contin if I am pregnant or breastfeeding?

You should not take MS Contin during pregnancy unless your doctor instructs you to and is aware that you are pregnant. Discuss with your doctor if you are pregnant or planning to become pregnant while using MS Contin.

MS Contin is found in breast milk; you should not breastfeed while taking this medicine.

What should I do if I miss a dose of MS Contin?

You should not double your dose of MS Contin. Skip the missed dose and return to your normal dosing schedule.

How should I store MS Contin?

MS Contin should be stored at room temperature away from light.

Mupirocin See Bactroban, page 195.

Mycophenolate mofetil See Cellcept, page 276.

MYSOLINE

Generic name: Primidone

What is Mysoline?

Mysoline is a medication that is used to help control seizures. Mysoline may be taken alone or in combination with other medications to treat grand mal, psychomotor, and focal epileptic type seizures.

What is the most important information I should know about Mysoline?

You should not suddenly stop taking Mysoline unless your doctor instructs you to as this may cause you to experience seizures. Mysoline may take several weeks to reach its full effect.

Who should not take Mysoline?

You should not take Mysoline if you have a disorder known as "porphyria" or if you are allergic or sensitive to phenobarbital or any ingredient in Mysoline.

What should I tell my doctor before I take the first dose of Mysoline?

Tell your doctor about all prescription, over-the-counter, and herbal medications you are taking before beginning treatment with Mysoline. Also, talk to your doctor about your complete medical history, especially if you are pregnant, plan to become pregnant, are breastfeeding, or are taking any other type of anti-seizure medications.

What is the usual dosage?

The information below is based on the dosage guidelines your doctor uses. Depending on your condition and medical history, your doctor may prescribe a different regimen. Do not change the dosage or stop taking your medication without your doctor's approval.

Adults and children ages 8 and older:

Patients who are not taking other seizure medications: The initial daily dosage is as follows: Days 1-3, take 100-125 milligrams (mg) at bedtime; Days 4-6, take 100-125 mg twice daily; Days 7-9, take 100-125 mg three times daily; Day 10 and on for maintenance, 250 mg taken 3-4 times daily. Daily doses should not exceed 500 mg taken 4 times daily

Patients who are not taking other seizure medications: The usual starting dose is 100-125 mg taken at bedtime, and the dose is then gradually increased as the dose of the other medication is gradually decreased over the course of several weeks.

Children age 8 and younger: The initial daily dosage is as follows: Days 1-3; take 50 mg at bedtime; Days 4-6; take 50 mg twice daily; Days 7-9 take 100 mg twice daily; Day 10 and on for maintenance; 125-250 mg taken 3 times daily.

How should I take Mysoline?
Mysoline should be taken at the same time every day and can be taken with or without food.

What should I avoid while taking Mysoline?
You should avoid suddenly stopping Mysoline therapy unless your doctor instructs you to.

What are possible food and drug interactions associated with Mysoline?
If Mysoline is taken with certain other drugs, the effects of either could be increased, decreased, or altered. It is especially important to check with your doctor before combining Mysoline with any other medications.

What are the possible side effects of Mysoline?
Side effects cannot be anticipated. If any develop or change in intensity, tell your doctor as soon as possible. Only your doctor can determine if it is safe for you to continue taking this drug.

Side effects may include: unstable balance, dizziness, nausea, vomiting, irritability, loss of appetite, mood swings, sexual dysfunction, drowsiness, or blistering rash.

Can I receive Mysoline if I am pregnant or breastfeeding?
The effects of Mysoline during pregnancy are unknown. Tell your doctor immediately if you are pregnant or plan to become pregnant. Mysoline is excreted in breast milk; you should not breastfeed while taking Mysoline unless otherwise instructed by your doctor.

What should I do if I miss a dose of Mysoline?
If you miss a dose of Mysoline, do not double your next dose. Skip the dose you missed and return to your normal dosing schedule.

How should I store Mysoline?
Mysoline should be stored at room temperature

Nabilone *See Cesamet, page 281.*

Nadolol *See Corgard, page 342.*

Naltrexone *See Vivitrol, page 1404.*

NAMENDA
Generic name: Memantine hydrochloride

What is Namenda?
Namenda is a medication that blocks certain receptors in the brain thought to contribute to the symptoms of Alzheimer's disease. Namenda is used to treat moderate-to-severe dementia in patients with Alzheimer's disease.

What is the most important information I should know about Namenda?
If you are taking Namenda or are the caretaker of a patient who is taking Namenda, you should know that doses of greater than 5 milligrams (mg) a day should be split into two doses. Also, wait at least 1 week between dosage increases (see "What is the usual dosage?" below).

Namenda should not be taken with other medications known as "NMDA antagonists," such as amantadine, ketamine, or dextromethorphan.

You should use caution when eating certain foods or taking other drugs (sodium bicarbonate, carbonic anhydrase inhibitors) that can change the pH of your urine to be more alkaline.

You should also be cautious taking Namenda if you have a condition of the kidney called "renal tubular necrosis," or if you have a severe urinary tract infection.

Who should not take Namenda?
You should not take Namenda if you are allergic or sensitive to memantine or any other ingredient in Namenda.

What should I tell my doctor before I take the first dose of Namenda?
Tell your doctor about all prescription, over-the-counter, and herbal medications you are taking before beginning treatment with Namenda. Also, talk to your doctor about your complete medical history, especially if you have kidney or liver disease, or any condition that can change the pH of your urine.

What is the usual dosage?
The information below is based on the dosage guidelines your doctor uses. Depending on your condition and medical history, your doctor may prescribe a different regimen. Do not change the dosage or stop taking your medication without your doctor's approval.

Adults: The usual starting dose is 5 milligrams (mg) taken once daily. Your doctor may then increase your dose up to 10 mg a day, taken in two doses. Next, your dose may be further increased to 15 mg, and then 20 mg daily (taken as two 10 mg doses). You should wait at least 1 week in between dosage increases, and do not increase your daily dose by more than 5 mg at one time.

How should I take Namenda?
Namenda may be taken with or without food and should be taken at the same time every day.

What should I avoid while taking Namenda?
You should not engage in activities that require mental alertness, such as driving an automobile, until you know how Namenda will affect you.

What are possible food and drug interactions associated with Namenda?
If Namenda is taken with certain other drugs, the effects of either could be increased, decreased, or altered. It is especially important to check with your doctor before combining Namenda with the following: cimetidine, hydrochlorothiazide, metformin, nicotine, NMDA antagonists such as amantadine, ketamine, or dextromethorphan, quinidine, ranitidine, Triamterene.

What are the possible side effects of Namenda?
Side effects cannot be anticipated. If any develop or change in intensity, tell your doctor as soon as possible. Only your doctor can determine if it is safe for you to continue taking this drug.

Side effects may include: headache, high blood pressure, dizziness, confusion, hallucinations, pain, tiredness, constipation, vomiting, cough, back pain, or shortness of breath

Can I receive Namenda if I am pregnant or breastfeeding?
Namenda is a pregnancy category B medication. This means studies in animals have not shown adverse effects of Namenda on animal newborns, however adequate studies in humans have not yet been done. You should not use Namenda during pregnancy unless your doctor instructs you to and is aware that you are pregnant. It is not known whether Namenda is excreted in breast milk. Tell your doctor immediately if you are pregnant, plan to become pregnant, or are breastfeeding.

What should I do if I miss a dose of Namenda?
You should not double your dose of Namenda. Skip the missed dose and return to your normal dosing schedule.

How should I store Namenda?
You should store Namenda at room temperature.

NAPROSYN
Generic name: Naproxen

What is Naprosyn?
Naprosyn is a non-steroidal anti-inflammatory drug (NSAID) used to treat pain, swelling, and inflammation from medical conditions such as arthritis, tendonitis, acute gout, and menstrual cramps.

What is the most important information I should know about Naprosyn?
NSAIDs may increase the chance of a heart attack or stroke that can lead to death. This chance increases with longer use of NSAIDs and in people who have heart disease.

   NSAIDs should never be used right before or after a heart surgery called a coronary artery bypass graft (CABG).

   NSAIDs can cause ulcers and bleeding in the stomach and intestines at any time during treatment.

   NSAIDs should only be used exactly as prescribed, at the lowest dose possible for your treatment, for the shortest time needed.

Who should not take Naprosyn?
If you had an asthma attack, hives, or other allergic reactions with aspirin or with any other NSAID, you should not take this medication. NSAIDs should not be used for pain right before or after heart bypass surgery.

What should I tell my doctor before I take the first dose of Naprosyn?
Tell your doctor about all prescription, over-the-counter, and herbal medications you are taking before beginning treatment with Naprosyn. Talk to your doctor about your complete medical history, especially if you have asthma or if you are pregnant or breastfeeding. You should also notify your doctor if you smoke, use alcohol, have liver or kidney dysfunction, heart failure, or if you have had a serious reaction to either aspirin or other NSAIDs in the past.

What is the usual dosage?
The information below is based on the dosage guidelines your doctor uses. Depending on your condition and medical history, your doctor may prescribe a different regimen. Do not change the dosage or stop taking your medication without your doctor's approval.

Rheumatoid Arthritis, Osteoarthritis and Ankylosing Spondylitis
Adults: The usual dose of Naprosyn is 250mg, 375mg, or 500mg twice daily.

Acute Gout
Adults: The recommended starting dose is 750mg of Naprosyn followed by 250mg every 8 hours until the attack has subsided.

Management of Pain, Menstrual Cramps,
and Acute Tendonitis and Bursitis
Adults: The recommended starting dose is 500mg every 12 hours or 250mg every 6-8 hours as required.

Juvenile Arthritis
Children: The recommended total daily dose is approximately 10 mg per 2.2 pounds of body weight given in 2 divided doses. The use of Naprosyn suspension is recommended for juvenile arthritis in children 2 years or older because it allows for more flexible dosing changes based on the child's weight.

How should I take Naprosyn?
To avoid upset stomach, you may take Naprosyn with food and with a full glass of water. Do not break, crush, or chew Naprosyn tablets.

If you take Naprosyn for arthritis, take it regularly and exactly as your doctor recommends.

What should I avoid while taking Naprosyn?
Avoid taking antacids, aspirin, or other NSAIDs while taking Naprosyn.

What are possible food and drug interactions associated with Naprosyn?
If Naprosyn is taken with certain other drugs, the effects of either could be increased, decreased, or altered. It is especially important to check with your doctor before combining Naprosyn with the following: ACE-inhibitors, antacids and sucralfate, aspirin, beta-blockers (propranolol), cholestyramine, diuretics, lithium, methotrexate, NSAIDs, sulphonyl-ureas, antidepressant medications known as SSRIs, and warfarin.

What are the possible side effects of Naprosyn?
Side effects cannot be anticipated. If any develop or change in intensity, tell your doctor as soon as possible. Only your doctor can determine if it is safe for you to continue taking this drug.

Serious side effects may include: heart attack, stroke, high blood pressure, heart failure from body swelling (fluid retention), kidney problems including kidney failure, bleeding and ulcers in the stomach and intestine, low red blood cells (anemia), life-threatening skin reactions, life-threatening allergic reactions, liver problems including liver failure, asthma attacks in people with asthma

Other side effects may include: stomach pain, constipation, diarrhea, gas, heartburn, nausea, vomiting, and dizziness

Get immediate medical attention if you experience any of the following: shortness of breath or trouble breathing, chest pain, weakness in one part or side of your body, slurred speech, swelling of the face or throat, nausea, fatigue or weakness, itching, yellowing of your skin or eyes, stomach pain, blood in your vomit, blood in your bowel movement (or it is black and sticky like tar), unusual weight gain, skin rash or blistering with fever, swelling of the arms, legs, hands, and feet

Can I receive Naprosyn if I am pregnant or breastfeeding?

Tell your doctor immediately if you are pregnant, plan to become pregnant, or you are breastfeeding. Naprosyn, like all NSAIDs, should be avoided during pregnancy, particularly in late pregnancy. Naprosyn should be not be used if breastfeeding.

What should I do if I miss a dose of Naprosyn?

If you take Naprosyn on a regular schedule for relief of arthritis pain, take the missed dose as soon as you remember. Do not take two doses at once.

How should I store Naprosyn?

Store Naprosyn at room temperature in a well-closed, light-resistant container.

Naproxen *See Anaprox, page 101, or Naprosyn, page 860.*

Naratriptan hydrochloride *See Amerge, page 82.*

NARDIL

Generic name: Phenelzine sulfate

What is Nardil?

Nardil is used to treat depression. Nardil is often used in the treatment of depression associated with anxiety, phobias, or neurotic behaviors.

What is the most important information I should know about Nardil?

Antidepressant medicines may increase suicidal thoughts or actions in some children, teenagers, and young adults when the medicine is first started. Depression and other serious mental illnesses are the most important causes of suicidal thoughts and actions. Some people may have a particularly high risk of having suicidal thoughts or actions. These include people who have (or have a family history of) bipolar disorder (also called manic-depressive illness) or suicidal thoughts or actions.

Pay close attention to any changes, especially sudden changes, in mood, behaviors, thoughts, or feelings. This is very important when an antidepressant medicine is first started or when the dose is changed.

Call the doctor right away to report new or sudden changes in mood, behavior, thoughts, or feelings. Signs to watch for include new or worsening depression, new or worsening anxiety, agitation, insomnia, hostility, panic attacks, restlessness, extreme hyperactivity, and suicidal thinking or behavior.

Keep all follow-up visits as scheduled, and call the doctor between visits as needed, especially if you have concerns about symptoms.

Nardil is a monoamine oxidase inhibitor (MAOI). This class of drugs, including Nardil, can cause a sudden, large increase in blood pressure (hypertensive crisis) if you consume foods and drinks that contain high amounts of tyramine.

You should use caution when taking Nardil if you have diabetes, schizophrenia, or epilepsy.

Nardil may also cause low blood pressure, which can lead to dizziness, lightheadedness, or fainting.

Nardil should be discontinued at least 10 days before undergoing any type of surgery that requires anesthesia or numbing agents.

You should wait at least 14 days between the discontinuation of Nardil and starting therapy with another antidepressant of any class.

Who should not take Nardil?
You should not take Nardil if you are allergic or sensitive to phenelzine sulfate or any other ingredient in Nardil; if you have a condition known as pheochromocytoma, congestive heart failure, severe kidney impairment or disease, liver disease, or abnormal liver function tests.

What should I tell my doctor before I take the first dose of Nardil?
Tell your doctor about all prescription, over-the-counter, and herbal medications you are taking before beginning treatment with Nardil. Also, talk to your doctor about your complete medical history, especially if you have a history or family history of suicide or suicidal thoughts, bipolar disorder, liver or kidney disease, heart disease, epilepsy, or schizophrenia.

What is the usual dosage?
The information below is based on the dosage guidelines your doctor uses. Depending on your condition and medical history, your doctor may prescribe a different regimen. Do not change the dosage or stop taking your medication without your doctor's approval.

Adults: The usual starting dose is 15 milligrams (mg) taken three times a day. Your doctor will likely increase your daily dose over the course of several weeks to 60 mg to 90 mg per day in divided daily doses. After maximum benefit from Nardil is achieved, dosage should be reduced slowly over several weeks. Maintenance dose may be as low as one tablet, 15 mg, a day or every other day, and should be continued for as long as required.

How should I take Nardil?

Nardil can be taken with or without food (see the next section for a list of foods to avoid) and should be taken at the same time every day.

What should I avoid while taking Nardil?

While on Nardil, avoid tyramine-rich foods such as dried or aged meats (sausages/salami), fava beans, aged cheeses, beer on tap, yeast, sauerkraut, and soybean products.

Avoid taking any cold and cough preparations (including those containing dextromethorphan); nasal decongestants (tablets, drops, or spray); allergy, sinus and asthma medications; weight-loss drugs; or products containing L-tryptophan.

Avoid the concurrent use of sympathomimetic drugs (including amphetamines, cocaine, methylphenidate, dopamine, epinephrine, and norepinephrine) or related compounds (including methyldopa, L-dopa, L-tryptophan, L-tyrosine, and phenylalanine).

What are possible food and drug interactions associated with Nardil?

If Nardil is taken with certain other drugs, the effects of either could be increased, decreased, or altered. It is especially important to check with your doctor before combining Nardil with the following: allergy medicines, amitriptyline, amoxapine, appetite suppressants, asthma medicines, carbamazepine, citalopram, clomipramine, cold and cough preparations, cyclobenzaprine, decongestants, desipramine, dexfenfluramine, dextromethorphan, doxepin, fluoxetine, fluvoxamine, guanethidine, imipramine, products containing L-tryptophan, maprotiline, meperidine, mirtazapine, nortriptyline, paroxetine, perphenazine and amitriptyline, protriptyline, rauwolfia alkaloids, sertraline, trimipramine, and venlafaxine.

Nardil should be used with caution in combination with antihypertensive drugs, including thiazide diuretics and beta blockers, since low blood pressure may result.

What are the possible side effects of Nardil?

Side effects cannot be anticipated. If any develop or change in intensity, tell your doctor as soon as possible. Only your doctor can determine if it is safe for you to continue taking this drug.

Side effects may include: dizziness, headache, drowsiness, trouble sleeping, fatigue, muscle twitching, trouble balancing, psychosis, decreased sexual ability, dry mouth, constipation, weight gain, trouble urinating, rash, itching skin, weakness, blurred vision, glaucoma, sweating, liver injury

Can I receive Nardil if I am pregnant or breastfeeding?
The effects of Nardil during pregnancy and breastfeeding are unknown. Tell your doctor immediately if you are pregnant, plan to become pregnant, or are breastfeeding.

What should I do if I miss a dose of Nardil?
You should not double your dose of Nardil. Skip the missed dose and return to your normal dosing schedule.

How should I store Nardil?
Store at room temperature.

NASONEX
Generic name: Mometasone furoate monohydrate

What is Nasonex?
Nasonex nasal spray prevents and relieves the runny, stuffy nose that accompanies hay fever and year-round allergies. It contains a steroid medication that fights inflammation. Nasonex is also used to treat a condition called nasal polyps.

What is the most important information I should know about Nasonex?
A long-term treatment for allergies, Nasonex does not provide immediate relief. To be effective, it must be used regularly once a day. It starts working within 2 days after the first dose, but takes 1 to 2 weeks to yield its maximum benefits. If you suffer from hay fever, you should begin taking it 2 to 4 weeks before the start of pollen season.

You should use caution when switching from medications called oral corticosteroids to using a topical corticosteroid such as Nasonex. If you use excessive amounts of Nasonex you may experience side effects such as acne, water retention, or menstrual irregularities. If you notice any of these symptoms contact your doctor right away.

You may be more prone to getting infections when using Nasonex. Report any new or existing infections to your doctor immediately. You should use caution in using Nasonex if you have active or latent tuberculosis, and any type of infection caused by bacteria, fungi, or viruses.

Who should not take Nasonex?
You should not use Nasonex if you are sensitive or allergic to any ingredient in Nasonex.

What should I tell my doctor before I take the first dose of Nasonex?

Tell your doctor about all prescription, over-the-counter, and herbal medication you are taking before beginning treatment with Nasonex. Also, talk to your doctor about your complete medical history, especially if you have tuberculosis, any other type of local or systemic infection, or intranasal ulcerations.

What is the usual dosage?

The information below is based on the dosage guidelines your doctor uses. Depending on your condition and medical history, your doctor may prescribe a different regimen. Do not change the dosage or stop taking your medication without your doctor's approval.

Allergic Rhinitis
Adults and children 12 years of age and older: The usual dosage is 2 sprays (50 micrograms of mometasone furoate per spray) in each nostril once daily.

Children 2 to 11 years of age: The usual dosage is 1 spray in each nostril once daily.

Nasal Polyps
Adults and children 18 years of age and older: The usual dosage is 2 sprays in each nostril twice daily, however, 2 sprays in each nostril once daily is also effective in some patients.

How should I take Nasonex?

Take Nasonex regularly at the same time each day. Do not use more than the prescribed amount, and do not take it more than once a day.

Shake the bottle thoroughly before each use. Before the first use, prime the pump by pressing it repeatedly until a fine mist appears. If more than a week passes between uses, you'll need to prime the pump again. Avoid spraying the mist into your eyes. Administer the spray as follows:

1. Gently blow your nose to clear the nostrils.
2. Press one nostril closed, tilt your head slightly forward, and insert the nasal applicator into the other nostril.
3. For each spray, press once on the shoulders of the applicator with your forefinger and middle finger, while supporting the base of the bottle with your thumb. Do not spray directly into the wall separating your two nostrils.
4. Breathe in through the nostril, then breathe out through your mouth.
5. Repeat in the other nostril.
6. Wipe the nasal applicator with a clean tissue and replace the cap.

Discard the bottle after 120 sprays. Any medication remaining in it will not be dispensed at the correct dosage.

What should I avoid while taking Nasonex?

You should avoid exposure to anyone who has chicken pox or measles. You should also avoid using more than the recommended dose of Nasonex.

What are possible food and drug interactions associated with Nasonex?

No interactions have been reported.

What are the possible side effects of Nasonex?

Side effects cannot be anticipated. If any develop or change in intensity, tell your doctor as soon as possible. Only your doctor can determine if it is safe for you to continue taking this drug.

Side effects may include: Coughing, flu-like symptoms, headache, muscle and bone pain, nosebleed, painful menstruation, sinus inflammation, sore throat, upper respiratory tract infection, viral infection

Can I receive Nasonex if I am pregnant or breastfeeding?

The effects of Nasonex during pregnancy are unknown. Tell your doctor immediately if you are pregnant, plan to become pregnant, or are breastfeeding.

It is not known whether Nasonex appears in breast milk. However, other steroids do appear in breast milk. Your doctor may suggest discontinuing Nasonex if you are going to breastfeed your baby.

What should I do if I miss a dose of Nasonex?

Take it as soon as you remember. If it is time for your next dose, skip the missed dose and go back to your regular schedule. Do not take 2 doses at the same time.

How should I store Nasonex?

Store at room temperature, away from direct light.

Nateglinide See Starlix, page 1222.

Natural thyroid hormones See Armour Thyroid, page 127.

NAVANE

Generic name: Thiothixene

What is Navane?

Navane is an antipsychotic medication that is used to treat schizophrenia.

What is the most important information
I should know about Navane?

Navane can cause tardive dyskinesia, a serious, sometimes irreversible movement disorder that causes involuntary movements of muscles. The risk for tardive dyskinesia is higher in the elderly and for women. Tell your doctor immediately if you experience any involuntary muscle movements while taking Navane.

Navane can also cause another serious sometime fatal disorder known as neuroleptic malignant syndrome, characterized by muscle stiffness, increased body temperature, sweating, changes in mood or consciousness, and a rapid or irregular heartbeat. If you experience any of these symptoms while taking Navane, seek emergency medical attention immediately.

Navane should be used with caution in patients who might be exposed to extreme heat or who are receiving atropine. Navane should also be used with caution in patients with cardiovascular disease. Careful adjustment of dosage is indicated when Navane is used with other CNS depressants.

Who should not take Navane?

You should not take Navane if you are sensitive or allergic to any ingredient in Navane.

Navane should not be administered to anyone in a comatose state.

Do not take Navane if you are taking a sleep aid or any other substance that slows your central nervous system.

If you have had circulatory system collapse or if you have an abnormal bone marrow or blood condition, you should not take Navane.

What should I tell my doctor before
I take the first dose of Navane?

Tell your doctor about all prescription, over-the-counter, and herbal medications you are taking before beginning treatment with Navane. Also, talk to your doctor about your complete medical history, especially if you have a history of tardive dyskinesia or neuroleptic malignant syndrome (see "What is the most important information I should know about this medication?").

Let your doctor know if you have liver disease, breast cancer, seizures, high or low blood pressure, depression, lupus, heart disease, or if you are or have been alcohol dependent. Also, let your doctor know if you are pregnant, plan to become pregnant, or are breastfeeding.

What is the usual dosage?

The information below is based on the dosage guidelines your doctor uses. Depending on your condition and medical history, your doctor may prescribe a different regimen. Do not change the dosage or stop taking your medication without your doctor's approval.

The use of Navane in children under 12 years of age is not approved.

The usual daily dose is 20-30 milligrams (mg) once daily. Dosage is individually adjusted depending on the severity of the patient's disease state. Initially, small doses are used. Further gradual increase is based on patient response and the optimal effect of the drug.

For Milder Conditions
Adults and children 12 years and older: The usual starting dosage is 2 mg taken 3 times a day. Your doctor may increase the dose to a total of 15 mg a day.

For More Severe Conditions
Adults and children 12 years and older: The usual starting dosage is 5 mg taken two times a day. Your doctor may increase this dose to a total of 60 mg a day. Exceeding a total daily dose of 60mg rarely increases the beneficial response.

How should I take Navane?
Navane can be taken with or without food and should be taken at the same time(s) every day. Take Navane as prescribed by your doctor.

What should I avoid while taking Navane?
You should not drive a car or operate heavy machinery until you know how Navane will affect you.

When taking Navane, avoid becoming dehydrated and exposing yourself to very hot environments.

When taking Navane, you should avoid consumption of alcohol as it may intensify the side effects of the drug.

What are possible food and drug interactions associated with Navane?
If Navane is taken with certain other drugs, the effects of either could be increased, decreased, or altered. It is especially important to check with your doctor before combining Navane with the following: anticholinergic medications such as atropine, antihistamines, barbiturates, blood pressure medications, carbamazepine, opiates, and tricyclic antidepressants.

What are the possible side effects of Navane?
Side effects cannot be anticipated. If any develop or change in intensity, tell your doctor as soon as possible. Only your doctor can determine if it is safe for you to continue taking this drug.

Side effects may include: allergic rash, blurred vision, dizziness, drowsiness, dry mouth, immobility, increased heart rate, involuntary muscle contractions, involuntary muscle movements, liver damage, low blood pressure, menstrual irregularities, muscle restlessness, muscle stiffness, muscle tremors, blood disorders

Navane may cause damage to your liver or your eyes. Some of the warning signs of liver damage include nausea, vomiting, fatigue, loss of appetite, itching, yellow coloring of skin or eyes (jaundice), flu-like symptoms, and dark urine. If you experience any of these symptoms, call your doctor right away. Also, contact your doctor right away if you experience any changes in your vision.

Can I receive Navane if I am pregnant or breastfeeding?
The effects of Navane during pregnancy and breastfeeding are unknown. Tell your doctor immediately if you are pregnant, plan to become pregnant, or are breastfeeding.

What should I do if I miss a dose of Navane?
You should not double your dose of Navane. Skip the missed dose and return to your normal dosing schedule.

How should I store Navane?
Store at room temperature.

Nebivolol See Bystolic, page 236.

Nelfinavir mesylate See Viracept, page 1393.

Neomycin, polymyxin B sulfates, and hydrocortisone
  See Cortisporin Otic, page 344.

NEOPROFEN
Generic name: Ibuprofen lysine

What is NeoProfen?
NeoProfen is used to close a hole in the heart (patent ductus arteriosus, or PDA) in premature infants weighing between 500 grams (g) and 1500 g who are no more than 32 weeks gestational age when normal medical management is ineffective.

What is the most important information
I should know about NeoProfen?
NeoProfen, like other nonsteroidal anti-inflammatory drugs (NSAIDs), may lengthen bleeding time. The infant should be carefully observed for signs and symptoms of bleeding.

  This drug may also change the normal signs and symptoms of infection. The physician should use the drug with extra care when an infection is present or if an infant is at risk of infection.

  NeoProfen should be administered carefully to avoid extravascular injection or leakage of the medicine in surrounding tissue; the solution may be irritating to the tissue.

Who should not take NeoProfen?

Preterm infants should not begin treatment with NeoProfen if they have any of the following: a proven or suspected untreated infection, heart disease that requires opening of the patent ductus arteriosus (PDA) in order to maintain proper pulmonary or systemic blood flow (eg, pulmonary atresia, severe tetralogy of Fallot, severe narrowing of the aorta), bleeding problems (eg, bleeding within the brain, gastrointestinal bleeding), thrombocytopenia (a decrease of platelets in the blood), blood clotting problems, necrotizing enterocolitis (where portions of the bowel undergo tissue death), and kidney problems.

What should I tell my doctor before I take the first dose of NeoProfen?

Tell your doctor about all prescription, over-the-counter, and herbal medications your child is taking.

What is the usual dosage?

The information below is based on the dosage guidelines your doctor uses. Depending on your condition and medical history, your doctor may prescribe a different regimen. Do not change the dosage or stop taking your medication without your doctor's approval.

NeoProfen is first given at 10 milligrams (mg) per 2.2 pounds of body weight, followed by two doses of 5 mg per 2.2 pounds of body weight, after 24 and 48 hours. All doses should be based on birth weight.

How should I take NeoProfen?

NeoProfen will be given to your child in a hospital setting, through an IV.

If the PDA closes or is reduced in size after the first course of NeoProfen, no further doses are necessary. If the PDA does not close or re-opens, then a second course of NeoProfen, alternative therapy, or surgery may be necessary.

What should I avoid while taking NeoProfen?

Avoid administering Neoprofen in the same intravenous (IV) line as total parenteral nutrition (TPN). If it is necessary to give NeoProfen in the same line, then the TPN should be turned off 15 minutes prior to giving Neoprofen and should not be restarted until 15 minutes after NeoProfen has been administered. Your healthcare professional will inform you of any other precautions for your child.

What are possible food and drug interactions associated with NeoProfen?

There are currently no known drug interactions associated with NeoProfen. However, it is important to notify your physician of all prescription and nonprescription medications your infant is taking.

What are the possible side effects of NeoProfen?

Side effects cannot be anticipated. If any develop or change in intensity, tell your doctor as soon as possible. Only your doctor can determine if it is safe for you to continue taking this drug.

Side effects may include: anemia, bleeding, blood in urine, breathing problems, gastrointestinal disorders, kidney problems, low sugar levels in the blood, respiratory infection, skin lesions or irritation, septic infection, urinary tract infection

Can I receive NeoProfen if I am pregnant or breastfeeding?

NeoProfen is only used in infants. It is not indicated for pregnant or breastfeeding females.

What should I do if I miss a dose of NeoProfen?

You will not be administering the dose of NeoProfen to your infant. Your infant's healthcare professional will be responsible for giving the appropriate doses.

How should I store NeoProfen?

This medication is usually stored by a healthcare professional at room temperature and protected from light. NeoProfen vials should be stored in the carton until contents have been used.

Nepafenac ophthalmic suspension See Nevanac, page 875.

NEURONTIN
Generic name: Gabapentin

What is Neurontin?

Neurontin is used to treat nerve pain that follows shingles (herpes zoster) in adults. Neurontin is also used in combination with other medications to treat partial seizures with or without secondary generalization in patients over 12 years of age with epilepsy. Neurontin can also be used in combination with other drugs to treat partial seizures in pediatric patients 3 to 12 years of age.

What is the most important information I should know about Neurontin?

If you are taking Neurontin for seizures, do not suddenly stop taking Neurontin. Stopping Neurontin suddenly may bring on a seizure.

Neurontin sometimes leads to central nervous system side effects in children 3-12 years of age. Let your doctor know if you notice any of the following changes in your child's behavior: emotional liability (primarily behavior problems); hostility, including aggressive behaviors; thought disorder, including concentration problems and change in school performance; or restlessness and hyperactivity.

Do not drive or perform other possibly unsafe tasks until you know how you react to Neurontin; this medication may cause drowsiness, dizziness, or blurred vision. These effects may be worse if you take it with alcohol or certain medicines.

Neurontin may affect your blood sugar. Check blood sugar levels closely and discuss with your doctor before changing the dose of your diabetes medicine.

Who should not take Neurontin?
Do not take Neurontin if you are allergic to the medication or any or its ingredients.

What should I tell my doctor before I take the first dose of Neurontin?
Tell your doctor about all prescription, over-the-counter, and herbal medication you are taking before beginning treatment with Neurontin. Also, talk to your doctor about your complete medical history, especially if you have a history of mental or mood problems, suicidal thoughts, or you have kidney, liver, or heart disease. Tell your doctor if you have ever had an allergic reaction to any medicine.

What is the usual dosage?
The information below is based on the dosage guidelines your doctor uses. Depending on your condition and medical history, your doctor may prescribe a different regimen. Do not change the dosage or stop taking your medication without your doctor's approval.

If Neurontin dose is reduced, discontinued, or substituted with an alternative medication, this should be done gradually over a minimum of 1 week (a longer period may be needed at the discretion of the prescriber).

Pain Following Shingles
Adults: The usual starting dose is a single 300mg dose on the first day, followed by a total 600 mg dose on the second day (taken in two divided doses), and a total 900 mg on the third day (taken in three divided doses). Your doctor may increase your daily dose up to a total 1800 mg given in 3 divided doses.

Epilepsy
Adults and adolescents over age 12: The usual daily dose is between 900 and 1800 milligrams (mg). This dose is taken in divided doses 3 times each day using 300 or 400 mg capsules, or 600 or 800 mg tablets. The time between subsequent doses should not exceed 12 hours. Daily doses of 3600mg have been used and tolerated in clinical trials.

Children 3 to 12 years old: The usual dose is calculated based on weight and age. The starting daily dose should range from 10mg to15mg per kilogram, given in 3 divided doses. The effective daily dose of Neurontin in patients 5 years of age and older is 25mg to 35mg per kilogram given in divided doses (three times a day). The effective daily dose in pediatric patients ages 3 and 4 years is 40mg per kilogram given in divided doses (three times a day). The effective dose should be reached by slowly increasing the dose over a period of approximately 3 days. Daily doses up to 50 mg per kilogram have been well-tolerated in a long-term clinical study. The maximum time interval between doses should not exceed 12 hours.

How should I take Neurontin?

Neurontin is given orally with or without food. Take Neurontin at the same time each day. Take each dose of Neurontin with a full glass of water. If you are also taking antacids, wait 2 hours after taking antacids to then take Neurontin. If you need to break a Neurontin tablet in half, take the unused half-tablet as the next dose or as soon as possible. If you do not use half-tablets within a few days of breaking the full tablet, you should throw them away. You should plan ahead to have a refill on hand in case you run out of Neurontin. Take Neurontin only as prescribed by your doctor. Do not stop or change the dose of this medication without first speaking to your doctor.

What should I avoid while taking Neurontin?

Do not stop taking Neurontin unless your doctor tells you to. Stopping Neurontin suddenly may bring on a seizure. Your doctor will tell you when and how to stop taking Neurontin. Follow your doctor's directions. The dose will be decreased slowly, over a week or more.

Neurontin may cause dizziness or drowsiness. You should use caution when driving, operating machinery, or performing other hazardous activities. If you experience dizziness or drowsiness, you should avoid these activities.

What are possible food and drug interactions associated with Neurontin?

If Neurontin is taken with certain other drugs, the effects of either could be increased, decreased, or altered. It is especially important to check with your doctor before combining Neurontin with the following: antacids, hydrocodone, morphine, and naproxen.

What are the possible side effects of Neurontin?

Side effects cannot be anticipated. If any develop or change in intensity, tell your doctor as soon as possible. Only your doctor can determine if it is safe for you to continue taking this drug.

Side effects may include: back pain, clumsiness, constipation, diarrhea, dizziness, failure of muscular coordination, fever, hostility, nausea and/or vomiting, shaking or tremor, sleepiness or tiredness, stomach upset, swelling of hands and feet, viral infection, vision problems, weakness

Can I receive Neurontin if I am pregnant or breastfeeding?
The effects of Neurontin during pregnancy are unknown. Tell your doctor immediately if you are pregnant, plan to become pregnant, or are breastfeeding.

What should I do if I miss a dose of Neurontin?
If you miss a dose of Neurontin, take it as soon as you remember. If it is close to your next dose, just take your regular dose. Do not take more than 1 dose of Neurontin at a time.

How should I store Neurontin?
Store Neurontin Capsules at room temperature. Store away from heat, moisture, and light. Do not store in the bathroom. Keep Neurontin Capsules out of the reach of children.

NEVANAC
Generic name: Nepafenac ophthalmic suspension

What is Nevanac?
Nevanac is an ophthalmic suspension used to treat pain and inflammation associated with cataract surgery.

What is the most important information I should know about Nevanac?
Nevanac, like other nonsteroidal anti-inflammatory drugs (NSAIDs), may delay the healing process, or even increase bleeding.

Do not exceed the recommended dose or use Nevanac for longer than prescribed without checking with your doctor.

Using Nevanac more than 24 hours before surgery or for more than 14 days after surgery may increase your risk of side effects, some of which may be serious.

Do not wear contact lenses while you are using Nevanac. Sterilize contact lenses according to manufacturer's directions and check with your doctor before using them.

Who should not take Nevanac?
Do not take Nevanac if you are allergic to any of its ingredients or if you have an allergy to other nonsteroidal anti-inflammatory drugs (NSAIDs) such as ibuprofen.

What should I tell my doctor before I take the first dose of Nevanac?

Tell your doctor about all prescription, over-the-counter, and herbal medications you are taking to avoid a potential interaction with Nevanac. Also, discuss your complete medical history with your doctor, especially if you have had a severe allergic reaction to aspirin or phenylacetic acid, bleeding problems, diabetes, rheumatoid arthritis, or if have had repeated eye surgery within a short period of time.

What is the usual dosage?

The information below is based on the dosage guidelines your doctor uses. Depending on your condition and medical history, your doctor may prescribe a different regimen. Do not change the dosage or stop taking your medication without your doctor's approval.

The usual dose of Nevanac is one drop in the affected eye(s), 3 times per day. Treatment with Nevanac should begin the day before cataract surgery and be continued until 2 weeks after surgery.

How should I take Nevanac?

Shake the bottle well before each use. Wash your hands. Tilt your head back. Using your index finger, pull the lower eyelid away from the eye to form a pouch. Drop the medicine into the pouch and close your eye for 1 to 2 minutes. Remove excess medicine around your eye with a clean tissue, taking care not to touch your eye.

If more than one topical ophthalmic medication is being used, the medicines must be administered at least 5 minutes apart.

What should I avoid while taking Nevanac?

Do not wear contact lenses while you are using Nevanac. Sterilize contact lenses according to manufacturer's directions and check with your doctor before using them.

Do not exceed the recommended dose or use Nevanac for longer than prescribed without checking with your doctor.

Do not touch the applicator tip to any surface, including your eye, to avoid contaminating the medicine.

What are possible food and drug interactions associated with Nevanac?

If Nevanac is taken with certain other drugs, the effects of either could be increased, decreased, or altered. Nevanac may be used with other ophthalmic medicines; talk to your doctor about the medications you are on to make sure they are compatible with Nevanac. Tell your doctor if you are currently or have used anticoagulants (such as warfarin) in the past.

What are the possible side effects of Nevanac?
Side effects cannot be anticipated. If any develop or change in intensity, tell your doctor as soon as possible. Only your doctor can determine if it is safe for you to continue taking this drug.

Side effects may include: crusting of the eye lid, headache, high blood pressure, light sensitivity, nausea, pain in the eye, sinus infection, sticky sensation in the eye, tearing, vomiting, dry eye

Can I receive Nevanac if I am pregnant or breastfeeding?
The effects of Nevanac during pregnancy and breastfeeding are unknown. Talk with your doctor before taking this drug if you are pregnant, plan to become pregnant, or are breastfeeding.

What should I do if I miss a dose of Nevanac?
Take it as soon as you remember. If it is almost time for your next dose, skip the missed dose and go back to your regular schedule. Never take 2 doses at the same time.

How should I store Nevanac?
Store Nevanac in the refrigerator or at room temperature. Do not freeze. Store away from heat, moisture, and light. Keep Nevanac out of the reach of children.

Nevirapine *See Viramune, page 1395.*

NEXAVAR
Generic name: Sorafenib

What is Nexavar?
Nexavar is a cancer treatment for adults with kidney cancer (renal cell carcinoma) and liver cancer (hepatocellular carcinoma).

**What is the most important information
I should know about Nexavar?**
Nexavar may cause birth defects or death in unborn babies. Women should not get pregnant while taking Nexavar. Men and women should use effective birth control during treatment with Nexavar and for at least 2 weeks after stopping treatment. Talk with your doctor about effective birth control methods.

Nexavar may reduce the number of clot-forming cells (platelets) in your blood. To prevent bleeding, avoid situations in which bruising or injury may occur. Report unusual bleeding, bruising, blood in stools, or dark, tarry stools to your doctor.

Nexavar may lower your body's ability to fight infection. Prevent infection by avoiding contact with people with colds or other infections. Notify your doctor of any signs of infection, including fever, sore throat, rash, or chills.

Before you have any medical or dental treatments, emergency care, or surgery, tell the doctor or dentist that you are using Nexavar.

Do not suddenly stop taking Nexavar, even if you feel better.

Who should not take Nexavar?
Do not take Nexavar if you are allergic to sorafenib (the active ingredient) or any of the other ingredients.

What should I tell my doctor before I take the first dose of Nexavar?
Tell your doctor if you have kidney problems (in addition to cancer), liver problems (in addition to cancer), high blood pressure, bleeding problems, heart problems or chest pain, or if you are pregnant or breast-feeding.

Also, you should tell your doctor about all prescription, over-the-counter, and herbal medications you are on, to prevent an interaction with Nexavar. Tell your doctor if you are taking warfarin.

What is the usual dosage?
The information below is based on the dosage guidelines your doctor uses. Depending on your condition and medical history, your doctor may prescribe a different regimen. Do not change the dosage or stop taking your medication without your doctor's approval.

The recommended dose of Nexavar is 400 milligrams (mg) (2 tablets of 200 mg) taken twice daily. A total of 4 tablets should be taken daily.

How should I take Nexavar?
Take doses of Nexavar on an empty stomach (either 1 hour before or 2 hours after a meal). Swallow Nexavar whole. Do not break, crush, or chew before swallowing. Take Nexavar with a full glass of water (8 oz/240 mL). Treatment with this medication should continue until you are no longer benefiting from it.

What should I avoid while taking Nexavar?
While on Nexavar and for 2 weeks after stopping treatment, use appropriate birth control in order to prevent pregnancy.

Do not break, crush, or chew before swallowing; swallow Nexavar tablets whole.

Avoid situations in which bruising or injury may occur.

Do not suddenly stop taking Nexavar, even if you feel better.

What are possible food and drug interactions associated with Nexavar?
If Nexavar is taken with certain other drugs, the effects of either could be increased, decreased, or altered. It is especially important to check with

your doctor before combining Nexavar with the following: doxorubicin (Adriamycin, Doxil); irinotecan (Camptosar); and warfarin (Coumadin).

What are the possible side effects of Nexavar?
Side effects cannot be anticipated. If any develop or change in intensity, tell your doctor as soon as possible. Only your doctor can determine if it is safe for you to continue taking this drug.

Side effects may include: birth defects or fetal death, heart problems, high blood pressure, loss of appetite, mouth sores, nausea, numbness, skin problems, thinning hair, tingling on the hands or feet, vomiting, weakness

Nexavar may reduce the number of clot-forming cells (platelets) in your blood. To prevent bleeding, avoid situations in which bruising or injury may occur. Report unusual bleeding, bruising, blood in stools, or dark, tarry stools to your doctor.

Nexavar may lower your body's ability to fight infection. Prevent infection by avoiding contact with people with colds or other infections. Notify your doctor of any signs of infection, including fever, sore throat, rash, or chills.

Can I receive Nexavar if I am pregnant or breastfeeding?
Nexavar may cause birth defects or death to an unborn child. Do not take Nexavar if you are pregnant, plan to become pregnant, or are nursing. Do not breast feed while you are taking Nexavar because this drug may pass into breast milk. If you think you may be pregnant, contact your doctor.

What should I do if I miss a dose of Nexavar?
If you miss a dose of Nexavar, skip the missed dose and go back to your regular dosing schedule. Do not take 2 doses at once.

How should I store Nexavar?
Store Nexavar at 77 degrees F (25 degrees C). Brief storage at temperatures between 59 and 86 degrees F (15 and 30 degrees C) is permitted. Store away from heat, moisture, and light. Do not store in the bathroom. Keep Nexavar out of the reach of children.

NEXIUM
Generic name: Esomeprazole magnesium

What is Nexium?
Nexium is used to treat several acid-related problems. Nexium may be prescribed for gastroesophageal reflux disease (GERD), commonly known as acid reflux disease. Nexium is also used to treat erosive esophagitis, which is caused by acid rising up and eroding the lining of the esophagus over time.

Nexium may also be used to reduce the risk of gastric ulcers in people on continuous therapy with anti-inflammatory drugs that do not contain steroids. Nexium may also be prescribed in combination with amoxicillin and clarithromycin in order to treat *H. Pylori* infection and ulcers. Nexium can also be used as a long-term treatment for certain conditions involving excessive bodily secretions, including Zollinger-Ellison Syndrome.

What is the most important information I should know about Nexium?

Nexium capsules should be swallowed whole. Do not crush or chew the capsules.

Nexium may be prescribed to you in combination with amoxicillin and clarithromycin. Amoxicillin and clarithromycin can occasionally cause severe side effects. If you are pregnant, do not use clarithromycin, except if no alternative therapy is appropriate. Clarithromycin and amoxicillin may both cause an inflammatory disease of the colon that can range from mild to life-threatening. If you are taking amoxicillin, it is important to know that serious and occasionally fatal reactions have been reported in patients on penicillin therapy. If you have a history of penicillin allergies, and/or a history of sensitivity to multiple allergens, be sure to tell your doctor.

Take Nexium exactly as prescribed by your doctor. Do not change your dose or stop taking the medication without talking to your doctor.

Take this medication for the entire length of time prescribed by your doctor. Your symptoms may get better before your treatment is completed.

Who should not take Nexium?

Do not take Nexium if you are allergic to the medication or any of its ingredients. You should not take Nexium if you have been allergic to other protein pump inhibitors (PPIs) in the past.

What should I tell my doctor before I take the first dose of Nexium?

Tell your doctor about all prescription, over-the-counter, and herbal medication you are taking before beginning treatment with Nexium. Also, be sure to tell your doctor if you have any drug allergies; a history of liver problems; are pregnant, think you may be pregnant, or are planning to become pregnant; are breastfeeding or planning to breastfeed.

What is the usual dosage?

The information below is based on the dosage guidelines your doctor uses. Depending on your condition and medical history, your doctor may prescribe a different regimen. Do not change the dosage or stop taking your medication without your doctor's approval.

Erosive Esophagitis

Adults: The usual dose for healing erosive esophagitis is 20 milligrams (mg) or 40 mg taken 1 time each day for 4 to 8 weeks. Your doctor may recommend an additional 4-8 weeks of treatment if you do not heal after the initial 4-8 weeks of treatment. The usual dose for maintaining the healing of erosive esophagitis is 20 mg taken 1 time a day.

Gastroesophageal Reflux Disease (GERD)

Adults: The usual dose for relief of GERD symptoms is 20 mg taken 1 time each day for 4 weeks. Your doctor may recommend an additional 4 weeks of treatment if you do not heal after the initial 4 weeks of treatment.

Risk Reduction of Duodenal Ulcer Recurrence

Adults: This treatment involves taking three different medications. The usual dose for the triple therapy is: Nexium 40 mg taken 1 time each day for 10 days, Amoxicillin 1000 mg taken 2 times each day for 10 days, and Clarithromycin 500 mg taken 2 times each day for 10 days.

Risk Reduction of Gastric Ulcer

Adults: The usual dose is 20 mg or 40 mg taken 1 time each day for up to 6 months.

Treatment of Hypersecretory Conditions Including Zollinger-Ellison Syndrome

Adults: The usual dose is 40 mg taken 2 times each day. However, treatment of patients with these conditions varies with the individual patient. Doses up to 240 mg have been administered. Nexium can be used for long-term treatment in these patients.

Short-term Treatment of GERD

Adolescents 12 to 17 years old: The usual dose is 20 or 40 mg of taken 1 time each day for up to 8 weeks.

Short-term Treatment of Symptomatic GERD

Pediatrics 1 to 11 years old: The usual dose is 10 mg taken 1 time each day for up to 8 weeks.

Healing of Erosive Esophagitis

Pediatrics 1 to 11 years old: If the child weighs less than 20 kilograms, the usual dose is 10 mg taken once daily for up to 8 weeks. If the child weighs 20 kilograms or more, the usual dose is 10 mg to 20 mg taken once a day for up to 8 weeks.

Adults: Daily doses over 1 mg per kilogram have not been studied.

How should I take Nexium?

Nexium Delayed-Release Capsules should be swallowed whole and taken at least 1 hour before eating. If you have difficulty swallowing capsules, you can add 1 tablespoon of applesauce to an empty bowl and the Nexium Delayed-Release Capsule can be opened, and the granules inside the capsule carefully emptied onto the applesauce. Mix the granules with the applesauce and then swallow the mixture immediately. The applesauce used should not be hot and should be soft enough to be swallowed without chewing. Do not chew or crush the granules. Do not store the mixture of applesauce and granules for future use. Discard the empty capsule.

Nexium Delayed-Release Oral Suspension should be taken 1 hour before meals. To prepare the suspension, empty the contents of a 20 or 40 mg packet into a container with 1 tablespoon of water in it. Stir the suspension and let it sit for 2 to 3 minutes to thicken. Stir the suspension again and drink it within 30 minutes. If any suspension remains in the container after you drink it, add more water, stir, and drink immediately.

If you have a nasogastric or gastric tube in place, talk to your doctor about how you should take Nexium Delayed-Release Capsules or Oral Suspension.

Antacids may be used while taking Nexium.

Take Nexium exactly as prescribed by your doctor. Do not change your dose or stop taking the medication without talking to your doctor.

Take this medication for the entire length of time prescribed by your doctor. Your symptoms may get better before your treatment is completed.

What should I avoid while taking Nexium?

Avoid taking Nexium with food. Take Nexium at least 1 hour before meals.

Do not change your dose or stop taking the medication without talking to your doctor.

What are possible food and drug interactions associated with Nexium?

If Nexium is taken with certain other drugs, the effects of either could be increased, decreased, or altered. It is especially important to check with your doctor before combining Nexium with the following: atazanavir, digoxin, iron salts or products that contain iron, ketoconazole, voriconazole, and warfarin.

What are the possible side effects of Nexium?

Side effects cannot be anticipated. If any develop or change in intensity, tell your doctor as soon as possible. Only your doctor can determine if it is safe for you to continue taking this drug.

Side effects may include: abdominal pain, constipation, diarrhea, dry mouth, flatulence, headache, nausea

Can I receive Nexium if I am pregnant or breastfeeding?

The effects of Nexium during pregnancy are unknown. Tell your doctor immediately if you are pregnant, or plan to become pregnant.

You should not breastfeed while taking Nexium. It is unknown if the drug passes into breast milk or if it could harm your baby.

What should I do if I miss a dose of Nexium?
Take the missed dose as soon as you remember. If it is almost time for your next dose, skip the missed dose and take the medicine at the next regularly scheduled time. Do not take extra medicine to make up the missed dose.

How should I store Nexium?
Store Nexium at room temperature in a tightly closed container.

Niacin See Niaspan, below.

NIASPAN
Generic name: Niacin

What is Niaspan?
Niaspan is a medication that is used along with diet and exercise to improve cholesterol levels. Niaspan increases "good" HDL cholesterol in your body and also lowers the "bad" LDL cholesterol and triglycerides in your body. Niaspan is for people whose cholesterol has not come down enough with exercise and a low-fat diet alone.

Niaspan is also prescribed to combat clogged arteries, heart disease, and lower the chance of repeated heart attacks. Niaspan is often taken along with another drug called a bile acid binding resin. It can also be prescribed with statins. Niaspan is also used to reduce very high levels of the blood fats known as triglycerides, a condition that can cause inflammation of the pancreas.

What is the most important information I should know about Niaspan?
Taking Niaspan is not a substitute for following a healthy low-fat and low-cholesterol diet and exercising to lower your cholesterol.

Niaspan preparations should not be substituted for equivalent doses of immediate-release niacin. If you make such a substitution in your medications, it may lead to very severe liver problems. If you are switching from immediate-release niacin to Niaspan, which is delayed-release, therapy with Niaspan should start with low doses and the Niaspan dose should then be titrated to get the desired response. Your doctor will perform liver tests on you while you are taking Niaspan.

Use Niaspan with caution in patients who consume substantial quantities of alcohol and/or have a past history of liver disease due to the possible side effects that may occur.

If you are currently on both a HMG-CoA reductase inhibitor (also known as a "statin") and Niaspan, you should carefully monitor for any signs and symptoms of muscle pain, tenderness, or weakness, particularly during the initial months of therapy and when the dose of either drug is being increased. The potential benefits and risks should be weighed carefully before combining these medicines.

Do not drive or perform other possibly unsafe tasks until you know how you react to Niaspan; this drug may cause dizziness or lightheadedness. These effects may be worse if you take it with alcohol or certain medicines.

Niaspan may cause dizziness; alcohol, hot weather, exercise, or fever may increase this effect. To prevent it, sit up or stand slowly, especially in the morning. Sit or lie down at the first sign of this effect.

If you stop taking Niaspan for an extended period, contact your doctor before you start taking it again. Your dose may need to be adjusted.

Flushing occurs with Niaspan and may last for several hours. Talk with your doctor if flushing becomes bothersome. Take Niaspan at bedtime so that flushing will occur during sleep. If you are awakened by flushing at night, get up slowly, especially if you feel dizzy or faint or if you are taking blood thinners. Take aspirin or a nonsteroidal anti-inflammatory drug (NSAID) (such as ibuprofen) 30 minutes before taking Niaspan to lessen flushing.

Niaspan may cause the results of some tests for urine glucose to be wrong. Ask your doctor before you change your diet or the dose of your diabetes medicine.

Do not take large doses of vitamins while you use Niaspan unless your doctor tells you to.

Who should not take Niaspan?
Do not take Niaspan if you are allergic to the medication or any of its ingredients. Also, do not take Niaspan if you have liver disease, active peptic ulcer disease, or a history of arterial bleeding.

What should I tell my doctor before I take the first dose of Niaspan?
Tell your doctor about all prescription, over-the-counter, and herbal medication you are taking before beginning treatment with Niaspan. Also, talk to your doctor about your complete medical history, especially if you have heart, kidney, or liver problems. Tell your doctor if you have diabetes; muscle pain or disease; gallbladder problems; history of bleeding; consume large amounts of alcohol; have severe low blood pressure, gout, or a history of jaundice (yellowing of your skin or eyes related to liver problems).

What is the usual dosage?
The information below is based on the dosage guidelines your doctor uses. Depending on your condition and medical history, your doctor

may prescribe a different regimen. Do not change the dosage or stop taking your medication without your doctor's approval.

Adults 21 and older: The usual starting dose is 500 milligrams (mg) taken 1 time each day at bed time. Every 4 weeks, your doctor may increase your dosage by no more than 500 mg. The recommended maintenance dose is 1000 mg (two 500 mg tablets or one 1000 mg tablet) to a maximum of 2000 mg (two 1000 mg or four 500 mg tablets) daily. Women may respond to lower doses than men.

If Niaspan is discontinued for an extended period of time, the drug should be reintroduced with small increases in dose made over a period of time.

How should I take Niaspan?

Take each dose of Niaspan with a full glass of water at bedtime, after a low-fat snack (such as low-fat yogurt, banana, or crackers with a glass of milk). It is not recommended to take Niaspan on an empty stomach. Swallow Niaspan whole. Do not crush, chew, or break the tablets. To lessen the chance of side effects such as flushing, avoid alcohol, hot beverages, and spicy foods near the time you take Niaspan. Flushing is when your face, neck, chest, and back become red, warm, itchy, or if you feel a tingling sensation on any of these areas of your body. Your doctor may also tell you to take aspirin or a nonsteroidal anti-inflammatory drug 30 minutes before taking Niaspan in order to help prevent flushing.

If you are taking Niaspan with bile acid-binding resins, you should wait 4 to 6 hours, or as much time as possible, between the time when you take the bile acid-binding resins and the time when you take Niaspan.

What should I avoid while taking Niaspan?

Avoid hot or alcoholic beverages and do not eat spicy foods around the time when you take Niaspan. Do not break, crush, or chew Niaspan caplets.

Do not drive or perform other possibly unsafe tasks until you know how you react to Niaspan; this drug may cause dizziness or lightheadedness.

Avoid sitting or standing up too quickly when you are taking Niaspan, especially in the morning or in the middle of the night. Sit or lie down at the first sign of dizziness, a side effect of Niaspan.

Do not take large doses of vitamins while you use Niaspan unless your doctor tells you to.

What are possible food and drug interactions associated with Niaspan?

If Niaspan is taken with certain other drugs, the effects of either could be increased, decreased, or altered. It is especially important to check with your doctor before combining Niaspan with the following: alcohol or hot drinks, anticoagulants such as warfarin, antihypertensive therapy, aspirin, cholesterol-lowering drugs known as bile acid sequestrants, fibrates such as gemfibrozil, HMG-CoA reductase inhibitors such as lovastatin, or vitamins or other nutritional supplements containing large doses of niacin.

What are the possible side effects of Niaspan?
Side effects cannot be anticipated. If any develop or change in intensity, tell your doctor as soon as possible. Only your doctor can determine if it is safe for you to continue taking this drug.

Taking multivitamins containing large doses of niacin and related compounds may increase the chance of side effects from Niaspan.

Side effects may include: abdominal pain, chills, diarrhea, dizziness, fainting, flushing, headache, indigestion, itching, nasal inflammation, nausea, pain, rapid heartbeat, rash, shortness of breath, skipped beat during heartbeat, sweating, swelling, vomiting

In rare cases, it may be possible for people who take Niaspan along with cholesterol-lowering medications called statins, like lovastatin, to develop muscle aches and pains, muscle disintegration, or muscle disease. Tell your doctor if you experience any muscle pain, tenderness, or weakness.

Flushing occurs with Niaspan and may last for several hours. Talk with your doctor if flushing becomes bothersome. Take Niaspan at bedtime so that flushing will occur during sleep. If you are awakened by flushing at night, get up slowly, especially if you feel dizzy or faint or if you are taking blood thinners. Take aspirin or a nonsteroidal anti-inflammatory drug (NSAID) (such as ibuprofen) 30 minutes before taking Niaspan to lessen flushing.

Can I receive Niaspan if I am pregnant or breastfeeding?
The effects of Niaspan during pregnancy are unknown. Tell your doctor immediately if you are pregnant or plan to become pregnant. Talk to your doctor if you are breastfeeding; Niaspan is found in breast milk and may cause harm to your baby.

What should I do if I miss a dose of Niaspan?
If you miss a dose of Niaspan and you are taking 1 dose daily at bedtime, skip the missed dose. Do not take the dose in the morning or 2 doses at once. Continue your regular dosing regimen after the missed dose.

How should I store Niaspan?
Store Niaspan at room temperature. Store away from heat, moisture, and light. Do not store in the bathroom. Keep Niaspan out of the reach of children.

Nicardipine hydrochloride See Cardene/Cardene SR,
  page 252.

Nicotine See Nicotrol, below.

Nicotine nasal spray See Nicotrol NS, page 889.

NICOTROL
Generic name: Nicotine

What is Nicotrol?
Nicotrol inhaler is used as an aid to smoking cessation for the relief of
nicotine withdrawal symptoms.

What is the most important information
I should know about Nicotrol?
Do not use more than 16 cartridges per day unless directed to do so by
your doctor. Do not use longer than 6 months. Nicotine from any source
can be toxic and addictive.

  Smoking causes lung disease, cancer, and heart disease, and may ad-
versely affect pregnant women or the fetus. You should not continue to
smoke while using Nicotrol; you may experience adverse effects due to
peak nicotine levels higher than those experienced from smoking alone.

Who should not take Nicotrol?
You should not use Nicotrol if you are hypersensitive or allergic to nicotine or to menthol.

What should I tell my doctor before
I take the first dose of Nicotrol?
Tell your doctor about any medication you are taking. Check with your
doctor before taking any new medicine while using Nicotrol. Tell your
doctor if you have heart problems (recent heart attacks, irregular heartbeat, severe or worsening heart pain), stomach ulcers, overactive thyroid, high blood pressure, allergies to drugs, diabetes requiring insulin,
kidney or liver disease, wheezing or asthma.

What is the usual dosage?
**The information below is based on the dosage guidelines your doctor
uses. Depending on your condition and medical history, your doctor
may prescribe a different regimen. Do not change the dosage or stop
taking your medication without your doctor's approval.**

  For up to 12 weeks, the recommended number of cartridges per day
is 6-16.

How should I take Nicotrol?

Stop smoking completely during the Nicotrol treatment.

Take out cartridge tray, peel back to release 1 cartridge, insert cartridge into inhaler, and push hard on the cartridge until it pops down into place.

Line up the marking again and push the two pieces back together so they fit tight. Turn the top and bottom pieces so the markings do not line up and it is locked again. Store cartridges in plastic case when in use.

Inhale deeply into back of throat or puff in short breaths. As you inhale or puff through the mouthpiece, nicotine turns into a vapor and is inhaled.

Nicotine in cartridges is used up after about 20 minutes of active puffing.

When cartridge is empty, take off the top of mouthpiece and throw cartridge away. Wash mouthpiece with soap and water.

What should I avoid while taking Nicotrol?

You should not smoke while using Nicotrol.

What are possible food and drug interactions associated with Nicotrol?

If Nicotrol is used with certain other drugs, the effects of either could be increased, decreased, or altered. It is especially important to check with your doctor before combining Nicotrol with tricyclic antidepressants and theophylline.

What are the possible side effects of Nicotrol?

Many people experience mild irritation of the mouth or throat and cough when they first use Nicotrol. Stomach upset may occur.

Can I receive Nicotrol if I am pregnant or breastfeeding?

The specific effects of Nicotrol Inhaler therapy on fetal development are unknown. The safety of Nicotrol in nursing has not been examined, but nicotine passes freely into breast milk. Tell your doctor if you are pregnant, plan to become pregnant, or are breastfeeding.

What should I do if I miss a dose of Nicotrol?

Nicotrol is not used on a daily regimen. It is used as a therapy to stop patients from smoking. If you miss a dose, you do not have to double the next dose.

How should I store Nicotrol?

Store at room temperature. Protect from light.

NICOTROL NS
Generic name: Nicotine nasal spray

What is Nicotrol NS?
Nicotrol helps you quit smoking by providing low levels of nicotine, which may help you to quit by lessening physical signs of withdrawal symptoms.

What is the most important information I should know about Nicotrol NS?
It is possible to become dependent to Nicotrol . The product is less addictive than cigarettes but nearly a third of the people using it report some feelings of dependence, and 15% to 20% of patients use the product for longer than the recommended period. Nicotrol has not been studied for more than 6 months. Long-term use is not recommended.

For Nicotrol work effectively, you must be firmly committed to quitting smoking. Stop smoking as soon as you start using Nicotrol . Do not smoke or use any other tobacco product at any time while under treatment with Nicotrol; nicotine overdose can occur. (Symptoms include: bad headaches, dizziness, upset stomach, drooling, vomiting, diarrhea, cold sweat, blurred vision, hearing difficulties, mental confusion, weakness, and fainting.) If you experience any symptoms of nicotine overdose, call your doctor.

Nicotrol may cause dizziness, lightheadedness, or blurred vision. Do not drive, operate machinery, or do anything else that could be dangerous until you know how you react to Nicotrol . Using Nicotrol alone, with certain other medicines, or with alcohol may lessen your ability to drive or perform other potentially dangerous tasks.

Before you have any medical or dental treatments, emergency care, or surgery, tell your healthcare provider that you are using Nicotrol.

Be careful while opening and closing the container of medicine. The container may break if it is dropped. If this happens, clean the spill up immediately with an absorbent cloth or paper towel. Avoid contact with the skin. Pick up broken glass carefully, using a broom. Wash the area several times. The absorbent material may be thrown away as household waste. If even a small amount of Nicotrol contacts your skin, lips, eyes, ears, or the affected area, immediately rinse the area with water only.

Nicotrol may affect your blood sugar. Check blood sugar levels closely and ask your doctor before adjusting the dose of your diabetes medicine.

Do not suddenly stop taking Nicotrol without your doctor's approval. Stopping Nicotrol suddenly may cause serious withdrawal symptoms including: anxiety, craving, impaired concentration, increased appetite, irritability, nervousness, sleep disturbances, and weight gain. If you experience any of these symptoms, contact your doctor.

Who should not take Nicotrol NS?

Do not use Nicotrol NS Spray if you have had a recent heart attack, you have severe chest pain or a severely irregular heartbeat, you continue to smoke, chew tobacco, use snuff or any other nicotine containing products (nicotine overdose may occur); or if you are allergic to any ingredient in Nicotrol NS Spray.

Contact your doctor or healthcare provider right away if any of these apply to you.

What should I tell my doctor before I take the first dose of Nicotrol NS?

Tell your doctor about all prescription, over-the-counter, and herbal medications you are taking before beginning treatment with Nicotrol. Also, talk to your doctor about your complete medical history, especially if you have blood vessel problems; chronic nasal problems such as nasal allergies, inflammation, sinusitis, or nasal polyps (growths); diabetes requiring insulin; drug allergies; heart problems (recent heart attack, irregular heartbeat, severe or worsening heart pain); high blood pressure; kidney or liver disease; overactive thyroid; stomach ulcers; or wheezing or asthma.

What is the usual dosage?

The information below is based on the dosage guidelines your doctor uses. Depending on your condition and medical history, your doctor may prescribe a different regimen. Do not change the dosage or stop taking your medication without your doctor's approval.

Adults: The usual starting dose is 1 spray in each nostril (a total of 2 sprays). One or 2 doses per hour is recommended. Take no more than 5 doses per hour or 40 doses per day. During the treatment period, a minimum of 8 doses per day is usually needed for the drug to be effective.

The dose of Nicotrol should be individualized on the basis of your nicotine dependence and the occurrence of symptoms associated with nicotine excess. The success or failure of smoking cessation is influenced by the quality, intensity and frequency of supportive care. You are more likely to quit smoking if you frequently participate in formal smoking cessation programs. The goal of Nicotrol therapy is complete abstinence from smoking. If you are unable to stop smoking by the fourth week of therapy, treatment should probably be discontinued.

Recommended strategies for discontinuation of Nicotrol NS include: use only ½ a dose (1 spray) at a time, use the spray less frequently, keep a tally of daily usage, try to meet a steadily reducing usage target, skip a dose by not medicating every hour, or set a planned "quit date" for stopping use of the spray.

How should I take Nicotrol NS?

Nicotrol NS Spray comes with an additional patient leaflet. Read it carefully and reread it each time you get Nicotrol refilled.

Avoid contact with skin, eyes, and mouth. If the bottle breaks, wear rubber gloves, wipe up with paper towel and wash surfaces thoroughly. Do not let nicotine come in contact with your skin, mouth, or eyes. If it does, rinse with plain water immediately. Nicotine overdose can occur when nicotine is absorbed through the skin. If symptoms of overdose occur call your doctor.

Use as directed by your doctor. However, do not use more than 5 times an hour or 40 times in 24 hours. Stop smoking completely during Nicotrol treatment program.

To use Nicotrol, press in circles on the sides of the bottle and pull off the cap. Prime the pump before the first use. Get a tissue or paper towel. Hold the bottle so that your thumb is under the flat part (bottom) of the bottle and your index finger is at the base of the nozzle. (Do not touch the nozzle of the spray.) While holding the bottle, use your thumb to press up from the bottom of the bottle. Pump into a tissue until you see a fine spray (6 to 8 times). Throw the tissue away.

Blow nose if it is not clear. Tilt head back slightly. Insert tip of bottle into nostril as far as is comfortable. Breathe through mouth. Spray once in each nostril. Do not sniff or inhale while spraying. If nose runs, gently sniff to keep the medicine in nose. Wait 2 or 3 minutes before blowing nose.

Place cap back on bottle after use. If you don't use the Nasal Spray for 24 hours, prime the pump into a tissue 1 or 2 times.

What should I avoid while taking Nicotrol NS?

Do not sniff, swallow, or inhale through the nose while the spray is being used. Avoid contact with skin, eyes, and mouth. Avoid excessive priming.

Do not use more than 1 spray in each nostril for a dose without checking with your doctor.

Do not smoke or use any other tobacco product at any time while under treatment with Nicotrol because nicotine overdose can occur.

Do not stop taking Nicotrol without speaking to your doctor first; withdrawal symptoms may occur.

Do not drive, operate machinery, or do anything else that could be dangerous until you know how you react to Nicotrol. Nicotrol may cause dizziness, lightheadedness, or blurred vision.

What are possible food and drug interactions associated with Nicotrol NS?

If Nicotrol is used with certain other drugs, the effects of either could be increased, decreased, or altered. It is especially important to check with your doctor before combining Nicotrol with the following: airway-opening products such as Isuprel, Afrin, and Neo-Synephrine; acetaminophen-containing products; caffeine-containing products such as No-Doz; heart medications known as beta blockers; imipramine; insulin; labetalol; oxazepam; pentazocine; prazosin; theophylline; and tricyclic antidepressants such as amitriptyline.

What are the possible side effects of Nicotrol NS?

Side effects cannot be anticipated. If any develop or change in intensity, tell your doctor as soon as possible. Only your doctor can determine if it is safe for you to continue taking this drug.

Side effects may include: acne; back pain; burning or irritation of the mouth, nose, or eyes; changes in taste and smell; constipation; cough; earache; flushing of the face; gas; headache; hoarseness; indigestion; irritability; joint pain; mouth sores; nasal ulcers or blisters; nausea; nose bleed; numbness of the mouth; painful menstruation; runny nose; sinus irritation; sneezing; sore throat; stuffy nose; tingling; tooth disorder; watery eyes

Serious side effects may include: Severe allergic reactions (rash, hives, difficulty breathing, tightness in the chest, swelling of the mouth, face, lips, or tongue); fast or irregular heartbeat; lightheadedness; memory loss; severe dizziness or headache; shortness of breath; tightness in the chest; tremor. Seek medical attention right away if any of these occur.

Symptoms of nicotine overdose include: bad headaches, dizziness, upset stomach, drooling, vomiting, diarrhea, cold sweat, blurred vision, hearing difficulties, mental confusion, weakness, and fainting. Call your doctor if these occur.

Serious withdrawal symptoms include: anxiety, craving, impaired concentration, increased appetite, irritability, nervousness, sleep disturbances, and weight gain. Call your doctor if these occur.

Can I receive Nicotrol NS if I am pregnant or breastfeeding?

Nicotine from any source can harm a developing baby. If you're pregnant, it's best to quit without a nicotine replacement product.

Nicotine is found in breast milk. A nursing infant may be exposed to less nicotine from Nicotrol than from cigarette smoking, but the best course is to avoid nicotine entirely.

What should I do if I miss a dose of Nicotrol NS?

If you miss a dose of this medicine, use it as soon as possible. If it is almost time for your next dose, skip the missed dose and go back to your regular dosing schedule. Do not use 2 doses at once.

How should I store Nicotrol NS?

Store at room temperature away from heat, moisture, and light. Do not store in the bathroom.

Nifedipine *See Procardia, page 1076.*

Nisoldipine *See Sular, page 1229.*

Nitazoxanide *See Alinia, page 62.*

Nitrofurantoin macrocrystals *See Macrodantin, page 785.*

NITROGLYCERIN

What is Nitroglycerin?

Nitroglycerin is used to treat chest pain, or angina pectoris (ischemic heart disease). It is available in tablets, capsules, ointment, solution for intravenous use, transdermal patches (placed on the skin), or sprays administered sublingually (held under the tongue).

The patch and the ointment are for *prevention* of chest pain.

In the form of sublingual (held under the tongue) or buccal (held in the cheek) tablets, or in oral spray (sprayed on or under the tongue), nitroglycerin helps relieve chest pain that has already occurred. The spray can also prevent anginal pain. The type of nitroglycerin you use will depend on your condition.

What is the most important information I should know about Nitroglycerin?

Nitroglycerin may cause severe low blood pressure (possibly marked by dizziness or light-headedness), especially if you are in an upright position or have just gotten up from sitting or lying down. You may also find your heart rate slowing and your chest pain increasing. People taking diuretic medication (water pills), or who have low systolic blood pressure (less than 90 mm Hg), should use nitroglycerin with caution. This effect may be more frequent in patients who have also consumed alcohol.

Since nitroglycerin can cause dizziness, you should observe caution while driving, operating machinery, or performing other tasks that demand concentration.

Nitroglycerin tablets lose their effectiveness when exposed to air. If you are taking sublingual (held under the tongue) nitroglycerin, you may notice a burning or tingling sensation. This does not necessarily mean that tablets that have been exposed to air for a long period of time are still effective.

Daily headaches sometimes accompany treatment with nitroglycerin. Patients should resist the temptation to avoid headaches by altering the schedule of their treatment with nitroglycerin, since loss of headache may be associated with simultaneous loss of efficacy.

To avoid tooth and gum decay, vary location sites and brush your teeth after the tablet has completely dissolved.

Do not fall asleep with a tablet in your mouth.

Who should not take Nitroglycerin?

Do not take nitroglycerin if you are allergic to the medication or any of its ingredients.

The capsule form should not be used if you have closed-angle glaucoma (pressure in the eye). Do not take nitroglycerin spray if you are currently taking a phosphodiesterase type 5 inhibitor (such as Viagra) for erectile dysfunction; the concomitant use of these 2 medications may cause postural hypotension (dizziness upon standing up).

Do not use nitroglycerin patches if you are allergic to the adhesive.

What should I tell my doctor before I take the first dose of Nitroglycerin?

Tell your doctor about all prescription, over-the-counter, and herbal medications you are taking before beginning treatment with nitroglycerin. Also, talk to your doctor about your complete medical history, especially if you have had a recent heart attack, head injury, or stroke; or if you have anemia, low blood pressure, glaucoma (pressure in the eye), or heart, kidney, liver, or thyroid disease.

What is the usual dosage?

The information below is based on the dosage guidelines your doctor uses. Depending on your condition and medical history, your doctor may prescribe a different regimen. Do not change the dosage or stop taking your medication without your doctor's approval.

Adults: Sublingual or Buccal Tablets: At the first sign of chest pain, 1 tablet should be dissolved under the tongue or inside the cheek. You may repeat the dose every 5 minutes until the pain is relieved. If your pain continues after you have taken 3 tablets in a 15-minute period, notify your doctor or seek medical attention immediately. You may take sublingual or buccal nitroglycerin from 5 to 10 minutes before starting activities that may cause chest pain. *Patch:* A patch is applied to the skin for 12 to 14 hours. After this time, the patch is removed; it is not applied again for 10 to 12 hours (a "patch-off" period). Apply the patch as soon as you remove it from its protective pouch. Spray: At the first sign of chest pain, spray 1 or 2 premeasured doses onto or under the tongue. You should not use more than 3 sprays within a 15-minute period. If your chest pain continues, you should contact your doctor or seek medical attention immediately. The spray can be used 5 to 10 minutes before activity that might precipitate an attack, such as exercise. *Ointment:* The usual starting dose may be a daily total of 1 inch of ointment. Apply one-half inch on rising in the morning, and the remaining one-half inch 6 hours later. If needed, follow your doctor's instructions for increasing your dosage. Apply in a thin, uniform layer, regardless of the amount of your dosage. There should be a daily period where no ointment is applied. Usually, the "ointment-off" period will last from 10 to 12 hours. The dose could be doubled, and even doubled again, in patients tolerating this dose but failing to respond to it. Absorption varies with site of application; more is absorbed through the chest. *Sustained-Release Capsules or Tablets:* The smallest effective amount should be taken 2 or 3 times a day at 8- to 12-hour intervals.

Children: The safety and effectiveness of nitroglycerin have not been established for children.

How should I take Nitroglycerin?

If you use a patch, dispose of it carefully. There is enough drug left in a used patch to be harmful to children and pets.

Nitroglycerin is available in many forms. It is extremely important for you to follow your doctor's directions for taking the type of nitroglycerin prescribed for you. Never interchange brands.

For changes in dosage and frequency of application consult your physician. Dosage instructions should be obtained from your physician.

Ointment: One appropriate dosing schedule for the ointment would begin with two daily ½ inch (7.5 mg) doses, one applied on rising in the morning and one applied six hours later. The foilpac is intended as a unit dose package only and is equivalent to approximately 1 inch as squeezed from the tube. Use entire contents of foilpac to obtain full dose and discard immediately after use.

To apply, measure desired dosage of Nitroglycerin Ointment 2% by means of the dose measuring applicator supplied with the tube. Place the applicator on a flat surface, printed side down. Squeeze the necessary amount of ointment from the tube onto the applicator, and place the applicator (ointment side down) on the desired area of the skin.

Spread the ointment using the dose measuring applicator lightly onto the chest or other areas of skin if preferred. Do not rub into the skin. Coverage of an area approximately the size of the dose measuring applicator (3½" by 2¼") should be sufficient to obtain the desired clinical effects. A larger area may be used.

Tape the applicator into place. The ointment can stain clothing. Care should be taken to completely cover the dose measuring applicator with a plastic kitchen wrap.

Spray: At the first sign of chest pain, spray 1 or 2 premeasured doses onto or under the tongue. You should not use more than 3 sparys within a 15-minute period. If your chest pain continues, you should contact your doctor or seek medical attention immediately.

The spray can be used 5 to 10 minutes before activity that might precipitate an attack, such as exercise.

Patch: Nitroglycerin Patch comes with an additional patient leaflet. Read it carefully and reread it each time you get Nitroglycerin Patch refilled.

Nitroglycerin Patch is for external use only.

Wash your hands thoroughly before and after applying. Apply the patch to the chest, inner side of the upper arm, or shoulder. Clean and dry the skin before applying the patch. If necessary, hair may be removed by clipping.

Remove the patch from the package. Apply with a firm pressure to the skin. To avoid skin irritation, change the treatment site daily. Do not apply to irritated or damaged skin.

If the patch becomes loose, remove it and apply a new patch at a different site. After you remove the used patch, fold the sticky side together and throw away. This patch should only be worn for up to 12 to 14 hours a day, or as directed by your doctor, so that you will have a 10 to 12 hour "nitrate-free" period each day. Do not use more of Nitroglycerin Patch than prescribed. It is important to have a "nitrate-free" period of time each day for Nitroglycerin Patch to continue to work well and to decrease the risk of physical dependence.

Sublingual or Buccal Tablets: At the first sign of chest pain, 1 tablet should be dissolved under the tongue or inside the cheek. You may repeat the dose every 5 minutes until the pain is relieved. If your pain continues after you have taken 3 tablets in a 15-minute period, notify your doctor or seek medical attention immediately.

You may take sublingual or buccal nitroglycerin from 5 to 10 minutes before starting activities that may cause chest pain.

What should I avoid while taking Nitroglycerin?

Do not shake container before administering dose.

Daily headaches may be an indicator of the drug's activity. Do not change your dose to avoid the headache, because you may reduce the drug's effectiveness at the same time.

Avoid alcohol intake.

What are possible food and drug interactions associated with Nitroglycerin?

If Nitroglycerin is taken with certain other drugs, the effects of either could be increased, decreased, or altered. It is especially important to check with your doctor before combining nitroglycerin with the following: alcohol, alteplase, aspirin, blood vessel dilators such as Loniten, dihydroergotamine (D.H.E.), erectile dysfunction drugs such as Viagra, heart medications known as beta-blockers and calcium channel blockers, and salicylates.

What are the possible side effects of Nitroglycerin?

Side effects cannot be anticipated. If any develop or change in intensity, tell your doctor as soon as possible. Only your doctor can determine if it is safe for you to continue taking this drug.

Side effects may include: dizziness, flushed skin (neck and face), head-ache, heavy sweating, light-headedness, nausea, worsened angina (chest) pain.

Can I receive Nitroglycerin if I am pregnant or breastfeeding?
The effects of nitroglycerin during pregnancy and breastfeeding are un-known. Tell your doctor immediately if you are pregnant, plan to become pregnant, or are breastfeeding.

What should I do if I miss a dose of Nitroglycerin?
If you are using a skin patch or ointment, apply it as soon as you remem-ber. If it is almost time for your regular dose, skip the one you missed and go back to your regular schedule. Never apply 2 skin patches at the same time.

If you are taking oral tablets or capsules, never double your dose of nitroglycerin if you miss a dose. Skip the missed dose and return to your regular schedule.

How should I store Nitroglycerin?
Keep nitroglycerin in the container it came in, tightly closed. Store it at room temperature. Do not refrigerate.

Avoid puncturing the spray container and keep it away from excess heat.

Do not open the container of sublingual tablets until you need a dose. Close the container tightly immediately after each use. Do not put other medications, a cotton plug, or anything else in the container.

Keep the sublingual tablets handy at all times. Keep the patches in the protective pouches they come in until use.

NITROMIST
Generic name: Nitroglycerin

What is NitroMist?
NitroMist is a nitrate vasodilator which has effects on both arteries and veins. It is sprayed on or under the tongue at the onset of chest pain to prevent and treat an angina attack.

What is the most important information
I should know about NitroMist?
NitroMist may cause severe low blood pressure. Treatment with nitro-glycerin products such as NitroMist may be associated with lightheaded-ness, especially just after rising from a laying or seated position. This effect may be more frequent in patients who have consumed alcohol, since alcohol use contributes to hypotension. If possible, patients should

be seated when taking NitroMist. This reduces the likelihood of falling due to lightheadedness or dizziness.

Frequent use of NitroMist may cause you to have a decreased response to treatment.

Nitrate therapy may worsen angina and other heart-related diseases.

Who should not take NitroMist?
Do not take NitroMist if you are using erectile dysfunction drugs such as Viagra (sildenafil), Levitra (vardenafil), and Cialis (tadalafil).

Patients who have severe anemia or increased intracranial pressure should not receive NitroMist.

You cannot take NitroMist if you are hypersensitive to NitroMist or to other nitrates or nitrites. Hypersensitivity skin reactions have been observed with nitrates.

What should I tell my doctor before I take the first dose of NitroMist?
Tell your doctor about all prescription, over-the-counter, and herbal medication you are taking, before beginning treatment with NitroMist. Also, talk to your doctor about your complete medical history, especially if you are pregnant, plan to become pregnant, or are breastfeeding.

What is the usual dosage?
The information below is based on the dosage guidelines your doctor uses. Depending on your condition and medical history, your doctor may prescribe a different regimen. Do not change the dosage or stop taking your medication without your doctor's approval.

This product delivers 400 micrograms (mcg) of nitroglycerin per spray.

Onset of Attack
Adults: Spray 1 to 2 sprays on or under the tongue. One spray may be repeated approximately every 5 minutes as needed. No more than 3 sprays are recommended within a 15-minute period.

Prevention Treatment
Adults: 1 to 2 sprays on or under the tongue 5 to 10 minutes before the activity that may trigger an attack.

How should I take NitroMist?
At the onset of an attack, administer 1 or 2 sprays on or under tongue. Wait 5 minutes and repeat if needed. No more than 3 sprays are recommended within a 15 minutes period. Do not spit or rinse your mouth for 5 to 10 minutes following administration.

NitroMist may be used prophylactically (preventative treatment) 5 to 10 minutes before engaging in activities that might precipitate an acute attack.

During use, you should rest in a sitting position. The container should be held in an upright position. The dose should be sprayed into the mouth on or under the tongue by pressing the button firmly and the mouth should be closed immediately after each dose. The spray should not be inhaled.

If chest pain persists after a total of 3 sprays, quick medical attention is recommended.

Changes in NitroMist dosage may cause severe headaches.

If the product is not used for more than 6 weeks, re-prime the pump with 2 sprays.

What should I avoid while taking NitroMist?
Avoid activities requiring coordination until drug effects are realized, as drug may cause dizziness. Do not use this medication along with erectile dysfunction drugs such as sildenafil, vardenafil, and tadalafil.

What are possible food and drug interactions associated with NitroMist?
If NitroMist is taken with certain other drugs, the effects of either could be increased, decreased, or altered. It is especially important to check with your doctor before combining NitroMist with the following: alcohol, aspirin, calcium channel blockers such as amlodipine or diltiazem, ergotamine, heparin, labetolol, sildenafil, tadalafil, tissue-type plasminogen activator (t-PA) therapy, and vardenafil.

What are the possible side effects of NitroMist?
Side effects cannot be anticipated. If any develop or change in intensity, tell your doctor as soon as possible. Only your doctor can determine if it is safe for you to continue taking this drug.

Side effects may include: collapse, flushing, headache, low blood pressure and dizziness upon standing, nausea, pallor, palpitations, sweating, syncope, vomiting, weakness

Can I receive NitroMist if I am pregnant or breastfeeding?
The effects of NitroMist during pregnancy and breastfeeding are unknown. Tell your doctor immediately if you are pregnant, plan to become pregnant, or are breastfeeding.

What should I do if I miss a dose of NitroMist?
Nitromist is taken as needed. If the product is not used for more than 6 weeks, the canister can be re-primed with 2 sprays.

How should I store NitroMist?
Store at room temperature.

Nizatidine *See Axid, page 175.*

NIZORAL
Generic name: Ketoconazole

What is Nizoral?
Nizoral, a broad-spectrum antifungal drug available in tablet form, may be given to treat several fungal infections within the body, including oral thrush and candidiasis.

It may also be given to treat severe, hard-to-treat fungal skin infections that have not cleared up after treatment with creams, ointments or the oral antifungal drug *griseofulvin,* or in those individuals who are unable to take griseofulvin.

What is the most important information I should know about Nizoral?
In some people, Nizoral may cause serious or even fatal damage to the liver. Before starting to take Nizoral, and at frequent intervals while you are taking it, you should have blood tests to evaluate your liver function. Tell your doctor immediately if you experience any signs or symptoms that could mean liver damage: these include unusual fatigue, loss of appetite, nausea or vomiting, yellowing of the eyes or skin, dark urine, or pale stools.

In rare cases, people have had anaphylaxis (a life-threatening allergic reaction) after taking their first dose of Nizoral. Symptoms may include difficulty breathing; tightness in the chest; swelling of the eyelids, face, or lips; or rash or hives. If this happens, seek immediate medical care.

Do not drive or perform other possibly unsafe tasks until you know how you react to Nizoral; this drug may cause dizziness or drowsiness. These effects may be worse if you take it with alcohol or certain medicines.

Use of alcohol with Nizoral has rarely caused symptoms such as flushing, rash, swelling of the hands and feet, nausea, and headache. Talk with your doctor before drinking alcohol while taking Nizoral

Do NOT take more than the recommended dose or use for longer than prescribed without checking with your doctor.

Nizoral only works against fungi; it does not treat viral infections (eg, the common cold) or bacterial infections.

Be sure to use Nizoral for the full course of treatment. If you do not, the medicine may not clear up your infection completely. The infection could also become less sensitive to this or other medicines. This could make the infection harder to treat in the future.

Nizoral may increase the risk of low blood sugar from your diabetes medicine. Check blood sugar levels closely. Consult your doctor before changing the dose of your diabetes medicine.

Hormonal birth control (eg, birth control pills) may not work as well while you are using this medicine. To prevent pregnancy, use an extra form of birth control (eg, condoms).

Use of Nizoral along with certain other medicines may increase your risk of serious and sometimes fatal heart problems, including irregular heartbeat. Do not take Nizoral if you are also taking astemizole, cisapride, or terfenadine.

Who should not take Nizoral?

Do not take Nizoral if you are sensitive to it or have ever had an allergic reaction to it. Never take Nizoral together with astemizole, cisapride, terfenadine, or triazolam. Rare, but sometimes fatal reactions have been reported when these drugs are combined.

What should I tell my doctor before I take the first dose of Nizoral?

Tell your doctor about all prescription, over-the-counter, and herbal medication you are taking before beginning treatment with Nizoral. Also, talk to your doctor about your complete medical history, especially if you have low stomach acid, a history of liver disease, blood problems, or if you regularly use, abuse or are dependent on alcohol.

What is the usual dosage?

The information below is based on the dosage guidelines your doctor uses. Depending on your condition and medical history, your doctor may prescribe a different regimen. Do not change the dosage or stop taking your medication without your doctor's approval.

Adults: The usual starting dose is a single daily administration of 200 mg (one tablet). In very serious infections or if you are unresponsive within the expected time, the dose of Nizoral may be increased to 400 mg (two tablets) once daily.

Children over 2 years: The usual starting dose is a single daily dose of 3.3 to 6.6 mg/kg.

Nizoral has not been studied in children under 2 years of age.

How should I take Nizoral?

You should keep taking the drug until tests show that your fungal infection has subsided. If you stop too soon, the infection might return.

Nizoral can be taken with or without food. You may want to take Nizoral tablets with meals to avoid stomach upset.

Do not take an antacid within 1 hour before or 2 hours after you take Nizoral.

Hormonal birth control (eg, birth control pills) may not work as well while you are using this medicine. To prevent pregnancy, use an extra form of birth control (eg, condoms).

What should I avoid while taking Nizoral?

Avoid alcohol and do not take with antacids. If antacids are necessary, you should wait 2 to 3 hours before taking them.

Do not drive or perform other possibly unsafe tasks until you know how you react to Nizoral; this drug may cause dizziness or drowsiness.

Do NOT take more than the recommended dose or use for longer than prescribed without checking with your doctor.

Do not take Nizoral if you are also taking astemizole, cisapride, or terfenadine.

What are possible food and drug interactions associated with Nizoral?

If Nizoral is taken with certain other drugs, the effects of either could be increased, decreased, or altered. It is especially important to check with your doctor before combining Nizoral with the following: alcohol, antacids, anticoagulants (blood thinners), anti-ulcer medications, astemizole, cisapride, cyclosporine, digoxin, drugs that relieve spasms, isoniazid, methylprednisolone, midazolam, oral diabetes drugs, phenytoin, rifampin, tacrolimus, terfenadine, theophyllines, and triazolam.

What are the possible side effects of Nizoral?

Side effects cannot be anticipated. If any develop or change in intensity, tell your doctor as soon as possible. Only your doctor can determine if it is safe for you to continue taking this drug.

Side effects may include: nausea, stomach pain or upset, vomiting

In rare cases, people have had anaphylaxis (a life-threatening allergic reaction) after taking their first dose of Nizoral. Symptoms may include difficulty breathing; tightness in the chest; swelling of the eyelids, face, or lips; or rash or hives. If this happens, seek medical care at once.

In some people, Nizoral may cause serious or even fatal damage to the liver. Tell your doctor immediately if you experience any signs or symptoms that could mean liver damage. These include unusual fatigue, loss of appetite, nausea or vomiting, yellowing of the eyes or skin, dark urine, or pale stools.

Can I receive Nizoral if I am pregnant or breastfeeding?

The effects of Nizoral during pregnancy and breastfeeding are unknown. Tell your doctor immediately if you are pregnant, plan to become pregnant, or are breastfeeding. Nizoral is found in breast milk. Do not breastfeed while using Nizoral.

What should I do if I miss a dose of Nizoral?

Take the forgotten dose as soon as you remember. However, if it is almost time for your next dose, skip the one you missed and go back to your regular schedule. Do not take double doses.

How should I store Nizoral?

Store Nizoral between 59 and 77 degrees F (15 and 25 degrees C). Store away from heat, moisture, and light. Do not store in the bathroom. Keep Nizoral out of the reach of children.

Norethindrone acetate *See Aygestin, page 177.*

Norethindrone acetate and ethinyl estradiol *See Estrostep Fe, page 519, or Loestrin 24 FE, page 752.*

Norfloxacin *See Noroxin, page 905.*

NORGESIC

Generic name: Orphenadrine citrate, aspirin and caffeine

What is Norgesic?

Norgesic is used for the relief of mild-to-moderate pain of severe muscle disorders. Norgesic is used, along with rest and physical therapy, to treat discomfort associated with painful muscular conditions.

What is the most important information I should know about Norgesic?

Norgesic may impair your ability to drive a car or operate dangerous machinery. Do not participate in potentially hazardous activities until you know how you react to Norgesic.

Because Norgesic contains aspirin, you should be careful taking it if you have a peptic ulcer or problems with blood clotting.

The safety of continuous, long-term therapy with Norgesic has not been established, your doctor should monitor your blood, urine, and liver function if you use Norgesic for a prolonged period of time.

Confusion, anxiety and tremors have been reported in a few patients receiving propoxyphene and orphenadrine concomitantly. As these symptoms may be simply due to an additive effect, reduction of dosage and/or discontinuation of one or both agents is recommended in such cases.

Call your doctor immediately if you experience a rash, itching, a fever, or nasal congestion during treatment with Norgesic.

Watch for bloody, black, or tarry stools or bloody vomit. This could indicate damage to the stomach.

Do not take more of this medication than is prescribed. If the pain is not being adequately treated, talk to your doctor.

Who should not take Norgesic?

Do not take Norgesic if you are allergic to any of its ingredients.

Taking aspirin while you have chickenpox or flu may cause a rare but serious condition called Reye's syndrome; do not give Norgesic to anyone with these diseases. Call your doctor if fever or swelling develops.

Do not use Norgesic if you have an enlarged prostate or a blockage of the urinary tract (difficulty urinating), or myasthenia gravis.

What should I tell my doctor before I take the first dose of Norgesic?

Tell your doctor about all prescription, over-the-counter, and herbal medications you are taking before beginning treatment with Norgesic. Also, talk to your doctor about your complete medical history, especially if you have had an eye condition called glaucoma, a stomach or intestinal blockage, an enlarged prostate gland, a bladder obstruction, achalasia (failure of stomach or intestinal muscles to relax), or myasthenia gravis (muscle weakness and fatigue).

What is the usual dosage?

The information below is based on the dosage guidelines your doctor uses. Depending on your condition and medical history, your doctor may prescribe a different regimen. Do not change the dosage or stop taking your medication without your doctor's approval.

Adults: The usual starting dose is 1 to 2 tablets 3 to 4 times daily.

Children: The safety and effectiveness of Norgesic have not been established in children.

How should I take Norgesic?

If aspirin upsets your stomach, you may take Norgesic with food. Take it exactly as prescribed. Take each dose with a full glass of water. If the pain is not being adequately treated, talk to your doctor.

What should I avoid while taking Norgesic?

Avoid driving a car or operate dangerous machinery.

Do not take more of this medication than is prescribed.

Use alcohol cautiously. Alcohol may increase drowsiness and dizziness while taking aspirin/caffeine/orphenadrine. Also, in combination with aspirin, alcohol can be damaging to the stomach.

Do not take other over-the-counter and prescription products that contain aspirin. Too much aspirin could be dangerous. Talk to your doctor or pharmacist before taking any over-the-counter preparations.

What are possible food and drug interactions associated with Norgesic?

If Norgesic is taken with certain other drugs, the effects of either could be increased, decreased, or altered. It is especially important to check with your doctor before combining Norgesic with the following: coumadin, diclofenac, etodolac, fenoprofen, flurbiprofen, indomethacin, ketoprofen, ketorolac, nabumetone, naproxen, nonsteroidal anti-inflammatory drugs (NSAIDs), oxaprozin, piroxicam, propoxyphene, sulindac, and tolmetin.

What are the possible side effects of Norgesic?
Side effects cannot be anticipated. If any develop or change in intensity, tell your doctor as soon as possible. Only your doctor can determine if it is safe for you to continue taking this drug.

Side effects may include: Blurred vision, confusion (in the elderly), constipation, difficulty in urinating, dilation of the pupils, dizziness, drowsiness, dry mouth, fainting, hallucinations, headache, hives, light-headedness, nausea, palpitations, rapid heart rate, skin diseases, stomach and intestinal bleeding, vomiting, weakness

Call your doctor immediately if you experience a rash, itching, a fever, or nasal congestion during treatment with Norgesic.

Watch for bloody, black, or tarry stools or bloody vomit. This could indicate damage to the stomach.

Can I receive Norgesic if I am pregnant or breastfeeding?
The effects of Norgesic during pregnancy and breastfeeding are unknown. Tell your doctor immediately if you are pregnant, plan to become pregnant, or are breastfeeding.

What should I do if I miss a dose of Norgesic?
Take the missed dose as soon as you remember. However, if it is almost time for the next dose, skip the missed dose and take only the next regularly scheduled dose. Do not take a double dose of this medication.

How should I store Norgesic?
Store at room temperature. Keep away from moisture and heat.

Norgestimate and ethinyl estradiol *See Ortho Tri-Cyclen Lo, page 961.*

NOROXIN
Generic name: Norfloxacin

What is Noroxin?
Noroxin is a type of antibiotic known as a quinolone and is used to treat bacterial infections, such as urinary tract infections, gonorrhea, and prostate infections.

What is the most important information I should know about Noroxin?

The safety and efficacy of norfloxacin in children, adolescents (under the age of 18), pregnant women, and nursing mothers have not been established.

Seizures, severe and in some cases, fatal allergic reactions have been reported. If you develop rash while taking norfloxacin, stop taking it and call your doctor right away.

Quinolones, including norfloxacin, may worsen the signs of myasthenia gravis (neuromuscular disorder characterized by fluctuating muscle weakness), leading to difficulty breathing which may be life threatening.

Fluoroquinolones, like Noroxin, are associated with an increased risk of tendonitis (inflammation or irritation of a tendon) and tendon rupture in all ages. The risk is further increased in older patients usually over 60 years of age, in patients taking corticosteroid drugs, and in patients with kidney, heart and lung transplant patients.

Your symptoms may improve before the infection is completely treated, however, you should take this medication for the entire length of time prescribed by your doctor.

It is important to drink several glasses of water each day while you are taking Noroxin to protect your kidneys. Do not give this medication to anyone younger than 18 years old as it may interfere with bone development in growing children.

Who should not take Noroxin?

Do not use this medication if you are allergic to Noroxin, or if you have problems with your tendons or a history of tendon rupture while taking a medicine similar to norfloxacin, such as Avelox, Cipro, Floxin, Levaquin, Maxaquin, Tequin, Trovan, or Zagam. Also, do not use this medication if you have abnormal heart rhythms and are being treated with medications such as quinidine, procainamide, amiodarone or sotalol.

If you have low potassium levels in your blood or are taking medications known as diuretics such as furosemide or hydrochlorothiazide, or if you are pregnant, plan to become pregnant or are breastfeeding, do not take Noroxin.

What should I tell my doctor before I take the first dose of Noroxin?

Tell your doctor about all prescription, over-the-counter, and herbal medications you are taking before beginning treatment with Noroxin. Give your doctor your complete medical history, especially if you have myasthenia gravis, a personal or family history of long QT syndrome, low levels of potassium in your blood (hypokalemia), heart disease or heart rhythm disorder, liver disease, kidney disease, seizures or epilepsy.

What is the usual dosage?
The information below is based on the dosage guidelines your doctor uses. Depending on your condition and medical history, your doctor may prescribe a different regimen. Do not change the dosage or stop taking your medication without your doctor's approval.

Uncomplicated Urinary Tract Infections (UTIs) (cystitis)
Due to E. coli, K. pneumoniae, *or* P. mirabilis
Adults 18 years and older: The usual starting dose is 400 milligrams (mg) every 12 hours for 3 days.

Uncomplicated UTIs Due to Other Indicated Organisms
Adults 18 years and older: The usual staring dose is 400 mg every 12 hours for 7-10 days.

Complicated UTIs
Adults 18 years and older: The usual starting dose is 400 mg every 12 hours for 10-21 days.

Uncomplicated Gonorrhea
Adults 18 years and older: The usual starting dose is a single dose of 800 mg for one day.

Prostatitis, Acute or Chronic
Adults 18 years and older: The usual starting dose is 400 mg every 12 hours for 28 days.

For elderly patients or patients with kidney problems the dosage may be different. Contact your doctor for more information.

How should I take Noroxin?
Take Noroxin at least 1 hour before or at least 2 hours after a meal or drinking milk and/or other dairy products. Take Noroxin with a full glass of water (8 ounces). It is important to drink several glasses of water each day while you are taking Noroxin to protect your kidneys.

Multivitamins, other products containing iron or zinc, antacids containing magnesium and aluminum, sucralfate, or Videx (didanosine) chewable/buffered tablets or the pediatric powder for oral solution, should not be taken within 2 hours before or after taking Noroxin.

Take Noroxin at evenly spaced intervals. Follow your doctor's instructions.

Take Noroxin for the entire length of time prescribed by your doctor. Your symptoms may get better before the infection is completely treated. Noroxin will not treat a viral infection such as the common cold or flu.

What should I avoid while taking Noroxin?
Avoid exposure to sunlight or artificial UV rays (eg, sunlamps or tanning beds). Noroxin can make your skin more sensitive to sunlight and more

susceptible to sunburn. Use a sunscreen (minimum SPF 15) and wear protective clothing if you must be out in the sun.

Antibiotic medicines can cause diarrhea, which may be a sign of a new infection. If you have diarrhea that is watery or has blood in it, call your doctor. Do not use any medicine to stop the diarrhea unless your doctor instructs you to.

What are possible food and drug interactions associated with Noroxin?

If Noroxin is taken with certain other drugs, the effects of either could be increased, decreased, or altered. It is especially important to check with your doctor before combining Noroxin with any of the following: antibiotics known as quinolones; antidepressants; aspirin or other NSAIDs (nonsteroidal anti-inflammatory drugs); blood thinners such as warfarin; caffeine; cisapride; cyclosporine; heart rhythm medications such as quinidine, procainamide, amiodarone or sotalol; insulin or oral diabetes medications such as glyburide; multivitamins or other products containing iron or zinc; antacids or sucrafalte; nitrofurantoin; probenecid; psychiatric disorder medications such as clozapine; ropinirole; tacrine; tizanidine; theophylline; and videx (Didanosine).

What are the possible side effects of Noroxin?

Side effects cannot be anticipated. If any develop or change in intensity, tell your doctor as soon as possible. Only your doctor can determine if it is safe for you to continue taking this drug.

Side effects may include: dizziness, headache, nausea, stomach cramps, heartburn, vomiting, diarrhea, constipation, gas; changes in hearing and pain, burning, tingling, numbness, weakness in arms or legs, rash

If rash occurs, stop taking Noroxin and call your doctor right away.

Can I receive Noroxin if I am pregnant or breastfeeding?

The effects of Noroxin during pregnancy and breastfeeding are unknown. Tell your doctor immediately if you are pregnant, plan to become pregnant, or are breastfeeding.

What should I do if I miss a dose of Noroxin?

Take the missed dose as soon as you remember. If you are more than 2 hours late in taking your medicine, skip the missed dose and take the medicine at the next regularly scheduled time. Do not take extra medicine to make up the missed dose.

How should I store Noroxin?

Store Noroxin at room temperature. Keep the container tightly closed.

NORPACE

Generic name: Disopyramide phosphate

What is Norpace?

Norpace is used to treat severe irregular heartbeat. It relaxes an overactive heart and improves the efficiency of the heart's pumping action.

What is the most important information I should know about Norpace?

Norpace may cause or worsen congestive heart failure and can cause severe low blood pressure. If you have a history of heart failure, your doctor will carefully monitor your heart function while you are taking Norpace.

Do not stop taking Norpace without first consulting your doctor. Stopping suddenly can cause serious changes in heart function.

Your doctor should check your potassium levels before prescribing Norpace for you. Low potassium levels may make Norpace ineffective; high levels may increase its toxic effects.

Norpace can cause low blood sugar (hypoglycemia), especially if you have congestive heart failure; poor nutrition; or kidney, liver, or other diseases; or if you are taking beta-blocking blood pressure drugs such as Tenormin or if you drink alcohol.

Who should not take Norpace?

This drug should not be used if the blood output of your heart is inadequate (cardiogenic shock), or if you are sensitive to or have ever had an allergic reaction to Norpace.

Norpace can be used for only certain types of irregular heartbeat, and must not be used for others.

What should I tell my doctor before I take the first dose of Norpace?

Tell your doctor about all prescription, over-the-counter, and herbal medications you are taking before beginning treatment with Norpace. Also, talk to your doctor about your complete medical history, especially if you have a history of heart failure, structural heart disease, inflammation of the heart muscle, or other heart disorders, kidney or liver disease, glaucoma (increased eye pressure), myasthenia gravis (neuromuscular disorder characterized by fluctuating muscle weakness), or difficulty urinating (particularly if you have a prostate condition), or low or high levels of potassium in your blood.

What is the usual dosage?

The information below is based on the dosage guidelines your doctor uses. Depending on your condition and medical history, your doctor

may prescribe a different regimen. **Do not change the dosage or stop taking your medication without your doctor's approval.**

Treatment with Norpace should be started in the hospital.

Your doctor will adjust your dosage according to your own response to, and tolerance of, Norpace.

Adults: The usual dosage range of Norpace and Norpace controlled-release (CR) is 400 milligrams (mg) to 800 mg per day, divided into smaller doses.

There are very specific calculations for your starting dose and dosage increase schedule based on your age, weight, medical condition, and other medication that you are taking. Contact your doctor for more information.

Children: Dosage in children to age 18 is based on body weight. The total daily dosage should be divided into equal doses taken orally every 6 hours or at intervals that are best for the individual.

How should I take Norpace?
Take each dose with a full glass of water. Do not crush, chew, or break any CR forms of Norpace. Swallow them whole. Do not skip doses or change your dosing schedule without talking to your doctor. Changing your schedule could make your condition much worse.

What should I avoid while taking Norpace?
Avoid alcoholic beverages while taking Norpace.

Use caution when driving, operating machinery, or performing other potentially hazardous activities. Disopyramide may cause dizziness, drowsiness, or blurred vision. If you experience any of these conditions, avoid potentially hazardous activities.

What are possible food and drug interactions associated with Norpace?
If Norpace is taken with certain other drugs, the effects of either could be increased, decreased, or altered. It is especially important to check with your doctor before combining Norpace with the following: alcohol; clarithromycin; erythromycin; heart-regulating drugs such as quinidine, procainamide, lidocaine, propranolol; phenytoin; and verapamil.

What are the possible side effects of Norpace?
Side effects cannot be anticipated. If any develop or change in intensity, tell your doctor as soon as possible. Only your doctor can determine if it is safe for you to continue taking this drug.

Side effects may include: abdominal pain, aches and pains, bloating and gas, blurred vision, constipation, dizziness, dry eyes, nose, and throat, dry mouth, fatigue, headache, inability to urinate, increased urinary frequency and urgency, muscle weakness, nausea, vague feeling of bodily discomfort

Side effects other than those listed here may also occur. Talk to your doctor about any side effect that seems unusual or that is especially bothersome.

Can I receive Norpace if I am pregnant or breastfeeding?
The effects of Norpace during pregnancy and breastfeeding are unknown. Tell your doctor immediately if you are pregnant, plan to become pregnant, or are breastfeeding.

What should I do if I miss a dose of Norpace?
If you do miss a dose, take it as soon as you remember. However, if it is almost time for your next dose, skip the missed dose and take only your next regularly scheduled dose. Do not take a double dose of this medication.

How should I store Norpace?
Store Norpace at room temperature away from moisture and heat.

NORPRAMIN
Generic name: Desipramine hydrochloride

What is Norpramin?
Norpramin is used to treat the symptoms of depression.

What is the most important information
I should know about Norpramin?
Norpramin is not approved for use in children.

Antidepressant medicines may increase suicidal thoughts or actions in some children, teenagers, and young adults when the medicine is first started. Depression and other serious mental illnesses are the most important causes of suicidal thoughts and actions. Some people may have a particularly high risk of having suicidal thoughts or actions. These include people who have (or have a family history of) bipolar disorder (also called manic-depressive illness) or suicidal thoughts or actions.

Pay close attention to any changes, especially sudden changes, in mood, behaviors, thoughts, or feelings. This is very important when an antidepressant medicine is first started or when the dose is changed.

Call the doctor right away to report new or sudden changes in mood, behavior, thoughts, or feelings. Signs to watch for include new or worsening depression, new or worsening anxiety, agitation, insomnia, hostility, panic attacks, restlessness, extreme hyperactivity, and suicidal thinking or behavior.

Keep all follow-up visits as scheduled, and call the doctor between visits as needed, especially if you have concerns about symptoms.

Who should not take Norpramin?
Do not take Norpramin if you are allergic to it or any of its components.

Do not take Norpramin if you have recently had a heart attack.

If you are taking or have taken antidepressant medications known as monoamine oxidase inhibitors (MAOIs) within the last 14 days, do not take Norpramin.

If you are planning to have elective surgery, make sure that your doctor is aware that you are taking Norpramin. It should be discontinued as soon as possible prior to surgery.

What should I tell my doctor before I take the first dose of Norpramin?
Tell your doctor about all prescription, over-the-counter, and herbal medications you are taking before beginning treatment with Norpramin. Also, talk to your doctor about your complete medical history, especially if you have heart disease, a history of heart attack, stroke, seizures, bipolar disorder (manic-depression), schizophrenia or other mental illness, liver disease, overactive thyroid, high blood sugar, increased pressure in the eyes (glaucoma), or problems with urination.

What is the usual dosage?
The information below is based on the dosage guidelines your doctor uses. Depending on your condition and medical history, your doctor may prescribe a different regimen. Do not change the dosage or stop taking your medication without your doctor's approval.

Adults: The usual dose ranges from 100 to 200 milligrams (mg) per day, taken in one dose or divided into smaller doses. If needed, dosages may gradually be increased to 300 mg a day. Dosages above 300 mg per day are not recommended.

Older adults and adolescents: The usual dose ranges from 25 to 100 mg per day. If needed, dosages may gradually be increased to 150 mg a day. Doses above 150 mg per day are not recommended.

How should I take Norpramin?
Norpramin should be taken exactly as prescribed. Do not stop taking Norpramin if you feel no immediate effect. It can take up to 2 or 3 weeks for improvement to begin.

Norpramin can cause dry mouth. Sucking hard candy or chewing gum can help this problem.

What should I avoid while taking Norpramin?

Norpramin may increase your skin's sensitivity to sunlight. Overexposure could cause rash, itching, redness, or sunburn. Avoid direct sunlight or wear protective clothing.

This drug may impair your ability to drive a car or operate potentially dangerous machinery. Do not participate in any activities that require full alertness if you are unsure about your ability.

Avoid drinking alcohol. It can cause dangerous side effects when taken together with Norpramin.

What are possible food and drug interactions associated with Norpramin?

If Norpramin is taken with certain other drugs, the effects of either could be increased, decreased, or altered. It is especially important to check with your doctor before combining Norpramin with the following: alcohol, antidepressants (including MAOIs and SSRIs), cimetidine, drugs that improve breathing, muscle relaxants, guanethidine, sedatives/hypnotics, sertraline, and thyroid medications.

What are the possible side effects of Norpramin?

Side effects cannot be anticipated. If any develop or change in intensity, tell your doctor as soon as possible. Only your doctor can determine if it is safe for you to continue taking this drug.

Side effects may include: anxiety, confusion, dizziness, dry mouth, frequent urination or problems urinating, high blood pressure, hallucinations, hives, impaired coordination, irregular heartbeat, low blood pressure, numbness, rapid heartbeat, sensitivity to sunlight, sex drive changes, tingling, tremors

Can I receive Norpramin if I am pregnant or breastfeeding?

The effects of Norpramin during pregnancy and breastfeeding are unknown. Tell your doctor immediately if you are pregnant, plan to become pregnant, or are breastfeeding.

What should I do if I miss a dose of Norpramin?

If you do miss a dose, take it as soon as you remember. However, if it is almost time for your next dose, skip the missed dose and take only your next regularly scheduled dose. Do not take a double dose of this medication.

How should I store Norpramin?

Store at room temperature and protect from excessive heat.

Nortriptyline hydrochloride See Pamelor, page 973.

NORVASC

Generic name: Amlodipine besylate

What is Norvasc?

Norvasc is in a class of drugs called calcium channel blockers, which relax (widen) the blood vessels (veins and arteries), making it easier for the heart to pump and reducing its workload.

Norvasc is used to treat hypertension (high blood pressure) and to treat angina (chest pain).

What is the most important information I should know about Norvasc?

If you have high blood pressure, you must take Norvasc regularly for it to be effective. Since blood pressure declines gradually, it may be several weeks before you get the full benefit of Norvasc; and you must continue taking it even if you are feeling well. Norvasc does not cure high blood pressure; it merely keeps it under control.

Although very rare, if you have severe heart disease, you may experience an increase in frequency and duration of angina attacks (chest pain), or even have a heart attack, when you are starting on Norvasc or your dosage is increased.

Who should not take Norvasc?

If you are sensitive to or have ever had an allergic reaction to Norvasc, do not take Norvasc.

What should I tell my doctor before I take the first dose of Norvasc?

Tell your doctor about all prescription, over-the-counter, and herbal medications you are taking before beginning treatment with Norvasc. Also, talk to your doctor about your complete medical history, especially if you have heart conditions or liver disease.

What is the usual dosage?

The information below is based on the dosage guidelines your doctor uses. Depending on your condition and medical history, your doctor may prescribe a different regimen. Do not change the dosage or stop taking your medication without your doctor's approval.

Angina
Adults: The usual starting dose is 5 to 10 mg once daily. If you have liver disease, the lower 5mg dose will be used at the start.

Adults over 65 years: The usual starting dose is 5 mg. Your doctor may adjust the dose based on your response to the drug.

High Blood Pressure
Adults: The usual starting dose is 5 milligrams (mg) taken once a day. The most you should take in a day is 10 mg. If your doctor is adding Norvasc to other high blood pressure medications, the dose is 2.5 mg once daily. The lower 2.5-mg starting dose also applies if you have liver disease.

Children 6 to 17 years: The usual dose is 2.5 to 5 mg once a day. Doses exceeding 5 mg have not been studied in children.

Adults over 65 years: The usual starting dose is 2.5 mg.

How should I take Norvasc?
Norvasc may be taken with or without food. A once-a-day medication, Norvasc may be used alone or in combination with other drugs for high blood pressure or angina.

You should take Norvasc exactly as prescribed, even if your symptoms have disappeared. You will begin to see a drop in your blood pressure 24 hours after you start the medication.

What should I avoid while taking Norvasc?
Use caution when you stand or sit up from a lying position, especially if you wake up during the night. You may become dizzy when changing positions. Use alcohol cautiously. Alcohol may further lower blood pressure and increase drowsiness or dizziness while taking Norvasc.

What are possible food and drug interactions associated with Norvasc?
There are no known food or drug interactions with Norvasc.

What are the possible side effects of Norvasc?
Side effects cannot be anticipated. If any develop or change in intensity, tell your doctor as soon as possible. Only your doctor can determine if it is safe for you to continue taking this drug.

Side effects may include: dizziness, fatigue, flushing, fluid retention and swelling, headache, palpitations (fluttery or throbbing heartbeat)

Can I receive Norvasc if I am pregnant or breastfeeding?
The effects of Norvasc during pregnancy and breastfeeding are unknown. Tell your doctor immediately if you are pregnant, plan to become pregnant, or are breastfeeding.

What should I do if I miss a dose of Norvasc?
If you forget to take a dose, take it as soon as you remember. If it is almost time for your next dose, skip the one you missed and go back to your regular schedule. Never take 2 doses at the same time.

How should I store Norvasc?
Store at room temperature in a tightly closed container, away from light.

NORVIR
Generic name: Ritonavir

What is Norvir?
Norvir is an antiviral medication. It is in a group of drugs called protease inhibitors. Norvir keeps human immunodeficiency virus (HIV) cells from reproducing in your body.

Norvir treats HIV, which causes acquired immunodeficiency syndrome (AIDS). However, Norvir is not a cure for HIV or AIDS.

Norvir is used in combination with other HIV drugs called nucleoside analogues (Retrovir, Hivid, and others). These two types of drugs act against HIV in different ways.

What is the most important information I should know about Norvir?
Taking Norvir while taking certain other medications could cause serious and even life-threatening problems such as irregular heart beat, breathing difficulties, or excessive sleepiness. These medications include: alfuzosin hydrochloride, amiodarone, astemizole, bepridil, cisapride, dihydroergotamine, ergonovine, ergotamine, flecainide, methylergonovine, midazolam, pimozide, propafenone, quinidine, terfenadine, triazolam, and voriconazole.

Norvir is not a cure for AIDS or HIV infection. You may continue to experience symptoms and develop complications, including opportunistic infections (diseases that attack when the immune system falters, such as certain types of pneumonia, tuberculosis, and fungal infections).

Norvir does not reduce the danger of transmission of HIV to others through sexual contact or blood contamination. Therefore, you should continue to avoid practices that could give HIV to others.

Some patients taking Norvir can develop serious problems with their pancreas (pancreatitis), which may cause death. Tell your doctor if you have nausea, vomiting, or abdominal pain. These may be signs of pancreatitis.

When your Norvir supply starts to run low, get more from your doctor or pharmacy. This is very important because the amount of virus in your blood may increase if the medicine is stopped for even a short time. The virus may develop resistance to Norvir and become harder to treat.

Who should not take Norvir?
If you have ever had an allergic reaction to Norvir or any of its ingredients, do not take the drug.

What should I tell my doctor before I take the first dose of Norvir?

Tell your doctor about all prescription, over-the-counter, and herbal medications you are taking before beginning treatment with Norvir. Also, talk to your doctor about your complete medical history, especially if you have diabetes (high blood sugar), hemophilia (a bleeding disorder), high cholesterol, liver disease, and if you are pregnant, plan to become pregnant or are breastfeeding.

What is the usual dosage?

The information below is based on the dosage guidelines your doctor uses. Depending on your condition and medical history, your doctor may prescribe a different regimen. Do not change the dosage or stop taking your medication without your doctor's approval.

Adults: The recommended dose of Norvir is 600 milligrams (mg) twice a day with food.

Should you experience nausea when first starting on Norvir, your doctor may lower your starting dosage to 300 mg twice a day and increase it at 2 to 3 day intervals by 100 mg twice a day.

Your doctor may suggest taking Norvir alone at first and adding a second drug later in the first 2 weeks of therapy. This approach may cause fewer stomach problems.

If you are taking Norvir along with saquinavir, the dosage of both drugs may be reduced to 400 milligrams twice daily.

Adolescents and children 1 month old and over: The dosage of Norvir in children is based on the child's height and weight, and should not exceed 600 mg twice a day. Use of a special spoon or dosing syringe with measurements on it will help ensure that the child receives the proper dose.

How should I take Norvir?

Take Norvir with food, if possible, or the medication may not work properly.

Norvir is available in soft gelatin capsule and oral solution forms. If you are taking Norvir oral solution, shake well before each use. If you want to improve the taste, you can mix the liquid with 8 ounces of chocolate milk, Ensure, or Advera. Take this combination no later than an hour.

Use a measuring cup or spoon to measure each dose of the oral solution accurately. A household teaspoon may not hold the correct amount of oral solution.

What should I avoid while taking Norvir?

Avoid having unprotected sex (without a condom) or sharing intravenous needles with another person. Norvir will not cure HIV or AIDS, and you can still transmit the virus to others.

Do not change or stop taking Norvir without talking to your doctor first. Do not share this medication with anyone else.

What are possible food and drug interactions associated with Norvir?

If Norvir is taken with certain other drugs, the effects of either could be increased, decreased, or altered. It is especially important to check with your doctor before combining Norvir with any of the following: alfuzosin hydrochloride, amiodarone, astemizole, atorvastatin, bepridil, birth control medications, cisapride, dihydroergotamine, disulfiram, ergonovine, ergotamine, flecainide, fluticasone propionate, lovastatin, methylergonovine, metronidazole, midazolam, pimozide, propafenone, quinidine, rifabutin, rifampin, saquinavir, sildenafil, simvastatin, St. John's wort, tadalafil, terfenadine, triazolam, vardenafil, and voriconazole.

What are the possible side effects of Norvir?

Side effects cannot be anticipated. If any develop or change in intensity, tell your doctor as soon as possible. Only your doctor can determine if it is safe for you to continue taking this drug.

Side effects may include: abdominal pain, anxiety, bedwetting, confusion, diarrhea, dizziness, drowsiness, fatigue, fever, general feeling of illness, headache, indigestion, insomnia, loss of appetite, muscle aches, nausea, numbness or tingling sensation around the face or mouth, "pins and needles" sensation in the arms and legs, rash, sore or irritated throat, sweating, taste alteration, vomiting, weakness

Can I receive Norvir if I am pregnant or breastfeeding?

The effects of Norvir during pregnancy have not been adequately studied. If you are pregnant or plan to become pregnant, tell your doctor immediately.

You should not breast-feed while you are using Norvir. Women with HIV or AIDS should not breast-feed at all. Even if your baby is born without HIV, you may still pass the virus to the baby in your breast milk.

What should I do if I miss a dose of Norvir?

Take it as soon as possible. If it is almost time for the next dose, skip the one you missed and go back to your regular schedule. Never double the dose.

How should I store Norvir?

Capsules are best kept in the refrigerator, although they do not require refrigeration if used within 30 days and stored below 77°F. Protect from excessive heat or cold.

Do not refrigerate the oral solution. Store at room temperature. Shake before each use. Avoid exposure to excessive heat or cold and keep cap tightly closed.

Keep Norvir in its original container and use by the expiration date.

NOVOLIN
Generic name: Insulin

What is Novolin?
Novolin is a type of insulin used to control blood sugar in people with diabetes when diet modifications and oral medications failed to correct the condition. It comes in three forms: Novolin R PenFill, Novolin N PenFill, and Novolin 70/30 PenFill.

What is the most important information I should know about Novolin?
Any change of insulin should be made cautiously and only under medical supervision. Changes in purity, strength, brand (manufacturer), type (Regular, NPH, Lente, etc), species (beef, pork, beef-pork, human), and/or method of manufacture (recombinant DNA versus animal-source insulin) may result in the need for a change in dosage.

Special care should be taken when the transfer is from a standard beef or mixed species insulin to a purified pork or human insulin. A change in the type, strength, species or purity of insulin could require a dosage adjustment. Any change in insulin should be made under medical supervision. To avoid possible transmission of disease, PenFill cartridge should not be shared. Before use, check that the PenFill cartridge is intact (e.g. no cracks). Do not use if any damage is visible, or if the part of the rubber piston that you see is wider than the white bar code band.

You may have learned how to test your urine or your blood for glucose. It is important to do these tests regularly and to record the results for review with your physician or nurse educator. If you have an acute illness, especially with vomiting or fever, continue taking your insulin. If possible, stay on your regular diet. If you have trouble eating, drink fruit juices, regular soft drinks, or clear soups; if you can, eat small amounts of bland foods. Test your urine for glucose and ketones and, if possible, test your blood glucose. Note the results and contact your physician for possible insulin dose adjustment. If you have severe and prolonged vomiting, seek emergency medical care.

Insulin reaction (hypoglycemia) occurs when the blood glucose falls very low. This can happen if you take too much insulin, miss or delay a meal, exercise more than usual, or work too hard without eating, or become ill (specially with vomiting and fever).

You should always carry identification which states that you have diabetes. Do not try to refill a PenFill cartridge.

Who should not take Novolin?

Do not use Novolin if you are sensitive to or allergic to any of its ingredients.

What should I tell my doctor before I take the first dose of Novolin?

Tell your doctor about all prescription, over-the-counter, and herbal medication you are taking before beginning treatment with Novolin. Also, talk to your doctor about your complete medical history.

What is the usual dosage?

Your doctor will determine your correct dose based on the severity of your condition and your lifestyle.

How should I take Novolin?

The following areas are suitable for subcutaneous insulin injection: thighs, upper arms, buttocks, and abdomen. Do not change areas without consulting your physician.

Preparing the Injection: Never place a single-use disposable needle on your device until you are ready to give an injection, and remove the needle immediately after the injection. Follow the directions for use in the instruction manual for your insulin delivery device. PenFill cartridges may contain a small amount of air bubbles. To prevent an injection of air and to make certain a full dose of insulin is injected, an air shot must be done before each injection. Directions for performing an air shot are provided in your insulin delivery device instruction manual.

Giving the Injection: The following areas are suitable for subcutaneous insulin injection: thighs, upper arms, buttocks, and abdomen. Do not change areas without consulting your physician. The actual point of injection should be changed each time; injection sites should be about an inch apart.

The injection site should be clean and dry. Pinch up skin area to be injected and hold it firmly. Hold the device like a pencil and push the needle quickly and firmly into the pinched-up area. Release the skin and push the push-button all the way in to inject insulin beneath the skin. After the injection, the needle should remain under the skin for at least 6 seconds. Keep the push button fully depressed until the needle is withdrawn from the skin. This will ensure that the full dose has been injected.

Do not inject into a muscle unless your physician has advised it. You should never inject insulin into a vein. Follow the directions for use of your insulin delivery device.

Remove the needle. If slight bleeding occurs, press lightly with a dry cotton swab for a few seconds - do not rub.

Use the injection technique recommended by your physician.

What should I avoid while taking Novolin?

Avoid injecting Novolin into areas other than the ones indicated by your doctor. Also, avoid injecting in the same area twice. The actual injection points should be changed each time, and should be at least one inch apart.

What are possible food and drug interactions associated with Novolin?

If Novolin is taken with certain other drugs, the effects of either could be increased, decreased, or altered. It is especially important to check with your doctor before combining Novolin with any of the following: ACE inhibitors such as the blood pressure medications benazepril and quinapril; anabolic steroids.

Appetite suppressants such as diethylpropion; aspirin; beta-blocking blood pressure medicines such as atenolol and metoprolol; diuretics such as furosemide and hydrochlorothiazide; epinephrine; estrogens; isoniazid; major tranquilizers such as chlorpromazine and thioridazine; MAO inhibitors (drugs such as the antidepressants phenelzine and tranylcypromine); niacin; octreotide; oral contraceptives; oral drugs for diabetes such as chlorpropamide and tolbutamide; phenytoin; steroid medications such as prednisone; sulfa antibiotics such as sulfamethoxazole; and thyroid medications such as levothyroxine.

Use alcohol carefully, since excessive alcohol consumption can cause low blood sugar. Don't drink unless your doctor has approved it.

What are the possible side effects of Novolin?

Side effects cannot be anticipated. If any develop or change in intensity, tell your doctor as soon as possible. Only your doctor can determine if it is safe for you to continue taking this drug.

Side effects may include: local skin reaction (red, swollen and itchy skin where the insulin has been injected)

Although rare, if after injecting insulin you experience rash all over the body, shortness of breath, fast pulse, sweating, and low blood pressure, seek immediate emergency medical care.

Can I receive Novolin if I am pregnant or breastfeeding?

Novolin is not contraindicated in pregnancy or breastfeeding. However, it is particularly important to maintain good control of your diabetes during pregnancy. Special attention must be paid to your diet, exercise and insulin regimens. If you are pregnant, plan to become pregnant, or are breastfeeding, consult your physician or nurse educator.

What should I do if I miss a dose of Novolin?

Contact your doctor for advice if you miss an insulin injection or a meal.

How should I store Novolin?

Insulin should be stored in a cold place, preferably in a refrigerator, but not in the freezer. Do not let it freeze.

Keep Novolin R PenFill cartridges in the carton so that they will stay clean and protected from light. Be sure to protect cartridges from sunlight and extreme heat or cold.

The Novolin R PenFill cartridge that you are *currently* using should not be refrigerated but should be kept as cool as possible (below 86 degress) and away from direct heat and light. Unrefrigerated Novolin R PenFill cartridges must be discarded 28 days after the first use, even if they still contain Novolin R insulin.

Never use PenFill cartridges after the expiration date, which is printed on the label and carton.

Novolin N PenFill cartridges can be kept unrefrigerated for 14 days. Novolin 70/30 PenFill cartridges can be kept unrefrigerated for 10 days. Unrefrigerated cartridges must be used within this time period or discarded.

Never use any Novolin N PenFill cartridge or Novolin 70/30 if the precipitate (the white deposit) has become lumpy or granular in appearance or has formed a deposit of solid particles on the wall of the cartridge. This insulin should not be used if the liquid in the cartridge remains clear after it has been mixed.

NOXAFIL
Generic name: Posaconazole

What is Noxafil?

Noxafil is used to help prevent fungal infections caused by *Aspergillus* and *Candida*, in people who are13 years of age and older and have an immune system which is severely impaired.

Noxafil is also used to treat orthopharyngeal candidiasis (thrush).

What is the most important information I should know about Noxafil?

If you are allergic to other antifungals, you should talk to your doctor before taking Noxafil.

It is important to notify your physician of all prescription and nonprescription medications you are taking. It is especially important to notify your physician if you are taking any of the following medications: terfenadine, astemizole, cisapride, pimozide, halofantrine, quinidine, cimetidine, rifabutin, phenytoin, efavirenz, ergot alkaloids (eg, ergotamine, dihydroergotamine), sirolimus, cyclosporine, and tacrolimus.

Noxafil may cause you to develop heart arrhythmias or liver complications. It is important to notify your doctor if you have had any previous liver or heart arrhythmia problems. While on therapy with Noxafil, your doctor will perform periodic monitoring to try and prevent these conditions from occurring.

It is important to notify your doctor if you develop severe diarrhea or vomiting while on therapy with Noxafil, because this may decrease the effectiveness of Noxafil.

It is important to take Noxafil with a full meal or liquid nutritional supplement. If you cannot do this, then it is important to notify your physician who may want to switch you to a different therapy.

Who should not take Noxafil?
Do not take Noxafil if you are allergic to any of its ingredients, or if you are taking terfenadine, astemizole, pimozide, cisapride, quinidine, halofantrine, ergot alkaloids (eg, ergotamine, dihydroergotamine), and sirolimus.

What should I tell my doctor before I take the first dose of Noxafil?
Tell your doctor about all prescription, over-the-counter, and herbal medications you are taking to avoid an interaction with Noxafil. Also, talk to your doctor about your complete medical history, especially if you have a history of abnormal heart rate or rhythm or liver problems, are pregnant, plant to become pregnant, or are breastfeeding.

What is the usual dosage?
The information below is based on the dosage guidelines your doctor uses. Depending on your condition and medical history, your doctor may prescribe a different regimen. Do not change the dosage or stop taking your medication without your doctor's approval.

Prevention of Invasive Fungal Infections
Adults: Noxafil oral suspension should be given at 200 milligrams (mg) (5 milliliters [mL]) three times a day. The duration of therapy will be based on the recovery from your disease state.

Orapharyngeal Candidiasis
Adults: 100 mg (2.5 mL) twice a day on the first day, then 100 mg (2.5 mL) once a day for 13 days

Orapharyngeal Candidiasis Resistant to Other Antifungals
Adults: 400 mg (10 mL) twice a day. Duration of treatment is based on the severity of your condition and how well you respond.

How should I take Noxafil?
Shake Noxafil well before taking it; take each dose of Noxafil oral suspension with a full meal or liquid nutritional supplement. If you cannot eat a full meal or a nutritional supplement, a different type of antifungal therapy should be considered besides Noxafil.

What should I avoid while taking Noxafil?

While taking Noxafil, avoid taking terfenadine, astemizole, pimozide, cisapride, quinidine, halofantrine, ergot alkaloids (eg, ergotamine, dihydroergotamine), and sirolimus.

What are possible food and drug interactions associated with Noxafil?

If Noxafil is taken with certain other drugs, the effects of either could be increased, decreased, or altered. It is especially important to check with your doctor before combining Noxafil with any of the following: astemizole, atazanavir, calcium channel blockers, cimetidine, cisapride, cyclosporine, digoxin, efavirenz, ergot alkaloids (eg, ergotamine, dihydroergotamine), halofantrine, midazolam, phenytoin, pimozide, quinidine, rifabutin, ritonavir, sirolimus, statins, tacrolimus, terfenadine, and vinca alkaloids (eg, vincristine, vinblastine).

What are the possible side effects of Noxafil?

Side effects cannot be anticipated. If any develop or change in intensity, tell your doctor as soon as possible. Only your doctor can determine if it is safe for you to continue taking this drug.

Side effects may include: breathing problems, constipation, cough, diarrhea, dizziness, fever, headache, loss of appetite, nausea, shakiness, stomach pain, tiredness, upset stomach, vomiting, weakness

Can I receive Noxafil if I am pregnant or breastfeeding?

The effects of Noxafil during pregnancy and breastfeeding are unknown. Talk with your doctor before taking this drug if you are pregnant, planning to become pregnant, or are breastfeeding.

What should I do if I miss a dose of Noxafil?

Take the missed dose as soon as you remember it. However, if it is almost time for your next dose, skip the one you missed and return to your regular dosing schedule. Do not take a double dose.

How should I store Noxafil?

Store at room temperature; do not freeze. Keep container tightly closed.

NUVARING

Generic name: Etonogestrel and ethinyl estradiol

What is NuvaRing?

NuvaRing is a flexible combined contraceptive vaginal ring. It is used to prevent pregnancy.

What is the most important information I should know about NuvaRing?

NuvaRing does not protect against HIV infection (AIDS) and other sexually transmitted diseases (STD's) such as chlamydia, genital herpes, genital warts, gonorrhea, hepatitis B, and syphilis.

To make sure NuvaRing works properly, you must follow a strict schedule for insertion and removal. Each ring should be inserted and left in place for exactly 3 weeks, then removed. Exactly 1 week after removal, a new ring should be inserted for the following 3 weeks. Always insert and remove NuvaRing on the same day of the week, at approximately the same time of day.

Cigarette smoking increases the risk of serious cardiovascular side effects when you use combination oral contraceptives. This risk increases even more if you are over age 35 and if you smoke 15 or more cigarettes a day. Women who use combination hormonal contraceptives, including NuvaRing, are strongly advised not to smoke.

Do not breastfeed while using NuvaRing. Some of the medicine may pass through the milk to the baby and could cause yellowing of the skin (jaundice) and breast enlargement in your baby. NuvaRing could also decrease the amount and quality of your breast milk.

Who should not take NuvaRing?

Do not use NuvaRing if you have any of the following conditions: pregnancy or suspected pregnancy; a history of blood clots in your legs (thrombophlebitis), lungs (pulmonary embolism), or eyes; chest pain (angina pectoris); a history of heart attack or stroke; severe high blood pressure; diabetes with complications of the kidneys, eyes, nerves or blood vessels; headaches with neurological symptoms; known or suspected breast cancer or cancer of the lining of the uterus, cervix or vagina (now or in the past); unexplained vaginal bleeding (until a diagnosis is reached by your doctor); yellowing of the whites of the eyes or of the skin (jaundice) during pregnancy or during past use of birth control medications of any kind; liver tumors or active liver disease; heart valve or heart rhythm disorders associated with blood clots formation; need for a long period of bed rest following major surgery; an allergic reaction to any of the components of NuvaRing.

What should I tell my doctor before I take the first dose of NuvaRing?

Tell your doctor about all prescription, over-the-counter, and herbal medications you are taking before beginning treatment with NuvaRing. Also, talk to your doctor about your complete medical history, especially if you have any of the following conditions: a family history of breast cancer, breast nodules, fibrocystic disease, an abnormal breast x-ray, or abnormal mammogram, diabetes (high blood sugar), high blood pressure, high cholesterol or triglycerides, headaches or epilepsy (seizures), mental depression, gallbladder, liver, heart or kidney disease, scanty or irregular menstrual periods, major surgery (You may need to stop using NuvaRing for a while to reduce your chance of getting blood clots), any condition that makes the vagina get irritated easily, prolapsed (dropped) uterus, dropped bladder (cystocele), or rectal prolapse (rectocele), severe constipation, and history of toxic shock syndrome.

What is the usual dosage?
The information below is based on the dosage guidelines your doctor uses. Depending on your condition and medical history, your doctor may prescribe a different regimen. Do not change the dosage or stop taking your medication without your doctor's approval.

Adults: NuvaRing is inserted in the vagina once a month. It stays in the vagina continuously for three weeks. It must be removed exactly 21 days after insertion. A new ring is inserted precisely 7 days later.

The time to start use of NuvaRing depends on your previous contraceptive program:

If you did not use a hormonal contraceptive in the past month
Count the first day of your menstrual period as day 1. Insert the first ring between day 1 and day 5 of the cycle, even if you are still bleeding on day 5. During the first cycle, use an extra method of birth control such as male condoms or spermicide for the first 7 days of ring use.

If you are switching from a combination birth control pill
Insert NuvaRing any time during the first 7 days after the last tablet and no later than the day you would have started a new pill cycle. No extra birth control method is needed.

If you are switching from a progestin-only contraceptive
When you are switching from a progestin-only contraceptive, use an extra method of birth control, such as male condoms or spermicide, for the first 7 days after inserting NuvaRing.

If you are switching from the "mini-pill," you can start using NuvaRing on any day of the month. Do not skip days between your last pill and first day of NuvaRing use.

If you are switching from a progestin implant (Norplant), start using NuvaRing on the same day you have your implant removed.

If you are switching from an injectable contraceptive (Depo-Provera), start using NuvaRing on the day when your next injection is due.

If you are switching from a progestin intra-uterine device (IUD), start using NuvaRing on the same day you have your IUD removed.

Following a first trimester abortion or miscarriage
If you start using NuvaRing within 5 days after a complete first trimester abortion or miscarriage, you do not need to use an extra method of con-

traception. If more than 5 days have passed, proceed as you would if you had not used a hormonal contraceptive for the past month.

Following a second trimester abortion or miscarriage
You may start using NuvaRing 4 weeks after a complete second trimester abortion or miscarriage.

Following delivery
If you choose not to breastfeed your child, you may start using NuvaRing 4 weeks after a complete delivery. It is recommended to use an extra form of contraception such a male condoms or spermicide for the first 7 days. If you choose to breastfeed your child, do not use NuvaRing. Instead, use other forms of contraception until the child is weaned.

How should I take NuvaRing?

Wash and dry your hands and remove NuvaRing from its foil pouch. Choose the position that is most comfortable for you, such as lying down, squatting, or standing with one leg up. Hold NuvaRing between your thumb and index finger and press the opposite sides of the ring together. Gently push the folded ring into your vagina. The exact position of the ring is not important for it to work. If you feel discomfort, use your finger to gently push NuvaRing further into the vagina. Most women do not feel the ring once it is in place, although some are aware of it.

Leave the ring in place for exactly 3 weeks, and then remove it. Hook your index finger under the forward rim or hold the rim between your index finger and middle finger and pull the ring out. Place the used ring in the foil pouch it came in and dispose of it in the garbage, away from children and pets. Do not discard in the toilet.

Your menstrual period will usually start 2 to 3 days after the ring is removed and may not have finished before it's time to insert the next ring. For continued pregnancy protection, you need to insert the new ring exactly 1 week after the old one was removed, even if your period has not stopped.

What should I avoid while taking NuvaRing?

Do not smoke or breastfeed while using NuvaRing.

What are possible food and drug interactions associated with NuvaRing?

If NuvaRing is taken with certain other drugs, the effects of either could be increased, decreased, or altered. It is especially important to check with your doctor before combining NuvaRing with any of the following: acetaminophen, antibiotics such as ampicillin and tetracycline, anticonvulsants, antifungals, atorvastatin, clofibrate, cyclosporine, HIV drugs known as protease inhibitors, morphine, phenylbutazone, prednisolone, rifadin, St. John's wort, temazepam, theophylline, and vitamin C.

What are the possible side effects of NuvaRing?

Side effects cannot be anticipated. If any develop or change in intensity, tell your doctor as soon as possible. Only your doctor can determine if it is safe for you to continue taking this drug.

Side effects may include: abdominal cramps, allergic rash, bloating, blood clots, breakthrough bleeding and spotting, breast secretions, change in menstrual flow, changes in the breast such as tenderness or enlargement, dark pigmentation of the skin, decreased milk production in nursing mothers, depression, emotional instability, gallbladder disease, headaches, heart attack, high blood pressure, intolerance to contact lenses, liver disease, liver tumors, migraine headaches, missed periods, nausea, problems with the ring, sinus inflammation, stroke, swelling, temporary infertility after discontinuing NuvaRing, upper respiratory tract infections, vaginal inflammation or discharge, vision problems, vomiting, weight gain or loss, yeast infections, yellow tint to the skin

Can I receive NuvaRing if I am pregnant or breastfeeding?

NuvaRing should not be used during pregnancy or while nursing.

What should I do if I miss a dose of NuvaRing?

If NuvaRing slips out, you'll still be protected against pregnancy provided the ring is replaced within 3 hours. You can use the old ring (after rinsing it with cool or lukewarm water) or insert a new ring. Remove the ring according to your original schedule.

If you're unable to replace the ring within 3 hours, insert it as soon as possible and use an additional method of birth control for 7 days.

If you forget and leave the ring in place for an extra week, remove it, take a one-week break, and reinsert a new one on day 7. If you leave the ring in place for more than 4 weeks you may not be adequately protected against pregnancy.

If you miss a menstrual period, you should check to be sure you are not pregnant if any of the following circumstances apply: if NuvaRing was out of the vagina for more than 3 hours during the 3 weeks of ring use; if you waited longer than 1 week to insert a new ring after removing the old one; if you followed the instructions but miss 2 periods in a row; or if you have left NuvaRing in place for longer than 4 weeks.

How should I store NuvaRing?

Store NuvaRing at room temperature. Avoid direct sunlight or storing above 86°F (30°C).

NUVIGIL
Generic name: Armodafinil

What is Nuvigil?

Nuvigil is used to improve awakeness in adults who are very sleepy due to one of the following diagnosed sleep problems: shift work sleep disorder (SWSD), obstructive sleep apnea/hypopnea syndrome (OSAHS) or narcolepsy. Nuvigil is used along with other medical treatments for these sleep problems and is not a replacement for a continuous positive airway pressure (CPAP) machine. It is important that you continue to use your CPAP machine while sleeping.

What is the most important information I should know about Nuvigil?

Nuvigil may cause a serious allergic reaction. Stop Nuvigil and call your doctor right away or seek emergency treatment if you develop any of the following: swelling of your face, eyes, lips, tongue, or throat; trouble swallowing or breathing; skin rash; hives; sores in your mouth; blistering or peeling skin; or hoarse voice.

You should be diagnosed with a sleep disorder before taking Nuvigil. This drug will not cure any sleep disorder, but it may help improve wakefulness. Nuvigil does not take the place of getting enough sleep. Follow your doctor's advice about good sleep habits and using other treatments.

Nuvigil has not been studied in children less than 17 years old and should not be used in this age group.

Nuvigil is a controlled substance because it can be abused or lead to dependence. Keep it in a safe place to prevent misuse and abuse. Selling or giving away Nuvigil may harm others, and is against the law. Tell your doctor if you have ever abused or been dependent on alcohol, prescription medicines, or street drugs.

It is not known if Nuvigil is effective or safe to use in children less than 17 years old.

Who should not take Nuvigil?

Do not take Nuvigil if you are allergic to any of its ingredients or if you have had a rash or allergic reaction to modafinil, the active ingredient in Provigil.

What should I tell my doctor before I take the first dose of Nuvigil?

Tell your doctor about all prescription, over-the-counter, and herbal medication you are taking before beginning treatment with Nuvigil. Also, talk to your doctor about your complete medical history, especially if you have ever had a heart attack, mental health problems, high blood pressure, heart problems, liver or kidney problems, or a history of drug or alcohol addiction. You should also tell your doctor if you are pregnant, planning to become pregnant, or are breastfeeding.

Tell the doctor if you use a hormonal birth control method; Nuvigil can interfere with these types of birth control. Hormonal birth control methods include pills, shots, implants, patches, vaginal rings, and intrauterine devices (IUDs). Women using hormonal birth control with Nuvigil may have a higher chance of getting pregnant while taking Nuvigil, and for 1 month after stopping the drug. Talk to your doctor about birth control methods that are right for you while using Nuvigil.

What is the usual dosage?
The information below is based on the dosage guidelines your doctor uses. Depending on your condition and medical history, your doctor may prescribe a different regimen. Do not change the dosage or stop taking your medication without you're doctor's approval.

Obstructive Sleep Apnea/Hypopnea Syndrome (OSAHS) and Narcolepsy
Adults: The recommended dose is 150 milligrams (mg) or 250 mg given as a single dose in the morning. In patients with OSAHS, doses up to 250 mg a day, given as a single dose, have been well tolerated.

Shift Work Sleep Disorder (SWSD)
Adults: The recommended dose is 150 mg given daily approximately 1 hour before the start of a work shift.

How should I take Nuvigil?
Take it exactly as prescribed by your doctor. Do not change the dose or the time of day that you take Nuvigil without your doctor's approval. Your doctor will tell you the right time of day to take this medication. If you take Nuvigil too close to your bedtime, you may find it harder to go to sleep.

What should I avoid while taking Nuvigil?
Do not drive, operate dangerous machinery, or engage in potentially hazardous activities until you know how this drug affects you. You should also avoid drinking alcohol while taking this drug.

What are possible food and drug interactions associated with Nuvigil?
If Nuvigil is taken with certain other drugs, the effects of either could be increased, decreased, or altered. It is especially important to check with your doctor before combining Nuvigil with the following: hormonal birth control, cyclosporine, diazepam, ethinyl estradiol, midazolam, omeprazole, phenytoin, propranolol, and triazolam.

What are the possible side effects of Nuvigil?
Side effects cannot be anticipated. If any develop or change in intensity, tell your doctor as soon as possible. Only your doctor can determine if it

is safe for you to continue taking this drug. Stop taking Nuvigil and call your doctor immediately or seek emergency treatment if you experience any of the following: a serious allergic reaction or rash; swelling of the face, eyes, lips, tongue, or throat; mental (psychiatric) symptoms such as depression, anxiety, hallucinations, mania, or thoughts of suicide; or heart problems including chest pain.

Common side effects may include: headache, nausea, dizziness, trouble sleeping

Can I receive Nuvigil if I am pregnant or breastfeeding?
It is not known if Nuvigil is safe to use during pregnancy and breastfeeding. Tell your doctor immediately if you are pregnant, plan to become pregnant, or are breastfeeding.

How should I store Nuvigil?
Store at room temperature.

OCUFLOX
Generic name: Ofloxacin ophthalmic solution

What is Ocuflox?
Ocuflox is an antibiotic used in the treatment of bacterial eye infections, including conjunctivitis (pinkeye) and ulcers of the cornea (the transparent covering over the pupil).

What is the most important information I should know about Ocuflox?
Other forms of Ocuflox have been known to cause allergic reactions in a few patients. These reactions can be extremely serious, leading to loss of consciousness and cardiovascular collapse. Early warning signs include a skin rash, hives, and itching. Other symptoms may include swelling of the face or throat, shortness of breath, and a tingling feeling. If you develop any of these symptoms, stop using Ocuflox and seek emergency help immediately.

If you wear contact lenses, ask your doctor if you should wear them during treatment. Ocuflox ophthalmic can cause the development of crystals on contact lenses. After applying this medication, wait at least 15 minutes before inserting contact lenses, unless otherwise directed by your doctor.

Who should not take Ocuflox?
Do not use Ocuflox ophthalmic if you have a viral or fungal infection in your eye. It is used to treat infections caused by bacteria only.

If you've ever had an allergic reaction to a quinolone antibiotic you should not use Ocuflox.

What should I tell my doctor before I take the first dose of Ocuflox?

Tell your doctor about all prescription, over-the-counter, and herbal medications you are taking before beginning treatment with Ocuflox.

What is the usual dosage?

The information below is based on the dosage guidelines your doctor uses. Depending on your condition and medical history, your doctor may prescribe a different regimen. Do not change the dosage or stop taking your medication without your doctor's approval.

Bacterial Conjunctivitis (Pinkeye)
Adults: Apply 1 or 2 drops in the affected eye(s) every 2 to 4 hours for the first 2 days, then 4 times daily for the next 5 days.

Bacterial Corneal Ulcers
Adults: For the first 2 days, apply 1 or 2 drops to the affected eye every 30 minutes while awake; also get up 4 to 6 hours after retiring and apply 1 or 2 drops. On days 3 through 7, apply 1 or 2 drops hourly while awake. From days 7 to 9 onward, apply 1 or 2 drops 4 times a day.

Children: The safety and effectiveness have not been established in children under the age of 1 year.

How should I take Ocuflox?

Wash your hands before using the eye drops. To apply the eye drops, shake the drops gently to be sure the medicine is well mixed. Tilt your head back slightly and pull down on your lower eyelid. Position the dropper above your eye. Look up and away from the dropper. Squeeze out a drop and close your eye. Apply gentle pressure to the inside corner of your eye (near your nose) for about 1 minute to prevent the liquid from draining down your tear duct.

If you are using more than one drop in the same eye or drops in both eyes, repeat the process with about 5 minutes between drops.

What should I avoid while taking Ocuflox?

Do not touch the dropper to any surface, including your eyes or hands. The dropper is sterile. If it becomes contaminated, it could cause an infection in your eye.

Do not use any eye drop that is discolored or has particles in it.

Use caution when driving, operating machinery, or performing other potentially hazardous activities. Ocuflox ophthalmic may cause blurred vision. If you experience blurred vision, avoid these activities.

What are possible food and drug interactions associated with Ocuflox?

If Ocuflox is taken with certain other drugs, the effects of either could be increased, decreased, or altered. It is especially important to check with your doctor before combining Ocuflox with the following: caffeine, cyclosporine, theophylline, warfarin, and other forms of eyedrops.

What are the possible side effects of Ocuflox?
Side effects cannot be anticipated. If any develop or change in intensity, tell your doctor as soon as possible. Only your doctor can determine if it is safe for you to continue taking this drug.

Side effects may include: local burning or discomfort, allergic reaction, blurred vision, dizziness, dry eye, eye pain, feeling of a foreign body in the eye, inflammation, itching, nausea, redness, sensitivity to light, stinging, swelling of the eye or face, tearing

Can I receive Ocuflox if I am pregnant or breastfeeding?
The effects of Ocuflox during pregnancy and breastfeeding are unknown. Tell your doctor immediately if you are pregnant, plan to become pregnant, or are breastfeeding.

What should I do if I miss a dose of Ocuflox?
Use the missed dose as soon as you remember. However, if it is almost time for your next regularly scheduled dose, skip the missed dose and use the next one as directed. Do not use a double dose of this medication.

How should I store Ocuflox?
Store Ocuflox at room temperature.

Ofloxacin See *Floxin, page 568.*

Ofloxacin ophthalmic solution See *Ocuflox, page 931.*

OGEN
Generic name: Estropipate

What is Ogen?
Ogen is a form of estrogen. Estrogen is a female sex hormone necessary for many processes in the body. Ogen is used to treat symptoms of menopause; deficiency in ovary function (including underdevelopment of female sexual characteristics and some types of infertility); some types of breast cancer in men and in postmenopausal women; degeneration of the vagina and urethra; and prostate cancer. In addition, Ogen is used to prevent osteoporosis.

What is the most important information I should know about Ogen?
Because estrogens have been linked with increased risk of endometrial cancer (cancer in the lining of the uterus) in post-menopausal women, it

is essential to have regular check-ups and to report any unusual vaginal bleeding to your doctor immediately.

Treatment with estrogens long-term may increase the risk of heart attack, stroke, invasive breast cancer, and blood clots in lungs and legs. Because of these risks, you should contact your doctor or healthcare provider to discuss your individual risks and benefits before taking an estrogen long-term. You should also talk to your doctor or healthcare provider on a regular basis (for example, every 3-6 months) about whether you should continue this treatment.

Women who take estrogen after menopause are more likely to develop gallbladder disease, and are also at risk for developing dementia, and vision abnormalities.

Who should not take Ogen?

Estrogens should not be used if you know or suspect you have breast cancer or other cancers promoted by estrogen. Do not use estrogen if you are pregnant or think you may be pregnant. Also avoid estrogen if you have abnormal, undiagnosed vaginal bleeding, liver disease, or if you have blood clots or a blood clotting disorder or a history of blood clotting disorders associated with previous estrogen use.

Ogen should not be used if you are sensitive to or have ever had an allergic reaction to any of its components.

What should I tell my doctor before I take the first dose of Ogen?

Tell your doctor about all prescription, over-the-counter, and herbal medications you are taking before beginning treatment with Ogen. Also, talk to your doctor about your complete medical history, especially if you have a history of high blood pressure, angina (chest pain), heart disease, high levels of cholesterol or triglycerides in the blood, liver disease, kidney disease, asthma (wheezing), epilepsy (seizures), migraines, diabetes (high blood sugar), depression, gallbladder disease, uterine fibroids. Tell your doctor if you have had a hysterectomy (uterus removed) or if you have experienced a circulation bleeding or blood-clotting disorder, undiagnosed abnormal vaginal bleeding, or any type of breast, uterine, or cancer associated with the use of hormones.

What is the usual dosage?

The information below is based on the dosage guidelines your doctor uses. Depending on your condition and medical history, your doctor may prescribe a different regimen. Do not change the dosage or stop taking your medication without your doctor's approval.

Hot Flushes and Night Sweats

Adults: The usual dose ranges from one .625 milligram (mg) tablet to two 2.5 mg tablets per day. Tablets should be taken in cycles, according to your doctor's instructions.

Vaginal Inflammation and Dryness
Adults: *Tablets:* The usual dose ranges from one .625 mg tablet to two 2.5 mg tablets per day. Tablets should be taken in cycles, according to your doctor's instructions. *Vaginal* Cream: The usual dose is 2 to 4 grams daily. Cream should be used in cycles, and only for limited periods of time.

Estrogen Hormone Deficiency
Adults: The usual dose ranges from one 1.25 mg tablet to three 2.5 tablets per day, taken for 3 weeks, followed by a rest period of 8 to 10 days.

Ovarian Failure
Adults: The usual dose ranges from one 1.25 mg tablet to three 2.5 mg tablets per day for 3 weeks, followed by a rest period of 8 to 10 days. Your doctor may increase or decrease your dosage according to your response.

Prevention of Osteoporosis
Adults: The usual dose is one .625 mg tablet per day for 25 days of a 31-day monthly cycle.

How should I take Ogen?
Take each dose with a full glass of water. Take Ogen with food or milk to lessen stomach upset. Try to take each dose at the same time each day. You may be taking it every day, or you may be taking it every day for 3 weeks with 1 week off each month to mimic your body's natural cycle. Follow the directions on your prescription label.

If you are taking Ogen to treat cancer, you may be taking it several times a day in very large doses.

What should I avoid while taking Ogen?
There are no restrictions on food, beverages, or activity while taking Ogen unless your doctor directs otherwise.

What are possible food and drug interactions associated with Ogen?
If Ogen is taken with certain other drugs, the effects of either could be increased, decreased, or altered. It is especially important to check with your doctor before combining Ogen with any of the following: barbiturates such as phenobarbital; blood thinners; epilepsy drugs; grapefruit juice; inhibitors of CYP3A4 such as erythromycin, clarithromycin, ketoconazole, itraconazole, ritonavir; insulin; rifampin; St. John's wort; and tricyclic antidepressants.

What are the possible side effects of Ogen?
Side effects cannot be anticipated. If any develop or change in intensity, tell your doctor as soon as possible. Only your doctor can determine if it is safe for you to continue taking this drug.

Side effects may include: abdominal cramps, bloating, breakthrough bleeding, breast enlargement, breast tenderness and secretions, change in amount of cervical secretion, changes in sex drive, changes in vaginal bleeding patterns, chorea (irregular, rapid, jerky movements, usually affecting the face and limbs), depression, dizziness, enlargement of benign tumors (fibroids), excessive hairiness, fluid retention, hair loss, headache, inability to use contact lenses, menstrual changes, migraine, nausea, reduced ability to tolerate carbohydrates, spotting, spotty darkening of the skin, especially around the face, skin eruptions (especially on the legs and arms) with bleeding, skin irritation, skin redness and scaling, vaginal yeast infection, vision problems, vomiting, weight gain or loss, yellow eyes and skin

Can I receive Ogen if I am pregnant or breastfeeding?
Estrogens should not be used during pregnancy. If you are pregnant or plan to become pregnant, notify your doctor immediately. These drugs may appear in breast milk and could affect a nursing infant. If Ogen is essential to your health, your doctor may advise you to discontinue breastfeeding until your treatment is finished.

What should I do if I miss a dose of Ogen?
If you do miss a dose, take it as soon as you remember. However, if it is almost time for your next dose, skip the missed dose and take only your next regularly scheduled dose. Do not take a double dose of this medication.

How should I store Ogen?
Store Ogen at room temperature.

Olanzapine *See Zyprexa/Zyprexa Zydis/Zyprexa Intramuscular, page 1508.*

Olanzapine and fluoxetine hydrochloride *See Symbyax, page 1240.*

Olmesartan medoxomil *See Benicar, page 202.*

Olmesartan medoxomil and hydrochlorothiazide *See Benicar HCT, page 204.*

Olopatadine hydrochloride *See Patanol, page 979.*

Olsalazine sodium *See Dipentum, page 428.*

OLUX-E
Generic name: Clobetasol propionate

What is Olux-E?
Olux-E is a topical steroid used to treat the inflammation and itchiness in people age 12 and older.

What is the most important information I should know about Olux-E?
The propellant in Olux-E Foam is flammable. Avoid fire, flame or smoking during and immediately following application.

Systemic absorption of topical steroids may cause adrenal suppression (the inability of the adrenal gland to produce adequate amounts of cortisol). Topical corticosteroids may also cause the manifestations of Cushing's syndrome (high levels of cortisol in the body), high blood sugar/glucose, and glucose in urine.

Application over large surface areas, prolonged use, and use of a dressing over the site of application may increase absorption. Adrenal suppression should be monitored and if necessary the drug should be used less frequency or stopped.

If irritation develops, stop use and use proper treatment. If a skin infection develops while using Olux-E, use the proper antifungal or antibacterial. If there is no response, stop use until the infection is controlled.

Olux-E is for external use only. Unless otherwise prescribed, it should not be used on the face or in skin-fold areas (eg, underarms or groin). Avoid contact with eyes and other mucous membranes. Wash hands after use. Treated areas should not be wrapped or bandaged unless otherwise directed by your doctor.

Report any signs of an adverse reaction to your doctor. If undergoing surgery, let your doctor know that you are using Olux-E Foam. Stop use when improvement of condition is seen.

Tell your doctor if there is no improvement after 2 weeks. No more than 50 grams (21 capfuls) should be used per week.

Who should not take Olux-E?
Do not use Olux-E if you are allergic to any of its ingredients.

What should I tell my doctor before I take the first dose of Olux-E?
Tell your doctor about all prescription, over-the-counter, and herbal medications you are taking, before beginning treatment with Olux-E. Also, talk to your doctor about your complete medical history, especially if you have adrenal suppression, Cushing's disease, or high blood sugar/glucose.

What is the usual dosage?
The information below is based on the dosage guidelines your doctor uses. Depending on your condition and medical history, your doctor may prescribe a different regimen. Do not change the dosage or stop taking your medication without your doctor's approval.

Apply a thin layer of Olux-E to the affected skin twice daily, morning and evening. As with other corticosteroids, Olux-E should be discontinued when the inflammation goes away. If no improvement is seen within 2 weeks, consult your doctor.

How should I take Olux-E?
For proper dispensing of foam, shake the can, hold it upside down, and depress the actuator. Apply a small amount of the foam to the affected area (excluding the eyes, face, groin, and armpits) and rub in gently until the foam is absorbed. Do not use more than a dollop the size of a golf ball. Do not cover areas treated with Olux-E with a dressing.

What should I avoid while taking Olux-E?
Avoid fire, flame or smoking during and immediately following application.

Olux-E is for external use only. Unless otherwise prescribed, it should not be used on the face or in skin-fold areas (eg, underarms or groin). Avoid contact with eyes and other mucous membranes. Treated areas shouldn't be wrapped or bandaged unless otherwise directed by the doctor.

What are possible food and drug interactions associated with Olux-E?
There are currently no known food or drug interactions associated with Olux-E. However, discuss with your physician all prescription and nonprescription medications you are currently taking.

What are the possible side effects of Olux-E?
Side effects cannot be anticipated. If any develop or change in intensity, tell your doctor as soon as possible. Only your doctor can determine if it is safe for you to continue taking this drug.

Side effects may include: burning/stinging/itching at application site, infection of hair follicles, acne, loss of skin color, inflammation, infection, irritation, stretch marks, rash

Can I receive Olux-E if I am pregnant or breastfeeding?
The effects of Olux-E during pregnancy and breastfeeding are unknown. Talk with your doctor before using this medication if you are pregnant, plan to become pregnant, or are breastfeeding.

What should I do if I miss a dose of Olux-E?
Apply the missed dose as soon as you remember it. However, if it is almost time for your next dose, skip the dose you missed and return to your regular dosing schedule.

How should I store Olux-E?
Store at room temperature, away from excessive heat or temperatures above 120°F (49°C).

Omega-3-acid ethyl esters *See Lovaza, page 772.*

Omeprazole *See Prilosec, page 1065.*

Omeprazole and sodium bicarbonate *See Zegerid, page 1453.*

OMNICEF
Generic name: Cefdinir

What is Omnicef?
Omnicef is an antibiotic used to treat many different types of bacterial infections, such as pneumonia, bronchitis, sinus infections, tonsillitis, ear infections, and skin infections.

What is the most important information I should know about Omnicef?
Your symptoms may start to improve before the infection is completely treated. However, you still have to take all of the Omnicef that has been prescribed for you even if you begin to feel better. Skipping doses or not completing the full course of therapy may decrease the effectiveness of your treatment and increase the likelihood the bacteria will develop resistance and will not be treatable by Omnicef or other antibacterial drugs in the future.

Antacids containing magnesium or aluminum and iron supplements, including multivitamins that contain iron, interfere with the effectiveness of Omnicef. If you are required to take these products, you should take Omnicef at least 2 hours before or after taking them. The only exception to this rule is the iron-fortified infant formula.

Diarrhea is a common problem caused by antibiotics which usually ends when the antibiotic is discontinued. If you develop watery and bloody stools, with our without stomach cramps, and fever; contact your doctor right away.

Omnicef suspension contains 2.86 grams of sugar per teaspoonful. If a child is diabetic, this could cause an increase in blood sugar levels.

Who should not take Omnicef?

If you've ever had an allergic reaction to a cephalosporin antibiotic, you should not take Omnicef. Note, too, that if you are allergic to penicillin, you may also be allergic to cephalosporins. The reaction can be extremely severe. Be sure to let the doctor know about any allergies you may have.

What should I tell my doctor before I take the first dose of Omnicef?

Tell your doctor about all medications you are taking before beginning treatment with Omnicef. Also, talk to your doctor about your complete medical history, especially if you have colitis (inflammation of the bowel), diabetes, kidney problems, or seizures.

What is the usual dosage?

The information below is based on the dosage guidelines your doctor uses. Depending on your condition and medical history, your doctor may prescribe a different regimen. Do not change the dosage or stop taking your medication without your doctor's approval.

Flare-ups of Chronic Bronchitis
Adults and adolescents 13 years and older: The usual starting dose is 300 mg every 12 hours for 5 to 10 days or 600 mg once a day for 10 days.

Middle Ear Infections
Children 6 months to 12 years old: The usual starting dose is 7 mg per 2.2 pounds every 12 hours for 5 to 10 days or 14 mg per 2.2 pounds once a day for 10 days.

Pneumonia
Adults and adolescents 13 years and older: The usual starting dose is 300 mg every 12 hours for 10 days.

Sinus Infections
Adults and adolescents 13 years and older: The usual starting dose is 300 mg every 12 hours or 600 mg once a day for 10 days.

Children 6 months to 12 years old: The usual starting dose is 7 mg per 2.2 pounds every 12 hours or 14 mg per 2.2 pounds once a day for 10 days.

Skin Infections
Adults and adolescents 13 years and older: The usual starting dose is 300 mg every 12 hours for 10 days.

Children 6 months to 12 years old: The usual starting dose is 7 mg per 2.2 pounds every 12 hours for 10 days.

Throat and Tonsil Infections
Adults and adolescents 13 years and older: The usual starting dose is 300 mg every 12 hours for 5 to 10 days or 600 mg once a day for 10 days.

Children 6 months to 12 years old: The usual starting dose is 7 mg per 2.2 pounds every 12 hours for 5 to 10 days or 14 mg per 2.2 pounds once a day for 10 days.

The maximum daily dose is 600 milligrams (mg), regardless of the infection.

The dose of Omnicef Suspension is based on body weight. The suspension contains 125 mg per teaspoonful (5 ml). Dosage should never exceed 600 mg or 24 ml daily.

If you have kidney problems, your doctor will lower the dosage.

How should I take Omnicef?
Shake the oral suspension thoroughly before each use. The drug can be taken with or without food. Take each tablet or capsule with a full glass of water.

Be sure to finish your entire prescription, even if you begin to feel better. If you stop taking the drug too soon, some germs may survive and cause a relapse.

What should I avoid while taking Omnicef?
Do not take antacids that contain aluminum or magnesium, iron supplements, or multivitamins with iron, with a dose of Omnicef. Take these products at least 2 hours before or after a dose of Omnicef to prevent decreased effectiveness of the antibiotic.

What are possible food and drug interactions associated with Omnicef?
If Omnicef is taken with certain other drugs, the effects of either could be increased, decreased, or altered. It is especially important to check with your doctor before combining Omnicef with any of the following: antacids, iron supplements, multivitamins containing iron, and probenecid.

The combination of iron and Omnicef sometimes turns the stool red. This is not a cause for concern.

What are the possible side effects of Omnicef?
Side effects cannot be anticipated. If any develop or change in intensity, tell your doctor as soon as possible. Only your doctor can determine if it is safe for you to continue taking this drug.

Side effects may include: Capsules: Diarrhea, nausea, vaginal infection; Suspension: Diarrhea, rash

Can I receive Omnicef if I am pregnant or breastfeeding?
The effects of Omnicef during pregnancy and breastfeeding are unknown. Tell your doctor immediately if you are pregnant, plan to become pregnant, or are breastfeeding.

What should I do if I miss a dose of Omnicef?

Take it as soon as you remember. If it is almost time for your next dose, skip the one you missed and go back to your regular schedule. Do not take two doses at once.

How should I store Omnicef?

Capsules can be stored at room temperature. The suspension can be kept at room temperature for up to 10 days, after which any unused portion must be thrown away.

OPANA ER

Generic name: Oxymorphone hydrochloride

What is Opana ER?

Opana ER is an extended-release prescription medicine that contains the opioid (narcotic pain medicine) oxymorphone. Opana ER is used to treat adults with continuous moderate-to-severe pain when a continuous, around-the-clock opioid analgesic is needed for an extended period of time.

What is the most important information I should know about Opana ER?

Opana ER can cause trouble breathing (hypoventilation), which can lead to death, if used differently than the way you were told to use it by your doctor.

Swallow Opana ER tablets whole. Do not break, crush, dissolve, or chew Opana ER tablets before swallowing. Do not drink alcohol or take medicines that contain alcohol while you are using Opana ER. If you do not follow these instructions, you could die from an overdose. If you are unsure if any of your medicines contain alcohol, check with your doctor or pharmacist.

Opana ER can be abused in a manner similar to other opioids, legal or illicit. Do not abruptly stop taking Opana ER without talking to your doctor first.

Opana ER is not intended for use as an "as needed" analgesic.

Who should not take Opana ER?

Do not take this medication if you are allergic to Opana ER, or any of its ingredients, or if you have a known severe allergic reaction to medications similar to morphine such as codeine.

You should also not take this medication during the first 12 to 24 hours following surgery if you have not already been taking Opana ER prior to surgery, or if pain after surgery is mild or not expected to persist for an extended period of time; in situations where opioids are contraindicated, for example, if you have severe asthma or other breathing problems; if you have, or suspect you have, paralytic ileus (intestinal obstruction); or if you have moderate or severe liver disease.

What should I tell my doctor before I take the first dose of Opana ER?

Tell your doctor about all prescription, over-the-counter, and herbal medications you are taking before beginning treatment with Opana ER. Also, talk to your doctor about your complete medical history, especially if you have had breathing problems, liver or kidney problems, brain injury, Addison's disease, seizures, problems urinating, prostate problems, or if you have experienced drug- or alcohol-dependency. Also, be sure to tell your doctor if you are pregnant, plan to become pregnant, or are breast-feeding.

What is the usual dosage?

The information below is based on the dosage guidelines your doctor uses. Depending on your condition and medical history, your doctor may prescribe a different regimen. Do not change the dosage or stop taking your medication without your doctor's approval.

Adults: If you have never taken an opioid before: It is suggested that your first dose of Opana ER should be 5 milligrams (mg) every 12 hours. Thereafter, your doctor may slowly increase your dose at increments of 5-10 mg every 12 hours every 3-7 days, until adequate pain control has been achieved and side effects are minimal. *Switching from Opana to Opana ER:* If you are on Opana you may be converted to Opana ER by taking half the total daily oral Opana dose as Opana ER, every 12 hours.

How should I take Opana ER?

Opana ER should be taken on an empty stomach, at least one hour prior to a meal or two hours after a meal. Opana ER tablets are to be swallowed whole.

What should I avoid while taking Opana ER?

Avoid taking broken, dissolved or crushed Opana ER tablets.

Avoid drinking or eating anything with alcohol in it, including alcoholic beverages and medication, while taking Opana ER. Alcohol may cause an overdose of oxymorphone.

Opana ER may cause drowsiness, dizziness, or lightheadedness, and may impair mental and/or physical abilities required for the performance of potentially hazardous tasks, such as driving a car or operating machinery.

What are possible food and drug interactions associated with Opana ER?

If Opana ER is taken with certain other drugs, the effects of either could be increased, decreased, or altered. It is especially important to check with your doctor before combining Opana ER with the following: alcohol, general anesthetics, hypnotics, opioids, phenothiazines, sedatives, and tranquilizers.

What are the possible side effects of Opana ER?
Side effects cannot be anticipated. If any develop or change in intensity, tell your doctor as soon as possible. Only your doctor can determine if it is safe for you to continue taking this drug.

Side effects may include: constipation, dizziness (vertigo), feeling of tiredness, headache, itchiness, nausea, sleeplessness, sweating, vomiting

Can I receive Opana ER if I am pregnant or breastfeeding?
The effects of Opana ER during pregnancy and breastfeeding are unknown. Talk with your doctor before taking this drug if you are pregnant, plan to become pregnant, or are breastfeeding.

What should I do if I miss a dose of Opana ER?
If you miss a dose, take it as soon as possible. If it is almost time for your next dose, skip the missed dose and go back to your regular dosing schedule. Do not take 2 doses at once unless your doctor tells you to. If you are not sure about your dosing call your doctor.

How should I store Opana ER?
Store at room temperature, in a child-proof container.

OPTIVAR
Generic name: Azelastine hydrochloride, eye drops

What is Optivar?
Optivar is taken to relieve and prevent the itchy eyes brought on by seasonal allergies. The drug usually starts to work within 3 minutes of placing the drops in the eye, and its effects usually last for about 8 hours.

What is the most important information I should know about Optivar?
Optivar is for the eye only. It should not be taken by mouth or injected.

Do not touch the dropper to any surface, including your eyes or hands. The dropper is sterile. If it becomes contaminated, it could cause an infection in your eye.

If you wear soft contact lenses and your eyes are not red, wait at least 10 minutes after using Optivar before inserting your lenses. This will prevent them from absorbing the preservative in Optivar. You should not wear contact lenses if your eyes are red.

Who should not take Optivar?

Do not use Optivar if you have ever had an allergic reaction to it.

If you wear contact lenses, remember that Optivar should not be used to treat eye irritation caused by your lenses. Do not use Optivar to treat eye irritation that isn't caused by seasonal allergies.

What should I tell my doctor before I take the first dose of Optivar?

Tell your doctor about all prescription, over-the-counter, and herbal medication you are taking before beginning treatment with Optivar.

What is the usual dosage?

The information below is based on the dosage guidelines your doctor uses. Depending on your condition and medical history, your doctor may prescribe a different regimen. Do not change the dosage or stop taking your medication without your doctor's approval.

Adults: The usual dose is 1 drop in each affected eye twice a day.

Children: Optivar is not recommended for use in children younger than 3 years old.

How should I take Optivar?

Use Optivar solution only in the eyes; never swallow it. Optivar is packaged in a bottle with a dropper tip. Wash your hands before using your eye drops.

To apply the eye drops: Tilt your head back slightly and pull down on your lower eyelid. Position the dropper above your eye. Look up and away from the dropper. Squeeze out a drop and close your eye. Apply gentle pressure to the inside corner of your eye (near your nose) for about 1 minute to prevent the liquid from draining down your tear duct. If you are using more than one drop in the same eye, repeat the process with about 5 minutes between drops. Repeat the process in your other eye if directed to do so by your doctor.

What should I avoid while taking Optivar?

Do not use any eye drop that is discolored or has particles in it.

Do not wear contact lenses during treatment with Optivar ophthalmic if your eyes are red, unless otherwise directed by your doctor. If you wear soft contact lenses, and your eyes are not red, wait at least 10 minutes after using Optivar ophthalmic before inserting your contact lenses.

Do not use other eye medications during treatment with Optivar ophthalmic without first talking to your doctor.

What are possible food and drug interactions associated with Optivar?

No significant interactions with Optivar have been reported at this time. If while taking Optivar, you develop any allergic reaction, such as hives, itchiness, or trouble breathing, it is important to contact your doctor immediately. Avoid another dose until speaking with your doctor.

What are the possible side effects of Optivar?
Side effects cannot be anticipated. If any develop or change in intensity, tell your doctor as soon as possible. Only your doctor can determine if it is safe for you to continue taking this drug.

Side effects may include: bitter taste, headache, temporary eye burning or stinging

Can I receive Optivar if I am pregnant or breastfeeding?
The possibility of harm to a developing baby has not been completely ruled out. Before using Optivar, let your doctor know if you are pregnant or plan to become pregnant.

It is not known whether Optivar appears in breast milk. If you plan to breastfeed, discuss your medication options with your doctor.

What should I do if I miss a dose of Optivar?
If you do miss a dose, take it as soon as you remember. However, if it is almost time for your next dose, skip the missed dose and take only your next regularly scheduled dose. Do not take a double dose of Optivar.

How should I store Optivar?
Store upright at room temperature. Keep the bottle tightly closed.

ORACEA
Generic name: Doxycycline

What is Oracea?
Oracea is a prescription medicine to treat only the pimples or bumps on the face caused by a condition called rosacea in adult patients. Oracea may not lessen the facial redness caused by rosacea.

What is the most important information I should know about Oracea?
Oracea should not be given to infants and children 8 years or younger. It may cause stained teeth in infants and children. The yellow, gray, brown colored staining will not go away.

Oracea should not be used for the treatment of infections.

Birth control pills may not work as well when taken with Oracea. Speak to your doctor about other methods of birth control when you are taking Oracea.

While taking Oracea, avoid prolonged exposure to sunlight or sunlamps. Oracea may cause you to get severe sunburns (photosensitivity).

Oracea has not been studied for use longer than 9 months.

Who should not take Oracea?

Do not take Oracea if you are allergic to any medicine known as a tetracycline, including doxycycline and minocycline, or any of the ingredients of Oracea. Do not take Oracea if you are pregnant or planning to become pregnant; Oracea may harm your unborn baby. Do not take Oracea if you are breastfeeding your baby because it passes into your breast milk and may harm your baby.

What should I tell my doctor before I take the first dose of Oracea?

Tell your doctor about all prescription, over-the-counter, and herbal medications you are taking to avoid an interaction with Oracea. Also, talk to your doctor about your complete medical history, especially if you have a history or predisposition to yeast or fungal infections, are allergic to doxycycline or tetracyclines, if you have had an allergic reaction to doxycycline or other medicines known as tetracyclines, are pregnant or planning to become pregnant, are breastfeeding, have kidney problems, have liver problems, have had surgery on your stomach, have or had a yeast or fungal infection in your mouth or vagina, spend time in sunlight or artificial sunlight (such as a tanning booth or sunlamp).

What is the usual dosage?

The information below is based on the dosage guidelines your doctor uses. Depending on your condition and medical history, your doctor may prescribe a different regimen. Do not change the dosage or stop taking your medication without your doctor's approval.

Adults: One Oracea capsule should be taken once a day in the morning.

Oracea should not be used in children.

How should I take Oracea?

Take Oracea in the morning, unless otherwise prescribed by your doctor. Take Oracea on an empty stomach, preferably at least one hour before or two hours after a meal. Take Oracea with a full glass of water while sitting or standing. To prevent irritation to your throat, do not lay down right after you take Oracea.

What should I avoid while taking Oracea?

While taking Oracea, avoid prolonged exposure to sunlight or sunlamps. Do not take Oracea with or right after taking antacids or products containing calcium, aluminum, magnesium, or iron.

What are possible food and drug interactions associated with Oracea?

If Oracea is taken with certain other drugs, the effects of either could be increased, decreased, or altered. It is especially important to check with your doctor before combining Oracea with any of the following: antacids containing calcium, magnesium, or aluminum; barbiturates; bismuth subsalicylate; blood thinners (anticoagulants) such as warfarin or Coumadin; carbamazepine (Tegretol); isotretinoin; iron products; methoxyflurane; oral contraceptives; phenobarbital; phenytoin (Dilantin); proton pump inhibitors; psoriasis or acne medicines.

What are the possible side effects of Oracea?
Side effects cannot be anticipated. If any develop or change in intensity, tell your doctor as soon as possible. Only your doctor can determine if it is safe for you to continue taking this drug.

Side effects may include: coughing; darkening of skin, scars, teeth, or gums; diarrhea; dizziness; double vision; increased blood pressure; light sensitivity; nasal congestion; rash; runny nose; sinus infection; severe headaches; sneezing; sore throat and nose

If you notice any of the following, stop taking Oracea and notify your doctor: skin rash, redness or severe sunburn, swelling, difficulty swallowing, tightness in your throat, stomach cramps, high fever and bloody diarrhea, joint pain, or if you become pregnant

What should I do if I miss a dose of Oracea?
If you miss a dose of Oracea, skip that dose and take the next scheduled dose at the regular time. Do not double your dose.

Can I receive Oracea if I am pregnant or breastfeeding?
Oracea should not be used during pregnancy or breastfeeding.

How should I store Oracea?
Store Oracea at room temperature. Keep it away from light in a tightly closed container, and keep out of the reach of children.

ORAL CONTRACEPTIVES

What are Oral contraceptives?
Oral contraceptives are highly effective means of preventing pregnancy. Oral contraceptives consist of synthetic forms of two hormones produced naturally in the body: either progestin alone or estrogen and progestin. Estrogen and progestin regulate a woman's menstrual cycle, and the fluctuating levels of these hormones play an essential role in fertility.

To reduce side effects, oral contraceptives are available in a wide range of estrogen and progestin concentrations. Progestin-only products are usually prescribed for women who should avoid estrogens; however, they may not be as effective as estrogen/progestin contraceptives.

What is the most important information I should know about Oral contraceptives?

Cigarette smoking increases the risk of serious heart-related side effects (stroke, heart attack, blood clots, etc.) in women who use oral contraceptives. This risk increases with heavy smoking (15 or more cigarettes per day) and with age. There is an especially significant increase in heart disease risk in women over 35 years old who smoke and use oral contraceptives.

Oral contraceptives do not protect against HIV infection (AIDS) or any other sexually transmitted disease. If there is a danger of infection, use a latex condom and spermicide in addition to your oral contraceptive.

Who should not take Oral contraceptives?

Do not use oral contraceptives if you: have unusual vaginal bleeding; have a history of certain cancers, including breast or uterine; had a stroke or heart attack in the past year; have a history of blood clots; have a history of liver problems; have undiagnosed and/or unexplained abnormal vaginal bleeding; are allergic to hormones or any of the ingredients in the product; think you may be pregnant; have diabetes complications that affect your circulation; have headaches with aura symptoms; have chest pain; or have high blood pressure.

What should I tell my doctor before I take the first dose of Oral contraceptives?

Tell your doctor about all prescription, over-the-counter, and herbal medications you are taking before beginning treatment with any oral contraceptive. Also, talk to your doctor about your complete medical history, especially about any preexisting conditions such as a history of blood clots, high cholesterol, heart problems, diabetes, migraines or seizures, depression, gallbladder disease, irregular periods, or if you have any known or suspected cancers.

What is the usual dosage?

The information below is based on the dosage guidelines your doctor uses. Depending on your condition and medical history, your doctor may prescribe a different regimen. Do not change the dosage or stop taking your medication without your doctor's approval.

The dosage will depend on the brand you are taking. Oral contraceptives are usually supplied in 21-day and 28-day packages. If you have any questions about how you should take oral contraceptives, consult your doctor or the patient instructions that come in the drug package.

How should I take Oral contraceptives?

Oral contraceptives should be taken daily, no more than 24 hours apart, for the duration of the prescribed cycle (usually 21 or 28 days). Start the cycle according to package directions. Ideally, you should take your pill at the same time every day to reduce the chance of forgetting a dose; with progestin-only contraceptives, taking the pill at the same time each day is essential.

What should I avoid while taking Oral contraceptives?

Avoid smoking cigarettes while taking oral contraceptives.

Due to the risk of blood clots, you should not take oral contraceptives if you are having major surgery with a prolonged period of bed rest.

What are possible food and drug interactions associated with Oral contraceptives?

Certain drugs may interact with birth control pills and make them less effective in preventing pregnancy or may cause unscheduled bleeding. Always check with your doctor before combining an oral contraceptive with any other medication, especially the following: rifampin, antiseizure drugs, barbiturates, phenytoin, antibiotics, and herbal products containing St. John's wort.

What are the possible side effects of Oral contraceptives?

Side effects cannot be anticipated. If any develop or change in intensity, inform your doctor as soon as possible. Only your doctor can determine if it is safe for you to continue taking an oral contraceptive.

Side effects may include: breakthrough bleeding between menstrual periods (spotting), depression, loss of menstrual periods, migraine, nausea, vomiting, water retention, weight gain, yeast infection

Serious, and possibly life-threatening, side effects are also possible, especially for women who smoke. Seek medical attention immediately if you have any of the following: chest pain, coughing up blood, or shortness of breath (indicating a possible blood clot in the lung); pain in the calf (indicating a possible blood clot in the leg); crushing chest pain or heaviness (indicating a possible heart attack); sudden, severe headache or vomiting, dizziness, fainting, vision or speech problems, weakness, or numbness in an arm or leg (indicating a possible stroke); sudden partial or complete loss of vision (indicating a possible blood clot in the eye); breast lumps (indicating possible breast cancer or fibrocystic breast disease); severe pain or tenderness in the stomach (indicating a possible liver tumor); difficulty sleeping, lack of energy, fatigue, change in mood (possibly indicating depression); yellowing of the skin or whites of the eyes (jaundice), sometimes accompanied by fever, fatigue, loss of appetite, dark-colored urine, or light-colored bowel movements (indicating possible liver problems).

Can I receive Oral contraceptives if I am pregnant or breastfeeding?

If you are pregnant (or think you might be), you should not use oral contraceptives, since they are not safe during pregnancy. Nursing mothers should not use most oral contraceptives, since these drugs can appear in breast milk and may cause jaundice and enlarged breasts in nursing infants. Contact your doctor immediately if you suspect you may be pregnant or if you plan on breastfeeding.

What should I do if I miss a dose of Oral contraceptives?

If you neglect to take only one estrogen/progestin pill, take it as soon as you remember, take the next pill at your regular time, and continue taking the rest of the medication cycle. The risk of pregnancy is small if you miss only one combination pill per cycle. If you miss more than one tablet, call your doctor or check your product's patient information for instructions.

Missing a single progestin-only tablet increases the chance of pregnancy. Consult your doctor immediately if you miss a single dose or if you take it 3 or more hours late, and use another method of birth control until your next period begins or pregnancy is ruled out.

How should I store Oral contraceptives?

To help keep track of your doses, use the original container. Store at room temperature.

ORAPRED ODT

Generic name: Prednisolone sodium phosphate

What is Orapred ODT?

Orapred ODT is a prescription medicine used for a variety of conditions as determined by your doctor. Some may include: severe allergies that cannot be otherwise treated, in adults and children with asthma (or asthma caused by different medical conditions), skin diseases, kidney problems in people with lupus (such as proteinuria), stomach problems (such as ulcers), leukemia and lymphomas, multiple sclerosis, eye problems, rheumatologic issues (such as rheumatoid arthritis), tuberculosis, and meningitis.

What is the most important information I should know about Orapred ODT?

Do not stop your course of Orapred ODT treatment abruptly. Patients on immunosuppressive doses of corticosteroids should be warned to avoid exposure to chickenpox and measles. If you are exposed to chicken pox or measles, seek medical advice without delay. While being treated with Orapred ODT, live vaccines should not be given, as this drug may suppress your immune system. Killed or inactivated vaccines can be administered, but the body's response cannot be predicted.

Who should not take Orapred ODT?
Do not take Orapred ODT if you have a fungal infection or if you are allergic to the drug or any of its components. Do not take Orapred ODT if you are receiving live or live attenuated vaccines.

What should I tell my doctor before I take the first dose of Orapred ODT?
Tell your doctor about all prescription, over-the-counter, and herbal medications you are taking to avoid an interaction with Orapred ODT. Also, talk to your doctor about your complete medical history, especially if you have a history of high blood pressure, heart problems, including congestive heart failure, kidney problems, stomach ulcers, a stomach infection, eye problems, if you are going through menopause, if you are pregnant, plan to become pregnant, or are breastfeeding.

What is the usual dosage?
The information below is based on the dosage guidelines your doctor uses. Depending on your condition and medical history, your doctor may prescribe a different regimen. Do not change the dosage or stop taking your medication without your doctor's approval.

Adults: The initial dose of Orapred ODT may vary from 10 to 60 milligrams (mg) per day, depending on the specific disease entity being treated.

Multiple Sclerosis
The usual daily doses are 200 mg of prednisolone for a week, followed by 80 mg every other day or 4 to 8 mg dexamethasone every other day for one month.

Children: The initial dose of Orapred ODT may vary depending on the specific disease entity being treated. The range of initial doses is 0.14 to 2 mg per 2.2 pounds body weight per day in three or four divided doses.

Kidney Problems
The usual children's dosage is 60 mg/m^2/day given in three divided doses for 4 weeks, followed by 4 weeks of single dose alternate-day therapy at 40 mg/m^2/day.

Asthma Uncontrolled by an Inhaler
The usual children's dosage is 1-2 mg per 2.2 pounds of body weight per day in single or divided doses.

How should I take Orapred ODT?
Do not remove Orapred ODT from its blister package until you are ready to use it. The blister pack should be peeled open, and the oral disintegrating tablet placed on your tongue, where tablets may be swallowed whole, or allowed to dissolve in the mouth, with or without the assistance of water.

What should I avoid while taking Orapred ODT?

Do not go for skin tests while on Orapred ODT. Do not break or use partial Orapred ODT tablets. Do not remove the tablet from the blister pack until right before you plan to use it.

What are possible food and drug interactions associated with Orapred ODT?

If Orapred is taken with certain other drugs, the effects of either could be increased, decreased, or altered. It is especially important to check with your doctor before combining Orapred with any of the following: amphotericin-B, antidiabetic drugs, aspirin, barbiturates, cyclosporine, digitalis glycosides, diuretics, ephedrine, estrogens, ketoconazole, live or live attenuated vaccines, phenytoin, rifampin, warfarin.

What are the possible side effects of Orapred ODT?

Side effects cannot be anticipated. If any develop or change in intensity, tell your doctor as soon as possible. Only your doctor can determine if it is safe for you to continue taking this drug.

Side effects may include: blood in stool, congestive heart failure, convulsions, eye irritation, eyelid swelling, facial redness, headache, impaired wound healing, increased blood pressure, increased hair growth in areas that usually have minimal growth, itchy skin, loss of muscle mass, menstrual irregularities, muscle weakness, osteoporosis, nausea, stomach ulcers, sweating, swelling, tiredness, vertigo, weakness, weight gain

Can I receive Orapred ODT if I am pregnant or breastfeeding?

The effects of Orapred ODT during pregnancy and breastfeeding are unknown. Talk with your doctor before taking this drug if you are pregnant, plan to become pregnant, or are breastfeeding.

What should I do if I miss a dose of Orapred ODT?

If you miss a dose of Orapred ODT, skip that dose and take the next scheduled dose at the regular time. Do not double your dose.

How should I store Orapred ODT?

Store Orapred ODT at room temperature. Keep it away from light and moisture, and keep it out of the reach of children.

ORINASE

Generic name: Tolbutamide

What is Orinase?

Orinase is an oral antidiabetic medication used to treat type 2 (non-insulin-dependent) diabetes. Diabetes occurs when the body does not make enough insulin, or when the insulin that is produced no longer works properly. Insulin works by helping sugar get inside the body's cells, where it is then used for energy.

Insulin or metformin (Glucophage) may also be used in combination with Orinase, if necessary.

What is the most important information I should know about Orinase?

Always remember that Orinase is an aid to, not a substitute for, good diet and exercise. Failure to follow a sound diet and exercise plan can lead to serious complications, such as dangerously high or low blood sugar levels. Remember, too, that Orinase is not an oral form of insulin, and cannot be used in place of insulin.

Know the signs and symptoms of low blood sugar (hypoglycemia), which include headache, drowsiness, weakness, dizziness, fast heartbeat, sweating, tremor, and nausea. Carry a piece of hard candy or glucose tablets with you to treat episodes of low blood sugar.

If you are taking Orinase, you should check your blood or urine periodically for abnormal sugar (glucose) levels.

Who should not take Orinase?

You should not take Orinase if you have had an allergic reaction to it.

Orinase should not be taken if you are suffering from diabetic ketoacidosis (a life-threatening medical emergency caused by insufficient insulin and marked by excessive thirst, nausea, fatigue, pain below the breastbone, and fruity breath).

In addition, Orinase should not be used as the sole therapy in treating type 1 (insulin-dependent) diabetes.

What should I tell my doctor before I take the first dose of Orinase?

Tell your doctor about all prescription, over-the-counter, and herbal medication you are taking before beginning treatment with Orinase. Also, talk to your doctor about your complete medical history, especially if you have kidney disease, liver disease, thyroid disease, type 1 diabetes, diabetic ketoacidosis, a serious infection, illness, injury, or need surgery.

What is the usual dosage?

The information below is based on the dosage guidelines your doctor uses. Depending on your condition and medical history, your doctor may prescribe a different regimen. Do not change the dosage or stop taking your medication without your doctor's approval.

Dosage levels are based on individual needs.

Adults: Usually an initial daily dose of 1 to 2 grams is recommended. Maintenance therapy usually ranges from 0.25 to 3 grams daily. Daily doses greater than 3 grams are not recommended.

Children: Safety and effectiveness have not been established in children.

Older adults: Older, malnourished, or debilitated people, or those with impaired kidney or liver function, are usually prescribed lower initial and maintenance doses to minimize the risk of low blood sugar (hypoglycemia).

How should I take Orinase?
Take each dose with a full glass of water.

Orinase is usually taken before breakfast or the first main meal if it is taken once a day, or before meals if it is taken multiple times each day. Follow your doctor's instructions.

What should I avoid while taking Orinase?
Avoid alcohol. It lowers blood sugar and may interfere with your diabetes treatment.

What are possible food and drug interactions associated with Orinase?
If Orinase is taken with certain other drugs, the effects of either could be increased, decreased, or altered. It is especially important to check with your doctor before combining Orinase with the following: adrenal corticosteroids such as prednisone (Deltasone) and cortisone (Cortone); airway-opening drugs such as Proventil and Ventolin; alcohol; anabolic steroids such as testosterone; barbiturates such as Amytal, Seconal, and Phenobarbital; beta blockers such as Inderal and Tenormin; blood-thinning drugs such as Coumadin; calcium channel blockers such as Cardizem and Procardia; chloramphenicol (Chloromycetin); cimetidine (Tagamet); clofibrate (Atromid-S); colestipol (Colestid); epinephrine (EpiPen); estrogens (Premarin); fluconazole (Diflucan); furosemide (Lasix); isoniazid (Nydrazid); itraconazole (Sporanox); major tranquilizers such as Stelazine and Mellaril; MAO inhibitors such as Nardil and Parnate; methyldopa (Aldomet); miconazole (Monistat); niacin (Nicobid, Nicolar); nonsteroidal anti-inflammatory agents such as Advil, aspirin, ibuprofen, Naprosyn, phenylbutazone and Voltaren; oral contraceptives; phenytoin (Dilantin); probenecid (Benemid); rifampin (Rifadin); sulfa drugs such as Bactrim and Septra; thiazide and other diuretics such as Diuril and HydroDIURIL; and thyroid medications such as Synthroid.

What are the possible side effects of Orinase?
Side effects cannot be anticipated. If any develop or change in intensity, tell your doctor as soon as possible. Only your doctor can determine if it is safe for you to continue taking this drug.

Side effects may include: bloating, heartburn, nausea

Orinase, like all oral antidiabetics, may cause hypoglycemia (low blood sugar). The risk of hypoglycemia can be increased by missed meals, alcohol, other medications, fever, trauma, infection, surgery, or excessive exercise. To avoid hypoglycemia, you should closely follow the dietary and exercise plan suggested by your physician.

Symptoms of mild hypoglycemia may include cold sweat, drowsiness, fast heartbeat, headache, nausea, and nervousness.

Symptoms of more severe hypoglycemia may include coma, pale skin, seizures, and shallow breathing.

Contact your doctor immediately if these symptoms of severe low blood sugar occur.

Ask your doctor what you should do if you experience mild hypoglycemia. Severe hypoglycemia should be considered a medical emergency, and prompt medical attention is essential.

Can I receive Orinase if I am pregnant or breastfeeding?
The effects of Orinase during pregnancy are unknown. Tell your doctor immediately if you are pregnant, or plan to become pregnant. Orinase is excreted in small amounts in the breast milk of nursing mothers. Therefore, you should discuss with your doctor whether to discontinue Orinase or to stop breastfeeding.

What should I do if I miss a dose of Orinase?
Take the missed dose as soon as you remember. However, if it is almost time for the next dose, skip the missed dose and take only the next regularly scheduled dose. Do not take a double dose of this medication.

How should I store Orinase?
Store Orinase at room temperature.

Orlistat *See Xenical, page 1428.*

Orphenadrine citrate, aspirin, and caffeine *See Norgesic, page 903.*

ORTHO EVRA
Generic name: Ethinyl estradiol and norelgestromin

What is Ortho Evra?
Ortho Evra is a contraceptive skin patch. It contains estrogen and progestin, the same hormones found in many birth control pills. Fertility depends on regular fluctuations in the levels of these hormones. Contraceptives such as Ortho Evra reduce fertility by eliminating the fluctuations. Once applied to the skin, the Ortho Evra patch releases a steady supply of estrogen and progestin through the skin and into the bloodstream.

What is the most important information I should know about Ortho Evra?

Cigarette smoking increases the risk of serious heart-related side effects (stroke, heart attack, blood clots, etc.) in women who use hormonal contraceptives. This risk increases with heavy smoking (15 or more cigarettes per day) and with age. There is an especially significant increase in heart disease risk in women over 35 years old who smoke and use hormonal birth control. Therefore, women who use Ortho Evra are strongly advised not to smoke.

Hormonal contraceptives, including Ortho Evra, should be used with caution if you are over 40 years old; smoke tobacco; have liver, heart, gallbladder, or kidney disease; have high blood pressure, high cholesterol, diabetes, or epilepsy; or tend to be seriously overweight. Caution is also advised if you have blood circulation problems or have had a heart attack or stroke in the past. Be cautious, too, if you have problems with depression, migraine or other headaches, irregular menstrual periods, or visual disturbances.

There have been conflicting reports on whether using hormonal contraceptives increases the risk of breast cancer. It appears that using hormonal contraceptives may slightly increase the chance of breast cancer, particularly if they're used before age 20. After hormonal contraceptives are stopped, the risk begins to go back down. If you use Ortho Evra, you should examine your breasts monthly and have yearly breast exams by a doctor. Also tell your doctor if you have a family history of breast cancer or if you have had breast nodules, fibrocystic breast disease, or an abnormal mammogram.

If you develop a migraine or severe headache that does not let up or keeps recurring while you are taking Ortho Evra, check with your doctor. You may need to switch to a different form of birth control.

You should also be aware that hormonal contraceptives have been know to cause rare cases of noncancerous—but dangerous—liver tumors. In people prone to high cholesterol and similar problems, hormonal contraceptives have been known to raise triglyceride levels, leading to pancreatitis.

If you miss a menstrual period but have followed the Ortho Evra regimen correctly, contact your doctor but do not stop using the patches. If you miss a period and have not followed the regimen correctly, or if you miss two consecutive periods, you may be pregnant; stop using the patches and check with your doctor immediately to see if you are pregnant. Use another form of birth control while you're off the patch.

Ortho Evra may be less effective in women who weigh more than 198 pounds; if you fall into this category, ask your doctor which form of birth control is best for you.

Hormonal contraceptives do not protect against HIV infection (AIDS) or any other sexually transmitted disease. If there is a danger of infection, use a latex condom in addition to Ortho Evra.

Be sure to tell the doctor that you are taking Ortho Evra before having lab tests done, since certain blood tests may be affected by hormonal contraceptives. Hormonal contraceptives may affect tests for blood sugar levels and thyroid function and may cause an increase in blood triglyceride levels.

Who should not take Ortho Evra?

Do not use Ortho Evra if you are pregnant (or think you might be). Also avoid it if the ingredients give you an allergic reaction or you suffer from headaches with neurological symptoms such as visual disturbances (pulsing lights and blind spots) and temporary numbness.

If you have ever had breast cancer or cancer in the reproductive organs or liver tumors, you should not take Ortho Evra. Avoid it, too, if you have or have ever had a stroke, heart disease, liver disease, angina (severe chest pain), or blood clots. It is also not recommended for women with significant high blood pressure or diabetes-related complications of the kidneys, eyes, nerves, or blood vessels.

Women who have had pregnancy-related jaundice (yellowing of the skin or whites of eyes) or jaundice stemming from previous use of hormonal contraceptives should not take Ortho Evra. You should also avoid it if you have undiagnosed and/or unexplained abnormal vaginal bleeding, or if you need prolonged bed rest after major surgery.

Do not use Ortho Evra if you are already taking birth control pills. Avoid the drug, too, if you are breastfeeding.

What should I tell my doctor before I take the first dose of Ortho Evra?

Tell your doctor about all prescription, over-the-counter, and herbal medications you are taking before beginning treatment with this drug. Also, talk to your doctor about your complete medical history, especially if you have liver, heart, gallbladder, or kidney disease; high blood pressure or high cholesterol; circulation problems; a history of cancer; diabetes; epilepsy; depression; migraines or other headaches; irregular menstrual periods; vision problems; or if you smoke.

What is the usual dosage?

The information below is based on the dosage guidelines your doctor uses. Depending on your condition and medical history, your doctor may prescribe a different regimen. Do not change the dosage or stop taking your medication without your doctor's approval.

Adults: You should use three Ortho Evra patches during each 28-day cycle. Apply a new patch on the same day each week for 3 weeks (21 total days). Do not apply a patch during the fourth week. Your menstrual period should start during this patch-free week.

How should I take Ortho Evra?

If you have any questions about how you should use Ortho Evra, consult your doctor or the patient instructions that come in the drug package. The following is a partial list of instructions for using Ortho Evra; it should not be used as a substitute for consultation with your doctor.

Apply each new patch on the same day of the week. This will be your "patch change day." The patch can be applied on the first day of your menstrual cycle or on the first Sunday afterwards. The instructions below are for the first-Sunday schedule.

For a Sunday Patch Change Schedule

Apply your first patch on the first Sunday after your menstrual period starts. *You must use backup contraception for the first week of your cycle when starting Ortho Evra for the first time.*

Choose a place on your body to put the patch where it won't be rubbed by tight clothing. You can apply the patch to your buttock, abdomen, upper outer arm, or upper back. *Never put the patch on your breasts.* To avoid irritation, apply each new patch to a different place on your skin.

Open the foil pouch that contains the patch by tearing along the top edge and one side edge. Peel the foil pouch apart and open it flat.

You will see that the patch is covered by a layer of clear plastic. It is important to remove the patch and the plastic together from the pouch. Using your fingernail, lift one corner of the patch and peel the patch and plastic off the foil liner. Sometimes patches can stick to the inside of the pouch; be careful not to accidentally remove the clear liner as you remove the patch.

Peel away half of the clear plastic liner. Be careful not to touch the exposed sticky surface of the patch with your fingers.

Apply the sticky side of the patch to clean, dry skin, then remove the other half of the clear plastic. Press firmly on the patch with the palm of your hand for 10 seconds, making sure the edges stick well. Run your finger around the edge of the patch to make sure it is sticking properly. Check your patch every day to make sure all the edges are sticking.

Wear the patch for 7 days. On the next Sunday (day 8), remove the used patch. Apply a new patch immediately. The used patch still contains some medicine; carefully fold it in half so that it sticks to itself before throwing it away. Do not flush the used patch down the toilet.

Apply a new patch on the following Sunday (day 15). After 7 days, throw away the patch.

Do not wear a patch during the fourth week (day 22 through day 28). Your period should start during this week.

Begin your next 4-week cycle by applying a new patch on the Sunday after day 28, even if your period hasn't ended yet.

What should I avoid while taking Ortho Evra?

Since the blood's clotting ability may be affected by hormonal contraceptives, you should avoid prolonged bed rest. Your doctor may have you stop using Ortho Evra before major surgery.

What are possible food and drug interactions associated with Ortho Evra?

If hormonal contraceptives are taken with certain other drugs, the effects of either could be increased, decreased, or altered. It is especially important to check with your doctor before combining Ortho Evra with the following: acetaminophen, antibiotics such as ampicillin and rifampin, anticonvulsants, aspirin, atorvastatin, barbiturates (e.g., phenobarbital, secobarbital), clofibrate, cyclosporine, diabetes drugs, folic acid, griseofulvin, itraconazole, ketoconazole, morphine, phenylbutazone, prednisolone, protease inhibitors (HIV drugs such as indinavir and nelfinavir), St. John's wort, temazepam, and theophylline.

What are the possible side effects of Ortho Evra?

Side effects cannot be anticipated. If any develop or change in intensity, tell your doctor as soon as possible. Only your doctor can determine if it is safe for you to continue taking this drug.

Side effects may include: abdominal pain, application site reaction, breast tenderness or enlargement, headache, menstrual cramps, mood swings, nausea and/or vomiting, upper respiratory infection

Can I receive Ortho Evra if I am pregnant or breastfeeding?

If you are pregnant (or think you might be), you should not use hormonal contraceptives, since they are not safe during pregnancy. For safety's sake, switch to a nonhormonal method of contraception if you miss a period and have not followed your patch schedule correctly. In addition, wait at least 4 weeks after delivery before starting Ortho Evra.

Nursing mothers should not use most hormonal contraceptives, since these drugs can appear in breast milk and may cause jaundice and enlarged breasts in nursing infants. In this situation, your doctor may advise you to use a different form of contraception while you are nursing your baby.

What should I do if I miss a dose of Ortho Evra?

If your patch becomes loose or falls off for less than 1 day, try to stick it back on, or apply a new patch immediately. If it's been missing for more than 1 day, or you're not sure how long it's been off, there's a chance you could become pregnant and you should use a backup method of birth control. Check the Ortho Evra patient information for instructions.

If you forget to change your patch at any time during the 4-week cycle, check the Ortho Evra patient information for instructions.

How should I store Ortho Evra?

Keep patches in their protective pouches until you're ready to wear them. Store at room temperature. Do not store in the refrigerator or freezer.

Used patches still contain some active hormones. Fold each patch so that it sticks to itself before throwing it away. Do not flush the used patch down the toilet.

ORTHO TRI-CYCLEN LO

Generic name: Norgestimate and ethinyl estradiol

What is Ortho Tri-Cyclen Lo?

Ortho Tri-Cyclen Lo tablets are used to prevent pregnancy in women who elect to use oral contraceptives as a method of birth control.

What is the most important information I should know about Ortho Tri-Cyclen Lo?

Cigarette smoking increases the risk of serious cardiovascular side effects from oral contraceptive use. This risk increases with age, especially over 35 years and with heavy smoking (15 or more cigarettes per day). You should not smoke while you are taking oral contraceptives.

Oral contraceptive use is associated with increased risks of myocardial infarction, thromboembolism, stroke, hepatic neoplasia, and gallbladder disease. Although the risk of serious morbidity or mortality is very small in healthy women without underlying risk factors, the risk increases in the presence of hypertension, hyperlipidemia, obesity, diabetes, or if you have or have had clotting disorders, heart attack, stroke, angina pectoris, cancer of the breast or sex organs, or malignant or benign liver tumors.

Women who have or had breast cancer should not use oral contraceptives.

You may experience breakthrough bleeding or spotting while taking oral contraceptives, especially during the first 3 months of use. You may also have irregular periods. If you have missed more than 2 periods in a row, it is recommended to determine if you are pregnant. If you are pregnant, stop taking the pill.

Call your doctor immediately if you experience chest pain, cough up blood, or you experience sudden shortness of breath; pain the calf of your leg; severe headache or vomiting, dizziness or fainting; vision or speech disturbances; weakness, or numbness in the arm or leg; sudden partial or complete vision loss, breast lumps, severe pain in the stomach area, sleep difficulties, depressed or change in mood; lack of energy; yellowing of the skin or eyeballs with fever, dark urine, light bowel movements, loss of appetite. These signs and symptoms could be an indication of a serious medical condition.

Ortho Tri-Cyclen Lo does not protect against HIV infection (AIDS) and other sexually transmitted diseases.

Stop taking the drug if your skin turns yellow, as you may have developed jaundice.

Contact lens wearers who develop visual changes should contact an ophthalmologist.

Who should not take Ortho Tri-Cyclen Lo?

You should not use the pill if you are over the age of 35 and are a heavy smoker, have a history of heart attack or stroke, blood clots in the legs, lungs or eyes, a history of blood clots in the deep veins of your legs, chest pain, known or suspected breast cancer or cancer of the lining of the uterus, cervix or vagina, unexplained vaginal bleeding, yellowing of the whites of the eyes or of the skin during pregnancy or during previous use of the pill, liver tumor, known or suspected pregnancy.

Do not use this medication if you plan to have surgery with prolonged bedrest, if you have very high blood pressure, elevated cholesterol or triglycerides, or diabetes with complications of the kidneys, eyes, nerves, or blood vessels. Also, do not use this drug if you have migraines or other headaches, epilepsy, mental depression, gallbladder, liver, heart, or kidney disease, history of scanty or irregular menstrual periods, or if you are allergic to any of the ingredients in Ortho Tri-Cyclen Lo.

What should I tell my doctor before I take the first dose of Ortho Tri-Cyclen Lo?

Tell your doctor if you have ever had any of the conditions above and also about all prescription, over-the-counter, and herbal medication you are taking before beginning treatment with Ortho Tri-Cyclen Lo. Also, talk to your doctor about your complete medical history, especially if you have had a heart attack, stroke, blood clots, chest pain, gallbladder, liver, heart, or kidney disease, disease or cancer of the breast or sex organs, liver tumors, high blood pressure, high cholesterol or triglycerides, water retention, mental depression, migraines or headaches, diabetes, irregular menstrual bleeding or periods, wear contact lenses, smoke, will undergo surgery and need a long period of bed rest, or you are pregnant or planning to become pregnant, or breastfeeding.

What is the usual dosage?

The information below is based on the dosage guidelines your doctor uses. Depending on your condition and medical history, your doctor may prescribe a different regimen. Do not change the dosage or stop taking your medication without your doctor's approval.

Sunday Start: When taking Ortho Tri-Cyclen Lo the first white "active" tablet should be taken on the first Sunday after menstruation begins. If the menstrual period begins on Sunday, the first white "active" tablet should be taken that day. Take one white, light blue or dark blue "active" tablet daily for 21 days followed by one dark green "reminder" tablet daily for 7 days. After 28 tablets have been taken, a new course is started the next day (Sunday). For the first cycle of a Sunday Start regimen, another method of contraception should be used until after the first 7 consecutive days of administration.

Day 1 Start: The dosage of Ortho Tri-Cyclen Lo for the initial cycle of therapy is one white, light blue or dark blue "active" tablet administered daily from the 1st day through the 21st day of the menstrual cycle, counting the first day of menstrual flow as "Day 1" followed by one dark green "reminder" tablet daily for 7 days. Take the tablets without interruption for 28 days. After 28 tablets have been taken, start a new course the next day.

How should I take Ortho Tri-Cyclen Lo?
You should take Ortho Tri-Cyclen Lo once daily at the same time every day.

What should I avoid while taking Ortho Tri-Cyclen Lo?
Avoid smoking while taking Ortho Tri-Cyclen Lo. Also, avoid getting pregnant while taking Ortho Tri-Cyclen Lo.

What are possible food and drug interactions associated with Ortho Tri-Cyclen Lo?
If Ortho Tri-Cyclen Lo is taken with certain other drugs, the effects of either could be increased, decreased, or altered. It is especially important to check with your doctor before coming Ortho Tri-Cyclen Lo with the following: acetaminophen, antibiotics, ascorbic acid, atorvastatin, bosentan, carbamazepine, clofibric acid, cyclosporine, felbamate, griseofulvin, itraconazole, ketoconazole, morphine, oxcarbazepine, phenobarbital, phenylbutazone, phenytoin, prednisolone, protease inhibitors like ritonavir, rifampin, salicylic acid, St. John's wort (hypericum perforatum), temazepam, theophylline, and topiramate.

What are the possible side effects of Ortho Tri-Cyclen Lo?
Side effects cannot be anticipated. If any develop or change in intensity, tell your doctor as soon as possible. Only your doctor can determine if it is safe for you to continue taking this drug.

Side effects may include: vaginal bleeding, spotty darkening of the skin (especially on the face), weight changes, nausea, vomiting, change in appetite, headache, nervousness, depression, dizziness, loss of scalp hair, rash, vaginal bleeding, infections, water retention causing swelling of the fingers or ankles and raised blood pressure weight changes

Can I receive Ortho Tri-Cyclen Lo if I am pregnant or breastfeeding?
Oral contraceptives should not be used if you are pregnant or nursing.

What should I do if I miss a dose of Ortho Tri-Cyclen Lo?

If you miss 1 white, light blue, or dark blue "active" pill, take it as soon as you remember. Take the next pill at your regular time. This means you can take 2 pills in 1 day. You do not need a backup birth control method if you have intercourse.

If you miss 2 white or light blue "active" pills in a row in week 1 or week 2, take 2 pills on the day you remember and 2 pills the next day. Then take 1 pill a day until you finish the pack. You could become pregnant if you have intercourse in the 7 days after you miss pills. You must use another birth control method (such as condoms or spermicides) as a backup method for those 7 days.

If you miss 2 dark blue "active" pills in a row in week 3, follow these instructions: If you are a Sunday starter, keep taking 1 pill every day until Sunday. On Sunday, throw out the rest of the pack and start a new pack on that same day.

If you are a day 1 starter, throw out the rest of the pack and start a new pack that same day. You may not have your period this month; this is normal. If you miss your period 2 months in a row, call your doctor; you might be pregnant.

You could become pregnant if you have intercourse in the 7 days after you miss pills. You must use another birth control method (such as condoms or spermicides) as a backup method for those 7 days.

If you miss 3 or more white, light blue, or dark blue "active" pills in a row during the first 3 weeks: follow these instructions:

If you are a Sunday starter, keep taking 1 pill every day until Sunday. On Sunday, throw out the rest of the pack and start a new pack on that same day.

If you are a day 1 starter, throw out the rest of the pack and start a new pack that same day. You may not have your period this month, but this is normal. If you miss your period 2 months in a row, call your doctor because you might be pregnant.

You could become pregnant if you have sex in the 7 days after you miss pills. You must use another birth control method (such as condoms or spermicides) as a backup method for those 7 days.

If you forget any of the 7 dark green "reminder" pills in week 4, throw away the pills you missed. Keep taking 1 pill every day until the pack is finished. You do not need a backup contraceptive method.

If you are not sure what to do about your missed pills, use a backup method each time you have intercourse and keep taking 1 "active" pill every day until you consult your doctor.

How should I store Ortho Tri-Cyclen Lo?

Store at room temperature in its original package.

Oseltamivir phosphate *See Tamiflu, page 1257.*

Oxaprozin *See Daypro, page 377.*

Oxcarbazepine *See Trileptal, page 1336.*

Oxiconazole nitrate *See Oxistat, below.*

OXISTAT
Generic name: Oxiconazole nitrate

What is Oxistat?
Oxistat topical prevents fungus from growing on your skin. It is available as a cream or lotion. Oxistat cream and lotion are used to treat fungal skin infections such as athlete's foot (tinea pedis), jock itch (tinea cruris), and ringworm of the entire body (tinea corporis). Oxistat cream is also used for tinea versicolor, which appears as patches on the skin. Oxistat cream may also be used in pediatric patients for athlete's foot, jock itch, ringworm of the entire body, and tinea versicolor, but these conditions rarely occur in children under the age of 12 years.

What is the most important information I should know about Oxistat?
Oxistat should not be used in, on, or near the eyes, or applied to the vagina. Oxistat is for external use only.

Always wash your hands after you apply Oxistat.

Use Oxistat for the full course of therapy as directed by your doctor even though your symptoms may have improved. If no improvement is seen after 2-4 weeks, or if your condition worsens, call your doctor.

You should also call your doctor if the application site shows signs of increased irritation, itching, burning, blistering, swelling, or oozing.

Do not use bandages or dressings that prevent air from circulating to the affected area (occlusive dressings) unless otherwise directed by your doctor.

Do not use Oxistat for anything other than what it was prescribed for.

Who should not take Oxistat?
Do not use Oxistat if you have ever had an allergic reaction to or are sensitive to Oxistat or any other ingredients in the cream or lotion.

What should I tell my doctor before I take the first dose of Oxistat?
Tell your doctor about all prescription, over-the-counter, and herbal medications you are taking before beginning treatment with Oxistat.

What is the usual dosage?
The information below is based on the dosage guidelines your doctor uses. Depending on your condition and medical history, your doctor

may prescribe a different regimen. Do not change the dosage or stop taking your medication without your doctor's approval.

For Athlete's Foot, Jock Itch, or Ringworm of the Body
Adults and children: The usual daily dose of Oxistat cream or lotion is once or twice a day. Athlete's foot is treated for 1 month. Jock itch and ringworm of the body are treated for 2 weeks.

For Tinea Versicolor
Adults and children: The usual daily dose is one application a day of Oxistat cream for 2 weeks.

How should I take Oxistat?
Wash your hands before and after using this medication. Clean and dry the affected area. If you are using Oxistat lotion, shake the lotion well before using. Apply the cream or lotion once or twice daily to the affected area(s) and the areas surround the affected area(s) as directed for 2 to 4 weeks.

Use this medication for the full amount of time prescribed by your doctor or recommended in the package even if you begin to feel better. Your symptoms may improve before the infection is completely healed.

If the infection does not clear up in 2 weeks (or 4 weeks for athletes foot), or if it appears to get worse, see your doctor.

What should I avoid while taking Oxistat?
Avoid getting this medication in your eyes, nose, mouth, or other mucous membranes.

Avoid wearing tight-fitting, synthetic clothing that does not allow air circulation. Wear loose-fitting clothing made of cotton and other natural fibers until the infection is healed.

What are possible food and drug interactions associated with Oxistat?
No interactions have been reported.

What are the possible side effects of Oxistat?
Side effects cannot be anticipated. If any develop or change in intensity, tell your doctor as soon as possible. Only your doctor can determine if it is safe for you to continue taking this drug.

Side effects may include: allergic skin inflammation; burning; cracks in the skin; eczema; irritation; itching; pain; rash; scaling; skin redness; skin softening; small, firm, raised skin eruptions similar to those of chicken-pox; stinging; tingling

Can I receive Oxistat if I am pregnant or breastfeeding?
The effects of Oxistat during pregnancy are unknown. Tell your doctor immediately if you are pregnant, or plan to become pregnant.

Oxistat appears in breast milk and could affect a nursing infant. If Oxistat is essential to your health, your doctor may advise you to stop breastfeeding until your treatment is finished.

What should I do if I miss a dose of Oxistat?
Apply the cream or lotion when you remember, then return to your regular schedule.

How should I store Oxistat?
Store Oxistat at room temperature.

Oxybutynin chloride *See Ditropan, page 432.*

Oxybutynin transdermal system *See Oxytrol, page 970.*

Oxycodone hydrochloride *See OxyContin, below.*

Oxycodone and aspirin *See Percodan, page 1003.*

OXYCONTIN
Generic name: Oxycodone hydrochloride

What is OxyContin?
OxyContin is a controlled-release form of the narcotic painkiller oxycodone. It is prescribed for moderate to severe pain when continuous, around-the-clock relief is needed for an extended period of time. It contains enough medicine to last up to 12 hours.

What is the most important information I should know about OxyContin?
You should only use OxyContin exactly the way your doctor tells you to, and it should only be used for the condition for which it was prescribed.

Be sure to swallow OxyContin tablets whole or it will not work properly for 12 hours. If broken, crushed, or chewed, the tablets quickly release a potentially fatal overdose of oxycodone.

Abusing OxyContin by chewing the tablets, snorting crushed tablets, or dissolving and injecting their contents can slow down or stop breathing and lead to death. Injecting OxyContin can also kill the tissue around the injection site and trigger heart and lung problems.

OxyContin 80 mg and 160 mg tablets are only for those who are opioid-tolerant. If these tablets are given to patients who have never been exposed to opioids before, it may cause severe medical consequences, including death.

The empty shell of the OxyContin tablet sometimes appears in the stool. This is not a reason for concern.

Do not stop taking OxyContin suddenly if you have been taking it continuously for more than 5 to 7 days. Stopping suddenly could cause withdrawal symptoms and make you uncomfortable. Your doctor may want to gradually reduce the dose.

This drug is not intended for occasional "as needed" use, and should never be taken more often than directed. If you suffer episodes of increased pain, check with your doctor; do not change the dosage on your own.

Do not give OxyContin to other people, even if they have the same symptoms you have.

Sharing is illegal and may cause severe medical problems, including death. Make sure to keep your tablets in a secure place to prevent theft from others. OxyContin contains a narcotic painkiller that can be a target for prescription drug abusers. Selling or giving away OxyContin is dangerous and illegal.

Who should not take OxyContin?
Do not take OxyContin if: your doctor did not prescribe OxyContin for you; your pain is mild or will go away in a few days; your pain can be controlled by occasional use of other painkillers; you have severe asthma or severe lung problems; you have had a severe allergic reaction (includes a severe rash, hives, breathing problems, or dizziness) to codeine, hydrocodone, dihydrocodeine, or oxycodone (such as Tylox, Tylenol with Codeine, or Vicodin); you had surgery less than 12 to 24 hours ago and you were not taking OxyContin just before surgery; you have or are suspected to have a condition called paralytic ileus (paralysis of the intestine).

What should I tell my doctor before I take the first dose of OxyContin?
Tell your doctor about all prescription, over-the-counter, and herbal medication you are taking before beginning treatment with OxyContin. Also, talk to your doctor about your complete medical history, especially if you have trouble breathing or lung problems, head injury, liver or kidney problems, adrenal gland problems (such as Addison's disease), convulsions or seizures, alcoholism, hallucinations or other severe mental problems, past or present substance abuse or drug addiction.

What is the usual dosage?
The information below is based on the dosage guidelines your doctor uses. Depending on your condition and medical history, your doctor may prescribe a different regimen. Do not change the dosage or stop taking your medication without your doctor's approval.

Adults: OxyContin is taken every 12 hours. The tablets come in strengths of 10, 20, 40, 80, and 160 milligrams. The starting dose of OxyContin is determined by your physical condition, the type of painkillers you've been taking, and your tolerance for narcotics. The doctor will adjust the dose until you have little or no pain when OxyContin is supplemented with no more than 2 doses of a second painkiller. The dose of OxyContin can be increased every 1 or 2 days. If a higher dose has excessive side effects, the doctor will adjust it downward and increase the dosage of supplemental painkillers.

OxyContin is not for use in children.

How should I take OxyContin?

Take each dose with a full glass of water. OxyContin can be taken with food or milk if stomach upset occurs. Do not crush, chew, or break Oxy-Contin. Swallow OxyContin whole.

Do not abruptly stop taking OxyContin all at once if you have been taking it for more than a few days. Your doctor will instruct you on how to stop taking OxyContin slowly to avoid withdrawal symptoms.

What should I avoid while taking OxyContin?

Avoid alcohol while taking OxyContin. Alcohol will greatly increase the drowsiness and dizziness caused by OxyContin and could be dangerous. Also, avoid taking OxyContin with other medications that will make you sleepy because they can increase the drowsiness and dizziness caused by OxyContin and can be dangerous.

Use caution when driving, operating machinery, or performing other hazardous activities. If you experience drowsiness or dizziness, avoid these activities.

What are possible food and drug interactions associated with OxyContin?

If OxyContin is taken with certain other drugs, the effects of either could be increased, decreased, or altered. It is especially important to check with your doctor before combining OxyContin with the following: alcoholic beverages; antipsychotic drugs such as Compazine, Mellaril, Stelazine, and Thorazine Butorphanol (Stadol); centrally-acting antiemetics; general anesthetics (propofol, etomidate, thiopental); muscle relaxants such as Flexeril, Robaxin, and Skelaxin Nalbuphine (Nubain); narcotic painkillers such as Demerol, Percodan, and Vicodin Pentazocine (Talacen, Talwin NX); sleep aids such as Ambien, Halcion, and Sonata; sleep-inducing antihistamines such as Benadryl and Phenergan.; and tranquilizers such as Ativan, Librium, Valium, and Xanax.

What are the possible side effects of OxyContin?

Side effects cannot be anticipated. If any develop or change in intensity, tell your doctor as soon as possible. Only your doctor can determine if it is safe for you to continue taking this drug.

Side effects may include: constipation, dizziness, drowsiness, dry mouth, headache, itching, nausea, sweating, vomiting, weakness

Side effects other than those listed here may also occur. Talk to your doctor about any side effect that seems unusual or that is especially bothersome.

Can I receive OxyContin if I am pregnant or breastfeeding?
OxyContin should be used during pregnancy only if clearly needed. If you are pregnant or plan to become pregnant, inform your doctor immediately.

OxyContin makes its way into breast milk. Nursing is not recommended if you are taking OxyContin. It may harm your baby.

What should I do if I miss a dose of OxyContin?
Take it as soon as possible. If it is almost time for your next dose, skip the missed dose and go back to your regular dosing schedule. Do not take 2 doses at once unless your doctor tells you to.

How should I store OxyContin?
Store at room temperature in a secure place out of reach of children. Protect from light. Dispose of unused tablets by flushing them down the toilet. Protect from theft.

Oxymorphone hydrochloride *See Opana ER, page 942.*

OXYTROL
Generic name: Oxybutynin transdermal system

What is Oxytrol?
Oxytrol is a transdermal system (skin patch) used to treat overactive bladder. It delivers the active ingredient, oxybutynin, through your skin and into your bloodstream.

What is the most important information I should know about Oxytrol?
Oxytrol is indicated for the treatment of overactive bladder with symptoms of urge urinary incontinence, urgency, and frequency.

Oxytrol should be used in patients with gastrointestinal obstructive disorders, because of the risk of gastric retention, or bladder outflow obstruction, because of the risk of urinary retention.

Oxytrol may decrease gastrointestinal motility and should be used with caution in patients with conditions such as ulcerative colitis, intestinal atony, and myasthenia gravis.

Oxytrol should be used with caution in patients who have gastroesophageal reflux (GERD) and/or who are taking drugs (such as bisphosphanates to manage osteoporosis) that can cause or exacerbate esophageal irritation.

Oxytrol can cause drowsiness, dizziness, or blurred vision and should be used with caution. Using alcohol while taking Oxytrol can exacerbate drowsiness.

Who should not take Oxytrol?

Oxytrol should not be given to: infants and children less than 18 years old; individuals experiencing high fever, heat exhaustion, or heat stroke; individuals using other anticholinergic medications; or individuals with urinary retention (the bladder does not empty or empty completely when you urinate), gastric retention (the stomach empties slowly or does not empty completely after a meal), or uncontrolled narrow-angle glaucoma (high pressure in the eye).

Do not take Oxytrol if you are hypersensitive to any components of the product. Do not take Oxytrol if you are allergic to medical tape products or to other skin patches without first talking to your doctor.

What should I tell my doctor before I take the first dose of Oxytrol?

Tell your doctor about all prescription, over-the-counter, and herbal medication you are taking before beginning treatment Oxytrol, especially if you are using any medications that could cause dry mouth, constipation, or sleepiness. Also, talk to your doctor about your complete medical history, especially if you have any of the following: liver or kidney disease; bladder obstruction (blockage); esophagitis (inflamed esophagus); gastric reflux disease; gastrointestinal obstruction (blockage in the digestive system); myasthenia gravis (nerve weakness); or ulcerative colitis (inflamed bowels).

What is the usual dosage?

The information below is based on the dosage guidelines your doctor uses. Depending on your condition and medical history, your doctor may prescribe a different regimen. Do not change the dosage or stop taking your medication without your doctor's approval.

Adults and children age 18 and older: The usual starting dose of Oxytrol is a single-dose application which delivers 3.9 mg oxybutynin per day. Put on a new patch two times a week (every 3 to 4 days) according to your doctor's instructions.

How should I take Oxytrol?

When you are ready to apply the Oxytrol patch, tear open the pouch and remove the patch. Apply the patch to your skin right away. Put the patch on a clean, dry, and smooth (fold-free) area of skin on your abdomen (stomach area), hips, or buttocks. Avoid your waistline area, since tight clothing may rub against the patch.

The sticky adhesive side of the patch is covered by 2 strips of overlapping protective liner. Remove the first piece of the protective liner and apply the patch with the adhesive side down, firmly onto the skin. Bend the patch in half gently and roll the remaining part on your skin using your fingertips. The second piece of the protective liner will move off the patch as you roll the patch in place. Apply firm pressure to the patch with your fingers to make sure it stays on. Avoid touching the sticky side of the patch when you are applying it because it may cause the patch to fall off early.

Wear the patch at all times until it is time to apply a new one. You should only wear one patch at a time.

If the patch falls off or partially comes off, press it firmly back into place and continue your regular application schedule. If the patch does not stay on, throw it out and place a new patch in a different area. Continue to follow your regular application schedule.

Do not use the same area for the patch for at least one week. The areas you choose should not be oily, damaged (cut or scraped), irritated (rashes), or have any other skin problems. Do not put Oxytrol on areas that have been treated with oils, lotions, or powders that could keep the patch from sticking well to your skin.

You should try to change the patch on the same 2 days each week.

When you are ready to change your patch, remove the old patch slowly to avoid skin damage. Fold the old patch in half with the sticky sides together once it is taken off and throw it out. The patch will still have some medicine left in it so it may be dangerous if accidentally worn or swallowed by another person or pet.

If there is any adhesive that stays on your skin after removing the patch, gently wash the area with warm water and mild soap. A small amount of baby oil may be used to remove any excess residue. Dirty adhesive rings may require a medical adhesive removal pad. Do not use alcohol or other dissolving liquids like nail polish remover that could irritate your skin.

What should I avoid while taking Oxytrol?
Do not expose the patch to sunlight. Always wear it under clothing.

Avoid applying the patch on the same site each time. Avoid touching the sticky adhesive side when putting on the patch. Avoid rubbing the patch area during bathing, swimming, or exercising.

Caution should be used when driving or operating dangerous machinery because Oxytrol may cause sleepiness or blurred vision. Also, avoid drinking alcohol because the sleepiness that can be caused by Oxytrol could be increased.

Avoid hot and warm temperatures because Oxytrol could decrease sweating. This may cause you to overheat or have a fever or heat stroke.

What are possible food and drug interactions associated with Oxytrol?

The concomitant use of Oxytrol with other anticholinergic drugs or with other agents that produce dry mouth, constipation, drowsiness, or blurred vision may increase the frequency and/or severity of such effects.

Use of alcohol may enhance the drowsiness caused by Oxytrol.

What are the possible side effects of Oxytrol?

Side effects cannot be anticipated. If any develop or change in intensity, tell your doctor as soon as possible. Only your doctor can determine if it is safe for you to continue taking this medication.

Side effects may include: itching and redness where the patch is applied, dry mouth, constipation, abnormal vision, drowsiness, dizziness, headache

For more information on side effects, ask your doctor or pharmacist.

Can I receive Oxytrol if I am pregnant or breastfeeding?

Tell your doctor if you are pregnant or breastfeeding. The safety of Oxytrol for women who are or who may become pregnant has not been established. Oxytrol should be used only when the benefits outweigh the risks. Caution should be taken when administering Oxytrol to nursing mothers.

What should I do if I miss a dose of Oxytrol?

If you forget to change your patch after 3-4 days, remove the old patch, and apply a new patch to a different area. Continue to follow your regular application schedule.

How should I store Oxytrol?

Oxytrol should be stored at room temperature. Protect from moisture and humidity. Do not remove the patch from its pouch until you are ready to apply it.

Once off, dispose of the patch properly so it cannot be accidentally worn or swallowed by another person, especially a child, or a pet.

Paliperidone *See Invega, page 668.*

PAMELOR
Generic name: Nortriptyline hydrochloride

What is Pamelor?

Pamelor is prescribed for the relief of symptoms of depression.

What is the most important information
I should know about Pamelor?

Antidepressants can increase the risk of suicidal thinking and behavior in children and teenagers. Adult and pediatric patients taking antidepressants should be watched closely for changes in moods and actions, especially when their dose is increased or decreased. Patients and their families should contact the doctor immediately if new symptoms develop or seem to get worse. Signs to watch for include anxiety, hostility, insomnia, restlessness, impulsive or dangerous behavior, and thoughts about suicide or dying.

Who should not take Pamelor?

Do not use Pamelor Solution if you are allergic to any ingredient in Pamelor Solution or to similar medicines. Also, do not take Pamelor if you are recovering from a recent heart attack.

If you have taken furazolidone or a monoamine oxidase inhibitor (MAOI) like phenelzine within the last 14 days, or if you are taking astemizole, dofetilide, droperidol, terfenadine, or cisapride, you should not take Pamelor.

What should I tell my doctor before
I take the first dose of Pamelor?

Tell your doctor about all prescription, over-the-counter, and herbal medications you are taking before beginning treatment with Pamelor. Also, talk to your doctor about your complete medical history, especially if you have a history of suicidal thoughts or behavior; an overactive thyroid; bipolar disorder or any other mental disorder; diabetes; difficulty urinating; glaucoma; heart, kidney, or liver problems; seizures; or porphyria (a blood disorder).

Be sure to let your doctor know if you are undergoing electroshock therapy, if you are scheduled to have any surgery, if you drink alcohol-containing beverages daily, or if you have a history of alcohol abuse.

What is the usual dosage?

The information below is based on the dosage guidelines your doctor uses. Depending on your condition and medical history, your doctor may prescribe a different regimen. Do not change the dosage or stop taking your medication without your doctor's approval.

This medication is available in tablet and liquid form. Only tablet dosages are listed. Consult your doctor if you cannot take the tablet form of Pamelor.

Adults: The usual starting dosage is 25 milligrams (mg) taken 3 or 4 times per day. Alternatively, your doctor may prescribe that the total daily dose be taken once a day. Doses above 150 mg per day are not recommended. Your doctor will monitor your response to Pamelor carefully and will gradually increase or decrease the dose to suit your needs.

Elderly: The usual dose is 30 to 50 mg taken in a single dose or divided into smaller doses, as determined by your doctor.

How should I take Pamelor?

Take Pamelor exactly as prescribed. Pamelor Solution may be taken with or without food. Pamelor may make your mouth dry. Sucking on hard candy, chewing gum, or melting ice chips in your mouth can provide relief.

What should I avoid while taking Pamelor?

Pamelor may cause you to become drowsy or less alert. Do not drive or operate dangerous machinery or participate in any hazardous activity that requires full mental alertness until you know how Pamelor affects you.

Pamelor may make your skin more sensitive to sunlight. Try to stay out of the sun, wear protective clothing, and apply sunblock.

Avoid drinking alcohol or taking other medications that cause drowsiness, such as sedatives.

What are possible food and drug interactions associated with Pamelor?

If Pamelor is taken with certain other drugs, the effects of either could be increased, decreased, or altered. It is especially important to check with your doctor before combining Pamelor with the following: albuterol, alcohol, antiarrhythmics, antidepressants, antihistamines, antispasmodics, blood pressure medication, cimetidine, chlorpropamide, levodopa, MAO inhibitors (combination with Pamelor can be fatal), quinidine, reserpine, stimulants such as dextroamphetamine, thyroid medication, tranquilizers, and warfarin.

What are the possible side effects of Pamelor?

Side effects cannot be anticipated. If any develop or change in intensity, tell your doctor as soon as possible. Only your doctor can determine if it is safe for you to continue taking this drug.

Side effects may include: anxiety, blurred vision, confusion, dry mouth, hallucinations, heart attack or vascular heart blockage, heartbeat irregularities, high blood pressure, insomnia, loss of muscle coordination, low blood pressure, rapid heartbeat, sensitivity to sunlight, skin rash, stroke, tremors, weight loss

Side effects due to rapid decrease in dose or abrupt withdrawal from Pamelor after prolonged treatment include: headache, nausea, vague feeling of bodily discomfort

Can I receive Pamelor if I am pregnant or breastfeeding?

The effects of Pamelor during pregnancy and breastfeeding are unknown. Tell your doctor immediately if you are pregnant, plan to become pregnant, or are breastfeeding.

What should I do if I miss a dose of Pamelor?

Take it as soon as you remember. If it is almost time for the next dose, skip the dose you missed and go back to your regular schedule. If you take Pamelor once a day at bedtime and you miss a dose, do not take it in the morning, since disturbing side effects could occur. Never take two doses at once.

How should I store Pamelor?

Store at room temperature in a tightly closed container and away from light.

Pantoprazole *See Protonix, page 1095.*

Paricalcitol *See Zemplar, page 1457.*

PARNATE
Generic name: Tranylcypromine sulfate

What is Parnate?

Parnate is prescribed for the treatment of major depression. This medication is usually given after other antidepressants have been tried without successful treatment of symptoms.

What is the most important information I should know about Parnate?

Parnate is a potent antidepressant in the class of drugs called monoamine oxidase inhibitors (MAOIs). It works by increasing the concentration of chemicals in your brain such as epinephrine, norepinephrine, and serotonin. It can produce serious side effects. It is typically prescribed only if other antidepressants fail, and then only for adults who are under close medical supervision. It can interact with a long list of drugs and foods to produce life-threatening side effects (see "What are possible food and drug interactions associated with this medication?").

Antidepressants can increase the risk of suicidal thinking and behavior in children and teenagers. Adult and pediatric patients taking antidepressants should be watched closely for changes in moods or actions, especially when they first start therapy or when their dose is increased or decreased. Patients and their families should contact the doctor immediately if new symptoms develop or seem to get worse. Signs to watch for include anxiety, hostility, insomnia, restlessness, impulsive or dangerous behavior, and thoughts about suicide or dying.

Who should not take Parnate?

Do not take Parnate if you have any of the following medical conditions: heart, kidney, or liver disease; high blood pressure; a history of headaches; a type of tumor known as pheochromocytoma; or if you will be undergoing elective surgery requiring general anesthesia.

What should I tell my doctor before I take the first dose of Parnate?

Tell your doctor about all prescription, over-the-counter, and herbal medications you are taking before beginning treatment with Parnate. Also, talk to your doctor about your complete medical history (see "Who should not take this medication?" above).

What is the usual dosage?

The information below is based on the dosage guidelines your doctor uses. Depending on your condition and medical history, your doctor may prescribe a different regimen. Do not change the dosage or stop taking your medication without your doctor's approval.

Adults: The usual dosage is 30 milligrams (mg) per day, divided into smaller doses. If ineffective, the dosage may be slowly increased under your doctor's supervision to a maximum of 60 mg per day.

How should I take Parnate?

Take this medication exactly as it was prescribed for you. Follow the instructions on your prescription label. Your doctor will adjust the dosage of Parnate according to your individual needs and response. It will usually take 48 hours to 3 weeks for you to see the benefits of Parnate.

What should I avoid while taking Parnate?

While you are taking Parnate, avoid foods that are high in tyramine (see "What are possible food and drug interactions associated with this medication?").

Avoid alcohol and large amounts of caffeine while you are taking Parnate.

Avoid driving, operating machinery, or other dangerous tasks until you know how Parnate will affect you. Parnate may cause you to be very drowsy.

What are possible food and drug interactions associated with Parnate?

Never take Parnate with the following drugs; the combination can trigger seizures or a dangerous spike in blood pressure: dibenzapine-related and other drugs classified as tricyclic antidepressants, such as amitriptyline, amoxapine, carbamazepine, clomipramine, cyclobenzaprine, desipramine, doxepin, imipramine, maprotiline, nortriptyline, perphenazine and amitriptyline, protriptyline, trimipramine maleate; other MAOIs such as furazolidone, isocarboxazid, pargyline, procarbazine, and phenelzine.

When switching from one of these drugs to Parnate, or vice versa, allow an interval of at least 1 week between medications.

If Parnate is taken with certain other drugs, the effects of either could be increased, decreased, or altered. It is especially important to check with your doctor before combining Parnate with the following: alcohol, amphetamines, anesthetics, antidepressants classified as SSRIs, antihistamines, blood pressure medication, blood-vessel constricting medicines for colds, hay fever and weight loss, bupropion, buspirone, cocaine, cough remedies containing dextromethorphan, dexfenfluramine, disulfiram, diuretics (water pills), dopamine, guanethidine, meperidine and other narcotic painkillers, methyldopa, Parkinson's disease medications, reserpine, sedatives (such as triazolam, pentobarbital, and secobarbital), and tryptophan.

While taking Parnate, you should also avoid foods that contain a high amount of a substance called tyramine, including: anchovies, avocados, bananas, beer (including nonalcoholic beer), canned figs, caviar, cheese (especially strong and aged varieties), chianti wine, chocolate, dried fruits (including raisins, prunes), liqueurs, liver, meat extracts or meat prepared with tenderizers, overripe fruit, pickled herring, pods of broad beans like fava beans, raspberries, sauerkraut, sherry, sour cream, soy sauce, yeast extracts, and yogurt.

What are the possible side effects of Parnate?

Side effects cannot be anticipated. If any develop or change in intensity, tell your doctor as soon as possible. Only your doctor can determine if it is safe for you to continue taking this drug.

Side effects may include: abdominal pain, agitation, anxiety, blood disorders, blurred vision, chills, constipation, diarrhea, dizziness, drowsiness, dry mouth, headache, impotence, insomnia, muscle spasm, nausea, numbness, overstimulation, rapid or irregular heartbeat, restlessness, ringing in the ears, tremors, urinary retention, water retention, weakness, weight loss

Can I receive Parnate if I am pregnant or breastfeeding?

If you are pregnant or plan to become pregnant, inform your doctor immediately. Parnate should be used during pregnancy only if its benefits outweigh potential risks.

Parnate is found in breast milk. If the drug is essential to your health, your doctor may advise you to stop nursing until your treatment is finished.

What should I do if I miss a dose of Parnate?
Take the missed dose as soon as you remember. If it is almost time for your next dose, skip the missed dose and take the medicine at the next regularly scheduled time. Do not take extra medicine to make up for a missed dose.

How should I store Parnate?
Store at room temperature.

Paroxetine hydrochloride *See Paxil, page 981.*

Paroxetine mesylate *See Pexeva, page 1014.*

PATANOL
Generic name: Olopatadine hydrochloride

What is Patanol?
Patanol is an antihistamine that relieves the red, itchy eyes often caused by allergies.

What is the most important information I should know about Patanol?
Patanol should be used only for allergic conditions. It is not a remedy for irritation from contact lenses.

Use Patanol only in your eyes. Patanol should not be taken orally or by injection.

The safety and effectiveness of Patanol have not been established in children under 3.

Patanol is a sterile solution. Avoid allowing the tip of the bottle to touch your eye, fingers, or any other surface; serious eye infections may occur if the bottle becomes contaminated.

Do not wear contact lenses if your eyes are red. The preservative in Patanol may be absorbed by soft contact lenses. If you wear soft contact lenses and your eyes are not red, wait at least 10 minutes after applying Patanol before inserting your contact lenses.

Who should not take Patanol?
Do not take Patanol if you are allergic to the medication or any of its ingredients.

What should I tell my doctor before I take the first dose of Patanol?
Tell your doctor about all prescription, over-the-counter, and herbal medication you are taking before beginning treatment with Patanol. Also, talk

to your doctor about your complete medical history, especially if you have a bacterial, viral, or fungal infection in your eye.

What is the usual dosage?

The information below is based on the dosage guidelines your doctor uses. Depending on your condition and medical history, your doctor may prescribe a different regimen. Do not change the dosage or stop taking your medication without your doctor's approval.

Adults: The usual dose is 1 drop in each affected eye 2 times a day. Allow 6 to 8 hours between doses.

How should I take Patanol?

Use Patanol eyedrops exactly as directed by your doctor. Wash your hands before and after using your eyedrops.

To apply the eyedrops: Tilt your head back slightly and pull down on your lower eyelid. Position the dropper above your eye. Look up and away from the dropper. Squeeze out a drop and close your eye. Apply gentle pressure to the inside corner of your eye (near your nose) for about 1 minute to prevent the liquid from draining down your tear duct. If you are using more than one drop in the same eye, repeat the process with about 5 minutes between drops.

What should I avoid while taking Patanol?

Do not touch the dropper to any surface, including your eyes or hands. The dropper is sterile. If it becomes contaminated, it could cause an infection in your eye.

Do not use any eyedrop that is discolored or has particles in it.

Patanol contains a preservative (benzalkonium chloride); do not wear contact lenses while applying this medication. You can insert contact lenses about 10 minutes after you take a dose of Patanol.

What are possible food and drug interactions associated with Patanol?

If Patanol is taken with certain other drugs, the effects of either could be increased, decreased, or altered. Always check with your doctor before combining Patanol with any other drugs, herbs, or supplements.

What are the possible side effects of Patanol?

Side effects cannot be anticipated. If any develop or change in intensity, tell your doctor as soon as possible. Only your doctor can determine if it is safe for you to continue taking this drug.

Side effects may include: allergic reactions, bloodshot eyes, blurred vision, burning or stinging, changes in taste, cold-like symptoms, dry eye, headache, inflammation of the cornea, itching, nausea, runny nose, sensation of a foreign body in the eye, sinus inflammation, sore throat, swollen lids, weakness

Can I receive Patanol if I am pregnant or breastfeeding?
The effects of Patanol during pregnancy and breastfeeding are unknown. Tell your doctor immediately if you are pregnant, plan to become pregnant, or are breastfeeding.

What should I do if I miss a dose of Patanol?
Apply the missed dose as soon as you remember. However, if it is almost time for your next regularly scheduled dose, skip the missed dose and apply the next dose as directed. Do not use a double dose of this medication.

How should I store Patanol?
Store Patanol at room temperature, away from moisture and heat. Keep bottle tightly closed.

PAXIL
Generic name: Paroxetine hydrochloride

What is Paxil?
Paxil is used to treat depression, obsessive compulsive disorder, panic disorder, social anxiety disorder, generalized anxiety disorder, and post-traumatic stress disorder.

What is the most important information I should know about Paxil?
Paxil is not approved for use in pediatric patients.

Antidepressant medicines may increase suicidal thoughts or actions in some children, teenagers, and young adults when the medicine is first started. Depression and other serious mental illnesses are the most important causes of suicidal thoughts and actions. Some people may have a particularly high risk of having suicidal thoughts or actions. These include people who have (or have a family history of) bipolar disorder (also called manic-depressive illness) or suicidal thoughts or actions.

Pay close attention to any changes, especially sudden ones, in mood, behaviors, thoughts, or feelings. This is very important when an antidepressant medicine is first started or when the dose is changed.

Call the doctor right away to report new or sudden changes in mood, behavior, thoughts, or feelings. Signs to watch for include new or worsening depression, new or worsening anxiety, agitation, insomnia, hostility, panic attacks, restlessness, extreme hyperactivity, and suicidal thinking or behavior.

Keep all follow-up visits as scheduled, and call the doctor between visits as needed, especially if you have concerns about symptoms.

Who should not take Paxil?

You should not take Paxil if you are allergic to it or any of its components. It should also be avoided if you are currently taking monoamine oxidase inhibitors (MAOIs), linezolid, thioridazine, or pimozide.

What should I tell my doctor before I take the first dose of Paxil?

Tell your doctor about all prescription, over-the-counter, and herbal medications you are taking before beginning treatment with Paxil. Also, talk to your doctor about your complete medical history, especially if you intend on becoming pregnant or if you have a history of suicidal thoughts, panic attacks, insomnia, seizures, glaucoma, or severe kidney or liver impairment.

What is the usual dosage?

The information below is based on the dosage guidelines your doctor uses. Depending on your condition and medical history, your doctor may prescribe a different regimen. Do not change the dosage or stop taking your medication without your doctor's approval.

Depression
Adults: The recommended starting dose is 20 milligrams (mg) daily. Depending on how you respond to Paxil, your doses may be increased in 10 mg/day increments up to a maximum daily dose of 50 mg.

Obsessive Compulsive Disorder
Adults: The recommended starting dose is 20 mg daily. Depending on how you respond to Paxil, your doses may be increased in 10 mg/day increments up to a maximum daily dose of 60 mg.

Panic Disorder
Adults: The recommended starting dose is 10 mg daily. Depending on how you respond to Paxil, your doses may be increased in 10 mg/day increments up to a maximum daily dose of 60 mg.

Social Anxiety Disorder
Adults: The recommended starting dose is 20 mg daily. Depending on how you respond to Paxil, your doses may be increased up to a maximum daily dose of 60 mg.

Generalized Anxiety Disorder
Adults: The recommended starting dose is 20 mg daily. Depending on how you respond to Paxil, your doses may be increased up to a maximum daily dose of 50 mg.

Post-traumatic Stress Disorder
Adults: The recommended starting dose is 20 mg daily. Depending on how you respond to Paxil, your dose may be increased up to a maximum daily dose to 50 mg.

How should I take Paxil?
Paxil is taken once daily, usually in the morning, with or without food.

What should I avoid while taking Paxil?
Avoid drinking alcohol during treatment with Paxil. Avoid driving or operating dangerous machinery or participating in any hazardous activity that requires full mental alertness until you know how this drug affects you.

What are possible food and drug interactions associated with Paxil?
If Paxil is taken with certain other drugs, the effects of either could be increased, decreased, or altered. It is especially important to check with your doctor before combining Paxil with any of the following: alcohol, antidepressants such as amitriptyline, desipramine, fluoxetine, imipramine, and nortriptyline, aspirin, cimetidine, diazepam, digoxin, flecainide, linezolid, lithium, nonsteroidal anti-inflammatory drugs (NSAIDs) such as aspirin, ibuprofen, naproxen, and ketoprofen, phenobarbital, phenytoin, pimozide, procyclidine, propafenone, propranolol, quinidine, St. John's wort, sumatriptan, theophylline, thioridazine, tramadol, triptans (a class of medication used to treat migraines; examples include sumatriptan and zolmitriptan), tryptophan, and warfarin.

What are the possible side effects of Paxil?
Side effects cannot be anticipated. If any develop or change in intensity, tell your doctor as soon as possible. Only your doctor can determine if it is safe for you to continue taking this drug.

Side effects may include: abnormal ejaculation, abnormal orgasm, constipation, decreased appetite, decreased sex drive, diarrhea, dizziness, drowsiness, dry mouth, gas, impotence, male and female genital disorders, nausea, nervousness, sleeplessness, sweating, tremor, weakness, vertigo.

Can I receive Paxil if I am pregnant or breastfeeding?
For women who intend to become pregnant or are in their first trimester of pregnancy, Paxil should only be initiated after consideration of the other available treatment options. The effects of Paxil during breastfeeding are unknown; discuss your options with your doctor.

What should I do if I miss a dose of Paxil?
Skip the missed dose and go back to your regular schedule. Do not take a double dose to make up for the one you missed.

How should I store Paxil?
Store at room temperature.

PEDIAPRED
Generic name: Prednisolone sodium phosphate

What is Pediapred?
Pediapred, a steroid drug, is used to reduce inflammation and improve symptoms in a variety of disorders, including rheumatoid arthritis, acute gouty arthritis, and severe cases of asthma. It may be given to people to treat primary or secondary adrenal cortex insufficiency (lack of or insufficient adrenal cortical hormone in the body). It is also given to help treat the following disorders: blood disorders such as leukemia and various anemias, certain cancers (along with other drugs), connective tissue diseases such as systemic lupus erythematosus, digestive tract diseases such as ulcerative colitis, eye diseases of various kinds, fluid retention due to nephrotic syndrome (a condition in which damage to the kidneys causes a loss of protein in the urine), high blood levels of calcium associated with cancer, lung diseases such as tuberculosis, severe allergic conditions such as drug-induced allergic reactions, severe skin eruptions.

Studies have shown that high doses of Pediapred are effective in controlling severe symptoms of multiple sclerosis, although they do not affect the ultimate outcome or natural history of the disease.

What is the most important information I should know about Pediapred?
Pediapred decreases your resistance to infection. It may also mask some of the signs and symptoms of an infection, which makes it difficult for a doctor to diagnose the actual problem.

If you are taking Pediapred and are subjected to unusual stress, notify your doctor. The drug reduces the function of your adrenal glands, and they may be unable to cope. Your doctor may therefore increase your dosage of this rapidly acting steroid before, during, and after the stressful situation.

Prolonged use of steroids may produce posterior subcapsular cataracts (a disorder under the envelope-like structure at the back of the eye that causes the lens to become less transparent) or the eye disease glaucoma, and may intensify additional eye infections due to fungi or viruses.

Average and high doses of this medication may cause an increase in blood pressure, salt and water retention, and an increased loss of potassium. Your doctor may have you decrease your salt intake and increase your potassium intake.

The effects of Pediapred may be intensified if you have an underactive thyroid or long-term liver disease.

If you have ocular herpes simplex (painful blisters of the eye), you should be careful using this drug because of the possibility of corneal perforation (puncture of the outer, transparent part of the eye).

The use of Pediapred may cause mood swings, feelings of elation, insomnia, personality changes, severe depression, or even severe mental disorders.

If you are being treated for a blood clotting factor deficiency, use aspirin with caution when taking Pediapred. Do not use this drug for any disorder other than that for which it was prescribed.

If you should develop a fever or other signs of infection while taking Pediapred, notify your doctor immediately.

Who should not take Pediapred?
This drug should not be used for fungal infections within the body. Avoid it if it gives you an allergic reaction.

What should I tell my doctor before
I take the first dose of Pediapred?
Tell your doctor about all prescription, over-the-counter, and herbal medications you are taking before beginning treatment with this drug. Also, talk to your doctor about your complete medical history. Your doctor will prescribe this medication very cautiously if you have any of the following: ulcerative colitis (inflammation of the colon and rectum) where there is a possibility of a puncture, abscess, or other infection; diverticulitis (inflammation of a sac formed at weak points of the colon); recent intestinal anastomoses (a surgical connection between two separate parts of the colon); active or inactive peptic (stomach) ulcers; unsatisfactory kidney function; high blood pressure; osteoporosis (brittle bones that may fracture); and myasthenia gravis (a long-term disease characterized by abnormal fatigue and weakness of certain muscles).

What is the usual dosage?
The information below is based on the dosage guidelines your doctor uses. Depending on your condition and medical history, your doctor may prescribe a different regimen. Do not change the dosage or stop taking your medication without your doctor's approval.

Adults: The starting dosage of Pediapred may vary from 5 milliliters to 60 milliliters, depending on the specific disease being treated.

Your doctor will adjust the dose until the results are satisfactory. If your condition does not improve after a reasonable period of time, the doctor may switch you to another medication.

Once you've shown a favorable response, your doctor will gradually decrease the dosage to the minimum that maintains the effect.

If you stop taking Pediapred after long-term therapy, your doctor will have you withdraw slowly, rather than abruptly.

For acute flare-ups of multiple sclerosis, the usual dose is 200 milligrams per day of Pediapred for 1 week followed by 80 milligrams every other day or 4 to 8 milligrams of dexamethasone every other day for 1 month.

Children: The starting dosage ranges from 0.14 to 2 milligrams per 2.2 pounds of body weight per day, divided into 3 or 4 smaller doses. For asthma, the recommended dosage is 1 to 2 milligrams per 2.2 pounds of body weight per day, taken in a single or several smaller doses.

How should I take Pediapred?
Pediapred may cause stomach upset and should be taken with food. Take this medication exactly as prescribed.

What should I avoid while taking Pediapred?
Do not discontinue the use of Pediapred abruptly or without medical supervision.

You should not be vaccinated against smallpox while being treated with Pediapred. Avoid other immunizations as well, especially if you are taking Pediapred in high doses, because of the possible hazards of nervous system complications and a lack of natural immune response.

Because Pediapred reduces resistance to infection, people who have never had measles or chickenpox—or been vaccinated against them—should be careful to avoid exposure. These diseases can be severe, or even fatal, in people with lowered resistance. Likewise, an ordinary case of threadworm or other intestinal parasites can grow into a grave emergency when the immune system is weak. Symptoms of threadworm include stomach pain, vomiting, and diarrhea. If you suspect an infection, call your doctor immediately.

What are possible food and drug interactions associated with Pediapred?
If Pediapred is taken with certain other drugs, the effects of either could be increased, decreased, or altered. It is especially important to check with your doctor before combining Pediapred with the following: amphotericin B, aspirin, barbiturates such as phenobarbital and secobarbital, cyclosporine, diabetes drugs such as glipizide, ephedrine, estrogens, isoniazid, ketoconazole, nonsteroidal anti-inflammatory drugs such as ibuprofen, oral contraceptives, phenytoin, rifampin, warfarin, and diuretics.

What are the possible side effects of Pediapred?
Side effects cannot be anticipated. If any develop or change in intensity, tell your doctor as soon as possible. Only your doctor can determine if it is safe for you to continue taking this drug.

Side effects may include: allergic reactions, headache, hot flashes, increased appetite, nausea/stomach upset, rash, stomach/intestinal pain, sweating, swelling, tiredness

Can I receive Pediapred if I am pregnant or breastfeeding?

The effects of Pediapred during pregnancy have not been adequately studied. If you are pregnant or plan to become pregnant, inform your doctor immediately. This medication may appear in breast milk and could affect a nursing infant. If this drug is essential to your health, your doctor may advise you to discontinue breastfeeding until your treatment is finished.

What should I do if I miss a dose of Pediapred?

Take it as soon as you remember. If it is almost time for your next dose, skip the one you missed and go back to your regular schedule. Never take 2 doses at the same time.

How should I store Pediapred?

Store Pediapred in a cool place, and keep the bottle tightly closed. This medication may be refrigerated.

PEGANONE

Generic name: Ethotoin

What is Peganone?

Peganone is a drug used to control tonic-clonic (grand mal) and complex partial (psychomotor) seizures.

Tonic-clonic seizures are a type of seizure in which the individual experiences a sudden loss of consciousness immediately followed by generalized convulsions. Complex partial seizures are characterized by blank staring and repetitive movements. Peganone works by slowing down impulses in the brain that cause seizures.

What is the most important information I should know about Peganone?

Do not change the brand, generic formulation, or dosage of this medication without first talking to your doctor. If you have been taking Peganone regularly to prevent major seizures, do not stop abruptly. This may precipitate prolonged or repeated epileptic seizures without any recovery of consciousness between attacks—a condition called status epilepticus—that can be fatal if not treated promptly.

Blood abnormalities have occurred in some patients taking Peganone, although it is unknown whether the drug was the cause. Your doctor will do monthly blood tests when you first start therapy to guard against any such problems. Call your doctor immediately if you have symptoms such as sore throat, fever, malaise (marked by bodily discomfort, fatigue, or a general feeling of illness), easy bruising, small purple skin spots, nosebleeds, or any sign of infection or bleeding tendency.

Because Peganone may cause gum hypertrophy (excessive formation of the gums over the teeth), it's important to practice good dental hygiene while taking Peganone.

There is some evidence suggesting that medicines like Peganone may interfere with folic acid and can cause megaloblastic anemia. Folic acid supplementation may be necessary if this happens while you are pregnant.

Who should not take Peganone?
Do not take Peganone if you have liver problems or blood disorders. Also, do not take Peganone if you are allergic to the medication or any or its ingredients.

What should I tell my doctor before I take the first dose of Peganone?
Tell your doctor about all prescription, over-the-counter, and herbal medication you are taking before beginning treatment with Peganone. Also, talk to your doctor about your complete medical history, especially if you have liver problems, blood disorders, or a chronic autoimmune disease involving the internal organs known as systemic lupus erythematosus.

What is the usual dosage?
The information below is based on the dosage guidelines your doctor uses. Depending on your condition and medical history, your doctor may prescribe a different regimen. Do not change the dosage or stop taking your medication without your doctor's approval.

Dosage is tailored to each individual's needs. Your doctor will monitor blood levels of the drug closely. If you're switching from another anti-epileptic drug, the doctor will have you slowly taper off the dosage while increasing the dose of Peganone.

Adults: The recommended starting dose is 1,000 milligrams (mg) or less each day, taken in 4 to 6 divided doses spaced as evenly as possible. Depending on your response, the doctor may raise your dose. The usual effective maintenance dose is 2,000 to 3,000 mg a day.

Children: Dosage depends on the child's age and weight. The initial starting dose should not exceed 750 mg a day, taken in 4 to 6 divided doses spaced as evenly as possible. The usual maintenance dose is 500 to 1,000 mg a day, although occasionally doses as high as 3,000 mg a day may be necessary.

How should I take Peganone?
Take Peganone with food to avoid stomach upset. Depending on the type of seizure disorder, your doctor may give you another drug to take with Peganone.

It is important that you follow the prescribed dosage regimen strictly and tell your doctor about any condition that makes it impossible for you to take Peganone as prescribed.

What should I avoid while taking Peganone?

Use caution when driving, operating machinery, or performing other hazardous activities, as Peganone may cause dizziness or drowsiness. If you experience dizziness or drowsiness, avoid these activities.

Do not drink alcohol while taking this medication. Alcohol can cause deep sedation or sleepiness when taken with Peganone.

What are possible food and drug interactions associated with Peganone?

If Peganone is taken with certain other drugs, the effects of either could be increased, decreased, or altered. It is especially important to check with your doctor before combining Peganone with: blood-thinning drugs such as warfarin; drugs used to treat blood disorders; and phenacemide.

What are the possible side effects of Peganone?

Side effects cannot be anticipated. If any develop or change in intensity, tell your doctor as soon as possible. Only your doctor can determine if it is safe for you to continue taking this drug.

Side effects may include: chest pain, diarrhea, dizziness, double vision, fatigue, fever, gum overgrowth or thickening, headache, insomnia, involuntary or rapid eye movement, loss of or impaired muscle coordination, lymph node disease, nausea, numbness, skin rash, vomiting, sore throat

Can I receive Peganone if I am pregnant or breastfeeding?

If you are pregnant or plan to become pregnant, inform your doctor immediately. Because of the possibility of birth defects with Peganone, you may need to discontinue the drug. Do not, however, stop taking it without first consulting your doctor.

Because Peganone appears in breast milk, you should not breastfeed during treatment with the drug.

What should I do if I miss a dose of Peganone?

Take the missed dose as soon as you remember. However, if it is almost time for your next dose, skip the dose you missed and take only your next regularly scheduled dose. Do not take a double dose of this medication.

If you forget to take your medication 2 or more days in a row, check with your doctor.

How should I store Peganone?

Store at room temperature, but not above 77° F. Protect from light.

Pemirolast *See Alamast, page 55.*

Penciclovir *See Denavir, page 392.*

PENICILLIN V POTASSIUM

What is Penicillin V potassium?

Penicillin V potassium is a penicillin antibiotic. It works by interfering with the formation of the bacteria's cell wall while it is growing. This weakens the cell wall and kills the bacteria. Penicillin V potassium is used to treat infections, including dental infections, infections in the heart, middle ear infections, rheumatic fever, scarlet fever, skin infections, and respiratory tract infections.

Penicillin V potassium works against only certain types of bacteria; it is not effective against fungi, viruses, and parasites.

What is the most important information I should know about Penicillin V potassium?

If you are allergic to either penicillin or cephalosporin antibiotics in any form, consult your doctor before taking penicillin V potassium. There is a possibility that you are allergic to both types of medication; and if a reaction occurs, it could be extremely severe. If you take the drug and feel signs of a reaction, seek medical attention immediately.

Long-term or repeated use of penicillin V potassium may cause a second infection. Tell your doctor if signs of a second infection occur. Your medicine may need to be changed to treat this.

If you are diabetic and taking large doses of penicillin, you may get a false-positive result for sugar in your urine. Check with your doctor before you change your diet or the dose of your diabetic medicine.

Who should not take Penicillin V potassium?

Do not take penicillin V potassium if you are allergic to any of its ingredients or to other penicillins.

What should I tell my doctor before I take the first dose of Penicillin V potassium?

Tell your doctor about all prescription, over-the-counter, and herbal medication you are taking before beginning treatment with penicillin V potassium. Also, talk to your doctor about your complete medical history, especially if you have had asthma; colitis (inflammatory bowel disease); diabetes; kidney or liver disease; diarrhea or a stomach infection (especially in children 9 years of age or younger). Be sure to talk to your doctor about preventing pregnancy while you are taking penicillin V potassium.

Hormonal birth control such as contraceptive pills may not work as well and you may have to use another form of birth control.

What is the usual dosage?

The information below is based on the dosage guidelines your doctor uses. Depending on your condition and medical history, your doctor may prescribe a different regimen. Do not change the dosage or stop taking your medication without your doctor's approval.

Adults and children 12 years and older: Continue taking penicillin V potassium for the full time of treatment, even if you begin to feel better after a few days. Failure to take a full course of therapy may prevent complete elimination of the infection. It is best to take the doses at evenly spaced times.

Typical dosages for various infections are as follows:

Mild Staph Infections of the Skin
The usual dosage is 250 milligrams (mg) to 500 mg every 6 to 8 hours.

Mild to Moderately Severe Gum Infections
(Vincent's gingivitis)
The usual dosage is 250 mg to 500 mg every 6 to 8 hours.

Mild to Moderately Severe Pneumococcal Infections of the Respiratory Tract, Including Middle Ear Infections
The usual dosage is 250 mg to 500 mg taken every 6 hours until you have been without a fever for at least 2 days.

Mild to Moderately Severe Strep Infections of the Upper Respiratory Tract and Skin, and Scarlet Fever
The usual dosage is 125 to 250 mg taken every 6 to 8 hours for 10 days.

Prevention of Bacterial Endocarditis in People Undergoing Dental or Surgical Procedures
For oral therapy, the usual dose is 2 grams of Penicillin V Potassium (1 gram for children under 60 lbs) taken one-half to 1 hour before the procedure, then 1 gram 6 hours later.

Prevention of Recurring Rheumatic Fever and/or Chorea
The usual dosage is 125 mg to 250 mg taken 2 times a day on a continuing basis.

How should I take Penicillin V potassium?

Penicillin V potassium may be taken on a full or empty stomach, though it is better absorbed when the stomach is empty. Be sure to take it for the full time of treatment.

Doses of the oral solution of penicillin V potassium should be measured with a calibrated measuring spoon. Shake the solution well before using it.

What should I avoid while taking Penicillin V potassium?

This medication has been prescribed for your current condition only. Do not use it later for another infection unless told to do so by your doctor. A different medication may be necessary in those cases.

What are possible food and drug interactions associated with Penicillin V potassium?

If penicillin V potassium is taken with certain other drugs, the effects of either could be increased, decreased, or altered. It is especially important to check with your doctor before combining penicillin V potassium with the following: methotrexate, oral contraceptives, or tetracycline and other medicines in the same class (such as doxycycline, minocycline, and tigecycline).

What are the possible side effects of Penicillin V potassium?

Side effects cannot be anticipated. If any develop or change in intensity, tell your doctor as soon as possible. Only your doctor can determine if it is safe for you to continue taking this drug.

Side effects may include: anemia, black hairy tongue, diarrhea, fever, hives, nausea, skin eruptions, stomach upset or pain, swelling in throat, vomiting

Can I receive Penicillin V potassium if I am pregnant or breastfeeding?

The effects of penicillin V potassium during pregnancy are unknown. Tell your doctor immediately if you are pregnant, or plan to become pregnant. Since penicillin V potassium appears in breast milk, you should consult with your doctor if you plan to breastfeed your baby. If penicillin V potassium is essential to your health, your doctor may advise you to discontinue breastfeeding until your treatment is finished.

What should I do if I miss a dose of Penicillin V potassium?

Take it as soon as you remember. If it is almost time for the next dose, skip the missed dose and continue with your regular dosing schedule. Do not take a double dose to make up for a missed one.

How should I store Penicillin V potassium?

Store in a tightly closed container. The reconstituted oral solution must be refrigerated. Discard any unused solution after 14 days. Tablets and powder for oral solution may be stored at room temperature.

PENLAC
Generic name: Ciclopirox

What is Penlac?
Penlac is a nail lacquer used in the treatment of nail infections caused by the fungus *Trichophyton rubrum* (ringworm of the nails). It is prescribed only if the pale semicircle at the base of the nail is free of infection. It is part of a comprehensive treatment plan that includes professional removal of the unattached infected nails as frequently as monthly.

What is the most important information I should know about Penlac?
It can take 6 months of daily Penlac application and periodic nail removal by a healthcare professional before symptoms begin to abate. Treatment typically lasts up to 48 weeks, and the infected nails may not be completely clear when your treatment is finished.

Use Penlac nail lacquer on nails and immediately surrounding skin only. Penlac nail lacquer is not for ophthalmic, oral, or intravaginal use.

Do not use nail polish or other nail cosmetic products on the treated nails.

Avoid use near heat or open flame; the product is flammable.

Inform a healthcare professional if you have diabetes or problems with numbness in your toes or fingers.

Who should not take Penlac?
Do not take Penlac if you are allergic to the medication or any or its ingredients.

What should I tell my doctor before I take the first dose of Penlac?
Tell your doctor about all prescription, over-the-counter, and herbal medication you are taking before beginning treatment with Penlac. Also, talk to your doctor about your complete medical history, especially if you have diabetes; problems with numbness in your toes or fingers; or if you are immunosuppressed (for example, if you have received an organ transplant or if you have AIDS).

What is the usual dosage?
The information below is based on the dosage guidelines your doctor uses. Depending on your condition and medical history, your doctor may prescribe a different regimen. Do not change the dosage or stop taking your medication without your doctor's approval.

Adults: Apply once daily at bedtime, or eight hours before washing, to the entire surface of all infected nails.

How should I take Penlac?

Before starting treatment, remove any loose nail material with clippers or a file. Brush Penlac evenly over the entire surface of all affected nails once daily, preferably at bedtime. Where possible, also apply the lacquer to the underside of the nail and the skin beneath. Allow the lacquer to dry for 30 seconds before putting on socks or stockings. Wait 8 hours before taking a bath or shower.

Daily applications of the nail lacquer should be made over the previous coat and removed with alcohol every 7 days. When removing Penlac from the nail (using an emery board), file any loose nail material and trim away as much of the damaged nail as possible. Continue this cycle throughout the duration of therapy.

What should I avoid while taking Penlac?

Keep Penlac away from the eyes and mucous membranes. Avoid contact with any skin outside the immediate area of the nail. Penlac is for external use only.

Do not use nail polish or other cosmetic nail products on the treated nails.

Avoid using Penlac near heat or open flame; it is flammable.

What are possible food and drug interactions associated with Penlac?

If Penlac is taken with certain other drugs, the effects of either could be increased, decreased, or altered. It is especially important to check with your doctor before combining Penlac with oral antifungal medications such as griseofulvin, terbinafine, and itraconazole.

What are the possible side effects of Penlac?

Side effects cannot be anticipated. If any develop or change in intensity, tell your doctor as soon as possible. Only your doctor can determine if it is safe for you to continue taking this drug.

Side effects may include: rash or redness around the nail, change in shape of nail, discoloration, ingrown toenail, blistering, burning, oozing of the treated area

Can I receive Penlac if I am pregnant or breastfeeding?

The effects of Penlac during pregnancy and breastfeeding are unknown. Tell your doctor immediately if you are pregnant, plan to become pregnant, or are breastfeeding.

What should I do if I miss a dose of Penlac?

If you miss a dose of Penlac Solution and you are using it daily at bedtime, skip the missed dose. Do not use the medicine the following morning. If you do not use the dose at bedtime and you miss a dose, use it as soon as possible. If several hours have passed or it is nearing time for the next dose, skip the missed dose and return to your regular dosing schedule.

How should I store Penlac?

Store Penlac Solution at room temperature and protect from light. Keep away from heat and flame. Keep Penlac Solution out of the reach of children.

PENTACEL

Generic name: Diphtheria and tetanus toxoids and acellular pertussis adsorbed, inactivated poliovirus vaccine and Haemophilus b conjugate (tetanus toxoid conjugate) vaccine

What is Pentacel?

Pentacel is a five-in-one combination vaccine intended to prevent diphtheria, tetanus, pertussis (whooping cough), polio, and *Haemophilus* b infection. It is used in children 6 weeks through 4 years of age (prior to the fifth birthday).

What is the most important information I should know about Pentacel?

Pentacel should not be given to anyone with history of allergic reactions to any vaccine that protects against diphtheria, tetanus, pertussis, *H. influenza*e, or polio.

Pentacel should not be given to anyone who experienced a brain or nervous system disorder within 7 days of receiving pertussis-containing vaccine; who had Guillain-Barryé syndrome after receiving a vaccine containing tetanus toxoid; or who had any of the following problems within 48 hours after a dose of pertussis-containing vaccine: fever >105°F, shock-like state, persistent crying lasting 3 hours or more, seizures with or without fever within 3 days of vaccination.

Pentacel is a vaccine and, as with other vaccines, there is a risk of allergic reaction. Signs of severe allergic reactions may include hives, difficulty breathing, and swelling of the throat. If any of these events occur, seek immediate medical attention.

Who should not take Pentacel?

See "What is the most important information I should know about Pentacel?" above.

Additionally, Pentacel should not be given to children with progressive neurological damage; children who experienced encephalopathy (eg, coma, decreased level of consciousness, or prolonged seizures) within 7 days of a previous dose of pertussis-containing vaccine; or children <6 weeks of age or ≥5 years of age.

What should I tell my doctor before I take the first dose of Pentacel?

Tell your doctor about all vaccines and prescription, over-the-counter and herbal medications your child has received before beginning treatment with Pentacel. Also talk to your doctor about your child's complete medical history, especially if they have a history of seizures, a weakened immune system, or a history of allergic reactions to vaccines or latex.

What is the usual dosage?

The information below is based on the dosage guidelines your doctor uses. Depending on your condition and medical history, your doctor may prescribe a different regimen. Do not change the dosage or stop taking your medication without your doctor's approval.

Children ≥6 weeks to <5 years: Pentacel is administered as a single intramuscular injection.

How should I take Pentacel?

Pentacel will be injected by the nurse or doctor in the upper leg (thigh), upper arm, or buttocks.

What should I avoid while taking Pentacel?

There are no specific warnings regarding activities to avoid after receiving this vaccination.

What are possible food and drug interactions associated with Pentacel?

If Pentacel is taken with certain other drugs, the effects of either could be increased, decreased, or altered. It is especially important to check with your doctor before combining Pentacel with corticosteroids, cytotoxic drugs, and immunosuppressive therapies, including irradiation

What are the possible side effects of Pentacel?

As with any other vaccine, there is a risk of allergic reactions. Side effects cannot be anticipated. If any develop or change in intensity, tell your doctor as soon as possible.

Side effects may include: pain, redness, or swelling at the injection site, fever, inconsolable crying, decreased activity, lethargy, irritability

Signs of severe allergic reactions may include hives, difficulty breathing, and swelling of the throat. If any of these events occur, seek immediate medical attention.

Can I receive Pentacel if I am pregnant or breastfeeding?

The effects of Pentacel during pregnancy and breastfeeding are unknown. Pentacel is to be avoided in women of child bearing age.

What should I do if I miss a dose of Pentacel?
This is a one-time vaccine administered in your doctor's office.

How should I store Pentacel?
Pentacel will be administered in your doctor's office.

Pentoxifylline *See Trental, page 1328.*

PEPCID
Generic name: Famotidine

What is Pepcid?
Pepcid is in a class of drugs called histamine receptor antagonists. Pepcid works by decreasing the amount of acid the stomach produces. Pepcid is prescribed for the short-term treatment of active duodenal ulcer (in the upper intestine) for 4 to 8 weeks and for active, benign gastric ulcer (in the stomach) for 6 to 8 weeks. It is prescribed for maintenance therapy, at reduced dosage, after a duodenal ulcer has healed.

Pepcid is also used for short-term treatment of GERD (gastroesophageal reflux disease), a condition in which the acid contents of the stomach flow back into the food canal (esophagus), and for resulting inflammation of the esophagus. It is also prescribed for certain diseases that cause the stomach to produce excessive quantities of acid, such as Zollinger-Ellison syndrome.

What is the most important information I should know about Pepcid?
Do not stop taking this medication without first talking to your doctor. It may take up to 8 weeks for an ulcer to heal.

Pepcid may cause dizziness. This effect may be worse if you take it with alcohol or certain medicines. Do not drive or perform other possibly unsafe tasks until you know how you react to it.

Notify your doctor if you have any symptoms of a bleeding ulcer, such as black, tarry stools or vomit that looks like coffee grounds.

Do not take antacids within 1 hour of taking Pepcid. Antacids may decrease the effectiveness of Pepcid.

You can help avoid heartburn and acid indigestion by: not lying down soon after eating, keeping your weight down; if you smoke, quitting or at least cutting down; not eating just before bedtime.

Avoiding or limiting caffeine, chocolate, fatty foods, and alcohol.

Who should not take Pepcid?
If you are sensitive to or have ever had an allergic reaction to Pepcid, or a comparable H_2 blocker such as cimetidine, ranitidine, or nizatidine, you should not take Pepcid.

What should I tell my doctor before I take the first dose of Pepcid?

Tell your doctor about all prescription, over-the-counter, and herbal medication you are taking before beginning treatment with Pepcid. Also, talk to your doctor about your complete medical history, especially if you have kidney or liver disease, trouble or pain swallowing food, vomiting with blood, bloody or black stools. In addition, tell your doctor if you are pregnant, expect to become pregnant, or are breastfeeding.

What is the usual dosage?

The information below is based on the dosage guidelines your doctor uses. Depending on your condition and medical history, your doctor may prescribe a different regimen. Do not change the dosage or stop taking your medication without your doctor's approval.

Pepcid for Oral Suspension may be substituted for Pepcid Tablets in any of the below indications. Each five mL of the suspension contains 40 mg of famotidine after constitution of the powder with 46 mL of Purified Water.

Benign Gastric Ulcer

Adults: The usual dose is 40 milligrams (mg) or 5 milliliters (ml) (1 teaspoonful) once a day at bedtime.

Duodenal Ulcer

Adults: The usual starting dose is 40 mg or 5 ml once a day at bedtime. You should see results within 4 weeks, and Pepcid should not be used at full dosage longer than 6 to 8 weeks. Your doctor may have you take 20 mg or 2.5 ml (½ teaspoonful) twice a day. The normal maintenance dose after your ulcer has healed is 20 mg or 2.5 ml (half a teaspoonful) once a day at bedtime.

Excess Acid Conditions (such as Zollinger-Ellison Syndrome)

Adults: The usual starting dose is 20 mg every 6 hours, although some people need a higher dose. Doses of up to 160 mg every 6 hours have been given in severe cases.

If your kidneys are not functioning properly, your doctor will adjust the dosage.

Gastroesophageal Reflux Disease (GERD)

Adults: The usual dose is 20 mg or 2.5 ml (½ teaspoonful) twice a day for up to 6 weeks. For inflammation of the esophagus due to GERD, the dose is 20 or 40 mg or 2.5 to 5 ml twice a day for up to 12 weeks.

Children 1 to 16 years old: The usual daily dose is 1 mg per 2.2 pounds of body weight, divided and given in 2 smaller doses. Do not exceed 40 mg daily.

If your child's kidneys are not functioning properly, your doctor will adjust the dosage.

Infants under 12 months old: The usual starting dose of the oral suspension is 0.5 mg per 2.2 pounds of body weight once a day for infants under 3 months of age, and twice a day for infants 3 to 11 months of age. The dosage can be given for up to 8 weeks. Your doctor may also recommend additional measures to relieve the symptoms, such as thickening the child's food.

If your infant's kidneys are not functioning properly, your doctor will adjust the dosage.

Peptic Ulcer
Children 1 to 16 years old: The usual daily dose is 0.5 mg per 2.2 pounds of body weight. The entire dose may be given at bedtime, or divided and given in 2 smaller doses. Do not give more than 40 mg per day.

If your child's kidneys are not functioning properly, your doctor will adjust the dosage.

How should I take Pepcid?
Take Pepcid by mouth with or without food. It may take several days for Pepcid to begin relieving stomach pain. You can use antacids for the pain at the same time you take Pepcid.

If you are taking Pepcid suspension, prepare the suspension at the time you are going to take it. Slowly add 46mL of purified water and shake vigorously for 5 to 10 seconds immediately after adding the water and immediately before use. Any unused oral suspension that has been prepared should be discarded after 30 days.

Take Pepcid AC with water. To prevent symptoms, take it 1 hour before a meal you expect will cause you trouble.

What should I avoid while taking Pepcid?
Do not take antacids within 1 hour of taking Pepcid. Antacids may decrease the effectiveness of Pepcid.

Do not drive or perform other possibly unsafe tasks until you know how you react to Pepcid for it can potentially cause dizziness.

What are possible food and drug interactions associated with Pepcid?
If Pepcid is taken with certain other drugs, the effects of either could be increased, decreased, or altered. It is especially important to check with your doctor before combining Pepcid with the following: antacids, itraconazole, and ketoconazole.

What are the possible side effects of Pepcid?
Side effects cannot be anticipated. If any develop or change in intensity, tell your doctor as soon as possible. Only your doctor can determine if it is safe for you to continue taking this drug.

Side effects may include: Headache, constipation, diarrhea, dizziness

Can I receive Pepcid if I am pregnant or breastfeeding?

The effects of Pepcid during pregnancy are unknown. Tell your doctor immediately if you are pregnant, or plan to become pregnant. Pepcid may appear in breast milk and could affect a nursing infant. If Pepcid is essential to your health, your doctor may advise you to discontinue breastfeeding until your treatment with Pepcid is finished.

What should I do if I miss a dose of Pepcid?

Take the missed dose as soon as you remember. However, if it is almost time for the next dose, skip the missed dose and take only the next regularly scheduled dose. Do not take a double dose of this medication unless otherwise directed by your doctor.

How should I store Pepcid?

Store Pepcid at 77 degrees F (25 degrees C). Brief storage at temperatures between 59 and 86 degrees F (15 and 30 degrees C) is permitted. Store away from heat, moisture, and light. Pepcid for oral suspension should be protected from freezing. Do not store in the bathroom. Keep Pepcid out of the reach of children.

PERCOCET

Generic name: Acetaminophen and oxycodone hydrochloride

What is Percocet?

Percocet, a narcotic analgesic, is used to treat moderate to moderately severe pain. It contains two drugs—acetaminophen and oxycodone. Acetaminophen is used to reduce both pain and fever. Oxycodone, a narcotic analgesic, is used for its calming effect and for pain.

What is the most important information I should know about Percocet?

Percocet contains a narcotic and, even if taken in prescribed amounts, can cause physical and psychological dependence when taken for a long time. Because Percocet may be habit-forming, it should be used only by the person it was prescribed for. Percocet should never be given to another person, especially someone who has a history of drug abuse or addiction.

Keep the medication in a secure place. Keep track of how many pills have been used from each new bottle of this medicine. Percocet is a drug of abuse and you should be aware if any person in the household is using this medicine improperly or without a prescription.

Avoid alcohol or other mental depressant medicines (tranquilizers or sleeping pills) while taking Percocet. Alcohol use combined with acetaminophen (an ingredient of Percocet) may increase your risk for liver damage (symptoms include yellowing of skin or eyes, stomach pain, dark urine).

You should take Percocet cautiously and according to your doctor's instructions as you would take any medication containing a narcotic. If you have ever had a problem with alcohol addiction, make sure your doctor is aware of it.

Do not drive, operate machinery, or do anything else that could be dangerous until you know how you react to Percocet. Percocet may cause dizziness, lightheadedness, blurred vision, or drowsiness; these effects may be made worse if you take Percocet with other medicines or with alcohol. To minimize dizziness or lightheadedness, get up slowly when rising from a seated or lying position.

Before you have any medical or dental treatments, emergency care, or surgery, tell the doctor or dentist that you are using Percocet.

To prevent constipation, maintain a diet adequate in fiber, drink plenty of water, and exercise. If you become constipated while using Percocet, talk with your doctor or pharmacist; a stool softener or bulk laxative may help.

Percocet contains acetaminophen. Adults should not take more than a total of 4 grams (4,000 mg) of acetaminophen in a 24 hour period (3 grams [3,000 mg] per day if you have liver disease). Check with your doctor before taking other pain relievers, cough-and-cold medicines, or allergy medicines as they may also contain acetaminophen. Acetaminophen may cause liver damage.

You may have withdrawal symptoms when you stop using this medication after using it over a long period of time. Do not stop using Percocet suddenly without first talking to your doctor. You may need to use less and less before you stop the medication completely.

Who should not take Percocet?

You should not use Percocet if you are sensitive to acetaminophen, oxycodone, or any other component of this product. Percocet should not be used in any situation where opioids are not to be used. This includes patients with significant respiratory depression (inadequate ventilation), hypercarbia (excess amount of carbon dioxide in the blood), or severe asthma. Also, Percocet should not be used in patients with suspected or known disruption of normal intestinal movement (when intestinal contents including drugs and food cannot move forward).

What should I tell my doctor before I take the first dose of Percocet?

Tell your doctor about all prescription, over-the-counter, and herbal medication you are taking before beginning treatment with Percocet. Also, talk to your doctor about your complete medical history, especially if you have ever had liver, kidney, thyroid gland, or Addison's disease (a disease of the adrenal glands), heart disease, seizures, gallbladder problems, sever diarrhea, inflammatory bowel disease, difficulty urinating; an enlarged prostate; stomach problems such as an ulcer; a history of substance abuse or dependence, psychiatric problems, suicidal ideations, or if you have experienced a head injury.

What is the usual dosage?
The information below is based on the dosage guidelines your doctor uses. Depending on your condition and medical history, your doctor may prescribe a different regimen. Do not change the dosage or stop taking your medication without your doctor's approval.

Adults: The usual dose is 1 to 2 tablets of the lowest strength (2.5 milligrams [mg] oxycodone/325 mg acetaminophen) every 6 hours. Doctors sometimes prescribe a higher dose if necessary. The total daily dose of acetaminophen should not exceed 4 grams. The maximum daily dose recommended for each strength of Percocet (oxycodone/acetaminophen) is as follows: 2.5 mg/325 mg: 12 tablets; 5 mg/325 mg: 12 tablets 7.5 mg/500 mg: 8 tablets; 10 mg/650 mg: 6 tablets.

Elderly people or those in a weakened condition should take Percocet cautiously.

When discontinuing therapy, doses should be decreased gradually to prevent signs and symptoms of withdrawal in a physically dependent patient. (This usually occurs after at least a few weeks of treatment with Percocet.)

Children: The safety and effectiveness of Percocet have not been established in children.

How should I take Percocet?
Take Percocet with meals or with milk. Taking Percocet with food may reduce stomach upset but will also decrease the effectiveness of the medication.

What should I avoid while taking Percocet?
Do not drink alcohol or take other mental depressant medications while you are taking Percocet.

This drug may impair your ability to drive a car or operate potentially dangerous machinery. Do not participate in any activities that require full alertness if you are unsure about the drug's effect on you.

Do not abruptly discontinue treatment with Percocet or change your dose without first talking to your doctor.

Adults should not take more than a total of 4 grams (4,000 mg) of acetaminophen in a 24 hour period (3 grams [3,000 mg] per day if you have liver disease). Check with your doctor before taking other pain relievers, cough-and-cold medicines, or allergy medicines as they may also contain acetaminophen.

What are possible food and drug interactions associated with Percocet?

If Percocet is taken with certain other drugs, the effects of either could be increased, decreased, or altered. It is especially important to check with your doctor before combining Percocet with the following: alcohol anticoagulants such as warfarin antispasmodic drugs such as benztropine and dicyclomine; barbiturate anesthetics such as thiopental; betablockers such as propranolol; cimetidine; isoniazid; major tranquilizers such as chlorpromazine and thioridazine; oral contraceptives; other narcotic painkillers such as propoxyphene and meperidine; sedatives such as phenobarbital and secobarbital; sodium oxybate (GHB); sulfinpyrazone; and tranquilizers such as alprazolam and diazepam.

What are the possible side effects of Percocet?

Side effects cannot be anticipated. If any develop or change in intensity, tell your doctor as soon as possible. Only your doctor can determine if it is safe for you to continue taking this drug.

Side effects may include: constipation, dizziness, exaggerated feelings of well-being or sadness, light-headedness, nausea, sedation, skin rash or itching; vomiting

Can I receive Percocet if I am pregnant or breastfeeding?

The effects of Percocet during pregnancy and breastfeeding are unknown. Tell your doctor immediately if you are pregnant, plan to become pregnant, or are breastfeeding.

What should I do if I miss a dose of Percocet?

Since Percocet is sometimes used as needed, you may not be on a dosing schedule. If you are taking the medication regularly, take the missed dose as soon as you remember. If it is almost time for your next dose, skip the missed dose and wait until your next regularly scheduled dose. Do not use extra medicine to make up for a missed dose.

How should I store Percocet?

Store Percocet at room temperature between 59 and 86 degrees F (15 and 30 degrees C) in a tightly closed container away from heat, moisture, and light. Do not store in the bathroom. Keep Percocet out of the reach of children .

PERCODAN

Generic name: Oxycodone and aspirin

What is Percodan?

Percodan is prescribed for moderate to moderately severe pain. Percodan is a combination of two pain-killing drugs—oxycodone and aspirin.

Oxycodone (related to codeine) is in a class of drugs called narcotic analgesics; it relieves pain. Aspirin is a less potent pain reliever, as well as an anti-inflammatory and a fever reducer. Aspirin increases the effects of oxycodone.

What is the most important information I should know about Percodan?

The oxycodone in Percodan can cause physical and psychological dependence. Use this product with caution. Never take more Percodan than is prescribed for you because this may heighten your risk of serious breathing problems. If your pain is not being adequately treated, talk to your doctor.

The oxycodone in Percodan may also cause constipation. Drink plenty of water (six to eight full glasses a day) to lessen this side effect. Increasing the amount of fiber in your diet can also help to alleviate constipation.

Do not stop taking Percodan suddenly if you have been taking it continuously for more than 5 to 7 days. Stopping suddenly could cause withdrawal symptoms and make you very uncomfortable. Your doctor may want to gradually reduce your dose.

Do not drive or perform other possibly unsafe tasks until you know how you react to Percodan; the drug may cause drowsiness, dizziness, lightheadedness, or blurred vision.

Check with your doctor before you drink alcohol or use medicines that may cause drowsiness (eg, sleep aids, muscle relaxers) while you are using Percodan; it may add to their effects.

Percodan may cause dizziness, lightheadedness, or fainting; alcohol, hot weather, exercise, alcohol, or fever may increase these effects. To prevent them, sit up or stand slowly, especially in the morning. Sit or lie down at the first sign of any of these effects.

Percodan may cause stomach bleeding. Your risk may be greater if you drink alcohol while you are using Percodan.

Talk to your doctor before you take Percodan if you drink 3 or more drinks with alcohol per day.

Percodan may reduce the number of clot-forming cells (platelets) in your blood. Avoid activities that may cause bruising or injury. Tell your doctor if you have unusual bruising or bleeding. Tell your doctor if you have dark, tarry, or bloody stools.

Do not give Percodan to a child or teenager who has the flu, chickenpox, or a viral infection. Aspirin, an ingredient of Percodan, has been linked to a serious illness called Reye syndrome.

Tell your doctor or dentist that you take Percodan before you receive any medical or dental care, emergency care, or surgery.

Percodan may affect your blood sugar. Check blood sugar levels closely. Ask your doctor before you change the dose of your diabetes medicine.

Percodan may interfere with certain lab tests. Be sure your doctor and lab personnel now you are taking Percodan.

Who should not take Percodan?
If you are allergic to either aspirin or oxycodone you will not be able to take Percodan. Also, Percodan cannot be used in situations where opioids cannot be used such as severe asthma or an asthma attack, nasal swelling, high levels of carbon dioxide in the blood, or if you have blockage of your bowel or other stomach or bowel problems.

In children and teenagers who have a viral infection, the aspirin in Percodan can trigger a severe, and even fatal, disorder called Reye's syndrome. Do not give Percodan to any child with an illness such as flu or chickenpox.

What should I tell my doctor before I take the first dose of Percodan?
Tell your doctor about all prescription, over-the-counter, and herbal medication you are taking before beginning treatment with Percodan. Also, talk to your doctor about your complete medical history, especially if you have: a clotting disorder, a head injury, a thyroid condition, abdominal disorders, Addison's disease, an enlarged prostate, difficulty urinating, kidney problems, seizures, a history of lung or breathing problems such as asthma, emphysema, or bronchitis, heart problems, low blood pressure, a history of alcohol or substance abuse or dependence or if you drink alcohol regularly, a history of mental or mood problems, suicidal thoughts, or suicide attempts, liver problems, or peptic ulcer disease.

What is the usual dosage?
The information below is based on the dosage guidelines your doctor uses. Depending on your condition and medical history, your doctor may prescribe a different regimen. Do not change the dosage or stop taking your medication without your doctor's approval.

Adults: The usual dose is one tablet every 6 hours as needed for pain. Your doctor may adjust the dosage according to the severity of pain and your response to the drug. The maximum daily dose of aspirin should not exceed 4 grams or 12 tablets.

When stopping treatment with Percodan, after at least a few weeks of therapy, dosage should be gradually reduced to prevent symptoms of withdrawal in physically dependent patients.

Children: A special formulation of Percodan called Percodan Demi is available for children. Do not give full-strength Percodan to a child.

How should I take Percodan?
Take Percodan exactly as your doctor instructs. Never take more of this medication than is prescribed for you. Too much Percodan could be

harmful. Do not stop taking Percodan or change your dose without first contacting your doctor.

Take each dose of Percodan with a full glass of water. Take Percodan with food or milk if it upsets your stomach.

What should I avoid while taking Percodan?

Percodan can impair the skills you need to drive a car or operate machinery safely. Do not attempt to drive if you are not fully alert or until you know how you react to this medication.

Avoid alcohol while taking Percodan. Alcohol may increase the drowsiness and dizziness caused by Percodan and could be dangerous. Also, alcohol increases the risk of stomach bleeding when you are taking a medication that contains aspirin.

Do not give Percodan to a child or teenager who has the flu, chickenpox, or a viral infection. Contact your doctor with any questions or concerns.

Avoid activities that may cause bruising or injury.

Avoid sitting up or standing quickly, especially in the morning.

What are possible food and drug interactions associated with Percodan?

If Percodan is taken with certain other drugs, the effects of either could be increased, decreased, or altered. It is especially important to check with your doctor before combining Percodan with the following: acetazolamide; alcohol; angiotensin converting enzyme (ACE) inhibitors; antidepressants such as amitriptyline, phenelzine, nortriptyline, and tranylcypromine; anticoagulants such as warfarin, clopidogrel, and heparin; beta-blockers; blood-thinning drugs such as warfarin; gout medications such as probenecid; major tranquilizers such as prochlorperazine, trifluoperazine, and chlorpromazine; methotrexate; nonsteroidal anti-inflammatory drugs (NSAIDs); oral hypoglycemic agents; other narcotic pain killers such as meperidine and oxycodone; promethazine; sleep aids such as triazolam or secobarbital; tranquilizers such as alprazolam or diazepam; and water pills.

What are the possible side effects of Percodan?

Side effects cannot be anticipated. If any develop or change in intensity, tell your doctor as soon as possible. Only your doctor can determine if it is safe for you to continue taking this drug.

Side effects may include: constipation, dizziness, exaggerated feelings of well-being or sadness, itching, light-headedness, nausea, sedation, vomiting, drowsiness, stomach upset, bloody or black stools, dark urine, decreased urination, muscle pain, fever, chills, persistent sore throat, hoarseness, severe or persistent heartburn, trouble swallowing

Can I receive Percodan if I am pregnant or breastfeeding?

Percodan is not recommended for pregnant women under ordinary circumstances. Inform your doctor immediately if you become pregnant. Also, consult your doctor before using Percodan while breastfeeding. Percodan has been shown to cause harm to the fetus; avoid using Percodan in the last 3 months of pregnancy.

What should I do if I miss a dose of Percodan?

Since Percodan is sometimes used as needed, you may not be on a dosing schedule. If you are taking the medication regularly, take the missed dose as soon as you remember. If it is almost time for your next dose, skip the missed dose and wait until your next regularly scheduled dose. Do not take extra medicine to make up for a missed dose.

How should I store Percodan?

Store Percodan at 77 degrees F (25 degrees C). Brief storage at temperatures between 59 and 86 degrees F (15 and 30 degrees C) is permitted. Store away from heat, moisture, and light. Do not store in the bathroom. Keep Percodan out of the reach of children and away from pets. Once Percodan is not longer needed, dispose of it by flushing down the toilet.

PERFOROMIST

Generic name: Formoterol

What is Perforomist?

Perforomist Inhalation Solution is used long term, twice a day (morning and evening) to control symptoms of chronic obstructive pulmonary disease (COPD) in adults.

What is the most important information I should know about Perforomist?

In patients with asthma, long-acting beta-agonist medicines may increase the chance of death from asthma.

Perforomist does not relieve sudden symptoms.

Do not stop using Perforomist unless told to do so by your healthcare provider.

Who should not take Perforomist?

Do not take Perforomist if you are suffering from status asthmaticus or an acute attack of asthma, or if you are allergic to Perforomist or any of its ingredients.

What should I tell my doctor before I take the first dose of Perforomist?

Tell your doctor about all prescription, over-the-counter, and herbal medications you are taking before beginning treatment with Perforomist. Also, talk to your doctor about your complete medical history, especially if you have a history of status asthmaticus, have heart or liver problems, high blood pressure, diabetes, seizures, thyroid problems, are pregnant or planning to become pregnant, or are breastfeeding.

What is the usual dosage?

The information below is based on the dosage guidelines your doctor uses. Depending on your condition and medical history, your doctor may prescribe a different regimen. Do not change the dosage or stop taking your medication without your doctor's approval.

Adults: The usual dosage of Perforomist is one ready-to-use vial twice a day inhaled through a nebulizer.

How should I take Perforomist?

Perforomist Inhalation solution is only used in a standardized jet nebulizer machine connected to an air compressor. Make sure you know how to use your nebulizer machine before you use with Perforomist inhalation solution. Connect the nebulizer to the compressor. Sit in a comfortable upright position. Place the mouthpiece in your mouth or put on the face mask and turn the compressor on. Breathe in as calmly and deeply as possible through your mouth until no more mist is formed. The average nebulization time is 9 minutes.

What should I avoid while taking Perforomist?

Do not use to treat asthma. Do not use more than 2 vials of Perforomist per day.

What are possible food and drug interactions associated with Perforomist?

If Perforomist is used with certain other drugs, the effects of either could be increased, decreased, or altered. It is especially important to check with your doctor before combining Perforomist with the following: other long-acting beta$_2$-agonist drugs, adrenergic drugs, diuretics, MAO inhibitors, tricyclic antidepressants, and steroids.

What are the possible side effects of Perforomist?

Side effects cannot be anticipated. If any develop or change in intensity, tell your doctor as soon as possible. Only your doctor can determine if it is safe for you to continue taking this drug.

Side effects may include: allergic reactions, fast irregular heart beat, headache, high blood sugar, high blood acid, low blood potassium, nervousness, tremors

Signs of severe allergic reactions may include hives, dry mouth, diarrhea, difficulty breathing, and swelling of the throat. If any of these events occur, seek immediate medical attention.

Can I receive Perforomist if I am pregnant or breastfeeding?
Perforomist is to be avoided during pregnancy and breastfeeding.

What should I do if I miss a dose of Perforomist?
If you miss a dose of Perforomist, just skip that dose. Take the next regular dose. Do not take 2 doses at one time.

How should I store Perforomist?
Store Perforomist Inhalation Solution in a refrigerator in the protective foil pouch or at room temperature for up to 3 months. If not used within 3 months, discard.

PERIDEX
Generic name: Chlorhexidine gluconate

What is Peridex?
Peridex reduces bacteria in the mouth. It is an oral rinse used to treat gingivitis, a condition in which the gums become red and swollen, between dental visits. Peridex is also used to control gum bleeding caused by gingivitis.

What is the most important information I should know about Peridex?
Peridex may stain front-tooth fillings, especially those with a rough surface. These stains have no adverse effect on the gums, and usually can be removed by a professional cleaning. In addition to staining, Peridex can also cause an excess of tartar build-up on your teeth. It is recommended that you have your teeth cleaned at least every 6 months.

If you have both gingivitis and periodontitis (disease of the tissue that supports and attaches the teeth), remember that Peridex is used only for gingivitis. Periodontitis may require additional treatment by your doctor or dentist.

The use of Peridex may leave a bitter after-taste. Do not rinse with water or other mouthwashes after rinsing with Peridex solution. Make sure to use Peridex after you brush your teeth. Do not swallow the solution.

Who should not take Peridex?
Do not take Peridex if you are allergic to the medication or any or its ingredients.

What should I tell my doctor before I take the first dose of Peridex?

Tell your doctor about all prescription, over-the-counter, and herbal medication you are taking before beginning treatment with Peridex. Also, talk to your doctor about your complete medical history, especially if you have fillings or other dental work on your front teeth or if you have periodontitis (another dental disease).

What is the usual dosage?

The information below is based on the dosage guidelines your doctor uses. Depending on your condition and medical history, your doctor may prescribe a different regimen. Do not change the dosage or stop taking your medication without your doctor's approval.

Adults: The usual dose of undiluted Peridex is 15 milliliters (one-half fluid ounce or one tablespoon) taken twice daily, morning and evening after brushing your teeth. Rinse with Peridex for approximately 30 seconds after brushing your teeth. Spit Peridex out after rinsing. You should never swallow Peridex.

Children: The safety and effectiveness of Peridex have not been established in children less than 18 years of age.

How should I take Peridex?

You should get a thorough dental cleaning and examination before beginning treatment with Peridex. It is recommended that you have your teeth cleaned at least every 6 months.

After brushing, thoroughly rinsing, and flossing your teeth, rinse with Peridex by swishing one-half fluid ounce (marked in the cap) in your mouth for 30 seconds, and then spit it out. Do not swallow the mouthwash. Do not dilute Peridex and do not rinse your mouth with water or other mouthwashes after using Peridex, even if it leaves an unpleasant taste. Also, avoid eating or drinking for at least 1 hour to allow the medication to continue to work.

What should I avoid while taking Peridex?

Avoid eating, drinking, and rinsing your mouth for at least 1 hour after using Peridex.

While you are using Peridex, avoid other mouthwashes or rinses unless otherwise directed by your doctor. Avoid swallowing Peridex solution.

What are possible food and drug interactions associated with Peridex?

If Peridex is taken with certain other drugs, the effects of either could be increased, decreased, or altered. Always check with your doctor before combining Peridex with any other drugs, herbs, or supplements.

What are the possible side effects of Peridex?
Side effects cannot be anticipated. If any develop or change in intensity, tell your doctor as soon as possible. Only your doctor can determine if it is safe for you to continue taking this drug.

Side effects may include: Change in taste; increase in plaque; staining of teeth, mouth, tooth fillings, dentures, or other appliances in the mouth; mild irritation or sores in the mouth; numbness or tingling in the mouth

Can I receive Peridex if I am pregnant or breastfeeding?
The effects of Peridex during pregnancy and breastfeeding are unknown. Tell your doctor immediately if you are pregnant, plan to become pregnant, or are breastfeeding.

What should I do if I miss a dose of Peridex?
If you miss a dose of Peridex Solution, use it as soon as possible following proper procedure (see "**How should I take this medication?**"). If it is almost time for your next dose, skip the missed dose and go back to your regular dosing schedule. Do not use 2 doses at once.

How should I store Peridex?
Store Peridex Solution at room temperature, between 59 and 86 degrees F (15 and 30 degrees C). Do not freeze. Store away from heat, moisture, and light. Do not store in the bathroom. Keep Peridex Solution out of the reach of children.

Perindopril erbumine See Aceon, page 11.

PERSANTINE
Generic name: Dipyridamole

What is Persantine?
Persantine helps reduce the formation of blood clots in people who have had heart valve surgery. It is used in combination with blood thinners such as warfarin. It may also be used for other conditions as determined by your doctor.

**What is the most important information
I should know about Persantine?**
Persantine is sometimes used with aspirin to provide better protection against the formation of blood clots. However, the risk of bleeding may also be increased when these two drugs are taken together. To reduce this risk, take only the amount of aspirin prescribed by the same doctor who directed you to take Persantine. If you need a medication for pain

or a fever, do not take extra aspirin without first consulting your doctor. (Persantine is commonly given with the anticoagulant warfarin. It should be noted that aspirin should not be given at the same time as coumarin anticoagulants.)

Persantine has been known to cause liver problems, including liver failure. Contact your doctor immediately if you notice any of the following signs of liver trouble: nausea, fatigue, drowsiness, itching, yellowish skin, flu-like symptoms, and pain in the upper right abdomen.

Do not drive or perform other possibly unsafe tasks until you know how you react to Persantine. This medication may cause dizziness. These effects may be worse if you take it with alcohol or certain medicines.

Persantine may cause dizziness, lightheadedness, or fainting; alcohol, hot weather, exercise, or fever may increase these effects. To prevent them, sit up or stand slowly, especially in the morning. Sit or lie down at the first sign of any of these effects.

Tell your doctor or dentist that you take Persantine before you receive any medical or dental care, emergency care, or surgery.

Persantine should be used with caution in patients who have severe heart problems because symptoms such as chest pain may be aggravated while taking this medication. Persantine should also be used with caution in patients with hypotension (low blood pressure).

Who should not take Persantine?
Do not take Persantine if you are allergic to the medication or to any of its ingredients.

What should I tell my doctor before I take the first dose of Persantine?
Tell your doctor about all prescription, over-the-counter, and herbal medication you are taking before beginning treatment with Persantine. Also, talk to your doctor about your complete medical history, especially if you have heart problems, angina, recent heart attack, liver problems, or low blood pressure.

What is the usual dosage?
The information below is based on the dosage guidelines your doctor uses. Depending on your condition and medical history, your doctor may prescribe a different regimen. Do not change the dosage or stop taking your medication without your doctor's approval.

Adults: The usual recommended dose is 75 milligrams (mg) to 100 mg, taken 4 times a day. Persantine is usually taken as an adjunct to an anticoagulant such as warfarin. (Aspirin should not be given at the same time as coumarin anticoagulants.)

Children: The safety and effectiveness of Persantine have not been established in children less than 12 years of age.

How should I take Persantine?

Persantine must be taken exactly as your doctor prescribes it, at regularly scheduled times.

It is best to take Persantine on an empty stomach at least 1 hour before or 2 hours after eating, with a full glass of water. However, if this upsets your stomach, you can take the drug with food or milk.

Do not change from one brand of Persantine to another without consulting your doctor or pharmacist. Products manufactured by different companies may not be equally effective.

What should I avoid while taking Persantine?

Do not take aspirin or nonsteroidal anti-inflammatory drugs (NSAIDs) such as ibuprofen, naproxen, or ketoprofen during therapy with Persantine. The combination could lead to bleeding, especially in your stomach. Talk to your pharmacist or doctor before taking any over-the-counter or prescription medications for pain, inflammation (including arthritis), or fever.

Be careful when driving, operating machinery, or performing other hazardous activities. Persantine may make you dizziness. If you experience dizziness, avoid these activities.

Avoid standing or sitting up to quickly because Persantine may cause dizziness, lightheadedness, or fainting; alcohol, hot weather, exercise, or fever may increase these effects.

What are possible food and drug interactions associated with Persantine?

If Persantine is taken with certain other drugs, the effects of either could be increased, decreased, or altered. It is especially important to check with your doctor before combining Persantine with the following: adenosine; Alzheimer's drugs such as donepezil, tacrine, and rivastigmine; anticholinesterases such as neostigmine; aspirin; blood thinners such as warfarin; heart medications such as adenosine; indomethacin; ticlopidine; and valproic acid.

What are the possible side effects of Persantine?

Side effects cannot be anticipated. If any develop or change in intensity, tell your doctor as soon as possible. Only your doctor can determine if it is safe for you to continue taking this drug.

Side effects may include: abdominal distress, dizziness, diarrhea, flushing, headache, itching, vomiting, chest pain, fast heartbeat, swelling of the throat

Can I receive Persantine if I am pregnant or breastfeeding?

The effects of Persantine during pregnancy are unknown. Tell your doctor immediately if you are pregnant or plan to become pregnant. This drug appears in breast milk and may affect a nursing infant. If Persantine is essential to your health, your doctor may advise you to discontinue breastfeeding until your treatment with Persantine is finished.

What should I do if I miss a dose of Persantine?
If you miss a dose, take it as soon as you remember. However, if it is almost time for your next dose, skip the missed dose and take only your next regularly scheduled dose. Do not take a double dose of this medication.

How should I store Persantine?
Store at room temperature away from heat, moisture, and light. Do not store in the bathroom.

PEXEVA
Generic name: Paroxetine mesylate

What is Pexeva?
Pexeva is used to treat depression, obsessive compulsive disorder, panic disorder, and generalized anxiety disorder.

What is the most important information I should know about Pexeva?
Antidepressant medicines may increase suicidal thoughts or actions in some children, teenagers, and young adults when the medicine is first started. Depression and other serious mental illnesses are the most important causes of suicidal thoughts and actions. Some people may have a particularly high risk of having suicidal thoughts or actions. These include people who have (or have a family history of) bipolar disorder (also called manic-depressive illness) or suicidal thoughts or actions.

Individuals being treated with antidepressants and their caregivers can help reduce the risk of suicidal thoughts and actions by doing the following: Pay close attention to any changes, especially sudden ones, in mood, behaviors, thoughts, or feelings. This is very important when an antidepressant medicine is first started or when the dose is changed; Call the doctor right away to report new or sudden changes in mood, behavior, thoughts, or feelings. Signs to watch for include new or worsening depression, new or worsening anxiety, agitation, insomnia, hostility, panic attacks, restlessness, extreme hyperactivity, and suicidal thinking or behavior; Keep all follow-up visits as scheduled, and call the doctor between visits as needed, especially if you have concerns about symptoms.

Pexeva is not approved for use in pediatric patients.

Who should not take Pexeva?
You should not take Pexeva if you are allergic to it or any of its components. It should also be avoided if you are currently taking monoamine oxidase inhibitors (MAOIs), linezolid, thioridazine, or pimozide.

What should I tell my doctor before I take the first dose of Pexeva?

Tell your doctor about all prescription, over-the-counter, and herbal medication you are taking before beginning treatment with Pexeva. Also, talk to your doctor about your complete medical history, especially if you intend on becoming pregnant or if you have a history of suicidal thoughts, panic attacks, insomnia, seizures, glaucoma, or severe kidney or liver impairment.

What is the usual dosage?

The information below is based on the dosage guidelines your doctor uses. Depending on your condition and medical history, your doctor may prescribe a different regimen. Do not change the dosage or stop taking your medication without your doctor's approval.

Depression
Adults: The recommended starting dose is 20mg daily. Depending on you respond to Pexeva, your dose may be increased in 10 mg/day increments up to a maximum daily dose of 50mg.

Obsessive Compulsive Disorder
Adults: The recommended starting dose is 20mg daily. Depending on how you respond to Pexeva, your dose may be increased in 10 mg/day increments up to a maximum daily dose of 60mg.

Panic Disorder
Adults: The recommended starting dose is 10mg daily. Depending on how you respond to Pexeva, your dose may be increased in 10 mg/day increments up to a maximum daily dose of 60mg.

Generalized Anxiety Disorder
Adults: The recommended starting dose is 20mg daily. Depending on how you respond to Pexeva, your dose may be increased up to a maximum daily dose of 50mg.

How should I take Pexeva?

Pexeva is taken once daily, usually in the morning, with or without food. Pexeva should be swallowed whole, and never be chewed or crushed.

What should I avoid while taking Pexeva?

Avoid drinking alcohol during treatment with Pexeva. Driving or operating dangerous machinery or participating in any hazardous activity that requires full mental alertness should be avoided until you know how this drug affects you.

What are possible food and drug interactions associated with Pexeva?

If Pexeva is taken with certain other drugs, the effects of either could be increased, decreased, or altered. It is especially important to check with your doctor before combining Pexeva with any of the following: alcohol; antidepressants such as amitriptyline, desipramine, fluoxetine, imipramine, and nortriptyline; aspirin; cimetidine; diazepam; digoxin; flecainide; linezolid; lithium; nonsteroidal anti-inflammatory drugs (NSAIDs) such as aspirin, ibuprofen, naproxen, and ketoprofen; phenobarbital; phenytoin; pimozide; procyclidine; propafenone; propranolol; quinidine; st. John's wort; sumatriptan; theophylline; thioridazine; tramadol; triptans (a class of medication used to treat migraines, such sumatriptan and zolmitriptan); tryptophan; and warfarin.

What are the possible side effects of Pexeva?
Side effects cannot be anticipated. If any develop or change in intensity, tell your doctor as soon as possible. Only your doctor can determine if it is safe for you to continue taking this drug.

Side effects may include: abnormal ejaculation, abnormal orgasm, constipation, decreased appetite, decreased sex drive, diarrhea, dizziness, drowsiness, dry mouth, gas, impotence, male and female genital disorders, nausea, nervousness, sleeplessness, sweating, tremor, weakness, and vertigo

Can I receive Pexeva if I am pregnant or breastfeeding?
For women who intend to become pregnant or are in their first trimester of pregnancy, Pexeva should only be initiated after consideration of the other available treatment options. The effects of Pexeva during breastfeeding are unknown; discuss your options with your doctor.

What should I do if I miss a dose of Pexeva?
Skip the missed dose and go back to your regular schedule. Do not take a double dose to make up for the one you missed.

How should I store Pexeva?
Store at room temperature.

Phenazopyridine hydrochloride *See Pyridium, page 1110.*

Phenelzine sulfate *See Nardil, page 862.*

PHENOBARBITAL

What is Phenobarbital?
Phenobarbital, a barbiturate, is used in the treatment of certain types of epilepsy, including generalized or grand mal seizures and partial seizures. It is also used for short-term treatment of insomnia.

What is the most important information I should know about Phenobarbital?

Phenobarbital can be habit-forming. You may become tolerant and need more of the drug to achieve the same effect. You may become physically and psychologically dependent with continued use. Never increase the amount of phenobarbital you take without checking with your doctor.

Phenobarbital may cause excitement, depression, or confusion in elderly or weakened individuals, and excitement in children.

Barbiturates such as phenobarbital may cause you to become tired or less alert. Be careful driving, operating machinery, or doing any activity that requires full mental alertness until you know how this medication affects you.

Who should not take Phenobarbital?

Phenobarbital should not be used if you suffer from porphyria (a blood disorder), liver or lung disease, or if you have ever had an allergic reaction to or are sensitive to phenobarbital or other barbiturates.

Phenobarbital should be used with extreme caution, or not at all, by people who are depressed or who have a history of drug or alcohol dependence.

What should I tell my doctor before I take the first dose of Phenobarbital?

Tell your doctor about all prescription, over-the-counter, and herbal medications you are taking before beginning treatment with phenobarbital. Also, talk to your doctor about your complete medical history, especially if you have a history of depression, suicidal thoughts, drug or alcohol dependence, liver disease, adrenal gland problems, constant pain, or if you are pregnant, planning to become pregnant, or are breastfeeding.

What is the usual dosage?

The information below is based on the dosage guidelines your doctor uses. Depending on your condition and medical history, your doctor may prescribe a different regimen. Do not change the dosage or stop taking your medication without your doctor's approval.

Seizures
Adults: Phenobarbital dosage must be individualized on the basis of specific laboratory tests. Your doctor will determine the exact dose best for you. The typical doses are 50 to 100mg taken two to three times daily.

Children: The phenobarbital dosage must be individualized on the basis of specific laboratory tests. Your doctor will determine the exact dose best for your child.

Sedation
Adults: The usual dose is 30 to 120 milligrams a day, divided into 2 to 3 doses.

Insomnia
Adults: The usual dose is 100 to 320 milligrams, taken at bedtime.

People who are elderly, debilitated, or who have liver or kidney disease may require a lower dose of phenobarbital.

How should I take Phenobarbital?

Take this medication exactly as indicated by your doctor. You should never stop taking this medication without consulting your doctor first, especially if you are using this medication for seizures.

What should I avoid while taking Phenobarbital?

Avoid driving, operating machinery, or doing any activity that requires full mental alertness until you know how this medication affects you.

What are possible food and drug interactions associated with Phenobarbital?

If phenobarbital is taken with certain other drugs, the effects of either could be increased, decreased, or altered. It is especially important to check with your doctor before combining this medication with any the following: antidepressants known as MAOIs, antihistamines, blood-thinners, doxycycline, epilepsy drugs, griseofulvin, narcotic pain relievers, oral contraceptives, sedatives, steroids, and tranquilizers.

What are the possible side effects of Phenobarbital?

Side effects cannot be anticipated. If any develop or change in intensity, inform your doctor as soon as possible. Only your doctor can determine if it is safe for you to continue taking this drug.

Side effects may include: allergic reactions, drowsiness, headache, lethargy, nausea, oversedation, sleepiness, slowed or delayed breathing, vertigo, vomiting

Can I receive Phenobarbital if I am pregnant or breastfeeding?

Barbiturates such as phenobarbital may cause fetal damage. Withdrawal symptoms may occur in an infant whose mother took barbiturates during the last 3 months of pregnancy. If you are pregnant or plan to become pregnant, inform your doctor immediately.

Phenobarbital is excreted in breast milk. Talk to your doctor about whether you should stop breastfeeding while taking this medication.

What should I do if I miss a dose of Phenobarbital?

Take it as soon as you remember. If it is almost time for your next dose, skip the one you missed and go back to your regular schedule. Never take two doses at once.

How should I store Phenobarbital?
Store at room temperature in a tightly closed container and protect from light.

Phenobarbital, hyoscyamine sulfate, atropine sulfate, scopolamine hydrobromide See Donnatal, page 438.

Phentermine hydrochloride See Adipex-P, page 39.

Phenytoin sodium See Dilantin, page 421.

PHOSPHOLINE IODIDE
Generic name: Echothiophate iodide

What is Phospholine Iodide?
Phospholine Iodide is used to treat chronic open-angle glaucoma, a partial loss of vision or blindness resulting from a gradual increase in pressure of fluid in the eye. Because the vision loss occurs slowly, people often do not experience any symptoms and do not realize that their vision has declined. By the time the loss is noticed, it may be irreversible. Phospholine Iodide helps by reducing fluid pressure in the eye.

Phospholine Iodide is also used to treat secondary glaucoma (such as glaucoma following surgery to remove cataracts); subacute or chronic angle-closure glaucoma after iridectomy (surgical removal of a portion of the iris); or when someone cannot have surgery or refuses it. This drug is also prescribed for children with accommodative esotropia (cross-eye).

What is the most important information I should know about Phospholine Iodide?
Avoid exposure to certain pesticides or insecticides such as Sevin and Trolene. They can boost the side effects of Phospholine Iodide. If you work with these chemicals, wear a mask over your nose and mouth, wash and change your clothing frequently, and wash your hands often.

Contact your doctor immediately if you notice any decrease in vision or an increase in floaters in your visual field. Rarely, Phospholine Iodide may cause retinal detachment. Retinal detachment can lead to blind spots, floaters in your visual field, and even blindness. Your doctor will want to check your retina before you use this medicine to determine if you have an increased risk or a prior history of retinal detachment.

Stop taking the drug and notify your doctor immediately if you experience any of the following: breathing difficulties, diarrhea, inability to hold urine, muscle weakness, profuse sweating, or salivation. If you will be using Phospholine Iodide for a long time, your doctor should schedule regular examinations to make sure that Phospholine Iodide is not causing unwanted effects.

Phospholine Iodide Eye Drops is for use in the eye only. Do not get Phospholine Iodide Eye Drops in your nose or mouth.

Use caution when driving, operating machinery, or performing other hazardous activities. Phospholine Iodide may cause your vision to decrease at night. If you experience decreased vision, avoid these activities.

If you wear contact lenses, remove them before applying Phospholine Iodide ophthalmic. Ask your doctor if contact lenses can be reinserted after application of the medication. Do not use other eye medications during treatment with Phospholine Iodide, except under the direction of your doctor.

Phospholine Iodide eye drops may be stored in room temperature for up to four weeks.

See "How do I take this medication?" for proper procedures on how to prepare and apply Phospholine Iodide.

Who should not take Phospholine Iodide?

You should not use Phospholine Iodide if you have an inflammation in the eye.

Most people with angle-closure glaucoma (a condition in which there is a sudden increase in pressure of fluid in the eye) should not use Phospholine Iodide due to the possibility of increasing angle block. This condition is also known as narrow-angle glaucoma.

If you have ever had an allergic reaction to or are sensitive to Phospholine Iodide or any of its ingredients, you should not use Phospholine Iodide.

What should I tell my doctor before I take the first dose of Phospholine Iodide?

Tell your doctor about all prescription, over-the-counter, and herbal medication you are taking before beginning treatment with Phospholine Iodide. Also, talk to your doctor about your complete medical history, especially if you have had heart failure; high or low blood pressure; a heart attack; asthma; certain nerve problems; a stomach ulcer or stomach spasms; epilepsy; hyperthyroidism (an overactive thyroid); blockage of the urinary tract or difficulty urinating; or Parkinson's disease.

What is the usual dosage?

The information below is based on the dosage guidelines your doctor uses. Depending on your condition and medical history, your doctor may prescribe a different regimen. Do not change the dosage or stop taking your medication without your doctor's approval.

Glaucoma
Adults: A dose of 0.03 percent should be used 2 times a day, in the morning and at bedtime. Your doctor may increase the dose if necessary. Your doctor may have you take 1 dose a day or 1 dose every other day.

Accommodative Esotropia

Children: Place 1 drop of 0.125 percent solution in both eyes at bedtime for 2 or 3 weeks to diagnose the condition.

Your doctor may then change the schedule to 0.125 percent every other day or reduce the dose to 0.06 percent every day.

The maximum dose usually recommended is 0.125 percent solution once daily.

If the eye drops are slowly withdrawn after a year or two of treatment, and the eye problem returns, your doctor may want you to consider surgery.

How should I take Phospholine Iodide?

Use Phospholine Iodide ophthalmic eye drops exactly as directed by your doctor.

To prepare eyedrops: 1. Use aseptic technique (techniques which decrease the risk of contaminating the drug or the container which holds the drug); 2. Tear off the aluminum seals, remove and discard rubber plugs from both drug and diluent containers. (A diluent is an ingredient found in medicinal preparation that is used for the dissolution of a drug.); 3. Pour diluent into drug container; 4. Remove dropper assembly from its sterile wrapping. Holding dropper assembly by the screw cap and, **without compressing the rubber bulb,** insert into drug container and screw down tightly; 5. Shake for several seconds to ensure mixing; 6. Do not cover nor obliterate instructions to patient regarding storage of eyedrops.

To apply the eye drops: Tilt your head back slightly and pull down on the lower eyelid. Position the dropper above your eye. Look up and away from the dropper. Squeeze out a drop and close your eye. Apply gentle pressure to the inside corner of your eye (near the nose) for about 1 minute to prevent the liquid from draining down the tear duct. If you are using more than 1 drop in the same eye, repeat the process with about 5 minutes between drops. Repeat the process in your other eye if needed.

Wipe off any excess Phospholine Iodide around your eye with a tissue.

Wash off any Phospholine Iodide that may get onto your hands.

Do not touch the dropper to any surface, including the eyes or hands. The dropper is sterile. If it becomes contaminated, it could cause an infection in your eye.

What should I avoid while taking Phospholine Iodide?

Use caution when driving, operating machinery, or performing other hazardous activities. Phospholine Iodide may cause your vision to decrease at night. If you experience decreased vision, avoid these activities.

Do not touch the dropper to any surface, including the eyes or hands. The dropper is sterile. If it becomes contaminated, it could cause an infection in your eye.

If you wear contact lenses, remove them before applying Phospholine Iodide ophthalmic. Ask your doctor if contact lenses can be reinserted after application of the medication. Do not use other eye medications during treatment with Phospholine Iodide, except under the direction of your doctor.

Phospholine Iodide Eye Drops is for use in the eye only. Do not get Phospholine Iodide Eye Drops in your nose or mouth.

What are possible food and drug interactions associated with Phospholine Iodide?

If Phospholine Iodide is taken with certain other drugs, the effects of either could be increased, decreased, or altered. It is especially important to check with your doctor before combining Phospholine Iodide with other cholinesterase inhibitors such as edrophonium and pyridostigmine.

What are the possible side effects of Phospholine Iodide?

Side effects cannot be anticipated. If any develop or change in intensity, tell your doctor as soon as possible. Only your doctor can determine if it is safe for you to continue taking this drug.

Side effects may include: ache above the eyes, blurred vision, headache, twitching of eyelid, burning, clouded eye lens, cyst formation, decreased pupil size, decreased visual sharpness, excess tears, eye pain, heart irregularities, increased eye pressure, inflamed iris, lid muscle twitching, nearsightedness, red eyes, stinging

Can I receive Phospholine Iodide if I am pregnant or breastfeeding?

The effects of Phospholine Iodide during pregnancy are unknown. Tell your doctor immediately if you are pregnant or plan to become pregnant.

Phospholine Iodide should not be used by women who are breastfeeding.

What should I do if I miss a dose of Phospholine Iodide?

Apply the missed dose as soon as you remember. However, if it is almost time for the next regularly scheduled dose, skip the missed dose and apply the next dose as directed. Do not use a double dose of this medication.

How should I store Phospholine Iodide?

Store in the refrigerator. Do not freeze. Phospholine Iodide Eye Drops may be stored at room temperature for up to 4 weeks. Do not store in the bathroom.

PILOCARPINE HYDROCHLORIDE

What is Pilocarpine hydrochloride?

Pilocarpine causes constriction of the pupils (miosis) and reduces pressure within the eye. It is used to treat increased pressure due to open-angle glaucoma and to lower eye pressure before surgery for acute angle-closure glaucoma. It can be used alone or in combination with other medications.

What is the most important information I should know about Pilocarpine hydrochloride?

There is no cure for glaucoma. Pilocarpine and similar drugs can keep ocular pressure under control, but only as long as you take them. Be sure to take the medication regularly.

Who should not take Pilocarpine hydrochloride?

Pilocarpine should not be used if you are sensitive to or have ever had an allergic reaction to any of the components of this solution. Your doctor will not prescribe it for you if you have an eye condition in which your pupils should not be constricted.

What should I tell my doctor before I take the first dose of Pilocarpine hydrochloride?

Tell your doctor about all prescription, over-the-counter, and herbal medications you are taking before beginning treatment with pilocarpine. Also talk to your doctor about your complete medical history, especially if you have ever had asthma, intestinal disease, ulcers, high blood pressure, heart disease, an overactive thyroid gland, seizures, Parkinson's disease, or an obstruction in the urinary tract.

What is the usual dosage?

The information below is based on the dosage guidelines your doctor uses. Depending on your condition and medical history, your doctor may prescribe a different regimen. Do not change the dosage or stop taking your medication without your doctor's approval.

Adults: The usual starting dose is 1 or 2 drops up to 6 times a day, depending on the severity of the glaucoma and your response. During a severe attack, your doctor will tell you to put drops into the unaffected eye as well.

How should I take Pilocarpine hydrochloride?

Follow these steps to administer pilocarpine:

1. Wash your hands thoroughly.
2. Gently pull your lower eyelid down to form a pocket next to your eye.
3. Brace the eyedrop bottle on the bridge of your nose or your forehead.

4. Tilt your head back and squeeze the medication into your eye.
5. Close your eyes gently. Keep them closed for 1 to 2 minutes.
6. Do not rinse the dropper.
7. Wait for 5 to 10 minutes before using a second eye medication.

To avoid contaminating the dropper and solution, do not touch the eyelids or surrounding areas with the tip of the dropper. Do not use if the solution is discolored.

What should I avoid while taking Pilocarpine hydrochloride?
Pilocarpine may make it difficult for you to see in the dark. Be careful driving at night, or doing any hazardous activity in dim light.

What are possible food and drug interactions associated with Pilocarpine hydrochloride?
If pilocarpine is taken with certain other drugs, the effects of either could be increased, decreased, or altered. Always check with your doctor before combining pilocarpine with other medications.

What are the possible side effects of Pilocarpine hydrochloride?
Side effects cannot be anticipated. If any develop or change in intensity, inform your doctor as soon as possible. Only your doctor can determine if it is safe for you to continue using pilocarpine.

Side effects may include: cloudy vision, detached retina, headache over your eye, nearsightedness, reduced vision in poor light, spasms of the eyelids, tearing eyes

Can I receive Pilocarpine hydrochloride if I am pregnant or breastfeeding?
The effects of pilocarpine during pregnancy have not been adequately studied. If you are pregnant or plan to become pregnant, inform your doctor immediately. Pilocarpine may appear in breast milk and could affect a nursing infant. If this medication is essential to your health, your doctor may advise you to stop breastfeeding until your treatment with pilocarpine is finished.

What should I do if I miss a dose of Pilocarpine hydrochloride?
Apply it as soon as you remember. If it is almost time for your next dose, skip the one you missed and go back to your regular schedule. Do not take 2 doses at once.

How should I store Pilocarpine hydrochloride?
Store at room temperature.

Pimecrolimus *See Elidel, page 474.*

PINDOLOL

What is Pindolol?

Pindolol, a type of medication known as a beta-blocker, is used in the treatment of high blood pressure. It is effective alone or combined with other high blood pressure medications, particularly with a thiazide-type diuretic. Beta-blockers decrease the force and rate of heart contractions.

What is the most important information I should know about Pindolol?

Pindolol is only part of a complete program of treatment for hypertension that may also include diet, exercise, and weight control. Follow your diet, medication, and exercise routines very closely if you are being treated for hypertension. To be sure this medication is helping your condition; your blood pressure will need to be tested on a regular basis. It is important that you not miss any scheduled visits to your doctor.

You must take pindolol regularly for it to be effective. Since blood pressure declines gradually, it may be several weeks before you get the full benefit of pindolol; you may initially feel tired. You must continue taking pindolol even if you are feeling well. Pindolol does not cure high blood pressure; it merely keeps it under control. Pindolol should not be stopped suddenly. It can cause increased chest pain and heart attack. Dosage should be gradually reduced.

If you need to have any type of surgery, you may need to temporarily stop using pindolol. Be sure the surgeon knows ahead of time that you are using pindolol.

Do not drive, operate machinery, or do anything else that could be dangerous until you know how you react to pindolol; it may cause dizziness or lightheadedness.

Pindolol may cause dizziness, lightheadedness, or fainting. Alcohol, other medications, hot weather, exercise, and fever can increase these effects. To prevent them, sit up or stand slowly, especially in the morning. Also, sit or lie down at the first sign of dizziness, lightheadedness, or weakness.

Pindolol may mask signs of low blood sugar such as a rapid heartbeat. Other symptoms, such as sweating, may still occur. Pindolol may affect blood sugar levels. Your doctor may need to change the dose of diabetes medicine you take. Check blood glucose levels regularly.

Who should not take Pindolol?

If you have bronchial asthma; severe congestive heart failure; inadequate blood supply to the circulatory system (cardiogenic shock); heart block (a heart irregularity); or a severely slow heartbeat, you should not take pindolol. You should also not take pindolol if you are allergic to it or any ingredient in the medication.

What should I tell my doctor before I take the first dose of Pindolol?

Tell your doctor about all prescription, over-the-counter, and herbal medication you are taking before beginning treatment with pindolol. Also, talk to your doctor about your complete medical history, especially if you have: a heart problem such as heart block; a thyroid disorder; asthma; bronchitis, emphysema, or other lung or breathing diseases; emphysema; depression; diabetes; liver or kidney disease; low blood pressure; myasthenia gravis; pheochromocytoma ; problems with circulation such as Raynaud's syndrome; sick sinus syndrome; slow heart rate or congestive heart failure.

What is the usual dosage?

The information below is based on the dosage guidelines your doctor uses. Depending on your condition and medical history, your doctor may prescribe a different regimen. Do not change the dosage or stop taking your medication without your doctor's approval.

Adults: Your doctor will determine the dosage according to your specific needs.

The usual starting dose is 5 milligrams (mg), taken 2 times per day, alone or with other high blood pressure medication. Your blood pressure should be lower in 1 to 2 weeks. If blood pressure is not reduced sufficiently within 3 to 4 weeks, your doctor may increase your total daily dosage by 10 mg at a time, at 3 to 4 week intervals, up to a maximum of 60 mg a day.

The safety and effectiveness of pindolol have not been established in children.

How should I take Pindolol?

Pindolol can be taken with or without food.

Take pindolol exactly as prescribed, even if your symptoms have disappeared. Take pindolol at the same time every day. Try not to miss any doses. If you do not take pindolol regularly, your condition may worsen.

What should I avoid while taking Pindolol?

Pindolol can cause side effects that may impair your thinking or reactions. Be careful if you drive or do anything that requires you to be awake and alert. Avoid drinking alcohol, which could increase drowsiness and dizziness while you are taking pindolol. Avoid standing or sitting up too quickly, especially when you first start taking pindolol.

Do not suddenly stop taking pindolol. Do not stop taking the drug after you feel better.

What are possible food and drug interactions associated with Pindolol?

If pindolol is taken with certain other drugs, the effects of either could be increased, decreased, or altered. It is especially important to check with your doctor before combining pindolol with the following: airway-opening drugs such as albuterol; blood pressure drugs such as reserpine; beta-receptor agonists such as dobutamine, dopamine, or norepinephrine; cimetidine; clonidine; digoxin ; epinephrine ; insulin or oral antidiabetic agents such as glyburide; nonsteroidal anti-inflammatory drugs such as ibuprofen; ritodrine; theophylline; epinephrine; indomethacin; caclium channel blockers such as nifedipine and verapamil; thioames such as tapazole; thioridazine; and verapamil.

What are the possible side effects of Pindolol?

Side effects cannot be anticipated. If any develop or change in intensity, tell your doctor as soon as possible. Only your doctor can determine if it is safe for you to continue taking this drug.

Side effects may include: abdominal discomfort, chest pain, difficult or labored breathing, dizziness, fatigue, joint pain, muscle pain or cramps, nausea, nervousness, strange dreams, swelling due to fluid retention, tingling or pins and needles, trouble sleeping, weakness

Can I receive Pindolol if I am pregnant or breastfeeding?

The effects of pindolol during pregnancy are unknown. Tell your doctor immediately if you are pregnant or plan to become pregnant. Pindolol appears in breast milk and could affect a nursing infant. If pindolol is essential to your health, your doctor may advise you to discontinue breast-feeding until your treatment with pindolol is finished.

What should I do if I miss a dose of Pindolol?

Take the missed dose as soon as you remember. If your next dose is less than 4 hours away, skip the missed dose and take pindolol at the next regularly scheduled time. Do not take extra medicine to make up for a missed dose.

How should I store Pindolol?

Store at room temperature away from heat, moisture, and light. Do not store in the bathroom.

Pioglitazone hydrochloride See ACTOS, page 32.

Pioglitazone hydrochloride and glimepiride See Duetact, page 448.

Pioglitazone hydrochloride and metformin hydrochloride See ACTOplus met, page 29.

Piroxicam *See Feldene, page 541.*

PLAN B
Generic name: Levonorgestrel

What is Plan B?
Plan B is an emergency contraception. Emergency contraception is a backup method of preventing pregnancy and is not for routine use. Drugs used for emergency contraception are called postcoital pills, or morning after pills. Plan B can reduce your chance of pregnancy after unprotected sex (if your regular birth control method fails or if you have had sex without birth control). For example, if you were using a condom and it broke, or if you forgot to take 2 or more of your birth control pills in a month, or if you did not use any birth control method, Plan B may work for you.

This drug works mainly by preventing ovulation (egg release). It may also prevent fertilization of a released egg (joining of sperm and egg) or attachment of a fertilized egg to the uterus (implantation).

What is the most important information I should know about Plan B?
Plan B is used as an emergency contraceptive. The first tablet should be taken as soon as possible following unprotected intercourse. The first dose must be taken within 72 hours of intercourse; the second tablet must be taken 12 hours later. (For women age 17 and younger, Plan B is a prescription only medication.)

Plan B does not protect against the AIDS virus (HIV) or other sexually transmitted diseases (STDs). Plan B should not be used as a regular birth control method. It does not work as well as most other forms of birth control when they are used consistently and correctly. Plan B is not effective in terminating an existing pregnancy. Plan B is a backup or emergency method of contraception.

Do not drive or perform other possibly unsafe tasks until you know how you react to Plan B; this medication may cause dizziness. This effect may be worse if you take Plan B with alcohol or certain medicines.

Plan B may affect your blood sugar. Check blood sugar levels closely. Ask your doctor before you change the dose of your diabetes medicine.

Who should not take Plan B?
Do not take Plan B if you are already pregnant (because it will not work), or you are allergic to levonorgestrel or any of its ingredients.

What should I tell my doctor before I take the first dose of Plan B?
Tell your doctor about all prescription, over-the-counter, and herbal medication you are taking before taking Plan B. Also, talk to your doctor about

your medical history especially if you have diabetes, a history of ectopic pregnancy (when the fertilized egg implants anywhere other than the uterine wall) or you are premenstrual.

What is the usual dosage?
The information below is based on the dosage guidelines your doctor uses. Depending on your condition and medical history, your doctor may prescribe a different regimen. Do not change the dosage or stop taking your medication without your doctor's approval.

Adults: The usual dosage of Plan B (for women 18 years and older) is to take the first tablet as soon as possible but not later than 72 hours (3 days) after unprotected sex, then take the second tablet 12 hours after you take the first tablet. If you vomit within 1 hour of taking either dose of medication, call your doctor to discuss whether to repeat the dose. A prescription is necessary only for patients 17 years and younger (see your doctor for more information).

How should I take Plan B?
Take Plan B as soon as possible after suspected birth control failure or after you have unprotected sexual intercourse. The first dose must be taken within 72 hours. Take the second tablet 12 hours after the first tablet. However, your doctor may instruct you to take Plan B in a different way. Follow the directions provided by your doctor.

Plan B can be used any time during the menstrual cycle.

If vomiting occurs within 1 hour after taking either tablet of Plan B, talk with your health care provider to discuss whether to repeat that dose.

What should I avoid while taking Plan B?
Try to avoid vomiting within 1 hour of taking Plan B. If you happen to vomit within 1 hour of taking either dose, call your doctor to discuss if you should repeat the dosage.

Do not drive or perform other possibly unsafe tasks until you know how you react to Plan B; this medication may cause dizziness. This effect may be worse if you take it with alcohol or certain medicines.

What are possible food and drug interactions associated with Plan B?
If Plan B is taken with certain other drugs, the effects of either could be increased, decreased, or altered. It is especially important to check with your doctor before combining Plan B with the following: anticoagulants such as warfarin; antifungals such as ketoconazole; barbiturates such as Phenobarbital; beta-adrenergic blockers such as metoprolol; carbamazepine; corticosteroids such as prednisone; felbamate; HIV protease inhibitors such as indinavir; hydantoins such as Phenytoin; Lamotrigine; modafinil; nevirapine; penicillins such as amoxicillin; Rifampin; selegi-

line; St. John's wort; tetracyclines such as doxycycline; theophylline; and topiramate.

What are the possible side effects of Plan B?

Side effects cannot be anticipated. If any develop or change in intensity, tell your doctor as soon as possible. Only your doctor can determine if it is safe for you to continue taking this drug.

Side effects may include: breast pain or tenderness, diarrhea, dizziness, headache, menstrual changes, nausea, stomach pain, tiredness, vomiting, lower stomach pain, spotting during your usual menstrual cycle

Can I receive Plan B if I am pregnant or breastfeeding?

Plan B does not end existing pregnancies. Do not use Plan B if you are pregnant. Plan B is found in breast milk; contact your doctor if you are breastfeeding and have currently taken Plan B.

What should I do if I miss a dose of Plan B?

If you miss a dose of Plan B, contact your doctor immediately to find out the best way to prevent pregnancy.

How should I store Plan B?

Store at room temperature away from heat, moisture, and light. Do not store in the bathroom.

PLAQUENIL

Generic name: Hydroxychloroquine sulfate

What is Plaquenil?

Plaquenil is prescribed for the prevention and treatment of certain forms of malaria.

Plaquenil is also used to treat the symptoms of rheumatoid arthritis such as swelling, inflammation, stiffness, and joint pain. It is also prescribed for lupus erythematosus, a chronic inflammation of the connective tissue.

What is the most important information I should know about Plaquenil?

Disorders of the retina causing impairment or loss of vision may be related to the length of time and the dose of Plaquenil given for lupus and rheumatoid arthritis. Problems have occurred several months to several years after beginning daily therapy. When you are on prolonged therapy, your doctor will perform eye examinations at the beginning of treatment and every 3 months after that. If you have any problem with your vision or your eyes, notify your doctor immediately.

All people on long-term therapy with Plaquenil should have a physical examination periodically, including testing of knee and ankle reflexes to detect any evidence of muscular weakness. Your doctor will also conduct periodic blood cell counts if you are on prolonged therapy with Plaquenil.

Children are especially sensitive to Plaquenil. Relatively small doses of Plaquenil have caused fatalities. Keep Plaquenil in a child-proof container and out of the reach of children.

Do not drive or perform other possibly unsafe tasks until you know how you react to Plaquenil; this medication may cause dizziness or blurred vision. These effects may be worse if you take it with alcohol or certain medicines.

If your symptoms do not improve after several months or if they become worse, check with your doctor.

Plaquenil may cause you to become sunburned more easily. Avoid the sun, sunlamps, or tanning booths until you know how you react to Plaquenil. Use a sunscreen or wear protective clothing if you must be outside for more than a short time.

Contact your healthcare provider if you notice any muscle weakness or problems with vision or hearing. Your knee and ankle reflexes will be tested periodically.

Who should not take Plaquenil?

If you are sensitive to or have ever had an allergic reaction to Plaquenil or similar drugs, such as chloroquine, you should not take Plaquenil. Make sure your doctor is aware of any drug reactions you have experienced.

Plaquenil should not be prescribed if you have suffered partial or complete loss of vision in small areas while taking Plaquenil or similar drugs. Notify your doctor of any past or present visual changes you have experienced.

This drug should not be used for long-term therapy in children.

What should I tell my doctor before I take the first dose of Plaquenil?

Tell your doctor about all prescription, over-the-counter, and herbal medication you are taking before beginning treatment with Plaquenil. Also, talk to your doctor about your complete medical history, especially the following: alcohol abuse, central nervous system disease, digestive system disease, elevated blood acid levels, eye damage or visual changes due to hydroxychloroquine or chloroquine, glucose-6-phosphate dehydrogenase deficiency, kidney problems, liver disease, psoriasis (a recurrent skin disorder characterized by patches of red, dry, scaly skin), or porphyria (an inherited metabolic disorder affecting the liver or bone marrow).

What is the usual dosage?

The information below is based on the dosage guidelines your doctor uses. Depending on your condition and medical history, your doctor

may prescribe a different regimen. Do not change the dosage or stop taking your medication without your doctor's approval.

Adults: One tablet of hydroxychloroquine sulfate, 200 mg, is equivalent to 155 mg base.

Children: One tablet of hydroxychloroquine sulfate, 200 mg, is equivalent to 155 mg base.

Acute Attack of Malaria
Adults: The usual starting dose is 800 milligrams (mg), to be followed by 400 mg in 6 to 8 hours and 400 mg on each of 2 consecutive days.
   Alternatively, your doctor may prescribe a single dose of 800 mg.

Children 10 years and older: A total dose representing 25mg of base per kg of body weight is administered as follows:
   First dose: 10 mg base per kg (but not exceeding a single dose of 620 mg base).
   Second dose: 5 mg base per kg (but not exceeding a single dose of 310 mg base) 6 hours after first dose.
   Third dose: 5 mg base per kg 18 hours after second dose.
   Fourth dose: 5 mg base per kg 24 hours after third dose.

Lupus Erythematosus
Adults: The usual starting dose for adults is 400 mg once or twice daily. You will continue to take this dose for several weeks or months, depending on your response. For longer-term maintenance therapy, your doctor may reduce the dose to 200 to 400 mg per day.

Restraint or Prevention of Malaria
Adults: The usual dose is 400 mg taken once every 7 days on exactly the same day of each week. If circumstances permit, preventive therapy should begin 2 weeks prior to exposure. If this is not possible, your doctor will have you take a starting dose of 800 mg, which may be divided into 2 doses taken 6 hours apart. You should continue this suppressive therapy for 8 weeks after leaving the area where malaria occurs.

Rheumatoid Arthritis
Adults: The usual starting dose for adults is 400 to 600 mg a day taken with a meal or a glass of milk. If your condition improves, usually within 4 to 12 weeks, your doctor will reduce the dose to a maintenance level of 200 to 400 milligrams daily.
   Should a relapse occur after medication is withdrawn, therapy must be resumed or continued on an intermittent schedule if there is no other reason why Plaquenil cannot be used in this particular patient.

Suppression of Malaria
Children 10 years and older: The weekly suppressive dosage is 5mg, calculated as base, per kg of body weight, but should not exceed the adult dose regardless of weight. Suppressive therapy should begin 2

weeks prior to supposed exposure. If suppressive therapy does not begin 2 weeks prior to exposure, 10mg base per kg should be taken in two divided doses 6 hours apart. Suppressive therapy should be continued for 8 weeks after leaving the area where malaria is present.

This drug has not been proved safe for treatment of juvenile arthritis.

How should I take Plaquenil?

Take Plaquenil exactly as prescribed for the full course of therapy.

If you have been prescribed Plaquenil for rheumatoid arthritis, it will take several weeks (4 to 12 weeks) for beneficial effects to appear. Take each dose with a meal or a glass of milk.

Take Plaquenil by mouth with food or a glass (8oz. or 240ml) of milk. If possible, preventative measure for malaria should begin 2 weeks prior to exposure and be continued for 8 weeks following your departure from the infected area.

What should I avoid while taking Plaquenil?

Use caution when driving or performing other hazardous activities until you know how this medication affects you. Plaquenil may cause visual disturbances such as blurred vision, misty vision, and difficulty focusing. Report any vision or hearing changes to your doctor.

Avoid the sun, sunlamps, or tanning booths until you know how you react to Plaquenil. Plaquenil may cause you to become sunburned more easily. Use a sunscreen or wear protective clothing if you must be outside for more than a short time.

What are possible food and drug interactions associated with Plaquenil?

If Plaquenil is taken with certain other drugs, the effects of either could be increased, decreased, or altered. It is especially important to check with your doctor before combining Plaquenil with the following: any medication that may cause liver damage, aurothioglucose, cimetidine, and digoxin.

What are the possible side effects of Plaquenil?

Side effects cannot be anticipated. If any develop or change in intensity, tell your doctor as soon as possible. Only your doctor can determine if it is safe for you to continue taking this drug.

Side effects of treatment for an acute malarial attack may include: abdominal cramps, diarrhea, dizziness, heart problems, lack or loss of appetite, mild headache, nausea, vomiting

Side effects of treatment for lupus erythematosus and rheumatoid arthritis may include: abdominal cramps, abnormal eye pigmentation, acne, anemia, bleaching of hair, blind spots, blisters in mouth and eyes, blood disorders, blurred vision, convulsions, decreased vision, diarrhea, difficulty focusing the eyes, diminished reflexes, dizziness, emotional changes, excessive coloring of the skin, eye muscle paralysis, vision problems, headache, hearing loss, heart problems, hives, involuntary eyeball movement, irritability, itching, light flashes and streaks, light intolerance, liver problems or failure, loss of hair, loss or lack of appetite, muscle paralysis, muscle weakness and wasting, nausea, nervousness, nightmares, psoriasis (dry, scaly, red skin patches), reading difficulties, ringing in the ears, skin eruptions, skin inflammation and scaling, skin rash, vertigo, vomiting, extreme fatigue, weight loss

Can I receive Plaquenil if I am pregnant or breastfeeding?

Use of Plaquenil during pregnancy should be avoided except in the suppression or treatment of malaria when, in the judgment of your doctor, the benefit outweighs the possible risks. This drug may appear in breast milk and could affect a nursing infant. If Plaquenil is essential to your health, your doctor may advise you to discontinue breastfeeding until your treatment is finished.

What should I do if I miss a dose of Plaquenil?

Take the missed dose as soon as you remember. However, if it is almost time for your next dose, skip the missed dose and only take your next regularly scheduled dose. Do not take a double dose of this medication.

How should I store Plaquenil?

Store at room temperature in a tightly closed container, away from heat, moisture, and light. Do not store in the bathroom.

PLAVIX

Generic name: Clopidogrel bisulfate

What is Plavix?

Plavix is used to treat people who have recently had a heart attack, stroke, or arterial disease; this drug will reduce the probability of experiencing these events again.

Plavix is also used to treat Acute Coronary syndrome; it will reduce the probability of experiencing a heart attack, or stoke.

What is the most important information I should know about Plavix?

Thrombotic thrombocytopenic purpura (TTP) has been reported in people being treated with Plavix. TTP is a very serious condition in which red blood cells burst and platelets form blood clots, potentially blocking blood supply to organs. TTP feels like the flu, with symptoms such as fever, tiredness, and aching joints.

Who should not take Plavix?

Do not take Plavix if you are allergic to any of its ingredients.

Plavix should not be used in patients with active bleeding such as stomach ulcer or brain hemorrhage.

What should I tell my doctor before I take the first dose of Plavix?

Tell your doctor about all prescription, over-the-counter, and herbal medications you are taking before beginning treatment with Plavix. Also, talk to your doctor about your complete medical history, especially if you have a stomach ulcer or any other type of internal bleeding, or if you have liver or kidney problems. If you are going to have surgery, it is recommended that treatment with Plavix is stopped 5 days before the surgery.

What is the usual dosage?

The information below is based on the dosage guidelines your doctor uses. Depending on your condition and medical history, your doctor may prescribe a different regimen. Do not change the dosage or stop taking your medication without your doctor's approval.

Recent MI, Recent Stroke, or Established Peripheral Arterial Disease
Adults: The recommended daily dose of Plavix is 75 milligrams (mg) once daily.

Acute Coronary Syndrome
Adults: The recommended daily dose of Plavix is a single 300 mg loading dose and then continued at 75 mg once daily. Aspirin (75 mg-325 mg once daily) should be started and continued in combination with Plavix.

How should I take Plavix?

Plavix can be taken with or without food. There are no dosage adjustments for the elderly with liver problems.

What should I avoid while taking Plavix?

You should avoid aspirin or aspirin-containing products during drug therapy unless approved by your healthcare professional.

What are possible food and drug interactions associated with Plavix?

If Plavix is taken with certain other drugs, the effects of either could be increased, decreased, or altered. It is especially important to check with your doctor before combining Plavix with nonsteroidal anti-inflammatory drugs (NSAIDs) or warfarin. Plavix may interfere with the metabolism of phenytoin, tamoxifen, tolbutamide, warfarin, torsemide, and fluvastatin.

What are the possible side effects of Plavix?

Side effects cannot be anticipated. If any develop or change in intensity, tell your doctor as soon as possible. Only your doctor can determine if it is safe for you to continue taking this drug.

Side effects may include: bruising easily, chest pain, increased blood pressure, coughing, depression, diarrhea, dizziness, flu-like symptoms, headache, itching, pain, joint pain/back pain, nasal infection, nausea, rash, sleepiness/tiredness, stomach pain

Can I receive Plavix if I am pregnant or breastfeeding?

Talk to your doctor if you are pregnant, planning to become pregnant, or are nursing, before taking Plavix, as you should only take this drug if it is necessary. Plavix may pass into your breast milk.

What should I do if I miss a dose of Plavix?

If you miss a dose of Plavix, take it as soon as you remember. If it is almost time for your next dose, skip the dose you missed and take your next regular dose. Do not double your next dose.

How should I store Plavix?

Store at room temperature.

PLENDIL

Generic name: Felodipine

What is Plendil?

Plendil is in a class of drugs called calcium channel blockers. Plendil relaxes (widens) your blood vessels (veins and arteries), which makes it easier for the heart to pump and reduces its workload.

Plendil is used to treat high blood pressure. It is effective alone or in combination with other high blood pressure medications.

What is the most important information I should know about Plendil?

If you have high blood pressure, you must take Plendil regularly for it to be effective. Since blood pressure declines gradually, it may be several weeks before you get the full benefit of Plendil; you must continue taking it even if you are feeling well. Plendil does not cure high blood pressure; it merely keeps it under control.

Plendil can cause your blood pressure to become too low. If you feel light-headed or faint, or if you feel your heart racing or you experience chest pain, contact your doctor immediately.

Your legs and feet may swell when you start taking Plendil, usually within the first 2 to 3 weeks of treatment. Your gums may become swollen and sore while you are taking Plendil. Good dental hygiene will help control this problem.

Who should not take Plendil?
If you are sensitive to or have ever had an allergic reaction to Plendil or other calcium channel blockers, such as verapamil and nifedipine, you should not take Plendil. Make sure your doctor is aware of any drug reactions you have experienced.

What should I tell my doctor before I take the first dose of Plendil?
Tell your doctor about all prescription, over-the-counter, and herbal medication you are taking before beginning treatment with Plendil. Also, talk to your doctor about your complete medical history, especially if you are pregnant, plan to become pregnant, or are breastfeeding, have liver disease, or another disease of the heart or blood vessels such as sick sinus syndrome, aortic stenosis (a condition in which the aortic valve has become narrowed or constricted and does not open normally), heart failure, low blood pressure, or coronary artery disease.

What is the usual dosage?
The information below is based on the dosage guidelines your doctor uses. Depending on your condition and medical history, your doctor may prescribe a different regimen. Do not change the dosage or stop taking your medication without your doctor's approval.

Adults: Your doctor will adjust the dosage according to your response to the drug. The usual starting dose is 5 milligrams (mg) taken once a day; but your doctor may adjust the dose at intervals of not less than 2 weeks.

The usual dosage range is 2.5 to 10 mg taken once daily.

Children 10 years and older: The safety and effectiveness of Plendil in children have not been established.

Adults over 65 years: The recommended dose is 2.5mg once a day.

People with liver problems usually require lower doses of Plendil and are carefully monitored while the dose is adjusted.

How should I take Plendil?
Plendil can be taken with a light meal which is low in fat and carbohydrates or without food. The tablets should be swallowed whole, not crushed or chewed.

Try not to miss any doses. If Plendil is not taken regularly, your blood pressure may increase.

What should I avoid while taking Plendil?

Grapefruit and grapefruit juice increases the amount of Plendil in your body. The interaction could lead to potentially dangerous effects and should be avoided.

What are possible food and drug interactions associated with Plendil?

If Plendil is taken with certain other drugs, the effects of either could be increased, decreased, or altered. It is especially important to check with your doctor before combining Plendil with the following: anticonvulsants such as phenytoin, carbamazepine, or phenobarbital; beta-blocking blood pressure medicines such as metoprolol, propranolol, and atenolol; cimetidine; epilepsy medications such as carbamazepine and phenytoin; erythromycin; grapefruit and grapefruit juice; itraconazole; ketoconazole; tacrolimus; and theophylline.

What are the possible side effects of Plendil?

Side effects cannot be anticipated. If any develop or change in intensity, tell your doctor as soon as possible. Only your doctor can determine if it is safe for you to continue taking this drug.

Side effects may include: flushing or a feeling of warmth, headache, swelling of the legs and feet, dizziness, a racing heartbeat, unusual tiredness

Can I receive Plendil if I am pregnant or breastfeeding?

The effects of Plendil during pregnancy and breastfeeding are unknown. Tell your doctor immediately if you are pregnant, plan to become pregnant, or are breastfeeding.

What should I do if I miss a dose of Plendil?

Take the missed dose as soon as you remember if it is within 12 hours then go back to your regular schedule. However, if it is more than 12 hours when you remember, skip the missed dose and take only the next regularly scheduled dose. Do not take a double dose of this medication.

How should I store Plendil?

Store at room temperature in a dry place.

Polyethylene glycol *See MiraLax, page 834.*

PONSTEL

Generic name: Mefenamic acid

What is Ponstel?

Ponstel, a nonsteroidal anti-inflammatory drug (NSAID), works by reducing hormones that cause inflammation and pain in the body. Ponstel is used for the relief of moderate pain (when treatment will not last for more than 7 days) and for the treatment of menstrual pain, also known as dysmenorrhea.

What is the most important information I should know about Ponstel?

You should have frequent checkups with your doctor if you take Ponstel regularly. Ulcers or internal bleeding can occur without warning.

This medicine can increase your risk of life-threatening heart or circulation problems, including heart attack or stroke. Seek emergency medical help if you have symptoms of heart or circulation problems, such as chest pain, weakness, shortness of breath, slurred speech, or problems with vision or balance.

Ponstel occasionally causes liver damage. If you develop warning signs such as nausea, fatigue, yellowing of the skin and eyes, itching, flu-like symptoms, and upper abdominal pain, stop taking Ponstel and seek medical attention immediately.

Who should not take Ponstel?

Do not take Ponstel if you are sensitive to or have ever had an allergic reaction to it. You should not take it, either, if you have had asthma attacks, hay fever, or hives caused by aspirin or other nonsteroidal anti-inflammatory drugs, including ibuprofen. Make sure your doctor is aware of any drug reactions you have experienced.

Do not use this medicine just before or after having heart bypass surgery (also called coronary artery bypass graft, or CABG).

Do not take Ponstel if you have ulcerations or frequently recurring inflammation of your stomach or intestines.

Avoid Ponstel if you have serious kidney disease.

What should I tell my doctor before I take the first dose of Ponstel?

Tell your doctor about all prescription, over-the-counter, and herbal medication you are taking before beginning treatment with Ponstel. Also, talk to your doctor about your complete medical history, especially if you have a history of heart attack, stroke, blood clot, heart disease, congestive heart failure, high blood pressure, liver or kidney disease, asthma, polyps in your nose, or if you smoke. Tell your doctor if you are pregnant, plan to become pregnant or are breastfeeding.

What is the usual dosage?

The information below is based on the dosage guidelines your doctor uses. Depending on your condition and medical history, your doctor may prescribe a different regimen. Do not change the dosage or stop taking your medication without your doctor's approval.

Menstrual Pain
Adults and and adolescents 14 years and older: The usual starting dose, once symptoms appear, is 500 milligrams (mg), followed by 250 mg every 6 hours for 2 to 3 days.

Moderate Pain
Adults and adolescents 14 years and older: The usual starting dose is 500 mg, followed by 250 mg every 6 hours, if needed, for 1 week.

The safety and effectiveness of Ponstel have not been established in children and adolescents under 14 years of age.

How should I take Ponstel?

Take Ponstel exactly as prescribed by your doctor.

Take Ponstel with food if possible. If it upsets your stomach, be sure to take it with food or with a full glass of milk.

What should I avoid while taking Ponstel?

Do not use any other over-the-counter cold, allergy, or pain medication without first asking your doctor or pharmacist. Many medicines available over the counter contain medicines similar to Ponstel (such as aspirin, ibuprofen, ketoprofen, or naproxen). Do not drink alcohol while taking Ponstel. Alcohol can increase the risk of stomach bleeding.

What are possible food and drug interactions associated with Ponstel?

If Ponstel is taken with certain other drugs, the effects of either could be increased, decreased, or altered. It is especially important to check with your doctor before combining Ponstel with the following: ACE inhibitors that are used to treat high blood pressure such as captopril and enalapril; alcohol; antacids; aspirin; blood-thinning medications such as warfarin; diuretics such as furosemide and hydrochlorothiazide; fluconazole; lithium; lovastatin; methotrexate; steroids such as prednisone and hydrocortisone; and trimethoprim.

What are the possible side effects of Ponstel?

Side effects cannot be anticipated. If any develop or change in intensity, tell your doctor as soon as possible. Only your doctor can determine if it is safe for you to continue taking this drug.

Side effects may include: bloating, constipation, diarrhea, dizziness, edema (swelling of any organ), gas, headache, mild heartburn or stomach pain, nervousness, ringing in your ears, skin itching or rash, upset stomach, vomiting

Can I receive Ponstel if I am pregnant or breastfeeding?
The effects of Ponstel during pregnancy have not been adequately studied. If you are pregnant or plan to become pregnant, inform your doctor immediately. You should not use Ponstel in late pregnancy because nonsteroidal anti-inflammatory drugs affect the heart and blood vessels of the developing baby. Ponstel may appear in breast milk and could affect a nursing infant. If Ponstel is essential to your health, your doctor may advise you to discontinue breastfeeding until your treatment is finished.

What should I do if I miss a dose of Ponstel?
Take the missed dose as soon as you remember. If it is almost time for your next dose, skip the missed dose and take the medicine at your next regularly scheduled time. Do not take extra medicine to make up for a missed dose.

How should I store Ponstel?
Store at room temperature away from moisture, heat, and light.

Posaconazole *See Noxafil, page 922.*

Potassium chloride *See Micro-K, page 823.*

Pramipexole dihydrochloride *See Mirapex, page 836.*

Pramlintide acetate *See Symlin, page 1244.*

PRANDIMET
Generic name: Repaglinide and metformin hydrochloride

What is PrandiMet?
PrandiMet is used along with diet and exercise to improve blood sugar control in adults with type 2 diabetes.

What is the most important information I should know about PrandiMet?
PrandiMet can cause a rare but potentially fatal condition called a lactic acidosis (a buildup of an acid in the blood). Lactic acidosis is a medical emergency. The most common symptoms of lactic acidosis are feeling very weak or tired, muscle pain, difficulty breathing, sleepiness, and abdominal pain with nausea, vomiting or diarrhea. If lactic acidosis is suspected, discontinue PrandiMet seek medical attention immediately.

You have a higher risk of lactic acidosis if you have kidney or liver problems, congestive heart failure, drink a lot of alcohol, or are dehydrated.

Who should not take PrandiMet?

You should not take PrandiMet if you have kidney or liver problems, are taking both gemfibrozil and itraconazole, have a condition called metabolic ketoacidosis, or are allergic to PrandiMet or any of its ingredients.

Do not take PrandiMet if you have a type 1 diabetes.

What should I tell my doctor before I take the first dose of PrandiMet?

Tell your doctor about all prescription, over-the-counter, and herbal medications you are taking before beginning treatment with PrandiMet. Also, talk to your doctor about your complete medical history, especially if you have kidney, liver or heart problems, drink a lot of alcohol, or if you are pregnant, planning to become pregnant or breastfeeding.

What is the usual dosage?

The information below is based on the dosage guidelines your doctor uses. Depending on your condition and medical history, your doctor may prescribe a different regimen. Do not change the dosage or stop taking your medication without your doctor's approval.

The dosage of PrandiMet should be adjusted based on your current regimen and your response to PrandiMet.

Adults: The usual starting dose of PrandiMet is as follows:

Patients inadequately controlled with metformin alone: 1 milligram (mg) repaglinide/500 mg metformin twice a day with gradual dose increases (based on your blood sugar levels).

Patients inadequately controlled with repaglinide alone: 500 mg of the metformin component twice daily with gradual dose increases (based on your blood sugar levels).

Patients currently using repaglinide and metformin together: dose similar to the current individual doses of repaglinide and metformin (but do not exceed the current dose).

The maximum daily dose of PrandiMet is 10 mg repaglinide/2500 mg metformin. You should not take more than 4 mg repaglinide/1000 mg metformin per meal.

How should I take PrandiMet?

PrandiMet should be taken within 15 minutes prior to meals, but the timing can vary from immediately preceding the meal up to 30 minutes before. If you skip a meal, you should not take PrandiMet for that meal. PrandiMet can be taken 2 to 3 times a day.

What should I avoid while taking PrandiMet?

Avoid drinking too much alcohol while on PrandiMet, since alcohol increases the chance of getting lactic acidosis. Also avoid rapidly increasing your dose to prevent stomach upset.

What are possible food and drug interactions associated with PrandiMet?

If PrandiMet is taken with certain other drugs, the effects of either could be increased, decreased, or altered. It is especially important to check with your doctor before combining PrandiMet with the following: amiloride, digoxin, gemfibrozil, itraconazole, ketoconazole, morphine, procainamide, quinidine, quinine, rifampin, ranitidine, triamterene, trimethoprim, and vancomycin.

What are the possible side effects of PrandiMet?

Side effects cannot be anticipated. If any develop or change in intensity, tell your doctor as soon as possible. Only your doctor can determine if it is safe for you to continue taking this drug.

Side effects may include: diarrhea, nausea, vomiting, low blood sugar

Can I receive PrandiMet if I am pregnant or breastfeeding?

The effects of PrandiMet during pregnancy are unknown. Talk to your doctor before taking this drug if you are pregnant or plan to become pregnant. PrandiMet is not recommended during breastfeeding because it may cause low blood sugar level in nursing infants.

What should I do if I miss a dose of PrandiMet?

Contact your doctor if you miss a dose of Prandimet.

How should I store PrandiMet?

Store at room temperature.

PRANDIN
Generic name: Repaglinide

What is Prandin?

Prandin is used to reduce blood sugar levels in people with type 2 diabetes (also known as non-insulin dependent diabetes mellitus or NIDDM). It is prescribed when diet and exercise alone fail to correct the problem. Prandin may be prescribed alone or in combination with other diabetes medications, such as metformin.

What is the most important information I should know about Prandin?

Chronically high glucose levels have been implicated in the kidney failure, blindness, and loss of sensation that plague many people with long-standing diabetes. A low-calorie diet, weight loss, and exercise are your first line of defense against these problems. Medications such as Prandin are prescribed only as a back-up when these other measures still leave your blood sugar too high. If diet, exercise, and a combination of Prandin and metformin all fail to do the job, your doctor may have to start you on insulin.

While taking Prandin, you should check your blood sugar regularly. Your doctor will also watch it; and to measure long-term glucose control, he will probably give you a glycosylated hemoglobin (HbA1C) test as well.

Too much Prandin can cause low blood sugar (hypoglycemia), which is marked by shaking; sweating; and cold, clammy skin. If you develop these symptoms, drink some orange juice or suck on a hard candy. The problem is more likely to surface if you are elderly, debilitated, or malnourished; have liver problems; or suffer from poor adrenal or pituitary function.

Who should not take Prandin?

If you have type 1 (insulin-dependent) diabetes, you cannot use Prandin. You cannot take Prandin for diabetic ketoacidosis (a life-threatening emergency first signaled by excessive thirst, nausea, fatigue, and fruity-smelling breath). This condition must be treated with insulin.

If you find that Prandin gives you an allergic reaction, you'll be unable to continue using it.

What should I tell my doctor before I take the first dose of Prandin?

Tell your doctor about all prescription, over-the-counter, and herbal medication you are taking before beginning treatment with Prandin. Also, talk to your doctor about your complete medical history, especially if you have kidney disease, liver disease, type 1 diabetes mellitus, diabetic ketoacidosis, a serious infection, illness, injury, or if you need surgery.

What is the usual dosage?
The information below is based on the dosage guidelines your doctor uses. Depending on your condition and medical history, your doctor may prescribe a different regimen. Do not change the dosage or stop taking your medication without your doctor's approval.

Adults: There is no fixed dosage regimen for the management of type 2 diabetes with Prandin.

Take Prandin before each meal. The recommended dose ranges from 0.5 milligram (mg) to 4 mg. If you have never taken a glucose-lowering medication before, you should start with the 0.5-mg dose. If you have taken these drugs in the past, the starting dose is 1 or 2 mg. Take no more than 16 mg a day.

Combination Therapy
Adults: If Prandin is being added to metformin therapy, you should begin with a 0.5-mg dose. Dosage will then be adjusted according to your blood glucose levels.

Dose Adjustment
Adults: Your dose of Prandin will be adjusted according to your fasting blood sugar levels. If your pre-meal glucose level appears normal and you are still experiencing glucose control problems, your doctor may test your glucose level after you have eaten a meal. Your doctor will wait at least a week after each change in dose to check your response.

Switching to Prandin
Adults : When Prandin replaces another oral glucose-lowering medicine, you should start taking it the day after your final dose or the previous drug. Be alert for signs of low blood sugar; effects of the drugs may overlap.

How should I take Prandin?

Prandin should be taken shortly before each meal. You can take it 30 minutes ahead of time or wait until just before starting to eat; a 15-minute period is typical. You can take Prandin 2, 3, or 4 times a day, depending on the number of meals you have. If you skip a meal (or add an extra meal), you should skip (or add) a dose of Prandin accordingly.

What should I avoid while taking Prandin?

Follow diet, medication, and exercise routines very closely. Changing any of these routines can affect your blood sugar levels.

Avoid alcohol; it lowers blood sugar and may interfere with your diabetes treatment.

What are possible food and drug interactions associated with Prandin?

If Prandin is taken with certain other drugs, the effects of either could be increased, decreased, or altered. It is especially important to check with your doctor before combining Prandin with the following: airway-opening medications such as metaproterenol and albuterol; alcohol; aspirin; barbiturates such as the sedatives secobarbital and pentobarbital; beta-blockers such as the blood pressure medications propranolol and atenolol; blood thinners such as dicumarol and anisindione; calcium channel blockers such as the blood pressure medications diltiazem and nifedipine; carbamazepine; chloramphenicol; clarithromycin; erythromycin; estrogens; ketoconazole; glucose-lowering agents such as glipizide and glyburide;isoniazid; itraconazole; major tranquilizers such as thioridazine and trifluoperazine; mao inhibitors such as the antidepressants isocarboxazid, phenelzine, and tranylcypromine; niacin; nonsteroidal anti-inflammatory drugs such as ibuprofen and naproxen; oral contraceptives; phenytoin; probenecid; rifampin; steroids such as prednisone; sulfa drugs such as sulfamethoxazole; thyroid medications such as levothyroxine; and diuretics such as hydrochlorothiazide.

Additionally, you should not start taking Prandin if you are already taking the triglyceride-lowering medication gemfibrozil. Conversely, you should not start taking gemfibrozil if you are already using Prandin. Combining the two drugs could lead to a dangerous drop in blood sugar. However, if you're already taking both drugs, the doctor will monitor your blood sugar levels closely and adjust the dosages as needed.

What are the possible side effects of Prandin?
Side effects cannot be anticipated. If any develop or change in intensity, tell your doctor as soon as possible. Only your doctor can determine if it is safe for you to continue taking this drug.

Side effects may include: back pain, bronchitis, chest pain, constipation, diarrhea, headache, indigestion, joint pain, low blood sugar, nasal inflammation, nausea, sinus inflammation, skin tingling, upper respiratory tract infection, urinary tract infection, vomiting

Can I receive Prandin if I am pregnant or breastfeeding?
The effects of Prandin during pregnancy and breastfeeding are unknown. Tell your doctor immediately if you are pregnant, plan to become pregnant, or are breastfeeding.

Because abnormal blood sugar during pregnancy can cause fetal defects, your doctor will probably prescribe insulin injections until the baby is born.

What should I do if I miss a dose of Prandin?
Wait until your next meal, and then take your regular dose. Do not take 2 doses at once.

How should I store Prandin?
Store at room temperature in a tightly closed container, away from moisture and heat.

PRAVACHOL
Generic name: Pravastatin sodium

What is Pravachol?
Pravachol is a cholesterol-lowering drug, also known as a "statin". Your doctor may prescribe it along with a cholesterol-lowering diet if your blood cholesterol level is dangerously high and you have not been able to lower it by diet alone.

Pravastatin is used to reduce the amounts of low-density lipoprotein (LDL) "bad" cholesterol, total cholesterol, triglycerides (another type of fat), and apolipoprotein B (a protein needed to make cholesterol) in your blood. These actions are important in reducing the risk of hardening of the arteries, which can lead to heart attacks, stroke, and peripheral vascular disease.

Pravachol can also be prescribed for children 8 years of age and older when diet alone fails to lower their cholesterol levels.

What is the most important information I should know about Pravachol?

Pravachol is usually prescribed only if diet, exercise, and weight-loss fail to bring your cholesterol levels under control. It's important to remember that Pravachol is a supplement—not a substitute—for those other measures. To get the full benefit of the medication, you need to stick to the diet and exercise program prescribed by your doctor. These efforts to keep your cholesterol levels normal are important because together they may lower your risk of heart disease.

Because Pravachol may cause damage to the liver, your doctor will probably do blood tests before you start taking the drug and whenever he plans a dosage increase. The doctor should monitor you very carefully if you've had liver disease recently, if you have any symptoms of liver disease, or if you're a heavy drinker.

Since Pravachol may cause damage to muscle tissue, promptly report to your doctor any unexplained muscle pain, tenderness, or weakness, especially if you also have a fever or you just generally do not feel well.

Who should not take Pravachol?

Do not take Pravachol if you are sensitive or have ever had an allergic reaction to it. Do not take Pravachol if you have liver disease. If you are pregnant or plan to become pregnant, you should not take Pravachol, since this medication may harm an unborn baby.

What should I tell my doctor before I take the first dose of Pravachol?

Tell your doctor about all prescription, over-the-counter, and herbal medication you are taking before beginning treatment with Pravachol. Also, talk to your doctor about your complete medical history, especially if you have liver disease, kidney disease, a chronic muscular disease, a blood disorder, or if you drink alcoholic beverages. Tell your doctor if you are pregnant, plan to become pregnant or are breastfeeding.

What is the usual dosage?

The information below is based on the dosage guidelines your doctor uses. Depending on your condition and medical history, your doctor may prescribe a different regimen. Do not change the dosage or stop taking your medication without your doctor's approval.

Adults: The usual starting dose is 40 milligrams (mg) once a day. If this does not reduce LDL levels sufficiently, your doctor may increase your dose to 80 mg once daily.

Children 14 to 18 years old: The recommended starting dose is 40 mg once a day. Doses greater than 40 mg have not been studied in this age group.

For people with kidney or liver problems and those taking a medication that suppresses the immune system, the starting dose is 10 mg. People on immunosuppressive drugs generally take no more than 20 mg of Pravachol daily.

Children 8 to 13 years old: The recommended starting dose is 20 mg once a day. Doses greater than 20 mg have not been studied in this age group.

How should I take Pravachol?

For an even greater cholesterol-lowering effect, your doctor may prescribe Pravachol along with a different kind of lipid-lowering drug such as cholestyramine or colestipol. However, you must not take Pravachol at the same time of day as the other cholesterol-lowering drug. Take Pravachol at least 1 hour before or 4 hours after taking the other drug.

Pravachol should be taken once daily. You may take it anytime, with or without food.

What should I avoid while taking Pravachol?

Avoid drinking alcohol while you are taking Pravachol. Alcohol and Pravachol can both damage the liver.

What are possible food and drug interactions associated with Pravachol?

If Pravachol is taken with certain other drugs, the effects of either could be increased, decreased, or altered. It is especially important to check with your doctor before combining Pravachol with the following: Cholestyramine, Cimetidine, Colestipol, Diltiazem, Drugs that suppress the immune system, such as cyclosporine, Erythromycin, Gemfibrozil, Itraconazole, Niacin.

What are the possible side effects of Pravachol?

Side effects cannot be anticipated. If any develop or change in intensity, tell your doctor as soon as possible. Only your doctor can determine if it is safe for you to continue taking this drug.

Side effects may include: abdominal pain, chest pain, constipation, cough, diarrhea, dizziness, fatigue, gas, headache, heartburn, inflammation of nasal passages, muscle aching or weakness, nausea, rash, stomach or intestinal discomfort, urinary problems, vomiting

Can I receive Pravachol if I am pregnant or breastfeeding?

Do not take Pravachol if you are pregnant, plan to become pregnant, or if you are nursing due to the harmful effects Pravachol may have on your unborn or breastfeeding baby. You should not take Pravachol if you are of a child-bearing age unless it is highly unlikely that you will become pregnant. If you do become pregnant while taking Pravachol, inform your doctor immediately.

What should I do if I miss a dose of Pravachol?
Take the missed dose as soon as you remember. However, if it is almost time for the next dose, skip the missed dose and take only the next regularly scheduled dose. Do not take a double dose of this medication.

How should I store Pravachol?
Store at room temperature away from moisture and heat.

Pravastatin sodium *See Pravachol, page 1046.*

Prazosin hydrochloride *See Minipress, page 830.*

PRED FORTE
Generic name: Prednisolone acetate ophthalmic suspension

What is Pred Forte?
Pred Forte is in a class of drugs called corticosteroids. It inhibits processes in the body that cause inflammation. Pred Forte is used for the treatment of redness, irritation, and swelling due to inflammation of the eye.

What is the most important information I should know about Pred Forte?
Do not use Pred Forte more often or for a longer period than your doctor orders. Overuse can increase the risk of side effects and can lead to eye damage. If you use Pred Forte eyedrops for 10 days or longer, an eye doctor should check your intraocular pressure (pressure inside the eyeball) frequently. If you have glaucoma, use Pred Forte cautiously. Chronic increased intraocular pressure may cause loss of vision.

If your eye inflammation or pain lasts longer than 48 hours or becomes worse, stop using Pred Forte and call your doctor.

If your eye problems return, do not use any leftover Pred Forte without first consulting your doctor.

Who should not take Pred Forte?
You should not take Pred Forte if you have herpes or other viral diseases of the eye, or certain bacterial or fungal diseases of the eye.

Do not use Pred Forte if you are allergic to prednisolone or other steroids.

What should I tell my doctor before I take the first dose of Pred Forte?

Tell your doctor about all prescription, over-the-counter, and herbal medication you are taking before beginning treatment with Pred Forte. Also, talk to your doctor about your complete medical history, especially if you have had viral, bacterial or fungal diseases of the eye.

What is the usual dosage?

The information below is based on the dosage guidelines your doctor uses. Depending on your condition and medical history, your doctor may prescribe a different regimen. Do not change the dosage or stop taking your medication without your doctor's approval.

Adults: Put 1 to 2 drops under the eyelid 2 to 4 times daily. During the first 24 to 48 hours, your doctor may want you to use more frequent doses.

How should I take Pred Forte?

Use Pred Forte exactly as directed by your doctor. Follow these steps to administer Pred Forte:

1. Wash your hands thoroughly.
2. Vigorously shake the dropper bottle.
3. Gently pull your lower eyelid down to form a pocket next to your eye.
4. Do not touch the applicator tip to any surface including your eye.
5. Brace the bottle against the bridge of your nose or your forehead.
6. Tilt your head back and squeeze Pred Forte into your eye.
7. Close your eyes gently. Keep them closed for 1 to 2 minutes.
8. Do not rinse the dropper.
9. Wait for 5 to 10 minutes before using a second eye medication.

What should I avoid while taking Pred Forte?

Pred Forte may increase the chance of infection from contact lenses. Your doctor may advise you to stop wearing your contacts while using Pred Forte.

Do not touch the dropper to any surface, including your eyes or hands. The dropper is sterile. If it becomes contaminated, it could cause an infection in your eye.

What are possible food and drug interactions associated with Pred Forte?

If Pred Forte is taken with certain other drugs, the effects of either could be increased, decreased, or altered. It is especially important to check with your doctor before combining Pred Forte with oral steroid medication such as prednisone, methylprednisolone, and others.

What are the possible side effects of Pred Forte?

Side effects cannot be anticipated. If any develop or change in intensity, tell your doctor as soon as possible.

Side effects may include: allergic reactions, blurred vision, burning/stinging, cataract formation, delayed wound healing, dilated pupils, drooping eyelid, increased pressure inside the eyeball, inflamed eyes, perforation of the eyeball, secondary infection, ulcers of the cornea

Occasionally, long-term use of Pred Forte eyedrops may cause side effects due to an overload of steroid hormone. Side effects may include a "moon-faced" appearance, obese trunk, humped upper back, wasted limbs, and purple stretch marks on the skin. These effects are likely to disappear once Pred Forte use stops.

Can I receive Pred Forte if I am pregnant or breastfeeding?

The effects of Pred Forte during pregnancy and breastfeeding are unknown. Tell your doctor immediately if you are pregnant, plan to become pregnant, or are breastfeeding.

What should I do if I miss a dose of Pred Forte?

Apply the missed dose as soon as you remember. However, if it is almost time for your next regularly scheduled dose, skip the missed dose and apply the next one as directed. Do not use a double dose of this medication.

How should I store Pred Forte?

Store away from heat and direct light. Keep the bottle tightly closed and protect from freezing.

Prednisolone acetate ophthalmic suspension *See Pred Forte, page 1049.*

Prednisolone sodium phosphate *See Orapred ODT, page 951, or Pediapred, page 984.*

PREDNISONE

What is Prednisone?

Prednisone, a steroid drug, is used to reduce inflammation and alleviate symptoms in a variety of disorders, including rheumatoid arthritis and severe cases of asthma. It may be given to treat primary or secondary adrenal cortex insufficiency (lack of sufficient adrenal hormone in the body).

What is the most important information I should know about Prednisone?

Prednisone may lower your resistance to infections and make them harder to treat. Prednisone may also mask some of the signs of an infection, making it difficult for your doctor to diagnose the infection.

A few people taking prednisone develop Kaposi's sarcoma, a form of cancer; it may disappear when the drug is stopped.

Do not get a smallpox vaccination or any other immunization while you are taking prednisone. Also avoid exposure to chickenpox or measles, which can be very serious and even fatal in both children and adults taking prednisone.

Prednisone may reactivate a dormant case of tuberculosis (TB). If you have inactive TB and must take prednisone for an extended time, take anti-TB medication as well.

Who should not take Prednisone?

Do not take prednisone if you have ever had an allergic reaction to it or have a body-wide fungus infection, such as candidiasis or cryptococcosis.

What should I tell my doctor before I take the first dose of Prednisone?

Tell your doctor about all prescription, over-the-counter, and herbal medication you are taking before beginning treatment with prednisone. Also, talk to your doctor about your complete medical history, especially if you have kidney disease, liver disease, high blood pressure, heart disease, eye herpes, ulcerative colitis (inflammation of the bowel), diverticulitis, stomach ulcers, hypothyroidism (low thyroid levels), a psychiatric condition, osteoporosis, myasthenia gravis (muscle weakness), or type 2 diabetes (high blood sugar).

What is the usual dosage?

The information below is based on the dosage guidelines your doctor uses. Depending on your condition and medical history, your doctor may prescribe a different regimen. Do not change the dosage or stop taking your medication without your doctor's approval.

Adults: Dosage is determined by the condition being treated and your response to the drug. Typical starting doses can range from 5 milligrams (mg) to 60 mg a day. Once you respond to the drug, your doctor will lower the dose gradually to the minimum effective amount.

Children: Dosage is determined by the condition being treated and their response to the drug.

Treatment of Acute Attacks of Multiple Sclerosis
Adults: The usual starting dose is as much as 200 mg per day may be given for a week, followed by 80 mg every other day for a month.

How should I take Prednisone?

Take prednisone exactly as prescribed. Take prednisone with food to avoid stomach upset.

If you are on alternate-day therapy or have been prescribed a single daily dose, take prednisone in the morning with breakfast (about 8 a.m.). If you have been prescribed several doses per day, take them at evenly spaced intervals around the clock.

If you have been taking prednisone for a period of time, you may need an increased dosage of the medication before, during, and after any stressful situation. Always consult your doctor if you are anticipating stress and think you may need a temporary dosage increase.

What should I avoid while taking Prednisone?

Avoid alcohol. Alcohol and prednisone may be damaging to the stomach.

Avoid sources of infection; your immune system may be weakened while taking prednisone. Wash your hands frequently and keep them away from your mouth and eyes.

Do not receive immunizations during treatment with prednisone without first talking to your doctor.

What are possible food and drug interactions associated with Prednisone?

If prednisone is taken with certain other drugs, the effects of either could be increased, decreased, or altered. It is especially important to check with your doctor before combining prednisone with the following: amphotericin B, aspirin, blood thinners, carbamazepine, cyclosporine, estrogen drugs, insulin, ketoconazole, oral contraceptives, oral diabetes medication, phenobarbital, phenytoin, potent diuretics, rifampin, and troleandomycin.

What are the possible side effects of Prednisone?

Side effects cannot be anticipated. If any develop or change in intensity, tell your doctor as soon as possible. Only your doctor can determine if it is safe for you to continue taking this drug.

Side effects may include: euphoria, insomnia, mood changes, personality changes, psychotic behavior, severe depression, or may worsen any existing emotional instability

At a high dosage, prednisone may cause fluid retention and high blood pressure.

With prolonged prednisone treatment, eye problems may develop (e.g., a viral or fungal eye infection, cataracts, or glaucoma). Also, the buildup of adrenal hormones in your body may cause a condition called Cushing's syndrome, marked by weight gain, a moon-faced appearance, thin, fragile skin, muscle weakness, brittle bones, and purplish stripe marks on the skin. Women are more vulnerable to this problem than men. Alternate-day therapy may help prevent the development of Cushing's syndrome.

Can I receive Prednisone if I am pregnant or breastfeeding?
If you are pregnant or plan to become pregnant, inform your doctor immediately. Prednisone should be taken during pregnancy or while breastfeeding only if clearly needed and only if the benefit outweighs the potential risks to the child.

What should I do if I miss a dose of Prednisone?
Take the missed dose as soon as you remember. If it is almost time for your next dose, skip the missed dose and take the medicine at the next regularly scheduled time. Do not take a double dose of the medication.

How should I store Prednisone?
Store at room temperature.

Pregabalin *See Lyrica, page 782.*

PREMARIN
Generic name: Conjugated estrogens

What is Premarin?
Premarin is a medicine that contains a mixture of estrogens. Premarin is used after menopause to reduce moderate to severe symptoms of menopause, including feelings of warmth in the face, neck, and chest, and the sudden intense episodes of heat and sweating known as "hot flashes."

Premarin is also used to treat moderate to severe menopausal changes, such as dryness, itching, and burning, in and around the vagina, or painful intercourse caused by menopausal changes; help reduce your chances of getting osteoporosis (thin, weak bones) after menopause; treat certain conditions in women before menopause if their ovaries do not make enough estrogen naturally; and ease symptoms of certain cancers that have spread through the body, in men and women.

What is the most important information I should know about Premarin?
Estrogens increase your risk of developing cancer of the uterus. Report any unusual bleeding immediately to your healthcare provider while you are taking Premarin. Vaginal bleeding after menopause may be a warning sign of uterine cancer.

Do not use estrogens with or without progestins to prevent heart disease, heart attacks, strokes, or dementia. Using estrogens with or without progestins may increase your chances of getting heart attacks, strokes, breast cancer, and blood clots. It may also increase your risk of dementia, based on a study of women age 65 years or older. Talk regularly with your doctor about whether you still need treatment with Premarin.

Premarin vaginal cream can weaken latex condoms, diaphragms, and cervical caps.

Who should not take Premarin?
Do not take Premarin if you currently have or have had stroke or heart attack in the last year, blood clots, liver problems, unusual vaginal bleeding, or certain cancers, including cancer of the breast and uterine. Do not take Premarin if you are hypersensitive to it.

What should I tell my doctor before I take the first dose of Premarin?
Tell your doctor about all prescription, over-the-counter, and herbal medication you are taking before beginning treatment with Premarin. Also, talk to your doctor about your complete medical history, especially if you have asthma (wheezing), epilepsy (seizures), migraine, endometriosis, lupus, problems with your heart, liver, thyroid, kidneys, or have high calcium levels in your blood. Also, tell your doctor if you are going to have surgery or will be on bedrest.

What is the usual dosage?
The information below is based on the dosage guidelines your doctor uses. Depending on your condition and medical history, your doctor may prescribe a different regimen. Do not change the dosage or stop taking your medication without your doctor's approval.

Adults: Your doctor will start therapy with Premarin at a low dose and adjust the dosage according to your response. He or she will want to check you periodically at 3- to 6-month intervals to determine the need for continued therapy.

PREMARIN TABLETS
The usual starting dosage is 0.3 milligrams daily. However, this may vary depending upon the condition being treated. Your doctor will prescribe the correct regimen for your treatment needs.

PREMARIN VAGINAL CREAM
Given cyclically for short-term use only.

Degeneration of Genital Tissue or Severe Itching in the Genital Area
Adults: The recommended dosage is one-half to 2 grams daily, inserted into the vagina, depending on the severity of the condition. You will use the cream for 3 weeks, then stop for 1 week. Tell your doctor if you notice any unusual bleeding.

How should I take Premarin?

Take one Premarin tablet at the same time each

Estrogens should be used at the lowest dose possible for your treatment only as long as needed. You and your healthcare provider should talk regularly (for example, every 3 to 6 months) about the dose you are taking and whether you still need treatment with Premarin.

If you are using Premarin vaginal cream, apply it as follows:

1. Remove cap from tube.
2. Screw nozzle end of applicator onto tube.
3. Gently squeeze tube from the bottom to force sufficient cream into the barrel to provide the prescribed dose. Use the marked stopping points on the applicator as a guide.
4. Unscrew applicator from tube.
5. Lie on back with knees drawn up. Gently insert applicator deeply into the vagina and press plunger downward to its original position.

To cleanse the applicator, pull the plunger to remove it from the barrel, then wash with mild soap and warm water. Do not boil or use hot water.

What should I avoid while taking Premarin?

Do not smoke while using this medication. Smoking can increase your risk of blood clots, stroke, or heart attack caused by conjugated estrogens. Avoid taking estrogen along with grapefruit juice.

What are possible food and drug interactions associated with Premarin?

If Premarin is taken with certain other drugs, the effects of either could be increased, decreased, or altered. It is especially important to check with your doctor before combining Premarin with the following: barbiturates such as phenobarbital; blood thinners such as warfarin; carbamazepine; clarithromycin; drugs used for epilepsy; erythromycin; itraconazole; ketoconazole; major tranquilizers; oral diabetes drugs; rifampin; ritonavir; St. John's wort; steroid medications; thyroid preparations; tricyclic antidepressants; and vitamin C.

What are the possible side effects of Premarin?

Side effects cannot be anticipated. If any develop or change in intensity, tell your doctor as soon as possible. Only your doctor can determine if it is safe for you to continue taking this drug.

Side effects may include: headache, breast pain, irregular vaginal bleeding or spotting, stomach/abdominal cramps, bloating, nausea and vomiting, hair loss, high blood pressure, liver problems, high blood sugar, fluid retention, enlargement of benign tumors of the uterus (fibroids), vaginal yeast infections

Serious side effects may include: breast cancer, cancer of the uterus, stroke, heart attack, blood clots, dementia, gallbladder disease, ovarian cancer

Warning signs of serious side effects include: breast lumps, unusual vaginal bleeding, dizziness and faintness, changes in speech, severe headaches, chest pain, shortness of breath, pains in your legs, changes in vision, vomiting

Call your doctor right away if you get any of these warning signs or any other unusual symptom that concerns you.

Can I receive Premarin if I am pregnant or breastfeeding?
If you are pregnant or plan to become pregnant, notify your doctor immediately. Premarin and conjugated estrogens should not be taken during pregnancy because of the possibility of harm to the fetus.

If you are breastfeeding, the hormones in Premarin can pass into your milk. Your doctor may advise you not to breastfeed while you are taking Premarin.

What should I do if I miss a dose of Premarin?
If you miss a dose, take it as soon as possible. If it is almost time for your next dose, skip the missed dose and go back to your normal schedule. Do not take 2 doses at the same time.

How should I store Premarin?
Store at room temperature.

PREVACID
Generic name: Lansoprazole

What is Prevacid?
Prevacid is a medicine that blocks the production of stomach acid. Prevacid belongs to a class of drugs known as proton-pump inhibitors (PPIs). It is prescribed for the short-term treatment of stomach ulcers, duodenal ulcers, erosive esophagitis (inflammation of the esophagus), and heartburn or other symptoms of gastroesophageal reflux disease (GERD).

Prevacid is also used to prevent a relapse of duodenal ulcer or esophagitis; to reduce the risk of stomach ulcers in people who develop ulcers while taking nonsteroidal anti-inflammatory drugs (NSAIDs); for long-term treatment of certain diseases marked by excessive acid production, such as Zollinger-Ellison syndrome; and as part of a combination treatment to eliminate the *Helicobacter pylori* infection that causes most cases of duodenal ulcer.

What is the most important information I should know about Prevacid?

Take Prevacid for the full length of treatment your doctor prescribes. Continue to take the drug and see your doctor even if you begin to feel better. Do not take Prevacid any longer than your doctor has prescribed.

Prevacid should not be used for long-term therapy of duodenal ulcer or erosive esophagitis. Prevacid has no effect on stomach cancer, which may be present even if Prevacid relieves your symptoms.

Who should not take Prevacid?

Do not take Prevacid if you've ever had an allergic reaction to it, or if you've ever had an allergic reaction to penicillin or macrolide antibiotics, such as clarithromycin or erythromycin.

Avoid Prevacid if you're taking cisapride, pimozide, astemizole, or terfenadine. Combining Prevacid with these drugs could cause dangerous, and even fatal, heartbeat irregularities.

What should I tell my doctor before I take the first dose of Prevacid?

Tell your doctor about all prescription, over-the-counter, and herbal medications you are taking before beginning treatment with Prevacid. Also, talk to your doctor about your complete medical history, especially if you have liver disease or phenylketonuria, a genetic disorder.

What is the usual dosage?

The information below is based on the dosage guidelines your doctor uses. Depending on your condition and medical history, your doctor may prescribe a different regimen. Do not change the dosage or stop taking your medication without your doctor's approval.

*Eradication of Ulcer-Causing Bacteria (*H. pylori*)*
Adults: To eliminate the *H. pylori* bacteria that cause most duodenal ulcers, Prevacid is taken with amoxicillin alone or amoxicillin and Biaxin. When combined with amoxicillin only, the usual dosage is 30 mg of Prevacid and 1 gram of amoxicillin 3 times daily for 14 days. If all 3 drugs are used, the usual dosage is 30 milligrams of Prevacid, 1 gram of amoxicillin, and 500 mg of Biaxin twice daily for 10 to 14 days.

Prevention of Stomach Ulcer Due to Nonsteroidal Anti-inflammatory Drugs
Adults: The usual dose is 15 mg once a day for up to 12 weeks.

Prevention of Duodenal Ulcer Relapse
Adults: Take 15 mg once a day.

Short-Term Treatment of Duodenal Ulcer
Adults: The usual dose is 15 milligrams (mg) once daily, before eating, for 4 weeks.

Short-Term Treatment of Erosive Esophagitis
Adults: The usual dose is 30 mg daily, before eating, for up to 8 weeks. Depending on your response to the medication your doctor may suggest another 8-week treatment regimen.

Children 12 to 17 years: The usual dose is 30 mg once a day for up to 8 weeks.

Children 1 to 11 years: Dosage is based on the child's weight. For children weighing <66 pounds, the usual dose is 15 mg once a day for up to 12 weeks. For children weighing >66 pounds, the usual dose is 30 mg once a day for up to 12 weeks. If the child's symptoms don't improve after 2 or more weeks, the doctor may increase the dose up to a maximum of 30 mg twice a day. Children with severe liver problems will need their dosage adjusted.

Short-Term Treatment of Gastroesophageal Reflux Disease (GERD)
Adults: Take 15 mg once a day for up to 8 weeks.

Children 12 to 17 years: The usual dose is 15 mg once a day for up to 8 weeks.

Children 1 to 11 years: Dosage is based on the child's weight. For children weighing <66 pounds, the usual dose is 15 mg once a day for up to 12 weeks. For children weighing >66 pounds, the usual dose is 30 mg once a day for up to 12 weeks. If the child's symptoms don't improve after 2 or more weeks, the doctor may increase the dose up to a maximum of 30 mg twice a day. Children with severe liver problems will need their dosage adjusted.

Short-Term Treatment of Stomach Ulcer
Adults: The usual dose is 30 mg once a day for up to 8 weeks.

Zollinger-Ellison Syndrome (and Other Excess Acid Conditions)
Adults: The usual starting dose is 60 mg once daily. This dose can be adjusted upward by your doctor, depending on your response. Dosages totaling more than 120 mg a day should be divided into smaller doses.
  Safety and effectiveness have not been studied in children <1 year old.

How should I take Prevacid?
Prevacid should be taken before meals. If you're having trouble swallowing the regular delayed-release capsules, you may sprinkle the contents onto a tablespoon of applesauce; swallow immediately without chewing or crushing the granules. You may also mix the granules with 2 ounces of orange juice or tomato juice. (Rinse the glass with an additional 4 ounces of juice to make sure you get the entire dose.)
  For the delayed-release Prevacid SoluTabs, place each tablet on the

tongue. The dissolved particles may be swallowed with or without water. The SoluTabs should not be chewed or swallowed whole. If you or your child has trouble swallowing the SoluTabs, you may dissolve the tablet in water and administer the solution with an oral syringe or through a nasogastric tube.

For specific instructions, talk to your doctor. The general steps are as follows: Place the tablet in an oral syringe. Follow your doctor's directions on the amount of water you need to draw up into the syringe. Gently shake the syringe to dissolve the tablet. Administer the solution within 15 minutes. This can be done directly, with the oral syringe, or by injecting the syringe into a nasogastric tube. To be sure you have taken all of the drug, rinse out any remaining residue by refilling the syringe with water and shaking gently; then administer the remaining contents.

Alternatively, you may use Prevacid for Delayed-Release Oral Suspension. Empty the packet into 2 tablespoonfuls of water, stir well, and swallow immediately. Do not use any other liquid; and avoid chewing or crushing the granules. If any material remains in the glass, add more water, stir, and drink immediately.

What should I avoid while taking Prevacid?

If you also take sucralfate, avoid taking it at the same time you take Prevacid. Wait at least 30 minutes after taking Prevacid before you take sucralfate.

What are possible food and drug interactions associated with Prevacid?

If Prevacid is taken with certain other drugs, the effects of either could be increased, decreased, or altered. It is especially important to check with your doctor before combining Prevacid with the following: ampicillin, digoxin, iron salts, ketoconazole, sucralfate, theophylline, warfarin

What are the possible side effects of Prevacid?

Side effects cannot be anticipated. If any develop or change in intensity, tell your doctor as soon as possible. Only your doctor can determine if it is safe for you to continue taking this drug.

Side effects may include: abdominal pain, constipation, diarrhea, dizziness or headache (more common in children), nausea

Can I receive Prevacid if I am pregnant or breastfeeding?

The effects of Prevacid during pregnancy and breastfeeding are unknown. Tell your doctor immediately if you are pregnant, plan to become pregnant, or are breastfeeding.

What should I do if I miss a dose of Prevacid?
Take it as soon as you remember. If it is almost time for your next dose, skip the one you missed and go back to your regular schedule. Do not take 2 doses at once.

How should I store Prevacid?
Store at room temperature in a tightly closed container. Keep away from moisture.

PREVPAC
Generic name: Amoxicillin, clarithromycin, and lansoprazole

What is Prevpac?
Prevpac is a prepackaged combination of drugs designed to treat duodenal ulcers caused by *Helicobacter pylori* bacteria, the most common cause of ulcers. Prevpac is made up of 3 medications: amoxicillin and clarithromycin (Biaxin) are the antibiotic components and lansoprazole (Prevacid) is a proton-pump inhibitor that reduces the production of gastric acid.

What is the most important information
I should know about Prevpac?
Take Prevpac exactly as prescribed and finish your entire course of therapy. If you stop too soon, the ulcer may not heal completely and your symptoms may return.

Serious and occasionally fatal allergic reactions have occurred in people taking antibiotics similar to those in Prevpac. Seek emergency medical treatment if you develop hives, swelling, itching, fainting, breathing difficulties, or chest pain. Also, if you develop severe diarrhea while taking Prevpac, call your doctor.

Who should not take Prevpac?
Prevpac therapy is not recommended if you have severe kidney disease. Use Prevpac with caution if you are over 65 years old.

Do not take Prevpac if you've ever had an allergic reaction to antibiotics such as amoxicillin, clarithromycin, erythromycin, or penicillin. Also, avoid Prevpac if you've had a reaction to any cephalosporin-type antibiotic.

What should I tell my doctor before
I take the first dose of Prevpac?
Tell your doctor about all prescription, over-the-counter, and herbal medications you are taking before beginning treatment with Prevpac. Also, talk to your doctor about your complete medical history, especially if you have kidney or liver disease.

What is the usual dosage?
The information below is based on the dosage guidelines your doctor uses. Depending on your condition and medical history, your doctor may prescribe a different regimen. Do not change the dosage or stop taking your medication without your doctor's approval.

Adults: The recommended dosage is 1 capsule of lansoprazole (Prevacid), 2 capsules of amoxicillin, and 1 tablet of clarithromycin (Biaxin) taken together twice a day (morning and evening) for 10 or 14 days.

How should I take Prevpac?
Each pack contains a full day's supply of medication, consisting of two 30-milligram (mg) capsules of lansoprazole (Prevacid), four 500-mg capsules of amoxicillin, and two 500-mg tablets of clarithromycin (Biaxin). Take half the supply in the morning and the remainder at night.

Prevpac can be taken with or without food. Swallow each pill whole; do not crush or chew.

What should I avoid while taking Prevpac?
There are no restrictions on food, beverages, or activity while you are taking the medications contained in Prevpac, unless your doctor directs otherwise.

What are possible food and drug interactions associated with Prevpac?
If Prevpac is taken with certain other drugs, the effects of either could be increased, decreased, or altered. It is especially important to check with your doctor before combining Prevpac with drugs used to treat HIV infection as well as the following: alfentanil, alprazolam, ampicillin, antiarrhythmics (such as quinidine and disopyramide), astemizole, blood thinners, bromocriptine, carbamazepine, cholesterol-lowering drugs (such as lovastatin and simvastatin), cilostazol, cisapride, cyclosporine, digoxin, disopyramide, ergotamine-based drugs for migraine, ketoconazole, hexobarbital, iron supplements, methylprednisolone, midazolam, probenecid, phenytoin, pimozide, rifabutin, sildenafil, sucralfate, tacrolimus, terfenadine, theophylline, triazolam, valproic acid

What are the possible side effects of Prevpac?
Side effects cannot be anticipated. If any develop or change in intensity, tell your doctor as soon as possible. Only your doctor can determine if it is safe for you to continue taking this drug.

Side effects may include: diarrhea, headache, taste disturbances

Can I receive Prevpac if I am pregnant or breastfeeding?
The effects of Prevpac during pregnancy and breastfeeding are unknown. Tell your doctor immediately if you are pregnant, plan to become pregnant, or are breastfeeding.

What should I do if I miss a dose of Prevpac?
Take it as soon as you remember. If it is almost time for your next dose, skip the one you missed and go back to your regular schedule. Do not take 2 doses at the same time.

How should I store Prevpac?
Store Prevpac at room temperature, away from light and moisture.

PREZISTA
Generic name: Darunavir

What is Prezista?
Prezista is an oral tablet used for the treatment of HIV (human immunodeficiency virus) infection in adults. HIV is the virus that causes AIDS (acquired immune deficiency syndrome). Prezista is a type of anti-HIV drug called a protease inhibitor. Prezista does not cure HIV or AIDS. It will be used with another drug called ritonavir (Norvir) to slow the progress of the disease.

What is the most important information I should know about Prezista?
Prezista does not cure HIV or AIDS. Prezista does not reduce the risk of passing HIV to others through sexual contact, sharing needles, or being exposed to your blood.

Who should not take Prezista?
Do not take Prezista if you are allergic to darunavir, or any of the other ingredients in Prezista, or to ritonavir.

What should I tell my doctor before I take the first dose of Prezista?
Tell your doctor about all prescription, over-the-counter, and herbal medications you are on to prevent a harmful interaction. Tell your doctor about all of your medical conditions, including if you are allergic to sulfa medicines, or have diabetes. In general, anti-HIV medicines, such as Prezista, might increase sugar levels in the blood. Also, tell your doctor if you have liver problems or hemophilia as Prezista might increase the risk of bleeding.

What is the usual dosage?
The information below is based on the dosage guidelines your doctor uses. Depending on your condition and medical history, your doctor may prescribe a different regimen. Do not change the dosage or stop taking your medication without your doctor's approval.

Adults: The recommended adult dose is 600 milligrams (mg) (two 300-mg tablets) twice daily taken with ritonavir 100 mg twice daily.

How should I take Prezista?
Take with food.

Your doctor will tell you how much of this medicine to use and how often. Do not use more medicine or use it more often than your doctor tells you to. Prezista and ritonavir should be taken together. It is best to take this medicine with food or milk. Swallow the tablet whole. Do not crush, break, or chew it. If you also use didanosine (Videx), take it 1 hour before or 2 hours after taking Prezista.

What should I avoid while taking Prezista?
Prezista does not reduce the risk of passing HIV to others through sexual contact, sharing needles, or being exposed to your blood. For your health and the health of others, it is important to always practice safe sex by using a latex or polyurethane condom or other barrier methods to lower the chance of sexual contact with any body fluids such as semen, vaginal secretions, or blood. Never reuse or share needles.

What are possible food and drug interactions associated with Prezista?
If Prezista is taken with certain other drugs, the effects of either could be increased, decreased, or altered. It is especially important to check with your doctor before combining Prezista with any medications, including antiarrhythmics, anti-anxiety drugs, antibiotics, antidepressants, anti-fungals, antiseizure drugs, asthma drugs, blood thinners, cholesterol-lowering drugs, drugs to prevent organ rejection, drugs to treat heart disease, St. John's wort, erectile dysfunction drugs

What are the possible side effects of Prezista?
Side effects cannot be anticipated. If any develop or change in intensity, tell your doctor as soon as possible. Only your doctor can determine if it is safe for you to continue taking this drug.

Side effects may include: changes in body fat, common cold, diarrhea, headache, high blood sugar, increased bleeding, nausea

Side effects may occur if you are taking allergy, migraine/headache, digestive, psychotropic, or sleep/anxiety medications.

Can I receive Prezista if I am pregnant or breastfeeding?
Talk to your doctor if you are pregnant, or planning to become pregnant, while taking Prezista. Also, ask your doctor about how you can be included in the Antiretroviral Pregnancy Registry. Do not breastfeed if you are taking Prezista. You should not breastfeed if you have HIV because of

the chance of passing HIV to your baby. Talk with your doctor about the best way to feed your baby.

What should I do if I miss a dose of Prezista?
If you miss a dose of Prezista or ritonavir by more than 6 hours, wait and then take the next dose of Prezista and ritonavir at the regularly scheduled time. If you miss a dose of Prezista or ritonavir by less than 6 hours, take your missed dose of Prezista and ritonavir immediately. Then take your next dose of Prezista and ritonavir at the regularly scheduled time.

How should I store Prezista?
Store at room temperature.

PRILOSEC
Generic name: Omeprazole

What is Prilosec?
Prilosec is prescribed for the short-term treatment of stomach ulcer, duodenal ulcer, erosive esophagitis (inflammation of the esophagus), heartburn, and other symptoms of gastroesophageal reflux disease (GERD).

Prilosec is also used to treat patients whose ulcers are caused by infection with *Helicobacter pylori;* to maintain healing of erosive esophagitis; and for the long-term treatment of conditions in which too much stomach acid is secreted, including Zollinger-Ellison syndrome.

Prilosec OTC, an over-the-counter product, is approved only for frequent heartburn (occurring 2 or more days a week).

What is the most important information I should know about Prilosec?
Long-term use of Prilosec may cause severe stomach inflammation. Prilosec may mask the signs of stomach cancer.

Who should not take Prilosec?
Do not take Prilosec if you are sensitive to or have ever had an allergic reaction to Prilosec or any of its ingredients. Avoid the Prilosec/Biaxin combination treatment if you are allergic to certain antibiotics called macrolides, or if you are taking Orap. Do not take amoxicillin if you are allergic to any of the penicillin drugs.

What should I tell my doctor before I take the first dose of Prilosec?
Tell your doctor about all prescription, over-the-counter, and herbal medications you are taking before beginning treatment with Prilosec. Also, talk to your doctor about your complete medical history, especially if you have liver disease.

What is the usual dosage?
The information below is based on the dosage guidelines your doctor uses. Depending on your condition and medical history, your doctor may prescribe a different regimen. Do not change the dosage or stop taking your medication without your doctor's approval.

Gastric Ulcer
Adults: The usual dose is 40 mg once a day for 4 to 8 weeks.

Gastroesophageal Reflux Disease (GERD)
Adults: The usual dose for people with symptoms of GERD is 20 mg daily for up to 4 weeks. For erosive esophagitis accompanied by GERD symptoms, the usual dose is 20 mg day for 4 to 8 weeks. The dose may be continued to maintain healing.

Children 1 to 16 years: For children weighing 11 to 22 pounds, the usual dose is 5 mg a day; for children weighing 22 to 44 pounds, the usual dose is 10 mg a day. For those weighing 44 pounds or more, the usual dose is 20 mg a day. For children with erosive esophagitis, your doctor will determine the correct dose based on the child's weight.

Short-Term Treatment of Active Duodenal Ulcer
Adults: The usual dose is 20 milligrams (mg) once a day. Most people heal within 4 weeks, although some require an additional 4 weeks of Prilosec therapy.

Treatment of Duodenal Ulcers Caused by H. Pylori
Adults: In combination therapy with Biaxin alone, the usual dosage is 40 mg of Prilosec once daily and 500 mg of Biaxin 3 times a day for 14 days, followed by 20 mg of Prilosec once daily for an additional 14 days.

   If amoxicillin is included in the treatment, the recommended dosage is 20 mg of Prilosec, 500 mg of Biaxin, and 1,000 mg of amoxicillin twice a day for 10 days, followed by 20 mg of Prilosec once daily for an additional 18 days.

Zollinger-Ellison Syndrome (and Other Pathological Hypersecretory Conditions)
Adults: The usual starting dose is 60 mg once a day. If you take more than 80 mg a day, your doctor will divide the total into smaller doses. The dosing will be based on your needs.

The safety and effectiveness of Prilosec have not been studied in children <1 year old.

How should I take Prilosec?
Prilosec works best when taken before meals. It may be taken with an antacid.

   Swallow the capsule whole. It should not be opened, chewed, or crushed. You may also empty the contents of the Prilosec capsule onto a tablespoonful of applesauce, mix, and swallow with a glass of cool water.

Use cool, soft applesauce. Do not chew or crush the pellets. Use the mixture immediately. Do not store it.

It may take several days for Prilosec to begin relieving stomach pain. Continue taking the drug exactly as prescribed.

What should I avoid while taking Prilosec?
Avoid excessive amounts of caffeine while taking Prilosec.

What are possible food and drug interactions associated with Prilosec?
If Prilosec is taken with certain other drugs, the effects of either could be increased, decreased, or altered. It is especially important to check with your doctor before combining Prilosec with the following: ampicillin-containing drugs, atazanavir, cyclosporine, diazepam, disulfiram, iron, ketoconazole, phenytoin, tacrolimus, warfarin

What are the possible side effects of Prilosec?
Side effects cannot be anticipated. If any develop or change in intensity, tell your doctor as soon as possible. Only your doctor can determine if it is safe for you to continue taking this drug.

Side effects may include: abdominal pain, diarrhea, headache, nausea, vomiting

When taken with Biaxin, side effects may also include: flu symptoms, nasal inflammation, sore throat, taste alteration, tongue discoloration

When taken with amoxicillin and Biaxin, side effects may also include: diarrhea, headache, taste alteration

Can I receive Prilosec if I am pregnant or breastfeeding?
The effects of Prilosec during pregnancy have not been adequately studied. If you are pregnant or plan to become pregnant, inform your doctor immediately. Avoid combined therapy with Biaxin unless there is no alternative. Prilosec (and Biaxin) may appear in breast milk and could affect a nursing infant. If Prilosec is essential to your health, your doctor may advise you to discontinue breastfeeding until your treatment with Prilosec is finished.

What should I do if I miss a dose of Prilosec?
Take it as soon as you remember. If it is almost time for your next dose, skip the one you missed and go back to your regular schedule. Do not take 2 doses at once.

How should I store Prilosec?
Store at room temperature in a tightly closed container, away from light and moisture.

Primidone *See Mysoline, page 856.*

PRIMSOL
Generic name: Trimethoprim

What is Primsol?
Primsol is a liquid antibiotic prescribed to treat acute ear infections in children over 6 months old, and uncomplicated urinary tract infections in adults. Your doctor will order tests to make sure Primsol is effective against the bacteria that caused your infection. Primsol is not recommended in cases of chronic infection due to the risks associated with long-term use.

What is the most important information I should know about Primsol?
Primsol can cause a serious blood cell disorder, especially if taken in high doses or for a long period of time. This condition requires prompt medical treatment. Notify your doctor immediately if you develop fever, pale skin, sore throat, or small red or purple spots on the skin. Your doctor may order blood tests to monitor your health while taking Primsol.

Primsol should not be used for the prevention or long-term treatment of ear infection or urinary tract infection.

Primsol should be used with caution if you have a blood or bone marrow disorder, liver or kidney disease, or you have ever had vitamin deficiencies. Primsol interferes with your body's ability to absorb folic acid (folate, vitamin B9), an important B-vitamin. Your doctor may have you take extra vitamins during treatment with Primsol.

Primsol should not be given to infants under 2 months of age.

Who should not take Primsol?
Primsol should not be taken if you have an allergic reaction to it or to other drugs that contain the same ingredient, trimethoprim. Do not take Primsol if you have been diagnosed with megaloblastic (pernicious) anemia, a blood cell disorder caused by a B-vitamin deficiency.

What should I tell my doctor before I take the first dose of Primsol?
Tell your doctor about all prescription, over-the-counter, and herbal medications you are taking before beginning treatment with this drug. Also, talk to your doctor about your complete medical history, especially if you have liver or kidney disease, vitamin deficiencies, or a blood disorder.

What is the usual dosage?
The information below is based on the dosage guidelines your doctor uses. Depending on your condition and medical history, your doctor

may prescribe a different regimen. Do not change the dosage or stop taking your medication without your doctor's approval.

Adults: The usual adult dose is 100 milligrams taken twice a day, or 200 milligrams taken once a day for 10 days. For adults with impaired kidney function, the recommended dose of Primsol will be half the usual dose.

Children: For children aged 6 months and older, the recommended daily dose is 10 milligrams per 2.2 pounds of body weight every 12 hours for 10 days. Follow the directions that come with the prescription carefully and if you have questions, call your doctor or pharmacy. For children with impaired kidney function, the recommended dose of Primsol will be half the usual dose.

How should I take Primsol?

Primsol liquid is taken by mouth with or without food, twice daily, 12 hours apart. When Primsol is prescribed in just one daily dose, take it at about the same time each day.

What should I avoid while taking Primsol?

Avoid becoming pregnant or breastfeeding while using Primsol.

What are possible food and drug interactions associated with Primsol?

When Primsol is used with certain other drugs, the effects of either drug could be increased, decreased, or altered. It is especially important to check with your doctor before combining Primsol with methotrexate or phenytoin.

What are the possible side effects of Primsol?

Side effects cannot be anticipated. If any develop or change in intensity, tell your doctor as soon as possible. Only your doctor can determine if it is safe for you to continue taking this drug. Side effects may include diarrhea and/or skin rash.

Can I receive Primsol if I am pregnant or breastfeeding?

Primsol can interfere with the absorption of important vitamins that are vital to your baby's development during pregnancy. It is not recommended for pregnant women unless your doctor determines the benefit to your health outweighs the risk to your unborn baby. Tell your doctor immediately if you are pregnant or plan to become pregnant while taking Primsol.

Primsol appears in breast milk and can harm your nursing infant. Your doctor may advise you to stop breastfeeding if Primsol is essential to your health.

What should I do if I miss a dose of Primsol?
Take the forgotten dose as soon as you remember. However, if it is almost time for your next dose, skip the one you missed and return to your regular schedule. Do not take two doses at once.

How should I store Primsol?
Store at room temperature, away from light.

PRISTIQ
Generic name: Desvenlafaxine succinate

What is Pristiq?
Pristiq is used to treat major depression.

What is the most important information I should know about Pristiq?
Antidepressants can increase the risk of suicidal thinking and behavior in children and teenagers. Adult and pediatric patients taking antidepressants should be watched closely for changes in moods or actions, especially when they first start therapy or when their dose is increased or decreased. Patients and their families should contact the doctor immediately if new symptoms develop or seem to get worse. Signs to watch for include anxiety, hostility, sleeplessness, restlessness, impulsive or dangerous behavior, and thoughts about suicide or dying.

Pristiq is not approved for use in pediatric patients.

Who should not take Pristiq?
Do not take Pristiq if you are allergic to any of its ingredients, or if you are allergic to venlafaxine hydrochloride, the active ingredient in Effexor.

Do not take monoamine oxidase inhibitors (MAOIs) within 2 weeks before or after treatment with this medication. In some cases a serious, possibly fatal, reaction may occur. Examples of MAOIs include selegiline and the antidepressants phenelzine and tranylcypromine.

What should I tell my doctor before I take the first dose of Pristiq?
Tell your doctor about all prescription, over-the-counter, and herbal medication you are taking before beginning treatment with Pristiq. Also, talk to your doctor about your complete medical history, especially if you have high blood pressure, heart problems, high cholesterol or high triglycerides, history of stroke, glaucoma, kidney or liver problems, bleeding problems, seizures or convulsions, mania or bipolar disorder, or low sodium levels in your blood.

What is the usual dosage?

The information below is based on the dosage guidelines your doctor uses. Depending on your condition and medical history, your doctor may prescribe a different regimen. Do not change the dosage or stop taking your medication without your doctor's approval.

Adults: The recommended dose is 50 milligrams once daily with or without food. If you have poor kidney or liver function, your doctor may prescribe a different dose.

How should I take Pristiq?

Take Pristiq at the same time each day. You can take it with or without food. Tablets should be taken whole; do not crush, chew, dissolve, or divide them. When you take Pristiq, you may see something in your stool that looks like a tablet. This is the empty shell from the tablet after the medicine has been absorbed in your body.

What should I avoid while taking Pristiq?

Do not drive or operate dangerous machinery until you know how Pristiq affects you. You should also avoid alcohol.

What are possible food and drug interactions associated with Pristiq?

If Pristiq is taken with certain drugs, the effects of either could be increased, decreased, or altered. It is important to check with your doctor before combining Pristiq with the following: drugs that affect the central nervous system, lithium, migraine medications known as triptans, narcotic painkillers, sleep aids, weight-loss products such as phentermine, tranquilizers, antipsychotic medicines, antidepressants that affect serotonin such as fluoxetine and paroxetine, MAOIs, nonsteroidal anti-inflammatory drugs, blood thinners such as aspirin and warfarin, alcohol, ketoconazole, and desimipramine.

What are the possible side effects of Pristiq?

Side effects cannot be anticipated. If any develop or change in intensity, tell your doctor as soon as possible. Only your doctor can determine if it is safe for you to continue taking this drug.

Side effects may include: abnormal bleeding or bruising, anxiety, constipation, decreased sex drive, delayed orgasm and ejaculation, dilated pupils, dizziness, dry mouth, glaucoma, headache, high blood pressure, increased cholesterol and triglyceride levels, low sodium levels, seizures, serotonin syndrome (including restlessness, increased blood pressure, diarrhea, nausea, vomiting, increased body temperature, fast heartbeat, hallucinations, and loss of coordination), sleepiness, tiredness, tremor

Can I receive Pristiq if I am pregnant or breastfeeding?
Tell your doctor immediately if you are pregnant, plan to become pregnant, or are breastfeeding. It is not known if Pristiq is safe to use during pregnancy. Pristiq can pass into breast milk and may harm your baby. Talk with your doctor about the best way to feed your baby while taking this drug.

How should I store Pristiq?
Store at room temperature.

PRIVIGEN
Generic name: Immune globulin intravenous (human)

What is Privigen?
Privigen is obtained from human plasma and is used to treat primary immunodeficiency (PI) associated with defects in humoral immunity. It is also used to treat chronic immune thrombocytopenic purpura (ITP) to rapidly raise platelet counts to prevent bleeding.

What is the most important information I should know about Privigen?
Privigen is made from human plasma and therefore may carry a risk of transmitting viruses and other infections, such as Creutzfeldt-Jacob ("mad cow") disease. Immune globulins have been associated with kidney problems, kidney failure, and even death.

Who should not take Privigen?
Do not take Privigen if you have had an anaphylactic (fatal allergic reaction) or severe systemic reaction to the administration of human immune globulin or if you have selective Ig A deficiency.

What should I tell my doctor before I take the first dose of Privigen?
Tell your doctor about all prescription, over-the-counter, and herbal medications you are taking before beginning treatment with Privigen. Also, talk to your doctor about your complete medical history especially if you had experienced a severe allergic reaction to Privigen or if you have any kidney problems or diabetes.

What is the usual dosage?
The information below is based on the dosage guidelines your doctor uses. Depending on your condition and medical history, your doctor may prescribe a different regimen. Do not change the dosage or stop taking your medication without your doctor's approval.

Primary Immunodeficiency
Adults: The recommend dose is 200-800 milligrams (mg) per kilogram (kg) of body weight every 3 to 4 weeks.

Immune Thrombocytopenic Purpura
Adults: The recommend dose is 1 gram per kg for 2 consecutive days.

How should I take Privigen?
Privigen is administered via an intravenous infusion by your healthcare provider.

What should I avoid while taking Privigen?
Avoid getting dehydrated.
   Avoid receiving any live vaccines while being treated with Privigen.

What are possible food and drug interactions associated with Privigen?
If Privigen is used with certain other drugs, the effects of either could be increased, decreased, or altered. It is especially important to check with your doctor before combining Privigen with the following: live vaccines or drugs can damage the kidneys.

What are the possible side effects of Privigen?
Side effects cannot be anticipated. If any develop or change in intensity, tell your doctor as soon as possible. Only your doctor can determine if it is safe for you to continue taking this drug.

Side effects may include: headache, destruction of red blood cells, hyperthermia (raised body temperature), impairment of live virus vaccines, kidney failure, transfusion-related acute lung injury (characterized by fluid in the lungs, breathing difficulty, hypoxia)

Can I receive Privigen if I am pregnant or breastfeeding?
Privigen is to be avoided during pregnancy and breastfeeding.

What should I do if I miss a dose of Privigen?
If you miss your appointment, call your doctor to schedule your next dose.

How should I store Privigen?
Privigen is administered in your doctor's office.

Procainamide hydrochloride *See Procanbid, page 1074.*

PROCANBID

Generic name: Procainamide hydrochloride

What is Procanbid?

Procanbid is used to treat severe irregular heartbeats (arrhythmias). Arrhythmias are often caused by drugs or disease but can occur in otherwise healthy people with no history of heart disease or other illness.

What is the most important information I should know about Procanbid?

Procanbid may cause serious blood disorders, especially during the first 3 months of treatment. Notify your doctor if you notice any of the following: joint or muscle pain, dark urine, yellowing of skin or eyes, muscular weakness, chest or abdominal pain, appetite loss, diarrhea, hallucinations, dizziness, depression, wheezing, cough, easy bruising or bleeding, tremors, palpitations, rash, soreness or ulcers in the mouth, sore throat, nausea, vomiting, fever, and chills.

Antiarrhythmic agents may sometimes cause or worsen heartbeat irregularities and certain heart conditions, such as heart failure (the inability of the heart to sustain its workload of pumping blood). Your condition will be monitored throughout your treatment.

Procanbid has been known to trigger a disorder similar to lupus erythematosus. Notify your doctor if you develop any of the following lupus-like symptoms: joint pain or inflammation, abdominal or chest pain, fever, chills, muscle pain, skin lesions.

Who should not take Procanbid?

Do not take Procanbid if you have the heart irregularity known as complete heart block or incomplete heart block without a pacemaker, or if you have ever had an allergic reaction to procaine or similar local anesthetics.

Your doctor will not prescribe Procanbid if you have been diagnosed with the connective-tissue disease lupus erythematosus or the heartbeat irregularity known as torsades de pointes.

What should I tell my doctor before I take the first dose of Procanbid?

Tell your doctor about all prescription, over-the-counter, and herbal medications you are taking before beginning treatment with Procanbid. Also, talk to your doctor about your complete medical history, especially if you ever had congestive heart failure or other types of heart disease, kidney disease, liver disease, or myasthenia gravis (a disease that causes muscle weakness, especially in the face and neck).

What is the usual dosage?

The information below is based on the dosage guidelines your doctor uses. Depending on your condition and medical history, your doctor

may prescribe a different regimen. Do not change the dosage or stop taking your medication without your doctor's approval.

Adults: Your dosage will be based on your doctor's assessment of the degree of underlying heart disease, your age and weight, and the way your kidneys are functioning. The following is a general guide for determining the dose of Procanbid by body weight: 88 to 110 pounds: 1000 milligrams (mg); 132 to 154 pounds: 1500 mg; 176 to 198 pounds: 2000 mg; >220 pounds: 2500 mg

Your dose may be higher or lower, depending on your individual circumstances. Doses are usually taken every 12 hours.

Older people (especially those >50 years) or those with reduced kidney, liver, or heart function, will be prescribed lower doses or take a longer period between doses.

The safety and effectiveness of Procanbid have not been established in children.

How should I take Procanbid?

Take only your prescribed doses of Procanbid; never take more. Swallow Procanbid whole. Do not break or chew the tablet. You may see remnants of the tablet in your stool, since it does not disintegrate following release its active ingredient.

Try not to miss any doses. Skipping doses, changing the intervals between doses, or "making up" missed doses by doubling up later may cause your condition to worsen and may be dangerous.

What should I avoid while taking Procanbid?

Procanbid may cause dizziness, drowsiness, or blurred vision. Use caution when driving, operating machinery, or performing other hazardous activities.

Avoid the use of alcohol. Alcohol may decrease the effects of Procanbid.

What are possible food and drug interactions associated with Procanbid?

If Procanbid is taken with certain other drugs, the effects of either could be increased, decreased, or altered. It is especially important to check with your doctor before combining Procanbid with alcohol or with the following: amiodarone, antiarrhythmics such as quinidine and mexiletine, cimetidine, drugs that ease muscle spasms, lidocaine, ranitidine, trimethoprim

What are the possible side effects of Procanbid?

Side effects cannot be anticipated. If any develop or change in intensity, tell your doctor as soon as possible. Only your doctor can determine if it is safe for you to continue taking this drug.

Side effects may include: abdominal pain, bitter taste, blood disorders, chest pain, chills, diarrhea, dizziness, fever, flushing, giddiness, hallucinations, hives, itching, joint pain or inflammation, loss of appetite, low blood pressure, mental depression, muscle pain, nausea, rash, skin lesions, swelling, vague feeling of illness, vomiting, weakness

Can I receive Procanbid if I am pregnant or breastfeeding?
The effects of Procanbid during pregnancy are unknown. Tell your doctor immediately if you are pregnant, or plan to become pregnant. Procanbid appears in breast milk and may affect a nursing infant. If Procanbid is essential to your health, your doctor may advise you to discontinue breastfeeding until your treatment is finished.

What should I do if I miss a dose of Procanbid?
Take it as soon as you remember. If it is almost time for your next dose, skip the one you missed and go back to your regular schedule. Never take 2 doses at the same time.

How should I store Procanbid?
Store at room temperature in a tightly closed container, away from heat, light, and moisture.

PROCARDIA
Generic name: Nifedipine

What is Procardia?
Procardia and Procardia XL are used to treat angina. Procardia XL is also used to treat high blood pressure. Procardia and Procardia XL are calcium channel blockers, drugs that help the heart work better by relaxing the muscles in the walls of the arteries, allowing them to dilate. This improves blood flow through the heart and throughout the body, reduces blood pressure, and helps prevent angina. Procardia XL is taken once a day and provides a steady rate of medication over a 24-hour period.

What is the most important information I should know about Procardia?
Procardia XL controls blood pressure; it does not cure high blood pressure. If you have high blood pressure, take Procardia XL regularly. Since blood pressure declines gradually, it may be several weeks before you get the full benefit of Procardia XL. Continue taking the medication even if you are feeling well.

Procardia and Procardia XL may cause your blood pressure to become too low, which may make you feel light-headed or faint. Your doctor should check your blood pressure when you start taking Procardia or Procardia XL and continue monitoring it while your dosage is being adjusted.

Contact your doctor immediately if you experience increased angina (chest pain caused by lack of oxygen to the heart) when you start taking Procardia or Procardia XL, when your dosage is increased, or if you suddenly stop taking beta blockers when beginning Procardia therapy.

Notify your doctor and dentist that you are taking Procardia before you have surgery or dental treatment, or if you have a medical emergency.

Who should not take Procardia?

Procardia should not be used if you have ever had an allergic reaction to it or you are sensitive to it or to other calcium channel blockers. Make sure your doctor is aware of any drug reactions you have experienced.

Do not take Procardia for the first week or two following a heart attack, or if you are in danger of a heart attack.

What should I tell my doctor before I take the first dose of Procardia?

Tell your doctor about all prescription, over-the-counter, and herbal medication you are taking before beginning treatment with Procardia. Also, talk to your doctor about your complete medical history; especially if you have kidney disease, liver disease, stomach or intestinal narrowing, another disease of the heart or blood vessels such as sick sinus syndrome, aortic stenosis (a narrowing of the aortic valve that obstructs blood flow from the heart to the body), heart failure, low blood pressure, or coronary artery disease.

What is the usual dosage?

The information below is based on the dosage guidelines your doctor uses. Depending on your condition and medical history, your doctor may prescribe a different regimen. Do not change the dosage or stop taking your medication without your doctor's approval.

Adults: The usual starting dose of Procardia is one 10 milligram (mg) capsule, 3 times a day. The usual range is 10 to 20 mg 3 times a day. Some people may need 20 to 30 mg, 3 or 4 times a day. Usually you will not take more than 120 mg in a day and should take no more than 180 mg.

The starting dose of Procardia XL is usually a 30 or 60 mg tablet, taken once daily. Your doctor may increase the dose over 1 to 2 weeks if not satisfied with the way the drug is working. Doses above 120 mg per day are not recommended.

Although no serious side effects have been reported when Procardia or Procardia XL is stopped, your doctor will probably have you lower the dose gradually under close supervision.

Children: The safety of Procardia in children has not been established. This drug is not recommended for use in children.

How should I take Procardia?

Take Procardia and Procardia XL exactly as prescribed by your doctor, even if your symptoms have disappeared. Take Procardia XL once a day, the same time each day, with or without food.

Procardia XL tablets are designed to release the medication into your bloodstream slowly. If something that looks like a tablet appears in your stool, this is normal and means that the medication has been released, and the shell that contained the medication has been eliminated from your body.

Procardia and Procardia XL tablets should be swallowed whole. Do not break, crush, or chew. Do not substitute another brand of nifedipine for Procardia or Procardia XL unless your doctor directs.

What should I avoid while taking Procardia?

Do not combine Procardia with grapefruit juice, which can dramatically increase the effect of the drug.

What are possible food and drug interactions associated with Procardia?

If Procardia is taken with certain other drugs, the effects of either could be increased, decreased, or altered. It is especially important to check with your doctor before combining Procardia with the following: cimetidine, digoxin, quinidine

What are the possible side effects of Procardia?

Side effects cannot be anticipated. If any develop or change in intensity, tell your doctor as soon as possible. Only your doctor can determine if it is safe for you to continue taking this drug.

Side effects may include: Constipation, cough, dizziness, fatigue, flushing, giddiness, headache, heartburn, heat sensation, light-headedness, mood changes, muscle cramps, nasal congestion, nausea, sore throat, swelling of arms, legs, hands, and feet, tremors, wheezing

Can I receive Procardia if I am pregnant or breastfeeding?

The effects of Procardia during pregnancy and breastfeeding are unknown. Tell your doctor immediately if you are pregnant, plan to become pregnant, or are breastfeeding.

What should I do if I miss a dose of Procardia?

Take the forgotten dose as soon as you remember. If it is almost time for your next dose, skip the one you missed. Never take 2 doses at the same time.

How should I store Procardia?

Store Procardia at room temperature. Protect from moisture, light, humidity, and excessive heat.

PROMETHAZINE HYDROCHLORIDE

What is Promethazine hydrochloride?

Promethazine is used for relieving allergy symptoms including hives and nasal congestion. It is used to prevent and control pain and nausea during and after surgery. It is also used to help produce light sleep, and for the prevention of motion sickness.

Promethazine is a phenothiazine antihistamine. It works by blocking the sites where histamine acts.

What is the most important information I should know about Promethazine hydrochloride?

Promethazine should not be used in children younger than 2 years old. Serious and sometimes fatal side effects (difficult or slowed breathing, drowsiness leading to coma) have occurred when promethazine has been used in children in this age group. Promethazine should be used with extreme caution in children 2 years of age and older. The lowest effective dose should be used in this age group.

Do not drive or perform other possibly unsafe tasks until you know how you react to promethazine; this drug may cause dizziness, drowsiness, or blurred vision. These effects may be worse if you take it with alcohol or certain medicines.

Do not drink alcohol or use medicines that may cause drowsiness (such as sleep aids and muscle relaxers) while you are using promethazine; it may add to their effects.

Neuroleptic malignant syndrome (NMS) is a possibly fatal syndrome that can be caused by promethazine. Symptoms may include fever; stiff muscles; confusion; abnormal thinking; fast or irregular heartbeat; and sweating. Contact your doctor at once if you have any of these symptoms.

Promethazine may cause you to become sunburned more easily. Avoid the sun, sunlamps, or tanning booths until you know how you react to promethazine. Use sunscreen or wear protective clothing if you must be outside for more than a short time.

Promethazine should be used with caution in patients who have seizures or are on other medications which may lower seizure threshold.

Promethazine should be avoided or used with extreme caution in patients with compromised respiratory function (COPD or sleep apnea) due to the risk of serious side effects.

Promethazine should be used with caution in patients with bone marrow suppression due to the risk of serious side effects.

If you experience any involuntary muscle movements report them to your doctor.

Who should not take Promethazine hydrochloride?

Promethazine should not be used in pediatric patients less than 2 years old.

Promethazine is not to be used in patients who have severe central nervous system depression or are in a coma. Do not use promethazine in individuals known to be hypersensitive or to have had allergic reaction to other phenothiazines.

Antihistamines are not for use in the treatment of lower respiratory tract symptoms including asthma.

What should I tell my doctor before I take the first dose of Promethazine hydrochloride?

Tell your doctor about all prescription, over-the-counter, and herbal medication you are taking before beginning treatment with promethazine. Also, talk to your doctor about your complete medical history, especially if you have nervous system problems, bone marrow depression, heart problems, low blood pressure, blood disease, glaucoma, increased eye pressure, liver problems, prostate problems, Parkinson's disease, seizures, Reye's syndrome, or if you consume large amounts of alcohol.

What is the usual dosage?

The information below is based on the dosage guidelines your doctor uses. Depending on your condition and medical history, your doctor may prescribe a different regimen. Do not change the dosage or stop taking your medication without your doctor's approval.

Allergy
Adults: The average oral dose is 25 mg taken before going to sleep; however, 12.5 mg may be taken before meals and before going to sleep, if necessary. Single 25-mg doses at bedtime or 6.25 to 12.5 mg taken three times daily will usually suffice. After initiation of treatment, dosage should be adjusted to the smallest amount adequate to relieve symptoms. The administration of promethazine in 25-mg doses will control minor transfusion reactions of an allergic nature.

Children 2 years and older: The average oral dose is 25 mg taken before going to sleep; however, 12.5 mg may be taken before meals and before going to sleep, if necessary. Single 25-mg doses at bedtime or 6.25 to 12.5 mg taken three times daily will usually suffice. After initiation of treatment, dosage should be adjusted to the smallest amount adequate to relieve symptoms. The administration of promethazine in 25-mg doses will control minor transfusion reactions of an allergic nature.

Motion Sickness
Adults: The average adult dose is 25 mg taken twice daily. The initial dose should be taken one-half to one hour before anticipated travel and be repeated 8 to 12 hours later, if necessary. On succeeding days of travel, it

is recommended that 25 mg be given at breakfast or when you first wake up and again before the evening meal.

Children 2 years and older: The recommended dose is 12.5 mg to 25 mg twice daily. The initial dose should be taken one-half to one hour before anticipated travel and be repeated 8 to 12 hours later, if necessary. On the succeeding days of travel, the total daily dose should be given in 2 divided doses; one at breakfast or when the child first awakes and the other before the evening meal.

Nausea and Vomiting

Adults: The average effective dose of promethazine for the active therapy of nausea and vomiting is 25 mg. When oral medication cannot be tolerated, the dose should be given by injection (cf. promethazine injection) or by rectal suppository. Doses of 12.5- to 25-mg may be repeated, as necessary, at 4- to 6-hour intervals. For prevention of nausea and vomiting, during surgery and the postoperative period, the average dose is 25 mg repeated at 4- to 6-hour intervals, as necessary.

Children 2 years and older: The usual dose is 0.5 mg per pound of body weight, and the dose should be adjusted to the age and weight of the patient and the severity of the condition being treated. Antiemetics should not be used in vomiting of unknown cause in children and adolescents.

Pre- and Postoperative Use

Adults: Promethazine in 50-mg doses for adults the night before surgery relieves apprehension and produces a quiet sleep. Usual adult dosage of promethazine is 50 mg with an appropriately reduced dose of narcotic, barbiturate, and the required amount of a belladonna alkaloid. Postoperative sedation and adjunctive use with analgesics may be obtained by the administration of 25- to 50-mg doses in adults.

Children 2 years and older: Promethazine in 12.5- to 25-mg doses for children the night before surgery relieves apprehension and produces a quiet sleep.

For preoperative medication, children require doses of 0.5 mg per pound of body weight in combination with an appropriately reduced dose of narcotic, barbiturate, and appropriate dose of an atropine-like drug. Postoperative sedation and adjunctive use with analgesics may be obtained by the administration of 12.5mg to 25 mg of promethazine in children.

Sedation

Adults: This product relieves apprehension and induces a quiet sleep from which the patient can be easily aroused. Adults usually require 25 to 50 mg for nighttime, pre-surgical, or obstetrical sedation.

Children 2 years and older: This product relieves apprehension and induces a quiet sleep from which the patient can be easily aroused. Administration of 12.5 to 25 mg promethazine by the oral route or by rectal suppository at bedtime will provide sedation in children.

How should I take Promethazine hydrochloride?

Promethazine is taken by mouth with or without food daily. If stomach upset occurs, take this medication with food to reduce stomach irritation. If you are using promethazine for motion sickness, take your first dose at least 30 to 60 minutes before you begin travel; your second dose should be repeated 8 to 12 hours later, if necessary.

What should I avoid while taking Promethazine hydrochloride?

Promethazine should not be used in children younger than 2 years old.

Do not drive or perform other possibly unsafe tasks until you know how you react to promethazine; this drug may cause dizziness, drowsiness, or blurred vision.

Do not drink alcohol or use medicines that may cause drowsiness (such as sleep aids and muscle relaxers) while you are using promethazine; it may add to their effects.

Avoid the sun, sunlamps, or tanning booths until you know how you react to promethazine. Promethazine may cause you to become sunburned more easily. Use sunscreen or wear protective clothing if you must be outside for more than a short time.

What are possible food and drug interactions associated with Promethazine hydrochloride?

If promethazine is taken with certain other drugs, the effects of either could be increased, decreased, or altered. It is especially important to check with your doctor before combining promethazine with the following: angiotensin-converting enzyme (ACE) inhibitors such as enalapril, astemizole, bromocriptine, charcoal, cisapride, epinephrine, haloperidol, levodopa, lithium, meperidine, methyldopa, monoamine oxidase inhibitors (MAOIs) such as phenelzine, naltrexone, pergolide, polypeptide antibiotics such as actinomycin, terfenadine, thiopental, tramadol, and trazodone.

What are the possible side effects of Promethazine hydrochloride?

Side effects cannot be anticipated. If any develop or change in intensity, tell your doctor as soon as possible. Only your doctor can determine if it is safe for you to continue taking this drug.

Side effects may include: dizziness; drowsiness; dry mouth; increased or decreased blood pressure; nausea; occasional blurred vision; rash; sleepiness; vomiting; sensitivity to light; uncontrolled muscle movements; yellowing of skin or eyes; severe allergic reactions (rash; hives; itching; difficulty breathing; tightness in the chest; swelling of the mouth, face, lips or tongue)

Neuroleptic malignant syndrome (NMS) is a possibly fatal syndrome that can be caused by promethazine. Symptoms may include fever; stiff muscles; confusion; abnormal thinking; fast or irregular heartbeat; and sweating. Contact your doctor at once if you have any of these symptoms.

Can I receive Promethazine hydrochloride if I am pregnant or breastfeeding?

If you become pregnant, contact your doctor. You will need to discuss the benefits and risks of using promethazine while you are pregnant. This medication should only be used during pregnancy if the potential benefits outweigh the risks.

Promethazine is found in breast milk. If you are or will be breastfeeding while you use promethazine, check with your doctor. Discuss any possible risks to your baby.

What should I do if I miss a dose of Promethazine hydrochloride?

If you miss a dose of promethazine and you are using it regularly, take it as soon as possible. If it is almost time for your next dose, skip the missed dose and go back to you regular dosing schedule. Do not take 2 doses at once.

If you are using promethazine on a need only basis, skip the missed dose.

How should I store Promethazine hydrochloride?

Store this medicine at room temperature, away from heat, moisture, and light. Do not store in the bathroom.

Propafenone hydrochloride *See Rythmol, page 1173.*

PROMETHAZINE HYDROCHLORIDE AND CODEINE PHOSPHATE

What is Promethazine hydrochloride and codeine phosphate?

Promethazine, when combined with codeine, is used to relieve coughs and other symptoms of allergies and the common cold, including hives and nasal congestion. Promethazine is a phenothiazine antihistamine. It works by blocking the sites where histamine acts. Codeine, a narcotic analgesic, helps relieve pain and stops coughing.

What is the most important information I should know about Promethazine hydrochloride and codeine phosphate?

This product should not be used in children younger than 16 years old. Serious and sometimes fatal side effects (difficult or slowed breathing, drowsiness leading to coma) have occurred when promethazine has been used in children.

Do not drive or perform other possibly unsafe tasks until you know how you react to this medicaton; this drug may cause dizziness, drowsiness, or blurred vision. These effects may be worse if you take it with alcohol or certain medicines.

Do not drink alcohol or use medicines that may cause drowsiness (such as sleep aids and muscle relaxers) while you are using this drug; it may add to their effects.

Neuroleptic malignant syndrome (NMS) is a possibly fatal syndrome that can be caused by promethazine. Symptoms may include fever; stiff muscles; confusion; abnormal thinking; fast or irregular heartbeat; and sweating. Contact your doctor at once if you have any of these symptoms.

Promethazine may cause you to become sunburned more easily. Avoid the sun, sunlamps, or tanning booths until you know how you react to promethazine. Use sunscreen or wear protective clothing if you must be outside for more than a short time.

Promethazine should be used with caution in patients who have seizures or are on other medications which may lower seizure threshold.

Promethazine should be avoided or used with extreme caution in patients with compromised respiratory function (COPD or sleep apnea) due to the risk of serious side effects.

Promethazine should be used with caution in patients with bone marrow suppression due to the risk of serious side effects.

If you experience any involuntary muscle movements report them to your doctor.

It is possible to develop psychological and physical dependence on codeine. Although the likelihood of this is quite low with oral codeine, be cautious if you have a history of drug abuse or dependence.

Never take more cough syrup than has been prescribed. If your cough does not seem better within 5 days, check back with your doctor.

Who should not take Promethazine hydrochloride and codeine phosphate?

This product should not be used in pediatric patients less than 16 years old.

Promethazine is not to be used in patients who have severe central nervous system depression or are in a coma. Do not use this medication if you have a known hypersensitivity or allergic reaction to phenothiazines or codeine.

Antihistamines are not for use in the treatment of lower respiratory tract symptoms including asthma.

What should I tell my doctor before I take the first dose of Promethazine hydrochloride and codeine phosphate?

Tell your doctor about all prescription, over-the-counter, and herbal medication you are taking before beginning treatment with promethazine.

Also, talk to your doctor about your complete medical history, especially if you have nervous system problems, bone marrow depression, heart problems, low blood pressure, blood disease, glaucoma, increased eye pressure, liver problems, prostate problems, Parkinson's disease, seizures, Reye's syndrome, or if you consume large amounts of alcohol.

What is the usual dosage?
The information below is based on the dosage guidelines your doctor uses. Depending on your condition and medical history, your doctor may prescribe a different regimen. Do not change the dosage or stop taking your medication without your doctor's approval.

Adults and adolescents 16 years and older: The usual dosage is 1 teaspoon (5 milliliters) every 4 to 6 hours, not to exceed 6 teaspoons, or 30 milliliters, in 24 hours.

How should I take Promethazine hydrochloride and codeine phosphate?
Take with or without food, exactly as prescribed by your doctor.

What should I avoid while taking Promethazine hydrochloride and codeine phosphate?
Do not drive or perform other possibly unsafe tasks until you know how you react to this medication; this drug may cause dizziness, drowsiness, or blurred vision.

Do not drink alcohol or use medicines that may cause drowsiness (such as sleep aids and muscle relaxers) while you are using this medication; it may add to their effects.

Avoid the sun, sunlamps, or tanning booths until you know how you react to promethazine. Promethazine may cause you to become sunburned more easily. Use sunscreen or wear protective clothing if you must be outside for more than a short time.

What are possible food and drug interactions associated with Promethazine hydrochloride and codeine phosphate?
If this product is taken with certain other drugs, the effects of either could be increased, decreased, or altered. It is especially important to check with your doctor before combining it with the following: alcohol, angiotensin-converting enzyme (ACE) inhibitors such as enalapril, antidepressants, astemizole, bromocriptine, charcoal, cisapride, epinephrine, haloperidol, levodopa, lithium, meperidine, methyldopa, monoamine oxidase inhibitors (MAOIs) such as phenelzine, naltrexone, narcotic pain relievers, pergolide, polypeptide antibiotics such as actinomycin, terfenadine, thiopental, tramadol, trazodone, sedatives, and tranquilers.

What are the possible side effects of Promethazine hydrochloride and codeine phosphate?

Side effects cannot be anticipated. If any develop or change in intensity, tell your doctor as soon as possible. Only your doctor can determine if it is safe for you to continue taking this drug.

Side effects may include: constipation, dizziness; drowsiness; dry mouth; increased or decreased blood pressure; nausea; occasional blurred vision; rash; sleepiness; vomiting; sensitivity to light; uncontrolled muscle movements; yellowing of skin or eyes; severe allergic reactions (rash; hives; itching; difficulty breathing; tightness in the chest; swelling of the mouth, face, lips or tongue)

Neuroleptic malignant syndrome (NMS) is a possibly fatal syndrome that can be caused by promethazine. Symptoms may include fever; stiff muscles; confusion; abnormal thinking; fast or irregular heartbeat; and sweating. Contact your doctor at once if you have any of these symptoms.

Can I receive Promethazine hydrochloride and codeine phosphate if I am pregnant or breastfeeding?

If you become pregnant, contact your doctor. You will need to discuss the benefits and risks of using this product while you are pregnant. This medication should only be used during pregnancy if the potential benefits outweigh the risks. This drug appears in breast milk; talk to your doctor if you plan on breastfeeding.

What should I do if I miss a dose of Promethazine hydrochloride and codeine phosphate?

If you miss a dose, take it as soon as possible. If it is almost time for your next dose, skip the missed dose and go back to you regular dosing schedule. Do not take 2 doses at once.

How should I store Promethazine hydrochloride and codeine phosphate?

Store at room temperature, away from heat, moisture, and light. Do not store in the bathroom.

PROPECIA

Generic name: Finasteride

What is Propecia?

Propecia treats baldness in men with mild to moderate hair loss on the top of the head and the front of the midscalp area (male-pattern baldness). It increases hair growth, improves hair regrowth, and slows down hair loss. It works only on scalp hair and does not affect hair on other parts of the body.

Propecia is a low-dose form of Proscar, a drug prescribed for prostate enlargement.

What is the most important information I should know about Propecia?

Propecia is NOT to be used by women. Taken during pregnancy, Propecia may cause abnormal development of a baby's organs. Women who may be pregnant should avoid handling a crushed or broken Propecia tablet.

Propecia lowers readings of the prostate-specific antigen (PSA) screening test for prostate cancer. If you're scheduled to have your PSA level checked, make sure the doctor knows you're taking Propecia.

Who should not take Propecia?

Women should not take Propecia and should avoid handling Propecia if there is a chance that they may be pregnant.

Do not use Propecia if it gives you an allergic reaction, or if you've had an allergic reaction to Proscar.

What should I tell my doctor before I take the first dose of Propecia?

Tell your doctor about all prescription, over-the-counter, and herbal medications you are taking before beginning treatment with Propecia. Also, talk to your doctor about your complete medical history, especially if you have liver problems.

What is the usual dosage?

The information below is based on the dosage guidelines your doctor uses. Depending on your condition and medical history, your doctor may prescribe a different regimen. Do not change the dosage or stop taking your medication without your doctor's approval.

Adult men: The recommended dosage, for men only, is 1 milligram tablet daily.

Propecia is not approved for use in women or children.

How should I take Propecia?

For maximum benefit, take Propecia regularly once a day. It can be taken with or without food.

What should I avoid while taking Propecia?

There are no restrictions on food, beverages, or activities during treatment with finasteride unless your doctor directs otherwise.

What are possible food and drug interactions associated with Propecia?

No significant drug interactions have been reported.

What are the possible side effects of Propecia?

Side effects cannot be anticipated. If any develop or change in intensity, tell your doctor as soon as possible. Only your doctor can determine if it is safe for you to continue taking this drug.

Side effects may include: decreased amount of semen per ejaculation, decreased sex drive, impotence

Can I receive Propecia if I am pregnant or breastfeeding?

Propecia is not for use in pregnant or breastfeeding women. Women should not handle crushed or broken Propecia tablets when they are pregnant or may be pregnant because of the possibility of absorption of Propecia and the subsequent potential risk to a male fetus.

What should I do if I miss a dose of Propecia?

Take it as soon as you remember. If it is almost time for your next dose, skip the dose you missed and go back to your regular schedule. Do not take 2 doses at the same time.

How should I store Propecia?

Store at room temperature in a closed container away from moisture.

Propoxyphene napsylate and acetaminophen

See Darvocet-N, page 375.

PROPRANOLOL HYDROCHLORIDE

What is Propranolol hydrochloride?

Propranolol is used alone or in combination with other drugs to treat high blood pressure. It is also used to treat angina pectoris (chest pain usually caused by lack of oxygen to the heart due to clogged arteries), changes in heart rhythm, familial or hereditary essential tremor (involuntary, rhythmic movements, usually limited to the arms), hypertrophic aortic stenosis (a condition related to exertion-related angina), and tumors of the adrenal gland.

Propranolol is also used to prevent migraine headaches and to reduce the risk of dying after a severe heart attack.

What is the most important information I should know about Propranolol hydrochloride?

Do not suddenly stop taking propranolol without speaking to your doctor. Worsening of chest pain, and in some cases, heart attacks have been reported.

If you have high blood pressure, you must take propranolol regularly to be effective. Since blood pressure declines gradually, it may be several weeks before you get the full benefit of propranolol. You must continue taking it even if you are feeling well. Propranolol does not cure high blood pressure; it only keeps it under control.

Who should not take Propranolol hydrochloride?
Do not use propranolol if you are sensitive to the drug, or have asthma, inadequate blood supply to the circulatory system (cardiogenic shock), certain types of irregular heartbeat, a slow heartbeat, or chronic heart failure.

What should I tell my doctor before
I take the first dose of Propranolol hydrochloride?
Tell your doctor about all prescription, over-the-counter, and herbal medications you are taking before beginning treatment with propranolol. Also, talk to your doctor about your complete medical history, especially if you have chronic heart failure, diabetes, an overactive thyroid, certain types of irregular heartbeat, kidney or liver disease, tumors of the adrenal gland, asthma, or are scheduled for major surgery.

What is the usual dosage?
The information below is based on the dosage guidelines your doctor uses. Depending on your condition and medical history, your doctor may prescribe a different regimen. Do not change the dosage or stop taking your medication without your doctor's approval.

High Blood Pressure
Adults: The usual starting dose is 40 milligrams (mg) 2 times daily. This dose may be in combination with a diuretic. The usual maintenance dose is 120 to 240 mg per day. In some cases, a dose of 640 mg per day may be needed.

Chest Pain
Adults: The usual total daily dose is 80 to 320 mg divided into 2 to 4 smaller doses a day.

Irregular Heartbeat
Adults: The recommended dose is 10 to 30 mg 3 to 4 times daily before meals and at bedtime.

Heart Attack
Adults: The initial dose is 40 mg 3 times daily. After 1 month, the dose may be increased to 60 to 80 mg 3 times a day, as tolerated.

Migraine
Adults: The initial dose is 80 mg daily divided into smaller doses. The dosage may be increased gradually to achieve best results. The usual effective dose range is 160 to 240 mg per day. If you do not respond to the maximum dose of 240 mg after 4 to 6 weeks, propranolol should be stopped gradually over a period of several weeks.

Tremors
Adults: The initial dose is 40 mg 2 times daily. Best results are achieved with a dose of 120 mg per day, although it may be necessary to take 240 to 320 mg per day.

Hypertrophic Subaortic Stenosis
Adults: The usual dose is 20 to 40 mg 3 to 4 times daily before meals and at bedtime.

Before Adrenal Gland Surgery
Adults: The usual dose is 60 mg daily divided into smaller doses for 3 days before surgery in combination with an alpha-blocker drug.

Inoperable Tumors
Adults: The usual dose is 30 mg daily divided into smaller doses in combination with an alpha-blocking drug.

How should I take Propranolol hydrochloride?
Take propranolol at the same time every day, with or without food.

Do not crush, chew, break, or open the long-acting or extended-release capsules. Swallow capsules whole.

What should I avoid while taking Propranolol hydrochloride?
Avoid driving, operating machinery, or performing other hazardous activities until you know how this medication affects you. Propranolol may cause drowsiness, dizziness, and blood pressure changes.

What are possible food and drug interactions associated with Propranolol hydrochloride?
If propranolol is taken with certain other drugs, the effects of either could be increased, decreased, or altered. It is especially important to check with your doctor before combining propranolol with the following: adrenocorticotropic hormone, alcohol, amiodarone, antiarrhythmic drugs (such as lidocaine, propafenone, or quinidine), antidepressants(such as fluoxetine, fluvoxamine, and paroxetine), calcium-blocking blood pressure drugs (such as nicardipine, nifedipine, and nisoldipine), cigarette smoking, chlorpromazine, cholesterol-lowering drugs (such as cholestyramine or colestipol), cimetidine, ciprofloxacin, diazepam, fluconazole, HIV drugs (such as delavirdine or ritonavir), imipramine, isoniazid, phenobarbital, phenytoin, rifampin, rizatriptan, tenioposide, theophylline, thioridazine, tolbutamide, warfarin, zileuton, and zolmitriptan.

What are the possible side effects of Propranolol hydrochloride?
Side effects cannot be anticipated. If any develop or change in intensity, tell your doctor as soon as possible. Only your doctor can determine if it is safe for you to continue taking this drug.

Side effects may include: allergic reactions, chronic heart failure, depression, lightheadedness, low blood pressure, nausea, slow heartbeat

Can I receive Propranolol hydrochloride if I am pregnant or breastfeeding?
The effects of propranolol during pregnancy and breastfeeding are unknown. Tell your doctor immediately if you are pregnant, plan to become pregnant, or are breastfeeding.

What should I do if I miss a dose of Propranolol hydrochloride?
Take it as soon as you remember. If it is within a couple hours of your next scheduled dose, skip the one you missed and go back to your regular schedule. Never take 2 doses at the same time.

How should I store Propranolol hydrochloride?
Store at room temperature in a tightly closed, light-resistant container. Protect from freezing or excessive heat.

PROQUIN XR
Generic name: Ciprofloxacin hydrochloride

What is Proquin XR?
Proquin XR is an antibiotic in the class known as quinolones that is used to treat adults with uncomplicated urinary tract infections (also known as bladder infections) caused by bacteria.

What is the most important information I should know about Proquin XR?
Proquin XR is only used to treat bacterial infections and will not work if taken for a viral infection, such as a common cold.

Skipping doses or not completing the full course of Proquin XR therapy may decrease the effectiveness of the treatment and increase the likelihood that bacteria will develop resistance. If the bacteria develop resistance, they may not be treatable by Proquin XR or other antibacterial drugs in the future.

Fluoroquinolones, including Proquin XR, are associated with an increased risk of tendonitis (inflammation or irritation of a tendon) and tendon rupture in all ages. The risk is greater in older patients, usually >60 years of age, in patients taking corticosteroid drugs, and in patients with kidney, heart and lung transplants.

Who should not take Proquin XR?
Do not take Proquin XR if you are allergic to, or have ever had a severe reaction to, ciprofloxacin or to any other quinolone antibiotics.

What should I tell my doctor before I take the first dose of Proquin XR?

Tell your doctor about all prescription, over-the-counter, and herbal medications you are taking before beginning treatment with Proquin XR. Also, talk to your doctor about your complete medical history, especially if you have or ever had seizures (epilepsy), asthma, or liver or kidney problems.

What is the usual dosage?

The information below is based on the dosage guidelines your doctor uses. Depending on your condition and medical history, your doctor may prescribe a different regimen. Do not change the dosage or stop taking your medication without your doctor's approval.

Adults: Proquin XR should be taken once a day for 3 days shortly after a main meal of the day, preferably the evening meal. Proquin XR does not work as well if you take it without a meal. Your exact dosage of this medication will be prescribed by your doctor.

How should I take Proquin XR?

Take Proquin XR at least 4 hours before or 2 hours after antacids containing magnesium or aluminum, sucralfate, didanosine, chewable/buffered tablets or pediatric powder, metal cations such as iron, and multivitamin preparations containing zinc.

You should try to take Proquin XR at about the same time each day.

What should I avoid while taking Proquin XR?

Do not crush, split or chew Proquin XR tablets. Also, avoid taking this drug with dairy products.

What are possible food and drug interactions associated with Proquin XR?

If Proquin XR is taken with certain other drugs, the effects of either could be increased, decreased, or altered. It is especially important to check with your doctor before combining Proquin XR with the following: antacids or vitamins that contain magnesium, calcium, aluminum, iron, or zinc, chewable buffered tablets or pediatric powder, dairy products, didanosine, glyburide, phenytoin, sucralfate, warfarin

What are the possible side effects of Proquin XR?

Side effects cannot be anticipated. If any develop or change in intensity, tell your doctor as soon as possible. Only your doctor can determine if it is safe for you to continue taking this drug.

Side effects may include: diarrhea, dizziness, headache, nausea, stomach pain, vaginal yeast infection

Can I receive Proquin XR if I am pregnant or breastfeeding?

The effects of Proquin XR during pregnancy and breastfeeding are unknown. Talk with your doctor before taking this drug if you are pregnant, plan to become pregnant, or are breastfeeding.

What should I do if I miss a dose of Proquin XR?

If you miss a dose, take it as soon as you remember. If it is close to the time of your next dose, skip it and resume your scheduled dose. Do not take 2 doses at once.

How should I store Proquin XR?

Store at room temperature away from heat and direct light.

PROSCAR

Generic name: Finasteride

What is Proscar?

Proscar is prescribed to treat benign prostatic hyperplasia (BPH), an enlarged prostate gland. Proscar is used to shrink an enlarged prostate, which can lead to a gradual improvement in urine flow and symptoms.

What is the most important information I should know about Proscar?

Pregnant women and those who may be pregnant should not use Proscar and should avoid handling a crushed or broken Proscar tablet, because the active ingredient may be absorbed through the skin. Contact with the active ingredient in Proscar may cause the male baby to be born with abnormalities of the sex organs.

Proscar is not a treatment for prostate cancer. See your doctor regularly while taking Proscar. Promptly report any changes in your breasts such as lumps, pain or nipple discharge.

Who should not take Proscar?

Pregnant women and those who may be pregnant should avoid Proscar.

Do not take Proscar if you are sensitive to it or have ever had an allergic reaction to it.

What should I tell my doctor before I take the first dose of Proscar?

Tell your doctor about all prescription, over-the-counter, and herbal medication you are taking before beginning treatment with Proscar. Also, talk to your doctor about your complete medical history, especially if you have liver disease.

What is the usual dosage?

The information below is based on the dosage guidelines your doctor uses. Depending on your condition and medical history, your doctor may prescribe a different regimen. Do not change the dosage or stop taking your medication without your doctor's approval.

Adults: The recommended dosage, for men only, is one 5 milligram tablet per day.

Children: Proscar is not indicated for use in children.

How should I take Proscar?

You may take Proscar either with a meal or between meals.

What should I avoid while taking Proscar?

There are no restrictions on food, beverages, or activities during treatment with Proscar unless your doctor directs otherwise.

What are possible food and drug interactions associated with Proscar?

No significant drug interactions have been reported.

What are the possible side effects of Proscar?

Side effects cannot be anticipated. If any develop or change in intensity, tell your doctor as soon as possible. Only your doctor can determine if it is safe for you to continue taking this drug.

Side effects may include: Decreased amount of semen per ejaculation, decreased sex drive, impotence

Can I receive Proscar if I am pregnant or breastfeeding?

Proscar is not indicated for use in women. Pregnant women and those who may be pregnant should avoid touching the active ingredient in Proscar.

What should I do if I miss a dose of Proscar?

Take it as soon as you remember. If it is almost time for your next dose, skip the one you missed and go back to your regular schedule. Never take 2 doses at the same time.

How should I store Proscar?

Store at room temperature in a tightly closed container. Protect from light.

PROTONIX

Generic name: Pantoprazole

What is Protonix?

Protonix is used to treat and maintain healing of erosive acid reflux disease, also known as erosive GERD (breaks in the lining of the esophagus) and to relieve associated symptoms that may include frequent and persistent heartburn and stomach acid backup. Protonix reduces the amount of acid your stomach produces

Protonix is also prescribed to maintain healing and to prevent a relapse of GERD. It is also used in the treatment of conditions marked by constant overproduction of stomach acid, such as Zollinger-Ellison syndrome.

What is the most important information I should know about Protonix?

Swallow Protonix tablets whole. Do not crush, chew, or split the tablets. They are formulated to release the medication slowly in the body.

Who should not take Protonix?

Do not take Protonix if you are allergic to the medication or any or its ingredients.

What should I tell my doctor before I take the first dose of Protonix?

Tell your doctor about all prescription, over-the-counter, and herbal medications you are taking before beginning treatment with Protonix. Also, talk to your doctor about your complete medical history, especially if you have liver disease.

What is the usual dosage?

The information below is based on the dosage guidelines your doctor uses. Depending on your condition and medical history, your doctor may prescribe a different regimen. Do not change the dosage or stop taking your medication without your doctor's approval.

Erosive Esophagitis
Adults: The usual dose is 40 milligrams (mg) once a day for up to 8 weeks. If your esophagus hasn't healed in that time, your doctor may prescribe an additional 8-week course of therapy. The same dose is used to maintain healing.

Zollinger-Ellison Syndrome (Overproduction of Stomach Acid)
Adults: The usual starting dose is 40 mg twice a day. The doctor may increase the dose if necessary. Doses as high as 240 mg per day have been used. Treatment may continue for years.

The safety and effectiveness of Protonix in children has not been established.

How should I take Protonix?
Protonix may be taken with or without food. Do not chew, crush, or split the delayed-release tablets. If patients are unable to swallow a 40-mg tablet, two 20-mg tablets may be taken.

Protonix Delayed-Release Oral Suspension should be administered in applesauce or apple juice approximately 30 minutes prior to a meal. To administer with applesauce, open packet and sprinkle intact granules on 1 teaspoonful of applesauce. Swallow within 10 minutes of preparation.

To administer in apple juice, open packet, empty intact granules into a small cup containing 5 mL of apple juice (approximately 1 teaspoonful). Stir for 5 seconds and swallow immediately. To ensure complete delivery of the dose, rinse the container once or twice with apple juice to remove any remaining granules and swallow immediately.

What should I avoid while taking Protonix?
There are no restrictions on food, beverages, or activity while taking Protonix, unless otherwise directed by your doctor.

What are possible food and drug interactions associated with Protonix?
If Protonix is taken with certain other drugs, the effects of either could be increased, decreased, or altered. It is especially important to check with your doctor before combining Protonix with ampicillin, iron, ketoconazole, or warfarin.

What are the possible side effects of Protonix?
Side effects cannot be anticipated. If any develop or change in intensity, tell your doctor as soon as possible. Only your doctor can determine if it is safe for you to continue taking this drug.

Side effects may include: abdominal pain, diarrhea, gas, headache, rash

Can I receive Protonix if I am pregnant or breastfeeding?
The effects of Protonix during pregnancy are unknown. Tell your doctor immediately if you are pregnant, or plan to become pregnant. There is a possibility that Protonix may appear in breast milk, causing serious side effects in the nursing infant. If you have to take the drug, you should not plan on breastfeeding.

What should I do if I miss a dose of Protonix?
Take it as soon as you remember. If it is almost time for your next dose, skip the one you missed and go back to your regular schedule. Never take 2 doses at once.

How should I store Protonix?
Store Protonix at room temperature.

Protriptyline hydrochloride See *Vivactil, page 1402.*

PROVENTIL HFA
Generic name: Albuterol sulfate

What is Proventil HFA?
Proventil HFA is used to treat and prevent wheezing and shortness of breath brought about by breathing problems such as asthma. It is also used in the prevention of exercise-induced asthma. Proventil HFA relaxes muscles in the airways to improve breathing.

What is the most important information I should know about Proventil HFA?
Increasing the number of doses of Proventil can be dangerous and may actually worsen asthma symptoms. Do not take Proventil more frequently than your doctor recommends.

   If the dose your doctor recommends does not provide relief of your symptoms, or if your symptoms become worse, consult your doctor immediately.

Who should not take Proventil HFA?
Do not take Proventil if you are allergic to the medication or any or its ingredients.

What should I tell my doctor before I take the first dose of Proventil HFA?
Tell your doctor about all prescription, over-the-counter, and herbal medications you are taking before beginning treatment with Proventil. Also, talk to your doctor about your complete medical history, especially if you have a heart condition, seizure disorder, high blood pressure, abnormal heartbeat, overactive thyroid gland, or diabetes.

What is the usual dosage?
The information below is based on the dosage guidelines your doctor uses. Depending on your condition and medical history, your doctor may prescribe a different regimen. Do not change the dosage or stop taking your medication without your doctor's approval.

Adults and children >4 years: For treatment of acute episodes of bronchospasm or prevention of asthmatic symptoms, the usual dosage for adults and children >4 years is 2 inhalations repeated every 4 to 6 hours.

How should I take Proventil HFA?
Speak with your doctor about the correct way to use the Proventil HFA inhaler and refer to the detailed instructions the accompanied the drug.

   As with all aerosol medications, it is recommended to prime the inhaler before using for the first time and in cases where the inhaler has not been used for more than 2 weeks. Prime by releasing 4 "test sprays" into the air, away from your face.

Keeping the plastic mouthpiece clean is extremely important to prevent medication buildup and blockage. The mouthpiece should be washed, shaken to remove excess water and air dried thoroughly at least once a week. The inhaler may stop spraying if not properly cleaned.

The correct amount of medication in each inhalation cannot be assured after 200 actuations, even though the canister is not completely empty. Discard the canister when the labeled number of actuations have been used. Before you reach the specific number of actuations, you should consult your physician to determine whether a refill is needed.

Just as you should not take extra doses without consulting your physician, you also should not stop using Proventil HFA Inhalation Aerosol without consulting your physician.

What should I avoid while taking Proventil HFA?
Avoid puncturing the inhaler.

What are possible food and drug interactions associated with Proventil HFA?
If Proventil is taken with certain other drugs, the effects of either could be increased, decreased, or altered. It is especially important to check with your doctor before combining Proventil with the following: antidepressants classified as MAO inhibitors and tricyclics, beta blockers, digoxin, drugs similar to albuterol and epinephrine, drugs that lower potassium levels, other inhaled medications.

What are the possible side effects of Proventil HFA?
Side effects cannot be anticipated. If any develop or change in intensity, tell your doctor as soon as possible. Only your doctor can determine if it is safe for you to continue taking this drug.

Side effects may include: bronchitis, cough, difficulty in breathing, dizziness, dry mouth, headaches, hives, nausea, nervousness, rash, swelling of mouth and throat, taste sensation on inhalation, throat irritation, tremors

Can I receive Proventil HFA if I am pregnant or breastfeeding?
The effects of Proventil during pregnancy and breastfeeding are unknown. Tell your doctor immediately if you are pregnant, plan to become pregnant, or are breastfeeding.

What should I do if I miss a dose of Proventil HFA?
Take the forgotten dose as soon as you remember; then take any remaining doses for that day at equally spaced intervals. Never take 2 doses at once.

How should I store Proventil HFA?
Proventil should be stored at room temperature.

PROVERA
Generic name: Medroxyprogesterone acetate

What is Provera?
Provera is used to treat menstrual periods that have stopped and abnormal uterine bleeding when these conditions are due to a hormone imbalance and not caused by fibroids or cancer. Provera is also used to reduce the risk of overgrowth of the lining of the uterus in women who are being treated with estrogen.

What is the most important information I should know about Provera?
Vaginal bleeding after menopause may be a warning sign of cancer of the uterus. Your doctor should check any unusual vaginal bleeding to find out the cause.

Do not use estrogens with progestins to prevent heart disease, heart attacks, or strokes. Using estrogens with or without progestins may increase your chance of getting heart attacks, strokes, breast cancer, and blood clots.

Do not use estrogens with progestins to prevent dementia. Using estrogens with or without progestins may increase your risk of dementia.

You and your healthcare provider should talk regularly about whether you still need treatment with Provera.

Who should not take Provera?
Do not take Provera if you have liver disease; a history of known or suspected cancer of the breast or reproductive organs, or hormone-sensitive tumors; unusual vaginal bleeding; history of blood clots in the legs, lungs, eyes, brain, or elsewhere; history of stroke or heart attack; may be having a miscarriage; are allergic to progesterone or any of the ingredients in the tablets; or are pregnant or think you might be pregnant.

Do not use Provera as a test for pregnancy.

What should I tell my doctor before I take the first dose of Provera?
Tell your doctor about all prescription, over-the-counter, and herbal medications you are taking before beginning treatment with Provera. Also, talk to your doctor about your complete medical history, especially if you have asthma (wheezing), epilepsy (seizures), migraine headaches, endometriosis (severe pelvic pain), lupus, problems with your heart, liver, thyroid, or kidneys, or if you have low calcium levels in your blood. Tell

your doctor if you are breastfeeding, or if you are going to have surgery or will be on bed rest.

What is the usual dosage?
The information below is based on the dosage guidelines your doctor uses. Depending on your condition and medical history, your doctor may prescribe a different regimen. Do not change the dosage or stop taking your medication without your doctor's approval.

To Accompany Estrogen Replacement Therapy
Adults: The recommended regimen is 5 or 10 mg of Provera a day for 12 to 14 consecutive days each month, beginning on either Day 1 or Day 16 of your cycle.

Abnormal Uterine Bleeding Due to Hormonal Imbalance
Adults: Beginning on the 16th or 21st day of your menstrual cycle, you will take 5 to 10 mg daily for 5 to 10 days. Make sure you discuss with your doctor what effect this will have on your menstrual cycle. You should have bleeding 3 to 7 days after you stop taking Provera.

To Restore Menstrual Periods
Adults: Provera Tablets are taken in dosages of 5 to 10 milligrams (mg) daily for 5 to 10 days. Make sure you discuss with your doctor what effect this will have on your menstrual cycle. You should have bleeding 3 to 7 days after you stop taking Provera.

The safety and effectiveness of Provera Tablets in children has not been established.

How should I take Provera?
Start at the lowest dose and talk to your healthcare provider about how well that dose is working for you. The lowest effective dose of Provera has not been determined. You and your healthcare provider should talk regularly (every 3-6 months) about your response to Provera and whether you still need treatment.

What should I avoid while taking Provera?
Avoid smoking while taking Provera. Smoking can increase the risk of developing a blood clot.

What are possible food and drug interactions associated with Provera?
If Provera is taken with certain other drugs, the effects of either could be increased, decreased, or altered. It is important to inform your doctor of all medications, vitamins, and herbal supplements you are taking while on Provera.

What are the possible side effects of Provera?

Side effects cannot be anticipated. If any develop or change in intensity, tell your doctor as soon as possible. Only your doctor can determine if it is safe for you to continue taking this drug.

Side effects may include: breast tenderness, breast milk secretion, breakthrough bleeding or spotting (minor vaginal bleeding), irregular periods, absence of menstrual periods, vaginal secretions, headache, nervousness, dizziness, depression, insomnia, sleepiness, fatigue, premenstrual syndrome-like symptoms, thrombophlebitis (inflammation cause by blood clots), itching, hives, skin rash, acne, hair loss, hair growth, abdominal discomfort, nausea, bloating, fever, increase in weight, swelling, changes in vision and sensitivity to contact lenses

These are not all the possible side effects of Provera. For more information, ask your healthcare provider or pharmacist.

Can I receive Provera if I am pregnant or breastfeeding?

You should not take Provera during pregnancy. If you are pregnant or plan to become pregnant, tell your doctor immediately. There is an increased risk of minor birth defects in children whose mothers take this drug during the first 4 months of pregnancy.

Provera appears in breast milk. Do not take this medication without first talking to your doctor if you are breast-feeding a baby.

What should I do if I miss a dose of Provera?

Take it as soon as you remember. If it is almost time for your next dose, skip the one you missed and resume your regular schedule. Never take 2 doses at the same time.

How should I store Provera?

Store at room temperature.

PROVIGIL

Generic name: Modafinil

What is Provigil?

Provigil is used to treat narcolepsy, obstructive sleep apnea/hypopnea syndrome, and shift work sleep disorder.

What is the most important information I should know about Provigil?

Provigil may cause a rash or a serious allergic reaction. Stop Provigil and call your doctor right away or get emergency treatment if you have any of the following: skin rash or skin that blisters and peels; hives; sores in your mouth; swelling of your face, eyes, lips, tongue, or throat; trouble swallowing or breathing; or hoarse voice.

Provigil is not approved for use in children.

Provigil is a controlled substance because it can be abused or lead to dependence. Keep Provigil in a safe place to prevent misuse and abuse.

Who should not take Provigil?
Do not take Provigil if you are allergic to any of its ingredients.

It is not known if Provigil is safe for children under the age of 16. Reduced levels of white blood cells (cells that fight infections) have occurred in some children who have taken Provigil.

What should I tell my doctor before I take the first dose of Provigil?
Tell your doctor about all prescription, over-the-counter, and herbal medications you are taking before beginning treatment with Provigil. Also, talk to your doctor about your complete medical history, especially if you have high blood pressure or problems with your heart, liver, or kidneys. Also tell your doctor if you have used stimulant medications or if you have or have had a mental disorder known as psychosis.

What is the usual dosage?
The information below is based on the dosage guidelines your doctor uses. Depending on your condition and medical history, your doctor may prescribe a different regimen. Do not change the dosage or stop taking your medication without your doctor's approval.

Adults: The usual dose of Provigil is 200 milligrams (mg) taken as a single dose in the morning. Adults 65 years and older may need a lower dose if they have liver or kidney disease, which reduces the body's ability to metabolize Provigil. For patients with narcolepsy or obstructive sleep apnea/hypopnea syndrome, Provigil should be taken as a single dose in the morning. For patients with shift work sleep disorder, Provigil should be taken approximately 1 hour prior to the start of their work shift.

How should I take Provigil?
Take Provigil exactly as prescribed by your doctor. Your doctor will tell you the right time of day to take Provigil. You can take Provigil with or without food.

If you take more than your prescribed dose, or take Provigil too late in your waking day, you may find it harder to go to sleep. Call your doctor if you have any concerns.

What should I avoid while taking Provigil?
Avoid driving or operating hazardous machinery until you know how Provigil affects you.

Avoid drinking alcohol while taking Provigil.

What are possible food and drug interactions associated with Provigil?

If Provigil is taken with certain other drugs, the effects of either could be increased, decreased, or altered. It is especially important to check with your doctor before combining Provigil with the following: antidepressants, carbamazepine, clomipramine, cyclosporine, diazepam, itraconazole, ketoconazole, MAOIs, methylphenidate, oral contraceptives and hormonal implants, phenobarbital, phenytoin, propranolol, rifampin, theophylline, and warfarin.

What are the possible side effects of Provigil?

Side effects cannot be anticipated. If any develop or change in intensity, tell your doctor as soon as possible. Only your doctor can determine if it is safe for you to continue taking this drug.

Side effects may include: headache, nausea, nervousness, stuffy nose, diarrhea, back pain, anxiety, trouble sleeping, dizziness, upset stomach

Serious side effects may include: chest pain, mental problems, allergic reactions such as rash or hives

Can I receive Provigil if I am pregnant or breastfeeding?

The effects of Provigil during pregnancy and breastfeeding are unknown. Tell your doctor immediately if you are pregnant, plan to become pregnant, or are breastfeeding.

What should I do if I miss a dose of Provigil?

Take it as soon as possible. If you don't remember until the next day, skip the dose you missed and go back to your regular schedule. Do not take two doses at the same time.

How should I store Provigil?

Store at room temperature.

PROZAC

Generic name: Fluoxetine hydrochloride

What is Prozac?

Prozac belongs to a class of drugs called selective serotonin reuptake inhibitors (SSRIs). It is used in adults for the treatment of major depressive disorder, panic disorder, obsessive-compulsive disorder, and bulimia. In children and adolescents, Prozac is used to treat major depression and obsessive-compulsive disorder. Prozac Weekly is approved for treating major depression.

What is the most important information I should know about Prozac?

Antidepressant medicines may increase suicidal thoughts or actions in some children, teenagers, and young adults within the first few months of treatment.

Individuals being treated with Prozac and their caregivers should watch for any change in symptoms or any new symptoms that appear suddenly—especially agitation, anxiety, hostility, panic, restlessness, extreme hyperactivity, and suicidal thinking or behavior—and report them to the doctor immediately. Be especially observant at the beginning of treatment or whenever there is a change in dose.

If you get a rash or hives while taking Prozac, call your doctor right away because this can be a sign of a serious medical condition.

Who should not take Prozac?

Do not take Prozac while using a medication known as a monoamine oxidase inhibitor (MAOI). You should also not use Prozac if you are taking thioridazine. You should not start thioridazine within 5 weeks of stopping Prozac. You should not take Prozac if you are taking pimozide.

If you are allergic to or have ever had an allergic reaction to Prozac or similar drugs, you should not take Prozac. Make sure that your doctor is aware of any drug reactions that you have experienced.

What should I tell my doctor before I take the first dose of Prozac?

Tell your doctor about all prescription, over-the-counter, and herbal medication you are taking before beginning treatment with Prozac. Also, talk to your doctor about your complete medical history, especially if you have liver disease, kidney disease, diabetes, seizures or epilepsy, bipolar disorder (manic depression) or a history of drug abuse or suicidal thoughts.

What is the usual dosage?

The information below is based on the dosage guidelines your doctor uses. Depending on your condition and medical history, your doctor may prescribe a different regimen. Do not change the dosage or stop taking your medication without your doctor's approval.

Depression
Adults: It may take 4 weeks before the full antidepressant effect of Prozac is seen.

The recommended starting dose is 20 milligrams (mg) a day, usually taken in the morning. If needed, the doctor may gradually increase the dose up to a maximum of 80 mg a day. The usual daily dose ranges from 20 to 60 mg. Daily doses above 20 mg should be taken in the morning or in two smaller doses taken in the morning and at noon.

Prozac Weekly: You need to wait at least 7 days after stopping your daily dose of Prozac before switching to the once-weekly formulation. One Prozac Weekly capsule contains 90 milligrams of medication.

Children 8 years and older: The usual starting dose is 10 or 20 mg a day. Children starting at 10 mg will have their dose increased to 20 mg a day after 1 week. Underweight children may need to remain at the 10-mg dose.

Obsessive-Compulsive Disorder

Adults: It may take 5 weeks before the full effects of Prozac are seen.

The recommended starting dose is 20 mg a day, usually taken in the morning. If needed, the doctor may gradually increase the dose up to a maximum of 80 mg a day. The usual daily dose ranges from 20 to 60 mg. Daily doses above 20 mg should be taken in the morning or in two smaller doses taken in the morning and at noon.

Children 7 years and older: The recommended starting dose is 10 mg a day. After 2 weeks, the doctor will increase the dose to 20 mg. If needed, the doctor may further increase the dose up to a maximum of 60 mg a day. The recommended dosage range for underweight children is 10 to 30 mg a day.

Bulimia

Adults: The recommended dose is 60 mg day taken in the morning. The doctor may start you at a lower dose and gradually increase it over a period of several days.

Panic Disorder

Adults: The recommended starting dose is 10 mg a day. After 1 week, the doctor will increase the dose to 20 mg. If no improvement is seen after several weeks, the doctor may increase the dose to a maximum of 60 mg a day.

How should I take Prozac?

Prozac should be taken exactly as prescribed by your doctor. Do not stop taking Prozac suddenly without first talking to your doctor.

Prozac usually is taken once or twice a day, at the same time each day. To be effective, it should be taken regularly.

What should I avoid while taking Prozac?

Prozac may cause you to become drowsy or less alert and may affect your judgment. Therefore, driving or operating dangerous machinery or participating in any hazardous activity that requires full mental alertness is not recommended.

Do not drink alcohol while taking Prozac.

What are possible food and drug interactions associated with Prozac?

If Prozac is taken with certain other drugs, the effects of either could be increased, decreased, or altered. It is especially important to check with your doctor before combining Prozac with the following: alcohol, alprazolam, other antidepressants, antipsychotics, carbamazepine, clozapine, desipramine, diazepam, digitoxin, drugs that affect the central nervous system, flecainide, haloperidol, imipramine, linezolid, lithium, narcotic painkillers, nonsteroidal anti-inflammatory drugs (such as aspirin, ibuprofen, naproxen, and ketoprofen), phenytoin, pimozide, propafenone, sleep aids, St. John's wort, sumatriptan, terfenadine, tryptophan, tramadol, vinblastine, and warfarin.

Never take Prozac with MAO inhibitors or thioridazine.

What are the possible side effects of Prozac?

Side effects cannot be anticipated. If any develop or change in intensity, tell your doctor as soon as possible. Only your doctor can determine if it is safe for you to continue taking this drug.

Side effects may include: abnormal dreams, abnormal ejaculation, abnormal vision, anxiety, chest pain, chills, confusion, diarrhea, diminished sex drive, dizziness, dry mouth, flu-like symptoms, flushing, gas, headache, hives, impotence, impaired thinking, insomnia, itching, loss of appetite, nausea, nervousness, rash, seizures, sex-drive changes, sinusitis, sleepiness, sore throat, sweating, tremors, upset stomach, vomiting, weakness, yawning

Can I receive Prozac if I am pregnant or breastfeeding?

Tell your doctor immediately if you are pregnant, or plan to become pregnant. Prozac given late in the third trimester of pregnancy was associated with complications. If you are receiving Prozac during pregnancy, speak to your doctor about switching to other treatment options or lowering the dose.

This medication appears in breast milk, and breastfeeding is not recommended while you are taking Prozac.

What should I do if I miss a dose of Prozac?

Take it as soon as possible. If you don't remember until the next day, skip the dose you missed and go back to your regular schedule. Do not take a double dose.

How should I store Prozac?

Store at room temperature.

PULMICORT TURBUHALER
Generic name: Budesonide inhalation powder

What is Pulmicort Turbuhaler?

Pulmicort Turbuhaler is an anti-inflammatory steroid medication. Inhaled on a regular basis, Pulmicort helps prevent asthma attacks. It is sometimes prescribed in addition to oral steroids, and may reduce or eliminate the need for them.

Pulmicort Turbuhaler is a preventive medicine used to treat asthma in adults and children over age 6. It will not relieve an acute or life-threatening episode of asthma.

What is the most important information I should know about Pulmicort Turbuhaler?

If you are switching to Pulmicort from an oral steroid medication, your doctor will reduce your oral dosage very gradually. Taking oral steroids suppresses the natural production of steroids by the adrenal gland; it takes months for production to return to normal after oral steroids are stopped. In the meantime, the body will be unusually vulnerable to stress.

There have been reports of death during and immediately after transfer from oral steroids to inhaled steroids; your doctor will monitor you carefully during this period. People who have been taking high doses of oral steroids for an extended period of time are especially at risk, particularly when the oral steroids have been almost completely stopped. At that point, any stress from trauma, surgery, or infection (especially stomach or intestinal inflammation) is more likely to trigger adverse events.

If you experience a period of stress or a severe asthma attack during your switch to Pulmicort, begin taking your oral medication again (in large doses) and contact your doctor immediately. Carry a medical identification card indicating that you may need additional medication during periods of stress or a severe asthma attack.

Like other inhaled asthma medications, Pulmicort occasionally triggers an asthma attack. If this occurs, immediately use a fast-acting inhaled bronchodilator, stop using Pulmicort, and contact your doctor.

Steroid medications may stunt growth in children and teenagers. Your doctor will prescribe the lowest effective dose of Pulmicort and monitor the child's growth carefully.

Who should not take Pulmicort Turbuhaler?

If you are allergic to budesonide, you cannot use Pulmicort.

What should I tell my doctor before I take the first dose of Pulmicort Turbuhaler?

Tell your doctor about all prescription, over-the-counter, and herbal medication you are taking before beginning treatment with Pulmicort Turbuhaler. Also, talk to your doctor about your complete medical history, especially if you have liver disease.

What is the usual dosage?
The information below is based on the dosage guidelines your doctor uses. Depending on your condition and medical history, your doctor may prescribe a different regimen. Do not change the dosage or stop taking your medication without your doctor's approval.

Adults: The usual dosage depends on your previous treatments for asthma.

If you have previously been using only fast-acting bronchodilators, the usual starting dose is 200 to 400 micrograms (mcg) twice a day. The maximum long-term dosage is 400 mcg twice daily.

If you have previously been using inhaled steroids, the usual starting dose is 200 to 400 mcg twice a day (or once daily in the morning or evening if your asthma has been well controlled). The maximum long-term dosage is 800 mcg twice daily.

If you have previously been taking oral steroids, the usual starting dose is 400 to 800 mcg twice a day. The maximum long-term dosage is 800 mcg twice daily.

If you are taking oral steroids, you will continue to do so while starting Pulmicort Turbuhaler. After one week, the doctor will lower your dose of oral steroids, then gradually lower it further at one- or two-week intervals.

Children age 6 and older: As with adults, the child's usual dosage depends on previous treatments.

If the child has previously been using only a fast-acting bronchodilator the usual starting dose is 200 mcg twice a day. The maximum long-term dosage is 400 mcg twice daily.

If the child has previously been using inhaled steroids, the usual starting dose is 200 mg twice daily. (A once-a-day dose of 200 or 400 mcg may be prescribed instead.) The maximum long-term dosage is 400 mcg twice daily.

If the child has previously been taking oral steroids, the highest recommended dose is 400 mcg taken twice a day. As with adults, the dosage of oral steroids will be gradually reduced while the child continues to take Pulmicort.

How should I take Pulmicort Turbuhaler?
Use Pulmicort Turbuhaler exactly as directed. The effectiveness of Pulmicort Turbuhaler depends on its regular use. When starting therapy, carefully read the instructions that come with the inhaler. Asthma symptoms may begin to improve in 24 hours; you may not see the maximum benefit for 1 to 2 weeks or longer. If your symptoms worsen or fail to improve, contact your doctor.

Pulmicort Turbuhaler delivers a dose of medication in dry powder form. To assure the correct dose, the inhaler must be held in an upright position, with the mouthpiece on top, during priming and loading.

Before its first use, each new inhaler must be primed. To prime the inhaler, hold it upright and turn the brown grip fully to the right, then fully to the left until it clicks. Repeat this procedure a second time. The unit is now primed.

The inhaler must be loaded with medication immediately prior to each use. Turn the brown grip fully to the right, then fully to the left until it clicks.

During inhalation, the inhaler must be held in an upright (mouthpiece up) or horizontal position. Do not shake the inhaler. Place the mouthpiece between your lips and inhale forcefully and deeply. The Pulmicort powder is then delivered to the lungs. Do not exhale through the inhaler.

You may not taste or sense any medication entering the lungs when inhaling from the Turbuhaler. This lack of sensation is not a cause for concern.

To decrease the risk of developing a fungus infection in the mouth, rinse it with water, without swallowing, after each dose. Do not use the inhaler with a spacer. Do not bite or chew the mouthpiece.

What should I avoid while taking Pulmicort Turbuhaler?

Avoid exposing the eyes to the medication. To decrease the risk of developing a fungus infection in the mouth, rinse with water, without swallowing, after each dose.

Avoid exposure to infectious diseases such as chickenpox and measles. If you are exposed, contact your doctor immediately.

What are possible food and drug interactions associated with Pulmicort Turbuhaler?

If Pulmicort Turbuhaler is taken with certain other drugs, the effects of either could be increased, decreased, or altered. It is especially important to check with your doctor before combining Pulmicort Turbuhaler with the following: clarithromycin, erythromycin, itraconazole, ketoconazole.

What are the possible side effects of Pulmicort Turbuhaler?

Side effects cannot be anticipated. If any develop or change in intensity, tell your doctor as soon as possible. Only your doctor can determine if it is safe for you to continue taking this drug.

Side effects may include: Aching joints, back pain, cough, fever, flu-like symptoms, fungal infection in mouth, headache, indigestion, nasal and sinus inflammation, pain, respiratory infection, sore throat, weakness

Can I receive Pulmicort Turbuhaler if I am pregnant or breastfeeding?

Pulmicort does not appear to harm the developing infant during pregnancy. Nevertheless, the possibility for harm cannot be ruled out. This medication should be used during pregnancy only if it is clearly needed.

Steroids make their way into breast milk. Because they could affect the nursing infant, discuss with your doctor whether to discontinue breast-feeding or stop taking Pulmicort Turbuhaler.

What should I do if I miss a dose of Pulmicort Turbuhaler?
Take it as soon as you remember. If it is almost time for your next dose, skip the one you missed. Do not take two doses at once.

How should I store Pulmicort Turbuhaler?
Keep the Pulmicort Turbuhaler clean at all times. Replace the cover securely after each opening. Store with the cover tightened in a dry place at room temperature. Discard the unit when a red mark appears in the indicator window.

PYRIDIUM
Generic name: Phenazopyridine hydrochloride

What is Pyridium?
Pyridium is an analgesic used to relieve the pain, burning, urgency, frequency, and irritation caused by infection, trauma, catheters, or various surgical procedures in the lower urinary tract. Pyridium is indicated for short-term use and can only relieve symptoms; it is not a treatment for the underlying cause of symptoms.

What is the most important information I should know about Pyridium?
Pyridium produces an orange-to-red color in urine and may stain fabric. Staining of contact lenses has also been reported; do not wear contact lenses while on this medication.

If your skin or the whites of your eyes develop a yellowish tone, it may indicate that your kidneys are not eliminating the medication as they should. Notify your doctor immediately. If you are older, your doctor will monitor you more closely.

Who should not take Pyridium?
Pyridium should be avoided if you have kidney disease or if you are sensitive to or have ever had an allergic reaction to Pyridium. Do not use in children >12 years.

What should I tell my doctor before I take the first dose of Pyridium?
Tell your doctor about all prescription, over-the-counter, and herbal medications you are taking before beginning treatment with Pyridium. Also, talk to your doctor about your complete medical history, especially if you have kidney disease.

What is the usual dosage?
The information below is based on the dosage guidelines your doctor uses. Depending on your condition and medical history, your doctor may prescribe a different regimen. Do not change the dosage or stop taking your medication without your doctor's approval.

Adults: The usual dose is two 100-milligram (mg) tablets or one 200-mg tablet 3 times a day after meals. You should not take Pyridium for more than 2 days if you are also taking an antibiotic for the treatment of a urinary tract infection.

How should I take Pyridium?
Take Pyridium after meals, exactly as prescribed.

What should I avoid while taking Pyridium?
Avoid wearing contact lenses while taking Pyridium.

What are possible food and drug interactions associated with Pyridium?
No food or drug interactions have been reported.

What are the possible side effects of Pyridium?
Side effects cannot be anticipated. If any develop or change in intensity, tell your doctor as soon as possible. Only your doctor can determine if it is safe for you to continue taking this drug.

Side effects may include: headache, itching, rash, severe allergic reaction (rash, difficulty breathing, fever, rapid heartbeat, convulsions), upset stomach

Can I receive Pyridium if I am pregnant or breastfeeding?
The effects of Pyridium during pregnancy and breastfeeding are unknown. Tell your doctor immediately if you are pregnant, plan to become pregnant, or are breastfeeding.

What should I do if I miss a dose of Pyridium?
Take it as soon as you remember. If it is almost time for your next dose, skip the one you missed and go back to your regular schedule. Never take 2 doses at the same time.

How should I store Pyridium?
Store at room temperature.

Quazepam *See Doral, page 440.*

QUESTRAN

Generic name: Cholestyramine

What is Questran?

Questran is used to lower cholesterol levels in the blood of people with primary hypercholesterolemia (too much LDL cholesterol). Hypercholesterolemia is a genetic condition characterized by a lack of the LDL receptors that remove cholesterol from the bloodstream. This drug can be used to lower cholesterol levels in people who also have hypertriglyceridemia, a condition in which an excess of fat is stored in the body. This drug may also be prescribed to relieve itching associated with gallbladder obstruction.

It is available in two forms: Questran and Questran Light. The same instructions apply to both.

What is the most important information I should know about Questran?

It's important to remember that Questran is a supplement to—not a substitute for—diet, exercise, and weight loss. To get the full benefit of the medication, you need to stick to the diet and exercise program prescribed by your doctor. All these efforts to keep your cholesterol levels normal are important because together they may lower your risk of heart disease.

If you are being treated for any disease that contributes to increased blood cholesterol, such as hypothyroidism (reduced thyroid function), diabetes, nephrotic syndrome (kidney and blood vessel disorder), dysproteinemia, obstructive liver disease, or alcoholism, or if you are taking any drugs that may raise cholesterol levels, consult your doctor before taking this medication. Caution is also in order if your kidney function is poor.

The use of this medication may produce or worsen constipation and aggravate hemorrhoids. If this happens, inform your doctor. To prevent constipation, the doctor may increase your dosage very slowly, and ask you to drink more fluids, take more fiber, or take a stool softener. If severe constipation develops anyway, the doctor may switch to a different drug.

The prolonged use of Questran may change acidity in the bloodstream, especially in younger and smaller individuals in whom the doses are relatively higher. It is important that you or your child be checked by your doctor on a regular basis.

Who should not take Questran?

If you are sensitive to or have ever had an allergic reaction to Questran or similar drugs, you should not take this medication. Make sure that your doctor is aware of any drug reactions that you have experienced. Unless you are directed to do so by your doctor, do not take this medication if you are being treated for gallbladder obstruction.

What should I tell my doctor before I take the first dose of Questran?

Tell your doctor about all prescription, over-the-counter, and herbal medications you are taking before beginning treatment with this drug. Also, talk to your doctor about your complete medical history, especially if you have reduced thyroid function, diabetes, nephrotic syndrome (kidney and blood vessel disorder), obstructive liver disease, or if you drink a lot of alcohol or take any drugs that may raise cholesterol levels.

If you have phenylketonuria, a genetic disorder, check with your doctor before taking Questran Light because this product contains phenylalanine.

What is the usual dosage?

The information below is based on the dosage guidelines your doctor uses. Depending on your condition and medical history, your doctor may prescribe a different regimen. Do not change the dosage or stop taking your medication without your doctor's approval.

Adults: The recommended starting dose is 1 single-dose packet or 1 level scoopful, 1 to 2 times daily. The usual maintenance dosage is a total of 2 to 4 packets or scoopfuls daily divided into 2 doses preferably at mealtime (usually before meals). The maximum daily dose is 6 packets or scoopfuls. Although the recommended dosing schedule is 2 times daily, your doctor may ask you to take Questran in up to 6 smaller doses per day.

Children: The dosage will be based on your child's weight. Follow your doctor's recommended dosing schedule.

How should I take Questran?

Never take Questran in its dry form. Always mix it with water or other liquids *before* taking it. For Questran, use 2 to 6 ounces of liquid per packet or level scoopful; for Questran Light, use 2 to 3 ounces. Soups or fruits with a high moisture content, such as applesauce or crushed pineapple, can be used in place of beverages.

What should I avoid while taking Questran?

Avoid sipping Questran or holding it in your mouth for a long period, as this can lead to tooth discoloration, enamel erosion, or decay. Be sure to brush and floss regularly.

What are possible food and drug interactions associated with Questran?

If Questran is taken with certain other drugs, the effects of either could be increased, decreased, or altered. It is especially important to check with your doctor before taking questran with the following: digitalis, estrogens and progestins, oral diabetes drugs, penicillin G, phenobarbital, phenylbutazone, propranolol, spironolactone, tetracycline, thiazide-type diuretic pills, thyroid medication, and warfarin.

Your doctor may recommend that you take other medications at least 1 hour before or 4 to 6 hours after you take Questran.

If you are taking a drug such as digitalis, stopping Questran could be hazardous, since you might experience exaggerated effects of the other drug. Consult your doctor before discontinuing Questran.

This drug may interfere with normal digestion and absorption of fats, including fat-soluble vitamins such as A, D, E, and K. If supplements of vitamins A, D, E, and K are essential to your health, your doctor may prescribe an alternative form of these vitamins.

What are the possible side effects of Questran?

Side effects cannot be anticipated. If any develop or change in intensity, tell your doctor as soon as possible. Only your doctor can determine if it is safe for you to continue taking this drug.

Side effects may include: constipation, heartburn, nausea, vomiting, abdominal pain, flatulence, diarrhea, loss of appetite, osteoporosis, rash, vitamin A and D deficiency, vitamin K deficiency

Can I receive Questran if I am pregnant or breastfeeding?

The effects of Questran during pregnancy have not been adequately studied. If you are pregnant or plan to become pregnant, inform your doctor immediately. Because this medication can interfere with vitamin absorption, you may need to increase your vitamin intake before the baby is born and while nursing an infant.

What should I do if I miss a dose of Questran?

Take the forgotten dose as soon as you remember. If it is almost time for the next dose, skip the one you missed and go back to your regular schedule. Never double the dose.

How should I store Questran?

Store at room temperature. Protect from moisture and high humidity.

Quetiapine fumarate See Seroquel, page 1186.

Quetiapine fumarate, extended-release See Seroquel XR, page 1189.

Quinapril hydrochloride See Accupril, page 5.

Quinapril hydrochloride and hydrochlorothiazide See Accuretic, page 7.

QUINIDINE SULFATE

What is Quinidine sulfate?
Quinidine sulfate is used to correct certain types of irregular heart rhythms and to slow an abnormally fast heartbeat. It can also be used to treat malaria.

What is the most important information I should know about Quinidine sulfate?
Quinidine sulfate is associated with an increased risk of death when used to treat non-life-threatening irregular heartbeat. This risk may be greater if you have structural heart disease.

Quinidine sulfate is reserved for certain kinds of dangerously rapid heart irregularities. It works well for some people, providing them with significant relief of symptoms. However, it has not been shown to improve chances of long-term survival. Under certain conditions (slow heart rate, low potassium or magnesium levels), quinidine sulfate may cause certain types of heart irregularity. It may cause the condition known as heart block, and should be used with caution if you have partial heart block.

Who should not take Quinidine sulfate?
Do not take quinidine sulfate if you have ever had an allergic reaction to quinidine. Also avoid quinidine sulfate if quinine or quinidine causes you to bruise easily.

Quinidine sulfate is prescribed for specific types of heart irregularity, and should be avoided when other irregularities are present. It should also be avoided in patients whose heart rhythms are dependent on a pacemaker. It could also prove harmful if you have myasthenia gravis (abnormal muscle weakness) or a similar condition.

What should I tell my doctor before I take the first dose of Quinidine sulfate?
Tell your doctor about all prescription, over-the-counter, and herbal medications you are taking before beginning treatment with quinidine sulfate. Also, talk to your doctor about your complete medical history, especially if you have myasthenia gravis, kidney or liver disease, congestive heart failure, heart block, QT prolongation, or other heart problems; low blood pressure, high or low blood calcium levels, decreased blood platelets, or digitalis intoxication.

What is the usual dosage?
The information below is based on the dosage guidelines your doctor uses. Depending on your condition and medical history, your doctor may prescribe a different regimen. Do not change the dosage or stop taking your medication without your doctor's approval.

Adults: Depending on your individual goals of therapy, your doctor will prescribe a dose specific for your condition.

How should I take Quinidine sulfate?
Take quinidine sulfate exactly as prescribed. If you experience stomach upset you may take this medication with food.

What should I avoid while taking Quinidine sulfate?
Avoid activities that require mental alertness until you know how your body reacts to this medication. Try to avoid antacids, grapefruit juice, and herbal products; speak to your doctor before using them with this medication.

What are possible food and drug interactions associated with Quinidine sulfate?
If quinidine sulfate is taken with certain other drugs, the effects of either could be increased, decreased, or altered. It is especially important to check with your doctor before combining quinidine sulfate with the following: amiodarone, antidepressants, antacids containing magnesium, antispasmodic drugs, aspirin, beta-blocking blood pressure medications, blood thinners, diuretics, cimetidine, codeine, decamethonium, digoxin, digitoxin, diltiazem, disopyramide, felodipine, grapefruit juice, haloperidol, hydrocodone, ketoconazole, major tranquilizers, mexiletine, nicardipine, nifedipine, nimodipine, phenobarbital, phenytoin, physostigmine, procainamide, reserpine, rifampin, sodium bicarbonate, sucralfate, thiazide diuretics, verapamil.

A decrease in your salt intake can lead to a higher blood level of quinidine sulfate. Try to keep the salt in your diet constant.

What are the possible side effects of Quinidine sulfate?
Side effects cannot be anticipated. If any develop or change in intensity, tell your doctor as soon as possible. Only your doctor can determine if it is safe for you to continue taking this drug.

Side effects may include: abdominal pain, change is sleep habits, chest pain, diarrhea, eye problems, headache, hepatitis, light headedness, inflammation of the esophagus, loss of appetite, nausea, rash, vomiting, weakness

Another possible side effect is a sensitivity reaction called cinchonism. Symptoms include blurred or double vision, confusion, delirium, diarrhea, headache, intolerance to light, hearing loss, ringing in the ears, vertigo, and vomiting.

Can I receive Quinidine sulfate if I am pregnant or breastfeeding?
There are no adequate studies on the effects of quinidine sulfate during pregnancy, so it should be given to a pregnant woman only if clearly

needed. Tell your doctor immediately if you are pregnant or plan to become pregnant.

Quinidine sulfate appears in breast milk and can affect a nursing infant. If this drug is essential to your health, your doctor may advise you to discontinue breastfeeding until your treatment is finished.

What should I do if I miss a dose of Quinidine sulfate?
Take it as soon as you remember. However, if it is within 4 hours of your next dose, skip the missed dose and continue with your normal dosing schedule. Do not take 2 doses at once.

How should I store Quinidine sulfate?
Store at room temperature in a tightly closed container, away from light.

Rabeprazole sodium *See AcipHex, page 16.*

Raloxifene hydrochloride *See Evista, page 526.*

Raltegravir *See Isentress, page 671.*

Ramelteon *See Rozerem, page 1171.*

Ramipril *See Altace, page 74.*

RANEXA
Generic name: Ranolazine

What is Ranexa?
Ranexa is used in adults for the treatment of chronic angina. It is sometimes used in combination with beta-blockers, nitrates, calcium channel blockers, anti-platelet therapy, lipid-lowering therapy, ACE inhibitors, and angiotensin receptor blockers.

What is the most important information I should know about Ranexa?
Ranexa may cause QT interval prolongation, an irregularity of the electrical activity within the heart.

Who should not take Ranexa?
Do not take Ranexa if you are taking any of the following drugs: carbamazepine, clarithromycin, indinavir, itraconazole, ketoconazole, nefazodone, nelfinavir, phenobarbital, phenytoin, rifampin, rifabutin, rifapentin, ritonavir, saquinavir, and St. John's wort. In addition, do not take Ranexa if you have problems with your liver.

What should I tell my doctor before I take the first dose of Ranexa?

Tell your doctor about all prescription, over-the-counter, and herbal medications you are taking before beginning treatment with Ranexa. Also, talk to your doctor about your complete medical history, especially if you are pregnant, breastfeeding, have liver or kidney problems, if you have a history or family history of QTc prolongation or congenital long QT syndrome, are taking drugs that prolong the QTc interval (eg, quinidine, dofetilide, sotalol, amiodarone, erythromycin, thioridazine, ziprasidone), or if you are taking any of the following drugs: carbamazepine, clarithromycin, indinavir, itraconazole, ketoconazole, nefazodone, nelfinavir, phenobarbital, phenytoin, rifampin, rifabutin, rifapentin, ritonavir, saquinavir, and St. John's wort.

What is the usual dosage?
The information below is based on the dosage guidelines your doctor uses. Depending on your condition and medical history, your doctor may prescribe a different regimen. Do not change the dosage or stop taking your medication without your doctor's approval.

Adults: The usual dosage of Ranexa is 500 milligrams (mg) twice a day, which may be increased to 1000 mg twice a day as needed.

How should I take Ranexa?
Ranexa may be taken with or without food. Do not crush, break, or chew the tablets.

What should I avoid while taking Ranexa?
While taking Ranexa, you should avoid treatment with carbamazepine, clarithromycin, indinavir, itraconazole, ketoconazole, nefazodone, nelfinavir, phenobarbital, phenytoin, rifampin, rifabutin, rifapentin, ritonavir, saquinavir, and St. John's wort. Also, avoid eating or drinking any grapefruit-containing products.

What are possible food and drug interactions associated with Ranexa?
If Ranexa is taken with certain other drugs, the effects of either could be increased, decreased, or altered. It is especially important to check with your doctor before combining Ranexa with the following: aprepitant, carbamazepine, clarithromycin, cyclosporine, diltiazem, erythromycin, fluconazole, grapefruit juice or grapefruit-containing products, indinavir, itraconazole, ketoconazole, nefazodone, nelfinavir, phenobarbital, phenytoin, rifampin, rifabutin, rifapentin, ritonavir, saquinavir, St. John's wort, and verapamil

What are the possible side effects of Ranexa?
Side effects cannot be anticipated. If any develop or change in intensity, tell your doctor as soon as possible. Only your doctor can determine if it is safe for you to continue taking this drug.

Side effects may include: dizziness, nausea, weakness, constipation, headache

Can I receive Ranexa if I am pregnant or breastfeeding?
The effects of Ranexa on pregnancy have not been adequately studied. It is important to notify your physician if you are pregnant or planning to become pregnant prior to beginning therapy with Ranexa.

It is not known if Ranexa is found in breast milk. You should not breastfeed while on therapy with Ranexa.

What should I do if I miss a dose of Ranexa?
If you miss a dose of Ranexa, skip the dose you missed and take your next dose at your regular scheduled time. Do not take a double dose.

How should I store Ranexa?
Store Ranexa at room temperature.

Ranitidine *See Zantac, page 1445.*

Ranolazine *See Ranexa, page 1117.*

RAPTIVA
Generic name: Efalizumab

What is Raptiva?
Raptiva belongs to a class of drugs called immunosuppressives. These drugs decrease the activity of the immune system. Raptiva is prescribed for patients with severe plaque psoriasis (a skin disease that is caused, in part, by an overactive immune system) who can no longer control their disease with topical medicines.

What is the most important information I should know about Raptiva?
Raptiva, like other immunosuppressive agents, has the potential to increase the risk of serious infections and cancer. Also, Raptiva likely increases the risk of getting progressive multifocal leukoencephalopathy (PML), a rare brain disease caused by a virus. Call your doctor immediately if you are diagnosed with cancer or if your psoriasis worsens. Also contact your doctor if you develop an infection, excessive bleeding, or unusual bruising.

Many people experience a reaction the first time they receive a dose of Raptiva. Symptoms include headache, fever, nausea, vomiting, muscle aches, and chills, which usually occur within two days following the first two injections.

Your psoriasis may worsen or new forms of psoriasis may appear while you're using Raptiva or after treatment has stopped. Tell your doctor right away if your symptoms worsen or if a new rash appears.

Raptiva may affect the ability of your blood to clot. Inform your doctor immediately if you develop bleeding gums, unusual bruising, or purplish-red spots on your skin.

Raptiva may increase the breakdown of your red blood cells and cause very low blood counts. Call your doctor right away if you feel lightheaded and weak, your skin and eyes turn yellow in color, or your urine turns red or dark.

Some patients have also had worsening or new arthritis while taking Raptiva. Tell your doctor if you have severe redness, pain, swelling, or stiffness of joints such as hands, knees, and ankles.

Cases of disorders that affect the nervous system have been reported in people taking Raptiva. Tell you doctor right away if these types of symptoms develop.

You should not receive vaccines while using Raptiva; because Raptiva may prevent vaccines from working.

Who should not take Raptiva?
Do not use Raptiva if you have ever had an allergic reaction to the medication.

What should I tell my doctor before I take the first dose of Raptiva?
Tell your doctor about all prescription, over-the-counter, and herbal medications you are taking before beginning treatment with Raptiva. Also, talk to your doctor about your complete medical history, especially if you have active or chronic viral, bacterial, or fungal infections; immune system problems; or if you are pregnant or breastfeeding.

What is the usual dosage?
The information below is based on the dosage guidelines your doctor uses. Depending on your condition and medical history, your doctor may prescribe a different regimen. Do not change the dosage or stop taking your medication without your doctor's approval.

Adults: To avoid an allergic reaction the first time you inject Raptiva, the recommended initial dose is 0.7 milligrams (mg) per 2.2 pounds of body weight. Thereafter, the recommended dose is 1 mg per 2.2 pounds of body weight, injected once a week. Individual doses should not exceed a total of 200 mg. Raptiva should be injected on the same day each week.

Children: The safety and effectiveness of Raptiva in children has not been established.

How should I take Raptiva?

Raptiva is administered once a week, the same day each week, as an injection under the skin. If you will be giving the injection to yourself or another person, the doctor will instruct you on how to prepare and inject the medication. The usual sites for injection are the upper leg, upper arm, abdomen, or buttocks. The injection site should be rotated each week. Do not change the dose or stop taking Raptiva without first talking to your doctor.

Once Raptiva has been mixed, it should be used right away. If you are unable to inject the medication immediately, you may let the mixture sit at room temperature for up to eight hours before injecting it. Do not use the mixture once eight hours have passed.

What should I avoid while taking Raptiva?

You should not receive vaccines while using Raptiva. Raptiva may prevent a vaccine from working. Talk to your healthcare provider if you need to receive a vaccine while using Raptiva.

Do not undergo phototherapy while taking Raptiva.

Throw away all syringes and needles after one use. Do not save them for later.

Do not use the solution if it appears discolored or has particles floating in it. Throw it out and mix a new solution instead.

You should not take other medications that are known as immunosuppressives.

What are possible food and drug interactions associated with Raptiva?

If Raptiva is taken with certain other drugs, the effects of either could be increased, decreased, or altered. It is especially important to check with your doctor before combining Raptiva with vaccines or immunosuppressive drugs such as cyclosporine or methotrexate.

What are the possible side effects of Raptiva?

Side effects cannot be anticipated. If any develop or change in intensity, tell your doctor as soon as possible. Only your doctor can determine if it is safe for you to continue taking this drug.

Side effects may include: back pain, chills, fever, headache, nausea, muscle aches, swelling of the arms and legs

These are not all the side effects of Raptiva. If you experience a side effect that concerns you or if you get an infection, call your healthcare provider.

Can I receive Raptiva if I am pregnant or breastfeeding?
The effects of Raptiva during pregnancy and breastfeeding are unknown. Tell your doctor immediately if you are pregnant, plan to become pregnant, or are breastfeeding.

What should I do if I miss a dose of Raptiva?
Call your doctor to find out when to take your next dose and what schedule you should follow after that.

How should I store Raptiva?
Raptiva should be stored in its original carton in the refrigerator. Do not freeze the medication. Protect the vial from exposure to light. Throw away Raptiva vials that are out of date.

Rasagiline See *Azilect, page 182.*

RAZADYNE ER/RAZADYNE
Generic name: Galantamine hydrobromide

What is Razadyne ER/Razadyne?
Razadyne is used in Alzheimer's patients to treat mild to moderate dementia. It is thought to work by boosting levels of the chemical messenger acetylcholine in the brain. (In Alzheimer's disease, the cells that produce acetylcholine slowly deteriorate.)

What is the most important information I should know about Razadyne ER/Razadyne?
The use of Razadyne may cause you to develop a slow heart rate. You should notify your physician if you develop symptoms of dizziness or faintness.

Razadyne may also cause you to develop gastrointestinal symptoms such as nausea, vomiting, diarrhea, a loss of appetite, and weight loss.

While on therapy with Razadyne, it is important to drink an adequate amount of fluids.

It is important to avoid skipping doses of Razadyne. If you miss taking Razadyne for several days, it is important to contact your physician. He or she may have to give you a lower dose of Razadyne, and then gradually increase your dose back to the dose you were originally taking.

If you are planning to undergo surgery, it is important to notify your surgeon that you are on therapy with Razadyne.

Who should not take Razadyne ER/Razadyne?
Do not take Razadyne if you are allergic to it or any of its components.

What should I tell my doctor before I take the first dose of Razadyne ER/Razadyne?

Tell your doctor about all prescription, over-the-counter, and herbal medications you are taking before beginning treatment with Razadyne. Also, talk to your doctor about your complete medical history, especially if you have severe asthma or lung disease, have kidney disease, have liver problems, have a history of stomach ulcers, if you are using nonsteroidal anti-inflammatory drugs (NSAIDs), or if you have a heart condition.

What is the usual dosage?

The information below is based on the dosage guidelines your doctor uses. Depending on your condition and medical history, your doctor may prescribe a different regimen. Do not change the dosage or stop taking your medication without your doctor's approval.

Razadyne ER
Adults: The recommended starting dose of Razadyne ER capsules is 8 milligrams (mg) once a day. After four weeks, the dose should be increased to 16 mg once a day. After another four weeks, the dose should be further increased to 24 mg once a day. Your doctor will increase your dose based on how well you respond to therapy with Razadyne ER capsules.

Razadyne
Adults: The recommended starting dose of Razadyne tablets or oral solution is 4 mg twice a day. Four weeks later, the dose should be increased to 8 mg twice a day. After waiting an additional four weeks, the dose should be increased to 12 mg twice a day. Your doctor will increase your dose based on how well you respond to therapy with Razadyne tablets or oral solution.

How should I take Razadyne ER/Razadyne?

Razadyne ER capsules should be taken once a day, preferably in the morning with food.

Razadyne tablets or oral solution should be taken twice a day, preferably with morning and evening meals. If you are using the oral solution, draw the required amount into the measuring pipette that comes with the bottle. Empty the pipette into three to four ounces of a nonalcoholic beverage, then stir well and take immediately.

It is important to maintain adequate hydration while on therapy with Razadyne ER capsules/Razadyne tablets or oral solution.

What should I avoid while taking Razadyne ER/Razadyne?

It is important to avoid skipping doses of Razadyne. If Razadyne doses have been missed for several days, it is important to contact your physician; your dose may need to be lowered.

What are possible food and drug interactions associated with Razadyne ER/Razadyne?

If Razadyne is taken with certain other drugs, the effects of either could be increased, decreased, or altered. It is especially important to check with your doctor before combining Razadyne with the following: anticholinergic medications, cholinergic agonists (eg, bethanechol), cholinesterase inhibitors, cimetidine, erythromycin, ketoconazole, paroxetine, succinylcholine, and paroxetine.

What are the possible side effects of Razadyne ER/Razadyne?

Side effects cannot be anticipated. If any develop or change in intensity, tell your doctor as soon as possible. Only your doctor can determine if it is safe for you to continue taking this drug.

Side effects may include: blood in the urine, depression, diarrhea, dizziness, drowsiness, fatigue, headache, indigestion, loss of appetite, nausea, runny nose, sleeplessness, stomach pain, tremor, urinary tract infection, vomiting, weight loss

Can I receive Razadyne ER/Razadyne if I am pregnant or breastfeeding?

The effects of using Razadyne during pregnancy have not been adequately studied. It is not known if Razadyne is found in breast milk. It is important to notify your physician if you are pregnant, planning to become pregnant, or are breast feeding before beginning therapy with Razadyne.

What should I do if I miss a dose of Razadyne ER/Razadyne?

If you have missed taking a single dose of Razadyne, take it as soon as you remember. If it is almost time for your next dose, skip the missed dose and return to your normal dosing schedule. Do not take a double dose.

If you have missed taking Razadyne for several days, it is important to contact your physician before taking another dose. Your doctor may need to lower your dose.

How should I store Razadyne ER/Razadyne?

The tablets, extended-release capsules, and the oral solution may be stored at room temperature. Do not freeze the solution.

REGLAN

Generic name: Metoclopramide hydrochloride

What is Reglan?

Reglan increases the contractions of the stomach and small intestine, helping the passage of food. It is used to treat the symptoms of diabetic gastroparesis, a condition in which the stomach does not contract. These symptoms include vomiting, nausea, heartburn, feelings of indigestion, persistent fullness after meals, and appetite loss.

Reglan is also used for short periods to treat heartburn in people with gastroesophageal reflux disorder (GERD), in which stomach contents backflow into the esophagus. In addition, it is given to prevent nausea and vomiting caused by cancer chemotherapy and surgery.

What is the most important information I should know about Reglan?

Reglan may cause symptoms similar to those of Parkinson's disease, such as slow movements, rigidity, tremor, or a mask-like facial appearance.

Reglan may also cause tardive dyskinesia, a syndrome of jerky or writhing involuntary movements, particularly of the tongue, face, mouth, or jaw. Elderly people are at a higher risk for this condition. In children and adults >30, Reglan may cause involuntary movements of the arms and legs, and sometimes loud or labored breathing, usually in the first day or two of treatment.

Reglan may cause intense restlessness with associated symptoms such as anxiety, agitation, foot-tapping, pacing, inability to sit still, jitteriness, and insomnia. These symptoms may disappear as your body gets used to Reglan, or if your dosage is reduced.

Who should not take Reglan?

You should not take Reglan if you: have an obstruction, perforation, or hemorrhage of the stomach or small bowel that might be aggravated by increased stomach and small-bowel movement; have pheochromocytoma (a nonmalignant tumor that causes hypertension), since taking Reglan could trigger a dangerous jump in blood pressure; have epilepsy, since taking Reglan could increase the frequency and severity of seizures; are taking a drug that is likely to cause side effects such as tremors, jerks, grimaces, or writhing movements, since taking Reglan could make such symptoms more severe; are >18 years of age; are allergic to or sensitive to Reglan

What should I tell my doctor before I take the first dose of Reglan?

Tell your doctor about all prescription, over-the-counter, and herbal medications you are taking before beginning treatment with Reglan. Also, talk to your doctor about your complete medical history, especially if you have kidney disease, cirrhosis (chronic liver disease), a history of depression, Parkinson's disease, diabetes, high blood pressure, heart disease, stomach problems or if you have recently had stomach surgery.

What is the usual dosage?
The information below is based on the dosage guidelines your doctor uses. Depending on your condition and medical history, your doctor may prescribe a different regimen. Do not change the dosage or stop taking your medication without your doctor's approval.

Symptoms of GERD
The usual dose is 10 milligrams (mg) to 15 mg of Reglan, up to 4 times a day, 30 minutes before each meal and at bedtime, depending upon the symptoms being treated and the effectiveness of the dose. Treatment usually lasts no longer than 12 weeks. If symptoms occur only intermittently or at specific times of the day, your doctor may give you a single dose of up to 20 mg as a preventive measure.

Elderly: Older patients may need only 5 mg per dose

Symptoms Associated with Diabetic Gastroparesis or Gastric Stasis
Adults: The usual dose is 10 mg taken 30 minutes before each meal and at bedtime for 2 to 8 weeks.

How should I take Reglan?
Reglan is usually taken 30 minutes before a meal. If you suffer from heartburn that occurs only intermittently or only at certain times of day, your doctor may want you to schedule your Reglan therapy around those times.

   You will probably take Reglan for only 4 to 12 weeks. Continuous treatment beyond 12 weeks is not recommended.

   If you have diabetic "lazy stomach" (gastric stasis) that tends to recur, your doctor may want you to take Reglan at the first sign of a recurrence.

What should I avoid while taking Reglan?
Reglan may make you drowsy and impair your coordination. You should not drive, climb, or perform hazardous tasks until you know how the medication affects you.

What are possible food and drug interactions associated with Reglan?
If Reglan is taken with certain other drugs, the effects of either could be increased, decreased, or altered. It is especially important to check with your doctor before combining Reglan with the following: acetaminophen, alcohol, antispasmodic drugs, cimetidine, cyclosporine, digoxin, insulin, MAO inhibitor antidepressants, levodopa, narcotic painkillers, sleeping pills, tetracycline, tranquilizers.

What are the possible side effects of Reglan?

Side effects cannot be anticipated. If any develop or change in intensity, tell your doctor as soon as possible. Only your doctor can determine if it is safe for you to continue taking this drug.

Side effects may include: drowsiness, fatigue, restlessness, weakness, insomnia, headache, confusion, dizziness

Can I receive Reglan if I am pregnant or breastfeeding?

The effects of Reglan during pregnancy are unknown. Tell your doctor immediately if you are pregnant, or plan to become pregnant. Reglan appears in breast milk. Your doctor may recommend that you discontinue Reglan while you are breastfeeding your baby.

What should I do if I miss a dose of Reglan?

Take it as soon as you remember. If it is almost time for your next dose, skip the one you missed and go back to your regular schedule. Do not take 2 doses at once.

How should I store Reglan?

Store at room temperature in a tight, light-resistant container.

RELENZA

Generic name: Zanamivir

What is Relenza?

Relenza is used to treat influenza A and B viruses (the flu) in adults and children 7 years of age and older. Also, Relenza is used to prevent the flu in adults and children 5 years of age and older.

What is the most important information I should know about Relenza?

Relenza should not be used to treat the flu in people with airway disease, such as asthma or chronic obstructive pulmonary disease. This drug should be stopped immediately if it begins to cause breathing problems.

Relenza may cause you to develop serious allergic reactions such as rash or difficulty breathing. If this occurs, stop using Relenza and immediately notify your physician.

Relenza is not a substitute for the annual flu shot.

Relenza will help to treat influenza A and B (the flu). However, others around you will remain at risk for becoming infected with influenza A or B while you are infected with it.

The use of Relenza may cause you to develop signs of abnormal behavior. If this develops, notify your physician.

Who should not take Relenza?

Do not take Relenza if you are allergic to any of its ingredients, which include lactose (a milk protein).

What should I tell my doctor before I take the first dose of Relenza?

Tell your doctor about all prescription, over-the-counter, and herbal medications you are taking before beginning treatment with Relenza. Also, talk to your doctor about your medical history, especially if you have asthma, chronic obstructive pulmonary disease, are pregnant, or are nursing.

What is the usual dosage?

The information below is based on the dosage guidelines your doctor uses. Depending on your condition and medical history, your doctor may prescribe a different regimen. Do not change the dosage or stop taking your medication without your doctor's approval.

Treatment of the Flu

Adults and children ≥7 years of age: The recommended dose of Relenza is 10 milligrams (mg) twice daily (approximately 12 hours apart) for 5 days. Two doses should be taken on the first day of treatment whenever possible as long as at least 2 hours elapse between doses. On the following days, doses should be about 12 hours apart (eg, (morning and evening) and given at approximately the same time each day.

For Prevention of the Flu When Others in the Household Have It

Adults and children ≥5 years of age: The recommended dose is 10 mg taken once daily for 10 days. The dose should be taken at approximately the same time each day.

For Prevention of the Flu When There is a Community Outbreak

Adults and children ≥5 years of age: The recommended dose is 10 mg taken once daily for 28 days. The dose should be taken at approximately the same time each day.

How should I take Relenza?

Relenza is for use only with the Diskhaler inhalation device provided. Follow the patient instructions included within the Relenza packaging.

What should I avoid while taking Relenza?

If you are receiving treatment for asthma with an inhaler, it is important to avoid using the asthma inhaler at the same time as Relenza. Use your asthma inhaler before taking your dose of Relenza.

What are possible food and drug interactions associated with Relenza?

If Relenza is used with certain other drugs, the effects of either could be increased, decreased, or altered. It is especially important to check with your doctor before combining Relenza with a live attenuated influenza vaccine (LAIV).

What are the possible side effects of Relenza?

Side effects cannot be anticipated. If any develop or change in intensity, tell your doctor as soon as possible. Only your doctor can determine if it is safe for you to continue taking this drug.

Side effects may include: allergic reactions (difficulty breathing, serious skin rash); bronchitis; cough; diarrhea; dizziness; ear, nose, and throat infections; nasal symptoms; nausea; sinusitis; vomiting.

Can I receive Relenza if I am pregnant or breastfeeding?

The effects of using Relenza during pregnancy have not been adequately studied. Notify your physician if you are pregnant or planning to become pregnant prior to beginning therapy with Relenza.

It is not known if Relenza is found in breast milk. Notify your physician if you are breastfeeding prior to beginning therapy with Relenza.

What should I do if I miss a dose of Relenza?

If you miss a dose of Relenza, take it as soon as you remember. If it is almost time for your next dose, skip the dose you missed and return to your normal dosing schedule. Do not take a double dose.

How should I store Relenza?

Store Relenza at room temperature, away from children. Do not puncture any Relenza Rotadisk blisters until you take a dose using the diskhaler.

RELPAX

Generic name: Eletriptan hydrobromide

What is Relpax?

Relpax is used to treat migraine headaches with or without the presence of auras (visual disturbances that precede an attack, such as halos or flickering lights). It shortens the duration of the headache but will not prevent attacks.

What is the most important information I should know about Relpax?

Relpax should only be used during a genuine attack of classic migraine. Do not attempt to prevent migraines with this drug, and do not use it for tension headaches, cluster headaches, or unusual types of migraine such as hemiplegic or basilar migraine.

In rare cases, medications similar to Relpax have caused heart attack, stroke, and certain types of ischemia (restricted blood flow to an area). Call your doctor immediately if you experience chest pains, shortness of breath, sudden numbness or weakness on one side of the body, trouble speaking or seeing, loss of balance, bloody diarrhea, or stomach pain.

If you are at risk for stroke or heart disease, your doctor may perform cardiovascular tests to be sure it is safe for you to take Relpax. Your doctor may ask you to take the first dose of Relpax in the office, where you can be monitored for cardiac side effects.

Relpax can cause a slight increase in blood pressure, especially in people with kidney problems and the elderly. Your doctor will monitor you closely to make sure your blood pressure stays at a safe level. If you develop high blood pressure that can't be controlled, you'll have to stop taking Relpax.

Who should not take Relpax?

If Relpax causes an allergic reaction, you will not be able to use it. You should not use Relpax if you have ever had a heart attack or if you have ever had any of the following vascular problems: angina, cardiovascular disease, coronary artery vasospasm, ischemic bowel disease, ischemic heart disease, peripheral vascular disease, Prinzmetal's angina, stroke, transient ischemic attacks, or uncontrolled high blood pressure.

You cannot take Relpax if you have severe liver impairment.

Relpax should never be taken within 24 hours of other migraine or headache medication (see "What are possible food and drug interactions associated with Relpax?").

What should I tell my doctor before I take the first dose of Relpax?

Tell your doctor about all prescription, over-the-counter, and herbal medications you are taking before beginning treatment with this drug. Also, talk to your doctor about your complete medical history, especially if you have kidney or liver problems, heart problems, high blood pressure, or a history of stroke.

What is the usual dosage?

The information below is based on the dosage guidelines your doctor uses. Depending on your condition and medical history, your doctor may prescribe a different regimen. Do not change the dosage or stop taking your medication without your doctor's approval.

Adults: When a headache begins, take one 20-milligram or 40-milligram tablet. If the first dose does not relieve the headache, check with your doctor before taking a second one. If the headache goes away but returns later, a second dose may be taken if 2 hours have elapsed since the first dose. Do not take more than 80 milligrams of Relpax in a 24-hour period.

How should I take Relpax?
Take Relpax exactly as prescribed by your doctor.

What should I avoid while taking Relpax?
Since Relpax can make you drowsy or dizzy, do not participate in activities that require full alertness until you are certain of the drug's effect.

What are possible food and drug interactions associated with Relpax?
If Relpax is taken with certain other drugs, the effects of either could be increased, decreased, or altered. Never take Relpax within 24 hours of using another migraine or headache drug, including: almotriptan, dihydroergotamine, ergotamine, frovatriptan, methysergide, naratriptan, rizatriptan, sumatriptan, and zolmitriptan.

You should also refrain from using Relpax within 72 hours of taking the following: clarithromycin, itraconazole, ketoconazole, nefazodone, nelfinavir, ritonavir, and troleandomycin.

What are the possible side effects of Relpax?
Side effects cannot be anticipated. If any develop or change in intensity, tell your doctor as soon as possible. Only your doctor can determine if it is safe for you to continue taking this drug.

Side effects may include: chest tightness or pressure, dizziness, dry mouth, headache, nausea, sleepiness, tingling, weakness

Can I receive Relpax if I am pregnant or breastfeeding?
The effects of Relpax in pregnancy have not been adequately studied. If you are pregnant or plan to become pregnant, inform your doctor immediately. Relpax is excreted in breast milk. If you are nursing an infant, discuss your treatment options with your physician.

What should I do if I miss a dose of Relpax?
Relpax is not intended for regular use and should be taken only to relieve an acute migraine attack.

How should I store Relpax?
Store at room temperature.

REMERON

Generic name: Mirtazapine

What is Remeron?

Remeron is a tetracyclic antidepressant used for the treatment of major depressive disorder.

What is the most important information I should know about Remeron?

Antidepressant medicines may increase suicidal thoughts or actions in some children, teenagers, and young adults when the medicine is first started. Depression and other serious mental illnesses are the most important causes of suicidal thoughts and actions. Some people may have a particularly high risk of having suicidal thoughts or actions. These include people who have (or have a family history of) bipolar disorder (also called manic-depressive illness) or suicidal thoughts or actions.

Pay close attention to any changes, especially sudden changes, in mood, behaviors, thoughts, or feelings. This is very important when an antidepressant medicine is first started or when the dose is changed.

Call the doctor right away to report new or sudden changes in mood, behavior, thoughts, or feelings. Signs to watch for include new or worsening depression, new or worsening anxiety, agitation, insomnia, hostility, panic attacks, restlessness, extreme hyperactivity, and suicidal thinking or behavior.

Keep all follow-up visits as scheduled, and call the doctor between visits as needed, especially if you have concerns about symptoms.

Do not use this medication if you have used an MAO inhibitor (such as isocarboxazid, phenelzine, rasagiline, selegiline, or tranylcypromine) within the past 14 days.

If you of your family member develops signs and symptoms of fever, sore throat, stomatitis, or other signs of infection, contact your doctor right away as this may be a sign of a serious side effect.

While you may notice improvements with Remeron therapy in 1 to 4 weeks, you should continue therapy as directed.

Never stop an antidepressant, such as Remeron, without first talking to a healthcare provider. Stopping an antidepressant medicine suddenly can cause other symptoms.

This drug may impair the mental and/or physical abilities required for performing potentially hazardous tasks such as driving or operating machinery. These effects may become worse if you combine Remeron with alcohol or certain medicines.

Who should not take Remeron?

Remeron should not be used if you are known to be hypersensitive to this medication or any of its ingredients.

Do not use Remeron if you have used an MAO inhibitor within the past 14 days.

What should I tell my doctor before I take the first dose of Remeron?

Tell your doctor about all prescription, over-the-counter, and herbal medications you are taking before beginning treatment with Remeron. Also, talk to your doctor about your complete medical history, especially if you have liver disease or kidney disease, a low white blood cell count, have recently taken an MAO inhibitor (such as isocarboxazid, phenelzine, rasagiline, selegiline, or tranylcypromine) within the past 14 days, or if you have attempted or thought about suicide in the past.

What is the usual dosage?

The information below is based on the dosage guidelines your doctor uses. Depending on your condition and medical history, your doctor may prescribe a different regimen. Do not change the dosage or stop taking your medication without your doctor's approval.

Adults: The recommended starting dose of Remeron is 15 milligrams (mg) daily taken as a single dose. Preferably, this dose is to be taken in the evening, prior to sleep. The effective dose range is 15 mg to 45 mg daily. Older adults and people with serious liver or kidney problems may require a lower dose. If dose changes are needed, they should not be made at intervals of less than 1-2 weeks in order to allow sufficient time for evaluation of the drug's effect.

How should I take Remeron?

Remeron should be taken exactly as prescribed. Follow the directions on your prescription label.

Take Remeron by mouth with or without food daily. Take Remeron in the evening before bedtime unless your doctor tells you otherwise.

Improvements should be noticed within 1 to 4 weeks of taking this medication. Continue to take Remeron even if you feel well, do not miss a dose.

What should I avoid while taking Remeron?

Avoid driving or operating potentially dangerous machinery. Do not participate in any activities that require full alertness until you know how this drug affects you.

Avoid drinking alcohol. It can cause dangerous side effects when taken with Remeron.

Do not use Remeron if you have used an MAO inhibitor (such as isocarboxazid, phenelzine, rasagiline, selegiline, or tranylcypromine) within the past 14 days.

What are possible food and drug interactions associated with Remeron?

If Remeron is taken with certain other drugs, the effects of either could be increased, decreased, or altered. It is especially important to check with your doctor before combining Remeron with the following: alcohol, clonidine, fluvoxamine, furazolidone, MAO inhibitors (including Nardil and Parnate), and hydantoins such as phenytoin.

What are the possible side effects of Remeron?

Side effects cannot be anticipated. If any develop or change in intensity, tell your doctor as soon as possible. Only your doctor can determine if it is safe for you to continue taking this drug.

Side effects may include: abnormal dreams, abnormal thinking, constipation, dizziness, drowsiness, dry mouth, flu symptoms, increased appetite, weakness, weight gain, decreased ability to fight infection (fever, chill, sore throat), mental or mood changes, mouth sores, thoughts or hurting yourself, tremors, worsening of depression

Can I receive Remeron if I am pregnant or breastfeeding?

The effects of Remeron during pregnancy and breastfeeding are unknown. Tell your doctor immediately if you are pregnant, plan to become pregnant, or are breastfeeding.

What should I do if I miss a dose of Remeron?

If you do miss a dose, take it as soon as you remember. However, if it is almost time for your next dose, skip the missed dose and take only your next regularly scheduled dose. Do not double the dose.

How should I store Remeron?

Store at room temperature away from heat, moisture, and light. Do not store in the bathroom.

Repaglinide See *Prandin, page 1043*.

Repaglinide and metformin hydrochloride See *PrandiMet, page 1041*.

REQUIP

Generic name: Ropinirole hydrochloride

What is Requip?

Requip is used to help relieve the signs and symptoms of Parkinson's disease. It is also used to treat restless legs syndrome (RLS).

What is the most important information I should know about Requip?

Skin cancer (melanoma) has been reported in people taking Requip. Be sure to see your doctor regularly for screenings.

There have been some reports of symptoms getting worse during therapy for restless legs syndrome. Contact your doctor if this occurs.

A few patients—especially older ones—also develop hallucinations. Let your doctor know if this occurs. You may have to stop Requip therapy.

Use Requip with caution if you have heart disease. There is also a slight chance of developing respiratory difficulties or problems with your eyesight. If you find it hard to breathe, have any swelling, or develop problems with your vision, alert your doctor at once.

If you are taking Sinemet with Requip, you may experience jerking muscle movements. Tell your doctor. He will need to decrease your dose of Sinemet.

With other Parkinson's medications, a sudden dose reduction has been known to cause high fever, muscle stiffness, and loss of consciousness. Although this has not happened with Requip, be alert for such problems and contact your doctor immediately if they occur.

Requip may also cause darkening of your skin and eye color. Tell your doctor if you notice any change.

Who should not take Requip?
If Requip gives you an allergic reaction, you cannot continue using it.

What should I tell my doctor before I take the first dose of Requip?
Tell your doctor about all prescription, over-the-counter, and herbal medications you are taking before beginning treatment with this drug. Also, talk to your doctor about your complete medical history, especially if you have a history of skin cancer, eye problems, kidney or liver problems, heart problems, or if you smoke or drink alcohol.

What is the usual dosage?
The information below is based on the dosage guidelines your doctor uses. Depending on your condition and medical history, your doctor may prescribe a different regimen. Do not change the dosage or stop taking your medication without your doctor's approval.

Parkinson's Disease
Adults: Requip is taken 3 times a day. During the first week of therapy, each dose is 0.25 milligram. During the second week, the amount rises to 0.5 milligram. In the third week, it increases to 0.75 milligram, and in the fourth week reaches 1 milligram (3 milligrams daily). If necessary, your doctor will gradually increase the dosage further, up to a maximum of 24 milligrams per day.

If you need to stop Requip therapy, the doctor will discontinue the drug gradually over a 7-day period, reducing the number of doses from 3 to 2 per day for the first 4 days, then to once a day for the remaining 3 days.

Restless Legs Syndrome
Adults: The usual starting dose is 0.25 milligrams taken 1 to 3 hours before bedtime. Depending on your response, the doctor may increase your dose in small increments up to a maximum of 4 milligrams daily.

How should I take Requip?

Take 3 doses a day, with or without food. If the drug upsets your stomach, combining it with food may relieve the problem. If you are also taking levodopa, its dosage may be gradually decreased when you start therapy with Requip.

What should I avoid while taking Requip?

Requip may cause drowsiness, and some people have reported falling asleep without warning during their daily activities. Do not drive a car or operate machinery until you know how the drug affects you. If you find that Requip makes you sleepy or that you're suddenly falling asleep in the middle of routine activities, tell your doctor immediately.

At the start of Requip therapy and whenever the dose is increased, you face a slightly increased risk of a fainting spell or other symptoms of low blood pressure such as dizziness, nausea, sweating, and light-headedness, particularly when you get up suddenly after sitting or reclining for a prolonged period. To avoid such symptoms, be careful to stand up slowly.

Avoid alcohol and other central nervous system depressants while taking this medication.

What are possible food and drug interactions associated with Requip?

If Requip is taken with certain other drugs, the effects of either can be increased, decreased, or altered. It is especially important to check with your doctor before combining Requip with the following: alcohol, benzodiazepines such as alprazolam, certain antidepressants, ciprofloxacin, drugs that contain Levodopa, estrogen medications such as ethinyl estradiol, metoclopramide, and tranquilizers.

What are the possible side effects of Requip?

Side effects cannot be anticipated. If any develop or change in intensity, tell your doctor as soon as possible. Only your doctor can determine if it is safe for you to continue taking this drug.

Side effects may include: abdominal pain, abnormal dreaming, abnormal muscle movements, abnormal vision, amnesia, anxiety, arthritis, bronchitis, chest pain, confusion, constipation, decreased muscle movements, diarrhea, difficulty breathing, dizziness, drowsiness, dry mouth, eye problems, fainting, falling, fatigue, hallucinations, headache, hot flashes, increased sweating, increase/decrease in blood pressure, indigestion, joint pain, leg swelling, muscle spasms, nausea, nervousness, pain, paralysis, respiratory tract infection, runny nose, sinus inflammation, skin tingling, sore throat, stomach discomfort, swelling, toothache, tremor, urinary tract infection, viral infections, vomiting, weakness

Can I receive Requip if I am pregnant or breastfeeding?

Although the effects of Requip during pregnancy have not been adequately studied in humans, birth defects have occurred in animals. If you are pregnant or plan to become pregnant, inform your doctor immediately. Requip may inhibit production of breast milk. There is also a possibility that it will appear in breast milk and affect the nursing infant. If this medication is essential to your health, your doctor may advise you to discontinue breastfeeding.

What should I do if I miss a dose of Requip?

Take it as soon as you remember. If it is almost time for your next dose, skip the one you missed and go back to your regular schedule. Do not take 2 doses at once.

How should I store Requip?

Store at room temperature away from light.

RESTASIS

Generic name: Cyclosporine

What is Restasis?

Restasis is a medicated eye drop that increases tear production. It is used to relieve the symptoms of dry eye syndrome, including burning, redness, dryness, grittiness, and the sensation of a foreign object stuck in the eye.

What is the most important information I should know about Restasis?

Restasis should not be used to treat eye dryness that is related to an infection.

Be sure to tell your doctor if you've ever had herpes in either eye. Restasis has not been studied in people who have a history of eye-related herpes infection.

Who should not take Restasis?

Do not use Restasis if you currently have an eye infection. Also avoid the drug if you've ever had an allergic reaction to it.

What should I tell my doctor before I take the first dose of Restasis?

Tell your doctor about all prescription, over-the-counter, and herbal medications you are taking before beginning treatment with Restasis. Also, talk to your doctor about your complete medical history, especially if you have eye-related herpes infection.

What is the usual dosage?

The information below is based on the dosage guidelines your doctor uses. Depending on your condition and medical history, your doctor may prescribe a different regimen. Do not change the dosage or stop taking your medication without your doctor's approval.

Adults: The usual dose is one drop in each affected eye twice a day, about 12 hours apart.

Children: The safety and effectiveness of Restasis have not been established in children below the age of 16.

How should I take Restasis?

Use Restasis solution only in the eyes; never swallow it. Turn each individual, single-use vial upside down a few times before use to mix the solution (it should look white with no streaks). After opening the vial, immediately insert the drops into one or both eyes, as directed by your doctor. Throw away each vial when you're done; the vials should only be used once, they are not meant for multiple uses.

If you wear contact lenses, wait at least 15 minutes after using Restasis before inserting your lenses. This will prevent your contacts from absorbing the medication. You may use lubricating eye drops or artificial tears during treatment with Restasis; however, wait 15 minutes after using one product before using another.

What should I avoid while taking Restasis?

To prevent contamination of the solution, do not touch the tip of the vial to any surface, to your eyelids, or to the surrounding area of the eye.

If you wear contact lenses, talk to your doctor before using Restasis. People with reduced tear production generally should not wear contact lenses.

What are possible food and drug interactions associated with Restasis?

No interactions with Restasis have been reported.

What are the possible side effects of Restasis?

Side effects cannot be anticipated. If any develop or change in intensity, tell your doctor as soon as possible. Only your doctor can determine if it is safe for you to continue taking this drug.

Side effects may include: burning in the eye, discharge, pain, itching, redness, stinging, tearing, visual blurring

Can I receive Restasis if I am pregnant or breastfeeding?
The effects of Restasis during pregnancy and breastfeeding are unknown. Tell your doctor immediately if you are pregnant, plan to become pregnant, or are breastfeeding.

What should I do if I miss a dose of Restasis?
Take it as soon as you remember. If it is almost time for your next dose (within 6 hours), skip the dose you missed and go back to your regular schedule. Do not take two doses at once.

How should I store Restasis?
Store Restasis at room temperature.

RESTORIL
Generic name: Temazepam

What is Restoril?
Restoril is used for the relief of insomnia.

What is the most important information
I should know about Restoril?
Sleep problems are usually temporary, requiring treatment for only a short time, usually 1 or 2 days and no more than 2 to 3 weeks. Insomnia that lasts longer than this may be a sign of another medical problem. If you find you need this medicine for more than 7 to 10 days, be sure to check with your doctor.

After you stop taking Restoril, you may have more trouble sleeping than you did before you started taking it. This is called "rebound insomnia" and should clear up after one or two nights.

When you first start taking Restoril, until you know how this medicine affects you, try to avoid activities that require alertness, such as driving a car, or operating heavy machinery.

While taking Restoril, you may get up out of bed while not being fully awake and perform an activity that you do not know you are doing—nor remember the next morning. You have a greater chance of this if you drink alcohol or take other medicines that make you sleepy.

If you take Restoril every night for more than a few weeks, it loses its effectiveness to help you sleep. You can also develop physical dependence on this drug, especially if you take it regularly for more than a few weeks, or if you take more than is prescribed.

Who should not take Restoril?

If you are pregnant or plan to become pregnant, you should not take this medicine. It poses a potential risk to the developing baby.

What should I tell my doctor before I take the first dose of Restoril?

Tell your doctor about all prescription, over-the-counter, and herbal medications you are taking before beginning treatment with Restoril. Also, talk to your doctor about your complete medical history, especially if you are, or have been diagnosed with depression in the past, have kidney or liver problems, or if you have chronic lung disease. Let your doctor know if you have a history of alcohol or drug abuse.

What is the usual dosage?

The information below is based on the dosage guidelines your doctor uses. Depending on your condition and medical history, your doctor may prescribe a different regimen. Do not change the dosage or stop taking your medication without your doctor's approval.

Adults: The usual recommended dose is 15 milligrams (mg) at bedtime; however, 7.5 mg may be adequate. Your doctor will tailor your dose depending on your needs.

How should I take Restoril?

Take Restoril exactly as prescribed; do not take more than is prescribed by your doctor.

Take Restoril right before you get into bed, not sooner.

Do not take Restoril unless you are able to get a full night's sleep (7 to 8 hours) before you must be active again.

What should I avoid while taking Restoril?

Avoid drinking alcohol, or taking other medicines that can make you sleepy.

What are possible food and drug interactions associated with Restoril?

If Restoril is used with certain other drugs, the effects of either could be increased, decreased, or altered. It is especially important to check with your doctor before combining Restoril with the following: alcohol, antidepressants, antihistamines, benzodiazepines, and narcotic painkillers.

What are the possible side effects of Restoril?

Side effects cannot be anticipated. If any develop or change in intensity, tell your doctor as soon as possible. Only your doctor can determine if it is safe for you to continue taking this drug.

Side effects may include: drowsiness, headache, fatigue, nervousness, dizziness, nausea, "hangover" feeling the next morning

Side effects due to rapid decrease in dose or abrupt withdrawal from Restoril: abdominal and muscle cramps, convulsions, feeling of discomfort, inability to fall asleep or stay asleep, sweating, tremors, vomiting

Side effects due to overdose: coma, confusion, diminished reflexes, low blood pressure, difficulty breathing

Can I receive Restoril if I am pregnant or breastfeeding?
Do not take Restoril if you are pregnant or planning to become pregnant. There is an increased risk of birth defects. This drug may appear in breast milk and could affect a nursing infant. If this medication is essential to your health, your doctor may advise you to stop breastfeeding until your treatment with this medication is finished.

What should I do if I miss a dose of Restoril?
Take this medicine only when you need it.

How should I store Restoril?
Store at room temperature in a tightly sealed container. Do not share this medicine with anyone.

Retapamulin *See Altabax, page 71.*

RETIN-A AND RENOVA
Generic name: Tretinoin

What are Retin-A and Renova?
Retin-A and Renova contain the skin medication tretinoin. Retin-A is used in the treatment of acne. Renova is prescribed to reduce fine wrinkles, discoloration, and roughness on facial skin as part of a comprehensive skin care and sun-avoidance program.

What is the most important information I should know about Retin-A and Renova?
While using Retin-A or Renova, keep exposure to sunlight and sunlamps to a minimum. If you have sunburn, do not use Retin-A and Renova until you have fully recovered. Use sunscreen products (at least SPF 15) and wear protective clothing over treated areas when exposure to the sun cannot be avoided. Weather extremes, such as wind and cold, may be irritating and should also be avoided while using these products.

The medication may cause a brief feeling of warmth or a slight stinging when applied. If it causes an abnormal irritation, redness, blistering, or peeling of the skin, notify your doctor. You may need to use the medication less frequently, discontinue use temporarily, or discontinue use altogether.

During the early weeks of acne therapy, a worsening of the condition may occur due to the action of Retin-A on deep, previously unseen areas of inflammation. This is not a reason to discontinue therapy, but do notify your doctor if it occurs.

Who should not take Retin-A and Renova?

If you are sensitive to or have ever had an allergic reaction to either of these products, avoid using them.

What should I tell my doctor before I take the first dose of Retin-A and Renova?

Tell your doctor about all prescription, over-the-counter, and herbal medications you are taking before beginning treatment with Retin-A or Renova, especially if you are taking certain diuretics ("water pills") or antibiotics. You should also talk to your doctor about your complete medical history, especially if you have eczema or other chronic skin conditions.

What is the usual dosage?

The information below is based on the dosage guidelines your doctor uses. Depending on your condition and medical history, your doctor may prescribe a different regimen. Do not change the dosage or stop taking your medication without your doctor's approval.

Retin-A

Adults: Apply once a day in the evening. Once acne has responded satisfactorily, it may be possible to maintain the improvement with less frequent applications or other dosage forms. However, any change in formulation, drug concentration, or dose frequency should be closely monitored by your doctor to determine your tolerance and response.

Renova

Adults: Apply just enough to lightly cover the affected area once daily at bedtime. Do not apply more than the recommended amount; it will not improve results and may cause increased discomfort.

How should I take Retin-A and Renova?

Retin-A should be applied once a day, in the evening, to the skin where acne appears, using enough to lightly cover the affected area. The liquid form may be applied using a fingertip, gauze pad, or cotton swab. If you use gauze or cotton, avoid oversaturation, which might cause the liquid to run into areas where treatment is not intended.

Renova is applied once daily in the evening. Use only enough to lightly cover the affected area. Before you use Renova, wash your face with a mild soap, pat your skin dry, and wait 20 to 30 minutes. Then apply a dab of Renova cream the size of a pea and spread it lightly over your face, avoiding your eyes, ears, nostrils, mouth, and open wounds.

What should I avoid while taking Retin-A and Renova?

Be sure to keep these products away from the eyes, mouth, angles of the nose, and mucous membranes. Avoid sunlight and other medicines that may increase your sensitivity to sunlight.

What are possible food and drug interactions associated with Retin-A and Renova?

If Retin-A is taken with certain other drugs, the effects of either could be increased, decreased, or altered. It is especially important to check with your doctor before combining Retin-A with the following: preparations containing benzoyl peroxide or sulfur, resorcinol, salicylic acid. Use caution when using Retin-A or Renova in combination with other topical medications, medicated or abrasive soaps and cleansers, soaps and cosmetics that have a strong drying effect, products with high concentrations of alcohol, astringents, spices, or lime (especially the peel), permanent wave solutions, electrolysis, hair depilatories or waxes, or other preparations that may dry or irritate the skin.

Do not use Renova if you are taking other drugs that increase sensitivity to sunlight. These include: certain antibiotics, major tranquilizers, sulfa drugs, thiazide drugs.

What are the possible side effects of Retin-A and Renova?

Side effects cannot be anticipated. If any develop or change in intensity, tell your doctor as soon as possible. Only your doctor can determine if it is safe for you to continue taking this drug.

Side effects may include: burning, dry skin, itching, peeling, redness, and stinging.

An unusual darkening of the skin or lack of color of the skin may occur temporarily with repeated application of Retin-A.

Can I receive Retin-A and Renova if I am pregnant or breastfeeding?

The effects of Retin-A during pregnancy have not been adequately studied. If you are pregnant or plan to become pregnant, inform your doctor immediately. Do not use Renova during pregnancy or if there is a chance that you will become pregnant.

It is not known whether Retin-A or Renova appears in breast milk. Use with caution when breastfeeding and follow your doctor's instructions.

What should I do if I miss a dose of Retin-A and Renova?

Resume your regular schedule the next day. Do not apply a double dose.

How should I store Retin-A and Renova?

Store both Retin-A and Renova at room temperature and do not freeze. Retin-A gel is flammable and should be kept away from heat and flame.

RETROVIR

Generic name: Zidovudine (AZT)

What is Retrovir?

Retrovir is prescribed for adults and children >6 weeks of age infected with human immunodeficiency virus (HIV). Retrovir slows down the progress of HIV. Combining Retrovir with other drugs may help slow the progression of the disease. Retrovir is also prescribed for the prevention of the transmission of HIV from an HIV-infected mother to her unborn baby or newborn.

What is the most important information I should know about Retrovir?

The long-term effects of treatment with Retrovir are unknown. However, treatment with Retrovir may lead to blood diseases, including granulocytopenia (a severe blood disorder characterized by a sharp decrease of certain types of white blood cells called granulocytes) and severe anemia requiring blood transfusions. Retrovir may also cause an enlarged liver and the chemical imbalance known as lactic acidosis. This is especially true in women, individuals who are overweight, people who have been using Retrovir for an extended period, people with more advanced HIV, and people who start treatment later in the course of their infection.

Retrovir is not a cure for HIV infections or AIDS. Those who are infected may continue to develop complications, including opportunistic infections (infections that develop when the immune system weakens). Frequent blood counts by your doctor are strongly advised. Notify your doctor immediately of any changes in your general health.

Like other HIV drugs, Retrovir may cause a redistribution of body fat, resulting in added weight around the waist, a "buffalo hump" of fat on the upper back, breast enlargement, and wasting of the face, arms, and legs.

The use of Retrovir has not been shown to reduce the risk of transmission of HIV to others through sexual contact, blood contamination, or to nursing infants.

Who should not take Retrovir?

If you have ever had a life-threatening allergic reaction to Retrovir or any of its ingredients, you should not take Retrovir.

What should I tell my doctor before I take the first dose of Retrovir?

Tell your doctor about all prescription, over-the-counter, and herbal medications you are taking before beginning treatment with Retrovir. Also, talk to your doctor about your complete medical history, especially if you have kidney disease, liver disease, hepatitis C, pancreatitis, or bone marrow suppression.

What is the usual dosage?

The information below is based on the dosage guidelines your doctor uses. Depending on your condition and medical history, your doctor may prescribe a different regimen. Do not change the dosage or stop taking your medication without your doctor's approval.

All dosages of Retrovir must be very closely monitored by your physician. The following dosages are general; your physician will tailor the dose to your specific condition.

Tablets, Capsules, and Syrup

Adults: The usual dose of Retrovir, in combination with other HIV drugs, is 600 milligrams (mg) a day, divided into smaller doses. If you are pregnant, the usual dosage is 100 mg in capsules, tablets, or syrup 5 times a day, beginning at 14 weeks of pregnancy, until you go into labor. You will then be given the drug intravenously until the baby is born. The baby will get Retrovir every 6 hours until it is 6 weeks old.

Kidney impairment: In patients with end stage renal disease the recommended dose is 100 mg every 6 to 8 hours.

Children 6 weeks to 12 years: The usual starting dose is determined by body weight. While the dose should not exceed 200 mg every 8 hours, it must still be individually determined. The drug is given along with other HIV medications.

How should I take Retrovir?

Take Retrovir exactly as prescribed by your doctor. Do not share Retrovir with anyone and do not exceed your recommended dosage. Take it at even intervals around the clock as directed by your doctor.

What should I avoid while taking Retrovir?

Avoid having unprotected sex or sharing needles, razors, or toothbrushes. Taking this medication will not keep you from passing HIV to other people.

What are possible food and drug interactions associated with Retrovir?

If Retrovir is taken with certain other drugs, the effects of either could be increased, decreased, or altered. It is especially important to check with your doctor before combining Retrovir with the following: atovaquone, doxorubicin, fluconazole, ganciclovir, interferon, methadone, nelfinavir, phenytoin, probenecid, ribavirin, rifampin, ritonavir, stavudine, valproic acid.

Do not take Retrovir with other drugs that contain the same active ingredient (zidovudine).

What are the possible side effects of Retrovir?

Side effects cannot be anticipated. If any develop or change in intensity, tell your doctor as soon as possible. Only your doctor can determine if it is safe for you to continue taking this drug.

Side effects may include: cough, diarrhea, difficult or labored breathing, ear pain, discharge or swelling, enlarged liver, enlarged spleen, fever, general feeling of illness, headache, loss of appetite, mouth sores, nausea, nasal discharge or congestion, rash, swollen lymph nodes, vomiting

Can I receive Retrovir if I am pregnant or breastfeeding?

The effects of Retrovir during pregnancy are under study. Use during pregnancy has been shown to protect the developing baby from contracting HIV. If you are pregnant or plan to become pregnant, inform your doctor immediately. Since HIV can be passed on through breast milk to a nursing infant, do not breastfeed your baby.

What should I do if I miss a dose of Retrovir?

Take it as soon as you remember. If it is almost time for your next dose, skip the one you missed and go back to your regular schedule. Do not take 2 doses at once.

How should I store Retrovir?

Store Retrovir tablets, capsules, and syrup at room temperature. Keep capsules away from moisture.

REVATIO

Generic name: Sildenafil citrate

What is Revatio?

Revatio is used to treat pulmonary arterial hypertension (PAH). With PAH, the blood pressure in your lungs is too high. Your heart has to work hard to pump blood into your lungs. Revatio works to lower the blood pressure in your lungs and consequently helps to improve your ability to exercise.

What is the most important information I should know about Revatio?

It is important that Revatio is not combined with any type of nitrate medicines.

Revatio should also not be used if you are on therapy with ritonavir. Revatio may cause you to develop very low blood pressure levels. It is important to notify your physician if you have a history of having low blood pressure levels.

It is important to immediately notify your physician if you experience any type of hearing or vision problems while on therapy with Revatio.

Who should not take Revatio?

Revatio should not be taken by anyone who is allergic to it or any of its components. Revatio should also not be taken if you are taking nitrate medications.

What should I tell my doctor before I take the first dose of Revatio?

Tell your doctor about all prescription, over-the-counter, and herbal medications you are taking before beginning treatment with Revatio. Also, talk to your doctor about your complete medical history, especially if you are taking nitrate medications; are taking ritonavir; have a history of low blood pressure levels; have pulmonary veno-occlusive disease (PVOD); have experienced either a heart attack, stroke, or life threatening arrhythmia within the past 6 months; have coronary artery disease with angina (chest pain); have high blood pressure; have retinitis pigmentosa; are on therapy with bosentan; are on therapy with alpha-blockers; if you are a male and have penis deformities; if you have sickle cell anemia; have multiple myeloma; have leukemia; have a bleeding disorder; or if you have an active peptic ulcer..

What is the usual dosage?

The information below is based on the dosage guidelines your doctor uses. Depending on your condition and medical history, your doctor may prescribe a different regimen. Do not change the dosage or stop taking your medication without your doctor's approval.

Adults: The recommended dose of Revatio is 20 milligrams (mg) three times a day.

How should I take Revatio?

Revatio tablets should be taken 4-6 hours apart, at approximately the same time each day, with or without food.

What should I avoid while taking Revatio?

You must avoid using nitrate medications while you are taking Revatio. In addition, you should avoid taking Revatio if you are taking ritonavir.

What are possible food and drug interactions associated with Revatio?

If Revatio is taken with certain other drugs, the effects of either could be increased, decreased, or altered. It is especially important to check with your doctor before combining Revatio with the following: amlodipine, barbiturates, bosentan, carbamazepine, cimetidine, doxazosin, efavirenz, itraconazole, ketoconazole, nevirapine, nitrates, phenytoin, rifampin, rifabutin, ritonavir, and vitamin K antagonists.

What are the possible side effects of Revatio?
Side effects cannot be anticipated. If any develop or change in intensity, tell your doctor as soon as possible. Only your doctor can determine if it is safe for you to continue taking this drug.

Side effects may include: diarrhea, flushing, fever, headache, indigestion, insomnia, inflammation of the stomach, muscle pain, nose bleed, redness of the skin, runny nose, sinus inflammation, tingling or numbing of a body part, worsening shortness of breath

Can I receive Revatio if I am pregnant or breastfeeding?
The effects of Revatio during pregnancy and breastfeeding are unknown. Talk with your doctor before taking this drug if you are pregnant, plan to become pregnant, or are breastfeeding.

What should I do if I miss a dose of Revatio?
If you miss a dose of Revatio, take it as soon as you remember. If it is almost time for your next dose, skip the dose you missed and take your next dose at the regular scheduled time. Do not take a double dose.

How should I store Revatio?
Store Revatio at room temperature and keep out of the reach of children.

REYATAZ
Generic name: Atazanavir sulphate

What is Reyataz?
Reyataz is used to treat people who are infected with the human immunodeficiency virus (HIV); it is used in combination with other anti-HIV drugs. Reyataz is a protease inhibitor, and helps to block HIV protease, an enzyme that is needed for the virus to multiply.

What is the most important information I should know about Reyataz?
Reyataz does not cure HIV infection or AIDS. Reyataz does not lower your chance of passing HIV to other people through sexual contact, sharing needles, or being exposed to your blood.

Who should not take Reyataz?
You should not take Reyataz if you are allergic or sensitive to any of its ingredients.

See "What are possible food and drug interactions associated with this medication?" below for important information about what drugs you cannot take at the same time as Reyataz.

What should I tell my doctor before I take the first dose of Reyataz?
Tell your doctor about all the medications you take including prescription and nonprescription medication. Also talk to your doctor about your complete medical history, if you are pregnant or planning to become pregnant, or if you are breastfeeding. Also tell your doctor if you have liver problems or are infected with hepatitis B or C virus, or if you have end-stage kidney disease, diabetes, or hemophilia.

What is the usual dosage?
The information below is based on the dosage guidelines your doctor uses. Depending on your condition and medical history, your doctor may prescribe a different regimen. Do not change the dosage or stop taking your medication without your doctor's approval.

Patients Who Have Never Taken Anti-HIV Medication Before
Adults: The usual dose is 400 milligrams (mg) once daily with food.

Patients Who Have Taken Anti-HIV Medication Before
Adults: The usual dose is 300 mg plus 100 mg of Norvir (ritonavir) once daily with food.

Children 6 to 18 years: Dosing is based on body weight not to exceed the adult dose.

How should I take Reyataz?
Take Reyataz once every day, with food, exactly as instructed by your doctor.

What should I avoid while taking Reyataz?
You should avoid taking Reyataz with the medications listed in the next section as taking them in combination may cause serious, life-threatening side effects or death.

What are possible food and drug interactions associated with Reyataz?
If Reyataz is taken with certain drugs, the effects of either could be increased, decreased, or altered. It is especially important to check with your doctor before combining Reyataz with amiodarone, amitriptyline, atorvastatin, bepridil, cisapride, cyclosporine, desipramine, doxepin, ergot medicines (dihydroergotamine, ergonovine, ergotamine, and methylergonovine), fluticasone, imipramine, indinavir, irinotecan, lidocaine,

lovastatin, midazolam, pimozide, protyiptyline, quinidine, rifampin, rosuvastatin, sameterol, sildenafil, simvastatin, sirolimus, St. John's wort, tacrolimus, tadalafil, triazolam, trimipramine, trazodone, vardenafil, voriconazole, warfarin

What are the possible side effects of Reyataz?
Side effects cannot be anticipated. If any develop or change in intensity, tell your doctor as soon as possible. Only your doctor can determine if it is safe for you to continue taking this drug.

Side effects may include: nausea, headache, stomach pain, womiting, diarrhea, depression, fever, dizziness, trouble sleeping, and numbness, tingling or burning of hands or feet and muscle pain

If you develop a rash with any of the following symptoms, stop using Reyataz and call your doctor right away: shortness of breath, "flulike" symptoms, fever, muscle or joint aches, conjunctivitis (red or inflamed eyes, "pink eyes"), blisters, mouth sores, swelling of your face.

Can I receive Reyataz if I am pregnant or breastfeeding?
The effects of Reyataz during pregnancy are unknown. Only take Reyataz if the potential benefit justifies the potential risk to the fetus. You should not breastfeed if you are HIV-positive because of the chance of passing HIV to your baby. It is not known if Reyataz can pass into your breast milk or if it can harm your baby.

Your doctor should register you in the Antiretroviral Pregnancy Registry by calling 1-800-258-4263.

What should I do if I miss a dose of Reyataz?
If you miss a dose of Reyataz, take it as soon as possible and then take your next scheduled dose at its regular time. If it is within 6 hours of your next dose, do not take the missed dose. Wait and take the next dose at the regular time. Do not take 2 doses at one time. It is important that you do not miss any doses of Reyataz or your other anti-HIV medications.

How should I store Reyataz?
Store at room temperature.

RHINOCORT AQUA
Generic name: Budesonide

What is Rhinocort Aqua?
Rhinocort Aqua is an anti-inflammatory steroid nasal spray. It is prescribed for relief of the symptoms of hay fever and similar allergic nasal inflammations.

What is the most important information I should know about Rhinocort Aqua?

Because steroids can suppress the immune system, people taking Rhinocort Aqua may become more susceptible to infections, and their infections could be more severe. Anyone taking Rhinocort Aqua or other corticosteroids who has not had infections such as chickenpox and measles should avoid exposure to them. If you are taking Rhinocort Aqua and are exposed, tell your doctor immediately.

If you develop an infection of your nose and throat, stop using Rhinocort Aqua and call your doctor. If you already have tuberculosis or any other kind of infection, be sure your doctor knows about it.

If you have been taking a steroid in tablet form, such as prednisone, and are switched to Rhinocort Aqua, you may have symptoms of withdrawal, such as joint or muscle pain, lethargy, and depression. If you have been taking another steroid for a long time for asthma, your asthma may get worse if your medication is cut back too quickly. Using Rhinocort Aqua with another steroid drug can decrease the body's normal ability to make its own steroid chemicals.

Use this drug with caution in children and teenagers. It can affect their rate of growth.

Who should not take Rhinocort Aqua?

Do not use Rhinocort Aqua if you have recently had nasal ulcers, nasal surgery or a nasal injury; this drug would slow the healing process. You will also need to avoid Rhinocort if it gives you an allergic reaction.

What should I tell my doctor before I take the first dose of Rhinocort Aqua?

Tell your doctor about all prescription, over-the-counter, and herbal medications you are taking before beginning treatment with this drug. Also, talk to your doctor about your complete medical history, especially if you have liver problems or symptoms of an infection, or if you already take prednisone or any other steroid medication.

What is the usual dosage?

The information below is based on the dosage guidelines your doctor uses. Depending on your condition and medical history, your doctor may prescribe a different regimen. Do not change the dosage or stop taking your medication without your doctor's approval.

Adults: The recommended starting dose is 64 micrograms per day administered as 1 spray in each nostril once a day. The maximum recommended dose is 4 sprays per nostril once a day.

Children more than 12 years old: The recommended starting dose is 64 micrograms per day administered as 1 spray in each nostril once a day. The maximum recommended dose is 2 sprays per nostril once a day.

Children 6 to 12 years old: The recommended starting dose is 64 micrograms per day administered as 1 spray per nostril once a day. The maximum recommended dose is 2 sprays per nostril once a day.

How should I take Rhinocort Aqua?

Before using Rhinocort Aqua Nasal Spray, shake the container gently and prime the pump by spraying it 8 times. If used daily, the pump does not need to be reprimed. If not used for two consecutive days, reprime with one spray or until a fine mist appears. If not used for more than 14 days, rinse the applicator and reprime with two sprays or until a fine mist appears. Discard the bottle after 120 sprays, since the amount of drug in each spray will decline substantially after that point.

Relief may begin within 10 hours. Most improvement occurs during the first 1 or 2 days, but it may take as long as 2 weeks to achieve the maximum benefits. If symptoms do not improve after 2 weeks, or the condition grows worse, check with your doctor.

What should I avoid while taking Rhinocort Aqua?

Do not use doses that are larger than recommended. Avoid exposure to people who have infections such as chickenpox and measles.

What are possible food and drug interactions associated with Rhinocort Aqua?

If Rhinocort Aqua is taken with certain other drugs, its effects could be increased. It is especially important to check with your doctor before combining Rhinocort Aqua with the following: cimetidine, clarithromycin, erythromycin, itraconazole, and ketoconazole.

What are the possible side effects of Rhinocort Aqua?

Side effects cannot be anticipated. If any develop or change in intensity, tell your doctor as soon as possible. Only your doctor can determine if it is safe for you to continue taking this drug.

Side effects may include: nosebleeds, sore throat

Can I receive Rhinocort Aqua if I am pregnant or breastfeeding?

If you are pregnant or plan to become pregnant, inform your doctor immediately. Rhinocort Aqua should be used during pregnancy only if clearly needed. The effect of this drug on nursing infants is also unknown, although we do know that similar drugs have been found in breast milk. It should be used with caution by women who breastfeed.

What should I do if I miss a dose of Rhinocort Aqua?

Take the forgotten dose as soon as you remember. If it is almost time for your next dose, skip the one you missed and go back to your regular schedule. Never take two doses at the same time.

How should I store Rhinocort Aqua?
Store at room temperature with the valve up. Protect from light and do not freeze.

RIBAVIRIN

What is Ribavirin?
In combination with certain interferon drugs, ribavirin is prescribed to treat chronic hepatitis C. It is always used with another drug. By itself, ribavirin is not effective against hepatitis C.

What is the most important information I should know about Ribavirin?
Extreme care should be taken to avoid pregnancy when a woman or her partner is taking ribavirin. The drug poses a significant risk of serious harm to developing infants, even at lower doses, and it can also cause abnormalities in a man's sperm. The doctor will want to see a negative pregnancy report immediately before starting ribavirin therapy; and pregnancy tests should be done every month during therapy and for 6 months after it stops. Use at least two forms of birth control during treatment and for six months afterwards.

Within 2 weeks of starting treatment with ribavirin, about one patient in 10 develops a severe form of anemia. Your doctor will order blood tests periodically to check for this condition. Severe anemia is a serious condition that can lead to a potentially fatal heart attack. Ribavirin should be used with caution if you have a heart condition. Your doctor will perform heart tests such as an ECG before you begin treatment and will monitor your heart closely while you are taking ribavirin. You may have to discontinue therapy if you develop heart-related problems or if your heart condition gets worse.

Treatment with ribavirin and interferon drugs can have other serious side effects, including depression and suicidal thoughts (especially in adolescents), blood disorders, pancreas and lung problems, diabetes, autoimmune disorders, and infections. If you develop symptoms of these conditions, your doctor may have to discontinue treatment with ribavirin.

The risk of side effects is greater for individuals with poor kidney function. If you have this problem, your doctor will monitor you closely and adjust your dosage if necessary. Since many older adults have impaired kidney, liver, and heart function, the dosage of ribavirin is often decreased for these individuals.

The safety and effectiveness of ribavirin treatment have not been established for individuals with organ transplants, uncontrolled liver disease, and hepatitis B or unstable HIV infection. Your doctor will have your liver function tested before you begin taking ribavirin.

Who should not take Ribavirin?
Do not take ribavirin if you are pregnant or planning to become pregnant during treatment or during the 6 months after treatment has ended, are breastfeeding, or if you are a man and have a female partner who fits these criteria. In addition, you should not take ribavirin if you have hepatitis caused by your immune system attacking your liver (autoimmune hepatitis); have certain blood disorders, such as thalassemia major or sickle-cell anemia; have severe or unstable heart disease or liver disease; have severe kidney dysfunction; or have ever had an allergic reaction to any of the ingredients in this medication.

What should I tell my doctor before I take the first dose of Ribavirin?
Tell your doctor about all prescription, over-the-counter, and herbal medications you are taking before beginning treatment with this drug. Also, talk to your doctor about your complete medical history, especially if you have kidney or liver problems, heart problems, hepatitis B or unstable HIV infection, have had an organ transplant, or if you are pregnant, plan to become pregnant, or are breastfeeding.

What is the usual dosage?
The information below is based on the dosage guidelines your doctor uses. Depending on your condition and medical history, your doctor may prescribe a different regimen. Do not change the dosage or stop taking your medication without your doctor's approval.

Adults and children: Your doctor will determine the best dosage based on your condition, how much you weigh, and how your body responds to the drug. Your dosage will be lowered if you develop anemia while taking ribavirin.

How should I take Ribavirin?
Ribavirin is available in various forms, including tablets, capsules, and an oral solution.

Take it with food, and make sure you drink plenty of water while taking ribavirin, especially when you first begin treatment.

What should I avoid while taking Ribavirin?
Avoid becoming pregnant or breastfeeding while taking ribavirin.

Avoid becoming dehydrated; to reduce damage to teeth and oral membranes from dry mouth, brush your teeth and floss regularly.

What are possible food and drug interactions associated with Ribavirin?
If you are taking didanosine, treatment with ribavirin is not recommended. Serious and even fatal reactions have occurred.

If ribavirin is taken with certain other drugs, the effects of either could be increased, decreased, or altered. It is especially important to check with your doctor before combining ribavirin with HIV drugs known as nucleoside analogues, such as lamivudine and zidovudine.

What are the possible side effects of Ribavirin?

Side effects cannot be anticipated. If any develop or change in intensity, tell your doctor as soon as possible. Only your doctor can determine if it is safe for you to continue taking this drug.

Side effects may include: anxiety, anemia (possibly severe), blood disorders, chills, depression, dizziness, fatigue, fever, hair loss, headache, insomnia, irritability, joint or muscle pain, nausea, shortness of breath, skin problems, vomiting, weight loss

Can I receive Ribavirin if I am pregnant or breastfeeding?

Ribavirin may cause birth defects or death in the developing infant. Neither a woman nor her partner should take ribavirin while she is pregnant. Use two forms of contraception if either partner is taking ribavirin. Continue using two forms of contraception for 6 months after treatment is finished. If pregnancy occurs during ribavirin therapy or within 6 months afterwards, contact your doctor immediately.

It is not known whether ribavirin appears in breast milk. Because of the potential for serious adverse effects on the nursing infant, you should not breastfeed your baby while taking ribavirin.

What should I do if I miss a dose of Ribavirin?

Take it as soon as you remember. If it is almost time for your next dose, skip the one you missed and go back to your regular schedule. Never take two doses at once.

How should I store Ribavirin?

Store at room temperature.

Rifampin, isoniazid, and pyrizinamide See Rifater, below.

RIFATER

Generic name: Rifampin, isoniazid, and pyrizinamide

What is Rifater?

Rifater is a combination of the 3 drugs: rifampin, isoniazid, and pyrazinamide. It is an antibiotic used to treat the beginning phase of tuberculosis. After a 2-month period, your doctor may prescribe another combination of antituberculosis drugs, which may be continued for longer periods.

What is the most important information I should know about Rifater?

Isoniazid, one of the components of Rifater, may cause liver damage. Contact your doctor immediately if you develop yellowing of the eyes or skin, fatigue, weakness, loss of appetite, nausea, or vomiting. Rifater may cause your urine, sputum, sweat, and tears to turn a red-orange color. This is not harmful. The drug may also permanently discolor contact lenses. Since Rifater may cause eye problems, you should have a complete eye examination before starting therapy and periodically during Rifater treatment.

Who should not take Rifater?

Do not take Rifater if you have ever had an allergic reaction to or are sensitive to any of the ingredients in this product; if you have serious liver disease; or if you have ever had a severe side effect from isoniazid (such as fever, chills, and arthritis). Also avoid Rifater if you have had acute and painful joint swelling, including gout.

What should I tell my doctor before I take the first dose of Rifater?

Tell your doctor about all prescription, over-the-counter, and herbal medications you are taking before beginning treatment with Rifater. Also, talk to your doctor about your complete medical history, especially if you ever had an allergic reaction to medications, kidney disease, liver disease, porphyria, gout, or diabetes.

What is the usual dosage?

The information below is based on the dosage guidelines your doctor uses. Depending on your condition and medical history, your doctor may prescribe a different regimen. Do not change the dosage or stop taking your medication without your doctor's approval.

Adults: Take once a day, as follows: If you weigh <>97 pounds: 4 tablets; if you weigh 98 to 120 pounds: 5 tablets; if you weigh >121 pounds: 6 tablets

Safety and effectiveness in children under the age of 15 have not been established.

How should I take Rifater?

Take Rifater exactly as prescribed. Do not stop without consulting your doctor. It is important to take all of the drug prescribed for you, even if you feel better, and not to miss any doses.

Take Rifater on an empty stomach, either 1 hour before or 2 hours after a meal, with a full glass of water. Wait at least 1 hour before taking an antacid, as antacids may interfere with the drug.

If needed, your doctor may suggest taking vitamin B$_6$ while you are on Rifater therapy.

What should I avoid while taking Rifater?

Limit the amount of alcohol you drink while on this medicine. Daily alcohol intake may increase the risk for liver problems in certain individuals.

What are possible food and drug interactions associated with Rifater?

If Rifater is taken with certain other drugs, the effects of either could be increased, decreased, or altered. It is especially important to check with your doctor before combining Rifater with the following: antacids, anticonvulsants, barbiturates, blood pressure medicines, blood thinners, chloramphenicol, ciprofloxacin, clofibrate, cotrimoxazole, cycloserinem, cyclosporine, dapsone, diabetes medications, disulfiram, fluconazole, haloperidol, heart medications, itraconazole, ketoconazole, levodopa, narcotic analgesics, nortriptyline, probenecid, progestins, steroid drugs, sulfasalazine, theophylline, tranquilizers

Foods such as cheese, fish, and red wine may cause reactions if you are taking a medicine containing isoniazid. Call your doctor immediately if you experience a fast or fluttery heartbeat, flushing, sweating, headache, or light-headedness while you are taking Rifater.

What are the possible side effects of Rifater?

Side effects cannot be anticipated. If any develop or change in intensity, tell your doctor as soon as possible. Only your doctor can determine if it is safe for you to continue taking this drug.

Side effects may include: angina (chest pain), anxiety, bone pain, chest tightness, cough, coughing up blood, diabetic coma, diarrhea, difficult breathing, digestive pain, fast, fluttery heartbeat, headache, hepatitis, hives, itching, joint pain, nausea, numbness or tingling of the legs, rash, reddened skin, skin peeling or flaking, sleeplessness, sweating, swelling of the legs, vomiting, yellowing of skin and eyes

When rifampin, one of the drugs in Rifater, is taken at high doses (more than 600 milligrams) once or twice a week, it is likely that side effects may increase, including "flu-like" symptoms such as fever, chills, fatigue, weakness, upset stomach, and shortness of breath. Notify your doctor if you experience these symptoms.

Can I receive Rifater if I am pregnant or breastfeeding?

If you are pregnant or plan to become pregnant, tell your doctor immediately. You may need to discontinue the drug. If needed for preventive treatment, Rifater should be started after delivery. An ingredient in Rifater may cause uncontrollable bleeding after birth in the mother and baby when given during the last few weeks of pregnancy.

Rifater can pass into breast milk and may affect the nursing infant. Your doctor may recommend that you stop breastfeeding until your treatment with Rifater is finished.

What should I do if I miss a dose of Rifater?
Take it as soon as you remember. If it is almost time for the next dose, skip the one you missed and go back to your regular schedule. Never take 2 doses at once.

How should I store Rifater?
Store Rifater at room temperature. Protect from moisture.

Rifaximin See Xifaxan, page 1430.

Rimantadine See Flumadine, page 573.

Risedronate sodium See Actonel, page 24.

Risedronate sodium with calcium carbonate
See Actonel with Calcium, page 30.

RISPERDAL
Generic name: Risperidone

What is Risperdal?
Risperdal is an antipsychotic medication prescribed for the treatment of schizophrenia and for the short-term treatment of mania associated with bipolar disorder. It is also used in the treatment of irritability associated with autistic disorder in children.

What is the most important information I should know about Risperdal?
Risperdal may increase the risk of death when used to treat mental problems caused by dementia in elderly patients. Risperdal is not approved to treat mental problems caused by dementia.

Risperdal may cause tardive dyskinesia, a potentially irreversible condition that causes involuntary muscle spasms and twitches in the face and body. Elderly women appear to be at a higher risk for this condition. Tell your doctor immediately if you begin to have any involuntary movements. You may need to discontinue Risperdal therapy.

Risperdal may mask signs and symptoms of drug overdose and of conditions such as intestinal obstruction, brain tumor, and Reye's syndrome (a dangerous neurological condition that may follow viral infections, usually occurring in children). Risperdal may also cause difficulty when swallowing, which in turn can cause a type of pneumonia.

Risperdal may cause neuroleptic malignant syndrome (NMS), a potentially fatal condition marked by muscle stiffness or rigidity, fast heartbeat or irregular pulse, increased sweating, high fever, and blood pressure irregularities. Call your doctor immediately if you notice any of these symptoms.

Certain antipsychotic drugs, including Risperdal, are associated with an increased risk of developing high blood sugar, which on rare occasions has led to coma or death. See your doctor right away if you develop signs of high blood sugar, including dry mouth, unusual thirst, increased urination, and fatigue. If you have diabetes or have a high risk of developing it, see your doctor regularly for blood sugar testing.

Risperdal may cause dizziness, lightheadedness, or fainting; alcohol, hot weather, exercise, or fever may increase these effects. To prevent them, sit up or stand slowly, especially in the morning. Sit or lie down at the first sign of any of these effects. This effect may be more prominent when you first start taking Risperdal.

Do not drive or perform other possibly unsafe tasks until you know how you react to Risperdal.

Do not drink alcohol while you are using Risperdal.

Check with your doctor before taking medicines that may cause drowsiness (eg, sleep aids, muscle relaxers) while you are using Risperdal because the drug may add to their effects.

Risperdal may increase the amount of a certain hormone (prolactin) in your blood. Symptoms may include enlarged breasts, missed menstrual period, decreased sexual ability, or nipple discharge. Contact your doctor right away if you experience any of these symptoms.

Risperdal may rarely cause a prolonged, painful erection. This could happen even when you are not having sex. If this is not treated right away, it could lead to permanent sexual problems such as impotence. Contact your doctor right away if this happens.

Who should not take Risperdal?

If you are sensitive to or have ever had an allergic reaction to Risperdal or other major tranquilizers, you should not take Risperdal.

Risperdal should not be used to treat elderly patients who have dementia because the drug could increase the risk of stroke.

What should I tell my doctor before I take the first dose of Risperdal?

Tell your doctor about all prescription, over-the-counter, and herbal medications you are taking before beginning treatment with Risperdal. Also, talk to your doctor about your complete medical history, especially if you have breast cancer, liver, kidney or heart disease, high or low blood pressure, heart rhythm problems, a history of heart attack or stroke, seizures, epilepsy, alcohol or substance abuse or dependence, diabetes,

Alzheimer's disease, stomach or bowel problems, history of neuroleptic malignant syndrome, a history of suicidal thoughts, phenylketonuria, Parkinson's disease, or trouble swallowing. In addition, tell your doctor if you are pregnant, plan to become pregnant, or are breastfeeding.

What is the usual dosage?
The information below is based on the dosage guidelines your doctor uses. Depending on your condition and medical history, your doctor may prescribe a different regimen. Do not change the dosage or stop taking your medication without your doctor's approval.

Schizophrenia
Adults: Doses of Risperdal can be taken once a day, or divided in half and taken twice daily. The usual dose on the first day is 1 milligram (mg) taken twice a day. Incremental increases in dose are recommended. On the second day, the dose increases to 2 mg taken twice a day (for a second-day total of 4 mg). On the third day, the dose rises to 3 mg taken twice a day (for a third-day total of 6 mg). Further dosage adjustments can be made at intervals of 1 week. Over the long term, typical daily doses range from 2 to 8 mg. When dosage adjustments are necessary, small increases/decreases of 1 to 2 mg are recommended.

Bipolar Mania (Short-term Treatment of Acute Episodes)
Adults: The recommended starting dose is 2 to 3 mg per day, given as a single dose. If needed, the doctor will adjust the dose by 1 mg at intervals of at least 24 hours. The effective dosage range is 1 to 6 mg a day.

Debilitated, elderly, liver or kidney disease, or high risk for low blood pressure: The usual starting dose is 0.5 milligram (or 0.5 milliliter of oral solution) twice a day. The doctor may switch you to a once-a-day dosing schedule after the first 2 to 3 days of treatment. You may also need your Risperdal dose adjusted if you're taking certain medications. Dosage increases in these patients should be in increments of no more than 0.5 mg twice a day. Increases to dosages above 1.5 mg twice a day should generally occur at intervals of at least 1 week.

Irritability Associated with Autistic Disorder
Children 5 years and older: The recommended starting dose is 0.25 mg once a day for patients less than 44 pounds and 0.5 mg once a day for patients 44 pounds and over. The patient should continue on the starting dose for a minimum of 4 days. The dose can then be increased to the recommended dose of 0.5 mg per day for patients less than 44 pounds and 1 mg per day for patients 44 pounds and over. This dose should be maintained for a minimum of 14 days. If sufficient clinical response is not achieved, dose increases of 0.25 mg per day for patients less than 44 pounds and 0.5 mg per day for patients 44 pounds and over can be made at no less than 2-week intervals.

No dosing information is available in children under 33 pounds. Children who experience persistent drowsiness may benefit from a once-daily dose given at bedtime.

The safety and effectiveness of Risperdal have not been studied in autistic children less than 5 years old.

How should I take Risperdal?
Do not take more or less of Risperdal than prescribed. Higher doses are more likely to cause unwanted side effects.

Risperdal may be taken with or without food. Risperdal oral solution comes with a calibrated pipette to use for measuring. The oral solution can be taken with water, coffee, orange juice, and low-fat milk, but not with cola drinks or tea.

Take Risperdal on a regular schedule to get the most benefit from it. Taking Risperdal at the same time each day will help you remember to take it.

Continue to take Risperdal even if you feel well. Do not miss any doses.

What should I avoid while taking Risperdal?
Risperdal may make you sleepy. Avoid driving or operating potentially dangerous machinery. Do not participate in any activities that require full alertness until you know how this medication affects you.

Do not drink alcohol with Risperdal.

Check with your doctor before taking medicines that may cause drowsiness (eg, sleep aids, muscle relaxers) while you are using Risperdal; it may add to their effects.

What are possible food and drug interactions associated with Risperdal?
If Risperdal is taken with certain other drugs, the effects of either could be increased, decreased, or altered. It is especially important to check with your doctor before combining Risperdal with the following: blood pressure medicines, bromocriptine mesylate, carbamazepine, clozapine, fluoxetine, levodopa, paroxetine, phenobarbital, phenytoin, quinidine, rifampin, and valproic acid.

You may experience drowsiness and other potentially serious effects if Risperdal is combined with alcohol and other drugs that slow the central nervous system.

What are the possible side effects of Risperdal?
Side effects cannot be anticipated. If any develop or change in intensity, tell your doctor as soon as possible. Only your doctor can determine if it is safe for you to continue taking this drug.

Side effects may include: agitation, anxiety, constipation, dizziness, hallucinations, headache, indigestion, insomnia, rapid or irregular heartbeat, restlessness, runny nose, sleepiness, vomiting, weight change

Can I receive Risperdal if I am pregnant or breastfeeding?
The effects of Risperdal during pregnancy are unknown. Tell your doctor immediately if you are pregnant or plan to become pregnant. Because Risperdal is excreted in breast milk, do not use it if you are breastfeeding.

What should I do if I miss a dose of Risperdal?
Take it as soon as you remember. If it is almost time for your next dose, skip the one you missed and go back to your regular schedule. Do not take two doses at once.

How should I store Risperdal?
Store at room temperature. Protect the tablets from light and moisture; protect the oral solution from light and freezing.

Risperidone *See Risperdal, page 1158.*

RITALIN/RITALIN-SR/RITALIN LA
Generic name: Methylphenidate hydrochloride

What is Ritalin/Ritalin-SR/Ritalin LA?
Ritalin and other brands of methylphenidate are mild central nervous system stimulants used in the treatment of attention-deficit/hyperactivity disorder (ADHD) in children.

Ritalin is also used in adults to treat narcolepsy (an uncontrollable desire to sleep).

What is the most important information I should know about Ritalin/Ritalin-SR/Ritalin LA?
When given for ADHD, Ritalin should be an integral part of a total treatment program that includes psychological, educational, and social measures.

There are reports of heart and mental problems in patients taking Ritalin or other related stimulants. Some of the problems are sudden death in patients with previous heart problems, heart attacks in adults, increased blood pressure and heart rate, new or worsening symptoms of behavior problems, bipolar disorder, and aggressive or hostile behavior. Call your doctor right away if you or your child develop signs of heart problems such as chest pain, shortness of breath, or fainting while taking Ritalin.

Excessive doses of Ritalin over a long period of time may cause addiction. It is also possible to develop tolerance to the drug, so that larger doses are needed to produce the original effect. Be sure to check with your doctor before making any change in dosage; and stop the drug only under your doctor's supervision.

There is no information regarding the safety and effectiveness of long-term treatment in children. However, slowing of growth has been seen with the long-term use of stimulants, so your doctor will monitor your child carefully while he or she is taking Ritalin.

The use of Ritalin in children less than 6 years old is not recommended.

Who should not take Ritalin/Ritalin-SR/Ritalin LA?

This drug should not be prescribed for anyone experiencing anxiety, tension, and agitation, since the drug may aggravate these symptoms. Individuals sensitive or allergic to Ritalin should not take it.

This medication should not be taken by individuals with glaucoma, those who suffer from tics (repeated, involuntary twitches) or with a family history of Tourette's syndrome (severe and multiple tics).

This drug is not intended for use in children whose symptoms may be caused by stress or a psychiatric disorder.

This medication should not be used for the prevention or treatment of normal fatigue, nor should it be used for the treatment of severe depression.

Do not take Ritalin if you or your child are taking or have taken antidepressants known as monoamine oxidase inhibitors (MAOIs) in the last 14 days.

What should I tell my doctor before I take the first dose of Ritalin/Ritalin-SR/Ritalin LA?

Tell your doctor about all prescription, over-the-counter, and herbal medications you are taking before beginning treatment with Ritalin, especially if you are currently taking or have recently taken MAOIs. Also, talk to your doctor about your complete medical history, especially if you have a heart problems such as a congenital heart defect, heart failure, heart rhythm disorder or recent heart attack, high blood pressure, a personal or family history of mental illness, psychotic disorder, bipolar disorder, depression, suicide attempt, epilepsy or other seizure disorder, a history of drug or alcohol addiction, glaucoma, a personal or family history of tics or Tourette's syndrome, severe anxiety, tension, or agitation.

What is the usual dosage?

The information below is based on the dosage guidelines your doctor uses. Depending on your condition and medical history, your doctor may prescribe a different regimen. Do not change the dosage or stop taking your medication without your doctor's approval.

Ritalin tablets and capsules should not be given to children under 6 years of age.

Ritalin Tablets

Adults: The average dosage is 20 to 30 milligrams (mg) a day, divided into 2 or 3 doses, preferably taken 30 to 45 minutes before meals. Some people may need 40 to 60 mg daily, others only 10 to 15 mg. Your doctor will determine the best dose.

Children 6 years and older: The usual starting dose is 5 mg taken twice a day, before breakfast and lunch; your doctor may increase the dose by 5 to 10 mg a week. Your child should not take more than 60 mg in a day. If you do not see any improvement over a period of one month, check with your doctor.

Ritalin-SR Tablets

Adults: These are suspended-release tablets that keep working for 8 hours. They may be used in place of Ritalin tablets if they deliver a comparable dose over an 8-hour period.

Children 6 years and older: These tablets continue working for 8 hours. Your doctor will decide if they should be used in place of the regular tablets.

Ritalin LA Capsules

Children 6 years and older: The recommended starting dose is 20 mg once daily in the morning. At weekly intervals, your doctor may increase the dose by 10 mg, up to a maximum of 60 mg once a day.

How should I take Ritalin/Ritalin-SR/Ritalin LA?

Follow your doctor's directions carefully. Ritalin should be taken 30 to 45 minutes before meals. If the drug interferes with sleep, give the child the last dose before 6 p.m.

Ritalin-SR and Ritalin LA are long-acting forms of the drug and are taken less frequently. They should be swallowed whole, never crushed or chewed. Ritalin LA may also be given by sprinkling the contents of the capsule on a tablespoon of cool applesauce and administering immediately, followed by a drink of water.

What should I avoid while taking Ritalin/Ritalin-SR/Ritalin LA?

Some people have had visual disturbances such as blurred vision while being treated with Ritalin. Be careful if you drive or do anything that requires you to be awake and alert until you know how this drug affects you.

What are possible food and drug interactions associated with Ritalin/Ritalin-SR/Ritalin LA?

If Ritalin is taken with certain other drugs, the effects of either could be increased, decreased, or altered. It is especially important to check with your doctor before combining Ritalin with the following: antidepressants, antiseizure drugs, blood pressure drugs, blood thinners such as warfarin, clonidine, guanethidine, MAO inhibitors, and phenylbutazone.

What are the possible side effects of Ritalin/ Ritalin-SR/Ritalin LA?

Side effects cannot be anticipated. If any develop or change in intensity, tell your doctor as soon as possible. Only your doctor can determine if it is safe for you to continue taking this drug.

Side effects may include: inability to fall or stay asleep, nervousness
These side effects can usually be controlled by reducing the dosage and omitting the drug in the afternoon or evening.

More common side effects in children may include: loss of appetite, abdominal pain, weight loss during long-term therapy, inability to fall or stay asleep, abnormally fast heartbeat

Can I receive Ritalin/Ritalin-SR/Ritalin LA if I am pregnant or breastfeeding?
The effects of Ritalin during pregnancy and breastfeeding are unknown. Tell your doctor immediately if you are pregnant, plan to become pregnant, or are breastfeed

What should I do if I miss a dose of Ritalin/ Ritalin-SR/Ritalin LA?
Take it as soon as you remember. Take the remaining doses for the day at regularly spaced intervals. Do not take two doses at once.

How should I store Ritalin/Ritalin-SR/Ritalin LA?
Store at room temperature in a tightly closed, light-resistant container. Protect from moisture.

Ritonavir *See Norvir, page 916.*

RITUXAN
Generic name: Rituximab

What is Rituxan?
Rituxan is used to treat mild-to-moderate rheumatoid arthritis (RA) that has not responded to other therapy. It is also used in combination with chemotherapy to treat non-Hodgkin's Lymphoma (NHL).

What is the most important information I should know about Rituxan?
Rituxan may cause hives, swelling, dizziness, blurred vision, drowsiness, headache, cough, wheezing, or have trouble breathing while receiving or after receiving it. Also, this drug may cause severe skin reactions, such as painful sores, ulcers, blisters, or peeling of the skin.
Rituxan may cause Tumor Lysis syndrome (TLS); this is the quick breakdown of blood cancer, which may lead to kidney problems. People with non-Hodgkin's Lymphoma are more likely to develop TLS.

Who should not take Rituxan?
Do not take Rituxan if you are allergic to any of it ingredients.

What should I tell my doctor before I take the first dose of Rituxan?

Tell your doctor about all prescription, over-the-counter, and herbal medications you are taking before beginning treatment with Rituxan. Also, talk to your doctor about your complete medical history, including previous therapies used, especially if you have stomach/bowel problems, heart problems, kidney problems, or if you have/had hepatitis B.

What is the usual dosage?

The information below is based on the dosage guidelines your doctor uses. Depending on your condition and medical history, your doctor may prescribe a different regimen. Do not change the dosage or stop taking your medication without your doctor's approval.

Non-Hodgkin's Lymphoma
The recommended dose of Rituxan is 375 milligrams (mg)/m² IV infusion once weekly for 4 or 8 doses.

Rheumatoid Arthritis
The recommended dose Rituxan is two-1000 mg IV infusions separated by 2 weeks.

How should I take Rituxan?

This drug will be administered to you by your doctor. The Rituxan solution for IV infusion should be given at an initial rate of 50 mg/hr. Rituxan should not be mixed or diluted with any other drugs.

What are the possible side effects of Rituxan?

Side effects cannot be anticipated. If any develop or change in intensity, tell your doctor as soon as possible. Only your doctor can determine if it is safe for you to continue taking this drug.

Side effects for RA patients may include: Aching joints, chills, cough, fever, headache, hives, itching, nausea, shakes, sneezing, swelling, throat irritation or tightness, upper respiratory tract infection

Side effects for NHL patients may include: Fever, headache, nausea, shaking chills, tiredness

Can I receive Rituxan if I am pregnant or breastfeeding?

The effects of Rituxan during pregnancy and breastfeeding are unknown. Talk with your doctor before taking this drug if you are pregnant, plan to become pregnant, or are breastfeeding.

How should I store Rituxan?

Store in a refrigerator. Do not freeze or shake the vials.

Rituximab *See Rituxan, page 1165.*

Rivastigmine tartrate See Exelon, page 528.

Rizatriptan benzoate See Maxalt, page 790.

ROBAXIN
Generic name: Methocarbamol

What is Robaxin?
Robaxin is prescribed, along with rest, physical therapy, and other measures, for the relief of pain due to severe muscular injuries, sprains, and strains.

What is the most important information I should know about Robaxin?
Robaxin is not a substitute for the rest or physical therapy needed for proper healing.

Although the drug may temporarily provide relief from an injury, avoid pushing your recovery. Lifting or exercising too soon may further damage the muscle.

Who should not take Robaxin?
If you are sensitive to or have ever had an allergic reaction to Robaxin or other drugs of this type, you should not take Robaxin.

What should I tell my doctor before I take the first dose of Robaxin?
Tell your doctor about all prescription, over-the-counter, and herbal medication you are taking before beginning treatment with Robaxin. Also, talk to your doctor about your complete medical history, especially if you have kidney or liver disease.

What is the usual dosage?
The information below is based on the dosage guidelines your doctor uses. Depending on your condition and medical history, your doctor may prescribe a different regimen. Do not change the dosage or stop taking your medication without your doctor's approval.

Robaxin
Adults: The usual starting dose is 500 milligrams (mg) 3 tablets taken 4 times a day. The usual long-term dose is 2 tablets taken 4 times a day.

Robaxin-750
Adults: The usual starting dose is 750 mg 2 tablets taken 4 times a day. The usual long-term dose is 1 tablet taken every 4 hours or 2 tablets taken 3 times a day.

Children: The safety and effectiveness of Robaxin have not been established in children.

How should I take Robaxin?
Take Robaxin exactly as prescribed. Do not take a larger dose or use more often than directed.

What should I avoid while taking Robaxin?
Robaxin may cause drowsiness and dizziness. Do not drive a car or operate potentially dangerous machinery until you know how the drug affects you.

Avoid or be careful using alcoholic beverages.

What are possible food and drug interactions associated with Robaxin?
If Robaxin is taken with certain other drugs, the effects of either could be increased, decreased, or altered. It is especially important to check with your doctor before combining Robaxin with the following: alcohol, drugs for myasthenia gravis, narcotic pain relievers, sleep aids, tranquilizers.

What are the possible side effects of Robaxin?
Side effects cannot be anticipated. If any develop or change in intensity, tell your doctor as soon as possible. Only your doctor can determine if it is safe for you to continue taking this drug.

Side effects may include: Abnormal taste, allergic reaction, amnesia, blurred vision, confusion, double vision, dizziness, drop in blood pressure and fainting, drowsiness, fever, flushing, headache, hives, indigestion, insomnia, itching, light-headedness, nasal congestion, nausea, pinkeye, poor coordination, rash, seizures, slowed heartbeat, uncontrolled eye movement, vertigo, vomiting, yellow eyes and skin

Can I receive Robaxin if I am pregnant or breastfeeding?
The effects of Robaxin during pregnancy and breastfeeding are unknown. Tell your doctor immediately if you are pregnant, plan to become pregnant, or are breastfeeding.

What should I do if I miss a dose of Robaxin?
If only an hour or so has passed, take it as soon as you remember. If you do not remember until later, skip the dose and go back to your regular schedule. Do not take 2 doses at once.

How should I store Robaxin?
Store at room temperature in a tightly closed container.

Ropinirole hydrochloride See Requip, page 1134.

Rosiglitazone maleate See Avandia, page 162.

Rosiglitazone maleate and glimepiride See Avandaryl, page 160.

Rosiglitazone maleate and metformin hydrochloride
See Avandamet, page 157.

Rosuvastatin calcium See Crestor, page 354.

ROWASA
Generic name: Mesalamine

What is Rowasa?

Rowasa suspension enema is used to treat mild to moderate ulcerative colitis (inflammation of the large intestine and rectum), as well as inflammation of the lower colon and rectum.

What is the most important information I should know about Rowasa?

Mesalamine, the active ingredient in this product, has been known to cause side effects such as bloody diarrhea, cramping, fever, rash, severe headache, and severe stomach pain. If you develop any of these symptoms, stop taking this medication and consult your doctor.

Your doctor should check your kidney function while you are taking mesalamine, especially if you have a history of kidney disease or you are using other anti-inflammatory drugs. Because older adults tend to have weaker kidneys, mesalamine is more likely to trigger side effects within this age group. The drug also seems more prone to cause blood disorders in older adults. If you are 65 or older, be sure to tell the doctor about any change in your health.

You should use mesalamine cautiously if you are allergic to sulfasalazine. If you develop a rash or fever, you should stop using the medication and notify your doctor.

Some people using mesalamine have developed flare-ups of their colitis. Inflammation of the pancreas has also been reported.

Rare cases of pericarditis, in which the membrane surrounding the heart becomes inflamed, have been reported with products containing mesalamine. Symptoms may include chest, neck, and shoulder pain, and shortness of breath.

Rowasa contains a sulfite that may cause allergic reactions in some people. These reactions may include shock and severe, possibly fatal asthma attacks. Most people aren't sensitive to sulfites. However, some people with asthma might be sensitive and should take any medication containing sulfites cautiously.

Who should not take Rowasa?

Do not use Rowasa if you are allergic or sensitive to mesalamine or any other ingredients in the product.

What should I tell my doctor before I take the first dose of Rowasa?

Tell your doctor about all prescription, over-the-counter, and herbal medications you are taking before beginning treatment with this drug. Also, talk to your doctor about your complete medical history, especially if you have kidney or liver problems, heart problems, or you are allergic to sulfites or any medications.

What is the usual dosage?

The information below is based on the dosage guidelines your doctor uses. Depending on your condition and medical history, your doctor may prescribe a different regimen. Do not change the dosage or stop taking your medication without your doctor's approval.

Adults: The usual dose is 1 rectal enema (60 milliliters) per day, preferably used at bedtime and retained for about 8 hours. Treatment time usually lasts from 3 to 6 weeks, although improvement may be seen within 3 to 21 days.

How should I take Rowasa?

Rowasa suspension enema comes in boxes of 7 bottles each. After the foil on the box has been unwrapped, all Rowasa Suspension Enemas should be used promptly, following your doctor's instructions. The suspension enema is normally off-white to tan in color, but may darken over time once its foil cover is unwrapped. You may still use the enema if it is slightly discolored, but do not use Rowasa if it is dark brown. If you have any questions about using this product, contact your doctor.

Use Rowasa at bedtime. Shake the bottle thoroughly. Uncover the applicator tip. You may find it easier to use Rowasa if you lie down on your left side, extending your left leg and bending your right leg forward for a comfortable balance. An alternative position is on your knees with your hips in the air and your head and shoulders down on the bed. Pointing the applicator tip slightly towards the navel, gently insert the tip into the rectum. Tilt the bottle slightly towards the back, then squeeze it slowly to discharge the contents. Remain in position for at least 30 minutes to allow thorough distribution of the medicine. Retain the enema all night (8 hours) for best results.

What should I avoid while taking Rowasa?

Avoid getting the medication on clothes, fabrics, and similar surfaces, since it may leave a stain.

What are possible food and drug interactions associated with Rowasa?

If Rowasa is taken with certain other drugs, the effects of either could be increased, decreased, or altered. It is especially important to check with your doctor before combining Rowasa with sulfasalazine.

What are the possible side effects of Rowasa?
Side effects cannot be anticipated. If any develop or change in intensity, tell your doctor as soon as possible. Only your doctor can determine if it is safe for you to continue taking this drug.

Side effects may include: diarrhea, dizziness, flu-like symptoms, gas, headache, nausea, stomach pain

Can I receive Rowasa if I am pregnant or breastfeeding?
Pregnant women should use mesalamine only if clearly needed. Mesalamine has been found in breast milk. If this medication is essential to your health your doctor may advise you to discontinue breastfeeding until your treatment is finished.

What should I do if I miss a dose of Rowasa?
Take it as soon as you remember. If it is almost time for your next dose, skip the one you missed and go back to your regular schedule. Never take 2 doses at the same time.

How should I store Rowasa?
Store at room temperature.

ROZEREM
Generic name: Ramelteon

What is Rozerem?
Rozerem is used for the treatment of insomnia characterized by difficulty with sleep onset.

What is the most important information I should know about Rozerem?
If you experience worsening insomnia or any unusual thinking or behavior, see your doctor since this may signal an unrecognized disorder.

Rozerem is not approved for use in children.

Who should not take Rozerem?
Do not take Rozerem if you are allergic to the medication or any of its ingredients.

Rozerem should not be used in combination with fluvoxamine or if you have severe liver disease.

What should I tell my doctor before I take the first dose of Rozerem?
Tell your doctor about all prescription, over-the-counter, and herbal medications you are taking before beginning treatment with Rozerem. Also,

talk to your doctor about your complete medical history, especially if you have liver disease, sleep apnea (pauses in breathing during sleep), depression, or if you have suicidal thoughts.

What is the usual dosage?
The information below is based on the dosage guidelines your doctor uses. Depending on your condition and medical history, your doctor may prescribe a different regimen. Do not change the dosage or stop taking your medication without your doctor's approval.

Adults: The recommended dose is 8 milligrams (mg) taken within 30 minutes of going to bed. Do not take this medicine with, or immediately after a high-fat meal.

How should I take Rozerem?
Take Rozerem exactly as directed by your doctor. Take Rozerem within 30 minutes prior to going to bed and limit your activities to those necessary to prepare for bed.

You can take Rozerem with or without food, but for Rozerem to work best, do not take it with or immediately after a high-fat, heavy meal.

Do not crush or chew the tablets. Take each tablet whole.

What should I avoid while taking Rozerem?
Avoid using alcoholic beverages.

Use caution when driving, operating machinery, or performing other hazardous activities. Rozerem will cause drowsiness and may cause dizziness. If you experience drowsiness or dizziness, avoid these activities.

What are possible food and drug interactions associated with Rozerem?
If Rozerem is taken with certain other drugs, the effects of either could be increased, decreased, or altered. It is especially important to check with your doctor before combining Rozerem with the following: fluconazole, fluvoxamine, ketoconazole, and rifampin.

What are the possible side effects of Rozerem?
Side effects cannot be anticipated. If any develop or change in intensity, tell your doctor as soon as possible. Only your doctor can determine if it is safe for you to continue taking this drug.

Side effects may include: dizziness, fatigue, headache, nausea, drowsiness, upper respiratory tract infection

Can I receive Rozerem if I am pregnant or breastfeeding?
The effects of Rozerem during pregnancy and breastfeeding are unknown. Tell your doctor immediately if you are pregnant, plan to become pregnant, or are breastfeeding.

What should I do if I miss a dose of Rozerem?
Rozerem is usually taken only if you need it to help you sleep; missing a dose will not cause problems.

How should I store Rozerem?
Store at room temperature away from moisture and heat.

RYTHMOL
Generic name: Propafenone hydrochloride

What is Rythmol?
Rythmol is used to help correct certain life-threatening heartbeat irregularities (ventricular arrhythmias).

**What is the most important information
I should know about Rythmol?**
There is a possibility that Rythmol may cause new heartbeat irregularities or make existing ones worse. Rythmol is therefore used only for serious conditions, and should be accompanied by periodic electrocardiograms (EKGs) prior to and during treatment.

Rythmol may interfere with your body's normal ability to manufacture blood cells. Too few white blood cells may cause signs and symptoms that mimic infection. If you experience fever, chills, or sore throat while taking Rythmol—especially during the first 3 months of treatment—notify your doctor right away.

Rythmol may cause a lupus-like illness characterized by rashes and arthritic symptoms. If you have been taking Rythmol and tests shows that your blood contains ANA (antinuclear antibodies), your doctor may want to discontinue the medication.

Who should not take Rythmol?
Do not take Rythmol if you have ever had an allergic reaction to or are sensitive to it. Your doctor will not prescribe Rythmol if you are suffering from any of the following conditions: abnormally slow heartbeat; certain heartbeat irregularities, such as atrioventricular block or "sick sinus" syndrome, that have not been corrected by a pacemaker; cardiogenic shock (shock due to a weak heart); chronic bronchitis or emphysema; congestive heart failure that is not well controlled; mineral (electrolyte) imbalance; and severe low blood pressure.

**What should I tell my doctor before
I take the first dose of Rythmol?**
Tell your doctor about all prescription, over-the-counter, and herbal medication you are taking before beginning treatment with Rythmol. Also, talk to your doctor about your complete medical history, especially if you

have any other heart disease, heart problems, have a pacemaker, asthma, chronic obstructive pulmonary disease (COPD), any other breathing disorder, liver disease, kidney disease, or myasthenia gravis.

What is the usual dosage?
The information below is based on the dosage guidelines your doctor uses. Depending on your condition and medical history, your doctor may prescribe a different regimen. Do not change the dosage or stop taking your medication without your doctor's approval.

In most cases, treatment with Rythmol begins in the hospital. Your doctor will tailor your dosage according to your individual condition and the presence of other disorders.

Adults: The usual initial dose of Rythmol is 150 milligrams (mg) every 8 hours. Your doctor may increase the dosage at a minimum of 3-4 day intervals, depending on how you respond to the initial dosage. If you are an older adult, your doctor will increase the dosage more slowly at the beginning of treatment. The maximum recommended daily dosage of Rythmol is 900 mg.

How should I take Rythmol?
Rythmol may be taken with food or on an empty stomach.

Take Rythmol exactly as prescribed. It works best when there is a constant amount of the drug in the blood; take it at evenly spaced intervals.

What should I avoid while taking Rythmol?
Use caution when driving, operating machinery, or performing other hazardous activities that require mental alertness while taking Rythmol.

What are possible food and drug interactions associated with Rythmol?
If Rythmol is taken with certain other drugs, the effects of either could be increased, decreased, or altered. It is especially important to check with your doctor before combining Rythmol with the following: amiodarone, beta blockers, cimetidine, cyclosporine, digoxin, grapefruit juice, local anesthetics (including those used during dental procedures), quinidine, rifampin, theophylline, and warfarin.

There may be certain other psychiatric, antidepressant, antifungal, or antibiotic drugs that could possibly cause a reaction if combined with Rythmol. Be sure to tell your doctor if you are taking any of these types of medications.

What are the possible side effects of Rythmol?
Side effects cannot be anticipated. If any develop or change in intensity, tell your doctor as soon as possible. Only your doctor can determine if it is safe for you to continue taking this drug.

Side effects may include: constipation, blurred vision, dizziness, fatigue, headache, heartbeat abnormalities, nausea, unusual taste in the mouth, vomiting, weakness

Can I receive Rythmol if I am pregnant or breastfeeding?
The effects of Rythmol during pregnancy and breastfeeding are unknown. Tell your doctor immediately if you are pregnant, plan to become pregnant, or are breastfeeding.

What should I do if I miss a dose of Rythmol?
Take it as soon as you remember. If it is almost time for your next dose, skip the one you missed and go back to your regular schedule. Never take two doses at the same time.

How should I store Rythmol?
Keep Rythmol at room temperature in a tightly closed container away from direct light.

Salmeterol xinafoate *See Serevent, page 1182.*

SANCTURA
Generic name: Trospium chloride

What is Sanctura?
Sanctura is a smooth muscle relaxant. It relieves spasms of the bladder. Sanctura is used to treat overactive bladder with the symptoms of urinary frequency, urinary urgency, and urinary incontinence.

What is the most important information I should know about Sanctura?
Avoid becoming overheated in hot weather. Sanctura can reduce sweating, making you more susceptible to heat stroke.

Who should not take Sanctura?
Do not take Sanctura if you are allergic to the medication or any or its ingredients.

Sanctura should not be used if you have urinary retention (lack of ability to urinate), a blockage in the intestines, or uncontrolled narrow angle glaucoma (an eye disease).

What should I tell my doctor before I take the first dose of Sanctura?
Tell your doctor about all prescription, over-the-counter, and herbal medications you are taking before beginning treatment with Sanctura. Also,

talk to your doctor about your complete medical history, especially if you have kidney disease, liver disease, glaucoma, urinary retention, or gastrointestinal disorders.

What is the usual dosage?
The information below is based on the dosage guidelines your doctor uses. Depending on your condition and medical history, your doctor may prescribe a different regimen. Do not change the dosage or stop taking your medication without your doctor's approval.

Adults: Dosage is based on your medical condition and response to therapy.

The recommended dose is 20 milligrams (mg) twice daily.

For patients with severe kidney disease, the recommended dose is 20 mg once a day at bedtime.

Adults: The recommended dose is 20 mg once a day based on the patient's tolerability.

How should I take Sanctura?
Take Sanctura at least 1 hour before a meal or on an empty stomach.

What should I avoid while taking Sanctura?
Sanctura may produce dizziness or blurred vision. If you experience dizziness, drowsiness, or blurred vision, avoid activities that require mental alertness such as driving an automobile or operating machinery.

Do not drink alcohol while taking Sanctura.

Avoid becoming overheated in hot weather.

What are possible food and drug interactions associated with Sanctura?
If Sanctura is taken with certain other drugs, the effects of either could be increased, decreased, or altered. It is especially important to check with your doctor before combining Sanctura with the following: alcohol, anticholinergic agents, digoxin, metformin, morphine, procainamide, tenofovir, vancomycin.

What are the possible side effects of Sanctura?
Side effects cannot be anticipated. If any develop or change in intensity, tell your doctor as soon as possible. Only your doctor can determine if it is safe for you to continue taking this drug.

Side effects may include: blurred vision or large pupils, constipation, difficulty urinating, dizziness, drowsiness, dry mouth, dryness of the eyes, headache, upset stomach

Can I receive Sanctura if I am pregnant or breastfeeding?

The effects of Sanctura during pregnancy and breastfeeding are unknown. Tell your doctor immediately if you are pregnant, plan to become pregnant, or are breastfeeding.

What should I do if I miss a dose of Sanctura?

If you miss a dose take the next dose one hour prior to your next meal. Do not take a double dose.

How should I store Sanctura?

Store Sanctura at room temperature, away from moisture and heat.

SEASONIQUE

Generic name: Levonorgestrel and ethinyl estradiol

What is Seasonique?

Seasonique tablets are oral contraceptive pills used for the prevention of pregnancy in women.

What is the most important information I should know about Seasonique?

This product (like all oral contraceptives) is intended to prevent pregnancy. It does not protect against HIV infection (AIDS) and other sexually transmitted diseases such as chlamydia, genital herpes, genital warts, gonorrhea, hepatitis B, and syphilis.

If you miss your period when you are taking the yellow pills, call your healthcare provider because you may be pregnant.

Who should not take Seasonique?

You should not take the pill if you are pregnant. Although cardiovascular disease risks may be increased with oral contraceptive use after age 40 in healthy, nonsmoking women (even with the newer low-dose formulations), there are also greater potential health risks associated with pregnancy in older women. Also, do not take this medication if you have heart problems, have or had clotting disorders, have uncontrolled high blood pressure, are going to have a major surgery, or have a personal history of breast cancer.

What should I tell my doctor before I take the first dose of Seasonique?

Tell your doctor about all prescription, over-the-counter, and herbal medications you are taking before beginning treatment with Seasonique. Also, talk your doctor about your entire medical history, as well as issues you may be presently experiencing, including diabetes, high blood pressure, heart problems, high cholesterol, clotting disorders, undiagnosed genital bleeding, and if you have any known or suspected cancers.

What is the usual dosage?

The information below is based on the dosage guidelines your doctor uses. Depending on your condition and medical history, your doctor may prescribe a different regimen. Do not change the dosage or stop taking your medication without your doctor's approval.

The dosage of Seasonique is 1 light blue-green tablet for 84 consecutive days, followed by 7 days of yellow tablets.

How should I take Seasonique?

You should take 1 pill of Seasonique at the same time every day. If you miss pills you could get pregnant; this includes starting the pack late. The more pills you miss, the more likely you are to get pregnant. Do not skip pills even if you are spotting or have irregular bleeding. However, if this bleeding is persistent and prolonged, contact your healthcare provider.

What should I avoid while taking Seasonique?

Avoid smoking while taking Seasonique. Cigarette smoking increases the risk of serious heart problems and blood clots in the legs and lungs while on this medication. This risk increases with age and with the amount of smoking (15 or more cigarettes per day). Also, avoid using Seasonique before or during early pregnancy.

What are possible food and drug interactions associated with Seasonique?

If Seasonique is taken with certain other drugs, the effects of either could be increased, decreased, or altered. It is especially important to check with your doctor before combining Seasonique with the following: antibiotics, anticonvulsants, barbiturates, carbamazepine, felbamate, griseofulvin, oxcarbazepine, phenylbutazone, phenytoin, rifampin, St. John's wort, topiramate.

What are the possible side effects of Seasonique?

Side effects cannot be anticipated. If any develop or change in intensity, tell your doctor as soon as possible. Only your doctor can determine if it is safe for you to continue taking this drug.

Side effects may include: bleeding or spotting between menstrual periods, breast tenderness, difficulty wearing contact lenses, nausea, vomiting, weight gain

Can I receive Seasonique if I am pregnant or breastfeeding?

You should not take Seasonique if you are pregnant, planning to become pregnant, or are breastfeeding.

What should I do if I miss a dose of Seasonique?

If you miss 1 dose of Seasonique (light blue-green tablet):
Take the pill as soon as you remember, and continue your normal schedule. This means that you may take 2 pills in 1 day. You do not need to use a backup method of birth control.

If you miss 2 doses of Seasonique (light blue-green tablet):
Take 2 pills on the day you remember and 2 pills the day after. Continue taking 1 pill a day after that, until you finish the pack. You could become pregnant in the 7 days after you restart your pills so use a backup method of birth control for the 7 days after you restart your pills.

If you miss 3+ doses of Seasonique (light blue-green tablet):
Do not remove the missed pills from the pack, you will not take them. Continue taking 1 pill per day until the pack is finished. You may experience bleeding the week after you missed your pills. You may also become pregnant within the first 7 days of restarting your pills; use alternate forms of contraception (condoms) during this time.

If you miss any of the 7 yellow pills:
Throw away the missed pills. Keep taking the scheduled pills until the pack is finished. You do not need to use a backup method of birth control.

How should I store Seasonique?
Store Seasonique at room temperature.

SECTRAL
Generic name: Acebutolol hydrochloride

What is Sectral?
Sectral, a type of medication known as a beta blocker, is used in the treatment of high blood pressure and abnormal heart rhythms. When used to treat high blood pressure, it is effective used alone or in combination with other high blood pressure medications, particularly with a thiazide-type diuretic.

What is the most important information I should know about Sectral?
Sectral should not be stopped suddenly. This can cause increased chest pain and heart attack. Dosage should be gradually reduced. If you have had severe congestive heart failure in the past, Sectral should be used with caution.

If you experience difficulty breathing, or develop hives or large areas of swelling, seek medical attention immediately. You may be having a serious allergic reaction to the medicine. Sectral can also make other severe allergies worse.

If you suffer from asthma, seasonal allergies, other bronchial conditions, coronary artery disease, or kidney or liver disease, this medication should be used with caution.

Ask your doctor if you should check your pulse while taking Sectral. This medication can cause your heartbeat to become too slow.

This medication may mask the symptoms of low blood sugar or alter blood sugar levels. If you are diabetic, discuss this with your doctor.

Notify your doctor or dentist that you are taking Sectral if you have a medical emergency, or before you have any surgery.

Tell your doctor if you are taking over-the-counter cold medications and nasal drops. They may interact with Sectral.

Who should not take Sectral?

If you have heart failure, inadequate blood supply to the circulatory system (cardiogenic shock), heart block (a type of irregular heartbeat), or a severely slow heartbeat, you should not take this medication.

What should I tell my doctor before I take the first dose of Sectral?

Tell your doctor about all prescription, over-the-counter, and herbal medications you are taking before beginning treatment with this drug. Also, talk to your doctor about your complete medical history, especially if you have heart problems, allergies, asthma, or diabetes.

What is the usual dosage?

The information below is based on the dosage guidelines your doctor uses. Depending on your condition and medical history, your doctor may prescribe a different regimen. Do not change the dosage or stop taking your medication without your doctor's approval.

Hypertension
Adults: The usual initial dose for mild to moderate high blood pressure is 400 milligrams per day. It may be taken in a single daily dose or in 2 doses of 200 milligrams each. The usual daily dosage ranges from 200 to 800 milligrams.

People with severe high blood pressure may take up to 1,200 milligrams per day divided into 2 doses. Sectral may be taken alone or in combination with another high blood pressure medication.

Irregular Heartbeat
Adults: The usual starting dosage is 400 milligrams per day divided into 2 doses. Your doctor may gradually increase the dose to 600 to 1,200 milligrams per day. If your doctor wants you to stop taking this medication, he or she will have you taper off over a period of 2 weeks.

How should I take Sectral?

Sectral can be taken with or without food. Take it exactly as prescribed, even if your symptoms have disappeared.

What should I avoid while taking Sectral?
Avoid missing doses. If this medication is not taken regularly, your condition may worsen.

What are possible food and drug interactions associated with Sectral?
If Sectral is taken with certain other drugs, the effects of either could be increased, decreased, or altered. It is especially important to check with your doctor before combining Sectral with the following: albuterol, certain blood pressure medicines such as reserpine, certain over-the-counter cold remedies and nasal drops, nonsteroidal anti-inflammatory drugs, and oral diabetes drugs.

What are the possible side effects of Sectral?
Side effects cannot be anticipated. If any develop or change in intensity, tell your doctor as soon as possible. Only your doctor can determine if it is safe for you to continue taking this drug.

Side effects may include: abnormal vision, chest pain, constipation, cough, decreased sexual ability, depression, diarrhea, dizziness, fatigue, frequent urination, gas, headache, indigestion, joint pain, nasal inflammation, nausea, shortness of breath or difficulty breathing, strange dreams, swelling due to fluid retention, trouble sleeping, weakness

Can I receive Sectral if I am pregnant or breastfeeding?
The effects of Sectral during pregnancy have not been adequately studied. If you are pregnant or plan to become pregnant, inform your doctor immediately. Sectral appears in breast milk and could affect a nursing infant. If this medication is essential to your health, your doctor may advise you to discontinue breastfeeding until your treatment with Sectral is finished.

What should I do if I miss a dose of Sectral?
Take the forgotten dose as soon as you remember. If it's within 4 hours of your next scheduled dose, skip the one you missed and go back to your regular schedule. Never take 2 doses at the same time.

How should I store Sectral?
Store at room temperature, away from light. Keep the container tightly closed.

Selegiline hydrochloride See Eldepryl, page 467, or
   Zelapar, page 1455.

Selegiline patch See Emsam, page 479.

SEREVENT

Generic name: Salmeterol xinafoate

What is Serevent?

Serevent is used to prevent asthma attacks. Serevent relaxes the muscles in the walls of the bronchial tubes, allowing the passageways to expand and carry more air. It will not treat an asthma attack that has already begun. Serevent inhalation is also used to treat chronic obstructive pulmonary disease (COPD), including emphysema and chronic bronchitis.

What is the most important information I should know about Serevent?

Serevent is intended only for long-term prevention of symptoms, and should not be used more than twice a day. Do not use it to treat acute asthma attacks, and do not attempt to relieve worsening asthma by increasing the frequency of your doses. You should always have a short-acting bronchodilator with you for the relief of sudden asthma symptoms.

Asthma can be a life-threatening condition that needs immediate medical attention. Alert your doctor if your short-acting bronchodilator is becoming less effective. Tell your doctor if you need 4 or more inhalations of your short-acting bronchodilator daily for 2 days or more in a row, or you finish a 200-dose canister in <8 weeks.

A study found that the main ingredient in Serevent, salmeterol, may be associated with rare cases of serious asthma attacks or asthma-related death. Talk with your doctor about your options. Do not stop using Serevent without first consulting your doctor.

Who should not take Serevent?

Do not take Serevent if you are allergic to the medication or any of its ingredients.

What should I tell my doctor before I take the first dose of Serevent?

Tell your doctor about all prescription, over-the-counter, and herbal medications you are taking before beginning treatment with Serevent. Also, talk to your doctor about your complete medical history, especially if you have high blood pressure, heart disease, diabetes, an irregular heartbeat, seizure disorder, liver problems, or an overactive thyroid.

What is the usual dosage?

The information below is based on the dosage guidelines your doctor uses. Depending on your condition and medical history, your doctor may prescribe a different regimen. Do not change the dosage or stop taking your medication without your doctor's approval.

Asthma
Adults and children >4 years: The usual dose is 1 inhalation (50 micrograms) twice a day (morning and evening, approximately 12 hours apart).

Prevention of Exercise-Induced Asthma
Adults and children >4 years: Take 1 inhalation at least 30 minutes before exercise. Do not take another dose for 12 hours. (If you are on a twice-daily dosage schedule, do not take additional Serevent before exercise.)

Chronic Obstructive Pulmonary Disease
Adults: The usual dose is 1 inhalation twice a day (morning and evening, approximately 12 hours apart).

How should I take Serevent?

Use no more than the prescribed dose and follow package directions closely. Space your 2 daily doses approximately 12 hours apart, in the morning and evening. To be effective, the drug must be used regularly every day.

Serevent Diskus should never be used with a spacer. Always activate the Diskus device in a level, horizontal position. Never exhale into the Diskus device, and always keep it dry. Do not wash the mouthpiece or any other part of the device. Never attempt to take the Diskus apart.

What should I avoid while taking Serevent?

You may be able to taste or feel the medication delivered by the Diskus. Whether you can sense the delivery of a dose or not, never take more inhalations than your doctor has prescribed.

What are possible food and drug interactions associated with Serevent?

If Serevent is taken with certain other drugs, the effects of either could be increased, decreased, or altered. It is especially important to check with your doctor before combining Serevent with the following: airway-opening medications, atazanavir, beta blockers, clarithromycin, diuretics (water pills), itraconazole, ketoconazole, MAO inhibitors, nefazodone, nelfinavir, ritonavir, saquinavir, tricyclic antidepressants.

What are the possible side effects of Serevent?

Side effects cannot be anticipated. If any develop or change in intensity, tell your doctor as soon as possible. Only your doctor can determine if it is safe for you to continue taking this drug.

Side effects may include: asthma, back pain, bronchitis, chest congestion, cough, diarrhea, dizziness, headache, nasal inflammation, pallor, respiratory tract infection, sinus headache, sinus infection, sinus problems, sore throat, stomachache, tremor

Can I receive Serevent if I am pregnant or breastfeeding?

The effects of Serevent during pregnancy and breastfeeding are unknown. Tell your doctor immediately if you are pregnant, plan to become pregnant, or are breastfeeding.

What should I do if I miss a dose of Serevent?

Take it as soon as you remember. If it is almost time for your next dose, skip the one you missed and go back to your regular schedule. Never take 2 doses at once.

How should I store Serevent?

Store Serevent Diskus at room temperature away from direct sunlight, excessive heat, and freezing temperatures. Keep the Diskus in a dry place. Throw away the Diskus inhalation device after every blister has been used (when the dose indicator reads "0") or 6 weeks after the blisters have been removed from the foil pouch.

SEROPHENE

Generic name: Clomiphene citrate

What is Serophene?

Serophene is typically considered a beginning therapy for patients experiencing ovulatory failure or dysfunction. Serophene works by stimulating the body to release follicle stimulating hormone (FSH) and luteinizing hormone (LH), the hormones necessary for ovulation to occur.

What is the most important information I should know about Serophene?

As with other fertility medications, the use of Serophene is associated with multiple births (eg, twins, triplets). Do not use Serophene if you are already pregnant, as it may cause severe birth defects in your child, such as heart problems, Down syndrome, club foot, cleft palate, harelip, or webbed fingers/toes.

Prolonged use of this drug may increase the risk of developing ovarian cancer.

Serophene may cause you to have blurred vision and see spots. These symptoms may cause problems when driving a car or operating machinery.

Also, this drug may cause ovarian hyperstimulation syndrome (OHSS). (Please see "What are the possible side effects of this medication?" below for more information on the symptoms of OHSS.)

Who should not take Serophene?

Do not take Serophene if you are allergic to any of its ingredients. Also, do not use this drug if you are pregnant, as it may cause harm to your unborn baby. Serophene should not be used in patients with liver disease, abnormal uterine bleeding, ovarian cysts, and in patients with uncontrolled thyroid or adrenal dysfunction.

What should I tell my doctor before I take the first dose of Serophene?

Tell your doctor about all prescription, over-the-counter, and herbal medications you are taking before beginning therapy with Serophene. Also, talk to your doctor about your complete medical history; this includes any history of liver problems, abnormal uterine bleeding, ovarian cysts, and if you are pregnant or breastfeeding.

What is the usual dosage?

The information below is based on the dosage guidelines your doctor uses. Depending on your condition and medical history, your doctor may prescribe a different regimen. Do not change the dosage or stop taking your medication without your doctor's approval.

Adults: The usual dosage of Serophene begins low, at 50 milligrams (mg) daily (1 tablet) for 5 days. The dose should be increased to 100 mg for 5 days only in women who do not ovulate in response to 50 mg of Serophene.

How should I take Serophene?

Serophene tablets are taken only by mouth.

What should I avoid while taking Serophene?

Avoid activities that require your complete alertness, such as driving a car or operating heavy machinery, as Serophene may cause blurry vision and dizziness.

What are the possible side effects of Serophene?

Side effects cannot be anticipated. If any develop or change in intensity, tell your doctor as soon as possible. Only your doctor can determine if it is safe for you to continue taking this drug.

Side effects may include: abnormal uterine bleeding (such as spotting), blind spots, blurred vision, breast pain, double-vision, headache, light sensitivity, sensation of seeing light; stomach and lower-stomach discomfort/pain/bloating, vision problems

Symptoms of OHSS are: diarrhea, nausea, stomach pain and discomfort, vomiting, weight gain

Can I receive Serophene if I am pregnant or breastfeeding?

Do not take Serophene if you are pregnant, or nursing. This drug may cause severe birth defects in your child. Serophene and may pass into your breast milk.

What should I do if I miss a dose of Serophene?

If you miss a dose of this medication, take it as soon as you remember. If it is time for your next dose, then take the 2 doses together and go back to your regular dosing schedule. If you miss more than 1 dose, contact your doctor.

How should I store Serophene?

Store at room temperature, away from heat, light, and excessive humidity.

SEROQUEL
Generic name: Quetiapine fumarate

What is Seroquel?

Seroquel is an antipsychotic medication prescribed for the treatment of schizophrenia. It is also used for the treatment of mania associated with bipolar disorder as well as for the treatment of depressive episodes associated with bipolar disorder.

What is the most important information I should know about Seroquel?

The safety and effectiveness of Seroquel in children have not been established.

Antidepressants have increased the risk of suicidal thoughts and actions in children and teenagers. All patients starting treatment should be watched closely for worsening of depression, suicidal thoughts or actions, unusual changes in behavior, agitation, and irritability. Families and caregivers should watch patients daily and report these symptoms immediately to their physician.

Seroquel may increase the risk of death when used to treat mental problems caused by dementia in elderly patients and therefore should not be used in these patients. Most of the deaths were linked to heart problems or infection.

Seroquel may cause tardive dyskinesia, a potentially irreversible condition characterized by uncontrollable muscle spasms and twitches in the face and body. Older adults, especially women, appear to be at greater risk. Patients at risk of seizures should use Seroquel cautiously.

Seroquel may cause neuroleptic malignant syndrome (NMS), a serious, and potentially fatal, reaction to the drug. Call your doctor immediately if you develop muscle stiffness, confusion, irregular or rapid heartbeat, excessive sweating, and high fever. Be especially wary if you have a history of heart attack, heart disease, heart failure, circulation problems, or irregular heartbeat.

Certain antipsychotic drugs, including Seroquel, are associated with an increased risk of developing high blood sugar, which on rare occasions has led to coma or death. See your doctor right away if you develop signs of high blood sugar, including dry mouth, unusual thirst, increased urination, and tiredness. If you have diabetes or have a high risk of developing it, see your doctor regularly for blood sugar testing. In addition, Seroquel may affect cholesterol and triglyceride levels. Some patients have also experienced weight gain.

Seroquel may rarely cause a prolonged, painful erection. This could happen even when you are not having sex. If this is not treated right away, it could lead to permanent sexual problems, such as impotence. Contact your doctor right away if this happens.

Do not drink alcohol while you are using Seroquel.

Do not become overheated or dehydrated in hot weather or while you are being active; heatstroke, dizziness, or fainting may occur.

Seroquel may cause drowsiness, dizziness, or decreased vision. These effects may be worse if you take it with alcohol or certain medicines. Use Seroquel with caution. Do not drive or perform other possibly unsafe tasks until you know how you react to it.

Use Seroquel with particular caution if you have cardiovascular disease, cerebrovascular disease, or conditions that could lead to low blood pressure (dehydration, low blood volume, and treatment with blood pressure medications).

An eye exam for cataracts is recommended at the beginning of treatment and every six months.

Do not suddenly stop taking Seroquel without first talking with your doctor, as this may increase the risk of side effects. If you need to stop Seroquel or add a new medicine, your doctor will gradually lower the dose.

Rarely, Seroquel may lower the ability of your body to fight infection. Avoid contact with people who have colds or infections. Tell your doctor if you notice signs of infection like fever, sore throat, rash, or chills, especially if you have low white blood cell counts.

Who should not take Seroquel?
Do not take Seroquel if you are allergic to the medication or any of its ingredients.

What should I tell my doctor before I take the first dose of Seroquel?
Tell your doctor about all prescription, over-the-counter, and herbal medications you are taking before beginning treatment with Seroquel. Also, talk to your doctor about your complete medical history, especially if you have liver, kidney, or heart disease, high or low blood pressure, high cholesterol, heart rhythm problems, a history of heart attack or stroke, a thyroid disorder, seizures, epilepsy, Alzheimer's disease, obesity, breast

cancer, thyroid problems, cataracts, narrow-angle glaucoma, high blood prolactin levels, neuroleptic malignant syndrome, a personal or family history of diabetes, or trouble swallowing.

What is the usual dosage?
The information below is based on the dosage guidelines your doctor uses. Depending on your condition and medical history, your doctor may prescribe a different regimen. Do not change the dosage or stop taking your medication without your doctor's approval.

Bipolar Disorder
Adults: The usual dosage range is 300 to 800 milligrams (mg) a day. Doses above 800 mg a day have not been tested for safety. The dosage will be gradually increased over 4 to 6 days until the most effective dose is reached.

Schizophrenia
Adults: The usual dosage range is 300 to 400 mg a day, divided into two or three smaller doses. Doses as low as 150 mg a day sometimes prove effective; the dose rarely exceeds 750 mg per day. Doses above 800 mg per day have not been tested for safety. The dose is gradually increased over 4 days until the most effective dose is reached. If you have liver problems, you may be started at 25 mg a day. The doctor will increase the dose as needed.

Debilitated, elderly, or prone to low blood pressure: You may need your dose adjusted depending on your condition and response to the drug.

How should I take Seroquel?
Your doctor will increase your dose gradually until the drug takes effect. If you stop Seroquel for more than one week, you'll need to build up to your ideal dosage once again.

What should I avoid while taking Seroquel?
Seroquel tends to cause drowsiness, especially at the start of therapy, and can impair your judgment, thinking, and motor skills. Avoid driving or operating machinery until you know how the medication affects you.

Avoid exposure to extreme heat, strenuous exercise, and dehydration.

Avoid drinking alcohol while taking Seroquel. The drug increases the effects of alcohol.

When you first start treatment, avoid sitting up or standing up too quickly, especially in the morning. Seroquel may cause dizziness, light-headedness, or fainting due to a decrease in blood pressure. Alcohol, hot weather, exercise, or fever may increase these effects. Sit or lie down at the first sign of any of these effects.

Rarely, Seroquel may lower the ability of your body to fight infection. Avoid contact with people who have colds or infections. Tell your doctor if you notice signs of infection like fever, sore throat, rash, or chills.

What are possible food and drug interactions associated with Seroquel?

If Seroquel is taken with certain other drugs, the effects of either could be increased, decreased, or altered. It is especially important to check with your doctor before combining Seroquel with the following: alcohol, barbiturates such as phenobarbital, carbamazepine, cimetidine, divalproex, erythromycin, fluconazole, itraconazole, ketoconazole, levodopa, lorazepam, phenytoin, rifampin, steroids such as hydrocortisone and prednisone, and thioridazine.

What are the possible side effects of Seroquel?

Side effects cannot be anticipated. If any develop or change in intensity, tell your doctor as soon as possible. Only your doctor can determine if it is safe for you to continue taking this drug.

Side effects may include: abdominal pain, constipation, diminished movement, dizziness, drowsiness, dry mouth, excessive muscle tone, fatigue, headache, indigestion, low blood pressure (especially upon standing), nasal inflammation, neck rigidity, rapid or irregular heartbeat, rash, sleepiness, tremor, uncontrollable movements, vomiting, weakness, weight gain

Can I receive Seroquel if I am pregnant or breastfeeding?

The effects of Seroquel during pregnancy and breastfeeding are unknown. Tell your doctor immediately if you are pregnant, plan to become pregnant, or are breastfeeding. Seroquel should only be used during pregnancy if the potential benefit justifies the potential risk to the fetus.

What should I do if I miss a dose of Seroquel?

Take it as soon as you remember. If it is almost time for the next dose, skip the one you missed and go back to your regular schedule. Do not take two doses at once.

How should I store Seroquel?

Store at room temperature away from heat, moisture, and light. Do not store in the bathroom.

SEROQUEL XR

Generic name: Quetiapine fumarate, extended-release

What is Seroquel XR?

Seroquel XR is an antipsychotic medication prescribed for the treatment of schizophrenia. It is also used for the treatment of mania associated with bipolar disorder as well as for the treatment of depressive episodes associated with bipolar disorder.

What is the most important information I should know about Seroquel XR?

Seroquel XR is not approved for use in children.

Antidepressants have increased the risk of suicidal thoughts and actions in children and teenagers. All patients starting treatment should be watched closely for worsening of depression, suicidal thoughts or actions, unusual changes in behavior, agitation, and irritability. Families and caregivers should watch patients daily and report these symptoms immediately to their physician.

Seroquel XR may increase the risk of death when used to treat mental problems caused by dementia in elderly patients and therefore should not be used in these patients. Most of the deaths were linked to heart problems or infection.

Seroquel XR may cause tardive dyskinesia, a potentially irreversible condition characterized by uncontrollable muscle spasms and twitches in the face and body. Older adults, especially women, appear to be at greater risk. Patients at risk of seizures should use Seroquel XR cautiously.

Seroquel XR may cause neuroleptic malignant syndrome (NMS), a serious, and potentially fatal, reaction to the drug. Call your doctor immediately if you develop muscle stiffness, confusion, irregular or rapid heartbeat, excessive sweating, and high fever. Be especially wary if you have a history of heart attack, heart disease, heart failure, circulation problems, or irregular heartbeat.

Certain antipsychotic drugs, including Seroquel XR, are associated with an increased risk of developing high blood sugar, which on rare occasions has led to coma or death. See your doctor right away if you develop signs of high blood sugar, including dry mouth, unusual thirst, increased urination, and tiredness. If you have diabetes or have a high risk of developing it, see your doctor regularly for blood sugar testing. In addition, Seroquel XR may affect cholesterol and triglyceride levels. Some patients have also experienced weight gain.

Seroquel XR may rarely cause a prolonged, painful erection. This could happen even when you are not having sex. If this is not treated right away, it could lead to permanent sexual problems, such as impotence. Contact your doctor right away if this happens.

Do not drink alcohol while you are using Seroquel XR.

Do not become overheated or dehydrated in hot weather or while you are being active; heatstroke, dizziness, or fainting may occur.

Use Seroquel XR with particular caution if you have cardiovascular disease, cerebrovascular disease, or conditions that could lead to low blood pressure (dehydration, low blood volume, and treatment with blood pressure medications).

Do not suddenly stop taking Seroquel XR without first talking with your doctor, as this may increase the risk of side effects. If you need to stop Seroquel XR or add a new medicine, your doctor will gradually lower the dose.

Rarely, Seroquel XR may lower the ability of your body to fight infection. Avoid contact with people who have colds or infections. Tell your doctor if you notice signs of infection like fever, sore throat, rash, or chills, especially if you have low white blood cell counts.

Who should not take Seroquel XR?

Do not take Seroquel XR if you are allergic to the medication or any of its ingredients.

What should I tell my doctor before I take the first dose of Seroquel XR?

Tell your doctor about all prescription, over-the-counter, and herbal medications you are taking before beginning treatment with Seroquel XR. Also, talk to your doctor about your complete medical history, especially if you have liver, kidney or heart disease, high or low blood pressure, heart rhythm problems, high cholesterol, a history of heart attack or stroke, breast cancer, a thyroid disorder, seizures, epilepsy, Alzheimer's disease, dementia or mood problems, suicidal thoughts, obesity, history of alcohol or substance abuse, thyroid problems, cataracts, narrow-angle glaucoma, blood problems, a history of neuroleptic malignant syndrome, a personal or family history of diabetes, or trouble swallowing.

What is the usual dosage?

The information below is based on the dosage guidelines your doctor uses. Depending on your condition and medical history, your doctor may prescribe a different regimen. Do not change the dosage or stop taking your medication without your doctor's approval.

Bipolar Disorder

Adults: The usual dosage range is 300 to 800 milligrams (mg) a day. Doses above 800 mg a day have not been tested for safety. The dosage will be gradually increased over 4 to 6 days until the most effective dose is reached.

Schizophrenia

Adults: The recommended starting dose of Seroquel XR is 300 milligrams (mg) a day, preferably taken in the evening. The effective dose range is 400 mg to 800 mg daily depending on the response and tolerance of the individual patient. Dose increases can be made at 1-day intervals at increments of up to 300 mg per day. Individual dosage adjustments may be necessary. The safety of doses higher than 800 mg daily have not been studied in clinical trials.

How should I take Seroquel XR?

Seroquel XR sustained-release tablets are best taken in the evening. Take Seroquel XR by mouth on an empty stomach or with a light meal (approximately 300 calories). Continue the medication even if you start to feel better. Do not skip any doses, and do not suddenly stop taking Seroquel XR without first contacting your doctor.

What should I avoid while taking Seroquel XR?

Seroquel XR tends to cause drowsiness, especially at the start of therapy, and can impair your judgment, thinking, and motor skills. Until you are certain how the drug affects you, use caution when operating machinery or driving a car.

Avoid exposure to extreme heat, strenuous exercise, and dehydration.

Avoid drinking alcohol while taking Seroquel XR. The drug increases the effects of alcohol.

When you first start treatment, avoid sitting up or standing up too quickly, especially in the morning. Seroquel XR may cause dizziness, lightheadedness, or fainting due to a decrease in blood pressure. Alcohol, hot weather, exercise, or fever may increase these effects. Sit or lie down at the first sign of any of these effects.

Rarely, Seroquel XR may lower the ability of your body to fight infection. Avoid contact with people who have colds or infections. Tell your doctor if you notice signs of infection like fever, sore throat, rash, or chills.

What are possible food and drug interactions associated with Seroquel XR?

If Seroquel XR is taken with certain other drugs, the effects of either could be increased, decreased, or altered. It is especially important to check with your doctor before combining Seroquel XR with the following: alcohol, barbiturates such as phenobarbital, carbamazepine, cimetidine, divalproex, erythromycin, fluconazole, itraconazole, ketoconazole, levodopa, lorazepam, phenytoin, rifampin, steroids such as hydrocortisone and prednisone, and thioridazine.

What are the possible side effects of Seroquel XR?

Side effects cannot be anticipated. If any develop or change in intensity, tell your doctor as soon as possible. Only your doctor can determine if it is safe for you to continue taking this drug.

Side effects may include: constipation, dizziness, drowsiness, dry mouth, stomach upset, lightheadedness, weight gain, confusion, fainting, fever, chills, sore throat, increased saliva production or drooling, increased sweating, memory loss, menstrual changes, muscle pain, allergic reactions

Seek immediate medical attention if you experience allergic reactions such as rash, hives, itching, difficulty breathing, or swelling of the mouth, face, lips, or tongue.

Can I receive Seroquel XR if I am pregnant or breastfeeding?

The effects of Seroquel XR during pregnancy and breastfeeding are unknown. Tell your doctor immediately if you are pregnant, plan to become pregnant, or are breastfeeding.

Seroquel XR should only be used during pregnancy if the potential benefit justifies the potential risk to the fetus.

What should I do if I miss a dose of Seroquel XR?
Take it as soon as you remember. If it is almost time for the next dose, skip the one you missed and go back to your regular schedule. Do not take 2 doses at once. If you miss taking Seroquel XR for longer than 1 week, contact your doctor.

How should I store Seroquel XR?
Store at room temperature away from heat, moisture, and light. Do not store in the bathroom.

Sertraline hydrochloride *See Zoloft, page 1489.*

Sibutramine hydrochloride monohydrate *See Meridia, page 797.*

Sildenafil citrate *See Revatio, page 1146, or Viagra, page 1387.*

SILVADENE
Generic name: Silver sulfadiazine

What is Silvadene?
Silvadene Cream 1% is a cream to be applied to the skin. Silvadene is used along with other medications to prevent and treat wound infections in people with second- and third-degree burns. It is effective against a variety of bacteria and yeast.

What is the most important information I should know about Silvadene?
Silvadene is a sulfa derivative. If burn wounds cover extensive areas of the body, Silvadene may be absorbed into the bloodstream. If you have ever had an allergic reaction to sulfa drugs, this could lead to a similar reaction. Make sure your doctor is aware of any reactions you have experienced. There is a chance of fungal infection when using Silvadene.

Who should not take Silvadene?
You should not use Silvadene if you are allergic to sulfa drugs.

Do not use Silvadene at the end of pregnancy, on premature infants, or on newborn infants during the first two months of life.

What should I tell my doctor before I take the first dose of Silvadene?

Tell your doctor about all prescription, over-the-counter, and herbal medication you are taking before beginning treatment with Silvadene. Also, talk to your doctor about your complete medical history, especially if you have blood problems, glucose-6-phosphate dehydrogenase (G6PD) deficiency, porphyria, liver disease, or kidney disease.

What is the usual dosage?

The information below is based on the dosage guidelines your doctor uses. Depending on your condition and medical history, your doctor may prescribe a different regimen. Do not change the dosage or stop taking your medication without your doctor's approval.

Adults: Apply Silvadene Cream 1% to the affected area once or twice daily to a thickness of one-sixteenth of an inch. Treatment with Silvadene should be continued until your doctor is satisfied that healing has occurred or determines that the burn site is ready for grafting.

Children: The safety and effectiveness of Silvadene in children has not been established.

How should I take Silvadene?

Silvadene cream is for external use only. Clean your skin and apply Silvadene with a sterile, gloved hand. Apply a thin layer (about one-sixteenth of an inch) to the affected area.

Continue using Silvadene Cream until the area has healed or is ready for skin grafting.

What should I avoid while taking Silvadene?

Avoid exposure to sunlight or artificial ultraviolet light (e.g. sunlamps). Avoid getting Silvadene topical in the eyes.

What are possible food and drug interactions associated with Silvadene?

If Silvadene is taken with certain other drugs, the effects of either could be increased, decreased, or altered. It is especially important to check with your doctor before combining Silvadene with the following: topical enzyme preparations that contain collagenase, papain, or sutilains.

What are the possible side effects of Silvadene?

Side effects cannot be anticipated. If any develop or change in intensity, tell your doctor as soon as possible. Only your doctor can determine if it is safe for you to continue taking this drug.

Side effects may include: Areas of dead skin, burning sensation, red and raised rash on the body, skin discoloration

Can I receive Silvadene if I am pregnant or breastfeeding?
The effects of Silvadene during pregnancy and breastfeeding are unknown. Tell your doctor immediately if you are pregnant, plan to become pregnant, or are breastfeeding.

How should I store Silvadene?
Silvadene can be stored at room temperature.

Silver sulfadiazine *See Silvadene, page 1193.*

SIMCOR
Generic name: Simvastatin and niacin

What is Simcor?
Simcor is a combination drug used to treat elevated cholesterol in people who have an increased risk of atherosclerotic vascular disease (hardening of the arteries).

What is the most important information I should know about Simcor?
Simcor may cause skeletal muscle effects, liver enzyme abnormalities, and blood glucose level abnormalities.

Who should not take Simcor?
Do not take Simcor if you have active liver disease, a peptic ulcer, arterial bleeding, are pregnant or may become pregnant, are a nursing mother, or have a known hypersensitivity to any component to any component of this product

What should I tell my doctor before I take the first dose of Simcor?
Tell your doctor about all prescription, over the counter, and herbal medications you are taking before beginning treatment with Simcor. Also talk to your doctor about your complete medical history, especially if you have liver problems, an ulcer, or are pregnant, plan to become pregnant, or are breastfeeding.

What is the usual dosage?
The information below is based on the dosage guidelines your doctor uses. Depending on your condition and medical history, your doctor may prescribe a different regimen. Do not change the dosage or stop taking your medication without your doctor's approval.

Adults:. The dose of niacin extended-release should not be increased by more than 500 mg daily every 4 weeks.

The recommended maintenance dose for Simcor is 1000mg/20 mg to 2000mg/40 mg (two 1000mg/20 mg tablets) once daily depending on patient tolerability and lipid levels.

The maximum recommended dose is 2000mg/40 mg.

How should I take Simcor?

Simcor tablets should be taken at bedtime, after a low-fat snack. Do not crush or chew the tablet. Swallow whole. Do not take Simcor on an empty stomach.

What should I avoid while taking Simcor?

Avoid alcohol, hot beverages, and spicy food around the time you take Simcor to minimize flushing.

What are possible food and drug interactions associated with Simcor?

If Simcor is taken with certain other drugs, the effects of either could be increased, decreased, or altered. It is especially important to check with your doctor before combining Simcor with the following: amiodarone, clarithromycin, cyclosporine, danazol, erythromycin, fibrates, grapefruit juice (more than 1 quart daily); itraconazole, gemfibrozil, ketoconazole, nefazodone, protease inhibitors, telithromycin, and verapamil.

What are the possible side effects of Simcor?

Side effects cannot be anticipated. If any develop or change in intensity, tell your doctor as soon as possible. Only your doctor can determine if it is safe for you to continue taking this drug.

Side effects may include: flushing, headache, itching, back pain, diarrhea, muscle pain, changes in blood glucose levels, muscle break down, liver enzyme abnormalities

Can I receive Simcor if I am pregnant or breastfeeding?

Do not take Simcor if you are pregnant or breastfeeding.

What should I do if I miss a dose of Simcor?

If you miss a dose, take the next scheduled dose; do not double the dose.

How should I store Simcor?

Store at room temperature.

Simvastatin See Zocor, page 1484.

Simvastatin and niacin See Simcor, page 1195.

SINEMET CR

Generic name: Carbidopa and levodopa

What is Sinemet CR?

Sinemet CR is a controlled-release tablet that may be given to help relieve the muscle stiffness, tremor, and weakness caused by Parkinson's disease. It may also be given to relieve Parkinson-like symptoms caused by encephalitis, carbon monoxide poisoning, or manganese poisoning.

Sinemet CR contains two drugs, carbidopa and levodopa. The drug that actually produces the anti-Parkinson's effect is levodopa. Carbidopa prevents vitamin B_6 from destroying levodopa, thus allowing levodopa to work more efficiently.

What is the most important information I should know about Sinemet CR?

The carbidopa contained in Sinemet CR cannot eliminate side effects caused by levodopa. Since carbidopa helps levodopa reach your brain, Sinemet CR may, in fact, produce some levodopa side effects—particularly twitching, jerking, or writhing—sooner and at a lower dosage than levodopa alone. If such involuntary movements develop while you are taking Sinemet CR, you may need a dosage reduction.

Like levodopa, Sinemet CR may cause depression. Make sure your doctor knows if you have mental or emotional problems.

Muscle rigidity, high temperature, rapid heartbeat or breathing, sweating, blood pressure changes, and mental changes may occur when Sinemet CR is reduced suddenly or discontinued. If you stop taking this medication abruptly, your doctor should monitor your condition carefully.

Who should not take Sinemet CR?

Do not take Sinemet CR if you are sensitive to or have ever had an allergic reaction to its ingredients. Also avoid it if you have narrow-angle glaucoma; a suspicious, undiagnosed mole or a history of melanoma; or if you are taking or have taken an MAO inhibitor within the past 14 days.

What should I tell my doctor before I take the first dose of Sinemet CR?

Tell your doctor about all medications you are taking before beginning treatment with this drug. Also, talk to your doctor about your complete medical history, especially if you have bronchial asthma, cardiovascular or lung disease, endocrine (glandular) disorder, history of heart attack or heartbeat irregularity, history of active peptic ulcer, kidney or liver problems, skin lesions, a mental or emotional disorder, or wide-angle glaucoma (high pressure in the eye).

What is the usual dosage?

The information below is based on the dosage guidelines your doctor uses. Depending on your condition and medical history, your doctor may prescribe a different regimen. Do not change the dosage or stop taking your medication without your doctor's approval.

Adults: For patients with mild to moderate symptoms, the initial recommended dose is 1 tablet of Sinemet CR taken 2 times a day. Starting doses should be spaced out every 4 to 8 hours and then adjusted to each patient's individual response. The usual long-term dose is 2 to 8 tablets per day, taken in divided doses every 4 to 8 hours during the waking day.

How should I take Sinemet CR?

If you have been taking levodopa alone, you should stop taking levodopa for at least 12 hours before starting to take Sinemet CR. Take Sinemet CR after meals, rather than before or between meals. Swallow the tablets whole without chewing or crushing them. You may see a red, brown, or black coloration in your saliva, urine, or sweat. This is not harmful, but may stain your clothes. Too much stomach acid can interfere with absorption of the medication.

Sinemet CR releases its ingredients slowly over a period of 4 to 6 hours. It is important to follow a careful schedule, taking your doses at the same time every day. You should not change the prescribed dosage or add another product for Parkinson's disease without first consulting your doctor.

What should I avoid while taking Sinemet CR?

Avoid missing doses, and take them at evenly spaced intervals day and night. Do not chew or crush the tablets.

Avoid driving or operating machinery until you know how this drug affects you.

What are possible food and drug interactions associated with Sinemet CR?

If Sinemet CR is taken with certain other drugs, the effects of either could be increased, decreased, or altered. It is especially important to check with your doctor before combining Sinemet CR with the following: antacids, antiseizure drugs, antispasmodic drugs, blood pressure medications, high-protein foods, isoniazid, major tranquilizers such as haloperidol or risperidone, methionine, metoclopramide, papaverine, pyridoxine (vitamin B6), tranquilizers such as alprazolam, and tricyclic antidepressants.

If you have been taking an MAO inhibitor such as the antidepressants phenelzine and tranylcypromine or the Parkinson's drug selegiline, you must discontinue it at least 2 weeks before starting to take Sinemet CR.

A high-protein diet may impair the effectiveness of Sinement CR. Iron supplements can also reduce its effect.

What are the possible side effects of Sinemet CR?
Side effects cannot be anticipated. If any develop or change in intensity, tell your doctor as soon as possible. Only your doctor can determine if it is safe for you to continue taking this drug.

Side effects may include: confusion, hallucinations, nausea, uncontrollable twitching or jerking

Can I receive Sinemet CR if I am pregnant or breastfeeding?
If you are pregnant or plan to become pregnant, inform your doctor immediately. Sinemet CR should be used during pregnancy only if the benefit outweighs the potential risk to the unborn child. It is not known whether Sinemet CR appears in breast milk. If this medication is essential to your health, your doctor may advise you to stop nursing your baby until your treatment with this drug is finished.

What should I do if I miss a dose of Sinemet CR?
If you forget to take a dose, take it as soon as you remember. If it is almost time for your next dose, skip the one you missed and go back to your regular schedule. Do not take 2 doses at once.

How should I store Sinemet CR?
Store at room temperature in a tightly closed container.

SINGULAIR
Generic name: Montelukast sodium

What is Singulair?
Singulair is a medicine called a leukotriene receptor antagonist. It works by blocking substances in the body called leukotrienes. Blocking leukotrienes improves asthma and allergic rhinitis.

Singulair is prescribed for the treatment of asthma, the prevention of exercise-induced asthma, and allergic rhinitis (sneezing, stuffy nose, runny nose, itching of the nose, and outdoor and indoor allergies).

What is the most important information I should know about Singulair?
Singulair alleviates the on-going symptoms of asthma, but it won't stop an acute asthma attack.

If you have difficulty breathing while taking Singulair, or find that you need your orally inhaled bronchodilator more often than usual (or require more puffs than prescribed), notify your doctor.

If your asthma gets worse after exercise, continue using a short-acting inhaled airway opener to prevent the problem and relieve attacks.

Who should not take Singulair?
Do not take Singulair if you are allergic to any of its ingredients.

What should I tell my doctor before I take the first dose of Singulair?
Tell your doctor about all prescription, over-the-counter, and herbal medications you are taking before beginning treatment with Singulair. Also, talk to your doctor about your complete medical history, especially if you have phenylketonuria (an inability to process phenylalanine).

What is the usual dosage?
The information below is based on the dosage guidelines your doctor uses. Depending on your condition and medical history, your doctor may prescribe a different regimen. Do not change the dosage or stop taking your medication without your doctor's approval.

Asthma
Adults and children ≥15 years: The usual dose is one 10 milligram (mg) tablet once a day in the evening.

Children 6 to 14 years: The usual dose is one 5 mg chewable tablet once a day in the evening.

Children 2 to 5 years: The dosage is one 4 mg chewable tablet or 1 packet of 4 mg oral granules per day, taken in the evening.

Children 12 to 23 months: The dosage is 1 packet of 4 mg oral granules taken once a day in the evening.

The safety and effectiveness of Singulair for treating asthma in children <12 months have not been studied.

Seasonal Allergies in Adults and Children ≥2 years and Perennial (year-round) Allergies in Adults and Children ≥6 months
Adults and children ≥15 years: The usual dose is one 10 mg tablet once a day taken at any time.

Children 6 to 14 years: The usual dose is one 5 mg chewable tablet once a day taken at any time.

Children 2 to 5 years: The dosage is one 4 mg chewable tablet or 1 packet of 4 mg oral granules per day, taken at any time.

Children 6 to 23 months: The dosage is 1 packet of 4 mg oral granules per day, taken at any time.

Exercise-Induced Bronchoconstriction
Adults and children ≥15 years: The usual dose is one 10 mg tablet taken at least 2 hours before exercise. However, if you are already taking one tablet daily for your asthma or allergies, you do not need to take a second one before exercising. An additional dose should not be taken within 24 hours of a previous dose.

How should I take Singulair?
Take a Singulair tablet once daily, whether or not you have any symptoms. The tablet can be taken with or without food. If you have asthma, or asthma and allergies, take Singulair in the evening. If you have only allergies, you can take Singulair at any time.

For administration to children, place the oral granules directly in the child's mouth. The granules may also be mixed with a spoonful of one of the following soft foods: applesauce, carrots, rice, or ice cream. The food should be cold or at room temperature.

The granules can also be dissolved in 1 teaspoonful (5 milliliters) of cold or room temperature baby formula or breast milk. You should not use any other liquid to dissolve the granules. However, the child can drink liquids after the granules have been swallowed. Do not open the granules packet until your child is ready to take them. Once the packet is opened, give the full dose of medication within 15 minutes. Throw away any unused portion of the granules; do not store them for future use.

What should I avoid while taking Singulair?
If you have asthma and if your asthma is made worse by aspirin, continue to avoid aspirin or other medicines called nonsteroidal anti-inflammatory drugs while taking Singulair.

What are possible food and drug interactions associated with Singulair?
If Singulair is taken with certain other drugs, the effects of either could be increased, decreased, or altered. It is especially important to check with your doctor before combining Singulair with phenobarbital or rifampin.

What are the possible side effects of Singulair?
Side effects cannot be anticipated. If any develop or change in intensity, tell your doctor as soon as possible. Only your doctor can determine if it is safe for you to continue taking this drug.

Side effects may include: abdominal pain, abnormal dreams, allergic reaction, bronchitis, bruising, cough, dental pain, depression, diarrhea, difficulty breathing or swallowing, dizziness, drowsiness, ear infection, ear pain, eczema, eye inflammation, fatigue, feeling anxious, fever, flu, hallucinations, headache, hives, indigestion and other digestive problems, infection, insomnia, irritability, itching, joint pain, laryngitis, leg pain, muscle aches and cramps, nasal congestion, nausea, pancreatitis, pins and needles/numbness, pneumonia, rash, restlessness, runny nose, seizures, sinus pain, skin inflammation, sneezing, sore throat, suicidal thoughts and actions (including suicide), swelling due to fluid retention, swelling of the mouth or throat, upper respiratory infection, tendency to bleed easily, thirst, tremor, viral infection, vomiting

Can I receive Singulair if I am pregnant or breastfeeding?
The effects of Singulair during pregnancy and breastfeeding are unknown. Tell your doctor immediately if you are pregnant, plan to become pregnant, or are breastfeeding.

What should I do if I miss a dose of Singulair?
Take it as soon as you remember. If it is almost time for your next dose, skip the one you missed and go back to your regular schedule. Do not take 2 doses at once.

How should I store Singulair?
Store at room temperature, away from moisture and light.

Sitagliptin and metformin See *Janumet, page 676.*

Sitagliptin phosphate See *Januvia, page 678.*

SKELAXIN
Generic name: Metaxalone

What is Skelaxin?
Skelaxin, in addition to rest and physical therapy, is prescribed for the relief of severe and painful musculoskeletal conditions.

What is the most important information I should know about Skelaxin?
Skelaxin should be avoided by anyone with significant liver or kidney problems.

Who should not take Skelaxin?
Do not take Skelaxin if you are allergic to Skelaxin or any of its ingredients. Do not take it if you have a history of anemia or significant liver or kidney disease.

What should I tell my doctor before I take the first dose of Skelaxin?
Tell your doctor about all prescription, over-the-counter, and herbal medications you are taking before beginning treatment with Skelaxin. Also,

talk to your doctor about your complete medical history, especially if you have anemia, liver or kidney problems.

What is the usual dosage?
The information below is based on the dosage guidelines your doctor uses. Depending on your condition and medical history, your doctor may prescribe a different regimen. Do not change the dosage or stop taking your medication without your doctor's approval.

Adults and children ≥12 years: The usual is one 800 milligram (mg) tablet 3 to 4 times a day.

Safety and effectiveness in children <12 years have not been established.

How should I take Skelaxin?
Take exactly as prescribed.

What should I avoid while taking Skelaxin?
Skelaxin may impair mental and/or physical abilities required for performance of hazardous tasks, such as operating machinery or driving. Be careful in any activities that require you to be awake and alert until you know how this medication affects you.

Avoid drinking alcohol as it may increase some of the side effects of Skelaxin. Avoid using in combination with central nervous system depressants (such as cold medicine, pain medication, other muscle relaxers, and medicines to treat depression or anxiety). Concurrent use may make you sleepy.

What are possible food and drug interactions associated with Skelaxin?
If Skelaxin is taken with certain other drugs, the effects of either could be increased, decreased, or altered. It is especially important to check with your doctor before combining Skelaxin with any of the following: alcohol, barbiturates, central nervous system depressants

What are the possible side effects of Skelaxin?
Side effects cannot be anticipated. If any develop or change in intensity, tell your doctor as soon as possible. Only your doctor can determine if it is safe for you to continue taking this drug.

Side effects may include: dizziness, drowsiness, headache, irritability, nausea, nervousness, stomach upset, vomiting

Can I receive Skelaxin if I am pregnant or breastfeeding?
The effects of Skelaxin during pregnancy and breastfeeding are unknown. Tell your doctor immediately if you are pregnant, plan to become pregnant, or are breastfeeding.

What should I do if I miss a dose of Skelaxin?

Take the forgotten dose as soon as you remember. However, if it is almost time for your next dose, skip the one you missed and return to your regular schedule. Do not take 2 doses at once.

How should I store Skelaxin?

Store at room temperature.

Solifenacin succinate See VESIcare, page 1385.

SOMA

Generic name: Carisoprodol

What is Soma?

Soma is used, along with rest, physical therapy, and other measures, for the relief of acute, painful muscle strains and spasms.

What is the most important information I should know about Soma?

Soma alone will not heal your muscles. You need to follow the program of physical therapy, rest, or exercise that your doctor prescribes. Do not attempt any more physical activity than your doctor recommends, even though Soma temporarily makes it seem feasible.

In rare cases, the first dose of Soma may cause unusual symptoms that appear within minutes or hours of taking the medication. Symptoms reported include: agitation, confusion, disorientation, dizziness, double vision, enlargement of pupils, extreme weakness, exaggerated feeling of well-being, lack of coordination, speech problems, temporary loss of vision, and temporary paralysis of arms and legs. These symptoms usually subside within a few hours. If you experience any of them, contact your doctor immediately.

Who should not take Soma?

If you are sensitive to or have ever had an allergic reaction to Soma or drugs of this type, such as meprobamate, you should not take this medication. Make sure your doctor is aware of any drug reactions you have experienced.

Unless you are directed to do so by your doctor, do not take this medication if you have porphyria (an inherited blood disorder).

What should I tell my doctor before I take the first dose of Soma?

Tell your doctor about all prescription, over-the-counter, and herbal medications you are taking before beginning treatment with this drug. Also, talk to your doctor about your complete medical history, especially if you have kidney or liver problems or a history of drug dependence.

What is the usual dosage?
The information below is based on the dosage guidelines your doctor uses. Depending on your condition and medical history, your doctor may prescribe a different regimen. Do not change the dosage or stop taking your medication without your doctor's approval.

Adults and adolescents 16 years and older: The usual dosage is one 250-milligram or 350-milligram tablet, taken 3 times daily and at bedtime, for 2-3 weeks.

How should I take Soma?
Take Soma exactly as prescribed by your doctor.

What should I avoid while taking Soma?
Soma may impair the mental or physical abilities you need to drive a car or operate dangerous machinery. Do not participate in hazardous activities until you know how this drug affects you.

Avoid abruptly discontinuing treatment. Withdrawal symptoms, including abdominal cramps, chilliness, headache, insomnia, and nausea, have occurred in people who suddenly stop taking Soma.

Soma may intensify the effects of alcohol. Be careful drinking alcoholic beverages while you are taking this medication.

What are possible food and drug interactions associated with Soma?
If Soma is taken with certain other drugs, the effects of either could be increased, decreased, or altered. It is especially important to check with your doctor before combining Soma with the following: antidepressant drugs known as tricyclics or MAO inhibitors, major tranquilizers and antipsychotic drugs such as haloperidol, and other sedatives such as alprazolam and triazolam.

What are the possible side effects of Soma?
Side effects cannot be anticipated. If any develop or change in intensity, tell your doctor as soon as possible. Only your doctor can determine if it is safe for you to continue taking this drug.

Side effects may include: agitation, depression, dizziness, drowsiness, facial flushing, fainting, headache, hiccups, inability to fall or stay asleep, irritability, light-headedness upon standing up, loss of coordination, nausea, rapid heart rate, stomach upset, tremors, vertigo, vomiting

Allergic reactions usually seen between the first and fourth doses of Soma in patients who have never taken this drug before include: itching, red welts on the skin, and skin rash. A more severe allergic reaction may include symptoms such as asthmatic attacks, dizziness, fever, low blood pressure, shock, stinging of the eyes, swelling due to fluid retention, and weakness. If any of these occur, seek medical attention immediately.

Can I receive Soma if I am pregnant or breastfeeding?
The effects of Soma during pregnancy have not been adequately studied. If you are pregnant or plan to become pregnant, inform your doctor immediately. This drug appears in breast milk and could affect a nursing infant. If this medication is essential to your health, your doctor may advise you to discontinue breastfeeding until your treatment is finished.

What should I do if I miss a dose of Soma?
Take it as soon as you remember if only an hour or so has passed. If you do not remember until later, skip the dose you missed and go back to your regular schedule. Do not take 2 doses at once.

How should I store Soma?
Store at room temperature in a tightly closed container.

SONATA
Generic name: Zaleplon

What is Sonata?
Sonata is prescribed for people who have trouble falling asleep at bedtime. Because it has a short duration of action, it doesn't help those who suffer from frequent awakenings during the night or those who wake too early in the morning. It is intended only for short-term use.

What is the most important information I should know about Sonata?
Sonata is not approved for use in children.

Do not take Sonata unless you plan to be in bed for at least 4 hours after taking it. If you need to be alert and active in less than 4 hours, your performance could be impaired. Never attempt to drive a car or operate other dangerous machinery right after taking Sonata.

Problems with sleep are usually temporary and require only short-term treatment with medication. Call your doctor immediately if it seems the medication is making the problem worse, or if you notice any unusual changes in your thinking or behavior, such as hallucinations, amnesia, agitation, or a lack of inhibition.

Use Sonata only for temporary relief of insomnia; sleep medicines tend to lose their effect when taken for more than a few weeks. Taking sleeping pills for extended periods or in high doses can lead to physical dependence and the danger of a withdrawal reaction when the drug is abruptly stopped.

If you have worsening insomnia or the emergence of unusual thinking or behavior, see your doctor since this may signal an unrecognized disorder.

There have been reports of complex behaviors, such as "sleep driving" or "sleep eating" (driving or eating while not fully aware of what you are doing) in people taking medications such as Sonata. In general, people do not remember doing these things when they wake up in the morning. These activities can be dangerous, since people are not fully awake or alert.

Who should not take Sonata?
Sonata is not recommended for people with severe liver disease.

Do not take it if you are allergic to any of its ingredients. It contains the coloring agent FD&C Yellow No. 5, which causes a reaction in some individuals. This allergic reaction is more likely in people who are sensitive to aspirin.

What should I tell my doctor before I take the first dose of Sonata?
Tell your doctor about all prescription, over-the-counter, and herbal medications you are taking before beginning treatment with Sonata. Also, talk to your doctor about your complete medical history, especially if you have depression, liver disease, sleep apnea (stopping breathing for short periods while asleep), asthma, bronchitis, emphysema, or another respiratory disease, myasthenia gravis (a muscle weakness), or a history of drug or alcohol addiction.

What is the usual dosage?
The information below is based on the dosage guidelines your doctor uses. Depending on your condition and medical history, your doctor may prescribe a different regimen. Do not change the dosage or stop taking your medication without your doctor's approval.

Adults: The usual dose is 10 milligrams (mg) taken once daily at bedtime. Your doctor may adjust the dose to your individual need, especially if you are in a weakened condition or have a low body weight. A dose of 5 mg is recommended if you have liver disease or use the drug cimetidine. Doses above 20 mg have not been adequately evaluated and are not recommended.

Elderly: This population are more sensitive to the effects of Sonata and respond to 5 mg. Doses over 10 mg in the elderly are not recommended.

How should I take Sonata?

Sonata is very fast-acting and should be taken only at bedtime. Sonata should be taken immediately before bedtime or if you have difficulty falling asleep after you have gone to bed. Taking Sonata while still up and about may result in short-term memory impairment, hallucinations, impaired coordination, dizziness, and lightheadedness.

What should I avoid while taking Sonata?

Avoid alcoholic beverages when taking Sonata.

Never attempt to drive a car or operate other dangerous machinery right after taking Sonata.

What are possible food and drug interactions associated with Sonata?

If Sonata is taken with certain other drugs, the effects of either could be increased, decreased, or altered. It is especially important to check with your doctor before combining Sonata with the following: alcohol, carbamazepine, cimetidine, diphenhydramine, erythromycin, imipramine, ketoconazole, phenobarbital, promethazine, rifampin, and thioridazine.

Avoid high-fat meals immediately before taking Sonata; they tend to slow or reduce the drug's effect.

What are the possible side effects of Sonata?

Side effects cannot be anticipated. If any develop or change in intensity, tell your doctor as soon as possible. Only your doctor can determine if it is safe for you to continue taking this drug.

Side effects may include: abdominal pain, amnesia, back pain, chest pain, constipation, dizziness, drowsiness, dry mouth, eye pain, headache, memory loss, menstrual pain, migraine, muscle pain, nausea, sleepiness, tingling, weakness

Can I receive Sonata if I am pregnant or breastfeeding?

The effects of Sonata during pregnancy are unknown. Tell your doctor immediately if you are pregnant, or plan to become pregnant. Sonata is excreted in breast milk and may affect a nursing baby. Do not take this medication without first talking to your doctor if you are breastfeeding.

What should I do if I miss a dose of Sonata?

Take Sonata only when you're ready to sleep. Never double your dose.

How should I store Sonata?

Store at room temperature in a light-resistant container.

Sorafenib *See Nexavar, page 877.*

SORIATANE

Generic name: Acitretin

What is Soriatane?

Soriatane is a form of vitamin A that is prescribed for several types of severe psoriasis, a chronic skin condition that causes inflamed red patches with silvery scales. Soriatane is used when milder forms of treatment have failed.

What is the most important information I should know about Soriatane?

Soriatane must never be taken during pregnancy, as it can cause severe birth defects and physical abnormalities in a developing baby. You must not become pregnant while taking Soriatane and you must also avoid becoming pregnant for a full 3 years after you stop taking it.

Before starting Soriatane therapy, women of childbearing age must receive birth control counseling and sign a detailed consent form stating they understand the consequences of birth control failure, the risk of birth defects, and the warning not to use alcohol. You must have 2 negative pregnancy tests—1 when you and your doctor decide on a course of Soriatane therapy and 1 immediately before starting treatment. You must take monthly pregnancy tests and continue to receive regular birth control counseling while using Soriatane.

You must use 2 forms of reliable birth control for at least 1 month prior to starting treatment, as well as for the entire time you take Soriatane and for a full 3 years after discontinuing therapy. It may take 3 years for Soriatane to be eliminated from the body. If you accidentally become pregnant, miss a menstrual period, or have unprotected sex while taking Soriatane, stop taking the drug and call your doctor immediately.

Soriatane may cause mental and behavioral changes. If you start to have symptoms of depression or aggression while taking Soriatane, or if you have thoughts of suicide or self-injury, call the doctor immediately.

Soriatane does not cure psoriasis; it helps keep it under control. Your condition may return if you stop treatment.

Who should not take Soriatane?

Do not take Soriatane if it causes an allergic reaction or if you have ever had an allergic reaction to other drugs like it. Do not take Soriatane if you have kidney or liver disease, or if you have abnormally high cholesterol or triglyceride levels.

Do not take Soriatane if you are pregnant or if you plan to become pregnant within the next 3 years.

What should I tell my doctor before I take the first dose of Soriatane?

Tell your doctor about all prescription, over-the-counter, and herbal medications you are taking before beginning treatment with Soriatane. Also, talk to your doctor about your complete medical history, especially if you have kidney or liver disease, high blood sugar, high levels of cholesterol or triglycerides in your blood, heart disease, depression. Also inform your doctor if you drink alcohol, have a history of alcoholism, are pregnant, planning to become pregnant, or are breastfeeding.

What is the usual dosage?

The information below is based on the dosage guidelines your doctor uses. Depending on your condition and medical history, your doctor may prescribe a different regimen. Do not change the dosage or stop taking your medication without your doctor's approval.

Adults: The recommended dose is 25 to 50 milligrams (mg) once a day, taken with your main meal.

Safety and effectiveness of Soriatane in children have not been established.

How should I take Soriatane?

Take Soriatane with food, exactly as prescribed by your doctor, at about the same time each day.

What should I avoid while taking Soriatane?

Do not drink alcohol or take products containing alcohol while using Soriatane and for at least 2 months after discontinuing treatment. Combining alcohol with Soriatane causes a chemical change that makes it stay in your system longer.

Soriatane increases your sensitivity to sunlight. To prevent burning, do not stay in the sun for long periods, wear protective clothing, sunglasses, and sunscreen, and avoid using sunlamps or tanning beds.

Adults being treated with Soriatane may not give blood for at least 3 years.

What are possible food and drug interactions associated with Soriatane?

If Soriatane is taken with certain other drugs, the effects of either could be increased, decreased, or altered. It is especially important to check with your doctor before combining Soriatane with any of the following: alcohol, birth control pills containing progestin, demeclocycline, doxycycline, etretinate, methotrexate, minocycline, retinoids such as isotretinoin and tretinoin, phenytoin, tetracycline antibiotics

Avoid taking vitamin supplements that contain vitamin A without your doctor's approval. Soriatane is chemically related to vitamin A, and taking too much can cause harmful side effects or a toxic overdose.

If you take the herb St. John's wort, do not use hormonal estrogen/progestin pills, implants, or injections as a form of birth control. Women who take these products together can become pregnant. Make sure your doctor knows about any over-the-counter products you are taking.

What are the possible side effects of Soriatane?

Side effects cannot be anticipated. If any develop or change in intensity, tell your doctor as soon as possible. Only your doctor can determine if it is safe for you to continue taking this drug.

Side effects may include: abnormal bone growth or pain, abnormal skin changes (itching, peeling, rash, sensitivity, thinning), blood clots, changes in blood sugar or cholesterol and triglyceride (blood fat) levels, depression, eye problems (dryness, pain, redness, sensitivity), heart attack, joint pain, lip inflammation, liver disorders, muscle weakness, numbness or swelling of the hands or feet, inflammation of the pancreas, stroke, thoughts of suicide or self-injury, vision problems (blurring, difficulty seeing at night)

Can I receive Soriatane if I am pregnant or breastfeeding?

If taken during pregnancy, Soriatane can cause severe birth defects and physical abnormalities in a developing baby. Do not take Soriatane if you are pregnant or plan to become pregnant within 3 years after you stop taking it. Do not take Soriatane if you're breastfeeding, as it can harm a nursing baby.

What should I do if I miss a dose of Soriatane?

Take the forgotten dose as soon as you remember. However, if it is almost time for your next dose, skip the one you missed and return to your regular schedule. Do not take 2 doses at once.

How should I store Soriatane?

Store at room temperature, away from light and humidity, in a childproof container.

SPECTRACEF
Generic name: Cefditoren

What is Spectracef?

Spectracef is a cephalosporin antibiotic. It fights bacteria in the body. Spectracef cures mild-to-moderate bacterial infections of the skin, throat, and respiratory tract. Among these infections are pneumonia, strep throat, and tonsillitis. Spectracef is also prescribed for acute flare-ups of chronic bronchitis.

What is the most important information I should know about Spectracef?

Pseudomembranous colitis (an infection of the colon) has been reported with nearly all antibacterial agents, including Spectracef, and may range in severity from mild to life-threatening. Therefore, it is important to tell your doctor if you experience diarrhea during or after treatment with antibacterial agents such as Spectracef.

Who should not take Spectracef?

If you are sensitive to or have ever had an allergic reaction to penicillin, Spectracef or other cephalosporin antibiotics, do not take Spectracef.

Do not use Spectracef if you have a deficiency of the amino acid carnitine, or if you have a problem metabolizing carnitine. Also avoid the drug if you're allergic to milk protein, since Spectracef contains this substance. However, being lactose intolerant should not prevent you from using Spectracef.

What should I tell my doctor before I take the first dose of Spectracef?

Tell your doctor about all prescription, over-the-counter, and herbal medication you are taking before beginning treatment with Spectracef. Also, talk to your doctor about your complete medical history, especially if you have liver disease, kidney disease, decreased muscle mass, a history of gastrointestinal disease, or if you are malnourished.

What is the usual dosage?

The information below is based on the dosage guidelines your doctor uses. Depending on your condition and medical history, your doctor may prescribe a different regimen. Do not change the dosage or stop taking your medication without your doctor's approval.

For Acute Flare-ups of Chronic Bronchitis
Adults and children 12 years and older: The usual dose is 400 milligrams (mg) twice a day for 10 days.

For Pharyngitis, Tonsillitis, and Skin Infections
The usual dose is 200 mg twice a day for 10 days.

For Community-Acquired Pneumonia
The usual dose is 400 mg twice a day for 14 days.
If you have kidney disease, the dose may be lower.

Children less than 12 years old: Spectracef has not been studied in children less than 12 years old and should not be used in this age group.

How should I take Spectracef?

Spectracef should be taken with meals to enhance absorption. Take Spectracef only when directed to do so by your doctor.

To make certain your infection is completely cleared up, take all of the medication exactly as your doctor prescribes, even if you begin to feel better after the first few days.

What should I avoid while taking Spectracef?
Do not take it with antacids such as Tums or other medications that reduce stomach acid.

What are possible food and drug interactions associated with Spectracef?
If Spectracef is taken with certain other drugs, the effects of either could be increased, decreased, or altered. It is especially important to check with your doctor before combining Spectracef with the following: antacids, blood thinners such as warfarin, penicillins or other cephalosporin antibiotic, probenecid, ulcer drugs known as H_2 blockers such as famotidine.

What are the possible side effects of Spectracef?
Side effects cannot be anticipated. If any develop or change in intensity, tell your doctor as soon as possible. Only your doctor can determine if it is safe for you to continue taking this drug.

Side effects may include: Diarrhea, headache, nausea, vaginal infection

Can I receive Spectracef if I am pregnant or breastfeeding?
The effects of Spectracef during pregnancy are unknown. Tell your doctor immediately if you are pregnant, or plan to become pregnant. Spectracef can appear in breast milk. If Spectracef is essential to your health, your doctor may advise you to stop breastfeeding until your treatment is finished.

What should I do if I miss a dose of Spectracef?
Take it as soon as you remember. If it is almost time for your next dose, skip the one you missed and go back to your regular schedule. Do not take two doses at once.

How should I store Spectracef?
Store at room temperature; protect from light and moisture.

SPIRIVA HANDIHALER
Generic name: Tiotropium bromide

What is Spiriva HandiHaler?
Spiriva is a medicine used for the long-term, once-a-day treatment of bronchial spasms (wheezing) associated with chronic obstructive pul-

monary disease (COPD), which includes chronic bronchitis and emphysema. It comes as a capsule containing dry powder, which is inhaled through the mouth using the HandiHaler device. When inhaled, Spiriva opens up narrow air passages, allowing more oxygen to reach the lungs.

What is the most important information I should know about Spiriva HandiHaler?

Spiriva is not for initial use in sudden attacks of wheezing when fast action is needed. (Spiriva is not for "rescue therapy.")

An immediate allergic reaction (hives, swelling, or rash) is possible when you first use Spiriva HandiHaler. Inhaled medications such as Spiriva can also cause wheezing in some people. If you have an allergic reaction or you start wheezing, stop using Spiriva and contact your doctor.

Who should not take Spiriva HandiHaler?

You should not take Spiriva if you have an allergic reaction to it, or if you are allergic to atropine or any of its derivatives, including ipratropium.

What should I tell my doctor before I take the first dose of Spiriva HandiHaler?

Tell your doctor about all prescription, over-the-counter, and herbal medication you are taking before beginning treatment with Spiriva. Also, talk to your doctor about your complete medical history, especially if you have narrow angle glaucoma (high pressure inside the eye), an enlarged prostate, obstruction in the neck of the bladder, or kidney problems.

What is the usual dosage?

The information below is based on the dosage guidelines your doctor uses. Depending on your condition and medical history, your doctor may prescribe a different regimen. Do not change the dosage or stop taking your medication without your doctor's approval.

Adults: The recommended dose is the inhalation of the contents of one capsule, taken once a day, with the HandiHaler device.

Children: Spiriva has not been studied in children.

How should I take Spiriva HandiHaler?

Spiriva capsules are designed to be used only with the HandiHaler inhalation device. The capsules should not be swallowed. You should try to use the inhaler about the same time each day.

When removing a capsule from the blister card, peel back only the foil that is covering the capsule you are about to use. The capsule's effectiveness may be reduced if it is not used immediately after the foil is opened. If you accidentally remove the foil covering any of the other capsules, you must throw them away.

When you're ready to take the medication, use the HandiHaler device as follows:

1. Open the dust cap, and then open the mouthpiece.
2. Place the capsule in the center chamber. Close the mouthpiece until you hear a click. Leave the dust cap open.
3. Hold the HandiHaler device with the mouthpiece upward and press the piercing button that will make holes in the capsule to allow the powder to come out.
4. Before inhaling the powder, breathe out completely, but not into the mouthpiece.
5. Place the inhaler's mouthpiece in your mouth, make a seal with your lips, keep your head upright, and breathe in slowly and deeply with your mouth. Breathe in quickly enough that you hear the capsule vibrate.
6. Hold your breath for as long as is comfortable; at the same time, remove the HandiHaler from your mouth. Resume normal breathing.
7. When you're done, breathe out completely. Seal your lips around the mouthpiece again, and inhale a second time as before.
8. Remove the capsule from the inhaler and discard. A tiny amount of powder may still be left in the capsule; this is normal.

What should I avoid while taking Spiriva HandiHaler?
Avoid getting the Spiriva powder into your eyes. It may cause blurred vision.

Spiriva is for oral inhalation only. **Do not swallow Spiriva capsules.**

What are possible food and drug interactions associated with Spiriva HandiHaler?
The use of Spiriva together with other anticholinergic drugs has not been studied and is not recommended.

What are the possible side effects of Spiriva HandiHaler?
Side effects cannot be anticipated. If any develop or change in intensity, tell your doctor as soon as possible. Only your doctor can determine if it is safe for you to continue taking this drug.

Side effects may include: Abdominal pain, constipation, dry mouth, chest pain, common cold, indigestion, infection, muscle pain, nose bleeds, rash, runny nose or nasal inflammation, sinus infection, sore throat, swelling, urinary tract infection, vomiting, yeast infection

Can I receive Spiriva HandiHaler if I am pregnant or breastfeeding?
The effects of Spiriva during pregnancy and breastfeeding are unknown. Tell your doctor immediately if you are pregnant, plan to become pregnant, or are breastfeeding.

What should I do if I miss a dose of Spiriva HandiHaler?

Take it as soon as you remember. If it is almost time for your next dose, skip the one you missed and go back to your regular schedule. Do not take two doses at once.

How should I store Spiriva HandiHaler?

Store at room temperature. Do not store capsules in the HandiHaler. Keep capsules away from moisture and extreme temperatures, such as in the refrigerator or in direct sunlight.

Spironolactone *See Aldactone, page 60.*

Spironolactone and hydrochlorothiazide *See Aldactazide, page 58.*

SPORANOX

Generic name: Itraconazole

What is Sporanox?

Sporanox capsules are used to treat serious fungal infections: blastomycosis, histoplasmosis, and aspergillosis. Blastomycosis can affect the lungs, bones, and skin. Histoplasmosis can affect the lungs, heart, and blood. Aspergillosis can affect the lungs, kidneys, and other organs.

Sporanox capsules are also used to treat onychomycosis, which infects the toenails and fingernails.

Sporanox oral solution is used to treat candidiasis (fungal infection) of the mouth, throat, and esophagus, and for other fungal infections in people with weakened immunity and fever.

What is the most important information I should know about Sporanox?

Do not take Sporanox if you are taking cisapride, dofetilide, ergot alkaloids such as dihydroergotamine and ergometrine, levacetylmethadol, nisoldipine, pimozide, or quinidine. Combined with these drugs, Sporanox could cause serious—even fatal—problems.

In rare cases, Sporanox has caused severe liver damage, sometimes resulting in death. Tell your doctor immediately if you develop nausea, vomiting, abdominal pain, unusual tiredness, loss of appetite, yellow skin or eyes, itching, dark urine, or clay colored stools.

In rare cases, Sporanox has been associated with the onset of congestive heat failure (CHF). Contact your doctor if you develop symptoms that may indicate CHF, including shortness of breath, chest pain, or swelling during treatment with Sporanox.

Who should not take Sporanox?

If you are sensitive to or have ever had an allergic reaction to Sporanox or similar antifungal drugs such as ketoconazole, do not take Sporanox.

Sporanox can have a negative effect on the heart. It should not be used for fungal nail infections in people with heart problems such as congestive heart failure.

Serious heart problems, such as irregular heartbeats and even death, have occurred in people who have taken Sporanox at the same time as cisapride, dofetilide, midazolam, pimozide, quinidine, triazolam, or cholesterol-lowering drugs known as statins, such as lovastatin and simvastatin.

What should I tell my doctor before I take the first dose of Sporanox?

Tell your doctor about all prescription, over-the-counter, and herbal medication you are taking before beginning treatment with Sporanox. Also, talk to your doctor about your complete medical history, especially if you have kidney or liver disease, heart or heart valve disease, chronic obstructive pulmonary disease, or swelling or water retention.

What is the usual dosage?

The information below is based on the dosage guidelines your doctor uses. Depending on your condition and medical history, your doctor may prescribe a different regimen. Do not change the dosage or stop taking your medication without your doctor's approval.

Aspergillosis
Adults: The usual dose is 200-400 milligrams (mg) a day. Treatment usually continues for a minimum of 3 months, until tests indicate that the fungal infection has subsided.

Blastomycosis and Histoplasmosis
The usual dose is 2 100-mg capsules, taken after a full meal once a day. If you feel no improvement, or if there is evidence that the fungal disease has spread, your doctor will increase the dose to 100 mg at a time to a maximum of 400 mg a day. Daily dosages above 200 mg a day should be divided into 2 smaller doses.

Candidiasis, esophagus
The usual dose is 10 mL of oral solution a day for at least 3 weeks. You should continue the treatment for 2 weeks after your symptoms clear up. If necessary, the doctor may increase the dose to 20 mL a day.

Candidiasis, mouth and throat
The usual dose is 20 milliliters (mL) of oral solution a day for 1-2 weeks. If the infection does not go away, your dose will be changed to 10 mL twice a day.

Fungal Infections in People with
Weakened Immunity and Fever

Recommended treatment starts with 200 mg injections twice a day for 2 days followed by 200 mg injected once a day for up to 14 days. This may be followed by 20 mL of oral solution twice a day for up to a total of 28 days of treatment.

Onychomycosis

The usual dose for a toenail infection, whether or not fingernails are also involved, is 200 mg once a day for 12 weeks.

If only fingernails are infected, treatment is given in 2 7-day-long sessions during which you take 200 mg twice a day with a 3-week rest period between sessions.

Children: The safety and effectiveness of Sporanox in children have not been established.

How should I take Sporanox?

Take Sporanox exactly as prescribed. Be sure to take Sporanox for as long as your doctor prescribes. It will take 3 months or more to cure some infections completely. If you stop taking Sporanox too soon, the infection may return.

To make sure the capsules are properly absorbed, you should take them after a full meal. The oral solution should be taken without food. Do not take antacids within 1 hour before or 2 hours after taking Sporanox. The oral solution and capsules cannot be used interchangeably.

Swish the oral solution, 10 mL at a time, in your mouth for a few seconds before swallowing it.

What should I avoid while taking Sporanox?

Use alcohol with caution. Alcohol and Sporanox can both affect the liver.

Grapefruit and grapefruit juice may interact with Sporanox. The interaction could lead to potentially dangerous effects. Do not increase or decrease the amount of grapefruit products in your diet without first talking to your doctor.

What are possible food and drug interactions associated with Sporanox?

If Sporanox is taken with certain other drugs, the effects of either could be increased, decreased, or altered. It is especially important to check with your doctor before combining Sporanox with the following: acid-blocking drugs such as famotidine and ranitidine, alprazolam, amphotericin b, antacids such as cimetidine, ranitidine, esomeprazole, and pantoprazole, antiarrhythmics such as digoxin, dofetilide, and quinidine, antibiotics such as clarithromycin and erythromycin, antiseizure drugs such as carbamazepine, phenobarbital, and phenytoin, alfentanil, blood-thinners such as warfarin, buspirone, calcium-blocking drugs such as amlodipine and verapamil, cholesterol-lowering drugs such as atorvastatin, lovastatin, and simvastatin, cilostazol, cisapride, corticosteroids such as budesonide, dexamethasone, and methylprednisolone, cyclosporine, diabetes drugs such as glipizide and glyburide, diazepam, digoxin, dofetilide, drugs to treat cancer such as busulfan, docetaxel, and vinca alkaloids, eletriptan, fentanyl, halofantrine, HIV drugs such as indinavir, nevirapine, ritonavir, and saquinavir, isoniazid, midazolam, pimozide, rifabutin, rifampin, sirolimus, tacrolimus, triazolam, trimetrexate.

What are the possible side effects of Sporanox?

Side effects cannot be anticipated. If any develop or change in intensity, tell your doctor as soon as possible. Only your doctor can determine if it is safe for you to continue taking this drug.

Side effects may include: Abdominal pain, anxiety, bursitis, constipation, depression, diarrhea, dizziness, fatigue, fever, gas, headache, high blood pressure, indigestion, injury, itchiness, liver disorders, muscle pain, nasal and sinus inflammation, nausea, pain, rash, respiratory infection, swelling due to water retention, upper respiratory tract infection, upset stomach, urinary infection, vomiting

Additional side effects that may be seen with the oral solution are: Back pain, blood in the urine, chest pain, cough, dehydration, difficulty breathing, difficulty swallowing, hemorrhoids, hot flashes, impaired speech, inflamed mouth, insomnia, pneumonia, shivering, sweating, vision problems, weight loss

Can I receive Sporanox if I am pregnant or breastfeeding?

The effects of Sporanox during pregnancy and breastfeeding are unknown. Tell your doctor immediately if you are pregnant, plan to become pregnant, or are breastfeeding. You should not take Sporanox to treat fungal nail infections if you are or may become pregnant. Do not breastfeed while you are taking Sporanox.

What should I do if I miss a dose of Sporanox?

Take the forgotten dose as soon as you remember. If it is almost time for the next dose, skip the missed dose and go back to your regular schedule. Never take 2 doses at once.

How should I store Sporanox?

Store at room temperature. Protect the capsules from light and moisture. Do not freeze the oral solution.

STALEVO
Generic name: Carbidopa, levodopa, and entacapone

What is Stalevo?
Stalevo contains a combination of 3 drugs: carbidopa, levodopa, and entacapone. It is used to help relieve symptoms of Parkinson's disease, including tremors, muscle stiffness and rigidity, slowness of movement, and poor balance or coordination.

Stalevo can be used instead of carbidopa-levodopa or entacapone by people who are taking those medicines separately or when the benefits of levodopa are not lasting as long as they used to.

What is the most important information I should know about Stalevo?
You should never take Stalevo with certain antidepressants known as monoamine oxidase (MAO) inhibitors, such as phenelzine and tranylcypromine. Combining Stalevo with these drugs could cause serious—possibly life-threatening—side effects. MAO inhibitors should be stopped at least 2 weeks before starting therapy with Stalevo. However, Stalevo may be combined with the drugs rasagiline or selegiline. These drugs are a different type of MAO inhibitor that is often prescribed for Parkinson's disease. Always check with your doctor before taking any type of MAO inhibitor.

It is important to take Stalevo at regular intervals according to the schedule outlined by your doctor. Sometimes a weaning off effect may occur at the end of the dosing interval, where you may feel your Parkinson's symptoms. Contact your doctor if the medication is not controlling properly controlling your symptoms.

Your urine, salvia, or sweat may be discolored (dark color such as red, brown, or black) after taking Stalevo.

Who should not take Stalevo?
Do not take Stalevo if you are sensitive to any component of the drug; if you have glaucoma (high pressure in the eye); or if you have any suspicious, undiagnosed skin lesion or mole or a history of melanoma (skin cancer). Do not take Stalevo with certain MAO inhibitors such as phenelzine and tranylcypromine.

What should I tell my doctor before I take the first dose of Stalevo?
Tell your doctor about all prescription, over-the-counter, and herbal medication you are taking before beginning treatment with Stalevo. Also, talk to your doctor about your complete medical history, especially if you have: asthma, diabetes or thyroid disorders, glaucoma, liver or kidney

disease, severe heart or lung disease, or skin cancer. Also tell your doctor if you have a history of bile duct blockage, mental or emotional problems, or heart attacks or ulcers.

What is the usual dosage?
The information below is based on the dosage guidelines your doctor uses. Depending on your condition and medical history, your doctor may prescribe a different regimen. Do not change the dosage or stop taking your medication without your doctor's approval.

Your doctor will tailor your individual dosage carefully, depending on your response to previous therapy and symptoms. If you are already taking carbidopa/levodopa and entacapone as 2 separate medications, you will start a Stalevo regimen that matches what you were previously taking.

Adults: Stalevo may be taken up to 8 times a day. It is available in 3 different strengths: 12.5 milligrams (mg) carbidopa/50 mg levodopa/200 mg entacapone; 25 mg carbidopa/100 mg levodopa/200 mg entacapone; 37.5 mg carbidopa/150 mg levodopa/200 mg entacapone.

How should I take Stalevo?
Stalevo may be taken with or without food. Never chew, crush, or break the tablets. Do not increase or decrease the dose or add any other Parkinson's drugs without first talking to your doctor.

What should I avoid while taking Stalevo?
Low blood pressure may occur especially when starting therapy or when the dosage is increased. Use caution when rising rapidly after sitting or lying down. Give yourself plenty of time to understand how Stalevo affects you before you attempt to drive a car or operate machinery.

Avoid increasing the amount of protein in your diet. Do not take iron products or vitamin or mineral supplements that contain iron without first talking to your doctor. The effects of Stalevo may be reduced by iron.

What are possible food and drug interactions associated with Stalevo?
If Stalevo is taken with certain other drugs, the effects of either could be increased, decreased, or altered. It is especially important to check with your doctor before combining Stalevo with the following: ampicillin, antipsychotic drugs (such as chlorpromazine, droperidol, haloperidol, and perphenazine), apomorphine, bitolterol, blood-pressure drugs, chloramphenicol, cholestyramine, dobutamine, dopamine, epinephrine or norepinephrine, erythromycin, iron, isoniazid, isoproterenol, isoetherine, MAO inhibitors (such as phenelzine and tranylcypromine), methyldopa, metoclopramide, papaverine, phenytoin, probenecid, pyridoxine, rifampicin, risperidone, tricyclic antidepressants (such as amitriptyline and imipramine).

What are the possible side effects of Stalevo?
Side effects cannot be anticipated. If any develop or change in intensity, tell your doctor as soon as possible. Only your doctor can determine if it is safe for you to continue taking this drug.

Side effects may include: abdominal pain; constipation; diarrhea; dizziness; dyskinesia (unwanted or uncontrollable movements); fatigue; hallucinations; harmless discoloration of urine, sweat, and/or saliva; hyperkinesias (excessive muscle movements); hypokinesia (slow movements); nausea; pain, symptoms resembling neuroleptic malignant syndrome (a condition characterized by fever and muscle stiffness)

Stalevo may cause or worsen depression, hallucinations, psychosis, or suicidal thoughts. If you develop any of these symptoms, tell your doctor right away.

Can I receive Stalevo if I am pregnant or breastfeeding?
The effects of Stalevo during pregnancy and breastfeeding are unknown. Tell your doctor immediately if you are pregnant, plan to become pregnant, or are breastfeeding. Use caution if you are breastfeeding while you are taking Stalevo.

What should I do if I miss a dose of Stalevo?
Take it as soon as you remember. If it is almost time for your next dose, skip the missed dose and go back to your regular schedule. Do not take 2 doses at once.

How should I store Stalevo?
Store at room temperature.

STARLIX
Generic name: Nateglinide

What is Starlix?
Starlix can be used alone or in combination with another diabetes drug, such as metformin, pioglitazone, or rosiglitazone, to lower blood sugar in people who have type 2 diabetes. It is prescribed only when diet and exercise, or another diabetes drug alone, have failed to control blood sugar levels.

What is the most important information I should know about Starlix?
Starlix is an aid to, not a substitute for, good diet and exercise. Failure to follow a sound diet and exercise plan can lead to serious complications, such as dangerously high or low blood sugar levels. Starlix cannot be used in place of insulin.

Who should not take Starlix?

Do not take Starlix if you are sensitive to any component of the drug; if you have type 1 diabetes; or diabetic ketoacidosis (a life-threatening medical emergency caused by insufficient insulin and marked by excessive thirst, nausea, fatigue, pain below the breastbone, and fruity smelling breath).

What should I tell my doctor before I take the first dose of Starlix?

Tell your doctor about all prescription, over-the-counter, and herbal medications you are taking before beginning treatment with Starlix. Also, talk to your doctor about your complete medical history, especially if you have a serious infection, illness, or injury; kidney or liver disease; adrenal or pituitary disorders; type 1 diabetes (insulin-dependent diabetes); or need to have surgery.

What is the usual dosage?

The information below is based on the dosage guidelines your doctor uses. Depending on your condition and medical history, your doctor may prescribe a different regimen. Do not change the dosage or stop taking your medication without your doctor's approval.

Adults: Take Starlix 1 to 30 minutes prior to meals. The usual dose of Starlix, whether taken alone or in combination with other drugs, is 120 milligrams (mg) taken 3 times a day. If your doctor finds that your blood glucose (HbA1C) levels are near normal before you start taking the drug, you may take a lower dose of 60 mg 3 times a day.

The safety and effectiveness of Starlix in children have not been established.

How should I take Starlix?

Starlix should be taken before each meal, anywhere from 1-30 minutes before you begin to eat. If you skip a meal, skip your Starlix dose as well and wait until your next meal before taking Starlix.

What should I avoid while taking Starlix?

Starlix can cause hypoglycemia (low blood sugar). This risk is increased by missed meals, alcohol, other diabetes medications, and excessive exercise. It is more likely to occur in older or malnourished people and those with poorly functioning adrenal or pituitary glands. To avoid low blood sugar, take Starlix only with meals and closely follow the diet and exercise regimen suggested by your doctor.

Symptoms of mild low blood sugar may include blurred vision, cold sweats, dizziness, fast heartbeat, fatigue, headache, hunger, lightheadedness, nausea, and nervousness. Mild low blood sugar can usually be corrected by eating sugar or a sugar-based product. Symptoms of more severe low blood sugar may include coma, disorientation, pale skin, seizures, and shallow breathing. Severe low blood sugar should be considered a medical emergency that requires immediate medical attention.

What are possible food and drug interactions associated with Starlix?

If Starlix is taken with certain other drugs, the effects of either could be increased, decreased, or altered. It is especially important to check with your doctor before combining Starlix with the following: airway-opening drugs such as albuterol, aspirin, blood pressure medications such as atenolol and propranolol, corticosteroids, decongestants, MAO inhibitors such as phenelzine and tranylcypromine, NSAIDs such as ibuprofen and naproxen, salicylates, thiazide diuretics, thyroid medications.

What are the possible side effects of Starlix?

Side effects cannot be anticipated. If any develop or change in intensity, tell your doctor as soon as possible. Only your doctor can determine if it is safe for you to continue taking this drug.

Side effects may include: back pain, diarrhea, dizziness, flulike symptoms, joint infection, and upper respiratory tract infection

Can I receive Starlix if I am pregnant or breastfeeding?

The effects of Starlix during pregnancy and breastfeeding are unknown. Tell your doctor immediately if you are pregnant, plan to become pregnant, or are breastfeeding. It is not known whether Starlix appears in breast milk. Do not breastfeed while taking Starlix.

What should I do if I miss a dose of Starlix?

Wait until your next meal, then take your regular dose. Never take 2 doses at the same time.

How should I store Starlix?

Store at room temperature, in a tightly closed container.

Stavudine See Zerit, page 1459.

STAVZOR
Generic name: Valproic acid

What is Stavzor?

Stavzor is used to treat bipolar disorder (the manic episodes), epilepsy, and migraine.

What is the most important information I should know about Stavzor?

Stavzor can cause liver and pancreatic damage. Use of Stavzor during pregnancy can cause birth defects and malformations.

Who should not take Stavzor?

Do not take Stavzor if you: have liver problems and urea cycle disorders, have a known hypersensitivity to Stavzor, or if you are pregnant.

What should I tell my doctor before I take the first dose of Stavzor?

Tell your doctor about all prescription, over the counter, and herbal medications you are taking before beginning treatment with Stavzor. Also talk to your doctor about your complete medical history.

What is the usual dosage?

The information below is based on the dosage guidelines your doctor uses. Depending on your condition and medical history, your doctor may prescribe a different regimen. Do not change the dosage or stop taking your medication without your doctor's approval.

Manic Episodes of Bipolar Disorder
Adults: The initial starting dose is 750 milligrams (mg) per day, in divided doses. The maximum daily dose is 60 mg per kilogram (kg) of body weight per day.

Epilepsy
Adults: The starting dose is 10-15 mg per kg of body weight per day, and can be increased by 5-10 mg per kg of body weight per day.

Migraine
Adults: The starting dose is 250 mg twice a day, may be increased for some patients to 1000 mg per day.

How should I take Stavzor?

Stavzor is to be taken orally (by mouth). Swallow whole, do not chew or crush.

What should I avoid while taking Stavzor?

Avoid driving or operating machinery while on Stavzor until you know how this medication affects you.

What are possible food and drug interactions associated with Stavzor?

If Stavzor is taken with certain other drugs, the effects of either could be increased, decreased, or altered. It is especially important to check with your doctor before combining Stavzor with the following: alcohol, antidepressants, aspirin, carbamazepine, carbepenem antibiotics, felbamate, phenobarbital, phenytoin, rifampin.

What are the possible side effects of Stavzor?

Side effects cannot be anticipated. If any develop or change in intensity, tell your doctor as soon as possible. Only your doctor can determine if it is safe for you to continue taking this drug.

Side effects may include: liver damage, pancreatic damage, sedation, nausea, sleepiness, vomiting, dizziness, rash, increased or decreased blood pressure, chills, fever, neck rigidity, muscle pain, gastroenteritis, gas, loss of appetite

Can I receive Stavzor if I am pregnant or breastfeeding?

Stavzor is to be avoided if you are pregnant or breastfeeding.

What should I do if I miss a dose of Stavzor?

If you miss a dose of Stavzor, skip that dose. Take your next dose at the scheduled time. Do not take 2 doses at once.

How should I store Stavzor?

Store at room temperature.

STRATTERA

Generic name: Atomoxetine hydrochloride

What is Strattera?

Strattera is used to treat attention-deficit/hyperactivity disorder (ADHD). Strattera may help increase attention and decrease impulsiveness and hyperactivity. It should be used as part of a total treatment program for ADHD that may include counseling or other therapies.

What is the most important information I should know about Strattera?

In some children and teenagers, Strattera may increase the risk of suicidal thoughts. Call your doctor right away if your child has thoughts of suicide or sudden changes in mood or behavior, especially at the beginning of treatment or after a change in dose. New mental problems in children and teenagers may also occur. Call your doctor right away if your child has new psychotic symptoms (such as hearing voices, believing things that are not true, being suspicious), or new manic symptoms.

Strattera can cause liver damage. Call your doctor right away if you or your child has itching, right upper belly pain, dark urine, yellow skin or eyes, or unexplained flu-like symptoms.

Strattera use has been associated with heart-related problems, including sudden death in people who have heart problems or heart defects, stroke or heart attack in adults, and increased blood pressure and heart rate. Call your doctor right away if you or your child has any signs of heart problems such as chest pain, shortness of breath, or fainting.

Strattera has not been studied in children less than 6 years of age.

Who should not take Strattera?
Do not take Strattera within 14 days of taking antidepressants called monoamine oxidase inhibitors (MAOIs), including phenelzine, tranylcypromine, and selegiline. The combination of Strattera and an MAOI can cause severe, even fatal, reactions. If you experience high fever, rigid muscles, rapid changes in heart rate, delirium, and coma, call your doctor immediately.

You should not take Strattera if you have narrow-angle glaucoma (high pressure in the eye) or if you are allergic to anything in Strattera.

What should I tell my doctor before I take the first dose of Strattera?
Tell your doctor about all prescription, over-the-counter, and herbal medications you are taking before beginning treatment with Strattera. Also, talk to your doctor about your complete medical history, especially if there is a history of bipolar disorder or depression, heart problems, high or low blood pressure, irregular heart beat, liver disease, mental problems, psychosis, or suicidal thoughts or actions.

What is the usual dosage?
The information below is based on the dosage guidelines your doctor uses. Depending on your condition and medical history, your doctor may prescribe a different regimen. Do not change the dosage or stop taking your medication without your doctor's approval.

The daily dose of Strattera can be taken as a single dose in the morning, or divided into 2 equal doses taken in the morning and late afternoon or early evening.

Adults and teenagers over 154 pounds: The usual starting dosage is 40 milligrams (mg) per day. After at least 3 days, your doctor may increase the daily total to a recommended level of 80 mg. After another 2-4 weeks, dosage may be increased to a maximum of 100 mg daily. If you have liver problems, your dosage will be reduced.

Children and teenagers 154 pounds or less: the usual starting dosage is 0.5 mg per 2.2 pounds of body weight per day. After at least 3 days, the doctor may increase the daily total to a recommended level of 1.2 mg per 2.2 pounds. Daily doses should never exceed 1.4 mg per 2.2 pounds, or a total of 100 mg, whichever is less.

Strattera has not been tested in children less than 6 years of age.

How should I take Strattera?

Take Strattera exactly as prescribed by your doctor. Do not chew, crush, or open the capsules. Swallow the capsules whole with water or other liquids. Strattera can be taken with or without food. Take your dose at the same time each day to help you remember.

What should I avoid while taking Strattera?

Avoid touching a broken Strattera capsule. Wash hands and surfaces that touched an open capsule. If any powder gets in your eyes or your child's eyes, rinse them with water right away and call your doctor.

Use caution when driving, operating machinery, or performing other hazardous activities.

What are possible food and drug interactions associated with Strattera?

If Strattera is taken with certain other drugs, the effects of either could be increased, decreased, or altered. It is especially important to check with your doctor before combining Strattera with the following: albuterol and similar asthma medications, dopamine, dobutamine, fluoxetine, paroxetine, and quinidine.

What are the possible side effects of Strattera?

Side effects cannot be anticipated. If any develop or change in intensity, tell your doctor as soon as possible. Only your doctor can determine if it is safe for you to continue taking this drug.

Side effects in adults may include: constipation, decreased appetite, dizziness, dry mouth, menstrual cramps, nausea, problems urinating, sexual side effects, trouble sleeping

Side effects in children and teenagers may include: decreased appetite, dizziness, nausea or vomiting, mood swings, tiredness, upset stomach

Erections that won't go away (priapism) have occurred rarely during treatment with Strattera. If you have an erection that lasts more than 4 hours, seek medical help right away because of the potential for lasting damage, including the potential inability to have erections.

Can I receive Strattera if I am pregnant or breastfeeding?

The effects of Strattera during pregnancy and breastfeeding are unknown. Tell your doctor immediately if you are pregnant, plan to become pregnant, or are breastfeeding.

What should I do if I miss a dose of Strattera?

Take it as soon as remember on that day. If you miss a day of Strattera, do not double your dose. Just skip the day you missed.

How should I store Strattera?
Store at room temperature.

SULAR
Generic name: Nisoldipine

What is Sular?
Sular is used alone or with other medications to control high blood pressure.

**What is the most important information
I should know about Sular?**
You must take Sular regularly for it to be effective. Since blood pressure declines gradually, it may be several weeks before you get the full benefit of Sular, and you must continue taking it even if you are feeling well. Sular does not cure high blood pressure it only keeps it under control.

Who should not take Sular?
Do not take Sular if you are sensitive to it or to similar drugs such as felodipine or nifedipine.

**What should I tell my doctor before
I take the first dose of Sular?**
Tell your doctor about all prescription, over-the-counter, and herbal medication you are taking before beginning treatment with Sular. Also, talk to your doctor about your complete medical history, especially if you have heart disease, low blood pressure, congestive heart failure, or liver disease.

What is the usual dosage?
The information below is based on the dosage guidelines your doctor uses. Depending on your condition and medical history, your doctor may prescribe a different regimen. Do not change the dosage or stop taking your medication without your doctor's approval.

Adults: The usual starting dose is 20 milligrams (mg) once daily. Your doctor may increase the dose by 10 mg per week or longer intervals until your blood pressure is controlled.

The usual maintenance dosage is 20-40 mg once daily. The maximum dose should not exceed 60 mg daily.

If you are older than 65 or if you have liver disease the usual starting dose is 10 mg.

How should I take Sular?
Take Sular exactly as directed by your doctor.

What should I avoid while taking Sular?

Avoid taking Sular with high fat meals. Fatty foods may increase the amount of Sular in the blood.

Do not bite, divide, or crush Sular tablets. Swallow the tablets whole. The tablets are specially formulated to release the medication slowly in the body.

Use caution when you stand or sit up from a lying position. You may become dizzy when changing positions.

What are possible food and drug interactions associated with Sular?

If Sular is taken with certain other drugs, the effects of either could be increased, decreased, or altered. It is especially important to check with your doctor before combining Sular with the following: alcohol, atenolol, carbamazepine, cimetidine, grapefruit, high-fat foods, phenobarbital, phenytoin, rifampin, quinidine.

What are the possible side effects of Sular?

Side effects cannot be anticipated. If any develop or change in intensity, tell your doctor as soon as possible. Only your doctor can determine if it is safe for you to continue taking this drug.

Side effects may include: Dizziness, flushing, headache, heart palpitations, sinus inflammation, sore throat, swelling of the hands and feet

Sular may cause an excessive drop in blood pressure, especially when you are first taking the medication or when the dosage is increased. Low blood pressure can also become a problem if you are taking other blood pressure medications.

Can I receive Sular if I am pregnant or breastfeeding?

The effects of Sular during pregnancy and breastfeeding are unknown. Tell your doctor immediately if you are pregnant, plan to become pregnant, or are breastfeeding.

What should I do if I miss a dose of Sular?

Take it as soon as you remember. If is almost time for your next dose, skip the one you missed and go back to your regular schedule. Never take 2 doses at the same time.

How should I store Sular?

Store at room temperature in a tight, light-resistant container. Protect from moisture.

Sulfamethoxazole and trimethoprim *See Bactrim, page 193.*

Sulfasalazine *See Azulfidine, page 190.*

Sumatriptan and naproxen *See Treximet, page 1330.*

Sumatriptan succinate *See Imitrex, page 652.*

SUPRAX
Generic name: Cefixime

What is Suprax?
Suprax, a cephalosporin antibiotic, is prescribed for bacterial infections of the lungs, ears, urinary tract, and throat. It is also used to treat uncomplicated gonorrhea.

What is the most important information I should know about Suprax?
If you are allergic to either penicillin or cephalosporin antibiotics in any form, consult your doctor before taking Suprax. An allergy to either type of medication may signal an allergy to Suprax, and if a reaction occurs, it could be extremely severe. If you take the drug and feel signs of a reaction, seek medical attention immediately.

Who should not take Suprax?
Do not take Suprax if you are sensitive to or have ever had an allergic reaction to the drug or to other cephalosporin antibiotics.

What should I tell my doctor before I take the first dose of Suprax?
Tell your doctor about all prescription, over-the-counter, and herbal medications you are taking before beginning treatment with Suprax. Also, talk to your doctor about your complete medical history, especially if you have kidney or liver disease, a history of stomach or intestinal disease such as colitis (inflammation of the large intestine), or if you have ever had an allergic reaction to another cephalosporin or penicillin.

What is the usual dosage?
The information below is based on the dosage guidelines your doctor uses. Depending on your condition and medical history, your doctor may prescribe a different regimen. Do not change the dosage or stop taking your medication without your doctor's approval.

Infections Other Than Gonorrhea
Adults: The usual dose is 400 milligrams (mg) daily. If you have kidney disease, the dose may be lower.

Children >6 months: The usual dose is 8 mg of liquid per 2.2 pounds of body weight per day. This may be given as a single dose or in 2 half-doses every 12 hours. Children weighing >110 pounds or >12 years of age should be treated with an adult dose.

If your child has a middle ear infection (otitis media), your doctor will probably prescribe Suprax suspension. The tablet form is less effective against this type of infection.

Uncomplicated Gonorrhea
Adults: A single 400-mg dose is usually prescribed.

How should I take Suprax?
Suprax can be taken with or without food. If Suprax causes stomach upset, take it with meals.

If you are taking the liquid form of Suprax, use the specially marked measuring spoon to measure each dose accurately. Shake well before using.

Finish taking all of your medication even if you are feeling better in order to obtain the maximum benefit.

What should I avoid while taking Suprax?
Repeated use of Suprax may result in an overgrowth of bacteria that do not respond to Suprax and can cause a secondary infection. Do not save Suprax for use at another time.

What are possible food and drug interactions associated with Suprax?
If Suprax is taken with certain other drugs, the effects of either could be increased, decreased, or altered. It is especially important to check with your doctor before combining Suprax with the following: carbamazepine, blood thinners such as warfarin.

What are the possible side effects of Suprax?
Side effects cannot be anticipated. If any develop or change in intensity, tell your doctor as soon as possible. Only your doctor can determine if it is safe for you to continue taking this drug.

Side effects may include: abdominal pain, gas, indigestion, loose stools, mild diarrhea, nausea, vomiting

Can I receive Suprax if I am pregnant or breastfeeding?
The effects of Suprax during pregnancy and breastfeeding are unknown. Tell your doctor immediately if you are pregnant, plan to become pregnant, or are breastfeeding.

What should I do if I miss a dose of Suprax?
If you are taking Suprax once a day and you forget to take a dose, take it as soon as you remember. Wait at least 10 to 12 hours before taking your next dose, then return to your regular schedule.

If you are taking Suprax 2 times a day and you forget to take a dose, take it as soon as you remember and take your next dose 5 to 6 hours later. Then go back to your regular schedule.

If you are taking Suprax 3 times a day and you forget to take a dose, take it as soon as you remember and take your next dose 2 to 4 hours later. Then return to your regular schedule.

How should I store Suprax?

Suprax liquid may be kept for 14 days, either at room temperature or in the refrigerator. Keep the bottle tightly closed and do not store in damp places. Keep away from direct light and heat. Discard any unused Suprax after 14 days.

SURMONTIL

Generic name: Trimipramine maleate

What is Surmontil?

Surmontil is a tricyclic antidepressant used to treat depression.

What is the most important information I should know about Surmontil?

Never take Surmontil if you are taking an antidepressant drug called a monoamine oxidase inhibitor (MAOI) or if you have stopped taking an MAOI in the last 14 days. MAOI drugs include phenelzine, tranylcypromine, and isocarboxazid. Taking Surmontil close in time to an MAOI can result in serious—sometimes fatal—reactions, including high body temperature, coma, and seizures.

Antidepressants can increase the risk of suicidal thinking and behavior in children and teenagers. Adult and pediatric patients taking antidepressants should be watched closely for changes in moods or actions, especially when they first start therapy or when their dose is increased or decreased. Patients and their families should contact the doctor immediately if new symptoms develop or seem to get worse. Signs to watch for include anxiety, hostility, insomnia, restlessness, impulsive or dangerous behavior, and thoughts about suicide or dying.

Never stop an antidepressant medication without first talking to your healthcare provider. Abruptly stopping Surmontil can cause other symptoms.

Antidepressant medications have other side effects. Talk to your healthcare provider about the side effects of the medicine prescribed for you or your family member.

Who should not take Surmontil?

Surmontil should not be used if you are recovering from a recent heart attack or if you are sensitive to the drug.

What should I tell my doctor before I take the first dose of Surmontil?

Tell your doctor about all prescription, over-the-counter, and herbal medications you are taking before beginning treatment with Surmontil. Also, talk to your doctor about your complete medical history, especially if you have a family history of suicide, bipolar disorder, or depression. Also let your doctor know if you have a history of diabetes; glaucoma (increased pressure in the eye); heart, kidney, or liver disease; overactive thyroid; seizure disorder; or urinary retention.

What is the usual dosage?

The information below is based on the dosage guidelines your doctor uses. Depending on your condition and medical history, your doctor may prescribe a different regimen. Do not change the dosage or stop taking your medication without your doctor's approval.

Adults: The usual starting dose is 75 milligrams (mg) per day, divided into equal, smaller doses. Your doctor may gradually increase your dose to 150 mg per day, again, divided into smaller doses. Doses over 200 mg a day are not recommended. Doses for long-term therapy may range from 50 to 150 mg daily. You can take this total daily dosage at bedtime or spread it throughout the day.

Elderly or adolescents: Dosages usually start at 50 mg per day. Your doctor may increase the dose to 100 mg a day, if needed.

Surmontil is not approved for use in children.

How should I take Surmontil?

Surmontil is taken by mouth. Many people take one dose at bedtime. Others may find it works better to take Surmontil more than once a day.

It is important to take Surmontil exactly as prescribed, even if the drug seems to have no effect. It may take up to 4 weeks for its benefits to appear.

Surmontil can make your mouth dry. Sucking hard candy or chewing gum can help this problem.

What should I avoid while taking Surmontil?

Avoid driving a car, operating machinery, or participating in any activities that require full alertness if you are sure of the drug's effect on you.

Avoid using alcohol, which may increase drowsiness and dizziness while taking Surmontil.

What are possible food and drug interactions associated with Surmontil?

If Surmontil is taken with certain other drugs, the effects of either could be increased, decreased, or altered. It is especially important to check with your doctor before combining Surmontil with the following: antidepressants, antispasmodic drugs such as benztropine, atropine, cimetidine, decongestants, drugs for heart irregularities such as flecainide and propafenone, epinephrine, guanethidine, quinidine, tranquilizers, and thyroid medications.

What are the possible side effects of Surmontil?
Side effects cannot be anticipated. If any develop or change in intensity, tell your doctor as soon as possible. Only your doctor can determine if it is safe for you to continue taking this drug.

Side effects may include: allergic reactions, black tongue, blood disorders, blurred vision, breast development in men, confusion, dizziness, drowsiness, dry mouth, fluctuations in blood pressure, heartbeat irregularities, high or low blood pressure, insomnia, lack of coordination, stomach and intestinal problems, urination problems, vomiting

Can I receive Surmontil if I am pregnant or breastfeeding?
The effects of Surmontil during pregnancy and breastfeeding are unknown. Tell your doctor immediately if you are pregnant, plan to become pregnant, or are breastfeeding. There is no information on whether Surmontil appears in breast milk. The doctor may tell you to stop breastfeeding until your treatment is finished.

What should I do if I miss a dose of Surmontil?
Take it as soon as you remember. If it is almost time for the next dose, skip the missed dose and go back to your regular schedule. Do not take two doses at once. If you take Surmontil once a day at bedtime and you miss a dose, do not take it in the morning; it could cause disturbing side effects during the day.

How should I store Surmontil?
Store at room temperature in a tightly closed container, away from moisture.

SUSTIVA
Generic name: Efavirenz

What is Sustiva?
Sustiva is used to treat HIV (human immunodeficiency virus) infection in combination with other anti-HIV medications. Sustiva is not a cure for HIV infection.

What is the most important information I should know about Sustiva?
Though Sustiva can slow the progress of HIV, it is not a cure. You may continue to develop infections and other complications associated with

HIV. Sustiva does not reduce the risk of transmitting HIV to others through sexual contact or blood contamination. HIV-related infections remain a danger, so frequent checkups and tests are still advisable.

Who should not take Sustiva?
Do not take Sustiva if you are sensitive to any component of the drug.

Sustiva may cause serious and/or life-threatening side effects if taken with certain other medications, including astemizole, cisapride, ergotamine, dihydroergotamine, midazolam, or triazolam.

What should I tell my doctor before I take the first dose of Sustiva?
Tell your doctor about all prescription, over-the-counter, and herbal medications you are taking before beginning treatment with Sustiva. Also, talk to your doctor about your complete medical history, especially if you have liver disease, seizures, a history of mental illness or depression, or high blood levels of cholesterol or triglycerides.

What is the usual dosage?
The information below is based on the dosage guidelines your doctor uses. Depending on your condition and medical history, your doctor may prescribe a different regimen. Do not change the dosage or stop taking your medication without your doctor's approval.

Adults: The recommended dose is 600 milligrams (mg) daily in combination with other HIV medications.

Children >3 years: The recommended dose is based on weight. For children 22 to 32 lbs, the recommended dose is 200 mg; 33 to 43 lbs, 250 mg; 44 to 54 lbs, 300 mg; 55 to 71.5 lbs, 350 mg; 71.5 to 87 lbs, 400 mg. Children weighing more than 88 pounds receive the 600 mg adult dose.

How should I take Sustiva?
You should take Sustiva on an empty stomach, preferably at bedtime. Swallow Sustiva with water.

Taking Sustiva with food increases the amount of medicine in your body, which may increase the frequency of side effects. Taking Sustiva at bedtime may make some side effects less bothersome.

Sustiva must be taken in combination with other anti-HIV medicines. If you take only Sustiva, the medicine may stop working. Take the exact amount of Sustiva your doctor prescribes. Never change the dose on your own. Do not stop this medicine unless your doctor tells you to stop.

What should I avoid while taking Sustiva?
Avoid alcohol or use it with caution while taking Sustiva. Alcohol may increase dizziness and drowsiness while taking this medication. Sustiva may cause dizziness, problems concentrating, and/or drowsiness. Do not

drive or operate heavy machinery until you know how you will react to Sustiva.

Avoid high-risk activities such as unprotected sex and the sharing of needles. Sustiva does not cure HIV or AIDS. You can still transmit the virus to others during therapy with this medication.

What are possible food and drug interactions associated with Sustiva?

If Sustiva is taken with certain other drugs, the effects of either could be increased, decreased, or altered. It is especially important to check with your doctor before combining Sustiva with the following: alcohol, amprenavir, astemizole, atazanavir, carbamazepine, cisapride, clarithromycin, dihydroergotamine, ergotamine, indinavir, itraconazole, ketoconazole, methadone, midazolam, nelfinavir, oral contraceptives containing ethinyl estradiol, phenobarbital, phenytoin, rifabutin, rifampin, ritonavir, saquinavir, St. John's wort, triazolam, voriconazole, warfarin

What are the possible side effects of Sustiva?

Side effects cannot be anticipated. If any develop or change in intensity, tell your doctor as soon as possible. Only your doctor can determine if it is safe for you to continue taking this drug.

Side effects may include: abnormal dreaming, abnormal thinking, agitation, amnesia, confusion, cough, diarrhea, dizziness, drowsiness, fatigue, feelings of well-being, fever, hallucinations, headache, impaired concentration, insomnia, loss of identity, nausea, skin rash, vomiting

If you develop delusions, inappropriate behavior, severe depression, or suicidal thoughts, call your doctor immediately.

One of the most common side effects of Sustiva is skin rash. Most rashes usually clear up on their own. In rare cases, Sustiva can cause a severe rash associated with blistering, skin peeling, and fever. Call your doctor if you develop this type of rash.

Sustiva may cause a redistribution of body fat, leading to extra fat around the middle, a "buffalo hump" on the back, and wasting in the arms, legs, and face. It is not known if this is a long-term health problem or not.

In a few patients, Sustiva has toxic effects on the liver and can raise cholesterol levels in some patients. Your doctor will probably check your liver function and cholesterol regularly.

Can I receive Sustiva if I am pregnant or breastfeeding?

When taken in the first trimester, Sustiva may cause harm to a developing baby. Therefore, Sustiva should not be taken during pregnancy. Before you begin Sustiva therapy, your doctor will test to make sure that you're not pregnant. While taking the drug, you should use both a barrier type of contraceptive and a second method such as contraceptive pills.

Avoid breastfeeding. HIV infection can be passed to a nursing infant through breast milk.

What should I do if I miss a dose of Sustiva?
If you forget to take Sustiva, take the missed dose right away, unless it is almost time for your next dose. Do not take 2 doses at once.

How should I store Sustiva?
Store at room temperature.

SYMBICORT
Generic name: Budesonide and formoterol

What is Symbicort?
Symbicort combines two drugs —the inhaled corticosteroid budesonide and the long-acting beta$_2$ agonist formoterol—to control the symptoms of asthma.

What is the most important information I should know about Symbicort?
In patients with asthma, long-acting beta$_2$ agonists may increase the chance of death from asthma. Symbicort does not relieve sudden symptoms of asthma. Do not stop using Symbicort unless told to do so by your healthcare provider.

Who should not take Symbicort?
Do not take Symbicort if you are suffering from status asthmaticus or an acute attack of asthma.

Do not take if you are allergic to Symbicort or any of its ingredients.

Do not use if you are also using drugs that suppress the immune system or have chickenpox or measles.

What should I tell my doctor before I take the first dose of Symbicort?
Tell your doctor about all prescription, over-the-counter, and herbal medications you are taking before beginning treatment with Symbicort. Also talk to your doctor about your complete medical history, especially if you have a history of status asthmaticus, acute asthma attacks, are pregnant or breastfeeding. Tell your doctor if you are taking any drugs that suppress the immune system, are suffering from chickenpox or measles, cataracts, TB, if you have heart problems, high blood pressure, thyroid problems, diabetes, or osteoporosis..

What is the usual dosage?
The information below is based on the dosage guidelines your doctor uses. Depending on your condition and medical history, your doctor

may prescribe a different regimen. Do not change the dosage or stop taking your medication without your doctor's approval.

Adults: The usual dosage of Symbicort is 2 inhalations twice a day—once in the morning and once in the evening, 12 hours apart.

How should I take Symbicort?

Shake the inhaler well for 5 seconds before each use. Symbicort should be primed before using it for the first time or if you haven't used it for more than 7 days. Priming is done by releasing 2 test sprays. To use, exhale out fully, then place the white mouthpiece fully into your mouth and close your lips around it. While inhaling, press down firmly and fully on the counter on the inhaler. Continue to breathe in and hold your breath for 10 seconds or as long as you are comfortable. Take the prescribed number of puffs. After you are done, rinse your mouth with water.

What should I avoid while taking Symbicort?

Do not change or stop any of your medicines to control or treat your breathing problems. Do not swallow the medication.

What are possible food and drug interactions associated with Symbicort?

If Symbicort is used with certain other drugs, the effects of either could be increased, decreased, or altered. It is especially important to check with your doctor before combining Symbicort with any other drugs containing a long-acting beta$_2$ agonist, such as Advair Diskus or Serevent Diskus.

What are the possible side effects of Symbicort?

Side effects cannot be anticipated. If any develop or change in intensity, tell your doctor as soon as possible. Only your doctor can determine if it is safe for you to continue taking this drug.

Side effects may include: allergic reactions, cataracts, elevated intra-ocular pressure, fast irregular heartbeat, headache, reduced immunity, higher chance of infections, nervousness, tremors

Signs of severe allergic reactions may include hives, difficulty breathing, and swelling of the throat. If any of these events occur, seek immediate medical attention.

Can I receive Symbicort if I am pregnant or breastfeeding?

Symbicort is to be avoided during pregnancy and breastfeeding.

What should I do if I miss a dose of Symbicort?

Take it as soon as you remember. If it is almost time for your next dose, skip the one you missed and go back to your regular schedule. Do not take 2 doses at once.

How should I store Symbicort?

Store at room temperature.

SYMBYAX

Generic name: Olanzapine and fluoxetine hydrochloride

What is Symbyax?

Symbyax contains two medicines, olanzapine and fluoxetine. Symbyax is used to treat adults who have depressive episodes associated with bipolar disorder.

What is the most important information I should know about Symbyax?

Symbyax is not for use in dementia-related psychosis (decreased mental functioning complicated by seeing or hearing things or having irrational thoughts or fears). There is an increased risk of death in elderly patients with dementia-related psychosis who are treated with Symbyax.

A life-threatening condition called serotonin syndrome (serious changes in how your brain, muscles, and digestive system work) can happen when you take Symbyax with medicines known as triptans, which are used to treat migraine headaches. Signs and symptoms of serotonin syndrome include restlessness, diarrhea, hallucinations, coma, loss of coordination, nausea, fast heartbeat, vomiting, increased body temperature, rapid changes in blood pressure, and overactive reflexes. Serotonin syndrome may be more likely to occur when starting or increasing the dose of Symbyax or a triptan.

Antidepressants can increase the risk of suicidal thinking and behavior in children and teenagers. Adult and pediatric patients taking antidepressants should be watched closely for changes in moods or actions, especially when they first start therapy or when their dose is increased or decreased. Patients and their families should contact the doctor immediately if new symptoms develop or seem to get worse. Signs to watch for include anxiety, hostility, insomnia, restlessness, impulsive or dangerous behavior, and thoughts about suicide or dying.

Symbyax may cause drowsiness or dizziness. These effects may be worse if you take it with alcohol or certain medicines. Take Symbyax with caution. Do not drive or perform other possibly unsafe tasks until you know how you react to it.

Do not drink alcohol or use medicines that may cause drowsiness (eg, sleep aids, muscle relaxers) while you are using Symbyax; it may add to their effects.

Symbyax may cause dizziness, lightheadedness, or fainting; alcohol, hot weather, exercise, or fever may increase these effects. To prevent them, sit up or stand slowly, especially in the morning. Sit or lie down at the first sign of any of these effects.

Do not become overheated in hot weather or while you are being active; heatstroke may occur.

Several weeks may pass before your symptoms improve. Do NOT take more than the recommended dose, change your dose, or take Symbyax for longer than prescribed without checking with your doctor.

Symbyax may rarely cause a prolonged, painful erection. This could happen even when you are not having sex. If this is not treated right away, it could lead to permanent sexual problems such as impotence. Contact your doctor right away if this happens.

Symbyax may raise your blood sugar. High blood sugar may make you feel confused, drowsy, or thirsty. It can also make you flush, breathe faster, or have a fruit-like breath odor. If these symptoms occur, tell your doctor right away.

Neuroleptic malignant syndrome (NMS) is a potentially fatal syndrome that can be caused by Symbyax. Symptoms may include fever, stiff muscles, confusion, abnormal thinking, fast or irregular heartbeat, and sweating. Contact your doctor at once if you have any of these symptoms.

Some patients who take Symbyax may develop tardive dyskinesia, a potentially irreversible disorder characterized by involuntary muscle movements and twitches. Older people, especially women, appear to be at greater risk. The chance that this will happen or that it will become permanent is greater in those who take Symbyax in higher doses or for a long time. Tell your doctor at once if you have muscle problems with your arms, legs, tongue, face, mouth, or jaw (eg, tongue sticking out, puffing of cheeks, mouth puckering, chewing movements) while taking Symbyax.

Who should not take Symbyax?

Never take Symbyax if you are taking antidepressant drugs called monoamine oxidase inhibitors (MAOIs), or if you have stopped taking an MAOI in the last 14 days. Taking Symbyax close in time to an MAOI can result in serious—sometimes fatal—reactions, including high body temperature, coma, or seizures. Do not take an MAOI within 5 weeks of stopping Symbyax. MAOI drugs include isocarboxazid, phenelzine, and tranylcypromine.

Never take Symbyax while you are taking thioridazine and do not take thioridazine within 5 weeks of stopping Symbyax. Simultaneously taking these drugs can result in serious heart rhythm problems.

Do not take Symbyax if you are taking pimozide or if you are sensitive to any component of the drug.

What should I tell my doctor before I take the first dose of Symbyax?

Tell your doctor about all prescription, over-the-counter, and herbal medications you are taking before beginning treatment with Symbyax. Also talk to your doctor about your complete medical history, especially if you have any of the following: a history of certain cancers (breast, pancrease, pituitary) or if you are at risk for breast cancer; high blood sugar or diabetes or a family history of diabetes; a stomach problem called paralytic ileus; an enlarged prostate; narrow-angle glaucoma; history of heart attack; high or low blood pressure; liver, kidney, or heart problems; seizures; and strokes or mini-strokes.

Caregivers should tell the doctor if the patient has Alzheimer's disease or is older than 65 and has dementia.

Let the doctor know if you currently smoke, drink alcohol, exercise a lot, or are often in hot places.

You should especially tell your doctor if you are taking or plan to take Prozac, Prozac Weekly, Sarafem, olanzapine, Zyprexa, or Zyprexa Zydis. These medicines each contain an ingredient that is also found in Symbyax.

What is the usual dosage?
The information below is based on the dosage guidelines your doctor uses. Depending on your condition and medical history, your doctor may prescribe a different regimen. Do not change the dosage or stop taking your medication without your doctor's approval.

Adults: The usual starting dose is 1 capsule containing 6 milligrams (mg) of olanzapine and 25 mg of fluoxetine, taken once a day in the evening. If needed, your doctor may gradually increase the dose. The usual dose range is 6 to 12 mg of olanzapine and 25-50 mg of fluoxetine. The efficacy of Symbyax was demonstrated in a dose range of 6 mg to 12 mg of olanzapine and 25 mg to 50 mg of fluoxetine. The safety of doses above 18 mg olanzapine and 75 mg fluoxetine has not been evaluated in clinical studies.

Your doctor may adjust your dose if you have liver problems, a high risk of low blood pressure, or a combination of factors that may slow your body's processing of Symbyax (female, older age, nonsmoker).

How should I take Symbyax?
Take Symbyax exactly as instructed by your doctor. Your doctor will usually start you on a low dose of Symbyax. Your dose may be adjusted depending on your body's response to Symbyax. Do not stop taking Symbyax or change your dose even if you feel better. Do not suddenly stop taking Symbyax without checking with your doctor.

Symbyax is usually taken once a day in the evening. Take Symbyax at the same time each day.

You can take Symbyax with or without food.

What should I avoid while taking Symbyax?
Avoid driving, operating machinery, or performing other hazardous activities until you know how this medication affects you. If you experience

dizziness or drowsiness, avoid these activities. Dizziness may be more likely to occur when you rise from a sitting or lying position. Rise slowly to prevent dizziness and a possible fall.

Do not drink alcohol while taking Symbyax. The combination can cause a sudden drop in blood pressure.

Avoid becoming overheated while taking Symbyax. Drink plenty of fluid and use caution in hot weather and during exercise.

What are possible food and drug interactions associated with Symbyax?

If Symbyax is taken with certain other drugs, the effects of either could be increased, decreased, or altered. It is especially important to check with your doctor before combining Symbyax with the following: alprazolam, antidepressants known as MAOIs or tricyclics, blood pressure drugs, carbamazepine, clozapine, diazepam, dopamine, fluvoxamine, haloperidol, levodopa, lithium, omeprazole, phenytoin, pimozide, rifampin, St. John's wort, thioridazine, tramadol, triptans such as sumatriptan or eletriptan, tryptophan, and warfarin.

Be careful about combining Symbyax with aspirin or nonsteroidal antiinflammatory drugs (NSAIDs) such as ibuprofen, or with other drugs that affect blood clotting. The combination may increase the risk of bleeding.

What are the possible side effects of Symbyax?

Side effects cannot be anticipated. If any develop or change in intensity, tell your doctor as soon as possible. Only your doctor can determine if it is safe for you to continue taking this drug.

Side effects may include: diarrhea, constipation, decreased sexual desire or ability, dizziness, dry mouth, feeling weak, increased appetite, problems keeping your body temperature regulated, sleepiness, black or tarry stools, confusion, anxiety, memory problems, irritability, sore through, swelling of your hands and feet, tremors, trouble concentrating, weight gain, or allergic reactions

Seek immediate medical attention if you experience symptoms of an allergic reaction such as hives, rash, itching, difficulty breathing, or swelling of the lips, face, mouth, or tongue.

Can I receive Symbyax if I am pregnant or breastfeeding?

The effects of Symbyax during pregnancy and breastfeeding are unknown. Tell your doctor immediately if you are pregnant, plan to become pregnant, or are breastfeeding. Do not breastfeed while you are taking Symbyax.

Neonates exposed to fluoxetine, a component of Symbyax, late in the third trimester have developed complications requiring prolonged hospitalizations, respiratory support, and tube feeding. The risks and benefits of treatment should be carefully considered when using Symbyax during pregnancy.

What should I do if I miss a dose of Symbyax?
Take it as soon as you remember. However, if it is almost time for your next dose, skip the missed dose and take only your regularly scheduled dose. Do not take two doses at once.

How should I store Symbyax?
Store at room temperature away from heat, moisture, and light. Do not store in the bathroom.

SYMLIN
Generic name: Pramlintide acetate

What is Symlin?
Symlin is an injectable medication used with mealtime insulin to control blood sugar in adults with type 1 or type 2 diabetes. Symlin slows down the movement of food through your stomach, which affects how fast sugar enters your blood after eating. Symlin is always used with insulin to help lower blood sugar during the 3 hours after meals.

What is the most important information I should know about Symlin?
Even when Symlin is carefully added to your mealtime insulin therapy, your blood sugar may drop too low, especially if you have type 1 diabetes. If this low blood sugar (severe hypoglycemia) happens, it is seen within 3 hours after a Symlin injection. Severe low blood sugar makes it hard to think clearly, drive a car, operate heavy machinery, or perform other risky activities where you could hurt yourself or others. Symptoms include headache, hunger, irritability, sweating, tremor, difficulty concentrating, and can lead to more severe conditions including seizures, loss of consciousness, and coma.

Who should not take Symlin?
Do not use Symlin if you cannot tell when your blood sugar is low, have a stomach problem called gastroparesis (when your stomach does not empty as fast as it should), or are allergic to Symlin or any ingredients in Symlin.

What should I tell my doctor before I take the first dose of Symlin?
Tell your doctor about all prescription, over-the-counter, and herbal medications you are taking before beginning treatment with Symlin. Also, talk

to your doctor about your complete medical history, especially if you are pregnant, plan to become pregnant, or are breastfeeding.

What is the usual dosage?
The information below is based on the dosage guidelines your doctor uses. Depending on your condition and medical history, your doctor may prescribe a different regimen. Do not change the dosage or stop taking your medication without your doctor's approval.

When you first start Symlin, your healthcare professional should instruct you to reduce the dose of insulin you take before meals by 50%. Your doctor should direct future insulin changes based on blood sugar testing.

Type 1 Diabetes
Adults: The usual starting dose is 15 micrograms (mcg) injected into the thigh or abdomen immediately before meals at the same time as your insulin. Always inject Symlin in a different site than your insulin. Depending on your response, in time and with close monitoring, your doctor may adjust your dose in steps up to a maximum of 60 mcg. Only a healthcare professional skilled in the use of Symlin can monitor and recommend dose adjustments.

Type 2 Diabetes
Adults: The usual starting dose is 60 mcg injected into the thigh or abdomen immediately before meals at the same time as your insulin. Always inject Symlin in a different site than your insulin. Depending on your response, in time and with close monitoring, your doctor may adjust your dose up to a maximum of 120 mcg. Only a healthcare professional skilled in the use of Symlin can monitor and recommend dose adjustments.

Symlin has not been studied in children.

How should I take Symlin?
You must use Symlin exactly as prescribed. The amount of Symlin you use will depend on whether you have type 1 or type 2 diabetes.

Never mix insulin and Symlin. You should use different syringes for Symlin and insulin.

Injecting Symlin is similar to injecting insulin. Inject Symlin under the skin (subcutaneously) of your stomach area or thigh. Inject Symlin at a site that is more than 2 inches away from your insulin injection. Allow Symlin to warm to room temperature before injecting. Use a U-100 insulin syringe (best to use 0.3 mL size) to draw-up and inject Symlin. Always use a new syringe and needle for each Symlin injection. Do not use Symlin if the liquid in the vial looks cloudy.

Do not inject Symlin if you skip a meal. Do not use Symlin if: your blood sugar is too low; you plan to eat a meal with >250 calories or 30 grams of carbohydrate; you are sick and can't eat your usual meal; you are having surgery or a medical test where you cannot eat; you do not plan to eat.

What should I avoid while taking Symlin?
Do not drive or operate dangerous machinery until you know how Symlin affects your blood sugar. Low blood sugar makes it hard to think clearly, drive a car, operate heavy machinery, or perform other risky activities where you could hurt yourself or others.

Avoid alcohol. Alcohol may increase the risk of low blood sugar.

What are possible food and drug interactions associated with Symlin?
Symlin may slow the absorption of drugs taken by mouth. Your doctor may have you take your other medicines at least 1 hour before or 2 hours after your Symlin injection.

If Symlin is taken with certain other drugs, the effects of either could be increased, decreased, or altered. It is especially important to check with your doctor before combining Symlin with the following: antidepressants known as MAO inhibitors, blood pressure medications, clonidine, disopyramide, fibrates, fluoxetine, guanethidine, pentoxifylline, propoxyphene, reserpine, salicylates, sulfonamide antibiotics.

What are the possible side effects of Symlin?
Side effects cannot be anticipated. If any develop or change in intensity, tell your doctor as soon as possible. Only your doctor can determine if it is safe for you to continue taking this drug.

Side effects may include: decreased appetite, dizziness, indigestion, low blood sugar, nausea, stomach pain, or tiredness, injection-site reactions (eg, redness, minor bruising, or pain)

Can I receive Symlin if I am pregnant or breastfeeding?
The effects of Symlin during pregnancy and breastfeeding are unknown. Tell your doctor immediately if you are pregnant, plan to become pregnant, or are breastfeeding.

What should I do if I miss a dose of Symlin?
If you miss or forget a dose of Symlin, wait until the next meal and take your usual dose of Symlin at that meal. Do not take more than your usual dose of Symlin.

How should I store Symlin?
Store Symlin vials in the refrigerator until you open them. Opened vials can be refrigerated or kept at room temperature (>77°) for up to 28 days. Any opened vial should be thrown away after 28 days, even if it still has medicine in it. Symlin that has been frozen or heated must be thrown away.

Synthetic conjugated estrogens See Cenestin, page 278.

SYNTHROID

Generic name: Levothyroxine sodium

What is Synthroid?

Synthroid is a synthetic thyroid hormone that is used if your own thyroid gland is not making enough hormone; if you have an enlarged thyroid (a goiter) or are at risk of developing a goiter; if you have certain cancers of the thyroid; or if your thyroid production is low due to surgery, radiation, certain drugs, or disease of the pituitary gland or hypothalamus in the brain.

What is the most important information I should know about Synthroid?

If you are taking Synthroid to make up for a lack of natural hormone, it is important to take it regularly at the same time every day. You will probably need to take it for the rest of your life.

Who should not take Synthroid?

Do not take Synthroid if you are sensitive to thyroid hormone; if your thyroid gland is making too much thyroid hormone; if you have had a recent heart attack; or if your adrenal glands are not making enough corticosteroid hormone. If you are sensitive to dyes, you can take the Synthroid 50-microgram tablet, which is made without color additives.

Although Synthroid will speed up your metabolism, it is not effective as a weight-loss drug and should not be used as such. An overdose may cause life-threatening side effects, especially if you take Synthroid with an appetite-suppressant medication.

What should I tell my doctor before I take the first dose of Synthroid?

Tell your doctor about all prescription, over-the-counter, and herbal medications you are taking before beginning treatment with Synthroid. Also, talk to your doctor about your complete medical history, especially if you have: a history of blood clots, anemia (lack of red blood cells), angina (chest pain caused by a heart condition), diabetes, heart disease, high blood pressure, problems with your pituitary or adrenal glands, seizures.

What is the usual dosage?

The information below is based on the dosage guidelines your doctor uses. Depending on your condition and medical history, your doctor may prescribe a different regimen. Do not change the dosage or stop taking your medication without your doctor's approval.

Adults: The average full replacement dose of Synthroid is approximately 1.7 micrograms (mcg) per 2.2 pounds of body weight per day (eg, 100 to 125 mcg/day for a 154-pound adult). Older patients may require less than 1 mcg per 2.2 pounds of body weight per day.

Infants and Children: The usual recommended dose is based on body weight and decreases with age. For severe hypothyroidism, a starting dose of 25 mcg/day is recommended with increments of 25 mcg every 2-4 weeks until the desired effect is achieved.

Newborns: The recommended starting dose of Synthroid in newborn infants is 10 to 15 mcg per 2.2 pounds of body weight per day. A lower starting dose (eg, 25 mcg/day) may be given if your infant is at risk for heart failure; the dose should be increased in 4 to 6 weeks as needed based on your baby's response. If your newborn has very low amounts of thyroid hormone (serum T_4 concentrations), the recommended starting dose is 50 mcg/day.

How should I take Synthroid?
Take Synthroid as a single dose, preferably on an empty stomach, 30 minutes to 1 hour before breakfast. The drug is absorbed better on an empty stomach.

Take your daily dose of Synthroid at least 4 hours apart from taking any other medicines, supplements, or foods that may interact with Synthroid.

Synthroid tablets may swell quickly, resulting in choking or gagging. Be sure to take the pills with an entire glass of water to avoid this problem.

If an infant or child cannot swallow whole tablets, you may crush a Synthroid tablet and mix it into 1 to 2 teaspoonfuls of water. The suspension can be administered by spoon or by dropper. DO NOT STORE THE SUSPENSION.

Foods that decrease absorption of Synthroid, such as soybean infant formula, should not be used for administering Synthroid.

What should I avoid while taking Synthroid?
Do not stop taking Synthroid or change the way you take it unless your doctor tells you to do so. Do not stop taking Synthroid even if you feel fine. Stopping the medicine could lead to other health conditions, such as infertility, problems during pregnancy, and heart disease.

Do not change brands or change to a generic levothyroxine drug product without first asking your doctor. Different brands may not work in the same way.

Walnuts, dietary fiber, antacids, and iron and calcium supplements can decrease the amount of Synthroid your body absorbs. Take Synthroid at least 4 hours apart from these other food and medicines.

What are possible food and drug interactions associated with Synthroid?

If Synthroid is taken with certain other drugs, the effects of either could be increased, decreased, or altered. It is especially important to check with your doctor before combining Synthroid with the following: amiodarone, androgens (male hormones), antacids and antigas medications, antidepressants such as imipramine and sertraline, blood pressure drugs, blood-thinners such as heparin and warfarin, cancer drugs (such as 5-fluorouracil, 6-mercaptopurine, mitotane, and tamoxifen), chloral hydrate, cholesterol-lowering drugs, diabetes drugs such as glyburide and insulin, digoxin, estrogen products and oral contraceptives, furosemide, growth hormones, hormone inhibitors such as aminoglutethimide and methimazole, interferon, interleukin, iodide, iron supplements, kayexalate, ketamine, lithium, methadone and heroin, metoclopramide, nonsteroidal anti-inflammatory drugs such as ibuprofen and naproxen, Parkinson's drugs such as levodopa/carbidopa, propylthiouracil, seizure medications such as carbamazepine, phenobarbital, and phenytoin, steroids such as dexamethasone and hydrocortisone, stimulants such as epinephrine, sucralfate, tranquilizers, tuberculosis drugs, theophylline.

What are the possible side effects of Synthroid?

Side effects cannot be anticipated. If any develop or change in intensity, tell your doctor as soon as possible. Only your doctor can determine if it is safe for you to continue taking this drug.

Side effects may include: allergic reactions such as rash or hives, changes in appetite, initial and usually temporary hair loss, fatigue, headache, heat intolerance, diarrhea, vomiting, menstrual irregularities

In rare cases, infants taking Synthroid may experience increased pressure in the skull. Seizures are another rare side effect of Synthroid.

Excessive dosage or too rapid of an increase in dosage may lead to overstimulation of the thyroid gland.

Can I receive Synthroid if I am pregnant or breastfeeding?

If you need to take Synthroid because of a thyroid hormone deficiency, you can continue to take Synthroid during pregnancy. In fact, your doctor will test you regularly and may increase your dose. Once your baby is born, you may breastfeed while continuing to take carefully regulated doses of Synthroid, unless your doctor says otherwise.

What should I do if I miss a dose of Synthroid?

Take it as soon as you remember that day. If you do not remember until the next day, or if you miss more than one dose, call your doctor for advice on what you should do.

How should I store Synthroid?

Store at room temperature, away from light and moisture. Keep in a tightly closed container.

TACLONEX

Generic name: Calcipotriene and betamethasone dipropionate ointment

What is Taclonex?

Taclonex ointment is used on the skin to treat psoriasis in adults. It contains a strong corticosteroid (betamethasone) and a drug that is somewhat similar to vitamin D (calcipotriene hydrate).

What is the most important information I should know about Taclonex?

Taclonex can pass through your skin and possibly cause serious side effects if you use too much or use it for too long. Serious side effects may include adrenal gland problems or having too much calcium in your blood. The doctor may order special blood and urine tests to check your calcium levels and adrenal gland function while you are using Taclonex.

Do not apply Taclonex to your face, eyes, groin, or arm pit region. Also, do no apply Taclonex to areas where the skin appears to be thinning or peeling (skin atrophy).

Taclonex is not recommended for use in children. It has not been studied in people less than 18 years old.

Who should not take Taclonex?

Do not use Taclonex if you have a calcium metabolism disorder, or if you have erythrodermic psoriasis, exfoliative psoriasis, or pustular psoriasis. Also, you should not use Taclonex if you are allergic to any of its ingredients.

What should I tell my doctor before I take the first dose of Taclonex?

Tell your doctor about all prescription, over-the-counter, and herbal medications you are taking before beginning treatment with Taclonex. Also, talk to your doctor about your complete medical history, especially if you are taking any other corticosteroids or have a skin infection, which should be treated before you start using this medication. Also tell your doctor if you are receiving phototherapy for your psoriasis or if you have thin skin (atrophy) at the site that needs to be treated.

What is the usual dosage?

The information below is based on the dosage guidelines your doctor uses. Depending on your condition and medical history, your doctor

may prescribe a different regimen. Do not change the dosage or stop taking your medication without your doctor's approval.

Adults: Apply Taclonex ointment once a day to the areas of your skin affected by psoriasis. This medication is recommended for up to 4 weeks of treatment. Do not use it for more than 4 weeks unless prescribed by your doctor.

How should I take Taclonex?
Use Taclonex exactly as prescribed by your doctor. Do not use more than the maximum recommended weekly amount of 100 grams. Wash your hands well after using Taclonex.

Apply the ointment only on areas affected by psoriasis. Do not apply it to your face, armpits, or groin area. If you accidentally get the medication on your face or in your eyes, wash the area with water right away.

What should I avoid while taking Taclonex?
Avoid spending a long time in sunlight, and also avoid tanning booths and sunlamps. Use sunscreen and wear a hat when you are outside. Talk to your doctor if you get a sunburn.

What are possible food and drug interactions associated with Taclonex?
If Taclonex is used with certain other drugs, the effects of either could be increased, decreased, or altered. It is especially important to check with your doctor before combining it with other psoriasis treatments or a corticosteroid.

What are the possible side effects of Taclonex?
Side effects cannot be anticipated. If any develop or change in intensity, tell your doctor as soon as possible. Only your doctor can determine if it is safe for you to continue taking this drug.

Common side effects may include: itching, rash, skin burning

Other side effects may include: change in skin color at the site of application, inflamed hair pores (folliculitis), psoriasis, skin irritation or redness, thinning of the skin (atrophy), swollen fine blood vessels (makes the skin look red)

Serious side effects are more likely to happen if you use too much Taclonex, use it for too long, or use it with other topical medicines that contain corticosteroids, calcipotriene, or certain other ingredients.

Can I receive Taclonex if I am pregnant or breastfeeding?
Use this medication with caution if you are pregnant or breastfeeding, since the effects of Taclonex have not been studied in pregnant or nurs-

ing women. Before using this medication, let your doctor know if you are pregnant, plan to become pregnant, or are breastfeeding

What should I do if I miss a dose of Taclonex?
If you forget to use Taclonex, use it as soon as you remember. Then return to your normal dosing schedule.

How should I store Taclonex?
Store at room temperature.

Tadalafil See Cialis, page 285.

TAGAMET
Generic name: Cimetidine

What is Tagamet?
Tagamet is used to treat certain kinds of stomach and intestinal ulcers and related conditions. These related conditions include active duodenal (upper intestinal) ulcers; active benign stomach ulcers; erosive gastro-esophageal reflux disease (backflow of acid stomach contents); excess acid conditions such as Zollinger-Ellison syndrome (a form of peptic ulcer with too much acid); and prevention of upper abdominal bleeding in those who are critically ill.

Tagamet is also used for maintenance therapy of duodenal ulcer after active ulcers are healed.

Tagamet HB is an over-the-counter version of the drug used to relieve heartburn, acid indigestion, and sour stomach.

What is the most important information I should know about Tagamet?
Short-term treatment with Tagamet can result in complete healing of a duodenal ulcer. However, the ulcer can recur after Tagamet has been stopped. The rate of ulcer recurrence may be slightly higher in people healed with Tagamet rather than other forms of therapy. However, Tagamet is usually prescribed for more severe cases.

Who should not take Tagamet?
Do not use Tagamet if you are allergic to the active ingredient, cimetidine, or any other ingredient in it.

What should I tell my doctor before I take the first dose of Tagamet?
Tell your doctor about all prescription, over-the-counter, and herbal medications you are taking before beginning treatment with Tagamet. Also,

talk to your doctor about your complete medical history, especially if you have kidney or liver disease, chronic lung disease, diabetes, or a weakened immune system.

What is the usual dosage?
The information below is based on the dosage guidelines your doctor uses. Depending on your condition and medical history, your doctor may prescribe a different regimen. Do not change the dosage or stop taking your medication without your doctor's approval.

Active Benign Gastric Ulcer
Adults: The usual dose is 800 milligrams (mg) once a day at bedtime or 300 mg taken 4 times a day with meals and at bedtime.

Active Duodenal Ulcer
Adults: The usual dose is 800 mg once daily at bedtime. Other effective doses include: 300 mg 4 times a day with meals and at bedtime; 400 mg 2 times a day, in the morning and at bedtime; Most people heal in 4 weeks. If you require maintenance therapy, the usual dose is 400 mg at bedtime.

Erosive Gastroesophageal Reflux Disease (GERD)
Adults: The usual dosage is a total of 1600 mg daily divided into doses of 800 mg taken 2 times a day or 400 mg taken 4 times a day for 12 weeks.

Pathological Hypersecretory Condition
Adults: The usual dose is 300 mg taken 4 times a day with meals and at bedtime. Your doctor may adjust your dose based on your needs, but you should take no more than 2400 mg per day.

If you have kidney disease your doctor may adjust the dose.

Children: Safety and effectiveness have not been established in children under 16 years of age. However, your doctor may decide that the potential benefits of use may outweigh the potential risks. Doses of 20-40 mg per 2.2 pounds of body weight have been used.

How should I take Tagamet?
You can take Tagamet with or between meals. Do not take antacids within 1-2 hours of taking a dose of Tagamet. Avoid excessive amounts of caffeine while taking Tagamet.

It may take several days for Tagamet to begin relieving stomach pain. Be sure to continue taking the drug exactly as prescribed even if it seems to have no effect.

If you need to take an antifungal drug such as ketoconazole, you should take it at least 2 hours before you take Tagamet.

What should I avoid while taking Tagamet?
Avoid taking antacids at the same time as Tagamet. Antacids can reduce the effect of Tagamet when taken at the same time.

Ulcers may be more difficult to heal if you smoke cigarettes.

Avoid excessive amounts of caffeine while taking Tagamet.

Avoid alcoholic beverages while taking Tagamet. This drug increases the effects of alcohol.

What are possible food and drug interactions associated with Tagamet?

If Tagamet is taken with certain other drugs, the effects of either could be increased, decreased, or altered. It is especially important to check with your doctor before combining Tagamet with the following: antidiabetes drugs, antifungal drugs, aspirin, amoxicillin. antiarrhythmics, benzodiazepine tranquilizers, blood pressure drugs, chlorpromazine, cisapride, cyclosporine, digoxin, metoclopramide, metronidazole, narcotic pain relievers, nicotine, paroxetine, phenytoin, quinine, sucralfate, theophylline, warfarin.

What are the possible side effects of Tagamet?

Side effects cannot be anticipated. If any develop or change in intensity, tell your doctor as soon as possible. Only your doctor can determine if it is safe for you to continue taking this drug.

Side effects may include: breast development in men, headache, diarrhea, dizziness

Less commonly, agitation, anxiety, confusion, depression, disorientation, and hallucinations may occur in severely ill individuals who have been treated for 1 month or longer. These reactions are not permanent and have cleared up within 3 to 4 days of stopping the drug.

Can I receive Tagamet if I am pregnant or breastfeeding?

The effects of Tagamet during pregnancy have not been adequately studied. If you are pregnant or plan to become pregnant, notify your doctor immediately. Tagamet appears in breast milk and could affect a nursing infant. If this medication is essential to your health, your doctor may advise you to discontinue breastfeeding until treatment with this drug is finished.

What should I do if I miss a dose of Tagamet?

Take it as soon as you remember. If it is almost time for your next dose, skip the missed dose and go back to your regular schedule. Do not take 2 doses at once.

How should I store Tagamet?

Store at room temperature in a tightly closed container, away from light.

TAMBOCOR

Generic name: Flecainide acetate

What is Tambocor?

Tambocor is used to treat certain heart rhythm disturbances, including paroxysmal atrial fibrillation (a sudden attack or worsening of irregular heartbeat in which the upper chamber of the heart beats irregularly and very rapidly) and paroxysmal supraventricular tachycardia (a sudden attack or worsening of an abnormally fast but regular heart rate that occurs irregularly). Tambocor is also used to treat ventricular arrhythmias (an abnormal heart rhythm in which the lower chamber of the heart beats irregularly).

What is the most important information I should know about Tambocor?

Tambocor may sometimes cause or worsen heartbeat irregularities and certain heart conditions, such as heart failure. Tambocor should not be used if you have had a recent heart attack.

Who should not take Tambocor?

Do not take Tambocor if you are allergic to any of its ingredients, if you have heart block (without a pacemaker), or if your heart cannot supply enough blood to the body.

What should I tell my doctor before I take the first dose of Tambocor?

Tell your doctor about all prescription, over-the-counter, and herbal medications you are taking before beginning treatment with Tambocor. Also, talk to your doctor about your complete medical history, especially if you have a pacemaker, any other type of heart disease or heart problems, kidney or liver disease, or are pregnant or breastfeeding.

What is the usual dosage?

The information below is based on the dosage guidelines your doctor uses. Depending on your condition and medical history, your doctor may prescribe a different regimen. Do not change the dosage or stop taking your medication without your doctor's approval.

Treatment with Tambocor usually begins in the hospital.

Adults: The usual starting dose is 50 to 100 milligrams (mg) every 12 hours, depending on the condition under treatment. Every 4 days, your doctor my increase your dose by 50 mg every 12 hours until your condition is under control. The maximum recommended dose is 300 to 400 mg daily, depending on the condition being treated.

Children: The dosage is based on body surface area and is always supervised by a heart doctor specializing in arrhythmias in children. In children

<6 months of age, the usual initial dose is 50 mg/m² body surface area daily, divided into 2 or 3 equally spaced doses; >6 months of age, the initial starting dose may be increased to 100 mg/m² per day.

How should I take Tambocor?
Take Tambocor exactly as prescribed by your doctor. Serious heartbeat disturbances may result if you do not follow your doctor's instructions, if you miss any regular doses, or if you increase or decrease the dosage without consulting your doctor.

What should I avoid while taking Tambocor?
Smoking may reduce the amount of Tambocor in your body. Do not start or stop smoking without first talking to your doctor.

What are possible food and drug interactions associated with Tambocor?
If Tambocor is taken with certain other drugs, the effects of either could be increased, decreased, or altered. It is especially important to check with your doctor before combining Tambocor with the following: amiodarone, beta-blockers (such as atenolol, metoprolol, and propranolol), calcium-blocking drugs (such as diltiazem, nifedipine, and verapamil), carbamazepine, cimetidine, digoxin, disopyramide, phenobarbital, phenytoin, quinidine.

What are the possible side effects of Tambocor?
Side effects cannot be anticipated. If any develop or change in intensity, tell your doctor as soon as possible. Only your doctor can determine if it is safe for you to continue taking this drug.

Side effects may include: abdominal pain, chest pain, constipation, difficulty breathing, dizziness, faintness, fast heartbeat, fatigue, headache, lightheadedness, tremor, unsteadiness, visual disturbances, water retention

Tambocor may also cause new or worsened heartbeat abnormalities, heart attack, congestive heart failure, and heart block (an interference with contraction of the heart).

Can I receive Tambocor if I am pregnant or breastfeeding?
The effects of Tambocor during pregnancy and breastfeeding are unknown. Tambocor has been found to pass into human breast milk. Tell your doctor immediately if you are pregnant, plan to become pregnant, or are breastfeeding.

What should I do if I miss a dose of Tambocor?
Take Tambocor as soon as you remember if it is within 6 hours of your scheduled time. If you do not remember until later, skip the dose you

missed and go back to your regular schedule. Take the next dose as scheduled. Do not take 2 doses at once.

How should I store Tambocor?

Store Tambocor at room temperature in a tightly closed container, away from light.

TAMIFLU

Generic name: Oseltamivir phosphate

What is Tamiflu?

Tamiflu is used to treat adults and children with the flu whose flu symptoms (fevers, chills, muscle aches, sore throat, and runny or stuffy nose) started within the last day or two. Tamiflu can reduce the chance of getting the flu if there is a flu outbreak in the community, as well as in people who have a higher chance of getting the flu.

What is the most important information I should know about Tamiflu?

Tamiflu can prevent the flu as long as you take the medication correctly. Getting a yearly flu shot is still the best way of avoiding the disease entirely. For older adults, those in high-risk situations such as healthcare workers, and people with an immune deficiency or respiratory disease, vaccination is imperative.

Who should not take Tamiflu?

Do not take Tamiflu if you are allergic to any ingredient of the drug.

What should I tell my doctor before I take the first dose of Tamiflu?

Tell your doctor about all prescription, over-the-counter, and herbal medications you are taking before beginning treatment with Tamiflu. Also, talk to your doctor about your complete medical history, especially if you have kidney disease, heart disease, respiratory disease, or are pregnant or nursing.

What is the usual dosage?

The information below is based on the dosage guidelines your doctor uses. Depending on your condition and medical history, your doctor may prescribe a different regimen. Do not change the dosage or stop taking your medication without your doctor's approval.

Prevention of Influenza
Adults and children ≥13 years: The usual dose is 75 milligrams (mg) taken once a day for at least 7 days. If there is a general outbreak of the

flu in your community, your doctor may recommend that you continue taking Tamiflu for up to 6 weeks. If you have kidney disease, take one 75 mg capsule every other day, or 30 mg once a day.

Treatment of Influenza

Adults and children ≥13 years: The usual dosage is 75 mg taken twice daily (morning and evening) for 5 days. If you have kidney disease, take a 75 mg dose once a day.

Tamiflu's ability to prevent the flu in children under 13 years of age has not been established.

Children 1 to 12 years: Doses are given twice daily for 5 days using the dispenser that comes with the liquid suspension. Each dose is determined by the child's weight: >33 pounds: 30 mg; 33-55 pounds: 45 mg; 51-88 pounds: 60 mg; > 88 pounds: 75 mg

Tamiflu should not be used to treat flu in children <1 year of age.

How should I take Tamiflu?

It is important that you begin your treatment as soon as possible from the first appearance of flu symptoms or soon after you are exposed to the flu. If you feel worse, develop new symptoms during treatment with Tamiflu, or if your flu symptoms do not get better, talk to your doctor.

Take Tamiflu with or without food. If you experience stomach upset, take it with a light snack, milk, or a meal.

Shake the suspension (liquid) well for about 5 seconds before each use.

What should I avoid while taking Tamiflu?

Unless your doctor gives you specific directions, there are no restrictions on food, beverages, or activities while taking Tamiflu.

What are possible food and drug interactions associated with Tamiflu?

If Tamiflu is taken with certain other drugs, the effects of either could be increased, decreased, or altered. It is especially important to check with your doctor before combining Tamiflu with any other medications.

What are the possible side effects of Tamiflu?

Side effects cannot be anticipated. If any develop or change in intensity, tell your doctor as soon as possible. Only your doctor can determine if it is safe for you to continue taking this drug.

Side effects may include: bronchitis, diarrhea, dizziness, headache, nausea, stomach pain, vomiting, cough, fatigue

There have been reports of abnormal behavior in children taking Tamiflu. Children should be monitored for confusion, hallucinations, speech problems, or self-injury during treatment.

Can I receive Tamiflu if I am pregnant or breastfeeding?

The effects of Tamiflu during pregnancy and breastfeeding are unknown. Tell your doctor immediately if you are pregnant, plan to become pregnant, or are breastfeeding and follow your doctor's instructions.

What should I do if I miss a dose of Tamiflu?

Take it as soon as possible. If it is within 6 hours of your next dose, skip the missed dose and go back to your regular schedule. Never take 2 doses at once.

How should I store Tamiflu?

Store at room temperature. Keep the blister pack dry.

The liquid suspension should be refrigerated and used within 10 days. Do not freeze.

Tamsulosin hydrochloride See *Flomax, page 561.*

TARCEVA

Generic name: Erlotinib hydrochloride

What is Tarceva?

Tarceva is used to treat advanced non-small cell lung cancer (NSCLC) that is either only in the lung (localized) or spread throughout the body (metastatic).

It is also used in cancer patients who have not responded to other types of chemotherapy (medicine used to kill cancer).

What is the most important information I should know about Tarceva?

Some patients taking Tarceva have developed interstitial lung disease (ILD). ILD is a serious and life-threatening lung disease. The symptoms of ILD are a sudden or worsening cough, or shortness of breath and dry cough.

Women who are pregnant or breast-feeding should not take Tarceva. Women who can get pregnant should avoid pregnancy while taking Tarceva. Birth control should be used during Tarceva therapy and for 2 weeks after stopping Tarceva.

Who should not take Tarceva?

You should not begin treatment with Tarceva if you are pregnant, planning to become pregnant, or are breastfeeding.

What should I tell my doctor before I take the first dose of Tarceva?

Tell your doctor about your complete medical history, as well as problems that you are currently having, such as liver problems. Tarceva may cause liver damage called hepatotoxicity. If you have or had bleeding problems in your stomach or intestines such as ulcers, or you are pregnant, are trying to become pregnant, or are breastfeeding, tell your doctor before beginning therapy with Tarceva.

Also, talk to your doctor about all prescription, over-the-counter, and herbal medications you are taking to prevent a harmful interaction with Tarceva.

What is the usual dosage?
The information below is based on the dosage guidelines your doctor uses. Depending on your condition and medical history, your doctor may prescribe a different regimen. Do not change the dosage or stop taking your medication without your doctor's approval.

The usual dosage for NSCLC: The recommended daily dose of Tarceva is 150 milligrams (mg) taken at least one hour before or two hours after eating.

The usual dosage for pancreatic cancer: The recommended daily dose of Tarceva is 100 mg taken at least one hour before or two hours after eating, in combination with gemcitabine.

How should I take Tarceva?
Take prescribed dosage one hour before or two hours after eating.

What should I avoid while taking Tarceva?
Women who are taking Tarceva are advised to avoid pregnancy by taking the appropriate precautions during and 2 weeks after the treatment.

What are possible food and drug interactions associated with Tarceva?
Patients on Tarceva therapy and taking blood thinners (Coumadin) or other medicines called anticoagulants should have regular blood tests and watch for bleeding problems.

What are the possible side effects of Tarceva?
Side effects cannot be anticipated. If any develop or change in intensity, tell your doctor as soon as possible. Only your doctor can determine if it is safe for you to continue taking this drug.

Side effects may include: Cough, diarrhea, dry skin, eye problems, infection, itching, loss of appetite, nausea, rash, shortness of breath/trouble breathing, stomach pain, swollen mouth, tiredness, vomiting

Call your doctor right away if you have: Eye irritation, loss of appetite, nausea, new or worse trouble breathing or cough, severe or non-stop diarrhea, vomiting

Can I receive Tarceva if I am pregnant or breastfeeding?

Tarceva is not recommended if you are pregnant, planning to become pregnant, or are breastfeeding. This drug may cause harm to your unborn child or pass into breast milk.

How should I store Tarceva?

Store at room temperature.

TARKA

Generic name: Trandolapril and verapamil hydrochloride

What is Tarka?

Tarka is used to treat high blood pressure. It combines two blood pressure drugs: an ACE inhibitor (trandolapril) and a calcium channel blocker (verapamil hydrochloride).

What is the most important information I should know about Tarka?

When used in pregnancy during the second and third trimesters, Tarka can cause injury and even death to the developing fetus. Notify your doctor immediately if you think you might be pregnant.

Doctors usually prescribe Tarka for patients who have been taking one of its components—trandolapril or sustained-release verapamil—without showing improvement. Tarka must be taken regularly for it to be effective. Since blood pressure declines gradually, it may take a few weeks before you get the full benefit of Tarka. You must continue taking it even if you are feeling well. Tarka does not cure high blood pressure; it only keeps it under control.

Who should not take Tarka?

Do not take Tarka if you are sensitive to any component of this drug or to blood pressure medications known as ACE inhibitors, such as enalapril or lisinopril. You cannot use Tarka if you have low blood pressure, certain types of heart disease or an irregular heartbeat, or if you have ever developed a swollen throat and difficulty swallowing (angioedema) while taking an ACE inhibitor. Make sure your doctor is aware of any past trouble.

What should I tell my doctor before I take the first dose of Tarka?

Tell your doctor about all prescription, over-the-counter, and herbal medications you are taking before beginning treatment with Tarka. Also, talk to your doctor about your complete medical history, especially if you are undergoing surgery or if you have: a history of angioedema, collagen vascular disease (a connective tissue disorder), diabetes, Duchenne's dystrophy (the most common type of muscular dystrophy), heart disease or heart failure, kidney or liver disease.

What is the usual dosage?

The information below is based on the dosage guidelines your doctor uses. Depending on your condition and medical history, your doctor may prescribe a different regimen. Do not change the dosage or stop taking your medication without your doctor's approval.

Adults: Tarka comes in 4 strengths of trandolapril and sustained-release verapamil. Your doctor will prescribe a dose of Tarka that is close to the doses you were taking separately. Doses range from 1 to 4 milligrams (mg) of trandolapril and 180 to 480 mg of verapamil, given in a single daily dose or 2 divided doses.

Elderly or kidney or liver impairment: If you are over 65 years old, you may be more sensitive to Tarka. Your doctor will monitor your blood pressure more closely and adjust your medication dose accordingly. If you have liver or kidney disease, your doctor will adjust your dosage accordingly.

The safety and effectiveness of Tarka in children under 18 years of age have not been established.

How should I take Tarka?

Take each dose with food, exactly as prescribed. Do not break, crush, or chew this medication. Swallow the pills whole.

What should I avoid while taking Tarka?

Tarka may cause dizziness or drowsiness. Use caution when driving, operating machinery, or performing other hazardous activities. Avoid alcohol. Alcohol may further lower blood pressure and increase drowsiness and dizziness while you are taking Tarka.

Do not use salt substitutes or potassium supplements while taking Tarka.

Grapefruit and grapefruit juice may interact with Tarka and could lead to potentially dangerous effects.

Tarka sometimes causes a severe drop in blood pressure. The danger is especially great if you have been taking water pills (diuretics), or if you have heart disease, kidney disease, or a potassium or salt imbalance. Excessive sweating, severe diarrhea, and vomiting are also dangerous because they can deplete the body of water. This can cause a dangerous drop in blood pressure. If you feel lightheaded or faint, have chest pain, or feel your heart racing, lie down and contact your doctor immediately.

What are possible food and drug interactions associated with Tarka?

If Tarka is taken with certain other drugs, the effects of either could be increased, decreased, or altered. It is especially important to check with your doctor before combining Tarka with the following: beta-blockers (such as atenolol and propranolol), carbamazepine, cimetidine, cyclosporine, digoxin, disopyramide, diuretics (such as furosemide and hydrochlorothiazide), flecainide, lithium, phenobarbital, potassium-sparing diuretics (such as amiloride and spironolactone), potassium supplements, quinidine, rifampin, theophylline.

Because Tarka can increase the potassium level in your blood, you should avoid salt substitutes that contain potassium unless your doctor approves.

What are the possible side effects of Tarka?
Side effects cannot be anticipated. If any develop or change in intensity, tell your doctor as soon as possible. Only your doctor can determine if it is safe for you to continue taking this drug.

Side effects may include: constipation, cough, dizziness, headache, heartbeat irregularities, upper respiratory tract infection

Call your doctor right away if you experience swelling of the face, lips, tongue, or throat; swelling of the arms and legs; and difficulty swallowing or breathing.

Because another ACE inhibitor, captopril, has been known to cause serious blood disorders, your doctor will check your blood regularly while you are taking Tarka. If you develop signs of infection such as a sore throat or a fever, you should contact your doctor at once.

Can I receive Tarka if I am pregnant or breastfeeding?
Do not take Tarka during pregnancy. When taken during the final 6 months, the ACE inhibitor in Tarka can cause birth defects, premature birth, and death of the developing or newborn baby. If you are pregnant, tell your doctor immediately. Do not breastfeed while you are taking Tarka.

What should I do if I miss a dose of Tarka?
Take it as soon as you remember. If it is almost time for your next dose, skip the missed dose and go back to your regular schedule. Never take 2 doses at the same time.

How should I store Tarka?
Keep the container tightly closed. Store at room temperature.

TASMAR
Generic name: Tolcapone

What is Tasmar?
Tasmar is used together with a carbidopa/levodopa combination to treat Parkinson's disease. Tasmar helps to relieve the muscle stiffness, tremors, and weakness caused by Parkinson's disease.

What is the most important information I should know about Tasmar?

In rare cases, Tasmar has caused severe liver damage resulting in death. Tell your doctor immediately if you develop abdominal pain, clay colored stools, dark urine, itching, loss of appetite, nausea, unusual fatigue, vomiting, or yellow skin or eyes. These symptoms may be early signs of liver damage. Your doctor will want to monitor your liver function with blood tests.

Due to the risk of severe liver damage, Tasmar should only be used in combination with carbidopa/levodopa if you are not responding adequately to carbidopa/levodopa alone and cannot take other medicines for this condition.

Who should not take Tasmar?

Do not take Tasmar if you have liver disease or if you previously took Tasmar but had to stop therapy due to liver injury. Avoid Tasmar if you are allergic to it, or if you experience unexplained muscle tenderness or pain, high fever, or confusion.

What should I tell my doctor before I take the first dose of Tasmar?

Tell your doctor about all prescription, over-the-counter, and herbal medications you are taking before beginning treatment with Tasmar. Also, talk to your doctor about your complete medical history, especially if you have kidney or liver disease, are taking monoamine oxidase inhibitors (MAOIs) such as phenelzine and tranylcypromine, or have a history of rhabdomyolysis.

What is the usual dosage?

The information below is based on the dosage guidelines your doctor uses. Depending on your condition and medical history, your doctor may prescribe a different regimen. Do not change the dosage or stop taking your medication without your doctor's approval.

Adults: The usual dose is 100 milligrams (mg) 3 times a day (every 6 hours) in combination with carbidopa and levodopa.

Your doctor may increase your dose to 200 mg 3 times a day if necessary. If you do not benefit from the higher dose after 3 weeks of treatment, your doctor will stop therapy with Tasmar.

How should I take Tasmar?

Tasmar works by increasing the efficacy of carbidopa/levodopa, and will not work without it. It can be taken with either the immediate-release or controlled-release form of levodopa/carbidopa, with or without food.

Always take the first dose of Tasmar with your first dose of levodopa/carbidopa. Take your second and third doses of Tasmar 6 and 12 hours later. Your doctor will probably decrease your dose of levodopa/carbidopa when you start taking Tasmar.

What should I avoid while taking Tasmar?

Tasmar can cause drowsiness and affect mental and motor skills. Avoid operating machinery, driving, and performing other activities that require mental alertness until you know how the drug affects you.

Tasmar can cause severe low blood pressure marked by nausea, sweating, dizziness, or fainting. This usually occurs at the start of therapy. To avoid these symptoms, get up very slowly from a seated or reclining position.

Avoid drinking alcohol while taking Tasmar. Alcohol may increase drowsiness and dizziness.

What are possible food and drug interactions associated with Tasmar?

If Tasmar is taken with certain other drugs, the effects of either could be increased, decreased, or altered. It is especially important to check with your doctor before combining Tasmar with the following: apomorphine, desipramine, dobutamine, isoproterenol, MAO inhibitors (such as phenelzine and tranylcypromine), methyldopa, sedatives (such as phenobarbital and secobarbital), warfarin.

What are the possible side effects of Tasmar?

Side effects cannot be anticipated. If any develop or change in intensity, tell your doctor as soon as possible. Only your doctor can determine if it is safe for you to continue taking this drug.

Side effects may include: abnormal jerky movements, diarrhea, dizziness or fainting, hallucinations, sleep disorders

Serious side effects may include: confusion, death, extremely high fever, unexplained muscle tenderness or pain (rhabdomyolysis)

Tell your doctor if you experience persistent nausea, fatigue, loss of appetite, yellowing of the skin or eyes, dark urine, itchiness, and right-sided abdominal pain. Your doctor should do a blood test to check your liver function before you start Tasmar therapy, then every 2 weeks for the first year, every 4 weeks for the next 6 months, and every 8 weeks thereafter.

Hallucinations are most likely to occur within the first 2 weeks of therapy. If this problem occurs, tell your doctor right away.

Can I receive Tasmar if I am pregnant or breastfeeding?

The effects of Tasmar during pregnancy and breastfeeding are unknown. Tell your doctor immediately if you are pregnant, plan to become pregnant, or are breastfeeding.

What should I do if I miss a dose of Tasmar?
Take it as soon as you remember. If it is almost time for your next dose
(within 3 hours), skip the one you missed and go back to your regular
schedule. Do not take 2 doses at once.

How should I store Tasmar?
Store at room temperature in a tightly sealed container.

Tazarotene *See Tazorac, below.*

TAZORAC
Generic name: Tazarotene

What is Tazorac?
Tazorac is used to treat the type of psoriasis (a chronic disease of the skin
marked by red patches covered with red scales) that causes large plaques
on the skin. The 0.1% strength is also used to treat mild to moderate
facial acne.

**What is the most important information
I should know about Tazorac?**
Tazorac may cause severe birth defects. If you are a woman in your child-
bearing years, do not use Tazorac if there is any chance you are pregnant.
Your doctor should give you a pregnancy test within 2 weeks of starting
Tazorac therapy and you should use reliable birth control measures as
long as you are on Tazorac. If you accidentally become pregnant, stop
using Tazorac and call your doctor immediately.

Who should not take Tazorac?
Do not use Tazorac if you are or may become pregnant or if you are allergic to any component of the drug.

**What should I tell my doctor before
I take the first dose of Tazorac?**
Tell your doctor about all prescription, over-the-counter, and herbal medications you are taking before beginning treatment with Tazorac. Also,
talk to your doctor about your complete medical history, especially if you
are sunburned, sensitive to sunlight or are taking medications that might
make you more sensitive to sunlight, or have eczema or other chronic
skin conditions.

What is the usual dosage?
**The information below is based on the dosage guidelines your doctor
uses. Depending on your condition and medical history, your doctor**

may prescribe a different regimen. Do not change the dosage or stop taking your medication without your doctor's approval.

Adults: Apply to affected areas once a day in the evening.

How should I take Tazorac?

For psoriasis, apply a thin film of Tazorac to the affected areas each evening. Make sure your skin is dry before you begin. Keep Tazorac away from normal, healthy skin.

If you use a cream or lotion to soften or moisten your skin, wait at least an hour before applying Tazorac. Wash your hands after applying Tazorac.

To treat acne, first wash your face and dry it thoroughly. Then apply a thin film of Tazorac to the acne eruptions. Repeat every evening. Use enough to cover the entire affected area. Wash your hands after applying the medicine.

What should I avoid while taking Tazorac?

Keep Tazorac away from your eyes, eyelids, and mouth. If it gets in your eyes, wash them with large amounts of cool water. If eye irritation continues, contact your doctor.

Do not use Tazorac more often or use more than instructed. Using more Tazorac than recommended may cause more side effects and does not lead to better or faster results. Do not cover treated areas with dressings or bandages.

Avoid using other topical agents with a strong skin-drying effects, products with high concentrations of alcohol, astringents, spices, lime peels, medicated soaps or shampoos, permanent wave solutions, electrolysis, hair removers or waxes, or other preparations or processes that might dry or irritate the skin.

Avoid prolonged exposure to the sun or sunlamps while using Tazorac. Apply sunscreen (at least SPF 15) and wear protective clothing when you go into the sunlight.

What are possible food and drug interactions associated with Tazorac?

If Tazorac is taken with certain other drugs, the effects of either could be increased, decreased, or altered. It is especially important to check with your doctor before combining Tazorac with the following: quinolone antibiotics (such as ciprofloxacin and norfloxacin), sulfa drugs (such as sulfamethoxazole or sulfasalazine), tetracycline antibiotics (such as doxycycline and minocycline), thiazide-type diuretics (water pills), vitamin A supplements.

What are the possible side effects of Tazorac?

Side effects cannot be anticipated. If any develop or change in intensity, tell your doctor as soon as possible. Only your doctor can determine if it is safe for you to continue taking this drug.

Side effects may include: burning, dry skin, itching, peeling, red skin, stinging

Can I receive Tazorac if I am pregnant or breastfeeding?

Tazorac may cause birth defects and must never be used during pregnancy. Tazorac may appear in breast milk, so avoid use while breastfeeding.

What should I do if I miss a dose of Tazorac?

Skip the dose and continue on your normal schedule. Do not try to make up the missed dose of Tazorac. Do not apply extra Tazorac to make up for the missed dose.

How should I store Tazorac?

Store at room temperature.

TEGRETOL

Generic name: Carbamazepine

What is Tegretol?

Tegretol is used to treat seizures during which you lose awareness and may carry out actions such as walking, talking, or driving (complex partial seizures) and seizures in which loss of consciousness may occur (generalized seizures). It is also prescribed for trigeminal neuralgia (severe pain in the jaws) and pain in the tongue and throat.

What is the most important information I should know about Tegretol?

Tegretol can result in a very rare and potentially fatal blood abnormality (aplastic anemia) where the red blood cell count declines drastically. If you experience symptoms such as fever, sore throat, rash, ulcers in the mouth, easy bruising, or reddish or purplish spots on the skin, tell your doctor right away. Serious and sometimes fatal skin reactions have also been reported with use of Tegretol. At the first sign of a rash, inform your healthcare provider.

Who should not take Tegretol?

Do not use Tegretol if you have a history of bone marrow depression (reduced function), porphyria (an inherited metabolic disorder affecting the liver or bone marrow), are sensitive to Tegretol or tricyclic antidepressant drugs such as amitriptyline. You should not take Tegretol if you are on a monoamine oxidase inhibitor (MAOI) antidepressant such as phenelzine or tranylcypromine, or if you have taken this type of drug within the past 14 days.

What should I tell my doctor before I take the first dose of Tegretol?

Tell your doctor about all prescription, over-the-counter, and herbal medications you are taking before beginning treatment with Tegretol. Also, talk to your doctor about your complete medical history, especially if you have anemia, heart disease, kidney or liver disease, or glaucoma (increased pressure in the eyes).

What is the usual dosage?

The information below is based on the dosage guidelines your doctor uses. Depending on your condition and medical history, your doctor may prescribe a different regimen. Do not change the dosage or stop taking your medication without your doctor's approval.

Seizures

Adults and children over 12 years: The usual starting dose is 200 milligrams (mg) 2 times a day for tablets and extended-release tablets, or 1 teaspoon (tsp) 4 times a day for suspension. Your doctor may increase the dose at weekly intervals by adding 200-mg doses 2 times a day for Tegretol-XR or 3 to 4 times per day for the other forms. The dosage should generally not be more than 1000 mg daily in children 12 to 15 years old and 1200 mg daily for adults and children over 15. The usual daily maintenance dosage range is 800 to 1200 mg.

Children 6 to 12 years: The usual dose is 100 mg 2 times a day or ½ tsp 4 times a day. Your doctor may increase the dose at weekly intervals by adding 100 mg 2 times a day for Tegretol-XR or 3 to 4 times a day for the other forms. The total daily dosage should generally not exceed 1000 mg. The usual daily dosage range for maintenance is 400 to 800 mg.

Children <6 years: The usual daily starting dose for is 10 to 20 mg per 2.2 pounds of body weight per day. The total daily dose is divided into smaller doses taken 2 to 3 times a day for tablets or 4 times a day for suspension. Daily dosage should not exceed 35 mg per 2.2 pounds.

Trigeminal Neuralgia

Adults and children over 12 years: The usual dose is 100 mg 2 times a day for tablets and extended-release tablets, or ½ tsp 4 times a day for the suspension on the first day. Your doctor may increase this dose using increments of 100 mg every 12 hours or ½ tsp 4 times daily only as needed to achieve freedom from pain. Doses should not exceed 1200 mg daily and are usually in the range of 400 to 800 mg a day for maintenance.

How should I take Tegretol?

This medication should only be taken with meals, never on an empty stomach. Shake the Tegretol suspension well before using.

Tegretol-XR tablets must be swallowed whole. Do not crush or chew them and do not take tablets that have been damaged.

What should I avoid while taking Tegretol?

Tegretol may cause dizziness or drowsiness. Use caution when driving, operating machinery, or performing other activities that require mental alertness until you know how this medication affects you.

Do not drink alcohol while taking Tegretol. Alcohol may increase drowsiness caused by Tegretol and it may increase the risk of seizures.

Avoid prolonged exposure to artificial or natural sunlight. Tegretol may increase the sensitivity of your skin to sunlight, so use sunscreen and wear protective clothing when you are outside.

Grapefruit and grapefruit juice may interact with Tegretol and lead to potentially adverse effects. Do not increase or decrease the amount of grapefruit products in your diet without first talking to your doctor.

Do not stop taking Tegretol suddenly. It is possible that you can experience continuous epileptic attacks without return to consciousness, leading to possible severe brain damage and death. Only your doctor should determine if and when you should stop taking Tegretol.

What are possible food and drug interactions associated with Tegretol?

If Tegretol is taken with certain other drugs, the effects of either could be increased, decreased, or altered. It is especially important to check with your doctor before combining Tegretol with the following: acetaminophen, acetazolamide, aminophylline, amprenavir, antibiotics (such as azithromycin, clarithromycin, and erythromycin), antidepressants (such as bupropion, citalopram, clomipramine, fluoxetine, fluvoxamine, and trazodone), antifungals (such as fluconazole, itraconazole, and ketoconazole), antipsychotics (such as olanzapine, quetiapine, risperidone, and ziprasidone), antiseizure medications (such as felbamate, fosphenytoin, lamotrigine, oxcarbazepine, phenytoin, topiramate, and valproate), benzodiazepines (such as alprazolam, clonazepam, diazepam, and midazolam), blood thinners, calcium channel blocking drugs (such as diltiazem, felodipine, and verapamil), cimetidine, cisplatin, corticosteroids, danazol, dantrolene, doxorubicin, doxycycline, everolimus, haloperidol, ibuprofen, imatinib, isoniazid, levothyroxine, lithium, loratadine, methsuximide, niacinamide, nicotinamide, omeprazole, oral and other hormonal contraceptives, oxybutynin, pain relievers (such as methadone, propoxyphene, and tramadol), pancuronomium, phenobarbital, phensuximide, praziquantel, primidone, rifampin, ritonavir, terfenadine, ticlopidine, theophylline, tiagabine, tranquilizers (such as chlorpromazine, clozapine, and loxapine), water pills (diuretics), zonisamide.

Do not combine Tegretol suspension with other liquid medications such as chlorpromazine solution. The mixture may thicken inside your body.

What are the possible side effects of Tegretol?
Side effects cannot be anticipated. If any develop or change in intensity, tell your doctor as soon as possible. Only your doctor can determine if it is safe for you to continue taking this drug.

Side effects may include: allergic reactions, blood pressure changes, bone marrow suppression, dizziness, drowsiness, hives, rash, nausea, sensitivity to sunlight, unsteadiness, vomiting

Tegretol has been known to cause serious blood, liver, and skin reactions, both early in treatment and after extended use. Tell your doctor immediately if you develop warning signs such as fever, sore throat, rash, ulcers in the mouth, easy bruising or spots in the skin, swollen lymph glands, loss of appetite, nausea or vomiting, or yellowing of the skin and eyes.

Can I receive Tegretol if I am pregnant or breastfeeding?
Tegretol can cause birth defects and other serious fetal harm when used during pregnancy. Tell your doctor immediately if you are pregnant, plan to become pregnant, or are breastfeeding. Your doctor will determine if the benefit of using this medication outweighs the possible risk. Tegretol does pass into breast milk, so follow your doctor's instructions on whether or not you should use this medication while breastfeeding.

What should I do if I miss a dose of Tegretol?
If you miss a dose of Tegretol, take it as soon as your remember. If it is almost time for your next dose, skip the one you missed and go back to your regular schedule. Do not take 2 doses at once. If you miss more than one dose in a day, check with your doctor.

How should I store Tegretol?
Store at room temperature away from light and moisture.

TEKTURNA
Generic name: Aliskiren

What is Tekturna?
Tekturna is used to lower blood pressure. It may be used alone or in combination with other blood pressure-lowering medications.

What is the most important information I should know about Tekturna?
Tekturna is not to be used during pregnancy. If you become pregnant while on this medication, stop taking Tekturna and call your doctor

right away. Tekturna may harm an unborn baby, causing injury and even death.

Tekturna does not cure high blood pressure; it works to keep it under control. It is important to take Tekturna regularly for it to be effective. Since blood pressure declines gradually, it may take a few weeks before you see the full benefit of this medication; you must continue taking it even if you are feeling well.

Who should not take Tekturna?
You should not take this medication if you are pregnant, plan to become pregnant, or are breastfeeding. Also, you should not take Tekturna if you are allergic to any of its ingredients.

What should I tell my doctor before I take the first dose of Tekturna?
Tell your doctor about all prescription, over-the-counter, and herbal medications you are taking before beginning treatment with Tekturna. Also, talk to your doctor about your complete medical history, especially if you are pregnant, plan on becoming pregnant, are breastfeeding, have kidney problems, or are allergic to any of the ingredients in Tekturna.

What is the usual dosage?
The information below is based on the dosage guidelines your doctor uses. Depending on your condition and medical history, your doctor may prescribe a different regimen. Do not change the dosage or stop taking your medication without your doctor's approval.

Adults: The usual starting dose is 150 milligrams (mg) taken once daily. Your doctor may increase the dose to 300 mg daily if your blood pressure is not adequately controlled on the lower dose.

How should I take Tekturna?
Take Tekturna once a day, at the same time each day. It can be taken with or without food.

What should I avoid while taking Tekturna?
Avoid becoming pregnant while on this medication. It is not known whether Tekturna passes into breast milk; you may have to stop breast-feeding while on this medication or your doctor may want you to use another medication to lower your blood pressure instead. Speak to your doctor if you are breastfeeding.

What are possible food and drug interactions associated with Tekturna?
If Tekturna is taken with certain other drugs, the effects of either could be increased, decreased, or altered. It is especially important to check with your doctor before combining Tekturna with the following: anti-fungal drugs, cyclosporine, furosemide, diuretics, potassium-containing

medicines, potassium supplements, or salt substitutes containing potassium.

What are the possible side effects of Tekturna?

Side effects cannot be anticipated. If any develop or change in intensity, tell your doctor as soon as possible. Only your doctor can determine if it is safe for you to continue taking this drug.

Side effects may include: low blood pressure, diarrhea, cough, rash

Can I receive Tekturna if I am pregnant or breastfeeding?

You should not take this medication if you are pregnant. If you become pregnant while on this medication, inform your doctor as soon as possible. It is not known whether Tekturna passes into breast milk. There is potential for harm to the nursing infant, so your doctor will decide whether to discontinue nursing or whether to discontinue the medication.

What should I do if I miss a dose of Tekturna?

If you miss a dose, take it as soon as you remember. If it is within 12 hours of your next dose, do not take the missed dose. Just take the next dose at your regular time. Do not take 2 doses at the same.

How should I store Tekturna?

Store at room temperature in a dry place and in the original prescription bottle. Do not remove the drying agent from the bottle.

TEKTURNA HCT

Generic name: Aliskiren and hydrochlorothiazide

What is Tekturna HCT?

Tekturna HCT is used to lower blood pressure. It contains two medicines in one tablet: aliskiren and the diuretic hydrochlorothiazide. Tekturna HCT may be used alone or in combination with other blood pressure-lowering medications.

What is the most important information I should know about Tekturna HCT?

Do not use Tekturna HCT during pregnancy. If you become pregnant while on this medication, stop taking Tekturna HCT and call your doctor right away. Tekturna HCT may harm an unborn baby, causing injury and even death.

Tekturna HCT does not cure high blood pressure; it works to keep it under control. It is important to take Tekturna HCT regularly for it to be effective. Since blood pressure declines gradually, it may take a few weeks before you see the full benefit of this medication; you must continue taking it even if you are feeling well.

Who should not take Tekturna HCT?

You should not take this medication if you are pregnant, plan to become pregnant, or are breastfeeding. Also, you should not take Tekturna HCT if you are allergic to any of its ingredients or if you have urination problems due to kidney dysfunction.

What should I tell my doctor before I take the first dose of Tekturna HCT?

Tell your doctor about all prescription, over-the-counter, and herbal medications you are taking before beginning treatment with Tekturna HCT. Also, talk to your doctor about your complete medical history, especially if you have any of the following: kidney or liver problems, systemic lupus erythematosus (SLE), allergies or asthma, or if you have ever had a reaction called angioedema to an ACE inhibitor medicine. Signs of angioedema include difficulty breathing and swelling of the face, lips, tongue, throat, arms and legs.

Alert your doctor immediately if you are pregnant, plan on becoming pregnant, or are breastfeeding.

What is the usual dosage?

The information below is based on the dosage guidelines your doctor uses. Depending on your condition and medical history, your doctor may prescribe a different regimen. Do not change the dosage or stop taking your medication without your doctor's approval.

Adults: The usual starting dose is 150 milligrams (mg) of aliskiren/12.5 mg of hydrocholorothiazide taken once daily. Your doctor may increase the daily dose up to 300 mg of aliskiren/25 mg of hydrocholorothiazide if your blood pressure is not adequately controlled on a lower dose.

How should I take Tekturna HCT?

Take Tekturna HCT once a day, at the same time each day. It can be taken with or without food.

What should I avoid while taking Tekturna HCT?

Avoid becoming pregnant while on this medication. It is not known whether Tekturna HCT passes into breast milk; you may have to stop breastfeeding while on this medication or your doctor may want you to use another medication to lower your blood pressure instead. Speak to your doctor if you are breastfeeding.

What are possible food and drug interactions associated with Tekturna HCT?

If Tekturna HCT is taken with certain other drugs, the effects of either could be increased, decreased, or altered. It is especially important to check with your doctor before combining Tekturna HCT with the following: other medicines for high blood pressure or a heart problem, diuretics, medicines for treating fungus or fungal infections, cyclosporine, potassium-containing medicines, potassium supplements, salt substitutes containing potassium, cholestyramine, colestipol, medicines to treat diabetes including insulin, nonsteroidal anti-inflammatory drugs (NSAIDs), blood thinners, barbiturates, and narcotic medicines.

Do not use Tekturna HCT if you are taking lithium.

What are the possible side effects of Tekturna HCT?

Side effects cannot be anticipated. If any develop or change in intensity, tell your doctor as soon as possible. Only your doctor can determine if it is safe for you to continue taking this drug.

Side effects may include: dizziness, flu-like symptoms, diarrhea, cough, tiredness, low blood pressure, active or worsened systemic lupus erythematosus (SLE)

Serious side effects that require immediate medical attention include difficulty breathing and swelling of the face, lips, tongue, throat, arms and legs.

Can I receive Tekturna HCT if I am pregnant or breastfeeding?

You should not take this medication if you are pregnant. If you become pregnant while on this medication, inform your doctor as soon as possible. It is not known whether Tekturna HCT passes into breast milk; you may have to stop breastfeeding while on this medication or your doctor may want you to use another medication to lower your blood pressure instead. Tell your doctor immediately if you are breastfeeding.

What should I do if I miss a dose of Tekturna HCT?

If you miss a dose, take it as soon as you remember. If it is almost time for your next dose, skip the one you missed and return to your regular schedule. Never double the dose.

How should I store Tekturna HCT?

Store at room temperature in a dry place.

Telithromycin See Ketek, page 687.

Telmisartan See Micardis, page 819.

Telmisartan and hydrochlorothiazide See Micardis HCT, page 821.

Temazepam See Restoril, page 1139.

TEMOVATE

Generic name: Clobetasol propionate

What is Temovate?

Temovate is used to relieve the itching and inflammation of moderate to severe skin conditions. The scalp application is used for short-term treatment of scalp conditions. The cream, ointment, emollient cream, and gel are used for short-term treatment of skin conditions on the body.

What is the most important information I should know about Temovate?

Even though Temovate is used on the skin, some of the drug can be absorbed through your skin and into the bloodstream. Increased absorption can lead to unwanted side effects elsewhere in the body. To minimize this problem, avoid using Temovate over large areas and do not cover it with airtight dressings such as plastic wrap or adhesive bandages unless specifically directed by your doctor.

Who should not take Temovate?

Do not use Temovate if you are sensitive to any component of the preparation.

What should I tell my doctor before I take the first dose of Temovate?

Tell your doctor about all prescription, over-the-counter, and herbal medications you are taking before beginning treatment with Temovate. Also, talk to your doctor about your complete medical history, especially if you have a skin infection, rosacea (a skin condition characterized by redness, pimples, and broken blood vessels); or inflammation, redness, or pimples around the mouth.

What is the usual dosage?

The information below is based on the dosage guidelines your doctor uses. Depending on your condition and medical history, your doctor may prescribe a different regimen. Do not change the dosage or stop taking your medication without your doctor's approval.

Adults and children 12 years and older: Apply Temovate to the affected area 2 times a day, once in the morning and once at night. Treatment should not last for more than 2 weeks in a row. No more than 50 grams or 50 milliliters per week (approximately 1 large tube or bottle) should be used.

How should I take Temovate?

Use Temovate exactly as directed. Do not use it more often or for a longer time than ordered. Gently rub a thin layer of cream, ointment, or gel into the affected area.

What should I avoid while taking Temovate?

Do not cover or bandage the affected area after applying Temovate.

Temovate is for use only on the skin. Keep it out of your eyes. Do not use Temovate on the face, groin, or armpits. If the scalp application gets into your eyes, flush your eyes with a lot of water.

Do not use the scalp application near an open flame.

Avoid simultaneous use of cosmetics or skin care products on treated areas.

What are possible food and drug interactions associated with Temovate?

If Temovate is used with certain other drugs, the effects of either could be increased, decreased, or altered. Always check with your doctor before combining Temovate with any other medication.

What are the possible side effects of Temovate?

Side effects cannot be anticipated. If any develop or change in intensity, tell your doctor as soon as possible. Only your doctor can determine if it is safe for you to continue taking this drug.

Side effects may include: burning, cracking, irritation, itching, numbness of fingers, reddened skin, shrinking of the skin, stinging

Temovate is a strong corticosteroid that can be absorbed into the bloodstream. It has caused Cushing's syndrome, a disorder characterized by a moon-shaped face, emotional disturbances, high blood pressure, weight gain, changes in blood sugar, and abnormal growth of facial and body hair in women.

Can I receive Temovate if I am pregnant or breastfeeding?

The effects of Temovate during pregnancy and breastfeeding are unknown. Tell your doctor immediately if you are pregnant, plan to become pregnant, or are breastfeeding.

What should I do if I miss a dose of Temovate?

Apply it as soon as you remember. If it is almost time for the next dose, skip the one you missed and go back to your regular schedule.

How should I store Temovate?

Store at room temperature. Do not refrigerate the creams, gel, or scalp application.

Tenofovir disproxil fumarate *See Viread, page 1398.*

TENORETIC

Generic name: Atenolol and chlorthalidone

What is Tenoretic?

Tenoretic is used to treat high blood pressure. It is a combination of the beta-blocker drug atenolol and the diuretic chlorthalidone.

What is the most important information I should know about Tenoretic?

You must take Tenoretic regularly for it to be effective. Since blood pressure declines gradually, it may be several weeks before you get the full benefit of Tenoretic. You must continue taking it even if you are feeling well. Tenoretic does not cure high blood pressure; it only keeps it under control.

Tenoretic should not be stopped suddenly. It can result in increased chest pain and heart attack. When stopping the drug, your doctor will gradually reduce your dosage.

Who should not take Tenoretic?

Do not take Tenoretic if you have a slow heartbeat, a history of serious heart block (conduction disorder), inadequate blood supply to the circulatory system (cardiogenic shock), heart failure, or inability to urinate. Also, you should not begin treatment with Tenoretic if you are sensitive to its ingredients, or to other sulfonamide-derived drugs. Tenoretic should not be used if you have an untreated adrenal tumor.

What should I tell my doctor before I take the first dose of Tenoretic?

Tell your doctor about all prescription, over-the-counter, and herbal medications you are taking before beginning treatment with Tenoretic. Also, talk to your doctor about your complete medical history, especially if you have asthma, a heart condition, diabetes, gout, lupus, kidney or liver disease, thyroid disease, or will be undergoing surgery.

What is the usual dosage?

The information below is based on the dosage guidelines your doctor uses. Depending on your condition and medical history, your doctor may prescribe a different regimen. Do not change the dosage or stop taking your medication without your doctor's approval.

Adults: The dosage is always individualized.

The Tenoretic 50 tablet is made up of chlorthalidone 25 milligrams (mg) and atenolol 50 mg. The usual starting dosage of Tenoretic is 1 Tenoretic 50 tablet taken once a day. Your doctor may increase the dosage to 1 Tenoretic 100 tablet taken once a day. Your doctor may gradually add other high blood pressure medications.

Your doctor will adjust your dosage if you have kidney disease.

How should I take Tenoretic?
Tenoretic can be taken with or without food. Take this medication exactly as prescribed by your doctor, even if your symptoms have disappeared.

What should I avoid while taking Tenoretic?
Try not to miss any doses. If this medication is not taken regularly, your condition may worsen.

Avoid activities that require full mental alertness until you know how you respond to the drug. Tenoretic can make you drowsy or less alert.

What are possible food and drug interactions associated with Tenoretic?
If Tenoretic is taken with certain other drugs, the effects of either could be increased, decreased, or altered. It is especially important to check with your doctor before combining Tenoretic with the following: calcium blocking drugs (such as diltiazem and verapamil), clonidine, diabetes drugs, diuretics, lithium, nasal decongestants, Nonsteroidal anti-inflammatory drugs (such as ibuprofen and indomethacin), norepinephrine, reserpine, tubocurarine.

What are the possible side effects of Tenoretic?
Side effects cannot be anticipated. If any develop or change in intensity, tell your doctor as soon as possible. Only your doctor can determine if it is safe for you to continue taking this drug.

Side effects may include: dizziness, fatigue, nausea, slow heartbeat

Can I receive Tenoretic if I am pregnant or breastfeeding?
Tenoretic may cause harm to a developing baby. If you are pregnant, or plan to become pregnant, inform your doctor immediately. Tenoretic appears in breast milk and could affect a nursing infant. Do not breastfeed while you are taking Tenoretic.

What should I do if I miss a dose of Tenoretic?
Take the forgotten dose as soon as you remember. If it is within 8 hours of your next scheduled dose, skip the one you missed and go back to your regular schedule. Never take 2 doses at once.

How should I store Tenoretic?
Store at room temperature away from light in a tightly closed container.

TENORMIN

Generic name: Atenolol

What is Tenormin?

Tenormin is used to treat angina (chest pain caused by too little oxygen reaching the heart muscle), high blood pressure, and heart attack.

What is the most important information I should know about Tenormin?

You must take Tenormin regularly for it to be effective. Since blood pressure declines gradually, it may be several weeks before you get the full benefit of Tenormin. You must continue taking it even if you are feeling well. Tenormin does not cure high blood pressure. It only keeps it under control.

Tenormin should not be stopped suddenly. It can result in increased chest pain and heart attack. When stopping the drug, your doctor will gradually reduce your dosage.

Who should not take Tenormin?

Do not take Tenormin if you have a slow heartbeat, a history of serious heart block (conduction disorder), inadequate blood supply to the circulatory system (cardiogenic shock), heart failure, or if you are sensitive to any component of the drug.

What should I tell my doctor before I take the first dose of Tenormin?

Tell your doctor about all prescription, over-the-counter, and herbal medications you are taking before beginning treatment with Tenormin. Also, talk to your doctor about your complete medical history, especially if you have asthma, diabetes, kidney disease, heart failure, thyroid disease, diabetes, an adrenal gland tumor, or are undergoing major surgery.

What is the usual dosage?

The information below is based on the dosage guidelines your doctor uses. Depending on your condition and medical history, your doctor may prescribe a different regimen. Do not change the dosage or stop taking your medication without your doctor's approval.

High Blood Pressure

Adults: The usual starting dose is 50 milligrams (mg) daily either alone or in combination with a diuretic. Full effects should be seen in 1 to 2 weeks. If an optimal response is not achieved, your doctor may increase the dose to 100 mg daily.

Angina Pectoris
Adults: The usual starting dose is 50 mg daily. Full effects should be seen in 1 week. Your dose may be increased to 100 mg per day. In some cases, a single dose of 200 mg per day may be given.

Heart Attack
Adults: Your doctor will determine the proper dosage.

If you have kidney problems, the doctor will start you on a lower dose, usually 25 mg once a day up to a maximum of 50 mg daily.

How should I take Tenormin?
Tenormin is available as tablets, syrup, and as an injection.

It is very important to take this medicine as often as your doctor has told you to, even if you do not feel ill. This is because heart and blood pressure problems, if not treated, can get progressively worse.

Tenormin can be taken with or without food.

What should I avoid while taking Tenormin?
Try not to miss any doses. If this medication is not taken regularly, your condition may worsen.

Avoid activities that require full mental alertness until you know how you respond to the drug.

Avoid using alcohol because it may increase drowsiness and dizziness while taking this medication.

What are possible food and drug interactions associated with Tenormin?
If Tenormin is taken with certain other drugs, the effects of either could be increased, decreased, or altered. It is especially important to check with your doctor before combining Tenormin with the following: calcium blocking drugs (such as diltiazem and verapamil), clonidine, diabetes drugs, nonsteroidal anti-inflammatory drugs (such as ibuprofen or in-domethacin), reserpine.

What are the possible side effects of Tenormin?
Side effects cannot be anticipated. If any develop or change in intensity, tell your doctor as soon as possible. Only your doctor can determine if it is safe for you to continue taking this drug.

Side effects may include: dizziness, fatigue, nausea, slow heartbeat

Tenormin may mask the symptoms of low blood sugar or alter blood sugar levels.

Can I receive Tenormin if I am pregnant or breastfeeding?
Tenormin may cause harm to a developing baby. If you are pregnant or plan to become pregnant, inform your doctor immediately. Tenormin ap-

pears in breast milk and could affect a nursing infant. Do not breastfeed while you are taking Tenormin.

What should I do if I miss a dose of Tenormin?
Take the forgotten dose as soon as you remember. If it is within 8 hours of your next scheduled dose, skip the one you missed and go back to your regular schedule. Never take 2 doses at the same time.

How should I store Tenormin?
Store at room temperature away from light.

TERAZOL
Generic name: Terconazole

What is Terazol?
Terazol is an antifungal used to treat yeast infections of the vulva and vagina.

What is the most important information I should know about Terazol?
Use Terazol for as long as directed, even if the infection seems to have disappeared. If you stop too soon, the infection could return. You should continue using this medicine even during your menstrual period.

Who should not take Terazol?
Do not use Terazol if you are sensitive to any component of the medication.

What should I tell my doctor before I take the first dose of Terazol?
Mention all prescription, over-the-counter, and herbal medications you are taking before beginning treatment with Terazol. Also, talk to your doctor about your complete medical history, especially if you are using a diaphragm.

What is the usual dosage?
The information below is based on the dosage guidelines your doctor uses. Depending on your condition and medical history, your doctor may prescribe a different regimen. Do not change the dosage or stop taking your medication without your doctor's approval.

Terazol 3 and Terazol 7 Vaginal Cream
Adults: The recommended dose is 1 full applicator (5 grams) of cream inserted into the vagina once daily at bedtime. Apply Terazol 3 for 3 consecutive days and Terazol 7 for 7 consecutive days.

Terazol 3 Vaginal Suppositories
Adults: The recommended dose is 1 suppository inserted into the vagina once daily at bedtime for 3 consecutive days.

How should I take Terazol?

Follow these steps to apply Terazol Cream:

Filling the applicator:
1. Remove the cap from the tube.
2. Use the pointed tip on the top of the cap to puncture the seal on the tube.
3. Screw the applicator onto the tube.
4. Squeeze the tube from the bottom and fill the applicator until the plunger stops.
5. Unscrew the applicator from the tube.

Using the applicator:
1. Lie on your back with your knees drawn up toward your chest.
2. Holding the applicator by the ribbed end of the barrel, insert the filled applicator into the vagina as far as it will comfortably go.
3. Slowly press the plunger of the applicator to release the cream into the vagina.
4. Remove the applicator from the vagina.
5. Apply one full applicator each night at bedtime for as many days as directed by your doctor.

Cleaning the applicator (does not apply to sample applicators, which are for one-time use only):

After each use, you should thoroughly clean the applicator by following the procedure below:

1. Pull the plunger out of the barrel.
2. Wash the pieces with lukewarm, soapy water, and dry them thoroughly.
3. Put the applicator back together.

Follow these steps to use Terazol suppositories:

Filling the applicator:
1. Break off suppository from the plastic strip.
2. Pull the plastic completely apart at the notched end.
3. Place the flat end of the suppository into the open end of the applicator as shown. You are now ready to insert the suppository into the vagina.

Using the applicator:
1. Lie on your back with your knees drawn up toward your chest.
2. Holding the applicator by the ribbed end of the barrel, gently insert it into the vagina as far as it will comfortably go.
3. Press the plunger to release the suppository into the vagina.
4. Remove the applicator from the vagina.

Cleaning the applicator (does not apply to sample applicators, which are for one-time use only):

After each use, you should thoroughly clean the applicator by following the procedure below:

1. Pull the plunger out of the barrel.
2. Wash both pieces with lukewarm, soapy water, and dry them thoroughly.
3. Put the applicator back together by gently pushing the plunger into the barrel as far as it will go.

Insertion without the applicator:
1. Lie on your back with your knees drawn up toward your chest.
2. Place the suppository on the tip of your finger as shown.
3. Insert the suppository gently into the vagina as far as it will comfortably go.

To protect your clothing, wear a sanitary napkin. Do not use tampons because they will absorb the medicine. Wear cotton underwear and avoid synthetic fabrics such as nylon or rayon. Do not douche unless your doctor tells you to do so.

Dry the genital area thoroughly after a shower, bath, or swim. Change out of a wet bathing suit or damp workout clothes as soon as possible. Moisture encourages the growth of yeast.

What should I avoid while taking Terazol?

Avoid wearing tight-fitting, synthetic clothing that does not allow air circulation. Wear loose-fitting clothing made of cotton and other natural fibers until the infection is healed.

Avoid sexual intercourse if your doctor advises you to do so. The suppository formulation (not the cream) may damage the diaphragm. Therefore, use of the diaphragm during therapy with the suppository is not recommended. Consult your physician. If your partner has any penile itching, redness, or discomfort, he should consult his physician and mention that you are being treated for a yeast infection.

Try not to scratch. It can cause more irritation and can spread the infection.

What are possible food and drug interactions associated with Terazol?

No significant interactions have been reported at this time. However, always tell your doctor about any medicines you take, including over-the-counter drugs, vitamins, and herbal supplements.

If using Terazol suppositories, a component within the suppository may interact with certain rubber or latex products (such as those used in vaginal contraceptive diaphragms) and should not be used together.

What are the possible side effects of Terazol?

Side effects cannot be anticipated. If any develop or change in intensity, tell your doctor as soon as possible. Only your doctor can determine if it is safe for you to continue taking this drug.

Side effects may include: headache, menstrual pain, vaginal itching or burning, increased vaginal discharge, stomach discomfort, cramps, skin rash, headache

Can I receive Terazol if I am pregnant or breastfeeding?

Since Terazol is absorbed from the vagina, it should not be used during the first trimester (first 3 months) of pregnancy unless your doctor considers it essential to your health. Do not use Terazol while you are breastfeeding. Tell your doctor immediately if you are pregnant, plan to become pregnant, or are breastfeeding.

What should I do if I miss a dose of Terazol?

If you miss a dose of Terazol, apply it as soon as you remember. If it is almost time for your next dose, skip the one you missed and go back to your regular schedule. You should not use two doses at one time.

How should I store Terazol?

Store at room temperature, away from direct heat or light. Do not freeze.

Terazosin hydrochloride See Hytrin, page 647.

Terbinafine hydrochloride See Lamisil, page 702.

Terconazole See Terazol, page 1282.

TESSALON

Generic name: Benzonatate

What is Tessalon?

Tessalon is used for treating a cough. It works by reducing the reflex in the lungs that causes the urge to cough.

What is the most important information I should know about Tessalon?

Tessalon should be swallowed whole, not chewed, sucked, or dissolved in your mouth. Doing these may cause numbness in your mouth and throat or may cause choking or a severe allergic reaction.

Who should not take Tessalon?

Do not take Tessalon if you are sensitive to or have ever had an allergic reaction to the drug or similar drugs (such as local anesthetics).

What should I tell my doctor before I take the first dose of Tessalon?

Mention all prescription, over-the-counter, and herbal medications you are taking before beginning treatment with Tessalon. Also, talk to your doctor about your complete medical history, especially if you have ever had an allergic reaction to other anesthetic agents such as benzocaine or lidocaine.

What is the usual dosage?

The information below is based on the dosage guidelines your doctor uses. Depending on your condition and medical history, your doctor may prescribe a different regimen. Do not change the dosage or stop taking your medication without your doctor's approval.

Adults and children over 10 years old: The usual dose is 100 milligrams (mg) or 200 mg 3 times per day, as needed. The maximum dose is 600 mg a day.

How should I take Tessalon?

Tessalon perles (soft capsule form) should be swallowed whole. If chewed, they can produce a temporary numbness of the mouth and throat that may cause choking or a severe allergic reaction.

What should I avoid while taking Tessalon?

Do not suck or chew the capsules.

What are possible food and drug interactions associated with Tessalon?

There have been rare occurrences of bizarre behavior, including confusion and visual hallucinations when Tessalon is taken with other prescribed drugs. Check with your doctor before taking Tessalon with other medications.

What are the possible side effects of Tessalon?

Side effects cannot be anticipated. If any develop or change in intensity, tell your doctor as soon as possible. Only your doctor can determine if it is safe for you to continue taking this drug.

Side effects may include: allergic reactions, burning sensation in the eyes, confusion, constipation, dizziness, extreme calm (sedation), feeling cold, headache, itching, nausea, numbness in the chest, skin eruptions, stuffy nose, upset stomach, visual hallucinations

Can I receive Tessalon if I am pregnant or breastfeeding?

The effects of Tessalon during pregnancy and breastfeeding are unknown. Tell your doctor immediately if you are pregnant, plan to become pregnant, or are breastfeeding.

What should I do if I miss a dose of Tessalon?
Take the forgotten dose of Tessalon as soon as you remember. If it is almost time for you next dose, skip the one you missed and go back to your regular schedule. Never take two doses at once.

How should I store Tessalon?
Store at room temperature.

TESTOPEL
Generic name: Testosterone pellets

What is Testopel?
Testopel pellets contain testosterone, the sex hormone that is responsible for growth and maintenance of male physical characteristics. Testosterone is a member of the androgen family of steroids responsible for the growth spurt that happens during adolescence. Testopel is used to treat low testosterone levels caused by age, tumors, injury, radiation, or a condition present from birth. It also is used to stimulate puberty in boys who have a family history of delayed puberty.

In addition, testosterone is sometimes used to treat certain types of breast cancer.

What is the most important information I should know about Testopel?
If you are over 55 years of age and have prostate problems, make sure your doctor is aware of them. Supplementary testosterone may increase the risk of prostate cancer.

Who should not take Testopel?
You should not use this medicine if you have had an allergic reaction to testosterone, if you have breast cancer or prostate cancer, or if you have had an allergic reaction to anything that may be in the skin patch, such as alcohol or aluminum. A woman should never use this medicine, especially if she might be pregnant.

What should I tell my doctor before I take the first dose of Testopel?
Mention all prescription, over-the-counter, and herbal medications you are taking before beginning treatment with Testopel. Also, talk to your doctor about your complete medical history, especially if you have prostate cancer or suspected prostate cancer, diabetes, heart disease, or kidney or liver disease.

What is the usual dosage?
The information below is based on the dosage guidelines your doctor uses. Depending on your condition and medical history, your doctor

may prescribe a different regimen. **Do not change the dosage or stop taking your medication without your doctor's approval.**

The dosage of Testopel depends on the age of the patient and the condition being treated. The dosage is adjusted according to the medication's effectiveness and any adverse reactions it may trigger.

Testosterone Replacement Therapy in Men
The usual starting dose is 150-450 milligrams (mg) implanted by your doctor every 3-6 months.

Delayed Puberty in Adolescent Boys
The doctor may begin with a low dosage and gradually increase it as puberty progresses, or begin with a higher dose to induce puberty and then lower the dosage. The doctor will take into account the boy's age and stage in development when determining the dose. The Testopel pellets usually are implanted for only a limited period, such as 4-6 months.

How should I take Testopel?
Testopel pellets are implanted under the skin by your doctor. Their effects last for 3-4 months and sometimes for as long as 6 months.

What should I avoid while taking Testopel?
Due to its potentially serious side effects, Testopel should not be used to improve athletic performance.

What are possible food and drug interactions associated with Testopel?
If Testopel is taken with certain other drugs, the effects of either could be increased, decreased, or altered. It is especially important to check with your doctor before combining Testopel with the following: blood thinners (eg, warfarin), insulin, or oxyphenbutazone.

What are the possible side effects of Testopel?
Side effects cannot be anticipated. If any develop or change in intensity, tell your doctor as soon as possible. Only your doctor can determine if it is safe for you to continue taking this drug.

Side effects may include: abnormal hair growth, acne, anxiety, blood clotting disorders, decreased sperm count, depression, enlarged breasts in men, fluid retention and swelling, frequent and prolonged erections, headache, increased cholesterol levels, increased or decreased sex drive, inflammation and pain at the pellet site, liver disorders, male pattern baldness, nausea, prickling or tingling sensation, yellowing of skin and eyes

Can I receive Testopel if I am pregnant or breastfeeding?
Do not use Testopel if you are pregnant or breastfeeding. Testopel is not for use by women.

What should I do if I miss a dose of Testopel?
Testopel is implanted by your doctor at periodic intervals. Speak to your doctor regarding your next scheduled visit or if you think you missed a dose.

How should I store Testopel?
Testopel should be stored in a cool, dry place.

Testosterone gel *See AndroGel, page 102.*

TESTOSTERONE PATCHES

What are Testosterone Patches?
These patches are prescribed for men with low levels, or the absence of, the male hormone testosterone. Lack of testosterone can lead to declining interest in sex, impotence, fatigue, depression, and loss of masculine characteristics.

What is the most important information I should know about Testosterone Patches?
If you are over 55 years of age and have prostate problems, make sure your doctor is aware of them. Supplementary testosterone may increase the risk of prostate cancer.

Who should not take Testosterone Patches?
Do not use the patch if you have breast cancer or prostate cancer or if you are sensitive to any component of the drug. The patches are not for use by women.

What should I tell my doctor before I take the first dose of Testosterone Patches?
Tell your doctor about all prescription, over-the-counter, and herbal medications you are taking before beginning treatment with testosterone patches.

Also, talk to your doctor about your complete medical history, especially if you have prostate cancer or suspected prostate cancer, heart disease, or kidney or liver disease.

What is the usual dosage?
The information below is based on the dosage guidelines your doctor uses. Depending on your condition and medical history, your doctor may prescribe a different regimen. Do not change the dosage or stop taking your medication without your doctor's approval.

Androderm
Adults: The usual starting dose is one 5-mg patch or two 2.5-mg patches per day. Depending on results, your doctor may increase the dosage to 1 large and 1 small patch (or 3 small patches) daily, or reduce it to 1 small patch per day.

Testoderm
Adults: The usual dose is 1 patch per day. The larger patch delivers 6 milligrams (mg) of testosterone. The smaller patch delivers 4 mg.

How should I take Testosterone Patches?
Androderm
Apply Androderm at the same time every evening and replace the old one with a new one every 24 hours.

Apply Androderm patches to clean and dry areas. Avoid areas of the skin that are oily, prone to perspiration, or are covered with hair. Only apply the patch to the skin of the back, abdomen, upper arms, or thigh. Do NOT apply the patch to the scrotum. Avoid bony areas such as the shoulders and hips as well as areas that get the greatest pressure while you are sleeping or sitting. You should change the application site each day of the week, waiting 7 days before reusing a site.

Apply the patch(es) by pressing it firmly in place immediately after you take it out of the storage pouch. Leave the patch(es) in place for a full 24 hours.

If an Androderm patch falls off, try to reapply it. If it cannot be reapplied and it is before noon, apply a new patch. If it is after noon, wait until the evening and apply a new patch at the regularly scheduled time.

Testoderm
Testoderm patches are applied daily to the skin of the scrotum. For best results, the scrotal skin should be shaved, clean, and dry. Dry-shave the skin and avoid wet-shaving or chemical hair-removal products. The patch should be worn for 22-24 hours per day. Apply a new patch every 24 hours. Remove the patch during bathing, showering, or swimming.

Testoderm TTS patches should be applied at the same time every day, either during the day or night. Testoderm TTS patches should NOT be applied to the scrotum. Testoderm TTS patches can be applied to the arms, back, or upper buttocks. Avoid bony areas such as the shoulders and hips as well as areas that get the greatest pressure while you are sleeping or sitting. Leave the patch in place for 24 hours. If a Testoderm TTS patch falls off, try to reapply it. If it comes off after being worn for more than 12 hours and it cannot be reapplied, wait until the next scheduled application time to apply a new system.

What should I avoid while taking Testosterone Patches?
Avoid undergoing an MRI while wearing a testosterone patch. Burns have been reported at the patch site.

What are possible food and drug interactions associated with Testosterone Patches?

If the patch is taken with certain other drugs, the effects of either could be increased, decreased, or altered. It is especially important to check with your doctor before combining the patch with the following: blood-thinners such as warfarin, insulin, oxyphenbutazone.

What are the possible side effects of Testosterone Patches?

Side effects cannot be anticipated. If any develop or change in intensity, tell your doctor as soon as possible. Only your doctor can determine if it is safe for you to continue taking this drug.

Side effects may include: Blistering, burning, hardening of the skin, itching, and redness at the application site

In younger men being treated for delayed sexual development, supplementary testosterone can cause breast enlargement. In older men, it can increase the risk of prostate cancer. Among men with heart, kidney, or livery disease, it can lead to fluid retention and congestive heart failure.

Tell your doctor if you experience nausea, vomiting, swelling of the ankles, changes in skin color, too frequent or prolonged erections, breathing problems, or yellowing of the skin or eyes.

Some testosterone may be left on the skin after a patch is removed. Particularly with Testoderm, there is a possibility that your partner could absorb some of the hormone during sex and suffer unwanted changes. If she experiences increased hair growth or an aggravation of acne, tell your doctor.

Can I receive Testosterone Patches if I am pregnant or breastfeeding?

Testosterone is intended for use only by males and must not be used by women. If used during pregnancy, it can cause serious harm to the developing baby.

What should I do if I miss a dose of Testosterone Patches?

Apply it as soon as you remember. If it is almost time for the next application, skip the one you missed and go back to your regular schedule. Do not apply 2 patches at the same time unless instructed by your doctor.

How should I store Testosterone Patches?

Store at room temperature.

Testosterone pellets *See Testopel, page 1287.*

TETRACYCLINE

What is Tetracycline?
Tetracycline is an antibiotic used to treat bacterial infections such as Rocky Mountain spotted fever, typhus fever, tick fevers, pneumonia, gonorrhea, Chlamydia, urinary tract infections, trachoma (a chronic eye infection), conjunctivitis (pinkeye), acne, and others. Tetracycline is often an alternative drug for people who are allergic to penicillin.

What is the most important information I should know about Tetracycline?
Tetracycline should not be used in pregnancy or in children under the age of 8 years old. It may damage developing teeth and cause permanent discoloration.

Who should not take Tetracycline?
Do not take tetracycline if you are sensitive to or have ever had an allergic reaction to any tetracycline medication.

Do not take tetracycline if you are pregnant or breastfeeding.

What should I tell my doctor before I take the first dose of Tetracycline?
Mention all prescription, over-the-counter, and herbal medications you are taking before beginning treatment with tetracycline. Also, talk to your doctor about your complete medical history, especially if you are pregnant, plan to become pregnant, or are breastfeeding; have a history of allergy, asthma, hay fever, or hives; or if you have kidney or liver disease.

What is the usual dosage?
The information below is based on the dosage guidelines your doctor uses. Depending on your condition and medical history, your doctor may prescribe a different regimen. Do not change the dosage or stop taking your medication without your doctor's approval.

Adults: For most infections, the usual daily dose is 1 grams (g) divided as 500 milligrams (mg) twice a day or 250 mg four times daily. For more severe infections, a dose of 500 mg four times daily may be required.

Acne
In cases of severe acne, the recommended dose is 1 g daily in divided doses. When the acne improves, the dose may be reduced to 125-500 mg daily.

Brucellosis
The usual dose is 500 mg, four times daily for 3 weeks. Tetracycline use should be accompanied by streptomycin.

Gonorrhea
The usual dose is 500 mg, four times daily for 7 days.

Syphilis
Early syphilis (duration less than 1 year): 500 mg four times daily for 15 days

Syphilis (duration more than 1 year, except neurosyphilis): 500 mg four times daily for 30 days

*Urethral, Endocervical, or Rectal Infections
in Adults Due to* Chlamydia Trachomatis
The usual dose is 500 mg, four times daily, for at least 7 days.

Children 8 years of age and above: The usual daily dose is 10-20 mg per pound of body weight divided into 4 equal doses for at least 24-48 hours after symptoms and fever are gone.

How should I take Tetracycline?
Take each dose with a full glass of water (8 ounces). Adequate water should be taken with each dose to prevent irritation of the esophagus. Take tetracycline 1 hour before or 2 hours after meals, exactly as your doctor tells you to. Skipping doses or not taking all your tetracycline may decrease its effectiveness or increase the chance that bacteria will develop resistance to it.

What should I avoid while taking Tetracycline?
You should avoid becoming pregnant or breastfeeding. Avoid prolonged exposure to sunlight or artificial UV light (tanning beds). Tetracycline may increase the sensitivity of the skin to sunlight and you may be sunburned as a result. Use sunscreen and wear protective clothing when you are outside. Avoid simultaneous use of iron-containing preparations and aluminum-, calcium-, and magnesium-containing antacids or supplements because these can impair absorption of tetracycline.

What are possible food and drug interactions associated with Tetracycline?
If tetracycline is taken with certain other drugs, the effects of either could be increased, decreased, or altered. It is especially important to check with your doctor before combining tetracycline with the following: antacids containing aluminum, calcium, or magnesium; blood thinners, such as warfarin; dairy products; iron-containing products; methoxyflurane; oral contraceptives; or penicillin.

What are the possible side effects of Tetracycline?
Side effects cannot be anticipated. If any develop or change in intensity, tell your doctor as soon as possible. Only your doctor can determine if it is safe for you to continue taking this drug.

Side effects may include: anemia, blood disorders, blurred vision and headache (adults), bulging soft spot on the head (infants), diarrhea, difficult or painful swallowing, dizziness, extreme allergic reactions, genital or anal sores or rash, hives, inflammation of the large bowel, inflammation of the tongue, inflammation of the upper digestive tract, increased sensitivity to light, loss of appetite, nausea, ringing in the ears, swelling due to excess fluid retention, vision disturbances, vomiting

Can I receive Tetracycline if I am pregnant or breastfeeding?
Tetracycline is not recommended for use during pregnancy. Tetracycline may cause harm to an unborn infant or developing child under the age of 8. If you are pregnant or plan to become pregnant, tell your doctor right away. Tetracycline appears in breast milk. Do not breastfeed while you are taking tetracycline.

What should I do if I miss a dose of Tetracycline?
If you miss a dose, take it as soon as you can. If it is almost time for your next dose, wait until then to take the medicine and skip the missed dose. Do not use extra medicine to make up for a missed dose.

How should I store Tetracycline?
Store at room temperature in a closed container, away from heat, moisture, and direct light. Do not freeze the oral liquid.

TEVETEN
Generic name: Eprosartan mesylate

What is Teveten?
Teveten is used to treat high blood pressure, either alone or with other medications that help lower blood pressure, such as water pills (diuretics) or calcium channel blockers.

What is the most important information I should know about Teveten?
Do not use Teveten during the second or third trimesters of pregnancy. This drug can cause injury and even death to the developing baby. Tell your doctor immediately if you think you might be pregnant.

You must take Teveten regularly for it to be effective. Since blood pressure declines gradually, it may be several weeks before you get the full benefit of Teveten. You must continue taking it even if you are feeling well. Teveten does not cure blood pressure. It only keeps it under control.

Who should not take Teveten?

Do not take Teveten if you are pregnant or if you have ever had an allergic reaction to it or any of its ingredients.

What should I tell my doctor before I take the first dose of Teveten?

Mention all prescription, over-the-counter, and herbal medications you are taking before beginning treatment with Teveten. Also, talk to your doctor about your complete medical history, especially if you have kidney or liver disease, are on a salt-restricted diet or have high levels of potassium in your blood, or if you are taking potassium supplements.

What is the usual dosage?

The information below is based on the dosage guidelines your doctor uses. Depending on your condition and medical history, your doctor may prescribe a different regimen. Do not change the dosage or stop taking your medication without your doctor's approval.

Adults: The usual dose is 600 milligrams (mg) once daily. Teveten may also be taken once or twice daily with total daily doses ranging from 400-800 mg.

How should I take Teveten?

Teveten can be taken with or without food. Try to establish a regular routine by taking it at the same time each day—in the morning with breakfast, for example. This reduces the chance that you'll forget a dose.

What should I avoid while taking Teveten?

Teveten may cause dizziness or drowsiness. Use caution when driving, operating machinery, or performing other hazardous activities.

Use alcohol cautiously. Alcohol may increase drowsiness and dizziness while you are taking Teveten.

Avoid prolonged exposure to sunlight or artificial UV light (tanning beds). Teveten may increase the sensitivity of the skin to sunlight and you may be sunburned as a result. Use a sunscreen and wear protective clothing when you are outside.

What are possible food and drug interactions associated with Teveten?

If Teveten is taken with certain other drugs, the effects of either could be increased, decreased, or altered. It is especially important to check with your doctor before combining Teveten with any of the following: potassium-sparing diuretics (water pills), such as amiloride, spironolactone, or triamterene; or potassium supplements.

What are the possible side effects of Teveten?

Side effects cannot be anticipated. If any develop or change in intensity, tell your doctor as soon as possible. Only your doctor can determine if it is safe for you to continue taking this drug.

Side effects may include: cold, cough, runny nose, sore throat

Can I receive Teveten if I am pregnant or breastfeeding?

Teveten can cause injury or even death to an unborn child when used in the second or third trimester of pregnancy. Stop taking Teveten as soon as you know you are pregnant and be sure to tell your doctor if you are pregnant or plan to become pregnant. Teveten may appear in breast milk. Do not breastfeed while taking Teveten.

What should I do if I miss a dose of Teveten?

If you miss a dose of Teveten, take it as soon as possible. If it is almost time for your next dose, skip the one you missed and go back to your regular schedule.

How should I store Teveten?

Store at room temperature, away from moisture and heat.

TEVETEN HCT
Generic name: Eprosartan mesylate and hydrochlorothiazide

What is Teveten HCT?

Teveten HCT is a combination medication consisting of eprosartan and hydrochlorothiazide. It is used to treat high blood pressure, alone or in combination with other high blood pressure medications.

What is the most important information I should know about Teveten HCT?

Do not use Teveten HCT during the second or third trimesters of pregnancy. This drug can cause injury and even death to the developing baby. Tell your doctor immediately if you think you might be pregnant.

You must take Teveten HCT regularly for it to be effective. Since blood pressure declines gradually, it may be several weeks before you get the full benefit of Teveten HCT. You must continue taking it even if you are feeling well. Teveten HCT does not cure blood pressure; it only keeps it under control.

Teveten HCT can cause an excessive drop in blood pressure, especially when you first begin taking it. If you feel lightheaded or faint, let your doctor know about it. If you actually faint, stop taking Teveten HCT and see your doctor immediately. The problem is more likely if you suffer from a lack of fluids, due either to inadequate intake or to excessive sweating, diarrhea, or vomiting.

Excessive fluid loss can also lead to a chemical imbalance in the body. Warning signs include dry mouth, thirst, diminished urination, weakness, lack of energy, drowsiness, restlessness, confusion, seizures, muscle pain, muscle fatigue, nausea, vomiting, and rapid heartbeat. Alert your doctor if you develop any of these symptoms.

Who should not take Teveten HCT?

Do not take Teveten HCT if you are pregnant, if you have ever had an allergic reaction to it, or if you cannot urinate or are sensitive to other sulfa drugs.

What should I tell my doctor before I take the first dose of Teveten HCT?

Mention all prescription, over-the-counter, and herbal medications you are taking before beginning treatment with Teveten HCT. Also, talk to your doctor about your complete medical history, especially if you have a history of allergy, wheezing or breathing difficulties, kidney or liver disease, systemic lupus erythematosus (a chronic skin condition characterized by ulcerative lesions that spread over the body), joint inflammation, high blood sugar, or parathyroid disease.

What is the usual dosage?

The information below is based on the dosage guidelines your doctor uses. Depending on your condition and medical history, your doctor may prescribe a different regimen. Do not change the dosage or stop taking your medication without your doctor's approval.

Adults: Teveten HCT comes in two strengths: 600/12.5 and 600/25 (600 milligrams [mg] of eprosartan and either 12.5 mg or 25 mg of hydrochlorothiazide). The usual starting dose is one 600/12.5 tablet per day. If your blood pressure remains too high, the doctor may increase the dose to one 600/25 tablet per day.

How should I take Teveten HCT?

Teveten HCT can be taken with or without food. Try to establish a regular routine by taking it at the same time each day—in the morning with breakfast, for example. This reduces the chance that you'll forget a dose.

What should I avoid while taking Teveten HCT?

Teveten HCT may cause dizziness or drowsiness. Use caution when driving, operating machinery, or performing other hazardous activities.

Avoid prolonged exposure to sunlight or artificial UV light (tanning beds). Teveten HCT may increase the sensitivity of the skin to sunlight and you may be sunburned as a result. Use a sunscreen and wear protective clothing when you are outside.

Use alcohol cautiously. Alcohol may increase drowsiness and dizziness while you are taking Teveten HCT.

Avoid salt substitutes and do not take potassium supplements without first talking to your doctor.

What are possible food and drug interactions associated with Teveten HCT?

If Teveten is taken with certain other drugs, the effects of either could be increased, decreased, or altered. It is especially important to check with your doctor before combining Teveten with any of the following: barbiturates, such as phenobarbital or secobarbital; cholestyramine; colestipol; insulin; lithium; narcotic painkillers, such as meperidine or oxycodone; nonsteroidal anti-inflammatory medications, such as ibuprofen or naproxen; oral diabetes medications, such as glipizide or glucotrol; other blood pressure medications, such as atenolol or nifedipine; potassium-sparing diuretic (water pill), such as amiloride, spironolactone, or triamterene; potassium supplements; and steroid medications such as prednisone.

What are the possible side effects of Teveten HCT?

Side effects cannot be anticipated. If any develop or change in intensity, tell your doctor as soon as possible. Only your doctor can determine if it is safe for you to continue taking this drug.

Side effects may include: back pain, dizziness, fatigue, headache, upper respiratory tract infection

Can I receive Teveten HCT if I am pregnant or breastfeeding?

Teveten HCT can cause injury or even death to an unborn child when used in the second or third trimester of pregnancy. Stop taking Teveten HCT as soon as you know you are pregnant, and be sure to tell your doctor if you are pregnant or plan to become pregnant. Teveten HCT may appear in breast milk. Do not breastfeed while taking Teveten HCT.

What should I do if I miss a dose of Teveten HCT?

Take it as soon as possible. If it is almost time for your next dose, skip the one you missed and go back to your regular schedule. Do not take two doses at once.

How should I store Teveten HCT?

Store at room temperature, away from moisture and heat.

THALITONE
Generic name: Chlorthalidone

What is Thalitone?
Thalitone is a diuretic (water pill) used to treat high blood pressure and fluid retention associated with congestive heart failure, cirrhosis of the liver (a disease of the liver), corticosteroid and estrogen therapy, and kidney disease. Thalitone may be used alone or in combination with other high blood pressure medications.

What is the most important information I should know about Thalitone?
You must take Thalitone regularly for it to be effective. Since blood pressure declines gradually, it may be several weeks before you get the full benefit of Thalitone. You must continue taking it even if you are feeling well. Thalitone does not cure high blood pressure. It only keeps it under control.

Who should not take Thalitone?
Do not take Thalitone if you are unable to urinate or if you have ever had an allergic reaction to, or are sensitive to, Thalitone or other sulfa drugs.

What should I tell my doctor before I take the first dose of Thalitone?
Mention all prescription, over-the-counter, and herbal medications you are taking before beginning treatment with Thalitone. Also, talk to your doctor about your complete medical history, especially if you have kidney or liver disease, a history of allergies, wheezing or breathing difficulties, lupus (a chronic skin condition characterized by ulcerative lesions that spread over the body), joint inflammation, and high blood sugar.

What is the usual dosage?
The information below is based on the dosage guidelines your doctor uses. Depending on your condition and medical history, your doctor may prescribe a different regimen. Do not change the dosage or stop taking your medication without your doctor's approval.

High Blood Pressure
Adults: The usual starting dose is 15 milligrams (mg) once daily. Your doctor may increase your dose to 30 mg and then to 45-50 mg once daily.

Fluid Retention
Adults: The usual starting dose is 30-60 mg daily or 60 mg on alternate days. Some people may require up to 90-120 mg at these intervals. Your doctor may be able to lower the dose as treatment continues.

How should I take Thalitone?

Take Thalitone exactly as prescribed. Diuretics such as Thalitone increase urination. Take it in the morning, with or without food.

What should I avoid while taking Thalitone?

Thalitone may cause dizziness. Use caution when driving, operating machinery, or performing other hazardous activities.

Use alcohol cautiously. Alcohol may increase the side effects of Thalitone.

Avoid a diet high in salt. Too much salt may cause your body to retain water and may decrease the effects of Thalitone.

Avoid prolonged exposure to sunlight or UV light (tanning beds). Thalitone may increase the sensitivity of your skin to sunlight. Wear sunscreen and protective clothing when you are outside.

Avoid becoming overheated in hot weather and during exercise. Contact your doctor if you experience excessive thirst, tiredness, restlessness, drowsiness, muscle pains or cramps, nausea, vomiting, or increased heart rate or pulse.

What are possible food and drug interactions associated with Thalitone?

If Thalitone is taken with certain other drugs, the effects of either could be increased, decreased, or altered. It is especially important to check with your doctor before combining Thalitone with any of the following: blood pressure medications, such as clonidine and methyldopa; digoxin; insulin; lithium; norepinephrine; oral diabetes medications, such as glyburide; and tubocurarine.

What are the possible side effects of Thalitone?

Side effects cannot be anticipated. If any develop or change in intensity, tell your doctor as soon as possible. Only your doctor can determine if it is safe for you to continue taking this drug.

Side effects may include: allergic reaction, anemia, changes in blood sugar, change in potassium levels (causing such symptoms as dry mouth, excessive thirst, weak or irregular heartbeat, and muscle pain or cramps), constipation, cramping, diarrhea, dizziness (especially upon standing up), flaky skin, headache, hives, impotence, inflammation of a lymph or blood vessel, inflammation of the pancreas, itching, loss of appetite, low blood pressure, muscle spasms, nausea, rash, restlessness, sensitivity to light, stomach irritation, tingling or pins and needles, vision changes, vomiting, weakness, yellow eyes and skin

Can I receive Thalitone if I am pregnant or breastfeeding?

The effects of Thalitone during pregnancy and breastfeeding are unknown. Tell your doctor immediately if you are pregnant, plan to become pregnant, or are breastfeeding.

What should I do if I miss a dose of Thalitone?

Take it as soon as you remember. If it is almost time for the next dose, skip the one you missed and go back to your regular schedule. Do not take two doses at the same time.

How should I store Thalitone?

Store at room temperature.

THEOPHYLLINE

What is Theophylline?

Theophylline, an oral bronchodilator medication, is given to treat symptoms of asthma, chronic bronchitis, and emphysema. Theophylline is a chemical cousin of caffeine. It opens the airways by relaxing the smooth muscle that circles the tubes and blood vessels in the lungs.

What is the most important information I should know about Theophylline?

Theophylline is a controlled-release medication. For an acute attack you should take an immediate-release medication instead of more theophylline. If you develop status asthmaticus (a severe breathing difficulty that does not clear up with your usual medications), do not take extra theophylline; instead, seek medical treatment immediately. Since even a little extra theophylline may constitute an overdose, you should be treated in a place where close monitoring is possible.

Individual doses are determined by a person's response (a decrease in symptoms of asthma). In order to avoid overdosing or underdosing, your doctor will perform regular tests to determine the amount of theophylline in your bloodstream.

You should not change from one brand of theophylline to another brand without first consulting your doctor or pharmacist. Products manufactured by different companies may not be equally effective.

You should take theophylline cautiously and under close medical supervision if you are over age 60.

You should also take theophylline cautiously and under close supervision if you have had a sustained high fever, or if you have heart disease, liver disease, heartbeat irregularities, fluid in the lungs, an underactive thyroid gland, the flu or another viral illness, or the symptoms of shock.

Call your doctor immediately if you develop nausea, vomiting, a lasting headache, insomnia, restlessness, or a too-rapid heartbeat; if you develop a new illness, especially with a fever; or if an illness you already have gets worse.

Who should not take Theophylline?

Do not take theophylline if you have ever had an allergic reaction to it or similar drugs.

What should I tell my doctor before I take the first dose of Theophylline?

Tell your doctor about all prescription, over-the-counter, and herbal medications you are taking before beginning treatment with this drug. Also, talk to your doctor about your complete medical history, especially if you have breathing or lung problems, heart problems, thyroid problems, kidney or liver dysfunction, peptic ulcer, seizure disorders, heart rhythm problems, or if you smoke or have recently quit smoking.

What is the usual dosage?

The information below is based on the dosage guidelines your doctor uses. Depending on your condition and medical history, your doctor may prescribe a different regimen. Do not change the dosage or stop taking your medication without your doctor's approval.

Adults and adolescents 16 years and older: The usual initial dose is one 150-milligram tablet every 12 hours. If this is not effective, your doctor will gradually increase the dose until you respond. The usual dosage range is 400-600 milligrams per day. Depending on your condition and blood levels of the drug, the doctor may prescribed a higher dose.

Children and adolescents 12 to 15 years: The doctor will calculate the proper dosage based on the child's body weight.

How should I take Theophylline?

Take theophylline exactly as prescribed. Do not change the dose, the time you take it, or how often you take it without consulting your doctor.

The extended-release tablets should be swallowed whole, not crushed or chewed. The tablets of some brands are scored; if the doctor prescribes a partial dosage, these tablets should be broken only at the score. You may take the tablets with or without food. If you are taking them on a once-a-day basis, do not take the dose at night.

What should I avoid while taking Theophylline?

When taking theophylline, you should avoid large amounts of caffeine-containing beverages, such as tea or coffee.

What are possible food and drug interactions associated with Theophylline?

Theophylline interacts with a wide variety of drugs. Consult your doctor before combining any other medication with theophylline. Let your doctor know whenever another doctor starts you on a new medication or stops an old one. Let every doctor you deal with know you are taking theophylline.

What are the possible side effects of Theophylline?

Side effects cannot be anticipated. If any develop or change in intensity, tell your doctor as soon as possible. Only your doctor can determine if it is safe for you to continue taking this drug. Nausea and restlessness may occur when you first start to take theophylline, but will probably disappear as your body becomes used to the drug.

Side effects may include: convulsions, diarrhea, disturbances of heart rhythm, excitability, frequent urination, hair loss, headache, heart palpitations, insomnia, irritability, muscle twitching, rash, severe seizures, tremors, vomiting

Can I receive Theophylline if I am pregnant or breastfeeding?
If you are pregnant or plan to become pregnant, inform your doctor immediately. Theophylline should not be taken during pregnancy unless it is clearly needed, and unless the benefits to the mother outweigh the potential risk to the developing child. Theophylline appears in breast milk and may make a nursing baby irritable or harm the baby in other ways. If you are a new mother, you will probably need to choose between breastfeeding and taking theophylline.

What should I do if I miss a dose of Theophylline?
Take the next dose at the regular time. Do not try to make up the dose you missed.

How should I store Theophylline?
Store at room temperature in a tightly closed container. Protect from excessive heat, light, and moisture.

Thiothixene See Navane, page 867.

Tiagabine hydrochloride See Gabitril, page 604.

TIGAN
Generic name: Trimethobenzamide hydrochloride

What is Tigan?
Tigan is used to control nausea and vomiting.

What is the most important information I should know about Tigan?
Drugs that prevent or lessen nausea and vomiting (antiemetics) are not recommended for the treatment of simple vomiting in children. Use of Tigan in children should be limited to prolonged vomiting caused by a known disease. Tigan is thought to have an aggravating effect on Reye's syndrome (a potentially fatal childhood disease of the brain that sometimes strikes after a viral infection such as chickenpox). In addition, some of Tigan's side effects can actually be confused with the symptoms of Reye's syndrome.

Who should not take Tigan?

Do not take Tigan if you are allergic to any of its ingredients. Children should not receive the injectable form of Tigan.

What should I tell my doctor before I take the first dose of Tigan?

Mention all prescription, over-the-counter, and herbal medications you are taking before beginning treatment with Tigan. Also, talk to your doctor about your complete medical history, especially if you have a high fever, inflammation of the brain, inflammation of the digestive tract, or if you are dehydrated.

What is the usual dosage?

The information below is based on the dosage guidelines your doctor uses. Depending on your condition and medical history, your doctor may prescribe a different regimen. Do not change the dosage or stop taking your medication without your doctor's approval.

The dosage will be adjusted by your doctor according to your illness, the severity of your symptoms, and how well you do on the drug.

Adults: The usual dosage is one 300-milligram (mg) capsule taken 3-4 times per day.

How should I take Tigan?

Take Tigan exactly as directed by your doctor.

What should I avoid while taking Tigan?

Tigan may cause dizziness or drowsiness. Use caution when driving, operating machinery, or performing other activities that require mental alertness.

Use alcohol cautiously. Alcohol may increase drowsiness and dizziness while taking Tigan.

What are possible food and drug interactions associated with Tigan?

If Tigan is taken with certain other drugs, the effects of either could be increased, decreased, or altered. It is especially important to check with your doctor before combining Tigan with alcohol or central nervous system drugs, including phenothiazines such as chlorpromazine, barbiturates such as phenobarbital, and belladonna-type drugs.

What are the possible side effects of Tigan?

Side effects cannot be anticipated. If any develop or change in intensity, tell your doctor as soon as possible. Only your doctor can determine if it is safe for you to continue taking this drug.

Side effects may include: allergic-type skin reactions, blood disorders, blurred vision, coma, convulsions, depression, disorientation, dizziness, drowsiness, headache, muscle cramps, severe muscle spasm, tremors, yellowed eyes and skin

Can I receive Tigan if I am pregnant or breastfeeding?
The effects of Tigan during pregnancy and breastfeeding are unknown. Tell your doctor immediately if you are pregnant, plan to become pregnant, or are breastfeeding.

What should I do if I miss a dose of Tigan?
Take it as soon as you remember. If it is within 3 hours of your next dose, skip the one you missed and go back to your regular schedule. Do not take 2 doses at once.

How should I store Tigan?
Store at room temperature. Protect from excessive heat, light, and moisture.

Timolol maleate (ophthalmic) *See Betimol, page 212, or Timoptic, below.*

TIMOPTIC
Generic name: Timolol maleate (ophthalmic)

What is Timoptic?
Timoptic is an ophthalmic (applied directly in the eye) medication that reduces pressure in the eye. It is used to treat glaucoma (elevated pressure in the eye) alone or with other medications.

What is the most important information I should know about Timoptic?
Although Timoptic is applied only to the eye, the medication may be absorbed and may affect other parts of the body. If you have diabetes, asthma or other respiratory disease, or decreased heart function, make sure your doctor is aware of the problem.

Who should not take Timoptic?
Do not use Timoptic if you have bronchial asthma; a history of bronchial asthma or other serious breathing disorders, such as emphysema; if you have a slow heartbeat, heart block (conduction disorder), heart failure, or inadequate blood supply to the circulatory system (cardiogenic shock); or if you have ever had an allergic reaction or are sensitive to Timoptic or any of its ingredients.

What should I tell my doctor before I take the first dose of Timoptic?

Mention all prescription, over-the-counter, and herbal medications you are taking before beginning treatment with Timoptic. Also, talk to your doctor about your complete medical history, especially if you have diabetes, asthma, other respiratory diseases, overactive thyroid, decreased heart function, or if you have a medical emergency. You should also have a discussion with your doctor before surgery or before dental treatment.

What is the usual dosage?

The information below is based on the dosage guidelines your doctor uses. Depending on your condition and medical history, your doctor may prescribe a different regimen. Do not change the dosage or stop taking your medication without your doctor's approval.

Your doctor will tailor an individual Timoptic dosage depending on your medical condition and how you responded to any previous glaucoma treatment.

Adults: The usual recommended starting dose of the regular solution is to place 1 drop of 0.25% Timoptic in the affected eye(s) 2 times per day. If you do not respond satisfactorily to this dosage, your doctor may tell you to place 1 drop of 0.5% Timoptic in the affected eye(s) 2 times a day.

The usual dose of the gel-forming solution is 1 drop of either 0.25% or 0.5% in the affected eye(s) once a day. Invert the closed container and shake it once before you use it.

How should I take Timoptic?

Timoptic should be used exactly as prescribed by your doctor. If you need to use other eye medications along with Timoptic, use them at least 10 minutes before you instill Timoptic eye drops. If you wear contact lenses, remove them before using the drops and wait 15 minutes before reinserting them.

Handle the Timoptic solution carefully to avoid contamination. Do not let the tip of the dispenser actually touch the eye. Do not enlarge the hole in the dispenser tip. Do not wash the dispenser tip with water, soap, or any other cleanser.

To administer Timoptic eye drops, follow these steps:
1. Wash your hands thoroughly with soap and water.
2. Tilt your head back and gently pull your lower eyelid down to form a pocket.
3. Turn the bottle upside down, holding it with your thumb or index finger over the finger push area.
4. Press the bottle lightly until a single drop falls into the eye.
5. Repeat steps 3 and 4 with the other eye, if necessary.
6. Replace the cap firmly.

What should I avoid while taking Timoptic?
Do not touch the dropper to any surface. The dropper is sterile. If it becomes contaminated, it could cause an infection in the eye.

What are possible food and drug interactions associated with Timoptic?
If Timoptic is taken with certain other drugs, the effects of either could be increased, decreased, or altered. It is especially important to check with your doctor before combining Timoptic with the following: blood pressure drugs, such as atenolol or metoprolol; calcium-blocking drugs, such as diltiazem, nifedipine, or verapamil; clonidine; dioxin; epinephrine; quinidine; reserpine; and serotonin inhibitors, such as fluoxetine, paroxetine, and sertraline.

What are the possible side effects of Timoptic?
Side effects cannot be anticipated. If any develop or change in intensity, tell your doctor as soon as possible. Only your doctor can determine if it is safe for you to continue taking this drug.

Side effects may include: burning and stinging in the eye

Can I receive Timoptic if I am pregnant or breastfeeding?
The effects of Timoptic during pregnancy and breastfeeding are unknown. Tell your doctor immediately if you are pregnant, plan to become pregnant, or are breastfeeding. Do not breastfeed while you are using Timoptic.

What should I do if I miss a dose of Timoptic?
If you use Timoptic eye drops once a day, apply them as soon as you remember. If you do not remember until the next day, skip the dose you missed and go back to your regular schedule. Do not take 2 doses at once. If you use Timoptic eye drops 2 or more times a day, apply them as soon as you remember. If it is almost time for your next dose, skip the one you missed and go back to your regular schedule. Do not take 2 doses at once.

How should I store Timoptic?
Store at room temperature, protected from light. Keep from freezing.

TINDAMAX
Generic name: Tinidazole

What is Tindamax?
Tindamax is used to treat certain types of parasitic infections including trichomoniasis, giardiasis, intestinal amebiasis, amebic liver abscess, and bacterial vaginosis in nonpregnant women.

What is the most important information I should know about Tindamax?

Do not drink alcohol while taking Tindamax or for 3 days after you stop taking the drug. Combining alcohol with Tindamax can cause stomach cramps, nausea, vomiting, headaches, and flushing.

Take all of the Tindamax that has been prescribed for you even if you begin to feel better. Your symptoms may start to improve before the infection is completely treated.

Who should not take Tindamax?

Do not take Tindamax if you are sensitive to the drug or if you have ever had an allergic reaction to other drugs in the same class (known as "azoles"), such as metronidazole. Tindamax should not be used during the first 3 months of pregnancy or in nursing mothers unless breastfeeding is interrupted during treatment and for 3 days after the last dose of the drug.

What should I tell my doctor before I take the first dose of Tindamax?

Mention all prescription, over-the-counter, and herbal medications you are taking before beginning treatment with Tindamax. Also, talk to your doctor about your complete medical history, especially if you have a history of blood disorders, seizure disorder including epilepsy, central nervous system diseases, liver disease, or a yeast infection.

What is the usual dosage?

The information below is based on the dosage guidelines your doctor uses. Depending on your condition and medical history, your doctor may prescribe a different regimen. Do not change the dosage or stop taking your medication without your doctor's approval.

Trichomoniasis
Adults: The usual dose is a single dose of 2 grams (g) taken with food. Since trichomoniasis is a sexually transmitted disease, sexual partners should be treated with the same dose and at the same time.

Giardiasis
Adults: The usual dose is a single 2 g dose taken with food.

Children 3 years and older: The usual dose is a single dose of 50 milligrams (mg) per 2.2 pounds of body weight, up to a maximum of 2 g, taken with food.

Intestinal Amebiasis
Adults: The usual dose is 2 g daily for 3 days taken with food.

Children 3 years and older: The usual dose is 50 mg per 2.2 pounds of body weight, up to a maximum of 2 grams, taken for 3 days with food.

Amebic Liver Abscess
Adults: The usual dose is 2 g daily for 3-5 days taken with food.

Children 3 years and older: The usual dose is 50 mg per 2.2 pounds of body weight, up to a maximum of 2 g, taken for 3-5 days with food.

Bacterial Vaginosis
Adults: The usual dose is 2 g daily for 2 days taken with food or 1 g daily for 5 days taken with food.

Children who take Tindamax for more than 3 days must be closely monitored.

How should I take Tindamax?
Take Tindamax with food at about the same time each day. If you cannot swallow tablets, a pharmacist can make Tindamax into a syrup.

What should I avoid while taking Tindamax?
Avoid taking Tindamax if you have taken disulfiram within the last 2 weeks.

Do not drink alcohol while taking Tindamax and for 3 days after finishing the medication.

What are possible food and drug interactions associated with Tindamax?
If Tindamax is taken with certain other drugs, the effects of either could be increased, decreased, or altered. It is especially important to check with your doctor before combining Tindamax with the following: alcohol, blood thinners such as warfarin, cholestyramine, cimetidine, cyclosporine, disulfiram, fluorouracil, fosphenytoin, ketoconazole, lithium, oxytetracycline, phenobarbital, phenytoin, rifampin, and tacrolimus.

What are the possible side effects of Tindamax?
Side effects cannot be anticipated. If any develop or change in intensity, tell your doctor as soon as possible. Only your doctor can determine if it is safe for you to continue taking this drug.

Side effects may include: abdominal pain, loss of appetite, bitter or metallic taste, confusion, depression, difficulty breathing, drowsiness, fatigue, headache, loss of consciousness, nausea, skipped heartbeat, vaginal discharge, vomiting, weakness

Although rare, Tindamax has caused seizures and numbness or tingling in the arms, hands, legs, and feet. If you experience these symptoms stop taking Tindamax and call your doctor right away.

Can I receive Tindamax if I am pregnant or breastfeeding?
If you are pregnant or plan to become pregnant, tell your doctor immediately. Do not take Tindamax during the first 3 months of pregnancy or if

you are breastfeeding. Tindamax can be used during the last 6 months of pregnancy if your doctor decides the benefits outweigh the risks.

What should I do if I miss a dose of Tindamax?
Take the missed dose as soon as you remember. If it is almost time for your next dose, skip the one you missed and return to your regular schedule. Do not take 2 doses at once.

How should I store Tindamax?
Store Tindamax at room temperature and protect from light.

Tinidazole *See Tindamax, page 1307.*

Tiotropium bromide *See Spiriva HandiHaler, page 1213.*

Tipranavir *See Aptivus, page 118.*

Tizanidine *See Zanaflex, page 1443.*

Tobramycin *See Tobrex, below.*

TOBREX
Generic name: Tobramycin

What is Tobrex?
Tobrex is an antibiotic applied to the eye to treat bacterial infections.

What is the most important information I should know about Tobrex?
In order to clear up your infection completely, keep using Tobrex for the full time of treatment, even if your symptoms have disappeared.

Who should not take Tobrex?
Do not use Tobrex if you are sensitive to any component of the drug.

What should I tell my doctor before I take the first dose of Tobrex?
Mention all prescription, over-the-counter, and herbal medications you are taking before beginning treatment with Tobrex. Also, talk to your doctor about your complete medical history, especially if you have a viral or fungal infection in the eye.

What is the usual dosage?
The information below is based on the dosage guidelines your doctor uses. Depending on your condition and medical history, your doctor

may prescribe a different regimen. **Do not change the dosage or stop taking your medication without your doctor's approval.**

Adults using solution: If the infection is mild or moderate, place 1-2 drops into the affected eye(s) every 4 hours. In severe infections, place 2 drops into the eye(s) every hour until there is improvement. Then you will be instructed to use less medication before you stop using it altogether.

Adults using ointment: If the infection is mild to moderate, apply a ½-inch ribbon into the affected eye(s) 2-3 times per day. In severe infections, apply a ½-inch ribbon into the affected eye(s) every 3-4 hours until there is improvement. Then use less medication before stopping altogether.

How should I take Tobrex?

To apply Tobrex eye drops:
1. Wash your hands thoroughly with soap and water.
2. Gently pull down your lower eyelid to form a pocket between your eye and eyelid.
3. Brace the bottle on the bridge of your nose or your forehead.
4. Do not let the applicator tip touch your eye or any other surface.
5. Tilt your head back and squeeze the medication into the eye.
6. Keep your eyes closed for 1-2 minutes.
7. Do not rinse the dropper.
8. If you are using another eye drop wait 5-10 minutes before applying it.

To apply the ointment form of this medication:
1. Tilt your head back.
2. Place a finger on your cheek just under your eye and gently pull down until a "V" pocket is formed between your eyeball and your lower lid.
3. Place about a half an inch of Tobrex in the "V" pocket. Do not let the tip of the tube touch the eye.
4. Look downward before closing your eye.

What should I avoid while taking Tobrex?

Use Tobrex exactly as prescribed by your doctor. Do not touch the dropper or tube opening to any surface, including your eyes or hands. If it becomes contaminated it could cause an infection in the eye.

Do not wear contact lenses if you have an infection in your eye or when you are applying Tobrex eye drops or ointment.

Tobrex may cause blurred vision; use caution when driving, operating machinery, or performing other hazardous activities.

What are possible food and drug interactions associated with Tobrex?

If you are taking any other prescription antibiotics for your eyes, check with your doctor before using Tobrex.

What are the possible side effects of Tobrex?

Side effects cannot be anticipated. If any develop or change in intensity, tell your doctor as soon as possible. Only your doctor can determine if it is safe for you to continue taking this drug.

Side effects may include: abnormal redness of eye tissue, allergic reactions, lid itching, lid swelling

Can I receive Tobrex if I am pregnant or breastfeeding?

The effects of Tobrex during pregnancy and breastfeeding are unknown. Tell your doctor immediately if you are pregnant, plan to become pregnant, or are breastfeeding.

What should I do if I miss a dose of Tobrex?

Apply it as soon as you remember. If it is almost time for your next dose, skip the one you missed and go back to your regular schedule.

How should I store Tobrex?

Store at room temperature or in the refrigerator. Do not freeze and keep away from heat.

TOFRANIL/TOFRANIL-PM

Generic name: Imipramine

What is Tofranil/Tofranil-PM?

Tofranil and Tofranil-PM are used to treat depression. Tofranil is also used on a short-term basis, along with behavioral therapies, to treat bedwetting in children ages 6 and older.

What is the most important information I should know about Tofranil/Tofranil-PM?

Antidepressants can increase the risk of suicidal thinking and behavior in children and teenagers. Adult and pediatric patients taking antidepressants should be watched closely for changes in moods or actions, especially when they first start therapy or when their dose is increased or decreased. Patients and their families should contact the doctor immediately if new symptoms develop or seem to get worse. Signs to watch for include anxiety, hostility, insomnia, restlessness, impulsive or dangerous behavior, and thoughts about suicide or dying.

Never take Tofranil if you are taking another antidepressant drug called a monoamine oxidase inhibitor (MAOI) or if you have stopped taking an MAOI in the last 14 days. MAOI drugs include phenelzine, tranylcypromine, and isocarboxazid. Taking Tofranil within 2 weeks of an MAOI can result in serious—sometimes fatal—reactions, including high body temperature, coma, and seizures.

You should not take this medicine if you are recovering from a heart attack.

Who should not take Tofranil/Tofranil-PM?
Do not take Tofranil if you are recovering from a heart attack, if you are sensitive to the drug, or if you are using MAOI drugs or have used an MAOI in the last 14 days.

What should I tell my doctor before I take the first dose of Tofranil/Tofranil-PM?
Tell your doctor about all prescription, over-the-counter, and herbal medications you are taking before beginning treatment with Tofranil. Also, talk to your doctor about your complete medical history, especially if you have a history of heart disease, congestive heart failure, abnormal heart rhythm, have had a heart attack, stroke, rapid heartbeat, glaucoma (increased pressure in the eye), urinary retention, an enlarged prostate, overactive thyroid, seizure disorder, schizophrenia, bipolar disorder, kidney or liver disease, diabetes, if you will be undergoing surgery, or if you will be undergoing electroconvulsive therapy (ECT).

What is the usual dosage?
The information below is based on the dosage guidelines your doctor uses. Depending on your condition and medical history, your doctor may prescribe a different regimen. Do not change the dosage or stop taking your medication without your doctor's approval.

Depression
Adults: The usual dose is 75 milligrams (mg) a day. Your doctor may increase this to 150 mg a day. The maximum daily dose is 200 mg. People who need to take 75 mg or more a day may use Tofranil-PM capsules instead of the regular tablets.

Elderly and adolescents: The usual dose is 30 to 40 mg daily. Effective dosages usually do not exceed 100 mg a day.

Bedwetting
Children 6 years and older: The starting dose is 25 mg daily taken 1 hour before bedtime. If needed, this dose may be increased after 1 week to 50 mg (ages 6 to 11) or 75 mg (ages 12 and up), taken in one dose at bedtime or divided into 2 doses, 1 taken at mid-afternoon and 1 at bedtime.

The safety and effectiveness in children under the age of 6 have not been established. Tofranil-PM should not be used in children for any reason.

How should I take Tofranil/Tofranil-PM?
Take Tofranil exactly as prescribed by your doctor. Do not stop taking Tofranil if you feel no immediate effect. It can take anywhere from 1-3

weeks before you feel better. An abrupt decrease in dose could result in general feelings of illness, headache, and nausea.

Tofranil may be taken with or without food. It may be taken several times a day or in one daily dose at bedtime.

Tofranil can cause dry mouth. Sucking hard candy or chewing gum can help this problem.

What should I avoid while taking Tofranil/Tofranil-PM?
Do not drive or operate machinery, or participate in any activities that require full alertness until you know how this drug affects you.

Use alcohol cautiously. Alcohol may increase drowsiness and dizziness while taking Tofranil.

Tofranil can make you sensitive to light. Try to stay out of the sun as much as possible while you are taking it.

What are possible food and drug interactions associated with Tofranil/Tofranil-PM?
If Tofranil is taken with certain other drugs, the effects of either could be increased, decreased, or altered. It is especially important to check with your doctor before combining Tofranil with the following: albuterol, antidepressants, antipsychotic drugs, barbiturates such as phenobarbital, benztropine, blood pressure medications, carbamazepine, cimetidine, epinephrine, flecainide, guanethidine, methylphenidate, narcotic painkillers such as codeine and oxycodone, norepinephrine, phenytoin, propafenone, pseudoephedrine, quinidine, thyroid medications, and tranquilizers.

If you are switching from fluoxetine, wait at least 5 weeks after your last dose of fluoxetine before starting Tofranil.

What are the possible side effects of Tofranil/Tofranil-PM?
Side effects cannot be anticipated. If any develop or change in intensity, tell your doctor as soon as possible. Only your doctor can determine if it is safe for you to continue taking this drug.

Side effects may include: breast development in males, breast enlargement in females, breast milk production, confusion, diarrhea, dry mouth, hallucinations, hives, high blood pressure, low blood pressure upon standing, nausea, numbness, tremors, vomiting

Side effects in children being treated for bedwetting include: anxiety, collapse, constipation, convulsions, emotional instability, fainting, fatigue, nervousness, sleep disorders, stomach and intestinal problems

Can I receive Tofranil/Tofranil-PM if I am pregnant or breastfeeding?
The effects of Tofranil during pregnancy and breastfeeding are unknown. Tell your doctor immediately if you are pregnant, plan to become pregnant, or are breastfeeding.

What should I do if I miss a dose of Tofranil/Tofranil-PM?

If you take one dose a day at bedtime, contact your doctor. Do not take the dose in the morning because of possible side effects.

If you take two or more doses a day, take the forgotten dose as soon as you remember. If it is almost time for your next dose, skip the one you missed and go back to your regular schedule. Do not take two doses at once.

How should I store Tofranil/Tofranil-PM?

Store at room temperature in a tightly closed container.

Tolbutamide See Orinase, page 953.

Tolcapone See Tasmar, page 1263.

Tolterodine tartrate See Detrol, page 406.

Tolterodine tartrate, extended-release See Detrol LA, page 408.

TOPAMAX

Generic name: Topiramate

What is Topamax?

Topamax is an antiepileptic drug, prescribed to control both mild attacks known as partial seizures and severe tonic-clonic convulsions known as grand mal seizures. It is typically added to the treatment regimen when other drugs fail to fully control a patient's seizures.

Topamax is also prescribed for the prevention of migraine headaches. However, due to a lack of studies, it is not known whether the drug can treat a migraine once it has already started.

What is the most important information I should know about Topamax?

Topamax has been known to cause a potentially serious condition called metabolic acidosis (an increase of acid in the blood). In children, chronic metabolic acidosis may affect growth or cause rickets (a softening or weakness of the bones that can lead to bone deformities). Contact your doctor immediately if you experience symptoms of metabolic acidosis such as rapid breathing, an irregular heartbeat, confusion, lethargy, fatigue, or loss of appetite. Your doctor will decide if you should stop taking Topamax. Do not abruptly stop taking Topamax on your own; your doctor will gradually taper the dosage to avoid an increase in seizures.

Topamax has been known to trigger severe nearsightedness along with increased pressure inside the eye. The problem usually occurs within 1 month of starting treatment. If you develop blurred vision or eye pain, call your doctor immediately. You may have to stop taking the drug in order to prevent permanent vision loss.

Who should not take Topamax?

Do not take Topamax if you are allergic to the medication or any or its ingredients.

What should I tell my doctor before I take the first dose of Topamax?

Mention all prescription, over-the-counter, and herbal medications you are taking before beginning treatment with Topamax. Also, talk to your doctor about your complete medical history, especially if you have: asthma, bronchitis, emphysema, glaucoma, growth problems, kidney disease or a history of kidney stones, liver disease, metabolic acidosis (blood and body fluid abnormality), osteoporosis (weak or brittle bones) and/or soft bones (osteomalacia) or decreased bone density (osteopenia), or paresthesia.

Be sure to let your doctor know if you are on a high-fat diet, called a ketogenic diet, or if you have recently had surgery.

What is the usual dosage?

The information below is based on the dosage guidelines your doctor uses. Depending on your condition and medical history, your doctor may prescribe a different regimen. Do not change the dosage or stop taking your medication without your doctor's approval.

Adults: If you have liver or kidney problems, or are undergoing hemodialysis, the doctor may need to adjust the dosages listed below.

Prevention of Migraine Headaches
Adults: The recommended total daily dose is 100 milligrams (mg) a day, taken in two divided doses. Your doctor will increase the dose slowly over 4 weeks. The usual regimen is as follows:

Week 1: No morning dose; take 25 mg at night.
Week 2: Take 25 mg in the morning and another 25 mg at night.
Week 3: Take 25 mg in the morning and 50 mg at night.
Week 4: Take 50 mg in the morning and 50 mg at night.

Seizures
Adults: Topamax therapy usually begins with a dose of 25 mg twice a day during the first week. The daily dosage is then increased each week until you are taking 200 mg twice a day by the eighth week.

If you are also taking phenytoin or carbamazepine, the dosage of Topamax may need to be adjusted.

Children: The usual daily dose for children 2 to 16 years of age is 5 to 9 mg for every 2.2 pounds of body weight, divided into two doses. Topamax therapy usually begins with a dose of 25 mg (or less) once daily during the first week. The daily dosage is then increased each week until the doctor is satisfied with the response. It may take eight weeks to reach the ideal dose.

How should I take Topamax?

It is important to take Topamax exactly as prescribed. You can take it with or without food, but because of the medication's bitter taste, you should avoid breaking the tablets.

You can swallow Topamax capsules whole, or you can open the capsule and sprinkle its contents on a teaspoonful of soft food. To open the capsule, hold it so you can read the word "top" and carefully twist off the clear portion of the capsule. Do not chew the drug and food mixture; swallow it whole. Do not store the mixture for future use.

Topamax increases your risk of developing kidney stones. To prevent this problem, be sure to take Topamax with plenty of fluids.

What should I avoid while taking Topamax?

If you are taking Topamax or other antiepileptic drugs for epilepsy or seizures, you may need to avoid activities where loss of consciousness (passing out) could result in serious danger to yourself or those around you. Talk to your doctor before engaging in activities such as swimming, driving a car, and climbing in high places.

Do not drive a car or operate heavy machinery until you know how Topamax affects you. Topamax can impair your thinking, motor skills, and/or vision.

Avoid drinking alcoholic beverages with Topamax.

Unless prescribed by your healthcare professional, you should avoid other medicines like central nervous system depressants, which also impair or decrease your thinking, concentration, or muscle coordination.

Avoid becoming overheated or dehydrated during exercise and in hot weather. Drink extra fluids in these situations.

What are possible food and drug interactions associated with Topamax?

If Topamax is taken with certain other drugs, the effects of either could be increased, decreased, or altered. It is especially important to check with your doctor before combining Topamax with the following: acetazolamide, amitriptyline, carbamazepine, dichlorphenamide, digoxin, metformin, phenytoin, oral contraceptives, risperidone, or valproic acid.

Topamax can depress the central nervous system. Be extremely cautious about combining it with alcohol, sedatives, tranquilizers, and other central nervous system depressants.

What are the possible side effects of Topamax?

Side effects cannot be anticipated. If any develop or change in intensity, tell your doctor as soon as possible. Only your doctor can determine if it is safe for you to continue taking this drug.

Side effects may include: diarrhea, hair loss, loss of appetite, nausea, taste change, tingling in arms and legs, tiredness, upper respiratory tract infection, viral infection, weight loss

Can I receive Topamax if I am pregnant or breastfeeding?
The effects of Topamax during pregnancy and breastfeeding are unknown. Tell your doctor immediately if you are pregnant, plan to become pregnant, or are breastfeeding.

What should I do if I miss a dose of Topamax?
Take it as soon as you remember. If it is almost time for your next dose, skip the one you missed and go back to your regular schedule. Never take two doses at once.

How should I store Topamax?
Store at room temperature in a tightly closed container. Protect the tablets from moisture.

TOPICORT
Generic name: Desoximetasone

What is Topicort?
Topicort is a synthetic steroid medication that is used as an anti-inflammatory and anti-pruritic. It is available in cream, gel, and ointment forms.

What is the most important information I should know about Topicort?
When you use Topicort, some of the medication may be absorbed through your skin and into your bloodstream. Too much absorption can lead to unwanted side effects elsewhere in your body. To keep this problem to a minimum, avoid using large amounts of Topicort over large areas; do not use Topicort for extended periods of time; and do not cover areas to which you have applied Topicort with airtight dressings such as plastic wrap or adhesive bandages, unless your doctor specifically tells you to.

Who should not take Topicort?
Do not take Topicort if you are allergic to the medication or any of its ingredients.

What should I tell my doctor before I take the first dose of Topicort?
Mention all prescription, over-the-counter, and herbal medications you are taking before beginning treatment with Topicort. Also, talk to your doctor about your complete medical history.

What is the usual dosage?
The information below is based on the dosage guidelines your doctor uses. Depending on your condition and medical history, your doctor may prescribe a different regimen. Do not change the dosage or stop taking your medication without your doctor's approval.

Adults: Apply a thin film of Topicort cream, gel, or ointment to the affected area 2 times a day. Rub in gently.

Children: Use the least amount of Topicort necessary to relieve symptoms. Ask your doctor for specific instructions.

Topicort is not recommended for children under 10 years of age.

How should I take Topicort?
Topicort is only for use on the skin. Be sure to keep this medication out of your eyes.

Apply a thin coating of Topicort to the affected area. Rub in gently. The treated area should not be covered unless your doctor has told you to do so.

If Topicort is being used for an infant or toddler with a genital rash, make sure the diapers or plastic pants are not too tight, so that air can circulate.

What should I avoid while taking Topicort?
Avoid getting Topicort in your eyes. Do not use it to treat any condition other than the one for which it was prescribed.

Avoid covering a treated area with tight waterproof diapers or plastic pants. They can increase unwanted absorption of Topicort.

What are possible food and drug interactions associated with Topicort?
No interactions have been reported.

What are the possible side effects of Topicort?
Side effects cannot be anticipated. If any develop or change in intensity, tell your doctor as soon as possible. Only your doctor can determine if it is safe for you to continue taking this drug.

Side effects may include: acne-like pimples, blistering, burning of the skin, dryness, excessive hair growth, infection, inflammation of hair follicles, irritation, itching, loss of skin pigmentation, prickly heat, skin inflammation around the mouth, rash, redness, softening of the skin, stretch marks on the skin, thinning of the skin

Can I receive Topicort if I am pregnant or breastfeeding?
The effects of Topicort during pregnancy and breastfeeding are unknown. Tell your doctor immediately if you are pregnant, plan to become pregnant, or are breastfeeding.

What should I do if I miss a dose of Topicort?

Use Topicort only as needed, in the smallest amount required for relief. Do not apply Topicort twice in order to make up for a missed dose.

How should I store Topicort?

Store at room temperature.

Topiramate *See Topamax, page 1315.*

Torsemide *See Demadex, page 387.*

Tramadol hydrochloride *See Ultram, page 1351.*

Tramadol hydrochloride and acetaminophen *See Ultracet, page 1348.*

Trandolapril *See Mavik, page 787.*

Trandolapril and verapamil hydrochloride *See Tarka, page 1261.*

TRANXENE

Generic name: Clorazepate dipotassium

What is Tranxene?

Tranxene T-Tab and Tranxene tablets belong to a class of drugs known as benzodiazepines. Tranxene is used to treat anxiety disorders and for the short-term relief of anxiety symptoms. The drug is also used to relieve the symptoms of acute alcohol withdrawal and to help in treating certain convulsive disorders such as epilepsy.

What is the most important information I should know about Tranxene?

Tranxene may be habit-forming if taken regularly over a long period. You may experience withdrawal symptoms if you stop using this drug abruptly. Consult your doctor before discontinuing Tranxene or making any change in your dose.

This drug has not been studied in children less than 9 years old.

Who should not take Tranxene?

Do not use Tranxene if you have a known hypersensitivity to the drug or if you have an eye condition known as acute narrow-angle glaucoma.

What should I tell my doctor before I take the first dose of Tranxene?

Tell your doctor about all prescription, over-the-counter, and herbal medication you are taking before beginning treatment with Tranxene. Also, talk to your doctor about your complete medical history, especially if you are being treated for depression or anxiety or if you have a history of drug abuse or dependence.

What is the usual dosage?
The information below is based on the dosage guidelines your doctor uses. Depending on your condition and medical history, your doctor may prescribe a different regimen. Do not change the dosage or stop taking your medication without your doctor's approval.

Anxiety
Adults: Tranxene T-Tab is administered orally in divided doses. The usual daily dose is 30 milligrams (mg). The dose should be adjusted gradually within the range of 15-60 mg daily depending on your response. In elderly or debilitated patients, treatment may start at a daily dose of 7.5-15 mg. It can be given as a single dose at bedtime starting at 15 mg. Tranxene tablets may be given as a single dose every 24 hours after you are stable on a fixed dose divided throughout the day and can be switched to a once daily dose for convenience.

Alcohol Withdrawal Symptoms
Adults: The doctor will provide a schedule of reducing daily doses until your condition is stable.

Add-on Therapy with Antiepileptic Drugs
Adults and children over 12 years old: The starting dose is 7.5 milligrams (mg) 3 times a day. Your doctor may increase the dosage by 7.5 mg per week to a maximum of 90 mg a day.

Children 9-12 years old: The starting dose is 7.5 mg 2 times a day. Your doctor may increase the dosage by 7.5 mg per week to a maximum of 60 mg a day.

How should I take Tranxene?
Take Tranxene exactly as prescribed. Do not increase the amount you take or the number of doses per day without your doctor's approval.

What should I avoid while taking Tranxene?
Avoid driving a car or operating machinery until you know how Tranxene affects you. Also avoid alcohol and other central nervous system depressants while taking this drug.

What are possible food and drug interactions associated with Tranxene?
If Tranxene is taken with certain other drugs, the effects of either could be increased, decreased, or altered. Always check with your doctor before combining Tranxene T-Tabs with the following: antidepressants including monoamine oxidase inhibitors or tricyclics, antipsychotics, barbiturates,

narcotic pain relievers, and alcohol or other central nervous system depressants.

What are the possible side effects of Tranxene?

Side effects cannot be anticipated. If any develop or change in intensity, tell your doctor as soon as possible. Only your doctor can determine if it is safe for you to continue taking this drug.

Side effects may include: drowsiness, dizziness, stomach complaints, nervousness, blurred vision, dry mouth, headache, mental confusion

Can I receive Tranxene if I am pregnant or breastfeeding?

Tell your doctor if you are pregnant, plan to become pregnant, or are breastfeeding before taking this drug. Several studies have suggested an increased risk of birth defects associated with using minor tranquilizers during the first trimester of pregnancy. Because treatment with minor tranquilizers is rarely a matter of urgency, their use during this period should almost always be avoided. Tranxene should not be given to nursing mothers.

What should I do if I miss a dose of Tranxene?

Take it as soon as you remember. If it is almost time for your next dose, skip the one you missed and go back to your regular schedule. Never take 2 doses at the same time.

How should I store Tranxene?

Store at room temperature in a tightly closed, light-resistant container. Protect from moisture and excessive heat.

Tranylcypromine sulfate *See Parnate, page 976.*

TRAVATAN

Generic name: Travoprost

What is Travatan?

Travatan is an eyedrop that reduces excessive pressure in the eye (often a result of a condition called open-angle glaucoma). Travatan works by promoting drainage of the fluid that fills the eye. It is usually prescribed when you cannot use other remedies or when other drugs have not been effective.

What is the most important information I should know about Travatan?

Over a period of months or years, Travatan may permanently darken the color of your iris and eyelid. It may also increase the darkness, length, and thickness of your eyelashes. If you need Travatan in only one eye, this may cause a noticeable difference.

Contact your doctor immediately if you develop any adverse eye reactions while using Travatan, especially conjunctivitis (pinkeye) and eyelid reactions.

The safety and effectiveness of Travatan in children have not been established.

Who should not take Travatan?
You should avoid Travatan if you are allergic to travoprost, benzalkonium chloride, or any of the drug's other ingredients.

What should I tell my doctor before I take the first dose of Travatan?
Tell your doctor about all prescription, over-the-counter, and herbal medication you are taking before beginning treatment with Travatan. Also, talk to your doctor about your complete medical history, especially if you have an eye injury or infection, an inflammation of the iris, or swelling of the macular part of the eye.

What is the usual dosage?
The information below is based on the dosage guidelines your doctor uses. Depending on your condition and medical history, your doctor may prescribe a different regimen. Do not change the dosage or stop taking your medication without your doctor's approval.

Adults: Place one drop in the affected eye(s) once a day in the evening.

How should I take Travatan?
Gently pull your lower eyelid down to form a pocket, and then place a drop of Travatan in the pouch. Gently press your finger to the inside corner of the eye (near the nose) for about 1 minute to keep the liquid from draining into your tear duct.

Do not place Travatan in the eyes while wearing contact lenses. Remove the lenses before administering Travatan and wait 15 minutes before reinserting them.

If you need to use another eye medication along with Travatan, the drugs should be applied at least 5 minutes apart.

What should I avoid while taking Travatan?
Handle the Travatan solution carefully. Do not allow the tip of the bottle to come in contact with your eye or any surface. This could contaminate the solution and lead to an infection that seriously damages the eye.

Avoid using too much of this medication; overuse can actually make Travatan less effective in lowering the pressure inside your eye.

What are possible food and drug interactions associated with Travatan?
No interactions have been reported.

What are the possible side effects of Travatan?
Side effects cannot be anticipated. If any develop or change in intensity, tell your doctor as soon as possible. Only your doctor can determine if it is safe for you to continue taking this drug.

Side effects may include: decreased visual sharpness, eye discomfort, eye pain or itching, redness in the eye, sensation of a foreign body in the eye

Can I receive Travatan if I am pregnant or breastfeeding?
The effects of Travatan during pregnancy and breastfeeding are unknown. Tell your doctor immediately if you are pregnant, plan to become pregnant, or are breastfeeding.

What should I do if I miss a dose of Travatan?
Take it as soon as you remember. If it is almost time for your next dose, skip the dose you missed and go back to your regular schedule. Do not take 2 doses at once.

How should I store Travatan?
Store at room temperature. Throw away any unused medication after 6 weeks.

TRAVATAN Z
Generic name: Travoprost ophthalmic solution

What is Travatan Z?
Travatan Z is used to treat high intraocular pressure (IOP) in people who have glaucoma (high pressure in the eye) or ocular hypertension. This drug is used only when other drugs have failed to lower IOP.

What is the most important information I should know about Travatan Z?
Travatan Z may cause your iris (the colored part of the eye) and eyelid to become darker. Also, your eyelashes may become darker and longer. These changes may be permanent.

It takes about 2 hours for this medication to start working; do not take more then the recommend amount if relief is not immediate.

Who should not take Travatan Z?
Do not take Travatan Z if you are allergic to any of its ingredients.

What should I tell my doctor before I take the first dose of Travatan Z?

Tell your doctor about all prescription, over-the-counter, and herbal medications you are taking before beginning treatment with Travatan Z. Also, talk to your doctor about your complete medical history, especially if you have a history of eye-swelling or currently have it.

What is the usual dosage?

The information below is based on the dosage guidelines your doctor uses. Depending on your condition and medical history, your doctor may prescribe a different regimen. Do not change the dosage or stop taking your medication without your doctor's approval.

The recommended dosage of Travatan Z is one drop in the affected eye(s) once daily, in the evening.

How should I take Travatan Z?

Use the dispenser to put one drop of Travatan Z into the eye(s) each evening.

If you are using Travatan Z with another drug for your eyes, make sure that you separate the administration of the second drug by 5 minutes.

What should I avoid while taking Travatan Z?

While using Travatan Z, do not allow the tip of the dispenser to touch your eye; the dispenser may then have bacteria growth on it, which may lead to an infection in your eye.

The dosage of Travatan Z ophthalmic solution should not exceed once daily since it may not work as well if used more frequently.

What are possible food and drug interactions associated with Travatan Z?

No significant interactions have been reported at this time. However, always tell your doctor about any medicines you take, including over-the-counter drugs, vitamins, and herbal supplements.

What are the possible side effects of Travatan Z?

Side effects cannot be anticipated. If any develop or change in intensity, tell your doctor as soon as possible. Only your doctor can determine if it is safe for you to continue taking this drug.

Side effects may include: blurred vision, eye discomfort, foreign body sensation, itching, pain

Can I receive Travatan Z if I am pregnant or breastfeeding?

Talk to your doctor if you are pregnant, planning to become pregnant, or are nursing. The effects of Travatan Z are unknown on pregnancy, and it may pass into your breast milk.

What should I do if I miss a dose of Travatan Z?
If you miss a dose and it's less than 24 hours of your next dose, skip it and return to your normal scheduled time.. Do not exceed more than one dose in a 24 hour period. Never double your dose.

How should I store Travatan Z?
Store either at room temperature or in the refrigerator.

Travoprost See Travatan, page 1322.

Travoprost ophthalmic solution See Travatan Z, page 1324.

TRAZODONE HYDROCHLORIDE

What is Trazodone hydrochloride?
Trazodone is used to treat depression.

What is the most important information I should know about Trazodone hydrochloride?
Antidepressant medicines may increase suicidal thoughts or actions in some children, teenagers, and young adults when the medicine is first started. Depression and other serious mental illnesses are the most important causes of suicidal thoughts and actions. Some people may have a particularly high risk of having suicidal thoughts or actions. These include people who have (or have a family history of) bipolar disorder (also called manic-depressive illness) or suicidal thoughts or actions.

Pay close attention to any changes, especially sudden changes, in mood, behaviors, thoughts, or feelings. This is very important when an antidepressant medicine is first started or when the dose is changed.

Call the doctor right away to report new or sudden changes in mood, behavior, thoughts, or feelings. Signs to watch for include new or worsening depression, new or worsening anxiety, agitation, insomnia, hostility, panic attacks, restlessness, extreme hyperactivity, and suicidal thinking or behavior.

Keep all follow-up visits as scheduled, and call the doctor between visits as needed, especially if you have concerns about symptoms.

Who should not take Trazodone hydrochloride?
The safety and efficacy of trazodone in pediatric patients have not been established.

Trazodone is not recommended for use during the initial recovery phase of myocardial infarction (heart attack).

Caution should be used when administering trazodone to patients with cardiac disease, since antidepressants have been associated with the occurrence of cardiac arrhythmias.

What should I tell my doctor before I take the first dose of Trazodone hydrochloride?

Tell your doctor about all prescription, over-the-counter, and herbal medications you are taking before beginning treatment with trazodone. Also, talk to your doctor about your complete medical history, especially if you have been diagnosed with bipolar disorder in the past, have or had any heart problems, are currently taking other antidepressants, or have liver or kidney problems.

What is the usual dosage?

The information below is based on the dosage guidelines your doctor uses. Depending on your condition and medical history, your doctor may prescribe a different regimen. Do not change the dosage or stop taking your medication without your doctor's approval.

Adults: The usual starting dose is 150 milligrams (mg) daily in divided doses. The dose may be increased by 50 mg per day every three to four days if needed. The maximum daily dose should not exceed 400 mg. Although symptomatic relief may be seen during the first week of therapy, it is generally recommended that a course of antidepressant drug treatment should continue for several months.

How should I take Trazodone hydrochloride?

Take a major portion of the total daily dose at bedtime, preferably after a meal or light snack.

What should I avoid while taking Trazodone hydrochloride?

Since trazodone may cause drowsiness, avoid performing activities that require alertness, such as driving or operating machinery, until you learn how this medication affects you. Also avoid alcohol while on trazodone, since this may cause excessive sedation.

What are possible food and drug interactions associated with Trazodone hydrochloride?

If trazodone is used with certain other drugs, the effects of either could be increased, decreased, or altered. It is especially important to check with your doctor before combining trazodone with the following: aspirin and aspirin products, carbamazepine, digoxin, indinavir, itraconazole, keto-conazole, MAOIs, nefazodone, phenytoin, ritonavir, and warfarin.

What are the possible side effects of Trazodone hydrochloride?

Side effects cannot be anticipated. If any develop or change in intensity, tell your doctor as soon as possible. Only your doctor can determine if it is safe for you to continue taking this drug.

Side effects may include: changes in mood or behavior, dizziness, drowsiness, nausea, blurred vision, dry mouth, muscle aches, decreased libido, weight gain or loss, priapism (prolonged or painful erections)

Can I receive Trazodone hydrochloride if I am pregnant or breastfeeding?

The effects of trazodone during pregnancy and breastfeeding are unknown. Tell your doctor immediately if you are pregnant, plan to become pregnant, or are breastfeeding.

What should I do if I miss a dose of Trazodone hydrochloride?

Skip the dose and continue with your normal dosing schedule. Never double the dose.

How should I store Trazodone hydrochloride?

Store at room temperature.

TRENTAL

Generic name: Pentoxifylline

What is Trental?

Trental reduces the viscosity or stickiness of your blood, allowing it to flow more freely. It helps relieve the painful leg cramps caused by intermittent claudication, a condition that results when hardening of the arteries reduces the leg muscles' blood supply.

What is the most important information I should know about Trental?

Trental can ease the pain in your legs and make walking easier but should not replace other treatments, such as physical therapy or surgery.

Who should not take Trental?

Do not take Trental if you have recently had a stroke or bleeding in the retina of your eye.

If you are sensitive to or have ever had an allergic reaction to Trental, caffeine, theophylline (medication for asthma or other breathing disorders), or theobromine, do not take Trental. Make sure that your doctor is aware of any drug reactions that you have experienced.

What should I tell my doctor before I take the first dose of Trental?

Mention all prescription, over-the-counter, and herbal medications you are taking before beginning treatment with Trental. Also, talk to your doctor about your complete medical history, especially if you have an ulcer disease (stomach or duodenal ulcer), had any type of surgery (including dental), or if you have an irregular heartbeat because of heart disease and brain disorders. Make sure to let your doctor know if you have a bleeding disorder, liver disease, crushing chest pain, or low blood pressure.

What is the usual dosage?

The information below is based on the dosage guidelines your doctor uses. Depending on your condition and medical history, your doctor may prescribe a different regimen. Do not change the dosage or stop taking your medication without your doctor's approval.

Adults: The usual dosage of Trental in controlled-release tablets is one 400 milligram (mg) tablet 3 times a day with meals.

While the effect of Trental may be seen within 2 to 4 weeks, it is recommended that treatment be continued for at least 8 weeks.

Children: The safety and effectiveness of Trental in children have not been established.

How should I take Trental?

Trental comes in controlled-release tablets. Do not break, crush, or chew the tablets; swallow them whole. Take Trental exactly as prescribed.

What should I avoid while taking Trental?

Avoid using tobacco while you are taking Trental. Tobacco may worsen your condition or decrease the beneficial effects of Trental by narrowing your blood vessels.

What are possible food and drug interactions associated with Trental?

If Trental is taken with certain other drugs, the effects of either could be increased, decreased, or altered. It is especially important to check with your doctor before combining Trental with the following: blood pressure medications such as enalapril and diltiazem, blood-thinning medications such as warfarin, clot inhibitors such as dipyridamole, theophylline, or ulcer medicines such as cimetidine.

What are the possible side effects of Trental?

Side effects cannot be anticipated. If any develop or change in intensity, tell your doctor as soon as possible. Only your doctor can determine if it is safe for you to continue taking this drug.

Side effects may include: allergic reaction, anxiety, bad taste in the mouth, blind spot in vision, blurred vision, brittle fingernails, chest pain, confusion, pinkeye, constipation, depression, difficult or labored breathing, dizziness, dry mouth/thirst, earache, excessive salivation, flu-like symptoms, fluid retention, general body discomfort, headache, hives, indigestion, itching, laryngitis, loss of appetite, low blood pressure, nosebleeds, rash, seizures, sore throat/swollen neck glands, stuffy nose, tremor, vomiting, weight change

Can I receive Trental if I am pregnant or breastfeeding?

The effects of Trental during pregnancy are unknown. Tell your doctor immediately if you are pregnant, or plan to become pregnant.

Trental appears in breast milk and could affect a nursing infant. If Trental is essential to your health, your doctor may advise you to discontinue breastfeeding until your treatment with Trental is finished.

What should I do if I miss a dose of Trental?

Take it as soon as you remember. If it is almost time for your next dose, skip the dose you missed and go back to your regular schedule. Never take 2 doses at the same time.

How should I store Trental?

Store Trental in the container it came in, at room temperature. Keep the container tightly closed and away from light.

Tretinoin *See Atralin, page 146, or Retin-A and Renova, page 1141.*

TREXIMET

Generic name: Sumatriptan and naproxen

What is Treximet?

Treximet is used to treat migraine attacks in adults. It does not, however, prevent or reduce the number of migraines you have, nor is it used for other types of headaches.

What is the most important information I should know about Treximet?

Treximet contains sumatriptan and naproxen (a nonsteroidal anti-inflammatory drug, or NSAID). NSAIDs may increase the chance of heart attack or stroke, which can lead to death, especially during prolonged use and in patients with heart disease.

NSAIDs should never be used before or after heart bypass surgery.

NSAIDs can cause ulcers and bleeding in the stomach and intestines.

Who should not take Treximet?

Do not take Treximet for pain following heart surgery. You should not take Treximet if you have high blood pressure, liver problems, a history of stroke, asthma, or allergic reactions to aspirin, any other NSAID, or sumatriptan.

Do not take Treximet within 2 weeks of taking an antidepressant called a monoamine oxidase (MAO) inhibitor.

What should I tell my doctor before I take the first dose of Treximet?

Tell your doctor about all prescription, over-the-counter, and herbal medications you are taking before beginning treatment with Treximet. Also talk to your doctor about your complete medical history, especially if you have any known allergies to NSAIDS, are pregnant or breastfeeding, have chest pain, shortness of breath, or kidney or liver problems.

What is the usual dosage?

The information below is based on the dosage guidelines your doctor uses. Depending on your condition and medical history, your doctor may prescribe a different regimen. Do not change the dosage or stop taking your medication without your doctor's approval.

Adults: The recommended dose is 1 tablet. Do not take more than 2 tablets in 24 hours.

How should I take Treximet?

Take Treximet as prescribed. It can be taken with or without food. Tablets should not be crushed, split, or chewed.

What should I avoid while taking Treximet?

Avoid smoking, alcohol and taking with blood thinners or corticosteroids to reduce your risk of getting ulcers or bleeding.

Avoid taking other migraine medicines within 24 hours of taking Treximet.

What are possible food and drug interactions associated with Treximet?

If Treximet is taken with certain other drugs, the effects of either could be increased, decreased, or altered. It is especially important to check with your doctor before combining Treximet with ACE inhibitors, aspirin, blood thinners, cyclosporine, diuretics, lithium, methotrexate, or MAO inhibitors.

Serotonin syndrome is a serious, life-threatening problem that may occur with Treximet, especially if used with antidepressants known as selective serotonin reuptake inhibitors (SSRIs) or selective norepinephrine reuptake inhibitors (SNRIs).

What are the possible side effects of Treximet?

Side effects cannot be anticipated. If any develop or change in intensity, tell your doctor as soon as possible. Only your doctor can determine if it is safe for you to continue taking this drug.

Side effects may include: allergic reactions, heart attack, stroke, high blood pressure, heart failure, kidney problems, liver problems, asthma attacks in people who have asthma, stomach pain, diarrhea, gas

Call for emergency help if you have any of the following: shortness of breath, chest pain, slurred speech, swelling of face or throat, weakness on one part or side of the body.

Can I receive Treximet if I am pregnant or breastfeeding?
Treximet should be avoided during pregnancy and breastfeeding.

What should I do if I miss a dose of Treximet?
If you miss a dose, take it as soon as you remember. If it is within 12 hours of your next dose, do not take the missed dose. Just take the next dose at your regular time. Do not take 2 doses at the same.

How should I store Treximet?
Store at room temperature.

Triamcinolone acetonide *See Azmacort, page 185.*

Triazolam *See Halcion, page 634.*

TRICOR
Generic name: Fenofibrate

What is Tricor?
Tricor, in addition to an appropriate diet, is used to treat adults with high cholesterol, with or without elevated triglycerides. Tricor reduces elevated LDL-C (bad cholesterol), total cholesterol, triglycerides, and apolipoprotein B, and increases HDL-C (good cholesterol). Tricor is also used to treat adults with high triglycerides.

What is the most important information I should know about Tricor?
You should let your doctor know if you are taking any other drugs while taking Tricor. Tricor tablets may have an effect on drugs that help prevent blood clotting, such as the blood thinner warfarin. If you are taking Tricor tablets with a blood-thinning medication, your healthcare provider may want to monitor your blood-clotting tests more frequently. You should alert your healthcare provider about any cholesterol-lowering medications you may be taking as he or she will need to determine if the combination of Tricor tablets and one of those drugs is right for you.

Tricor may also affect liver function. Your doctor should perform periodic blood tests to monitor the health of your liver.

Who should not take Tricor?
You should not take Tricor if you have liver or gallbladder disease, severe kidney problems, or if you are allergic to it or any of its ingredients.

What should I tell my doctor before I take the first dose of Tricor?

Mention all prescription, over-the-counter, and herbal medications you are taking before beginning treatment with Tricor. Also, talk to your doctor about your complete medical history, especially if you have any type of liver disease, kidney disease, gallbladder disease, hypothyroidism (an underactive thyroid gland), or high blood sugar.

What is the usual dosage?

The information below is based on the dosage guidelines your doctor uses. Depending on your condition and medical history, your doctor may prescribe a different regimen. Do not change the dosage or stop taking your medication without your doctor's approval.

High Cholesterol Levels or a Combination of High Cholesterol and High Triglycerides
Adults: The initial dose of Tricor is 145 milligrams (mg) per day.

High Triglyceride Levels
Adults: The starting dose of Tricor ranges from 48 to 145 mg per day. The maximum dose of Tricor is 145 mg a day.

Children: Tricor has not been tested in children.

Older adults: The starting dose of Tricor for older adults and those with poor kidney function is 48 mg per day.

How should I take Tricor?

Tricor tablets can be taken with or without food.

What should I avoid while taking Tricor?

Avoid drinking alcohol while taking Tricor. Alcohol can raise triglyceride levels, and may also damage your liver while you are taking Tricor.

What are possible food and drug interactions associated with Tricor?

If Tricor is taken with certain other drugs, the effects of either could be increased, decreased, or altered. It is especially important to check with your doctor before combining Tricor with any of the following: blood thinners such as warfarin; cholesterol-lowering drugs colestipol and cholestyramine; cyclosporine; and cholesterol-lowering drugs known as statins, including fluvastatin, atorvastatin, lovastatin, pravastatin, and simvastatin.

What are the possible side effects of Tricor?

Side effects cannot be anticipated. If any develop or change in intensity, tell your doctor as soon as possible. Only your doctor can determine if it is safe for you to continue taking this drug.

Side effects may include: abdominal pain, back pain, headache, respiratory disorders

Can I receive Tricor if I am pregnant or breastfeeding?
The effects of Tricor during pregnancy and breastfeeding are unknown. Tell your doctor immediately if you are pregnant, plan to become pregnant, or are breastfeeding.

What should I do if I miss a dose of Tricor?
Take it as soon as you remember. If it is almost time for your next dose, skip the dose you missed and go back to your regular schedule. Never take 2 doses at the same time.

How should I store Tricor?
Store at room temperature and protect from moisture.

TRIGLIDE
Generic name: Fenofibrate

What is Triglide?
Triglide is a fenofibrate, and is used in combination with a healthy diet and exercise to lower LDL-cholesterol. LDL-cholesterol is known as the "bad" cholesterol, and stands for low-density lipoprotein.

What is the most important information I should know about Triglide?
Triglide should be used in combination with a healthy diet and exercise to reduce cholesterol levels. Triglide should not be used with blood thinners or statins.

Who should not take Triglide?
If you have kidney, liver, or gallbladder problems, do not take Triglide. Also, if you are allergic to one or more of the ingredients in Triglide, do not begin this type of cholesterol-lowering therapy.

What should I tell my doctor before I take the first dose of Triglide?
Mention all medications you are taking before beginning treatment with Triglide. Also, talk with your doctor about your complete medical history, especially if you are taking other cholesterol-lowering medications known as statins, or blood thinners.

What is the usual dosage?
The information below is based on the dosage guidelines your doctor uses. Depending on your condition and medical history, your doctor

may prescribe a different regimen. **Do not change the dosage or stop taking your medication without your doctor's approval.**

*High Cholesterol Levels or a Combination
of High Cholesterol and High Triglycerides*
Adults: The initial dose of Triglide is 160 milligrams (mg) per day.

High Triglyceride Levels
Adults: The starting dose of Triglide ranges from 50 to 160 mg per day.

Children: Triglide has not been tested in children.

Older adults: The starting dose of Triglide for older adults and those with poor kidney function is 50 mg per day.

How should I take Triglide?
Triglide may be taken with or without food.

What should I avoid while taking Triglide?
Do not start an exercise plan without talking to your doctor first.

What are possible food and drug interactions associated with Triglide?
If Triglide is taken with certain other drugs, the effects of either could be increased, decreased, or altered. It is especially important to check with your doctor before combining Triglide with blood thinners, cyclosporine, or other cholesterol-lowering medications known as statins.

What are the possible side effects of Triglide?
Side effects cannot be anticipated. If any develop or change in intensity, tell your doctor as soon as possible. Only your doctor can determine if it is safe for you to continue taking this drug.

Side effects may include: back pain, chest pain, constipation, diarrhea, flu-like symptoms, nausea, headache, stomach pain, weakness

Can I receive Triglide if I am pregnant or breastfeeding?
The effects of Triglide during pregnancy and breastfeeding are unknown. Tell your doctor immediately if you are pregnant, plan to become pregnant, or are breastfeeding.

What should I do if I miss a dose of Triglide?
Take the missed dose as soon as you remember it. However, if it is almost time for your next dose, skip the one you missed and return to your regular dosing schedule. Do not double the dose.

How should I store Triglide?
Store at room temperature away from light and moisture.

TRILEPTAL
Generic name: Oxcarbazepine

What is Trileptal?

Trileptal helps reduce the frequency of partial epileptic seizures, a form of epilepsy in which neural disturbances are limited to a specific region of the brain and the victim remains conscious throughout the attack. Trileptal may be prescribed by itself to treat this problem in adults, or it can also be used in combination with other seizure medications in adults and children as young as 4 years old.

What is the most important information I should know about Trileptal?

Trileptal can lead to a loss of sodium from the blood. This can result in a serious medical condition, which, if left untreated, could lead to convulsions, coma, and death. Your doctor should carefully monitor your blood sodium levels during treatment with Trileptal. Alert your doctor immediately if you develop warning signs such as nausea, headache, sluggishness, confusion, loss of feeling, or an increase in the frequency or severity of seizures.

Serious skin reactions and severe allergic reactions have been reported in association with Trileptal use. If you develop a skin reaction or symptoms such as swelling of the face, eyes, lips, or tongue or difficulty in swallowing or breathing while using Trileptal, contact your doctor immediately.

You should inform your doctor if you have used the epilepsy drug carbamazepine in the past. More than one quarter of patients who have had allergic reactions to carbamazepine may also experience allergic reactions to Trileptal.

Who should not take Trileptal?

Do not take Trileptal if you are allergic to the medication or any or its ingredients.

What should I tell my doctor before I take the first dose of Trileptal?

Mention all prescription, over-the-counter, and herbal medications you are taking before beginning treatment with Trileptal. Also, talk to your doctor about your complete medical history, especially if you have kidney disease.

What is the usual dosage?

The information below is based on the dosage guidelines your doctor uses. Depending on your condition and medical history, your doctor may prescribe a different regimen. Do not change the dosage or stop taking your medication without your doctor's approval.

Trileptal Combined with Another Antiepileptic Medication
Adults: The usual starting dose is 300 milligrams (mg) twice daily. Your doctor may increase the dose to 600 mg twice daily.

Children 4 to 16 years old (dosage based on body weight): After a 2-week buildup, the dosage typically ranges from 450 to 900 mg taken twice daily.

Trileptal Taken Alone
Adults: The usual starting dose is 300 mg twice daily. Your doctor may gradually increase the dose to 600 mg twice daily. In people with kidney disorders, the starting dose is 150 mg twice daily.

Children 4 to 16 years old (dosage based on body weight): Your child's doctor will gradually increase the dose every 3 days until the most effective dose is reached. The usual dose ranges from 300 to 1,050 mg taken twice daily.

When Changing from Another
Antiepileptic Medication to Trileptal
Adults: The usual starting dose is 300 mg twice daily. Your doctor will gradually increase the Trileptal dose over a period of 2 to 4 weeks, while reducing the other medication over a period of 3 to 6 weeks. The final dosage of Trileptal is typically 1,200 mg twice daily.

Children 4 to 16 years old (dosage based on body weight): Your child's doctor will gradually increase the dose of Trileptal while reducing the other medication over a period of 3 to 6 weeks. The doctor will increase the dose of Trileptal weekly until the most effective dose is reached. The usual dose ranges from 300 to 1,050 mg taken twice daily.

How should I take Trileptal?
Take Trileptal exactly as prescribed by your doctor. If you stop taking Trileptal suddenly your seizures could become more frequent. You can take it with or without food.

What should I avoid while taking Trileptal?
Trileptal can cause drowsiness, dizziness, and loss of coordination, which could impair your ability to drive a vehicle or operate dangerous machinery. Do not attempt hazardous activities until you know how the drug affects you.

Alcohol consumption may increase sleepiness. Avoid drinking alcohol while you are taking Trileptal.

What are possible food and drug interactions associated with Trileptal?
If Trileptal is taken with certain other drugs, the effects of either could be increased, decreased, or altered. It is especially important to check with your doctor before combining Trileptal with any of the following: calcium

channel blockers such as verapamil or felodipine, carbamazepine, phenobarbital, phenytoin, oral contraceptives, or valproic acid.

What are the possible side effects of Trileptal?

Side effects cannot be anticipated. If any develop or change in intensity,
tell your doctor as soon as possible. Only your doctor can determine if it
is safe for you to continue taking this drug.

Side effects may include: abdominal pain, abnormal vision, dizziness,
double vision, fatigue, indigestion, lack of coordination, nausea, sleepiness, tremor, unusual and uncontrollable problems with walking, vomiting

Can I receive Trileptal if I am pregnant or breastfeeding?

The effects of Trileptal during pregnancy are unknown. Tell your doctor
immediately if you are pregnant, or plan to become pregnant.

Trileptal appears in breast milk and could cause serious side effects
in a nursing infant. Your doctor may make a choice between whether
you should continue breastfeeding and continuing your Trileptal therapy.

What should I do if I miss a dose of Trileptal?

Take it as soon as you remember. If it is almost time for your next dose,
skip the dose you missed and go back to your regular schedule. Do not
take 2 doses at once. If you miss more than one dose in a day, check with
your doctor.

How should I store Trileptal?

Store at room temperature in a tightly closed container.

Trimethobenzamide hydrochloride *See Tigan, page 1303.*

Trimethoprim *See Primsol, page 1068.*

Trimipramine maleate *See Surmontil, page 1233.*

TRIZIVIR

Generic name: Abacavir, lamivudine, and zidovudine

What is Trizivir?

Trizivir combines three drugs used to fight HIV, the deadly virus that un-
dermines the immune system, leaving the body ever more vulnerable to
infection, and eventually leading to AIDS. The components of Trizivir are
all members of the category of HIV drugs known as nucleoside analogs.

Trizivir may be prescribed alone or in combination with other HIV
drugs. It reduces the amount of HIV in the bloodstream, but does not
completely cure the disease. You may still develop the rare infections and
other complications that accompany HIV.

What is the most important information I should know about Trizivir?

The abacavir component of Trizivir can cause a serious, possibly fatal, allergic reaction. You should stop taking Trizivir and seek immediate medical attention if you develop any of the following symptoms: abdominal pain, body aches, cough, diarrhea, extreme fatigue, fever, general ill feeling, nausea, shortness of breath, skin rash, severe peeling skin, sore throat, or vomiting. These symptoms usually appear during the first 6 weeks of therapy, but may occur any time during treatment. If they do occur, do not take another dose of Trizivir until you see your doctor.

Trizivir has been known to cause liver problems and a serious medical condition called lactic acidosis. This condition is more likely to develop in women, people who are overweight, those at risk of liver disease, and patients who have been taking nucleoside analogs for a long time. Be alert for warning signs of the problem, such as persistent nausea and fatigue, and notify your doctor if they occur. Be sure to let your doctor know if you've had liver problems in the past.

Treatment with Trizivir can cause serious blood disorders including anemia (low red blood cell count) and neutropenia (low white cell count). Prolonged treatment with Trizivir also has the potential to cause diseases of the muscles. Be sure to tell your doctor about any muscle pain or weakness you experience. Also, if you have the liver infection hepatitis B, there is a chance that it will get worse if treatment with Trizivir is discontinued.

Who should not take Trizivir?

Do not take Trizivir if you have ever had an allergic reaction to its abacavir component.

Also, you cannot take Trizivir if you weigh less than 90 pounds or have severe kidney disease.

Patients with hepatic impairment or kidney disease with CrCl less than 50 mL/min should not take Trizivir.

What should I tell my doctor before I take the first dose of Trizivir?

Mention all prescription, over-the-counter, and herbal medications you are taking before beginning treatment with Trizivir. Also, talk to your doctor about your complete medical history, especially if you have liver or kidney disease, have low blood cell counts, or are pregnant or breast-feeding.

What is the usual dosage?

The information below is based on the dosage guidelines your doctor uses. Depending on your condition and medical history, your doctor may prescribe a different regimen. Do not change the dosage or stop taking your medication without your doctor's approval.

Adults: The recommended dose of Trizivir is 1 tablet twice daily with or without food.

Children: Trizivir is not intended for children and adolescents who weigh less than 90 pounds. Teenagers who weigh more than 90 pounds receive the adult dose.

How should I take Trizivir?

Trizivir is usually taken twice a day, with or without food. It is important to take the medication exactly as prescribed and not to miss any doses. Be sure to refill your prescription before your supply runs out. If HIV drugs are stopped for even a short time, the virus can increase rapidly and may become harder to treat. If you miss a dose, take the missed dose right away, and the next dose at the usual scheduled time.

What should I avoid while taking Trizivir?

Avoid having unprotected sex or sharing needles, razors, or tooth-brushes. Remember, Trizivir does not reduce the risk of transmitting the virus to others. Talk with your doctor about safe methods of preventing HIV transmission during sex, such as using a condom and spermicide.

Avoid taking other medications that may already contain the combination of Trizivir, such as Combivir, Epivir, Epzicom, Retrovir, or Ziagen.

What are possible food and drug interactions associated with Trizivir?

If Trizivir is taken with certain other drugs, the effects of either could be increased, decreased, or altered. It is especially important to check with your doctor before combining Trizivir with the following: alcohol, atovaquone, doxorubicin, drugs used for bone marrow suppression and cancer therapy, fluconazole, ganciclovir, interferon-alpha, methadone, nelfinavir, probenecid, ribavirin, ritonavir, trimethoprim/sulfamethoxa-zole, valproic acid, or zalcitabine.

What are the possible side effects of Trizivir?

Side effects cannot be anticipated. If any develop or change in intensity, tell your doctor as soon as possible. Only your doctor can determine if it is safe for you to continue taking this drug.

Side effects may include: abdominal cramps, abdominal pain, allergic reaction, blisters in the mouth or eyes, blood and lymph disorders, breast enlargement in males, chills, cough, depression, diarrhea, dizziness, enlarged spleen, fatigue, fever, hair loss, headache, heart problems, high blood sugar, hives, ill feeling, indigestion, inflamed blood vessels, insomnia and other sleep problems, joint pain, liver problems, loss of appetite, mouth inflammation, muscle pain or weakness, nasal symptoms, nausea, pain or tingling in the hands or feet, pancreatitis, redistribution of body fat, seizures, severe peeling skin, skin rash, vomiting, weakness, wheezing

Can I receive Trizivir if I am pregnant or breastfeeding?
The effects of Trizivir during pregnancy are unknown. Tell your doctor immediately if you are pregnant, or plan to become pregnant.

Because the virus can be passed to a baby through breast milk, breast-feeding is not recommended for mothers with HIV.

What should I do if I miss a dose of Trizivir?
Take it as soon as you remember. If it is almost time for your next dose, skip the dose you missed and go back to your regular schedule. Do not double your dose.

How should I store Trizivir?
Store Trizivir tablets at room temperature.

Trospium chloride *See Sanctura, page 1175.*

TUSSIONEX
Generic name: Hydrocodone polistirex and
*   *chlorpheniramine polistirex*

What is Tussionex?
Tussionex Extended-Release Suspension is a cough suppressant/antihis-tamine combination used to relieve coughs and the upper respiratory symptoms of colds and allergies.

What is the most important information
I should know about Tussionex?
This medication can cause considerable drowsiness and make you less alert. You should not drive or operate machinery or participate in any activity that requires full mental alertness until you know how you react to Tussionex.

Tussionex contains a mild narcotic that can cause dependence and tolerance when the drug is used for several weeks. However, it is unlikely that dependence will develop when Tussionex is used for the short-term treatment of a cough.

Who should not take Tussionex?
Do not take Tussionex if you are sensitive to or have ever had an allergic reaction to hydrocodone or chlorpheniramine. Make sure your doctor is aware of any drug reactions you have experienced.

Tussionex is contraindicated in children less than 6 years of age due to increased risk of fatal respiratory depression.

What should I tell my doctor before I take the first dose of Tussionex?

Mention all prescription, over-the-counter, and herbal medications you are taking before beginning treatment with Tussionex. Also, talk to your doctor about your complete medical history, especially if you have an enlarged prostate gland, an eye condition known as narrow-angle glaucoma, an intestinal disorder, or an underactive thyroid gland. Make sure to let your doctor know if you have asthma, liver or kidney disease, lung disease or a breathing disorder, urinary difficulties, Addison's disease (a disorder of the adrenal glands), or if you have recently suffered a head injury.

What is the usual dosage?

The information below is based on the dosage guidelines your doctor uses. Depending on your condition and medical history, your doctor may prescribe a different regimen. Do not change the dosage or stop taking your medication without your doctor's approval.

Adults: The usual dose is 1 teaspoonful (5 milliliters) every 12 hours. Do not take more than 2 teaspoonfuls in 24 hours.

Children 6 to 12 years old: The usual dose is one-half teaspoonful every 12 hours. Do not take more than 1 teaspoonful in 24 hours.

Tussionex is not recommended for children under 6 years old.

How should I take Tussionex?

Tussionex should be taken exactly as prescribed. Do not dilute it with other liquids or mix it with other drugs. Shake well before using. Use an appropriate measuring device; a household teaspoon may not be an accurate dosage measurement.

What should I avoid while taking Tussionex?

Tussionex may increase the effects of alcohol. Do not drink alcohol while taking Tussionex.

What are possible food and drug interactions associated with Tussionex?

If Tussionex is taken with certain other drugs, the effects of either could be increased, decreased, or altered. It is especially important to check with your doctor before combining Tussionex with the following: alcohol, antihistamines (such as diphenhydramine), antispasmodic medications (such as dicyclomide and benztropine), major tranquilizers (such as chlorpromazine and prochlorpromazine), MAO inhibitor drugs (antidepressants such as phenelzine and tranylcypromine), medications for anxiety (such as alprazolam and diazepam), medications for depression (such as amitriptyline and fluoxetine), or narcotics (such as acetaminophen/oxycodone and meperidine).

What are the possible side effects of Tussionex?
Side effects cannot be anticipated. If any develop or change in intensity, tell your doctor as soon as possible. Only your doctor can determine if it is safe for you to continue taking this drug.

Side effects may include: anxiety, constipation, decreased mental and physical performance, difficulty breathing, difficulty urinating, dizziness, drowsiness, dry throat, emotional dependence, exaggerated feeling of depression, extreme calm, exaggerated sense of well-being, fear, itching, mental clouding, mood changes, nausea, rash, restlessness, sluggishness, tightness in chest, vomiting

Can I receive Tussionex if I am pregnant or breastfeeding?
The effects of Tussionex during pregnancy and breastfeeding are unknown. Tell your doctor immediately if you are pregnant, plan to become pregnant, or are breastfeeding.

What should I do if I miss a dose of Tussionex?
If you take Tussionex on a regular schedule, take the forgotten dose as soon as you remember. If it is almost time for your next dose, skip the dose you missed and go back to your regular schedule. Do not take 2 doses at once.

How should I store Tussionex?
Store at room temperature in a tightly closed container.

TUSSI-ORGANIDIN NR
Generic name: Guaifenesin and codeine phosphate

What is Tussi-Organidin NR?
Tussi-Organidin NR relieves cough due to minor sore throat and bronchial irritation that may occur with the common cold or inhaled irritants. Tussi-Organidin NR helps loosen phlegm (mucus) and thin bronchial secretions to rid the bronchial passageways of bothersome mucus, drain bronchial tubes, and make coughs more productive. This product helps loosen phlegm and thin bronchial secretions in patients with stable chronic bronchitis and helps suppress hyperactive or unproductive cough.

What is the most important information I should know about Tussi-Organidin NR?

If cough persists for more than one week, tends to recur, or is accompanied by fever, rash, persistent headache, or vomiting, consult a doctor. Do not take this product for persistent or chronic cough such as occurs with smoking, asthma, emphysema, or where excessive secretions accompany cough, except under the advice and supervision of a doctor.

Tussi-Organidin NR may cause you to be drowsy or less alert. Only take the drug for as long as it is prescribed, in the amount prescribed, and no more frequently than prescribed.

At high doses or in sensitive patients, Tussi-Organidin NR may slow your breathing or produce irregular and periodic breathing.

Who should not take Tussi-Organidin NR?

Do not use Tussi-Organidin NR if you have a known hypersensitivity to guaifenesin, codeine, other morphine derivatives, or any of its other components.

What should I tell my doctor before I take the first dose of Tussi-Organidin NR?

Mention all prescription, over-the-counter, and herbal medications you are taking before beginning treatment with Tussi-Organidin NR. Also, talk to your doctor about your complete medical history, especially if you have severe kidney or liver problems, an underactive thyroid gland, chronic lung disease or shortness of breath, Addison's disease, an enlarged prostate, urethral stricture (narrowing of the tube carrying urine from the bladder), a head injury, increased intracranial pressure, an abdominal condition, alcoholism, or if you are in a weakened condition.

What is the usual dosage?

The information below is based on the dosage guidelines your doctor uses. Depending on your condition and medical history, your doctor may prescribe a different regimen. Do not change the dosage or stop taking your medication without your doctor's approval.

Adults and children 12 years of age and older: The usual dose is 1 teaspoon (5 milliliters [mL]) every 4 hours, not to exceed 8 teaspoons in 24 hours.

Children 6 to under 12 years old: The usual dose is ½ teaspoon (2.5 mL) every 4 hours, not to exceed 4 teaspoons in 24 hours.

Children 2 to under 6 years old: Oral dosage is based on 1 milligram/kilogram/day of codeine administered in four equal divided doses. The average bodyweight for each age may also be used to determine codeine dosage.

Codeine is not recommended for children under 2 years of age.

How should I take Tussi-Organidin NR?

Take Tussi-Organidin NR exactly as prescribed. Do not increase the amount you take or the number of doses per day without your doctor's approval. Take this medication with a full glass of water after each dose to help loosen mucus in the lungs.

What should I avoid while taking Tussi-Organidin NR?

Avoid driving a car or operating machinery until you know how Tussi-Organidin NR affects you. Avoid alcohol and other central nervous system depressants while taking Tussi-Organidin NR.

What are possible food and drug interactions associated with Tussi-Organidin NR?

If Tussi-Organidin NR is taken with certain other drugs, the effects of either could be increased, decreased, or altered. Always check with your doctor before combining Tussi-Organidin NR with the following: antihistamines; antipsychotics; alcohol; anticholinergic drugs; antidepressants, including Monoamine Oxidase Inhibitors (MAOIs) or tricyclic antidepressants; anti-anxiety drugs; or central nervous system (CNS) depressants, including sedatives, tranquilizers, and narcotic painkillers.

What are the possible side effects of Tussi-Organidin NR?

Side effects cannot be anticipated. If any develop or change in intensity, tell your doctor as soon as possible. Only your doctor can determine if it is safe for you to continue taking this drug.

Side effects may include: lightheadedness, dizziness, shortness of breath, sedation, nausea, vomiting

Less frequent side effects may include: allergic reactions, mood disorders, constipation, abdominal pain, itching

Can I receive Tussi-Organidin NR if I am pregnant or breastfeeding?

Talk with your doctor before taking this drug if you are pregnant, plan to become pregnant, or are breastfeeding. Tussi-Organidin NR should be used during pregnancy only if the potential benefit justifies the potential risk to the fetus. Because many drugs are excreted in human milk and because of the potential for serious adverse reactions in nursing infants, a decision should be made whether to discontinue nursing or to discontinue the drug, taking into account the importance of the drug to the mother.

What should I do if I miss a dose of Tussi-Organidin NR?

Take it as soon as you remember. If it is almost time for your next dose, skip the one you missed and go back to your regular schedule. Never take 2 doses at the same time.

How should I store Tussi-Organidin NR?
Store at room temperature in a tightly sealed, light-resistant container.

TYLENOL WITH CODEINE
Generic name: Acetaminophen and codeine phosphate

What is Tylenol with Codeine?
Tylenol with Codeine, a narcotic analgesic, is used to treat mild to moderately severe pain. It contains two drugs—acetaminophen and codeine. Acetaminophen, a fever-reducing analgesic, is used to reduce pain and fever. Codeine, a narcotic analgesic, is used to treat pain that is moderate to severe.

What is the most important information I should know about Tylenol with Codeine?
Tylenol with Codeine contains a narcotic (codeine) and, even if taken in prescribed amounts, can cause physical and psychological addiction if taken for a long enough time.

Tylenol with Codeine tablets contain a sulfite that may cause allergic reactions in some people. These reactions may include shock and severe, possibly life-threatening, asthma attacks. People with asthma are more likely to be sensitive to sulfites.

Who should not take Tylenol with Codeine?
You should not use Tylenol with Codeine if you are sensitive to acetaminophen or codeine.

What should I tell my doctor before I take the first dose of Tylenol with Codeine?
Mention all prescription, over-the-counter, and herbal medications you are taking before beginning treatment with Tylenol with Codeine. Also, talk to your doctor about your complete medical history, especially if you have ever had liver, kidney, thyroid, or adrenal disease. Make sure your doctor knows if you have experienced a head injury, difficulty urinating, an enlarged prostate, or stomach problems such as a stomach ulcer.

What is the usual dosage?
The information below is based on the dosage guidelines your doctor uses. Depending on your condition and medical history, your doctor may prescribe a different regimen. Do not change the dosage or stop taking your medication without your doctor's approval.

Dosage will depend on how severe your pain is and how you respond to the drug.

To Relieve Pain
Adults: A single dose may contain from 15 milligrams (mg) to 60 mg of codeine phosphate and from 300 to 1,000 mg of acetaminophen. The maximum dose in a 24-hour period should be 360 mg of codeine phosphate and 4,000 mg of acetaminophen. Your doctor will determine the amounts of codeine phosphate and acetaminophen taken in each dose. Doses may be repeated up to every 4 hours.

Single doses above 60 mg of codeine do not provide sufficient pain relief to balance the increased number of side effects.

Adults may also take Tylenol with Codeine elixir (liquid). Tylenol with Codeine elixir contains 120 mg of acetaminophen and 12 mg of codeine phosphate per teaspoonful. The usual adult dose is 1 tablespoonful every 4 hours as needed.

Children 3 to 12 years old: The safety of Tylenol with Codeine elixir has not been established in children under 3 years old. Children 3 to 6 years old may take 1 teaspoonful 3 or 4 times daily. Children 7 to 12 years old may take 2 teaspoonfuls 3 or 4 times daily.

For tablets, the dose of codeine is 0.5 mg/kg.

How should I take Tylenol with Codeine?
Tylenol with Codeine may be taken with meals or with milk, but not with alcohol.

What should I avoid while taking Tylenol with Codeine?
If you generally drink 3 or more alcoholic beverages per day, check with your doctor before using Tylenol with Codeine and other acetaminophen-containing products, and never take more than the recommended dosage. There is a possibility of damage to the liver when large amounts of alcohol and acetaminophen are combined.

This drug may cause drowsiness and impair your ability to drive a car or operate potentially dangerous machinery. Do not participate in any activities that require full attention when using Tylenol with Codeine until you are sure of this medication's effect on you.

What are possible food and drug interactions associated with Tylenol with Codeine?
If Tylenol with Codeine is taken with certain other drugs, the effects of either could be increased, decreased, or altered. It is especially important to check with your doctor before combining Tylenol with Codeine with the following: antidepressants, such as amitriptyline, tranylcyromine, phenelzine, and imipramine; drugs that control spasms, such as benztropine; major tranquilizers, such as clozapine and chlorpromazine; narcotic painkillers, such as propoxyphene; or tranquilizers, such as alprazolam and diazepam.

What are the possible side effects of Tylenol with Codeine?

Side effects cannot be anticipated. If any develop or change in intensity, tell your doctor as soon as possible. Only your doctor can determine if it is safe for you to continue taking this drug.

Side effects may include: dizziness, light-headedness, nausea, sedation, shortness of breath, vomiting

At high doses, this medication may cause respiratory depression.

Can I receive Tylenol with Codeine if I am pregnant or breastfeeding?

The effects of Tylenol with Codeine during pregnancy are unknown. Tell your doctor immediately if you are pregnant, or plan to become pregnant.

Some studies, but not others, have reported that codeine appears in breast milk. Therefore, nursing mothers should talk to their doctor about using Tylenol with Codeine.

What should I do if I miss a dose of Tylenol with Codeine?

If you take Tylenol with Codeine on a regular schedule, take the forgotten dose as soon as you remember. If it is almost time for your next dose, skip the dose you missed and go back to your regular schedule. Do not take 2 doses at once.

How should I store Tylenol with Codeine?

Store away from heat, light, and moisture. Keep the liquid form from freezing.

ULTRACET

Generic name: Tramadol hydrochloride and acetaminophen

What is Ultracet?

Ultracet is used to treat moderate to moderately severe pain for a period of five days or less. It contains two pain-relieving agents—tramadol, known technically as an opioid analgesic, which is a narcotic pain reliever, and acetaminophen, a less potent pain reliever that increases the effects of tramadol.

What is the most important information I should know about Ultracet?

Take only the amount and number of doses prescribed. Exceeding the recommended dosage can lead to reduced breathing, liver damage, seizures, and death.

Ultracet poses a danger of mental and physical addiction. Never exceed the prescribed dosage. If you experience withdrawal symptoms, which can occur if you stop taking the drug abruptly, consult your doctor for a tapering regimen. Withdrawal symptoms include anxiety, chills, diarrhea, hallucinations, insomnia, nausea, pain, erection of hair, sweating, tremors, and upper respiratory symptoms.

Who should not take Ultracet?

Do not take Ultracet if you have had an allergic reaction to either of its active ingredients, or to any other narcotic pain reliever. Do not take Ultracet if you have been drinking, or have taken any other narcotic drug, sleep aid, tranquilizer, or antidepressant; your consciousness or breathing could be compromised. Avoid Ultracet if you've ever been dependent on other narcotic pain relievers.

What should I tell my doctor before I take the first dose of Ultracet?

Mention all prescription, over-the-counter, and herbal medications you are taking before beginning treatment with Ultracet. Also, talk to your doctor about your complete medical history, especially if you have a history of drug or alcohol addiction, depression, epilepsy or other seizure disorders, or head injury. Make sure to let your doctor know if you have a metabolic disorder; an infection of your brain or spinal cord, such as meningitis or encephalitis; kidney disease; liver disease; asthma or other breathing disorder; a stomach disorder; or mental illness or suicide attempt.

Tell your doctor if you are taking any antidepressants because Ultracet may increase your risk of getting a seizure.

What is the usual dosage?

The information below is based on the dosage guidelines your doctor uses. Depending on your condition and medical history, your doctor may prescribe a different regimen. Do not change the dosage or stop taking your medication without your doctor's approval.

Adults: The usual dose of Ultracet is two tablets every 4 to 6 hours as needed for pain relief, up to a maximum of 8 tablets per day for no more than 5 days.

If you have kidney problems, the doctor may reduce the dose to 2 tablets every 12 hours. Older adults may also receive a low dose.

Children: The safety and effectiveness of Ultracet have not been established in children under the age of 16 years.

How should I take Ultracet?

You should strictly follow your doctor's dosage recommendations, and stop taking the drug as soon as possible.

What should I avoid while taking Ultracet?

Do not take Ultracet if you will be driving a car or operating dangerous machinery. Ultracet may impair the mental and physical abilities needed for driving. Avoid alcohol.

What are possible food and drug interactions associated with Ultracet?

If Ultracet is taken with certain other drugs, the effects of either could be increased, decreased, or altered. It is especially important to check with your doctor before combining Ultracet with the following: acetaminophen-containing products; antidepressant drugs classified as MAO inhibitors, including phenelzine and tranylcypromine; antipsychotic drugs, such as chlorpromazine and haloperidol; carbamazepine; cyclobenzaprine; digoxin; narcotic pain relievers, such as aspirin/oxycodone and acetaminophen/hydrocodone; promethazine; quinidine; serotonin-boosting antidepressants, such as paroxetine and fluoxetine; sleep aids, such as triazolam and temazepam; tranquilizers, such as alprazolam and diazepam; tricyclic antidepressants, such as amitriptyline and imipramine; triptans such as sumatriptan, zolmitriptan, etc.; and warfarin.

What are the possible side effects of Ultracet?

Side effects cannot be anticipated. If any develop or change in intensity, tell your doctor as soon as possible. Only your doctor can determine if it is safe for you to continue taking this drug.

Side effects may include: blurry vision, constipation, diarrhea, dizziness, drowsiness, dry mouth, headache, nausea, sleepiness, sweating, vomiting

Can I receive Ultracet if I am pregnant or breastfeeding?

The effects of Ultracet during pregnancy are unknown. Tell your doctor immediately if you are pregnant or plan to become pregnant. Ultracet should be used in pregnancy only if the potential benefit justifies the potential risk to the fetus. Seizures, death, and stillbirths have been reported with tramadol.

Ultracet appears in breast milk and is not recommended for nursing mothers.

What should I do if I miss a dose of Ultracet?

Take Ultracet only as needed. Never take 2 doses at once.

How should I store Ultracet?

Store at room temperature in a tight container.

ULTRAM

Generic name: Tramadol hydrochloride

What is Ultram?

Ultram is used to manage mild to moderate pain in patients 17 years and older.

What is the most important information I should know about Ultram?

Ultram has been shown to cause seizures, especially in patients taking certain antidepressants (selective serotonin reuptake inhibitors and tricyclic antidepressants), some opioids, and MAO inhibitors. There is a greater risk of convulsions if you have a history of seizures, epilepsy, have drug/alcohol withdrawal, or a nervous system infection.

Ultram may cause dependence. You should not use it if you have previously been addicted to an opioid.

Who should not take Ultram?

Do not take Ultram if you are allergic to tramadol or any of its other ingredients. Also, do not take this drug if you are currently using alcohol, analgesics, narcotics, opioids, or other antidepressants.

What should I tell my doctor before I take the first dose of Ultram?

Mention all prescription, over-the-counter, and herbal medications you are taking before beginning treatment with Ultram. Also, talk to your doctor about your complete medical history, especially if you have a history of drug/alcohol abuse or depression and are currently being treated.

What is the usual dosage?

The information below is based on the dosage guidelines your doctor uses. Depending on your condition and medical history, your doctor may prescribe a different regimen. Do not change the dosage or stop taking your medication without your doctor's approval.

Adults: The usual starting dosage of Ultram for adults over the age of 17 is 25 milligrams (mg) a day. Approximately 25 mg of Ultram should be added every 3 days until you reach a total of 100 mg a day. After this, 50 mg may be added daily until you reach a total of 200 mg a day. After this step by step dose increase, Ultram 50 mg to 100 mg may be taken as needed for pain relief every 4 to 6 hours. Do not exceed 400 mg a day of Ultram.

How should I take Ultram?

Take your daily dose of Ultram in the morning. Only take the recommended dose, and not more. Overdosing may result in depression, seizures, or even death.

What should I avoid while taking Ultram?

Avoid using drugs/alcohol or antidepressants without consulting your doctor first. Usage of these products may cause seizures.

Avoid operating a car or heavy machinery while taking Ultram, as it is known to impair such abilities.

What are possible food and drug interactions associated with Ultram?

If Ultram is taken with certain other drugs, the effects of either could be increased, decreased, or altered. It is especially important to check with your doctor before combining Ultram with the following: carbamazepine; digoxin; MAO inhibitors; opioids; quinidine; SSRIs or tricyclic antidepressants, such as cyclobenzaprine and promethazine; triptans, such as sumatriptan, zolmitriptan, etc.; and warfarin.

What are the possible side effects of Ultram?

Side effects cannot be anticipated. If any develop or change in intensity, tell your doctor as soon as possible. Only your doctor can determine if it is safe for you to continue taking this drug.

Side effects may include: constipation, diarrhea, dizziness, dry mouth, headache, itchiness, nausea, sleeplessness, sweating, upset stomach, vomiting, weakness

Can I receive Ultram if I am pregnant or breastfeeding?

The effects of Ultram during pregnancy and breastfeeding are unknown. Tell your doctor immediately if you are pregnant, plan to become pregnant, or are breastfeeding.

What should I do if I miss a dose of Ultram?

Ultram is taken on an as-needed basis when you are experiencing pain. If you miss a dose and have pain, take the missed dose. Do not take a double dose.

How should I store Ultram?

Store at room temperature in an air-tight container.

ULTRAVATE

Generic name: Halobetasol propionate

What is Ultravate?

Ultravate is a high-potency steroid that relieves the itching and inflammation caused by a wide variety of skin disorders. It is available in cream and ointment formulations.

What is the most important information I should know about Ultravate?

Some of the medication in Ultravate is absorbed through the skin and into the bloodstream. If you apply Ultravate over a large area, or under an airtight dressing, the drug can cause a number of unwanted side effects, including increased sugar in your blood and urine, and a set of symptoms called Cushing's syndrome. Do not use more Ultravate than your doctor prescribes, and do not bandage or wrap the affected area unless your doctor specifically recommends it.

Use of steroid medications can lead to a slowdown in the body's production of natural steroids and result in a shortage when the medication is stopped. To reduce the likelihood of this problem, use Ultravate for no more than 2 weeks at a time, and apply it only to small areas.

When used on children, steroid creams and ointments have been known to stunt growth and raise pressure inside the skull, resulting in headaches, bulges on the head, and loss of vision.

Who should not take Ultravate?

Do not use Ultravate to treat red eruptions around the mouth (perioral dermatitis) or the red facial patches caused by rosacea. Avoid Ultravate if you are allergic to it or any of its ingredients.

What should I tell my doctor before I take the first dose of Ultravate?

Mention all prescription, over-the-counter, and herbal medications you are taking before beginning treatment with Ultravate. Also, talk to your doctor about your complete medical history.

What is the usual dosage?

The information below is based on the dosage guidelines your doctor uses. Depending on your condition and medical history, your doctor may prescribe a different regimen. Do not change the dosage or stop taking your medication without your doctor's approval.

Adults: Once or twice a day, gently and completely rub a thin layer of Ultravate into the affected skin. Do not use more than 50 grams per week, and do not continue treatment for more than 2 weeks.

Children: Ultravate is not recommended for children under 12 years of age.

How should I take Ultravate?

Only use Ultravate on the skin.

What should I avoid while taking Ultravate?

Do not apply Ultravate to the face, groin, or armpits. Be careful to keep it out of your eyes.

Avoid using bandages, coverings, or wrappings on the treated skin area unless otherwise directed by your doctor.

What are possible food and drug interactions associated with Ultravate?

No significant interactions have been reported at this time. However, always tell your doctor about any medicines you take, including over-the-counter drugs, vitamins, and herbal supplements.

What are the possible side effects of Ultravate?

Side effects cannot be anticipated. If any develop or change in intensity, tell your doctor as soon as possible. Only your doctor can determine if it is safe for you to continue taking this drug.

Side effects may include: burning, itching, stinging

Can I receive Ultravate if I am pregnant or breastfeeding?

The effects of Ultravate during pregnancy are unknown. Tell your doctor immediately if you are pregnant or plan to become pregnant. Ultravate should only be used during pregnancy if the possible benefits outweigh the possible risks to the baby.

Steroids do make their way into breast milk, and can cause harm to a nursing infant. Speak to your doctor if you are using Ultravate while breastfeeding.

What should I do if I miss a dose of Ultravate?

Apply the forgotten dose as soon as you remember. However, if it is almost time for your next dose, skip the dose you missed and return to your regular schedule.

How should I store Ultravate?

Store at room temperature, away from moisture and heat.

UNIRETIC

*Generic name: Moexipril hydrochloride and
    hydrochlorothiazide*

What is Uniretic?

Uniretic combines two types of blood pressure medication—moexipril hydrochloride and hydrochlorothiazide. Uniretic is used to treat high blood pressure, but it is not used for the initial treatment of high blood pressure. It is saved for later use, when a single blood pressure medication is not sufficient for the job.

What is the most important information I should know about Uniretic?

Blood pressure medications known as angiotensin converting enzyme (ACE) inhibitors, such as Uniretic, have been shown to cause injury and even death of the developing baby when used during the second and third trimesters of pregnancy. When pregnancy is confirmed, call your doctor right away for instructions on how to safely discontinue Uniretic.

Contact your doctor immediately if you develop swelling around your lips, tongue, or throat, or in your arms and legs, or if you begin to have difficulty breathing or swallowing while taking Uniretic. You may need emergency room treatment.

Uniretic can cause a severe drop in blood pressure if you lose too much liquid through excessive sweating, severe diarrhea, or vomiting. Contact your doctor immediately if you develop one of these problems.

You must take Uniretic regularly for it to be effective, and you must continue taking it even if you are feeling well. Like other blood pressure medications, Uniretic does not cure high blood pressure; it merely keeps it under control.

Who should not take Uniretic?

Do not take Uniretic if you have had a severe reaction called angioedema (swelling of the face, arms, legs, and throat) to any other ACE inhibitor, such as captopril or lisinopril. Avoid Uniretic, too, if you've had an allergic reaction to either of its ingredients, or to any sulfa drug. Allergic reactions to Uniretic are more likely if you have a history of allergies or wheezing or breathing difficulties.

If you have problems with urination, do not take Uniretic.

What should I tell my doctor before I take the first dose of Uniretic?

Mention all prescription, over-the-counter, and herbal medications you are taking before beginning treatment with Uniretic. Also, talk to your doctor about your complete medical history, especially if you have high blood sugar, inflammation of the pancreas or joints, high cholesterol, liver disease, kidney disease, or if you are on dialysis. Make sure to let your doctor know if you have a connective tissue disease, such as systemic lupus erythematosus. Tell your doctor if you have a blood or bone marrow disease, any type of heart disease, or if you have had a stroke.

What is the usual dosage?

The information below is based on the dosage guidelines your doctor uses. Depending on your condition and medical history, your doctor may prescribe a different regimen. Do not change the dosage or stop taking your medication without your doctor's approval.

Adults: Dosages of Uniretic are always tailored to your individual response. The doctor will probably start with a relatively low dosage, then after 2 or 3 weeks adjust it upward if necessary. In general, the daily dose of moexipril should not exceed 30 milligrams. For hydrochlorothiazide, the maximum is 50 milligrams a day.

Your doctor may prescribe other blood pressure medications along with Uniretic.

Children: The safety and effectiveness of Uniretic have not been established in children.

How should I take Uniretic?
Take Uniretic once a day, 1 hour before a meal. Try not to miss any doses. If you suddenly stop taking Uniretic, you could experience a rise in blood pressure.

What should I avoid while taking Uniretic?
While taking Uniretic, do not use potassium supplements, salt substitutes that contain potassium, or diuretics that leave potassium levels high (triamterene and amiloride hydrochloride/hydrochlorothiazide) unless your doctor recommends them.

Avoid a high-salt diet. Too much salt may cause your body to retain water and may decrease the effects of hydrochlorothiazide. Ask your doctor or nurse about low-salt diet alternatives.

Use caution when driving, operating machinery, or performing other hazardous activities.

Avoid prolonged exposure to sunlight. Uniretic may increase the sensitivity of your skin to sunlight. Use a sunscreen and wear protective clothing when exposure to the sun is unavoidable.

What are possible food and drug interactions associated with Uniretic?
If Uniretic is taken with certain other drugs, the effects of either could be increased, decreased, or altered. It is especially important to check with your doctor before combining Uniretic with the following: ACTH (adrenocorticotropic hormone); alcohol; barbiturates, such as phenobarbital or secobarbital sodium; cholestyramine; colestipol; diabetes medications, such as glyburide and insulin; guanabenz; lithium; narcotics, such as acetaminophen with oxycodone hydrochloride; nonsteroidal anti-inflammatory painkillers, such as ibuprofen and naproxen; potassium-sparing diuretics, such as triamterene or amiloride hydrochloride with hydrochlorothiazide; potassium supplements; propantheline; salt substitutes containing potassium; and steroid medications, such as prednisone.

What are the possible side effects of Uniretic?

Side effects cannot be anticipated. If any develop or change in intensity, tell your doctor as soon as possible. Only your doctor can determine if it is safe for you to continue taking this drug.

Side effects may include: abdominal pain, back pain, cramps, cough, diarrhea, upset stomach, dizziness, fatigue, fever, flu-like symptoms, headache, impotence, increased blood sugar

Can I receive Uniretic if I am pregnant or breastfeeding?

If you are pregnant, contact your doctor immediately for instructions on how to safely discontinue Uniretic. If you plan to become pregnant, discuss the situation with your doctor as soon as possible.

The effects of Uniretic during breastfeeding are unknown. If Uniretic is essential to your health, your doctor may advise you to stop breastfeeding while you are taking the drug.

What should I do if I miss a dose of Uniretic?

Take it as soon as you remember. If it is almost time for your next dose, skip the dose you missed and go back to your regular schedule. Never take 2 doses at the same time.

How should I store Uniretic?

Store at room temperature, away from moisture and in a tightly closed container.

UNIVASC

Generic name: Moexipril hydrochloride

What is Univasc?

Univasc is used in the treatment of high blood pressure. It is effective when used alone or with thiazide diuretics, which help rid the body of excess water.

What is the most important information I should know about Univasc?

Blood pressure medications known as angiotensin converting enzyme (ACE) inhibitors, such as Univasc, have been shown to cause injury and even death of the developing baby when used during the second and third trimesters of pregnancy. When pregnancy is confirmed, call your doctor right away Univasc.

Univasc can cause a severe drop in blood pressure if you lose too much liquid through excessive sweating, severe diarrhea, or vomiting. Contact your doctor immediately if you develop one of these problems.

You must take Univasc regularly for it to be effective. Since blood pressure declines gradually, it may be several weeks before you get the full benefit of Univasc, and you must continue taking it even if you are feeling well. Univasc does not cure high blood pressure; it merely keeps it under control.

If you develop swelling of your face, around the lips, tongue, or throat; swelling of your arms and legs; sore throat; or difficulty breathing or swallowing, stop taking the drug and contact your doctor immediately. You may need emergency treatment.

Who should not take Univasc?

If you have ever had an allergic reaction to Univasc or other angiotensin converting enzyme (ACE) inhibitors such as captopril, enalapril, and lisinopril, you should not take Univasc.

What should I tell my doctor before I take the first dose of Univasc?

Mention all prescription, over-the-counter, and herbal medications you are taking before beginning treatment with Univasc. Also, talk to your doctor about your complete medical history, especially if you have diabetes, liver disease, kidney disease, or if you are on dialysis. Make sure to also let your doctor know if you have a disease of connective tissue such as systemic lupus erythematosus, any type of heart disease, or if you have had a stroke.

What is the usual dosage?

The information below is based on the dosage guidelines your doctor uses. Depending on your condition and medical history, your doctor may prescribe a different regimen. Do not change the dosage or stop taking your medication without your doctor's approval.

Adults: For people not taking a diuretic drug, the usual starting dose is 7.5 milligrams (mg) taken once a day, an hour before a meal. The dosage after that can range from 7.5 to 30 mg per day, taken in either a single dose or divided into 2 equal doses. The maximum dose is 60 mg per day. Your doctor will closely monitor the effect of Univasc and adjust it according to your individual needs.

People already taking a diuretic should stop taking it, if possible, 2 to 3 days before starting Univasc. This reduces the possibility of fainting or light-headedness. If the diuretic cannot be discontinued, the starting dosage of Univasc should be 3.75 mg. If Univasc alone does not control your blood pressure, your doctor will have you start taking a diuretic again.

For people with kidney problems, the usual starting dose is 3.75 mg a day. Your doctor may gradually raise the dose to a maximum of 15 mg a day.

Children: The safety and effectiveness of Univasc have not been established in children.

How should I take Univasc?

Univasc should be taken 1 hour before a meal. Try to get in the habit of taking your medication at the same time each day, such as 1 hour before breakfast, so that it is easier to remember. Always take Univasc exactly as prescribed.

What should I avoid while taking Univasc?

Do not take potassium supplements or salt substitutes containing potassium without talking to your doctor first. In a medical emergency and before you have surgery, notify your doctor or dentist that you are taking Univasc.

Be careful if you are going to drive or do anything that requires you to be awake and alert while you are taking Univasc.

What are possible food and drug interactions associated with Univasc?

If Univasc is taken with certain other drugs, the effects of either could be increased, decreased, or altered. It is especially important to check with your doctor before combining Univasc with the following: diuretics (chlorothiazide, hydrochlorothiazide, furosemide), potassium supplements, potassium-sparing diuretics (spironolactone, amiloride hydrochloride/hydrochlorothiazide, hydrochlorothiazide/triamterene), or lithium.

What are the possible side effects of Univasc?

Side effects cannot be anticipated. If any develop or change in intensity, tell your doctor as soon as possible. Only your doctor can determine if it is safe for you to continue taking this drug.

Side effects may include: cough, diarrhea, dizziness, fatigue, flu-like symptoms, flushing, infection of the tonsils, muscle pain, rash

Can I receive Univasc if I am pregnant or breastfeeding?

If you are pregnant, contact your doctor immediately for instructions on how to safely discontinue Univasc. If you plan to become pregnant, discuss the situation with your doctor as soon as possible.

The effects of Univasc during breastfeeding are unknown. If Univasc is essential to your health, your doctor may advise you to stop breastfeeding while you are taking the drug.

What should I do if I miss a dose of Univasc?

Take the forgotten dose as soon as you remember. If it is almost time for the next dose, skip the dose you missed and go back to your regular schedule. Do not double the dose.

How should I store Univasc?

Store at room temperature in a tightly closed container, away from moisture.

UROXATRAL

Generic name: Alfuzosin hydrochloride

What is Uroxatral?

Uroxatral is used to treat the symptoms of an enlarged prostate—a condition technically known as benign prostatic hyperplasia or BPH. The walnut-sized prostate gland surrounds the urethra (the duct that drains the bladder). If the gland becomes enlarged, it can squeeze the urethra, interfering with the flow of urine. This can cause difficulty in starting urination, a weak flow of urine, and the need to urinate urgently or more frequently. Uroxatral doesn't shrink the prostate. Instead, it relaxes the muscle around it, freeing the flow of urine and decreasing urinary symptoms.

What is the most important information I should know about Uroxatral?

Benign enlargement of the prostate is not the only condition that can cause male urinary inefficiency and discomfort. Other possibilities include infection, obstruction, cancer of the prostate, and bladder disorders. Before prescribing Uroxatral, your doctor will want to do various tests to determine the cause of your urinary problems.

Stop taking Uroxatral immediately and call your doctor if symptoms of angina pectoris (chest pain due to a heart condition) start or get worse.

Who should not take Uroxatral?

If you have moderate or severe liver problems, are on antifungal drugs or HIV drugs, are under the age of 18, and if you are already taking an alpha blocker for either blood pressure or prostate problems, you should not take Uroxatral. You should also avoid the drug if you have ever had an allergic reaction to it. Make sure your doctor is aware of any drug reactions you might have experienced.

What should I tell my doctor before I take the first dose of Uroxatral?

Mention all prescription, over-the-counter, and herbal medications you are taking before beginning treatment with Uroxatral. Also, talk to your doctor about your complete medical history, especially if you have angina (chest pain), coronary artery disease (such as arteriosclerosis), electrical problems with your heart (QT prolongation), kidney or liver problems, low blood pressure, or prostate cancer.

What is the usual dosage?

The information below is based on the dosage guidelines your doctor uses. Depending on your condition and medical history, your doctor

may prescribe a different regimen. Do not change the dosage or stop taking your medication without your doctor's approval.

Adults: The recommended dosage is one 10-milligram tablet daily, taken immediately after the same meal each day.

Children: Uroxatral is not indicated for use in children.

How should I take Uroxatral?
Take Uroxatral with food, with the same meal each day.

What should I avoid while taking Uroxatral?
Uroxatral can cause dizziness and even fainting, especially in the first few hours after you take it. Be very careful about driving, operating machinery, or performing dangerous tasks during this period.

What are possible food and drug interactions associated with Uroxatral?
If Uroxatral is taken with certain other drugs, the effects of either could be increased, decreased, or altered. It is especially important to check with your doctor before combining Uroxatral with the following: alpha-blockers (used to treat high blood pressure or BPH), such as carvedilol, prazosin, doxazosin, and tamsulosin; atenolol; cimetidine; diltiazem; itraconazole; ketoconazole; and ritonavir.

What are the possible side effects of Uroxatral?
Side effects cannot be anticipated. If any develop or change in intensity, tell your doctor as soon as possible. Only your doctor can determine if it is safe for you to continue taking this drug.

Side effects may include: dizziness, fatigue, headache, upper respiratory tract infection

Can I receive Uroxatral if I am pregnant or breastfeeding?
Uroxatral is not to be used by women.

What should I do if I miss a dose of Uroxatral?
Take the forgotten dose as soon as you remember. However, if it is almost time for your next dose, skip the dose you missed and return to your regular schedule. Do not take 2 doses at once.

How should I store Uroxatral?
Store at room temperature and protect from heat, light, and moisture.

Ursodiol *See Actigall, page 19.*

VAGIFEM
Generic name: Estradiol

What is Vagifem?
Vagifem is a local estrogen therapy (inserted into the vagina) that can help to relieve the urinary and vaginal symptoms associated with the decline of your body's estrogen production during menopause.

What is the most important information I should know about Vagifem?
Vagifem may be associated with an increased risk of developing cancer of the endometrium (the lining inside of the uterus), marked by unusual vaginal bleeding. Vagifem may cause you to retain water, which can influence your condition if you have asthma, epilepsy, migraines, or heart or kidney problems.

If you have a family history of abnormal fat metabolism known as familial hyperlipoproteinemia, Vagifem may worsen your condition by increasing certain substances known as triglycerides in your blood. You should be cautious when using Vagifem if you have ever become jaundiced (yellowing of the skin) during pregnancy or if you have any type of liver injury, bone disease, or kidney disease. You should not begin using Vagifem if you currently have an untreated infection of the vaginal tract.

Who should not take Vagifem?
You should not use Vagifem if you are pregnant, have abnormal vaginal bleeding, have just given birth, are breastfeeding, or if you have a history of certain cancers. You should also not use Vagifem if you have blood disorders known as porphyria, thrombophlebitis, or any type of clotting disorder, especially if they were caused by previous estrogen usage. Do not take if you have an allergy to any components of Vagifem.

What should I tell my doctor before I take the first dose of Vagifem?
Mention all prescription, over-the-counter, and herbal medications you are taking before beginning treatment with Vagifem. Also, talk to your doctor about your complete medical history, especially if you have a history of cancer; abnormal vaginal bleeding; heart, liver, kidney, or bone disease; if you are planning on becoming pregnant; any type of blood disorder; or if you have had any type of adverse reaction to estrogen before.

What is the usual dosage?
The information below is based on the dosage guidelines your doctor uses. Depending on your condition and medical history, your doctor may prescribe a different regimen. Do not change the dosage or stop taking your medication without your doctor's approval.

Adults: The usual dosage is one tablet inserted inside the vagina once daily for 2 weeks. One tablet is inserted inside the vagina twice weekly thereafter.

How should I take Vagifem?

Vagifem tablets can be inserted into the vagina either when lying down or when standing. If the tablet has come out of the applicator before inserting it, do not try to replace it—use a fresh tablet-filled applicator instead. The applicator should be inserted inside the vagina until it cannot be comfortably inserted farther or until half the applicator is inside your vagina, whichever is less. Next, press the plunger until your hear a click.

What should I avoid while taking Vagifem?

You should not become pregnant while using Vagifem.

What are possible food and drug interactions associated with Vagifem?

To date, no drug or food interactions have been reported for Vagifem tablets.

What are the possible side effects of Vagifem?

Side effects cannot be anticipated. If any develop or change in intensity, tell your doctor as soon as possible. Only your doctor can determine if it is safe for you to continue taking this drug.

Side effects may include: allergic reaction, skin rash, vaginal discharge, vaginal spotting, headache, abdominal pain, back pain

Can I receive Vagifem if I am pregnant or breastfeeding?

Do not use Vagifem if you are pregnant, plan to become pregnant, or breastfeeding. This drug may cause birth defects.

What should I do if I miss a dose of Vagifem?

If you forget to insert a Vagifem tablet, insert one as soon as you remember. If it is closer to your next scheduled dose, skip the dose you missed and return to your normal dosing schedule.

How should I store Vagifem?

Store at room temperature.

Valacyclovir hydrochloride See Valtrex, page 1368.

VALCYTE

Generic name: Valganciclovir hydrochloride

What is Valcyte?

Valcyte is an antiviral medicine used to treat cytomegalovirus (CMV) in patients with acquired immunodeficiency syndrome (AIDS). CMV can also infect the eyes and is called CMV retinitis. Valcyte slows the growth of the CMV virus in your body and may prevent it from spreading to healthy cells.

In addition, Valcyte is used to prevent CMV in patients who have received a heart, kidney, or kidney-pancreas transplant from another patient infected with CMV.

What is the most important information I should know about Valcyte?

Valcyte can affect your blood cells and bone marrow, which may cause serious and life-threatening problems. Valcyte can lower the amount of your white blood cells, red blood cells, and platelets. Your doctor may do regular blood tests to check your blood cells while you are taking Valcyte. Based on these tests, the doctor may change your dose or tell you to stop taking this drug.

Valcyte causes cancer in animals. It is not known if Valcyte causes cancer in people.

Valcyte may cause birth defects, so it should not be taken during pregnancy. Tell your doctor immediately if you become pregnant while taking this drug. If you are of childbearing age, you should use effective birth control while using Valcyte. Men should use a condom during Valcyte treatment and 90 days after discontinuing treatment. Valcyte can lower the number of sperm in a man's body and may lead to fertility problems.

Valcyte changes into the medicine ganciclovir once it is in your body. You should not take other medicines that contain ganciclovir or valganciclovir while using Valcyte. In addition, Valcyte cannot be substituted for another drug that contains ganciclovir, since the dose of medicine is different.

Who should not take Valcyte?

You should not take Valcyte if you are pregnant or plan to become pregnant, receiving hemodialysis, are allergic to any component of the drug, or if you have ever had any reaction or sensitivity to a similar product such as ganciclovir.

What should I tell my doctor before I take the first dose of Valcyte?

Mention all prescription, over-the-counter, and herbal medications you are taking before beginning treatment with Valcyte. Also, talk to your doctor about your complete medical history, especially if you are pregnant or plan to become pregnant, are breastfeeding, have kidney or blood cell problems, or if you are undergoing radiation treatment or chemotherapy.

What is the usual dosage?
The information below is based on the dosage guidelines your doctor uses. Depending on your condition and medical history, your doctor may prescribe a different regimen. Do not change the dosage or stop taking your medication without your doctor's approval.

CMV Retinitis
Adults: The usual dosage is 900 milligrams (mg) taken twice a day for 21 days, then 900 mg taken once daily for maintenance.

Heart, Kidney, or Pancreas-Kidney Transplant
Adults: The usual dosage is 900 mg taken once daily starting within 10 days of the transplant, and continuing until 100 days after the transplant.

Children: The safety and effectiveness of Valcyte tablets in pediatric patients have not been established.

How should I take Valcyte?
Valcyte should be taken with food at the same time every day to maximize absorption. Do not break or crush the tablets. If your skin comes in contact with a broken tablet, wash off the area immediately.

Do not let your supply of Valcyte run out. Not taking Valcyte for even a short period of time may lead to an increase of the virus in your body.

Do not substitute Valcyte tablets for ganciclovir capsules.

What should I avoid while taking Valcyte?
You should not become pregnant or breastfeed while taking Valcyte. Men who take Valcyte should not get a partner pregnant during therapy or for 90 days after stopping the drug.

Do not operate heavy machinery or drive a car until you know how Valcyte will affect you.

What are possible food and drug interactions associated with Valcyte?
If Valcyte is taken with certain other drugs, the effects of either could be increased, decreased, or altered. It is especially important to check with your doctor before combining Valcyte with the following: cytovene, didanosine, ganciclovir, mycophenolate, probenecid, or zidovudine.

What are the possible side effects of Valcyte?
Side effects cannot be anticipated. If any develop or change in intensity, tell your doctor as soon as possible. Only your doctor can determine if it is safe for you to continue taking this drug.

Side effects may include: back pain, brain/nerve problems, constipation, diarrhea, fever, graft rejection, headache, high blood pressure, kidney problems, nausea, shaky movements (tremors), stomach pain, swelling of the legs, trouble sleeping, vomiting

Can I receive Valcyte if I am pregnant or breastfeeding?
No. Valcyte may harm your baby and should not be used during pregnancy or breastfeeding.

What should I do if I miss a dose of Valcyte?
Take it as soon as you remember. However, if it is almost time for your next dose, skip the one you missed and return to your normal dosing schedule. Do not double your doses.

How should I store Valcyte?
Store at room temperature.

Valganciclovir hydrochloride *See Valcyte, page 1364.*

VALIUM
Generic name: Diazepam

What is Valium?
Valium is used to treat anxiety disorders, the symptoms of sudden alcohol withdrawal, muscle spasms, and seizures.

What is the most important information I should know about Valium?
Due to the sleepiness and tiredness Valium can cause, you should not drive or operate dangerous machinery until you know how this drug affects you.

If you are taking Valium as part of seizure therapy, you should not suddenly stop taking it because this may worsen or even cause seizures.

You should not drink alcohol or take other medications that can make you tired or drowsy while you are taking Valium.

Some studies have shown that Valium may increase the risk of birth defects during the first trimester. You should tell your doctor immediately if you are pregnant or plan to become pregnant while taking Valium.

Use this drug with caution if you have any type of kidney or liver problems. If you take Valium for a long time, your doctor will likely perform blood tests to check your liver function and also the number of disease fighting cells in your blood.

You should talk to your doctor before increasing your Valium dose or before stopping therapy. Suddenly stopping Valium may cause you to experience symptoms of withdrawal that include shaking, stomach and muscle cramps, vomiting, sweating, insomnia, and seizures.

You may develop a physical or mental dependence on Valium, especially if you take it for a long time or if you have a history of alcohol or drug abuse.

Who should not take Valium?
You should not take Valium if you are pregnant, if you have an eye disorder known as acute narrow-angle glaucoma, or if you are allergic to diazepam or any other ingredient in Valium.

You should not use Valium if you have severe breathing problems, liver disease, sleep apnea, or a condition known as myasthenia gravis.

What should I tell my doctor before I take the first dose of Valium?
Tell your doctor about all prescription, over-the-counter, and herbal medications you are taking before beginning treatment with Valium. Also, talk to your doctor about your complete medical history, especially if you have kidney or liver problems, acute narrow-angle glaucoma, or if you drink alcohol regularly. Also tell your doctor if you have a history of drug abuse, breathing problems, or mental disorders.

What is the usual dosage?
The information below is based on the dosage guidelines your doctor uses. Depending on your condition and medical history, your doctor may prescribe a different regimen. Do not change the dosage or stop taking your medication without your doctor's approval.

Anxiety Disorders, Temporary Symptoms of Anxiety, Muscle Spasm, and Seizure Disorders
Adults: The usual dosage is 2-10 milligrams (mg) taken 2-4 times a day.

Children: Valium can be given to children 6 months and older. The usual dosage is 1-2.5 mg given 3-4 times a day.

Sudden Alcohol Withdrawal
Adults: The starting dose is 10 mg taken 3-4 times during the first 24 hours. The dose is then reduced to 5 mg, taken 3-4 times daily as needed.

How should I take Valium?
Take Valium at the same time every day. It may be taken with or without food.

What should I avoid while taking Valium?
Do not drink alcohol or take other medications that can make you tired or drowsy while you are taking Valium.

Avoid suddenly stopping Valium therapy without first talking to your doctor. Do not take more than is prescribed without your doctor's approval.

What are possible food and drug interactions associated with Valium?

If Valium is taken with certain other drugs, the effects of either could be increased, decreased, or altered. It is especially important to check with your doctor before combining Valium with the following: antidepressants, barbiturates, cimetidine, monoamine oxidase inhibitors (MAOIs), narcotics, and phenothiazines.

What are the possible side effects of Valium?

Side effects cannot be anticipated. If any develop or change in intensity, tell your doctor as soon as possible. Only your doctor can determine if it is safe for you to continue taking this drug.

Side effects may include: difficulty walking, drowsiness, tiredness, constipation, blurred vision

Can I receive Valium if I am pregnant or breastfeeding?

The effects of Valium during pregnancy and breastfeeding are unknown. Tell your doctor immediately if you are pregnant, plan to become pregnant, or are breastfeeding.

What should I do if I miss a dose of Valium?

Skip the dose you missed and return to your normal schedule.

How should I store Valium?

Store at room temperature away from light.

Valproic acid *See Depakene, page 393, or Stavzor, page 1224.*

Valsartan *See Diovan, page 424.*

Valsartan and hydrochlorothiazide *See Diovan HCT, page 426.*

VALTREX

Generic name: Valacyclovir hydrochloride

What is Valtrex?

Valtrex is a prescription antiviral medication that lowers the ability of herpes viruses to multiply in your body. It is used to treat cold sores, shingles, control (and treat) genital herpes infections in adults with healthy immune systems, control genital herpes infections in patients with HIV, and, along with safer sex practices, to help reduce the transmission of genital herpes. It can also be used to treat chickenpox for children ages 12-18 with healthy immune systems.

What is the most important information I should know about Valtrex?

Valtrex may cause life-threatening blood disorders, especially when taken at high doses and in patients with advanced HIV (human immunodeficiency virus) disease, or those undergoing allogenic bone marrow or kidney transplants. You should use caution when taking Valtrex if you have kidney problems or are elderly. It is not known if Valtrex can reduce the transmission of genital herpes if you have multiple sexual partners or in nonheterosexual couples. Valtrex does not cure genital herpes. You should avoid sexual contact if you have open lesions or an active outbreak; however, genital herpes may be spread even if you have no symptoms of an outbreak. You should always use a condom made of latex or polyurethane whenever you have sexual contact. If your doctor advises you to take Valtrex for recurrent outbreaks, start taking it at the first sign or symptom of an outbreak. If taking Valtrex to treat cold sores, you should take the first dose at the first sign or symptom, but not for longer than 1 day.

Who should not take Valtrex?

You should not take Valtrex if you are allergic to acyclovir or any ingredients in Valtrex.

What should I tell my doctor before I take the first dose of Valtrex?

Mention all prescription, over-the-counter, and herbal medications you are taking before beginning treatment with Valtrex. Also, talk to your doctor about your complete medical history, especially if you have had a bone marrow transplant or kidney transplant, or if you have advanced HIV disease or AIDS (Acquired Immunodeficiency Syndrome), if you have kidney problems, are over 65 years old, if you are pregnant or are planning to become pregnant, or if you are breastfeeding.

What is the usual dosage?

The information below is based on the dosage guidelines your doctor uses. Depending on your condition and medical history, your doctor may prescribe a different regimen. Do not change the dosage or stop taking your medication without your doctor's approval.

Herpes Zoster
Adults and adolescents 12 years and older: The usual dosage is 1 gram (g) taken 3 times a day for 7 days.

Genital Herpes, Initial Episodes
Adults: The usual dosage is 1 g taken 2 times a day for 10 days.

Genital Herpes, Recurrent Episodes
Adults: The usual dosage is 500 milligrams (mg) taken 2 times a day for 3 days.

Suppressive Therapy
Adults: The usual dosage is 1 g taken once daily. In patients with 9 or fewer recurrences a year, the alternative is 500 mg taken once daily. For patients with HIV who have a CD4 cell count of less than 100 cells/mm3, the usual dosage is 500 mg taken 2 times a day.

Reduction of Transmission
Adults: The usual dosage for patients with 9 or fewer episodes a year is 500 mg taken once daily.

Cold Sores (Herpes Labialis)
Adults: The usual dosage is 2 g taken 2 times a day for 1 day, each dose separated by 12 hours.

There are also a series of dosage recommendations for patients with kidney disease in the official Valtrex package insert.

Chickenpox
Children 2 years old to less than 18 years old: 20 mg/kg three times a day for 5 days; not to exceed more than 1 g three times a day.

How should I take Valtrex?
Valtrex should be taken as prescribed at the same time every day, and should not be discontinued unless directed by a healthcare provider. Valtrex may be taken with or without food. If you are taking Valtrex to treat shingles, cold sores, or genital herpes, you should start taking it as soon as you notice any symptoms of an outbreak. Do not take more Valtrex than prescribed. If you take too much, call your doctor right away.

What should I avoid while taking Valtrex?
You should avoid becoming dehydrated, so drink plenty of fluids while taking Valtrex. Do not have sexual intercourse during an outbreak. Always use a latex condom.

What are possible food and drug interactions associated with Valtrex?
If Valtrex is taken with certain other drugs, the effects of either could be increased, decreased, or altered. It is especially important to check with your doctor before combining Valtrex with antacids, cimetidine, digoxin, probenecid, or thiazide diuretics.

What are the possible side effects of Valtrex?
Side effects cannot be anticipated. If any develop or change in intensity, tell your doctor as soon as possible. Only your doctor can determine if it is safe for you to continue taking this drug.

Side effects may include: dizziness, headache, nausea, stomach pain, vomiting

Side effects in HIV-infected adults: headache, rash, tiredness

Can I receive Valtrex if I am pregnant or breastfeeding?
The effects of Valtrex during pregnancy and breastfeeding are unknown. Tell your doctor immediately if you are pregnant, plan to become pregnant, or are breastfeeding.

What should I do if I miss a dose of Valtrex?
If you miss a dose of Valtrex, take it as soon as you remember and then return to your normal dosing schedule. If it is almost time for your next dose, do not take the missed dose. Wait and take the next dose at the regular time.

How should I store Valtrex?
Store at room temperature in a child-resistant container.

VANDAZOLE
Generic name: Metronidazole

What is Vandazole?
Vandazole is an antibacterial agent (in the form of an intravaginal gel) used to treat bacterial vaginosis in nonpregnant women.

What is the most important information I should know about Vandazole?
Psychotic reactions have been reported in alcoholic patients who were using oral metronidazole along with disulfiram.

Seizures and peripheral neuropathy (numbness, tingling) have been reported with the use of oral metronidazole. If you experience any unusual neurological symptoms, discontinue the use of Vandazole and notify your doctor immediately.

Who should not take Vandazole?
Do not use Vandazole if you have a prior history of hypersensitivity to metronidazole, parabens, or other ingredients of the formulation.

What should I tell my doctor before I take the first dose of Vandazole?
Tell your doctor about all prescription, over-the-counter, and herbal medications you are taking before beginning treatment with Vandazole. Also talk to your doctor about your complete medical history, especially if have any liver problems.

What is the usual dosage?
The information below is based on the dosage guidelines your doctor uses. Depending on your condition and medical history, your doctor may prescribe a different regimen. Do not change the dosage or stop taking your medication without your doctor's approval.

Adults: The recommended dosage of Vandazole is one applicator full (approximately 5 grams) once or twice daily for 5 days.

How should I take Vandazole?
Vandazole is supplied with 5 vaginal applicators. For once-daily dosing, one applicator should be used per dose. For once-daily dosing, administer Vandazole at bedtime. For twice-daily dosing, the applicator should be washed, rinsed and dried following the morning application and reused for the evening dose. After the evening dose, the applicator should be discarded.

What should I avoid while taking Vandazole?
Avoid use of alcohol while being treated with Vandazole. Do not engage in vaginal intercourse or use other vaginal products such as tampons during treatment with this product.

What are possible food and drug interactions associated with Vandazole?
If Vandazole is used with certain other drugs, the effects of either could be increased, decreased, or altered. It is especially important to check with your doctor before combining Vandazole with the following: cimetidine, lithium, warfarin.

What are the possible side effects of Vandazole?
Side effects cannot be anticipated. If any develop or change in intensity, tell your doctor as soon as possible. Only your doctor can determine if it is safe for you to continue taking this drug.

Side effects may include: allergic reaction, breast pain, back pain, constipation, depression, fungal infections, headache, rash

Can I receive Vandazole if I am pregnant or breastfeeding?
Vandazole is to be avoided during pregnancy and breastfeeding.

What should I do if I miss a dose of Vandazole?
Take as soon as you remember. Do not double your dose.

How should I store Vandazole?
Store Vandazole at room temperature.

VANOS
Generic name: Fluocinonide 0.1%

What is Vanos?
Vanos cream is a corticosteroid that should be used to reduce inflammation and irritation of the skin in people with psoriasis and atopic dermatitis (eczema) who are age 12 and older.

What is the most important information I should know about Vanos?
Skin treated with Vanos cream should not be bandaged or otherwise covered. If you are using Vanos cream on a large portion of your body, you should be frequently checked by your doctor.

Who should not take Vanos?
Do not use Vanos if you are allergic to any of its ingredients. Also, Vanos should not be used at the same time as another topical corticosteroid cream.

What should I tell my doctor before I take the first dose of Vanos?
Mention all prescription, over-the-counter, and herbal medications you are taking. Also, talk to your doctor about your complete medical history, especially if you are planning on scheduling surgery.

What is the usual dosage?
The information below is based on the dosage guidelines your doctor uses. Depending on your condition and medical history, your doctor may prescribe a different regimen. Do not change the dosage or stop taking your medication without your doctor's approval.

Adults and children 12 years and older: For the treatment of atopic dermatitis, apply Vanos cream once daily for 2 weeks.

For the treatment of psoriasis, apply Vanos cream once or twice daily to the affected areas for 2 weeks.

For other skin conditions that Vanos is prescribed by your doctor for, apply a thin layer once or twice daily to the affected areas.

The use of Vanos should be limited to 2 consectuve weeks. The maximum amount of cream that should be applied weekly is 60 grams (g). Do not use more than have of the 120 g tube per week.

How should I take Vanos?
Vanos should be applied to the affected skin in a thin layer. Do not cover or bandage the area unless you are told to do so by your doctor.

For external use only. Wash your hands after each application. If no improvement is seen in 2 weeks, speak to your doctor.

What should I avoid while taking Vanos?
Avoid breastfeeding your child while using Vanos to treat your skin problem.

Avoid contact with the eyes. It should not be applied to the face, groin, or armpits.

What are possible food and drug interactions associated with Vanos?
If Vanos is taken with certain other drugs, the effects of either could be increased, decreased, or altered. It is especially important to check with your doctor before combining Vanos with another topical corticosteroid cream.

What are the possible side effects of Vanos?
Side effects cannot be anticipated. If any develop or change in intensity, tell your doctor as soon as possible. Only your doctor can determine if it is safe for you to continue taking this drug.

Side effects may include: burning, congestion, headache, nasal infection, sore throat

Can I receive Vanos if I am pregnant or breastfeeding?
The effects of Vanos during pregnancy and breastfeeding are unknown. Tell your doctor immediately if you are pregnant, plan to become pregnant, or are breastfeeding.

What should I do if I miss a dose of Vanos?
Apply it as soon as you remember. If it is almost time for your next dose, skip the missed dose and return to your normal dosing schedule. Do not apply a double dose.

How should I store Vanos?
Store at room temperature.

Vardenafil hydrochloride See Levitra, page 726.

Varenicline See Chantix, page 283.

VASERETIC
Generic name: Enalapril maleate and hydrochlorothiazide

What is Vaseretic?
Vaseretic is a combination product that contains two medicines: enalapril, known as an ACE (angiotensin converting enzyme) inhibitor, and hydro-chlorothiazide, a diuretic or water pill. These two medications work to-

gether to lower blood pressure in patients who may have not had enough blood pressure lowering from other medications.

What is the most important information I should know about Vaseretic?

If taken during the second or third trimester of pregnancy, Vaseretic can cause serious harm or even death to an unborn baby. If you become pregnant while taking Vaseretic, call your doctor right away for instructions on how to safely discontinue this medication.

Vaseretic can cause a rare but serious allergic reaction leading to extreme swelling of the face, lips, tongue, throat, or gut (causing severe abdominal pain). If you experience these symptoms, stop taking Vaseretic and contact your doctor or seek medical care right away.

Who should not take Vaseretic?

You should not take Vaseretic if you do not produce urine, you have a history of sensitivity or allergic reaction to ACE inhibitors, or you are allergic to sulfonamide-derived medications. You may be more at risk of experiencing sensitivity or an allergic reaction to Vaseretic if you have allergies or wheezing or breathing difficulties.

What should I tell my doctor before I take the first dose of Vaseretic?

Mention all prescription, over-the-counter, and herbal medications you are taking before beginning treatment with Vaseretic. Also, talk to your doctor about your complete medical history, especially if you are pregnant or plan on becoming pregnant, or if you have ever had an allergy or sensitivity to an ACE inhibitor or sulfonamide-derived medication.

What is the usual dosage?

The information below is based on the dosage guidelines your doctor uses. Depending on your condition and medical history, your doctor may prescribe a different regimen. Do not change the dosage or stop taking your medication without your doctor's approval.

Adults: The usual dose is 5/12.5 (5 milligrams [mg] of enalapril and 12.5 mg of hydrochlorothiazide) or 10/25 (10 mg of enalapril and 25 mg of hydrochlorothiazide).

How should I take Vaseretic?

You should take Vaseretic with or without food at the same time every day.

What should I avoid while taking Vaseretic?

Do not operate automobiles or heavy machinery until you know how Vaseretic will affect you. You should avoid becoming very dehydrated and drink adequate fluids while taking Vaseretic, because this could cause your blood pressure to drop too low. You should not take salt substitutes or supplements containing potassium unless otherwise directed by your doctor.

What are possible food and drug interactions associated with Vaseretic?

If Vaseretic is taken with certain other drugs, the effects of either could be increased, decreased, or altered. It is especially important to check with your doctor before combining Vaseretic with the following: cholestyramine; colestipol; corticosteroids; insulin; lithium; methenamine; nonsteroidal anti-inflammatory medications, such as ibuprofen or naproxen; norepinephrine; potassium-sparing diuretics, such as spironolactone, amiloride, and triamterene; potassium supplements; salt substitutes containing potassium; skeletal muscle relaxants; and thiazide-type diuretics, such as hydrochlorothiazide.

What are the possible side effects of Vaseretic?

Side effects cannot be anticipated. If any develop or change in intensity, tell your doctor as soon as possible. Only your doctor can determine if it is safe for you to continue taking this drug.

Side effects may include: cough, dizziness, fatigue, headache, muscle cramps, impotence

Can I receive Vaseretic if I am pregnant or breastfeeding?

Vaseretic should not be taken during pregnancy. Taking Vaseretic while you are pregnant could cause serious harm or even death to your unborn baby. Tell your doctor immediately if you are pregnant, plan to become pregnant, or are breastfeeding. Vaseretic is excreted in breast milk, and should not be taken if you are breastfeeding.

What should I do if I miss a dose of Vaseretic?

If you forget to take Vaseretic, do not double your next dose. Skip the dose you missed and then return to your normal dosing schedule.

How should I store Vaseretic?

Store at room temperature in a tightly closed container and protect from moisture.

VASOTEC

Generic name: Enalapril maleate

What is Vasotec?

Vasotec is a high blood pressure medication known as an ACE inhibitor. It works by preventing a chemical in your blood called angiotensin I from converting into a more potent form that increases salt and water retention in your body. It is effective when used alone or in combination with other medications, especially thiazide-type diuretics. It is also used in the treatment of congestive heart failure, usually in combination with diuretics and digitalis, and is prescribed as a preventive measure in certain conditions that could lead to heart failure.

What is the most important information I should know about Vasotec?

Vasotec may cause injury or death to an unborn baby if taken after the third month of pregnancy. If you think you may be pregnant, contact your doctor right away.

If you have high blood pressure, you must take Vasotec regularly for it to be effective. Since blood pressure declines gradually, it may be several weeks before you get the full benefit of Vasotec; you must continue taking it even if you are feeling well. Vasotec does not cure high blood pressure; it merely keeps it under control.

If you experience symptoms suggesting angioedema (swelling of the face, extremities, eyes, lips, tongue, difficulty in swallowing or breathing), consult with your prescribing physician before taking any more of the medication.

Do not drive or perform other possibly unsafe tasks until you know how you react to Vasotec; this medication may cause dizziness or light-headedness. These effects may be worse if you take it with alcohol or certain medicines.

Vasotec may cause you to become sunburned more easily. Avoid the sun, sunlamps, or tanning booths until you know how you react to Vasotec. Use sunscreen or wear protective clothing if you must be outside for more than a short time.

Check with your doctor before you use a salt substitute or a product that has potassium in it.

Avoid standing or sitting up too quickly when taking this medication, especially in the morning; light-headedness or dizziness may occur. Sit down at the first sign of these symptoms.

If vomiting or diarrhea occurs, you will need to take care not to become dehydrated. Contact your doctor for instructions.

Patients who take medications for high blood pressure often feel tired or run down for a few weeks after starting treatment. Be sure to take your medicine even if you may not feel "normal." Tell your doctor if you develop any new symptoms.

Vasotec may not work as well in black patients, who may also be at greater risk of side effects. Contact your doctor if your symptoms do not improve or if they become worse.

Tell your doctor or dentist that you take Vasotec before you receive any medical or dental care, emergency care, or surgery.

Who should not take Vasotec?

You should not take Vasotec if you have had a previous allergic reaction or are sensitive to Vasotec or any other ACE inhibitor.

What should I tell my doctor before I take the first dose of Vasotec?

Mention all prescription, over-the-counter, and herbal medications you are taking before beginning treatment with Vasotec. Also, talk to your doctor about your complete medical history, especially if you have liver or kidney disease, have bone marrow suppression, the blood disease porphyria, lupus, scleroderma, collagen vascular disease, narrowing or hardening of the arteries of the brain or heart, chest pain, or if you have ever had an allergy or sensitivity to an ACE inhibitor such as Vasotec. In addition, tell your doctor if you are pregnant or plan on becoming pregnant.

What is the usual dosage?

The information below is based on the dosage guidelines your doctor uses. Depending on your condition and medical history, your doctor may prescribe a different regimen. Do not change the dosage or stop taking your medication without your doctor's approval.

Hypertension
Adults: The usual dosage is 5 milligrams (mg) taken once a day. Your individual dose may be increased to 10-40 mg taken as one daily dose or in divided doses.

In patients who are currently being treated with a diuretic, a potentially dangerous decrease in blood pressure may occur following the initial dose of Vasotec. The diuretic should, if possible, be discontinued for two to three days before beginning therapy with Vasotec, to reduce the likelihood of hypotension (a blood pressure lower than the norm). If your blood pressure is not controlled with Vasotec alone, diuretic therapy may be resumed.

If the diuretic cannot be discontinued, an initial Vasotec dose of 2.5 mg should be used under medical supervision for at least two hours and until blood pressure has stabilized for at least an additional hour.

Heart Failure
Adults: The usual starting dose is 2.5 mg. Your doctor may increase your dose up to 20 mg taken twice a day depending on your individual response. Doses should be increased over a period of a few days or weeks based on how you respond to the medication and any possible side effects that may occur.

Asymptomatic Left Ventricular Dysfunction
Adults: The usual starting dose is 2.5 mg. Your doctor may increase your dose up to 20 mg a day (taken in divided doses) depending on your individual response.

Children: The usual starting dose is 0.08 mg per 2.2 pounds of body weight (up to 5 mg) taken once daily. Daily doses in excess of 40 mg have not been studied in pediatric patients.

How should I take Vasotec?

Vasotec can be taken with or without food and should be taken at the same time every day. If stomach upset occurs, take Vasotec with food.

Take this medication as prescribed by your doctor. Do not change the dose or suddenly stop taking this medication for any reason without first contacting your doctor.

What should I avoid while taking Vasotec?

Do not operate automobiles or heavy machinery until you know how Vasotec will affect you. Avoid being exposed to excessive heat; excessive sweating, dehydration, severe diarrhea, or vomiting could prompt you to lose too much water, causing your blood pressure to drop dangerously. You should not take salt substitutes or supplements containing potassium unless otherwise directed by your doctor.

Avoid the sun, sunlamps, or tanning booths until you know how you react to Vasotec. Use sunscreen or wear protective clothing if you must be outside for more than a short time.

Avoid standing or sitting up too quickly when taking this medication, especially in the morning; light-headedness or dizziness may occur.

What are possible food and drug interactions associated with Vasotec?

If Vasotec is taken with certain other drugs, the effects of either could be increased, decreased, or altered. It is especially important to check with your doctor before combining Vasotec with the following: dextran; diuretics, such as furosemide; lithium; nonsteroidal anti-inflammatory drugs (NSAIDs); oral diabetes medicine, such as glyburide; potassium-sparing diuretics, such as spironolactone, amiloride, and triamterene; potassium supplements; salt substitutes containing potassium; and thiazide-type diuretics, such as hydrochlorothiazide.

What are the possible side effects of Vasotec?

Side effects cannot be anticipated. If any develop or change in intensity, tell your doctor as soon as possible. Only your doctor can determine if it is safe for you to continue taking this drug.

Side effects may include: cough, dizziness, dizziness upon standing, fatigue, headache, low blood pressure, nausea, rash, vomiting, weakness, diarrhea

If you experience symptoms suggesting angioedema (swelling of the face, extremities, eyes, lips, tongue, difficulty in swallowing or breathing), consult with your prescribing physician before taking any more of the medication.

Can I receive Vasotec if I am pregnant or breastfeeding?

Vasotec should not be taken during pregnancy. Taking Vasotec during the second or third trimesters of your pregnancy could cause serious harm or even death to your unborn baby. Tell your doctor immediately if you are pregnant, plan to become pregnant, or are breastfeeding. Vasotec is found in breast milk, and should not be taken if you are breastfeeding.

What should I do if I miss a dose of Vasotec?

If you miss a dose of Vasotec, take it as soon as possible. If it is almost time for your next dose, skip the missed dose and go back to your regular dosing schedule. Do not take 2 doses at once.

How should I store Vasotec?

Store at room temperature below 86 degrees (30 degrees C). Store away from heat, moisture, and light. Do not store in the bathroom. Keep Vasotec out of the reach of children.

Venlafaxine hydrochloride See Effexor, page 463.

Venlafaxine hydrochloride, extended-release
   See Effexor XR, page 465.

VERAMYST
Generic name: Fluticasone furoate

What is Veramyst?

Veramyst is a medicine that treats seasonal and year-round allergy symptoms in adults and children 2 years old and older. Veramyst contains fluticasone furoate, which is a man-made (synthetic) corticosteroid. Corticosteroids are natural substances found in the body that reduce inflammation. When you spray Veramyst into your nose, it helps reduce the nasal symptoms of allergic rhinitis (inflammation of the lining of the nose), such as stuffy nose, runny nose, itching, and sneezing. Veramyst may also help red, itchy, and watery eyes in adults and teenagers with seasonal allergic rhinitis.

What is the most important information I should know about Veramyst?

Rare fungal infections may occur with treatment with Veramyst Nasal Spray. In addition, nasal corticosteroids are associated with nasal bleeding, nasal ulcerations, and nasal septal perforation and impaired wound healing.

   Patients who have experienced recent nasal ulcers, nasal surgery, or nasal trauma should not use Veramyst Nasal Spray until healing has occurred.

Glaucoma and cataracts are associated with nasal and inhaled corticosteroid use. You should have regular eye exams, and inform your health care provider if a change in vision is noted while using Veramyst Nasal Spray.

Immune system effects may increase the risk of infections with the use of Veramyst. Veramyst Nasal Spray should be used on a regular once-daily basis for optimal effect. Veramyst, like other corticosteroids, does not have an immediate effect on rhinitis symptoms. Although significant improvement is usually achieved within 24 hours with seasonal allergic rhinitis and 4 days with perennial allergic rhinitis, maximum benefit may not be reached for several days.

Long-term use of systemic corticosteroids may cause adrenal suppression.

Abrupt discontinuation may cause joint pain, muscular pain, and depression. Make sure to follow your healthcare provider's instructions when discontinuing this drug.

Make sure to tell you doctor if you have any form of liver disease.

Children taking Veramyst should have their growth checked regularly since corticosteroids may slow the growth of children.

Who should not take Veramyst?

You should not use Veramyst if you have had recent nasal surgery, nasal ulcers, or nasal trauma; if you've recently been exposed to chicken pox or measles; if you are pregnant or plan to become pregnant or are breast-feeding; if you have liver disease or you are allergic to any of the ingredients in Veramyst.

What should I tell my doctor before I take the first dose of Veramyst?

Tell your doctor about all prescription, over-the-counter, and herbal medication you are taking before beginning treatment with Veramyst, especially if you are taking a medicine that contains ritonavir (commonly used to treat HIV infection or AIDS). Also, talk to your doctor about your complete medical history, especially if you are pregnant or plan to become pregnant or you are breastfeeding; if you are allergic to any of the ingredients in Veramyst or any other nasal corticosteroid; if you have been exposed to chickenpox or measles; or if you are feeling unwell or have any symptoms that you do not understand.

What is the usual dosage?

The information below is based on the dosage guidelines your doctor uses. Depending on your condition and medical history, your doctor may prescribe a different regimen. Do not change the dosage or stop taking your medication without your doctor's approval.

Adults and children 12 years and older: The usual starting dosage is 2 sprays in each nostril, once a day. After you begin to feel better, your healthcare provider may recommend 1 spray in each nostril once a day.

Children 2 to 11 years: The usual starting dosage is 1 spray in each nostril, once a day. Your healthcare provider may tell you to take 2 sprays in each nostril once a day. After you begin to feel better, your healthcare provider may change the dosage to 1 spray in each nostril once a day.

How should I take Veramyst?

Before you use a new bottle the first time, you need to prime Veramyst Nasal Spray: With the cap on, shake the device well. Take the cap off by squeezing the finger grips and pulling it straight off. Do not press the button while you take off the cap. Hold the device with the nozzle pointing up and away from you. Place your thumb on the button. Then firmly press and release the button 6 times or until a fine mist is sprayed from the nozzle. Your Veramyst Nasal Spray is now ready to use.

Before taking a dose of Veramyst Nasal Spray, gently blow your nose to clear your nostrils. Tilt your head forward a little bit. Hold the device upright. Place the nozzle in one of your nostrils. Point the end of the nozzle toward the side of your nose, away from the center of your nose (septum). This helps get the medicine to the right part of your nose. Firmly press the button 1 time to spray the medicine in your nose while you are breathing in.

Do not get any spray in your eyes. If you do, rinse your eyes well with water.

Take the nozzle out of your nose. Breathe out through your mouth. Repeat these steps in the other nostril as well.

Put the cap back on the device after you have finished taking your dose. After each use, wipe the nozzle with a clean, dry tissue. Never try to clean the nozzle with a pin or anything sharp because this may damage the nozzle.

What should I avoid while taking Veramyst?

Avoid skipping doses of your medication. To get the best results with Veramyst you must be on top of your doses. Avoid giving this medication to a person that it is not prescribed for. Corticosteroids can be dangerous for some people who are not approved by a health care professional to take them. Keep this medication away from your eyes and mouth. Never leave your Veramyst device un-capped.

What are possible food and drug interactions associated with Veramyst?

If Veramyst is taken with certain other drugs, the effects of either or both drugs could be altered. It is especially important to check with your doctor before combining Veramyst with the following: ketoconazole, ritonavir.

What are the possible side effects of Veramyst?

Side effects cannot be anticipated. If any develop or change in intensity, tell your doctor as soon as possible. Only your doctor can determine if it is safe for you to continue taking this drug.

Side effects may include: cough and fever, nasal sores, nosebleeds, and headaches

Can I receive Veramyst if I am pregnant or breastfeeding?

The effects of Veramyst during pregnancy and breastfeeding are unknown. Tell your doctor immediately if you are pregnant, plan to become pregnant, or are breastfeeding.

What should I do if I miss a dose of Veramyst?

If you remember to take your dose within 12 hours of your scheduled time, go ahead and take the missed dose. If you remember to take your dose when it is more than 12 hours past your scheduled time, skip that dose and take the next one. Do not double the dose.

How should I store Veramyst?

Store Veramyst upright, at room temperature. Keep it out of the reach of children.

Verapamil hydrochloride See Calan, page 242.

VERDESO

Generic name: Desonide

What is Verdeso?

Verdeso foam is used to treat mild-to-moderate atopic dermatitis (eczema) in adults and children, age 3 months and older. Atopic dermatitis is a condition where the skin becomes extremely itchy; when scratched, it can result in redness, swelling, cracking, scaling, and crusting.

What is the most important information I should know about Verdeso?

The areas of your body being treated with Verdeso should not be covered with a bandage or dressing. This may cause an increase in blood sugar, sugar in urine, and, potentially, Cushing's syndrome. Cushing's syndrome is an increase in ACTH (adrenocorticotropic hormone), which can produce symptoms such as weight gain, fatigue, and increased blood pressure.

Who should not take Verdeso?

Do not use Verdeso if you are allergic to any of its ingredients.

What should I tell my doctor before I take the first dose of Verdeso?

Mention all prescription, over-the-counter, and herbal medications you are taking before beginning treatment with Verdeso. Also, talk to your doctor about your complete medical history, especially if you are going to have surgery.

What is the usual dosage?

The information below is based on the dosage guidelines your doctor uses. Depending on your condition and medical history, your doctor may prescribe a different regimen. Do not change the dosage or stop taking your medication without your doctor's approval.

Adults and children 3 months and older: A thin layer of Verdeso foam should be applied to the affected area(s) twice daily.

How should I take Verdeso?

Verdeso should not be put directly on the face. Squirt the foam into your hands and gently massage it into the affected areas of your face until the medication disappears. For areas other than the face, the medication may be applied directly on the affected area. Take care to avoid contact with the eyes. If no improvement is seen in 4 weeks, contact your doctor.

What should I avoid while taking Verdeso?

Avoid putting Verdeso directly on your face. Keep this medication away from your eyes.

What are possible food and drug interactions associated with Verdeso?

No significant interactions have been reported at this time. However, always tell your doctor about any medicines you take, including over-the-counter drugs, vitamins, and herbal supplements.

What are the possible side effects of Verdeso?

Side effects cannot be anticipated. If any develop or change in intensity, tell your doctor as soon as possible. Only your doctor can determine if it is safe for you to continue taking this drug.

Side effects may include: application site burning, asthma, cough, headache, irritability, itching, red skin blotches, redness

Can I receive Verdeso if I am pregnant or breastfeeding?

The effects of Verdeso during pregnancy and breastfeeding are unknown. Tell your doctor immediately if you are pregnant, plan to become pregnant, or are breastfeeding.

What should I do if I miss a dose of Verdeso?

Take the missed dose as soon as you remember. If it is almost time for your next dose, skip the missed dose and return to your normal dosing schedule. Do not double the dose.

How should I store Verdeso?

Store at room temperature.

VESICARE

Generic name: Solifenacin succinate

What is VESIcare?

VESIcare is prescribed for the treatment of overactive bladder (OAB). People with overactive bladder experience a strong and urgent need to urinate (urgency), a need to urinate more often than normal (frequency), or involuntary urine leakage (incontinence).

In OAB, the muscle in the bladder wall spasms, causing a need to urinate even when the bladder is not full. It can also result in accidental urination. VESIcare relaxes the muscle in the bladder wall, reducing spasms and restoring more normal bladder function.

What is the most important information I should know about VESIcare?

VESIcare can cause blurred vision. You must use caution when driving, operating machinery, or engaging in hazardous activities when taking this drug, to prevent injury to yourself and others.

Who should not take VESIcare?

Do not take VESIcare if you are not able to empty your bladder, have slow or delayed emptying of your stomach, have an untreated eye condition called narrow angle glaucoma, or if you are allergic or sensitive to VESIcare or any of its ingredients.

What should I tell my doctor before I take the first dose of VESIcare?

Mention all prescription, over-the-counter, and herbal medications you are taking before beginning treatment with VESIcare. Also, talk to your doctor about your complete medical history, especially if you have any stomach or intestinal problems, if you are currently constipated or have a history of constipation, if you have trouble emptying your bladder fully or you have a weak stream of urine, if you have liver or kidney problems, if you are pregnant, trying to become pregnant, or if you are breastfeeding.

What is the usual dosage?

The information below is based on the dosage guidelines your doctor uses. Depending on your condition and medical history, your doctor

may prescribe a different regimen. Do not change the dosage or stop taking your medication without your doctor's approval.

Adults: The usual starting dose of VESIcare is 5 mg once a day. Depending on your response, your doctor may increase the dose to 10 mg.

If you have severe kidney problems or moderate liver dysfunction, the maximum recommended dose is 5 mg a day. Using VESIcare is not recommended if you have severe liver dysfunction.

If you take antifungal or antiviral drugs, your dosage should not exceed 5 mg a day.

How should I take VESIcare?
You should take one VESIcare tablet once a day at the same time. You should swallow the tablet whole with a liquid, and you can take VESIcare with or without food.

What should I avoid while taking VESIcare?
You should not drive a car or operate heavy machinery until you know how VESIcare will affect you.

What are possible food and drug interactions associated with VESIcare?
If VESIcare is taken with certain other drugs, the effects of either could be increased, decreased, or altered. It is especially important to check with your doctor before combining VESIcare with the following: atazanavir, indinavir, itraconazole, ketoconazole, nelfinavir, ritonavir, saquinavir, and voriconazole.

What are the possible side effects of VESIcare?
Side effects cannot be anticipated. If any develop or change in intensity, tell your doctor as soon as possible. Only your doctor can determine if it is safe for you to continue taking this drug.

Side effects may include: blurred vision, constipation, dry mouth, nausea, upset stomach, urinary tract infection, heat prostration

Can I receive VESIcare if I am pregnant or breastfeeding?
The effects of VESIcare during pregnancy and breastfeeding are unknown. Tell your doctor immediately if you are pregnant, plan to become pregnant, or are breastfeeding.

What should I do if I miss a dose of VESIcare?
If you miss a VESIcare dose, do not double your next dose. Skip the dose you missed and return to your normal dosing schedule.

How should I store VESIcare?
Store at room temperature and away from children.

VIAGRA
Generic name: Sildenafil citrate

What is Viagra?
Viagra is an oral drug for male impotence, also known as erectile dysfunction (ED). It works by dilating blood vessels in the penis, allowing the inflow of blood needed for an erection.

What is the most important information I should know about Viagra?
Viagra causes erections only during sexual excitement. It does not work in the absence of arousal.

You should not take Viagra if you have been instructed by your doctor not to engage in sexual activity due to heart disease or other heart problems. Viagra may interact with your medications, and should never be taken with medications or foods containing nitrates.

Who should not take Viagra?
You should not take Viagra if you are also consuming other foods or medications that contain nitrates. You should also not take Viagra if you are allergic or sensitive to any of its ingredients.

What should I tell my doctor before I take the first dose of Viagra?
Mention all prescription, over-the-counter, and herbal medications you are taking before beginning treatment with Viagra. Also, talk to your doctor about your complete medical history, especially if you have heart disease; angina; recently suffered a heart attack, stroke or life-threatening arrhythmia; if you have a physical deformation of your penis; sickle cell anemia; an eye disease called retinitis pigmentosa; leukemia; or multiple myeloma.

What is the usual dosage?
The information below is based on the dosage guidelines your doctor uses. Depending on your condition and medical history, your doctor may prescribe a different regimen. Do not change the dosage or stop taking your medication without your doctor's approval.

Adults: The usual dosage is 50 milligrams (mg) taken as needed 1 hour before sexual activity.

How should I take Viagra?
Viagra may be taken anywhere from 30 minutes to 4 hours before sexual activity; however, 1 hour is usually most effective. You should not take more than 1 Viagra dose per day. Viagra may be taken with or without food, but should not be taken with anything that may contain nitrates.

What should I avoid while taking Viagra?

You should not eat food or take medications that contain nitrates such as nitroglycerin.

What are possible food and drug interactions associated with Viagra?

If Viagra is taken with certain other drugs, the effects of either could be increased, decreased, or altered. It is especially important to check with your doctor before combining Viagra with the following: blood pressure lowering medications, such as amlodipine or doxazosin; bosentan; cimetidine; erythromycin; itraconazole; ketoconazole; rifampin; ritonavir; and saquinavir.

What are the possible side effects of Viagra?

Side effects cannot be anticipated. If any develop or change in intensity, tell your doctor as soon as possible. Only your doctor can determine if it is safe for you to continue taking this drug.

Side effects may include: congestion, diarrhea, flushing (skin redness), headache, nasal congestion, urinary tract infection, eyes being more sensitive to light, blurred vision, upset stomach, dizziness

Can I receive Viagra if I am pregnant or breastfeeding?

Viagra is not for use in newborns, children, and women.

What should I do if I miss a dose of Viagra?

Viagra is not for regular use. Take it only before sexual activity. Do not take more than 1 dose in 24 hours.

How should I store Viagra?

Store at room temperature.

VICODIN

Generic name: Hydrocodone bitartrate and acetaminophen

What is Vicodin?

Vicodin is used to treat moderate to moderately severe pain.

What is the most important information I should know about Vicodin?

Vicodin may make cause irregular breathing patterns. This drug may also become habit-forming. Vicodin should be taken in the dose prescribed, only for the length of time your doctor recommends it.

Who should not take Vicodin?
Do not begin treatment with Vicodin if you are allergic to any of its ingredients.

What should I tell my doctor before I take the first dose of Vicodin?
Tell your doctor about all prescription, over-the-counter, and herbal medication you are taking before beginning treatment with Vicodin. Also, talk to your doctor about your complete medical history, especially if you have liver, kidney, or thyroid problems. Also, tell your doctor if you have a history of drug dependence.

What is the usual dosage?
The information below is based on the dosage guidelines your doctor uses. Depending on your condition and medical history, your doctor may prescribe a different regimen. Do not change the dosage or stop taking your medication without your doctor's approval.

Adults: The usual dosage is 1 or 2 tablets every 4-6 hours. Do not exceed 8 tablets per day.

How should I take Vicodin?
Take Vicodin exactly as your doctor prescribes it.

What should I avoid while taking Vicodin?
Avoid driving or operating machinery before you know how Vicodin will affect you.

What are possible food and drug interactions associated with Vicodin?
If Vicodin is taken with certain other drugs, the effects of either could be increased, decreased, or altered. It is especially important to check with your doctor before combining Vicodin with the following: MAO inhibitors and tricyclic antidepressants.

What are the possible side effects of Vicodin?
Side effects cannot be anticipated. If any develop or change in intensity, tell your doctor as soon as possible. Only your doctor can determine if it is safe for you to continue taking this drug.

Side effects may include: dizziness, lightheadedness, nausea, sleepiness, vomiting

Can I receive Vicodin if I am pregnant or breastfeeding?
The effects of Vicodin during pregnancy and breastfeeding are unknown. Tell your doctor immediately if you are pregnant, plan to become pregnant, or are breastfeeding.

How should I store Vicodin?
Store at room temperature.

VICOPROFEN
Generic name: Hydrocodone bitartrate and ibuprofen

What is Vicoprofen?
Vicoprofen is a non-steroidal anti-inflammatory drug (NSAID) used to treat pain and redness, swelling, and heat (inflammation).

**What is the most important information
I should know about Vicoprofen?**
Vicoprofen may increase the chance of a heart attack or stroke that can lead to death. It can also cause ulcers and bleeding in the stomach and intestines at any time during treatment.

Who should not take Vicoprofen?
Do not begin treatment with Vicoprofen if you had an asthma attack, hives, or other allergic reaction with aspirin or any other NSAID medicine for pain right before or after heart bypass surgery.

**What should I tell my doctor before
I take the first dose of Vicoprofen?**
Tell your doctor about all prescription, over-the-counter, and herbal medication you are taking before beginning treatment with Vicoprofen. Also, talk to your doctor about your complete medical history, especially if you heart problems, smoke, or drink alcohol regularly.

What is the usual dosage?
The information below is based on the dosage guidelines your doctor uses. Depending on your condition and medical history, your doctor may prescribe a different regimen. Do not change the dosage or stop taking your medication without your doctor's approval.

Adults: The recommended dose of Vicoprofen is one tablet every 4 to 6 hours, as necessary.

What should I avoid while taking Vicoprofen?
Avoid driving or operating heavy machinery while taking Vicoprofen, as it may cause drowsiness.

**What are possible food and drug interactions
associated with Vicoprofen?**
If Vicoprofen is taken with certain other drugs, the effects of either could be increased, decreased, or altered. It is especially important to check with your doctor before combining Vicoprofen with the following:

ACE-inhibitors, antianxiety medicines, antidepressants, antihistamines, antipsychotics, aspirin, buprenorphine, butorphanol, diuretics, lithium, methotrexate, nalbuphine, opioids, pentazocine, and warfarin.

What are the possible side effects of Vicoprofen?
Side effects cannot be anticipated. If any develop or change in intensity, tell your doctor as soon as possible. Only your doctor can determine if it is safe for you to continue taking this drug.

Side effects may include: fever, flu syndrome, headache, infection, pain, stomach pain, tiredness

Can I receive Vicoprofen if I am pregnant or breastfeeding?
The effects of Vicoprofen during pregnancy and breastfeeding are unknown. Tell your doctor immediately if you are pregnant, plan to become pregnant, or are breastfeeding.

How should I store Vicoprofen?
Store at room temperature.

VIDEX
Generic name: Didanosine

What is Videx?
Videx is one of the drugs used to fight human immunodeficiency virus (HIV)—the cause of AIDS. Over a period of years, HIV slowly destroys the immune system, leaving the body defenseless against infection. Videx disrupts reproduction of HIV, thereby staving off the immune system's collapse.

Signs and symptoms of advanced HIV infection include diarrhea, fever, headache, infections, nervous system problems, rash, sore throat, and significant weight loss.

What is the most important information I should know about Videx?
Although Videx can slow the progress of HIV, it is not a cure. You may continue to develop complications, including frequent infections. Even if you feel better, regular physical exams and blood counts are highly advisable. And notify your doctor immediately if you experience any changes in your general health.

Pancreatitis has occurred during therapy with Videx used alone or in combination regimens.

Who should not take Videx?
You should not take Videx if you have an allergy to Videx or any of its ingredients.

What should I tell my doctor before I take the first dose of Videx?

Mention all prescription, over-the-counter, and herbal medications you are taking before beginning treatment with Videx. Also, talk to your doctor about your complete medical history, especially if you have a history of pancreatitis (inflammation of the pancreas), kidney disease, hepatitis or other liver problems, alcohol abuse, or if you are pregnant or are planning to become pregnant.

What is the usual dosage?

The information below is based on the dosage guidelines your doctor uses. Depending on your condition and medical history, your doctor may prescribe a different regimen. Do not change the dosage or stop taking your medication without your doctor's approval.

Adults: If you weigh more than 132 pounds, the usual dose is 200 milligrams (mg) taken twice daily. If you weigh less than 132 pounds, the usual dose is

125 mg taken twice daily. A once daily dosing regimen is also available.

Children: The recommended dose of Videx in pediatric patients between 2 weeks and 8 months of age is 100 mg/m^2 twice daily, and the recommended Videx dose for pediatric patients older than 8 months is 120 mg/m^2 twice daily.

Dosing recommendations for Videx in patients less than 2 weeks of age cannot be made because the pharmacokinetics of didanosine in these children is too variable to determine an appropriate dose. There are no data on once-daily dosing of Videx in pediatric patients.

How should I take Videx?

Videx should be taken on an empty stomach, at least 30 minutes before or 2 hours after eating. You should swallow the capsule whole; do not open or crush the capsules.

What should I avoid while taking Videx?

You should not drink alcohol or become pregnant while taking Videx. You should also not take any other medications, vitamins, or supplements without first checking with your doctor.

What are possible food and drug interactions associated with Videx?

If Videx is taken with certain other drugs, the effects of either could be increased, decreased, or altered. It is especially important to check with your doctor before combining Videx with the following: allopurinol, ciprofloxacin, delavirdine, ganiciclovir, methadone, nelfinavir, ranitidine, rifabutin, ritonavir, stavudine, sulfamethoxazole, tenofovir, trimethoprim, and zidovudine.

What are the possible side effects of Videx?

Side effects cannot be anticipated. If any develop or change in intensity, tell your doctor as soon as possible. Only your doctor can determine if it is safe for you to continue taking this drug.

Side effects may include: changes in body fat, diarrhea, headache, nausea, pain/numbness/tingling in hands or feet, rash

Serious side effects include: lactic acidosis, liver failure, pancreatitis

Can I receive Videx if I am pregnant or breastfeeding?

Videx during pregnancy and breastfeeding are unknown. Tell your doctor immediately if you are pregnant, plan to become pregnant, or are breastfeeding.

The Centers for Disease Control and Prevention recommends that HIV-infected mothers not breastfeed their infants to avoid risking postnatal transmission of HIV.

What should I do if I miss a dose of Videx?

If you forget to take Videx, take the missed dose right away. If it is almost time for your next dose, do not take the missed dose. Instead, follow your regular dosing schedule by taking the next dose at its regular time.

How should I store Videx?

Store at room temperature and away from children.

VIRACEPT

Generic name: Nelfinavir mesylate

What is Viracept?

Viracept is a protease inhibitor used in combination with other antiretroviral drugs in the treatment of people with HIV infection. It can be used for adults and for children 2 years and older.

What is the most important information I should know about Viracept?

Viracept is not a cure for HIV infection or AIDS. People taking this medication may still develop opportunistic infections or other conditions associated with HIV infection. It does not reduce the risk of transmitting HIV to others through sexual contact or blood contamination. Continue to practice safe sex and do not use or share dirty needles.

Who should not take Viracept?

Do not take Viracept if you are taking certain medicines that are highly dependent on liver clearance, have an allergy to this medication, or if you have any known allergies to other medicines, foods, preservatives, or dyes. If you have phenylketonuria, the oral powder may not be suitable for you since it contains 11.2 mg of phenylalanine per gram of powder

What should I tell my doctor before I take the first dose of Viracept?
Tell your doctor about all prescription, over-the-counter, and herbal medications you are taking before beginning treatment with Viracept. Also talk to your doctor about your complete medical history, especially if you have liver or kidney disease, are pregnant, or plan to become pregnant.

What is the usual dosage?
The information below is based on the dosage guidelines your doctor uses. Depending on your condition and medical history, your doctor may prescribe a different regimen. Do not change the dosage or stop taking your medication without your doctor's approval.

Adults: The recommended dose is 1250 milligrams (mg) (five 250-mg tablets or two 625-mg tablets) 2 times daily or 750 mg (three 250-mg tablets) 3 times daily with meals

Children 2 to 13 years: The oral powder or 250 mg tablet dosage is 45 to 55 milligrams/kilogram (mg/kg) body weight 2 times daily or 25 to 35 mg/kg 3 times daily with meals. The maximum dose is 2500 mg per day.

How should I take Viracept?
You should stay under the care of a healthcare professional when taking Viracept. Do not change your treatment or stop treatment without first talking with your healthcare provider. You should take it every day exactly as directed with meals.

If you cannot swallow tablets, you may take Viracept oral powder or dissolve the tablets. Tablets can be dissolved in a small amount of water and mixed to form a cloudy liquid. It should be taken immediately, then rinse the glass with water and swallowed the remaining liquid to ensure the entire dose is consumed.

The oral powder may be mixed with a small amount of water, milk, formula, soy formula, soy milk, dietary supplement, or dairy foods such as pudding or ice cream. Once mixed, the entire amount must be taken to obtain the full dose. If the mixture is not consumed immediately, store in the refrigerator. It expires 6 hours after reconstitution.

What should I avoid while taking Viracept?
You should avoid having unprotected sex or sharing needles, razors, or toothbrushes as this drug does not reduce the risk of transmitting HIV to others. Talk with your doctor about safe methods of preventing HIV transmission during sex, such as using a condom and spermicide.

What are possible food and drug interactions associated with Viracept?

If Viracept is taken with certain other drugs, the effects of either could be increased, decreased, or altered. It is especially important to check with your doctor before combining it with the following: amiodarone, carbamazepine, dihydroergotamine, ergotamine, lovastatin, methylergonovine, midazolam, omeprazole, phenobarbital, pimozide, quinidine, rifampin, sildenafil, simvastatin, St. John's wort, tadalafil, triazolam, and vardenafil.

What are the possible side effects of Viracept?

Side effects cannot be anticipated. If any develop or change in intensity, tell your doctor as soon as possible. Only your doctor can determine if it is safe for you to continue taking this drug.

Side effects may include: diarrhea, nausea, flatulence, redistribution of fat

Can I receive Viracept if I am pregnant or breastfeeding?

The effects of Viracept during pregnancy are unknown. Tell your doctor immediately if you are pregnant, or plan to become pregnant. Because the virus can be passed to a baby through breast milk, breastfeeding is not recommended for mothers with HIV.

What should I do if I miss a dose of Viracept?

If you forget to take a dose, take it as soon as possible. However, if you skip the dose entirely, do not double the next dose. If you forget a number of doses, talk to your healthcare provider about how you should continue taking your medicine.

How should I store Viracept?

Store Viracept tablets at room temperature.

VIRAMUNE

Generic name: Nevirapine

What is Viramune?

Viramune is a medication used to treat Human Immunodeficiency Virus (HIV), the virus that causes AIDS (Acquired Immune Deficiency Syndrome). Viramune is a non-nucleoside reverse transcriptase inhibitor (NNRTI). Viramune must be taken in combination with other anti-HIV medications to reduce the amount of virus circulating in your blood, and increase the number of disease-fighting cells (CD4 cells) in the blood.

What is the most important information I should know about Viramune?

Viramune can also cause fatal or life-threatening skin reactions. These usually begin as a rash and then progress to more serious effects often involving one or more organs. Symptoms include swelling of the face, blisters, mouth sores, red or inflamed eyes, or flu-like symptoms. If you notice any of these while taking Viramune tell your doctor immediately. If your doctor has told you to stop taking Viramune due to any of the reactions described above, you should never begin treatment with it again. Liver damage has also been reported in the first 18 weeks of treatment.

Who should not take Viramune?
Do not take Viramune if you have an allergy or sensitivity to it or any of its ingredients. Do not take Viramune if you have ever had a serious side effect such as liver injury or severe skin reaction while taking it.

What should I tell my doctor before I take the first dose of Viramune?
Mention all prescription, over-the-counter, and herbal medications you are taking before beginning treatment with Viramune. Also, talk to your doctor about your complete medical history, especially if you have liver problems or have had hepatitis, are undergoing dialysis, have skin conditions such as a rash, are pregnant, plan on becoming pregnant, or if you are breastfeeding.

What is the usual dosage?
The information below is based on the dosage guidelines your doctor uses. Depending on your condition and medical history, your doctor may prescribe a different regimen. Do not change the dosage or stop taking your medication without your doctor's approval.

Adults: The usual initial dosage is one 200 milligram (mg) tablet taken once a day for 14 days. The dose is usually increased to 200 mg taken twice daily.

Children ages 2 months to 8 years: The usual dose is 4 mg per 2.2 pounds of body weight taken once daily for the first 14 days, then 7 mg per 2.2 pounds of body weight taken twice daily thereafter.

Children ages 8 years and older: The usual dose is 4 mg per 2.2 pounds of body weight taken once daily for the first 14 days, then 4 mg per 2.2 pounds of body weight taken twice daily thereafter.
 The total daily dose should not exceed 400 mg per day for any patient.

How should I take Viramune?
Take Viramune exactly as prescribed by your doctor: with water, milk, soda, or with or without food. If taking the Viramune suspension (liquid), shake it gently before use. Use an oral dosing syringe or dosing cup for precise measurements. After drinking the medicine, fill the dosing cup with water and drink it to make sure you get all the medicine. If the dose is less than 5 milliliters (one teaspoon), use the oral syringe with proper dose markers.

It is very important to take Viramune daily at the same time and not skip doses. Skipping or missing doses over time may make the virus in your body harder to treat.

What should I avoid while taking Viramune?

You should avoid engaging in behavior that may allow you to spread HIV to others. You should not share needles, razors, or other personal items that may have bodily fluids on them. You should always practice safe sex by using a latex or polyurethane condom.

What are possible food and drug interactions associated with Viramune?

If Viramune is taken with certain other drugs, the effects of either could be increased, decreased, or altered. It is especially important to check with your doctor before combining Viramune with the following: clarithromycin, efavirenz, fluconazole, indinavir, ketoconazole, lopinavir/ritonavir, methadone, nelfinavir, oral birth control pills, rifabutin, rifampin, saquinavir, and St. John's wort.

What are the possible side effects of Viramune?

Side effects cannot be anticipated. If any develop or change in intensity, tell your doctor as soon as possible. Only your doctor can determine if it is safe for you to continue taking this drug.

Side effects may include: abdominal pain, changes in body fat, diarrhea, fatigue, fever, muscle weakness, nausea, vomiting

Can I receive Viramune if I am pregnant or breastfeeding?

Viramune during pregnancy and breastfeeding are unknown. Tell your doctor immediately if you are pregnant, plan to become pregnant, or are breastfeeding.

The Centers for Disease Control and Prevention recommends that HIV-infected mothers not breastfeed their infants to avoid postnatal transmission of HIV.

What should I do if I miss a dose of Viramune?

If you forget to take Viramune, take the missed dose right away. If it is almost time for your next dose, do not take the missed dose. Instead, follow your regular dosing schedule by taking the next dose at its regular time. If you have not taken Viramune for more than 7 days, tell your doctor before you start taking Viramune again.

How should I store Viramune?

Store at room temperature and away from children.

VIREAD
Generic name: Tenofovir disproxil fumarate

What is Viread?
Viread is a medication used to treat HIV, the virus that causes AIDS. Viread must be taken in combination with other anti-HIV medications to reduce the amount of virus circulating in your blood, and increase the number of disease fighting cells (CD4 cells) in the blood. Viread is also used to treat hepatitis B.

What is the most important information I should know about Viread?
Viread does not completely eliminate HIV or totally restore the immune system. There is still a danger of serious infections, so you should be sure to see your doctor regularly for monitoring and tests. Notify your doctor immediately of any changes in your general health.

If you have Hepatitis B (HBV) infection or HIV and HBV infection together, you may have a "flare-up" of Hepatitis B, in which the disease suddenly returns in a worse way than before if you stop taking VIREAD. Do not stop taking VIREAD without your doctor's advice.

After stopping VIREAD, tell you doctor immediately about any new, unusual, or worsening symptoms that you notice after stopping treatment. After you stop taking VIREAD, your doctor will still need to check your health and take blood tests to check your liver for several months.

Lactic acidosis (a buildup in the blood of lactic acid, the same substance that causes your muscles to burn during heavy exercise) and severe hepatomegaly (enlargement of the liver) with steatosis, including fatal cases, have been reported. Treatment with VIREAD should be stopped in any patient who shows symptoms that suggest lactic acidosis or pronounced liver toxicity (including nausea, vomiting, unusual or unexpected stomach discomfort, and weakness).

Who should not take Viread?
You should not take Viread if you are allergic or sensitive to it or any of its ingredients. Do not take Viread if you are already taking Truvada or Atripla because Viread contains (tenofovir) one of the same active ingredients in these two medications. Also, do not take Viread if you have not already discontinued treatment with Hepsera (adefovir dipvoxil).

What should I tell my doctor before I take the first dose of Viread?
Tell your doctor about all prescription, over-the-counter, and herbal medication you are taking before beginning treatment with Viread. Also, talk to your doctor about your complete medical history, especially if you have

kidney or liver problems, including hepatitis B, HIV infection, bone problems, or if you are pregnant, breastfeeding, or plan to become pregnant.

What is the usual dosage?
The information below is based on the dosage guidelines your doctor uses. Depending on your condition and medical history, your doctor may prescribe a different regimen. Do not change the dosage or stop taking your medication without your doctor's approval.

Adults: The usual dosage is 300 milligrams (mg) taken once daily.

Dosages for HIV and hepatitis B patients are the same.

If you have kidney problems, your doctor may recommend that you take Viread less frequently.

How should I take Viread?
Viread should be taken at the same time every day and can be taken with or without food. You should take Viread exactly as your doctor has prescribed and you should not skip doses. Also make sure you are taking other anti-HIV medicines with Viread to prevent resistance.

What should I avoid while taking Viread?
You should not breastfeed while taking Viread.

Avoid running out of your medicine. This could cause the amount of virus in your blood to increase if you stop taking Viread for even a short time.

What are possible food and drug interactions associated with Viread?
If Viread is taken with certain other drugs, the effects of either could be increased, decreased, or altered. It is especially important to check with your doctor before combining Viread with the following: abacavir, atazanavir sulfate, didanosine, emtricitabine, indinavir, lamivudine, lopinavir/ritonavir, and saquinavir/ritonavir.

What are the possible side effects of Viread?
Side effects cannot be anticipated. If any develop or change in intensity, tell your doctor as soon as possible. Only your doctor can determine if it is safe for you to continue taking this drug.

Side effects may include: diarrhea, depression, dizziness, gas, headache, nausea, pain, rash, shortness of breath, vomiting, weakness

Can I receive Viread if I am pregnant or breastfeeding?
Viread. Tell your doctor immediately if you are pregnant, plan to become pregnant, or are breastfeeding.

What should I do if I miss a dose of Viread?
It is important that you do not miss any doses.

If you miss a dose of Viread, take it as soon as you remember and then take your next scheduled dose at its regular time. If it is almost time for your next dose, do not take the missed dose. Wait and take the next dose at the regular time. Do not double the next dose.

How should I store Viread?
Viread should be kept at room temperature, away from children. Do not store in places that are too hot or too cold. Do not keep medicine that is out of date.

VISTARIL
Generic name: Hydroxyzine pamoate

What is Vistaril?
Vistaril is used to treat anxiety, tension, and agitation caused by emotional stress. It is also prescribed as a sedative to alleviate anxiety and tension before or after certain medical procedures (eg, dental procedures or surgery). In addition, Vistaril is used to help control the following: nausea and vomiting (except during pregnancy), anxiety due to alcohol withdrawal, and extreme emotional distress associated with certain allergic conditions such as asthma, chronic hives, and severe itching.

What is the most important information I should know about Vistaril?
Vistaril should not be combined with other central nervous system depressants such as narcotics, barbiturates, or alcohol.

Who should not take Vistaril?
Vistaril should not be used during early pregnancy. Also, do not take Vistaril if you have ever had an allergic reaction to it.

What should I tell my doctor before I take the first dose of Vistaril?
Tell your doctor about all prescription, over-the-counter, and herbal medications you are taking before beginning treatment with Vistaril. Also talk to your doctor about your complete medical history, especially if you are pregnant, planning to become pregnant, or are breastfeeding.

What is the usual dosage?
The information below is based on the dosage guidelines your doctor uses. Depending on your condition and medical history, your doctor may prescribe a different regimen. Do not change the dosage or stop taking your medication without your doctor's approval.

Relief of Anxiety and Tension
Adults: 50-100 milligrams (mg) 4 times a day.

Children: Under 6 years old: 50 mg daily in divided doses. Over 6 years old: 50-100 mg daily in divided doses.

Relief of Itching Due to Allergic Reactions
Adults: 25 mg 3-4 times a day.

Children: Under 6 years old: 50 mg daily in divided doses. Over 6 years old: 50-100 mg daily in divided doses.

As a Sedative Before or After Surgery
Adults: 50-100 mg.

Children: The doctor will calculate an appropriate dose based on your child's weight.

How should I take Vistaril?
Take Vistaril exactly as prescribed by your doctor. It is usually taken in divided doses.

What should I avoid while taking Vistaril?
Avoid drinking alcohol or taking any other medications that may cause drowsiness or decrease your alertness.

This drug may cause drowsiness; be careful when engaging in activities that require alertness such as driving or operating heavy machinery.

What are possible food and drug interactions associated with Vistaril?
If Vistaril is taken with certain other drugs, the effects of either could be increased, decreased, or altered. It is especially important to check with your doctor before combining Vistaril with the following: barbiturates, other sedatives or nervous system depressants, narcotics, and non-narcotic painkillers.

What are the possible side effects of Vistaril?
Side effects cannot be anticipated. If any develop or change in intensity, tell your doctor as soon as possible. Only your doctor can determine if it is safe for you to continue taking this drug.

Side effects may include: dry mouth, drowsiness, tremor, convulsions

Can I receive Vistaril if I am pregnant or breastfeeding?
Tell your doctor immediately if you are pregnant, planning to become pregnant, or are breastfeeding. Vistaril should not be used during early pregnancy. It is not known whether Vistaril is excreted in breast milk. Since many drugs do appear in breast milk, you should not take Vistaril if you are nursing.

What should I do if I miss a dose of Vistaril?
Take it as soon as you remember. If it is almost time for your next dose, skip the one you missed and return to your normal schedule.

How should I store Vistaril?
Store at room temperature away from heat, light, and moisture.

VIVACTIL
Generic name: Protriptyline hydrochloride

What is Vivactil?
Vivactil is a tricyclic antidepressant used to treat depression in people who are under close medical supervision. It is particularly suitable for those who are inactive and withdrawn.

What is the most important information I should know about Vivactil?
Antidepressants can increase the risk of suicidal thinking and behavior in children and teenagers. Adult and pediatric patients taking antidepressants should be watched closely for changes in moods or actions, especially when they first start therapy or when their dose is increased or decreased. Patients and their families should contact the doctor immediately if new symptoms develop or seem to get worse. Signs to watch for include anxiety, hostility, sleeplessness, restlessness, impulsive or dangerous behavior, and thoughts about suicide or dying.

Because Vivactil can affect blood sugar levels, the doctor may monitor your blood sugar or change the dose of any diabetes medication you are taking.

Tell your doctor or dentist that you take Vivactil before receiving any medical or dental care, emergency treatment, or surgery.

Do not abruptly stop taking Vivactil without talking to your doctor first. Suddenly stopping this medication may cause withdrawal symptoms such as headache, nausea, and tiredness.

Who should not take Vivactil?
Do not take monoamine oxidase inhibitors (MAOIs) within 2 weeks before or after treatment with Vivactil. In some cases a serious, possibly fatal, reaction may occur. Examples of MAOIs include selegiline and the antidepressants phenelzine and tranylcypromine. Do not combine Vivactil with cisapride.

Vivactil should not be used during the recovery phase following a heart attack.

Do not use Vivactil if you are allergic to any of its ingredients.

What should I tell my doctor before I take the first dose of Vivactil?

Tell your doctor about all prescription, over-the-counter, and herbal medications you are taking before beginning treatment with Vivactil. Also, talk to your doctor about your complete medical history, especially if you have an overactive thyroid, glaucoma, heart problems, kidney or liver problems, diabetes, seizures, blood diseases, an enlarged prostate, difficulty urinating, and psychiatric disorders including bipolar disorder, schizophrenia, suicide attempts, or suicidal thoughts.

What is the usual dosage?

The information below is based on the dosage guidelines your doctor uses. Depending on your condition and medical history, your doctor may prescribe a different regimen. Do not change the dosage or stop taking your medication without your doctor's approval.

Adults: 15-40 milligrams (mg) taken in divided doses 3-4 times a day. Your doctor may increase the daily dose to 60 mg; daily doses above 60 mg are not recommended.

Adolescents and older patients: The usual starting dose is 5 mg 3 times a day with gradual increases if needed. In older patients, careful monitoring of the heart is necessary if the daily dose exceeds 20 mg.

How should I take Vivactil?

Take Vivactil at the same time every day, with or without food.

What should I avoid while taking Vivactil?

Do not drive or perform other possibly dangerous activities until you know how this drug affects you.

Do not drink alcohol while taking Vivactil, since this may increase the risk of side effects.

Vivactil may cause dizziness, lightheadedness, or fainting. Alcohol, hot weather, exercise, or fever may increase these effects. To prevent them, sit up or stand slowly, especially in the morning. Sit or lie down at the first sign of any of these side effects.

To prevent heatstroke while taking Vivactil, do not become overheated while doing physical activity outdoors.

Vivactil may increase sensitivity to the sun. Avoid exposure to the sun, sunlamps, or tanning booths until you know how this drug affects you. Always use sunscreen when you are outside.

What are possible food and drug interactions associated with Vivactil?

If Vivactil is taken with certain other drugs, the effects of either could be increased, decreased, or altered. It is especially important to check with your doctor before combining Vivactil with the following: other antidepressants, astemizole, antifungals such as fluconazole, barbiturates and other sedatives, cisapride, cimetidine, clonidine, duloxetine, guanethidine, MAOIs, quinolone antibiotics such as ciprofloxacin, dalfpristin and similar drugs, phenylephrine and similar drugs, terbinafine, and tramadol.

What are the possible side effects of Vivactil?
Side effects cannot be anticipated. If any develop or change in intensity, tell your doctor as soon as possible. Only your doctor can determine if it is safe for you to continue taking this drug.

Side effects may include: agitation, dizziness, drowsiness, headache, impotence, sweating, tiredness, upset stomach, weight loss or gain, pupil dilation, sensitivity to sunlight, excitement, anxiety, blurred vision, confusion, constipation, diarrhea, nausea, seizures, trouble urinating, vomiting

Can I receive Vivactil if I am pregnant or breastfeeding?
The effects of Vivactil during pregnancy and breastfeeding are unknown. Tell your doctor immediately if you are pregnant, plan to become pregnant, or are breastfeeding.

What should I do if I miss a dose of Vivactil?
Take it as soon as you remember. If it is almost time for your next dose, skip the one you missed and go back to your regular schedule. Do not take two doses at once. If you take one dose daily at bedtime, do not take the missed dose the next morning.

How should I store Vivactil?
Store at room temperature away from heat, moisture, and light. Do not store in the bathroom.

VIVITROL
Generic name: Naltrexone

What is Vivitrol?
Vivitrol is used to treat alcohol dependence.

What is the most important information I should know about Vivitrol?
Vivitrol may cause damage to your liver. If you already have liver problems, tell your doctor before beginning dependency treatment with this drug.

Vivitrol also may cause depression and suicidal thoughts.

Who should not take Vivitrol?

If you are taking an opioid (such as heroin), dependent on opioids, are in opiate withdrawal, or have tested positive for opiates in your urine, do not begin treatment with Vivitrol.

Also, if you are allergic to any of the ingredients in Vivitrol, or if you have liver problems, you should not begin therapy.

What should I tell my doctor before I take the first dose of Vivitrol?

Tell your doctor about all prescription, over-the-counter, and herbal medications you are currently taking. Also, talk to your doctor about your complete medical history, especially if you are opiate-dependent. Vivitrol is not for the treatment of opiate-dependency.

What is the usual dosage?

The information below is based on the dosage guidelines your doctor uses. Depending on your condition and medical history, your doctor may prescribe a different regimen. Do not change the dosage or stop taking your medication without your doctor's approval.

Adults: The recommended dosage of Vivitrol is 380 milligrams (mg) injected every 4 weeks by a doctor.

How should I take Vivitrol?

Vivitrol should be injected by your doctor into your buttocks, alternating sides with each injection.

What should I avoid while taking Vivitrol?

Vivitrol may make you feel dizzy. Do not engage in any potentially dangerous activities, such as driving a car, until you know how Vivitrol affects you.

Avoid nursing or becoming pregnant; if you become pregnant while on Vivitrol, contact your doctor immediately.

What are possible food and drug interactions associated with Vivitrol?

If Vivitrol is taken with certain other drugs, the effects of either could be increased, decreased, or altered. It is especially important to check with your doctor before combining Vivitrol with the following: antidiarrheals, antitussives, self-administered heroin can serious injury, coma, or death.

What are the possible side effects of Vivitrol?

Side effects cannot be anticipated. If any develop or change in intensity, tell your doctor as soon as possible. Only your doctor can determine if it is safe for you to continue taking this drug.

Side effects may include: Cramps, decreased appetite/anorexia, dizziness, dry mouth, fatigue, headache, injection-site reaction, nausea, stomach pain, suicidal thoughts, vomiting

Can I receive Vivitrol if I am pregnant or breastfeeding?
The effects of Vivitrol during pregnancy and breastfeeding are unknown. Tell your doctor immediately if you are pregnant, plan to become pregnant, or are breastfeeding.

What should I do if I miss a dose of Vivitrol?
If you miss a dose, see your doctor immediately for an injection.

How should I store Vivitrol?
Your doctor will store this medication.

VOLTAREN GEL
Generic name: Diclofenac sodium.

What is Voltaren Gel?
Voltaren Gel is used to relieve the pain of osteoarthritis in joints amenable to topical treatment, such as the knees and those of the hands.

What is the most important information I should know about Voltaren Gel?
NSAID medicines may increase the chance of heart attack or stroke, which can lead to death, especially on prolonged use and in patients with heart disease. NSAID medicines should never be used before a heart surgery called coronary artery bypass graft (CABG). NSAIDs can cause ulcers and bleeding in the stomach and intestines.

Who should not take Voltaren Gel?
Do not take NSAIDs if you have had an asthma attack, hives, or other allergic reaction to aspirin or any other NSAID medicine. Never take it for pain following heart surgery.

What should I tell my doctor before I take the first dose of Voltaren Gel?
Tell your doctor about all prescription, over-the-counter, and herbal medications you are taking before beginning treatment with Voltaren. Also, talk to your doctor about your complete medical history, especially if you are allergic to NSAIDs or are pregnant or breastfeeding.

What is the usual dosage?
The information below is based on the dosage guidelines your doctor uses. Depending on your condition and medical history, your doctor

may prescribe a different regimen. Do not change the dosage or stop taking your medication without your doctor's approval.

The maximum recommended dosage of Voltaren Gel is 32 grams (g) per day.

How should I take Voltaren Gel?

Use Voltaren Gel exactly as prescribed. The dose for your hands, elbows, or wrists is 2 g each time you apply it (total of 8 g) and 4 g for your knees, ankles, or feet (total of 16 g). Apply Voltaren Gel 4 times a day. Apply the gel to clean, dry skin. Do not use heating pads or apply bandages to where you have applied Voltaren Gel. Do not use sunscreens or any other cosmetics on the same skin area where the gel is applied, and do not expose the skin where the gel is applied to sunlight and artificial lights.

What should I avoid while taking Voltaren Gel?

Do not use Voltaren Gel while pregnant or during nursing. Do not substitute Voltaren Gel for corticosteroids. Minimize exposure to natural or artificial light and avoid exposure of Voltaren Gel to eyes and mucosa.

What are possible food and drug interactions associated with Voltaren Gel?

Voltaren Gel, when used with anticoagulants, increases the risk of gastrointestinal bleeding. Aspirin and diclofenac should not used together, to avoid increasing the risk of serious side effects. Avoid using Voltaren Gel with ACE inhibitors, diuretics, lithium, methotrexate, and cyclosporine.

What are the possible side effects of Voltaren Gel?

Side effects cannot be anticipated. If any develop or change in intensity, tell your doctor as soon as possible. Only your doctor can determine if it is safe for you to continue taking this drug.

Side effects may include: allergic reactions, heart attack, stroke, high blood pressure, heart failure, kidney problems, liver problems, asthma attacks in people who have asthma, stomach pain, diarrhea, gas. (Signs of severe allergic reactions may include hives, difficulty breathing, and swelling of the throat. If any of these events occur, seek immediate medical attention.)

Call for emergency help if you have any of the following: shortness of breath, chest pain, slurred speech, swelling of the face or throat, weakness on one part or side of the body

Can I receive Voltaren Gel if I am pregnant or breastfeeding?

Voltaren Gel should be avoided during pregnancy and in nursing mothers.

What should I do if I miss a dose of Voltaren Gel?

If you miss a dose of Voltaren Gel, continue with your next scheduled dose using the prescribed amount. Do not double the dose.

How should I store Voltaren Gel?

Store at room temperature.

VYTORIN

Generic name: Ezetimbe and simvastatin

What is Vytorin?

Vytorin is a cholesterol-lowering drug. It is used along with a special diet to lower the amount of fatty material in the blood—triglycerides and LDL (or "bad") cholesterol—that can build up on artery walls and block blood flow. At the same time, Vytorin raises HDL (or "good") cholesterol, which helps prevent fats from building up and clogging the arteries.

What is the most important information I should know about Vytorin?

LDL cholesterol is called "bad" cholesterol because it can build up in the wall of your arteries and form plaque. Over time, plaque buildup can cause a narrowing of the arteries. This narrowing can slow or block blood flow to your heart, brain, and other organs. High LDL cholesterol is a major cause of heart disease and one of the causes for stroke. HDL cholesterol is called "good" cholesterol because it keeps the bad cholesterol from building up in the arteries. Triglycerides also are fats found in your body.

Vytorin may cause a serious muscle condition called rhabdomyolysis, especially if you are taking a high dose or if you are taking certain other medicines with Vytorin. You should tell your doctor right away if you feel any muscle weakness, pain, or tenderness, especially with a fever.

It is important to remember that Vytorin is a supplement—not a substitute—for other measures to control your cholesterol. For the best results, Vytorin should be used along with exercise, a low-cholesterol/low-fat diet, and a weight-loss program if you are overweight. Follow the diet and exercise program given to you by your healthcare provider.

Keep taking Vytorin unless your doctor tells you to stop. If you stop taking it, your cholesterol may rise again. It may take several weeks for Vytorin to work.

If you also take a bile acid sequestrant (such as cholestyramine, colestipol, or colesevelam), do not take it within 2 hours before or 4 hours after taking Vytorin. Check with your doctor if you have questions.

Vytorin may harm your liver. Your risk may be greater if you drink alcohol while you are using Vytorin. Talk to your doctor before you take

Vytorin if you drink substantial amounts of alcohol per day (more than two alcoholic beverages per day).

Do not drive or perform other possibly unsafe tasks until you know how you react to Vytorin; this medication may cause drowsiness or change in vision. These effects may be worse if you take it with alcohol or certain medicines.

Proper dental care is important while you are taking Vytorin. Brush and floss your teeth and visit the dentist regularly.

Eating grapefruit or drinking grapefruit juice may increase the amount of Vytorin in your blood, which may increase your risk for serious side effects. The risk may be greater with large amounts of grapefruit or grapefruit juice (more than one quart daily). Talk with your doctor or pharmacist if you have questions about including grapefruit or grapefruit juice in your diet while you are taking Vytorin.

Who should not take Vytorin?

You should not take Vytorin if you are allergic or sensitive to ezetimbe, simvastatin, or any other ingredient in Vytorin. You should also not take Vytorin if you are pregnant or think you may be pregnant, planning to become pregnant, breastfeeding, or if you have active liver disease or liver problems.

What should I tell my doctor before I take the first dose of Vytorin?

Mention all prescription, over-the-counter, and herbal medications you are taking before beginning treatment with Vytorin. Also, talk to your doctor about your complete medical history, especially if you have kidney, thyroid, or liver problems; drink substantial amounts of alcoholic beverages per day (more than two alcoholic beverages); or have a history of muscle aches or weakness, low blood pressure, uncontrolled seizures, metabolic problems, electrolyte problems, or diabetes. In addition, tell your doctor if you have recently had major trauma, a severe infection, and if you recently had an organ transplant or are currently taking medication to suppress a rejection reaction.

What is the usual dosage?

The information below is based on the dosage guidelines your doctor uses. Depending on your condition and medical history, your doctor may prescribe a different regimen. Do not change the dosage or stop taking your medication without your doctor's approval.

Adults: The usual dosage is 10/10 milligrams (mg) (10 mg of ezetimbe and 10 mg of simvastatin) to 10/80 mg (10 mg of ezetimbe and 80 mg of simvastatin) taken once a day. The recommended staring dose is 10/20 mg (10 mg of ezetimbe and 20 mg of simvastatin) taken once a day. Two or more weeks after the initiation of Vytorin therapy lipid levels should be analyzed and, if necessary, the dose adjusted.

Patients with Homozygous Familial Hypercholesterolemia
Adults: The usual dosage is 10/40 mg to 10/80 mg taken once daily in the evening.

Vytorin has not been studied in children under 10 years of age.

How should I take Vytorin?
Vytorin should be taken once daily in the evening, with or without food.

Dosing of Vytorin should occur at least 2 hours before or 4 hours after administration of a bile acid sequestrant.

Keep taking Vytorin unless your doctor tells you to stop. If you stop taking it, your cholesterol may rise again. It may take some time to see the effects of Vytorin.

Continue to follow a cholesterol-lowering diet while taking Vytorin. Ask your doctor if you need diet information.

Eating grapefruit or drinking grapefruit juice may increase the amount of Vytorin in your blood, which may increase your risk for serious side effects. The risk may be greater with large amounts of grapefruit or grapefruit juice (more than one quart daily). Talk with your doctor or pharmacist if you have questions about including grapefruit or grapefruit juice in your diet while you are taking Vytorin.

Proper dental care is important while you are taking Vytorin. Brush and floss your teeth and visit the dentist regularly.

What should I avoid while taking Vytorin?
You should not become pregnant or breastfeed while taking Vytorin. You should also not drink more than 1 quart of grapefruit juice per day.

Do not drive or perform other possibly unsafe tasks until you know how you react to Vytorin; this medication may cause drowsiness or change in vision. These effects may be worse if you take it with alcohol or certain medicines.

What are possible food and drug interactions associated with Vytorin?
If Vytorin is taken with certain other drugs, the effects of either could be increased, decreased, or altered. It is especially important to check with your doctor before combining Vytorin with the following: amiodarone; antifungal agents, such as itraconazole or ketoconazole; clarithromycin; cyclosporine; danazol; erythromycin; fibric acid derivatives, such as gemfibrozil, bezafibrate, or fenofibrate; grapefruit juice (more than 1 quart daily); HIV protease inhibitors, such as indinavir, nelfinavir, ritonavir, and saquinavir; nefazodone; niacin or nicotinic acid; telithromycin; and verapamil.

What are the possible side effects of Vytorin?

Side effects cannot be anticipated. If any develop or change in intensity, tell your doctor as soon as possible. Only your doctor can determine if it is safe for you to continue taking this drug.

Side effects may include: headache, nausea, rash, flu-like symptoms, pain in the arms or legs, tiredness, upper respiratory tract infection

Serious side effects may include: hives, joint pain, muscle pain, swelling of the face/lips/tongue/throat

Vytorin may cause a serious muscle condition called rhabdomyolysis, especially if you are taking a high dose or if you are taking certain other medicines with Vytorin. You should tell your doctor right away if you feel any muscle weakness, pain, or tenderness, especially with a fever.

Can I receive Vytorin if I am pregnant or breastfeeding?

Do not take Vytorin if you are pregnant or breastfeeding. Vytorin can cause serious harm to your unborn baby. It is not known if Vytorin is found in breast milk. Tell your doctor immediately if you are pregnant, plan to become pregnant, or if you are breastfeeding.

What should I do if I miss a dose of Vytorin?

If you miss a dose of Vytorin, do not double your next dose. Skip the dose you missed and then return to your normal dosing schedule.

How should I store Vytorin?

Store at room temperature, away from heat, moisture, and light. Do not store in the bathroom.

VYVANSE

Generic name: Lisdexamfetamine dimesylate

What is Vyvanse?

Vyvanse is a central nervous system stimulant used for the treatment of attention-deficit/hyperactivity disorder (ADHD) in children 6-12 years old.

What is the most important information I should know about Vyvanse?

Because Vyvanse is an amphetamine stimulant, using it for a long period may lead to drug dependence. Misuse can lead to serious heart problems and sudden death.

Heart-related problems, hardening of the arteries, moderate to severe high blood pressure, hyperthyroidism, glaucoma, or if you are allergic to amphetamines.

Do not use Vyvanse while in agitated states or if you have a history of drug abuse.

Vyvanse may worsen behavior and thought disorders if you have a history of other mental illnesses, such as bipolar disorder. Aggressive behavior or hostility is often observed in children and adolescents with ADHD.

Growth should be monitored during treatment with Vyvanse, and patients who are not growing or gaining weight as expected may need to temporarily stop their treatment.

Vyvanse may increase the risk of having a seizure, especially if you have a history of seizures. Vyvanse may also worsen symptoms related to Tourette's syndrome.

Amphetamines may impair your ability to engage in potentially hazardous activities such as driving or operating machinery.

Who should not take Vyvanse?
Vyvanse should not be taken if you are suffering from advanced heart disease or other heart-related problems, hardening of the arteries, moderate to severe high blood pressure, hyperthyroidism, glaucoma, or if you are allergic to amphetamines.

Vyvanse should not be taken if you are in agitated states or if you have a history of drug abuse.

Do not take this medicine if you have been using drugs known as monoamine oxidase inhibitors (MAOIs) within the past 14 days.

What should I tell my doctor before I take the first dose of Vyvanse?
Tell your doctor about all prescription, over-the-counter, and herbal medications you are taking before beginning treatment with Vyvanse. Also, talk to your doctor about your complete medical history, especially if you have any heart conditions, an overactive thyroid, glaucoma, any psychiatric conditions, or if you have ever had a seizure.

What is the usual dosage?
The information below is based on the dosage guidelines your doctor uses. Depending on your condition and medical history, your doctor may prescribe a different regimen. Do not change the dosage or stop taking your medication without your doctor's approval.

Children: For children 6-12 years old, the recommended dose is 30 milligrams once daily in the morning. The doctor may want to increase the dose based on your child's condition.

How should I take Vyvanse?
Take this medicine in the morning. Afternoon doses should be avoided because of the potential for insomnia (difficulty sleeping). You can take Vyvanse with or without food.

If you are unable to swallow the capsule, you may open it and dissolve the contents in a glass of water. Drink the entire glass; do not store it for later use. Do not take less than one capsule per day.

What should I avoid while taking Vyvanse?
Use caution when driving or operating dangerous machinery while taking Vyvanse.

Avoid splitting the dose within a capsule; also avoid taking Vyvanse later in the day.

What are possible food and drug interactions associated with Vyvanse?
If Vyvanse is taken with certain other drugs, the effects of either could be increased, decreased, or altered. It is especially important to check with your doctor before combining Vyvanse with the following: antidepressants including monoamine oxidase inhibitors (MAOIs), antipsychotic medication, lithium, blood pressure medication, seizure medication, and narcotic painkillers.

What are the possible side effects of Vyvanse?
Side effects cannot be anticipated. If any develop or change in intensity, tell your doctor as soon as possible. Only your doctor can determine if it is safe for you to continue taking this drug.

Side effects may include: upper belly pains, decreased appetite, dizziness, dry mouth, irritability, trouble sleeping, nausea and vomiting, weight loss, slowing of growth, seizures (especially in patients with a history of seizures), blurred vision

Can I receive Vyvanse if I am pregnant or breastfeeding?
Talk with your doctor before taking this drug if you are pregnant, plan to become pregnant, or are breastfeeding. Amphetamines have been shown to cause birth defects in laboratory animals, but the effects in humans are unknown. Because amphetamines are excreted in breast milk, women should not breastfeed while using this drug.

What should I do if I miss a dose of Vyvanse?
Do not take an extra dose to make up for the one you missed. Wait and take your next dose at the regular time.

How should I store Vyvanse?
Store at room temperature.

Warfarin sodium See Coumadin, page 349.

WELCHOL

Generic name: Colesevelam hydrochloride

What is WelChol?

WelChol may be taken alone or with other medicines to lower the cholesterol in your blood. WelChol should be used as an adjunct to diet and exercise to reduce elevated low-density lipoprotein cholesterol (LDL-C) in patients with high cholesterol levels, or to control blood sugar in adults with type 2 diabetes mellitus.

Cholesterol is a fatty substance that may build up in the blood vessels and can lead to conditions such as heart disease, heart attacks, or strokes.

What is the most important information I should know about WelChol?

WelChol should be used with caution if you have any type of stomach or intestinal problems and if you have had major stomach or intestinal surgery. Promptly discontinue WelChol and seek medical attention if severe abdominal pain or severe constipation occurs while taking this medication.

Because of the tablet size, WelChol can cause esophageal obstruction and should be used with caution in patients who have trouble swallowing.

Do not use WelChol as a substitute for a healthy diet and exercise plan; the drug should be used as an adjunct to lower your cholesterol. You should still exercise and eat a diet low in cholesterol while taking WelChol to ensure its efficacy.

WelChol may cause low blood sugar. Low blood sugar may make you anxious, sweaty, weak, dizzy, drowsy, or faint. It may also make your heart beat faster; make your vision change; give you a headache, chills, or tremors; or increase your appetite. It is a good idea to carry a reliable source of glucose (eg, tablets or gel) to treat low blood sugar. If this is not available, you should eat or drink a quick source of sugar like table sugar, honey, candy, orange juice, or non-diet soda. This will raise your blood sugar level quickly. Tell your doctor right away if this happens. To prevent low blood sugar, eat meals at the same time each day and do not skip meals. Adhering to a diet, exercise program, and regularly testing your blood sugars may reduce the risk of these side effects.

If you also take glyburide (oral diabetic medication), birth control pills, phenytoin, or thyroid hormone replacements (eg, levothyroxine), take them at least 4 hours before you take WelChol.

Continue to take WelChol even if you feel well. Do not miss any doses. It may take several weeks for WelChol to begin working.

Discontinue WelChol and seek prompt medical attention if the hallmark symptoms of acute pancreatitis (inflammation of the pancreas) take place. These symptoms may include severe abdominal pain with or without nausea and vomiting.

Who should not take WelChol?

You should not take WelChol if you have a blockage in your intestines known as bowel obstruction or if you are allergic or sensitive to WelChol or any of its ingredients. WelChol should not be used in patients who have very high triglyceride levels (more than 500 mg/dL) or a history of inflammation of the pancreas (pancreatitis) caused by high triglyceride levels. WelChol should not be used for the treatment of type 1 diabetes or diabetic ketoacidosis.

What should I tell my doctor before I take the first dose of WelChol?

Mention all prescription, over-the-counter, and herbal medications you are taking before beginning treatment with WelChol. Also, talk to your doctor about your complete medical history, especially if you have diabetes or diabetic ketoacidosis, vitamin K deficiency, thyroid problems, liver or kidney disorders, alcoholism, trouble swallowing, or stomach or intestinal problems.

What is the usual dosage?

The information below is based on the dosage guidelines your doctor uses. Depending on your condition and medical history, your doctor may prescribe a different regimen. Do not change the dosage or stop taking your medication without your doctor's approval.

To Treat High Cholesterol Levels in the Blood Alone (Monotherapy) or in Combination with Another Cholesterol-Lowering Medicine
Adults: The usual dose is 1,875 milligrams (mg) taken as 3 tablets twice a day with a meal, or 3,750 mg taken as 6 tablets once a day with a meal and liquid.

After initiation of WelChol, lipid levels should be analyzed within 4 to 6 weeks.

To Control Blood Sugar in Patients with Type 2 Diabetes Mellitus
Adults: The usual dose is 1,875 milligrams (mg) taken as 3 tablets twice a day with a meal, or 3,750 mg taken as 6 tablets once a day with a meal and liquid.

How should I take WelChol?

WelChol should be taken with a plenty of fluids and a meal. WelChol can be taken at the same time as another cholesterol-lowering medicine known as an HMG-CoA reductase inhibitor.

If you also take glyburide (oral diabetic medication), birth control pills, phenytoin, or thyroid hormone replacements (eg, levothyroxine), take them at least 4 hours before you take WelChol.

Continue to take WelChol even if you feel well. Do not miss any doses.

What should I avoid while taking WelChol?

You should avoid eating foods that contain high amounts of cholesterol and fat to ensure you get the maximum cholesterol-lowering effect of WelChol.

The following medications should be administered at least 4 hours before you take WelChol: glyburide, birth control pills, phenytoin, or thyroid hormone replacements (eg, levothyroxine).

Do not change the dose or stop taking this medication without first talking to your doctor. Continue to take WelChol even if you feel well. Do not miss any doses.

What are possible food and drug interactions associated with WelChol?

If WelChol is taken with certain other drugs, the effects of either could be increased, decreased, or altered. It is especially important to check with your doctor before combining WelChol with verapamil (Calan SR).

What are the possible side effects of WelChol?

Side effects cannot be anticipated. If any develop or change in intensity, tell your doctor as soon as possible. Only your doctor can determine if it is safe for you to continue taking this drug.

Side effects may include: abdominal pain, accidental injury, back pain, constipation, diarrhea, flu syndrome, gas, headache, infection, nausea, runny nose, sinus pain, upset stomach, indigestion, muscle aches, weakness

WelChol may cause low blood sugar. Low blood sugar may make you anxious, sweaty, weak, dizzy, drowsy, or faint. It may also make your heart beat faster; make your vision change; give you a headache, chills, or tremors; or increase your appetite. Contact your doctor if any of these symptoms take place.

Discontinue WelChol and seek prompt medical attention if the hallmark symptoms of acute pancreatitis (inflammation of the pancreas) take place. These symptoms may include severe abdominal pain with or without nausea and vomiting.

Promptly discontinue WelChol and seek medical attention if severe abdominal pain or severe constipation occurs.

Tell your doctor if you are experiencing pain in your esophagus or if you have any problems swallowing the tablets.

Can I receive WelChol if I am pregnant or breastfeeding?

The effects of WelChol during pregnancy and breastfeeding are unknown. Tell your doctor immediately if you are pregnant, plan to become pregnant, or are breastfeeding. The drug should only be used during pregnancy if clearly needed.

What should I do if I miss a dose of WelChol?

If you miss a dose of WelChol, take it with a liquid at your next meal. If it is almost time for your next dose, skip the missed dose and go back to your regular dosing schedule. Do not take 2 doses at once.

How should I store WelChol?

Store WelChol at 77 degrees F (25 degrees C). Brief storage at temperatures between 59 and 86 degrees F (15 and 30 degrees C) is permitted. Store away from heat, moisture, and light. Do not store in the bathroom. Keep WelChol out of the reach of children.

WELLBUTRIN

Generic name: Bupropion hydrochloride

What is Wellbutrin?

Wellbutrin is used to treat major depression. Depression may be caused by an imbalance of brain chemicals called neurotransmitters. Wellbutrin helps balance the levels of two neurotransmitters called dopamine and norepinephrine.

What is the most important information I should know about Wellbutrin?

Antidepressants can increase the risk of suicidal thinking and behavior in children and teenagers. Adult and pediatric patients taking antidepressants should be watched closely for changes in moods or actions, especially when they first start therapy or when their dose is increased or decreased. Patients and their families should contact the doctor immediately if new symptoms develop or seem to get worse. Signs to watch for include anxiety, hostility, sleeplessness, restlessness, impulsive or dangerous behavior, and thoughts about suicide or dying.

Who should not take Wellbutrin?

Do not take Wellbutrin if you have a seizure disorder, anorexia or bulimia (eating disorders), or if you are going through alcohol recovery. Also, do not begin treatment with Wellbutrin if you are allergic to any of its ingredients.

Do not take monoamine oxidase inhibitors (MAOIs) within 2 weeks before or after treatment with this medication. In some cases a serious, possibly fatal, reaction may occur. Examples of MAOIs include selegiline and the antidepressants phenelzine and tranylcypromine.

Also, do not begin treatment with Wellbutrin if you are allergic to any of its ingredients.

What should I tell my doctor before I take the first dose of Wellbutrin?
Tell your doctor about all prescription, over-the-counter, and herbal medications you are taking before beginning treatment with Wellbutrin. Also, talk to your doctor about your complete medical history, especially if you have had seizure problems, eating disorders, or an addiction (eg, drug/alcohol problems).

What is the usual dosage?
The information below is based on the dosage guidelines your doctor uses. Depending on your condition and medical history, your doctor may prescribe a different regimen. Do not change the dosage or stop taking your medication without your doctor's approval.

Adults: The usual starting dose is 200 milligrams (mg) a day, taken as 100 mg twice a day. Depending on your response, the doctor may increase the dose to 300 mg a day, taken as 100 mg three times a day. The maximum daily dose for Wellbutrin is 450 mg. Taking doses greater than 450 mg a day may increase the risk of serious side effects, including seizures.

How should I take Wellbutrin?
Take Wellbutrin at the same time every day, at least 6 hours apart. You can take it with or without food.

What should I avoid while taking Wellbutrin?
Do not chew, cut, or crush Wellbutrin tablets.

What are possible food and drug interactions associated with Wellbutrin?
If Wellbutrin is taken with certain other drugs, the effects of either could be increased, decreased, or altered. It is especially important to check with your doctor before combining Wellbutrin with the following: amantadine, other antidepressants including MAOIs, antipsychotic medications, blood pressure medications known as beta-blockers, levodopa, phenelzine, and heart rhythm drugs such as propafenone and flecainide.

What are the possible side effects of Wellbutrin?
Side effects cannot be anticipated. If any develop or change in intensity, tell your doctor as soon as possible. Only your doctor can determine if it is safe for you to continue taking this drug.

Side effects may include: abnormal behavior, agitation, headaches, nausea and vomiting, neurological problems, seizures, sleeping problems, skin problems such as rashes, stomach problems

Can I receive Wellbutrin if I am pregnant or breastfeeding?
The effects of Wellbutrin during pregnancy and breastfeeding are unknown. Tell your doctor immediately if you are pregnant, plan to become pregnant, or are breastfeeding.

What should I do if I miss a dose of Wellbutrin?
Do not double your next dose. Skip the dose you missed and return to your regular dosing schedule. This is very important because taking too much Wellbutrin can increase your risk of having a seizure.

How should I store Wellbutrin?
Store at room temperature away from light and moisture.

WELLBUTRIN SR
Generic name: Bupropion hydrochloride, sustained-release

What is Wellbutrin SR?
Wellbutrin SR is used to treat major depression. Depression may be caused by an imbalance of brain chemicals called neurotransmitters. Wellbutrin SR helps balance the levels of two neurotransmitters called dopamine and norepinephrine.

What is the most important information I should know about Wellbutrin SR?
Antidepressants can increase the risk of suicidal thinking and behavior in children and teenagers. Adult and pediatric patients taking antidepressants should be watched closely for changes in moods or actions, especially when they first start therapy or when their dose is increased or decreased. Patients and their families should contact the doctor immediately if new symptoms develop or seem to get worse. Signs to watch for include anxiety, hostility, sleeplessness, restlessness, impulsive or dangerous behavior, and thoughts about suicide or dying.

Who should not take Wellbutrin SR?
Do not take Wellbutrin SR if you have a seizure disorder, anorexia or bulimia (eating disorders), or if you are going through alcohol recovery. In addition, you should not take Wellbutrin SR if you are taking Zyban or any other medicines that contain bupropion hydrochloride, such as Wellbutrin or Wellbutrin XL, or if you have suddenly stopped taking sedatives.

Do not take monoamine oxidase inhibitors (MAOIs) within 2 weeks before or after treatment with this medication. In some cases a serious, possibly fatal, reaction may occur. Examples of MAOIs include selegiline and the antidepressants phenelzine and tranylcypromine.

Also, do not begin treatment with Wellbutrin SR if you are allergic to any of its ingredients.

What should I tell my doctor before I take the first dose of Wellbutrin SR?
Tell your doctor about all prescription, over-the-counter, and herbal medications you are taking before beginning treatment with Wellbutrin SR. Also, talk to your doctor about your complete medical history, especially if you have seizure problems, eating disorders, liver or kidney problems, or an addiction (eg, drug or alcohol problems).

What is the usual dosage?
The information below is based on the dosage guidelines your doctor uses. Depending on your condition and medical history, your doctor may prescribe a different regimen. Do not change the dosage or stop taking your medication without your doctor's approval.

Adults: The usual dose is 150 milligrams (mg) once a day in the morning. Depending on your response, the doctor may increase your dose to 300 mg a day, taken as 150 mg twice a day.

How should I take Wellbutrin SR?
You should take Wellbutrin SR at the same time every day, at least 8 hours apart. You can take it with or without food.

What should I avoid while taking Wellbutrin SR?
You should not drink a lot of alcohol while taking Wellbutrin SR. If you currently drink a lot of alcohol and suddenly stop, you should tell your doctor, since this may increase your risk of having a seizure. You should also not drive a car or operate heavy machinery until you know how this drug affects you.

What are possible food and drug interactions associated with Wellbutrin SR?
If Wellbutrin SR is taken with certain other drugs, the effects of either could be increased, decreased, or altered. It is especially important to check with your doctor before combining Wellbutrin SR with the following: alcohol, amantadine, other antidepressants including MAOIs, antipsychotics, blood pressure drugs known as beta-blockers, carbamazepine, cimetidine, efavirenz, fluvoxamine, antiarrhythmics such as propafenone and flecainide, lamotrigine, levodopa, nelfinavir, nicotine patches, norfluoxetine, phenobarbital, phenytoin, ritonavir, steroids, and theophylline.

What are the possible side effects of Wellbutrin SR?

Side effects cannot be anticipated. If any develop or change in intensity, tell your doctor as soon as possible. Only your doctor can determine if it is safe for you to continue taking this drug.

Side effects may include: headache, infection, stomach or chest pains, dry mouth, nausea, diarrhea, constipation, loss of appetite, vomiting, difficulty sleeping (insomnia), dizziness, agitation, tremor, anxiety, nervousness, irritability, sore throat, sinus inflammation, sweating, rash, ringing in the ears, blurred vision

Can I receive Wellbutrin SR if I am pregnant or breastfeeding?

The effects of Wellbutrin SR during pregnancy and breastfeeding are unknown. Tell your doctor immediately if you are pregnant, plan to become pregnant, or are breastfeeding.

What should I do if I miss a dose of Wellbutrin SR?

Do not double your next dose. Skip the dose you missed and return to your regular dosing schedule. This is very important because taking too much Wellbutrin SR can increase your risk of having a seizure.

How should I store Wellbutrin SR?

Store at room temperature away from light and moisture.

WELLBUTRIN XL

Generic name: Bupropion hydrochloride, extended-release

What is Wellbutrin XL?

Wellbutrin XL is used to treat major depression and seasonal depression known as seasonal affective disorder (SAD). Depression may be caused by an imbalance of brain chemicals called neurotransmitters. Wellbutrin XL helps balance the levels of two neurotransmitters called dopamine and norepinephrine.

What is the most important information I should know about Wellbutrin XL?

Antidepressants can increase the risk of suicidal thinking and behavior in children and teenagers. Adult and pediatric patients taking antidepressants should be watched closely for changes in moods or actions, especially when they first start therapy or when their dose is increased or decreased. Patients and their families should contact the doctor immediately if new symptoms develop or seem to get worse. Signs to watch for include anxiety, hostility, sleeplessness, restlessness, impulsive or dangerous behavior, and thoughts about suicide or dying.

Who should not take Wellbutrin XL?

Do not take Wellbutrin XL if you have a seizure disorder, anorexia or bulimia (eating disorders), or if you are going through alcohol recovery. In addition, you should not take Wellbutrin XL if you are taking Zyban or any other medicines that contain bupropion hydrochloride, such as Wellbutrin or Wellbutrin SR, or if you have suddenly stopped taking sedatives.

Do not take monoamine oxidase inhibitors (MAOIs) within 2 weeks before or after treatment with this medication. In some cases a serious, possibly fatal, reaction may occur. Examples of MAOIs include selegiline and the antidepressants phenelzine and tranylcypromine.

Also, do not begin treatment with Wellbutrin XL if you are allergic to any of its ingredients.

What should I tell my doctor before I take the first dose of Wellbutrin XL?

Tell your doctor about all prescription, over-the-counter, and herbal medications you are taking before beginning treatment with Wellbutrin XL. Also, talk to your doctor about your complete medical history, especially if you have ever had a seizure, eating disorders, liver or kidney problems, or an addiction (e.g., drug/alcohol problems).

What is the usual dosage?

The information below is based on the dosage guidelines your doctor uses. Depending on your condition and medical history, your doctor may prescribe a different regimen. Do not change the dosage or stop taking your medication without your doctor's approval.

Depression
Adults: The usual dose is 150 milligrams (mg) once a day in the morning. Depending on your response, the doctor may increase the dose to 300 mg once a day.

Seasonal Affective Disorder
Adults: The usual dose is 150 mg once a day in the morning, starting in autumn before the onset of depressive symptoms. Depending on your response, the doctor may increase the dose to 300 mg once a day. If you are taking 300 mg a day, your doctor may taper the dose to 150 mg a day for 2 weeks before telling you to stop taking Wellbutrin XL in early spring.

How should I take Wellbutrin XL?

Wellbutrin XL is a once-daily tablet. Take it at the same time every day at least 24 hours apart. You can take Wellbutrin XL with or without food.

What should I avoid while taking Wellbutrin XL?

You should not drink a lot of alcohol while taking Wellbutrin XL. If you currently drink a lot of alcohol and suddenly stop, you should tell your doctor, since this may increase your risk of having a seizure. You should also not drive a car or operate heavy machinery until you know how this drug affects you.

What are possible food and drug interactions associated with Wellbutrin XL?

If Wellbutrin XL is taken with certain other drugs, the effects of either could be increased, decreased, or altered. It is especially important to check with your doctor before combining Wellbutrin XL with the following: alcohol, amantadine, other antidepressants including MAOIs, antipsychotics, blood pressure drugs known as beta-blockers, carbamazepine, cimetidine, efavirenz, fluvoxamine, antiarrhythmics such as propafenone and flecainide, lamotrigine, levodopa, nelfinavir, nicotine patches, norfluoxetine, phenobarbital, phenytoin, ritonavir, steroids, and theophylline.

What are the possible side effects of Wellbutrin XL?

Side effects cannot be anticipated. If any develop or change in intensity, tell your doctor as soon as possible. Only your doctor can determine if it is safe for you to continue taking this drug.

Side effects may include: dry mouth, nausea, constipation, gas, headache, dizziness, tremor (shakiness), upper respiratory tract infection, nasal or throat irritation, inflammation of the sinuses, trouble sleeping (insomnia), anxiety, abnormal dreams, pain in the hands or feet, muscle pain, feeling jittery, decreased appetite, rash, ringing in the ears

Can I receive Wellbutrin XL if I am pregnant or breastfeeding?

The effects of Wellbutrin XL during pregnancy and breastfeeding are unknown. Tell your doctor immediately if you are pregnant, plan to become pregnant, or are breastfeeding.

What should I do if I miss a dose of Wellbutrin XL?

Do not double your next dose. Skip the dose you missed and return to your regular dosing schedule. This is very important because taking too much Wellbutrin XL can increase your risk of having a seizure.

How should I store Wellbutrin XL?

Store at room temperature away from light and moisture.

XALATAN

Generic name: Latanoprost

What is Xalatan?

Xalatan is a prostaglandin eye drop that helps reduce the increased blood pressure of the eye(s) if you have open-angle glaucoma or hypertension of the eye.

What is the most important information I should know about Xalatan?

Xalatan eye solution has been reported to cause changes to colored tissues of the eyes, which may not become noticeable for several months to years, and are expected to increase as long as the eye drops are used. It can increase the color of the iris, eyelids, and eyelashes, and lengthen eyelashes. After stopping the use of the medication, the changes in the color of the iris are likely to be permanent while changes of the eyelids and eyelashes may be reversible in some patients. The effects of increased color changes beyond 5 years are not known.

Avoid allowing the tip of the dispensing container to contact the eye or surrounding structures because this could cause the tip to become contaminated by common bacteria known to cause eye infections. Serious damage to the eye and subsequent loss of vision may result from using contaminated solutions.

If you seem to continually get eye infections or irritation or have had ocular surgery, seek your physician's advice concerning the continued use of the multiple-dose container.

If any eye reactions occur, particularly conjunctivitis and lid reactions, seek immediate medical attention.

Who should not take Xalatan?

You should not use Xalatan if you have a known allergic reaction to latanoprost, benzalkonium chloride, or any other ingredients in this product.

What should I tell my doctor before I take the first dose of Xalatan?

Mention all prescription, over-the-counter, and herbal medications you are taking before beginning treatment with Xalatan. Also, talk to your doctor about your complete medical history, especially if you have diabetes, high blood pressure, eye surgery, or other eye disorders.

What is the usual dosage?

The information below is based on the dosage guidelines your doctor uses. Depending on your condition and medical history, your doctor may prescribe a different regimen. Do not change the dosage or stop taking your medication without your doctor's approval.

Adults: Instill one drop in the affected eye(s) once daily in the evening.

How should I take Xalatan?

Instill the directed number of drops in the affected eye in the evening. Remove contact lenses prior to administration; lenses may be reinserted after 15 minutes. Do not let the tip of the applicator touch the eye and avoid contamination of the applicator tip.

If more than one topical ophthalmic drug is being used, the drugs should be administered at least 5 minutes apart.

To instill the drop(s): 1. Wash your hands with soap and water. 2. Look toward the ceiling with both eyes open. 3. Pull your lower lid down—steady your hand on your forehead. 4. Put a drop of medicine in the sac behind the lashes of the lower lid. 5. Try to keep your eyes closed for 1 minute after instilling the drops to obtain the maximum benefit.

What should I avoid while taking Xalatan?

Avoid allowing the tip of the dropper from container to come in contact with your eye or any area surrounding your eye. If the tip of the dropper touches the eye or any other surface the medication can become contaminated, which can lead to an eye infection and possible damage to the eye.

Avoid simultaneously inserting Xalantan with any other eye medication. If you are taking an additional eye medication, separate the administration of one from the other by at least 5 minutes.

What are possible food and drug interactions associated with Xalatan?

If Xalatan is used with certain other drugs, the effects of either could be increased, decreased, or altered, and should be discussed with your doctor. Mixing certain thimerosol-containing eye drops with Xalatan may be harmful. Check with your doctor when using more than one eye drop; if such drugs are used, they should be administered at least five minutes apart.

What are the possible side effects of Xalatan?

Side effects cannot be anticipated. If any develop or change in intensity, tell your doctor as soon as possible. Only your doctor can determine if it is safe for you to continue taking this drug.

Side effects may include: changes in the color of the iris, eyelids, and texture of eyelashes; eye inflammation; increased fluid in certain parts of the eye(s)

Can I receive Xalatan if I am pregnant or breastfeeding?

The effects of Xalatan during pregnancy and breastfeeding are unknown. Tell your doctor immediately if you are pregnant, plan to become pregnant, or are breastfeeding. This medication should be used only if the benefits outweigh the risks.

What should I do if I miss a dose of Xalatan?

If you miss a dose, continue treatment with your next scheduled dose.

How should I store Xalatan?

Xalatan should be protected from light, and unopened bottles should be stored in the refrigerator. Once opened, the 2.5 mL container may be stored at room temperature up to 6 weeks.

XANAX

Generic name: Alprazolam

What is Xanax?

Xanax is a medicine known as a benzodiazepine; it works by slowing down the movement of chemicals in the brain. Xanax is used to treat anxiety and panic disorders.

What is the most important information I should know about Xanax?

If you take more than 4 milligrams (mg) of Xanax per day, you are at risk of extreme physical or mental dependence. You may also experience more severe withdrawal symptoms (including seizures) if you stop taking Xanax or if you lower the dose.

Even if you take Xanax for a short period of time, you may become mentally or physically dependent. Physical dependence could put you at risk for experiencing withdrawal symptoms if you stop taking Xanax. Withdrawal symptoms include seizures or a worsening of anxiety and associated symptoms.

Xanax binds to certain receptors in the brain that may cause you to become drowsy or sedated. Do not drive, operate machinery, or do anything else that could be dangerous until you know how this drug affects you.

You should not increase, decrease, or stop taking your Xanax doses without first talking to your doctor.

Avoid drinking alcohol or taking other medications that cause drowsiness (such as sedatives and tranquilizers) while taking Xanax. This medication will add to the effects of alcohol and other depressants.

Do not smoke while using Xanax. Cigarette smoking decreases blood levels of Xanax. Tell your doctor if you smoke or if you have recently stopped smoking.

Who should not take Xanax?

You should not take Xanax if you are pregnant, plan to become pregnant, or are breastfeeding.

Do not use this medication if you have an eye condition called acute narrow-angle glaucoma. (If you have open-angle glaucoma, Xanax may be used if you are receiving appropriate therapy.)

Do not take Xanax if you are allergic to any of its ingredients. Also avoid this drug if you are currently taking the medications itraconazole or ketoconazole.

What should I tell my doctor before I take the first dose of Xanax?

Tell your doctor about all prescription, over-the-counter, and herbal medications you are taking before beginning treatment with Xanax. Also, talk to your doctor about your complete medical history, especially if you have a history of alcohol abuse; liver, lung, or kidney problems; glaucoma; muscle problems; depression or suicidal tendencies; or if you have ever been physically or mentally dependent on a benzodiazepine medication.

What is the usual dosage?

The information below is based on the dosage guidelines your doctor uses. Depending on your condition and medical history, your doctor may prescribe a different regimen. Do not change the dosage or stop taking your medication without your doctor's approval.

Anxiety Disorders and Temporary Symptoms of Anxiety
Adults: The usual starting dose is 0.25-0.5 milligrams (mg), taken 3 times a day. You doctor may increase the dose up to a maximum of 4 mg per day, taken in divided doses (three to four times a day), depending on your condition. The risk of dependence may increase with more frequent doses and the length of treatment.

Panic Disorders
Adults: The usual dose is 1-10 mg per day, taken in divided doses. Treatment may be started with a dose of 0.5 mg 3 times daily and then adjusted based on your response

How should I take Xanax?

Xanax should be taken exactly as prescribed. You should not take more or stop the medication altogether without first talking to your doctor. Take Xanax at the same time every day, with or without food. If stomach upset occurs, take Xanax with food to reduce stomach irritation.

What should I avoid while taking Xanax?

Do not increase, decrease, or stop taking Xanax without first talking to your doctor.

You should not drink alcohol while taking Xanax. You should also not drive a car or operate heavy machinery until you know how this drug affects you.

Avoid eating grapefruit or drinking grapefruit juice while you are being treated with Xanax.

What are possible food and drug interactions associated with Xanax?

If Xanax is taken with certain other drugs, the effects of either could be increased, decreased, or altered. It is especially important to check with your doctor before combining Xanax with the following: alcohol, amiodarone, anticonvulsants, antihistamines, carbamazepine, cyclosporine, desipramine, diltiazem, ergotamine, fluoxetine, grapefruit juice, imipramine, isoniazid, itraconazole, ketoconazole, macrolide antibiotics such as erythromycin and clarithromycin, nicardipine, nifedipine, oral contraceptives, and propoxyphene.

What are the possible side effects of Xanax?
Side effects cannot be anticipated. If any develop or change in intensity, tell your doctor as soon as possible. Only your doctor can determine if it is safe for you to continue taking this drug.

Side effects may include: drowsiness, tiredness, fatigue, impaired coordination, irritability, memory impairment, dizziness, lightheadedness, headache, joint pain, trouble sleeping (insomnia), anxiety, abnormal involuntary movements, decreased or increased sexual drive, depression, confusion, muscle twitching, weakness, fainting, numbness, nausea, vomiting, diarrhea, increased or decreased salivation, stomach pain, upper respiratory tract infection, ringing in the ears, fast heartbeat, chest pain, blurred vision, rash, sweating, increased rate of breathing, change in appetite, weight loss or gain, menstrual disorders, trouble urinating, sexual dysfunction, water retention

Can I receive Xanax if I am pregnant or breastfeeding?
No. Xanax should not be taken if you are pregnant or breastfeeding due to the possible harm it may cause to an unborn or nursing infant. Tell your doctor immediately if you are pregnant, plan to become pregnant, or are breastfeeding.

What should I do if I miss a dose of Xanax?
If you miss a dose of Xanax and you are using it regularly, take it as soon as possible. If it is almost time for your next dose, skip the missed dose and go back to your regular dosing schedule. Do not take 2 doses at once.

How should I store Xanax?
Store at room temperature away from heat, moisture, and light. Do not store in the bathroom.

XENICAL
Generic name: Orlistat

What is Xenical?
Xenical is a prescription medication that helps people who are considerably overweight (have a body mass index, or BMI, of 30 or greater) lose weight. Xenical is also for people who are overweight (have a body mass index of 27 or greater) and also have other risk factors such as high blood pressure, high cholesterol, heart disease, or diabetes. Xenical blocks certain enzymes in the gut known as lipases, so your body cannot properly

digest fat and you absorb much less (about 30% less) of the fat that you eat. The undigested fat is eliminated in your bowel movements.

What is the most important information I should know about Xenical?

Xenical is not a substitute for healthy lifestyle changes needed to lose weight. Xenical should be taken with a nutritionally balanced, reduced-calorie diet containing no more than 30% of calories from fat.

Xenical may impair your body's ability to absorb some fat-soluble vitamins. You should take a multivitamin once a day that contains vitamins D, E, K, and beta-carotene, at least 2 hours before or after taking Xenical.

You will likely experience a change in your bowel movements, especially in the beginning of your treatment, and sometimes throughout your Xenical therapy. These changes include oily spotting, gas with discharge, oily or fatty stools, increased number of bowel movements, an urgency to have bowel movements, or an inability to control bowel movements. This may worsen if the total daily calories you consume contain more than 30% of fat.

The use of this medication longer than 4 years has not been studied.

Who should not take Xenical?

You should not take Xenical if you consistently have problems absorbing food, gallbladder problems, if you are pregnant or breastfeeding, or if you have ever had an allergy or sensitivity to Xenical or any of its ingredients.

What should I tell my doctor before I take the first dose of Xenical?

Mention all prescription, over-the-counter, and herbal medications you are taking before beginning treatment with Xenical. Also, talk to your doctor about your complete medical history, especially if you have allergies to any foods, medicines, or dyes; are taking any other weight loss medication; taking cyclosporine; planning to become pregnant; or if you have anorexia or bulimia.

What is the usual dosage?

The information below is based on the dosage guidelines your doctor uses. Depending on your condition and medical history, your doctor may prescribe a different regimen. Do not change the dosage or stop taking your medication without your doctor's approval.

Adults: The usual dosage is 120 milligrams (mg) taken at any meal that contains fat, up to 3 times a day.

How should I take Xenical?

You should take Xenical with a liquid during or up to 1 hour after any meal that contains fat (up to 3 times a day). Every time you take Xenical with a meal you should not consume more than 30% of your calories from fat.

What should I avoid while taking Xenical?

You should avoid eating very fatty foods when taking Xenical, as this may increase your risk of experiencing unpleasant side effects.

What are possible food and drug interactions associated with Xenical?

If Xenical is taken with certain other drugs, the effects of either could be increased, decreased, or altered. It is especially important to check with your doctor before combining Xenical with the following: cyclosporine, fat-soluble vitamins, levothyroxine (take at least 4 hours apart), warfarin, or other weight loss medications.

What are the possible side effects of Xenical?

Side effects cannot be anticipated. If any develop or change in intensity, tell your doctor as soon as possible. Only your doctor can determine if it is safe for you to continue taking this drug.

Side effects may include: oily spotting or oily discharge, gas with discharge, fatty or oily stools, increased number of bowel movements, inability to control bowel movements

Can I receive Xenical if I am pregnant or breastfeeding?

No. Xenical is not recommended to be taken during pregnancy or breastfeeding.

Tell your doctor immediately if you are pregnant, plan to become pregnant, or are breastfeeding.

What should I do if I miss a dose of Xenical?

If you forget to take Xenical with a meal, you may take it up to 1 hour after. If it has been longer than an hour, skip that dose and return to your normal dosing schedule. Do not double your Xenical doses.

How should I store Xenical?

Store at room temperature in a tightly closed container.

XIFAXAN

Generic name: Rifaximin

What is Xifaxan?

Xifaxan is an antibiotic-type medicine that is used to treat traveler's diarrhea caused by noninvasive strains of the bacteria *Escherichia coli (E. coli)* for patients 12 years of age and older.

What is the most important information I should know about Xifaxan?

Xifaxan is not effective in patients with diarrhea complicated by fever and/or blood in the stool or diarrhea due to bacteria other than *E. coli.* Seek immediate medical attention if you have blood in your bowel movements or if you have a fever.

You should not take Xifaxan if diarrhea symptoms get worse or persist more than 24-48 hours. Alternative antibiotic therapy should be considered.

Who should not take Xifaxan?

You should not take Xifaxan if you are allergic or sensitive to Xifaxan or any other rifamycin-type antibiotics. You should also not take Xifaxan if your diarrhea is caused by any bacteria other than *E. coli.*

What should I tell my doctor before I take the first dose of Xifaxan?

Mention all prescription, over-the-counter, and herbal medications you are taking before beginning treatment with Xifaxan. Also, talk to your doctor about your complete medical history, especially if you have a fever, blood in your bowel movements, or if you have been taking Xifaxan for more than 48 hours and your symptoms have not improved or have gotten worse.

What is the usual dosage?

The information below is based on the dosage guidelines your doctor uses. Depending on your condition and medical history, your doctor may prescribe a different regimen. Do not change the dosage or stop taking your medication without your doctor's approval.

Adults: The usual dosage is 200 milligrams (mg) taken 3 times a day for 3 days.

How should I take Xifaxan?

Xifaxan can be taken with or without food at the same time every day.

What should I avoid while taking Xifaxan?

You should not take Xifaxan for more than 48 hours, if your symptoms worsen, or if you have a fever or bloody bowel movements.

What are possible food and drug interactions associated with Xifaxan?

If Xifaxan is taken with certain other drugs, the effects of either could be increased, decreased, or altered. Always check with your doctor before combining Xifaxan with any other drugs, herbs, or supplements.

What are the possible side effects of Xifaxan?

Side effects cannot be anticipated. If any develop or change in intensity, tell your doctor as soon as possible. Only your doctor can determine if it is safe for you to continue taking this drug.

Side effects may include: gas, headache, stomach pain, muscle spasms in the rectum, frequent bowel movements, nausea, constipation, fever, vomiting

Can I receive Xifaxan if I am pregnant or breastfeeding?
The effects of Xifaxan during pregnancy and breastfeeding are unknown. Tell your doctor immediately if you are pregnant, plan to become pregnant, or are breastfeeding. You should only take Xifaxan during pregnancy if the benefits outweigh the risk to your unborn baby. A decision should be made whether to discontinue nursing or to discontinue the drug, taking into account the importance of the drug to the mother.

What should I do if I miss a dose of Xifaxan?
If you forget to take Xifaxan, take it as soon as you remember. If it is closer to your next scheduled dose, skip the dose you missed and take Xifaxan according to your regular dosing schedule. Do not double your doses.

How should I store Xifaxan?
Store at room temperature.

XOPENEX
Generic name: Levalbuterol

What is Xopenex?
Xopenex is a medicine that treats airway tightness (bronchospasm) in adults and in children ages 6 and older. Xopenex helps to relax the muscles that surround the airway passages in your lungs, to help you breathe easier.

What is the most important information I should know about Xopenex?
Rarely, instead of working the way it is intended, Xopenex can cause a closing of the airway. This may occur with the first use of a new canister or vial. If this type of reaction occurs, stop using Xopenex immediately and seek emergency medical attention.

If you notice that you need more Xopenex than usual, this may be a sign of your asthma worsening. If you experience this, contact your doctor right away.

Use caution when taking Xopenex if you have high blood pressure, heart arrhythmias (irregular heartbeats), heart disease, or any other heart-related problems due to the possible effects Xopenex may have on your heart or blood pressure.

Xopenex overdoses may be life-threatening. Do not take more Xopenex than your doctor has prescribed.

Xopenex can sometimes cause an allergic reaction the first time you take it. Signs of this include rash, itching, trouble breathing, fluid buildup on the airway, or airway closure. Although rare, if this occurs, you should seek immediate emergency medical attention.

High doses of Xopenex may worsen diabetes and lead to other diabetic complications. If you are a diabetic you should monitor your blood glucose and report any changes to your doctor while taking Xopenex.

Who should not take Xopenex?
You should not take Xopenex if you have ever had an allergic reaction or sensitivity to Xopenex or any of its ingredients.

What should I tell my doctor before I take the first dose of Xopenex?
Mention all prescription, over-the-counter, and herbal medications you are taking before beginning treatment with Xopenex. Also, talk to your doctor about your complete medical history, especially if you have a history of heart disease, heart arrhythmias (irregular heartbeats), convulsive disorders, hyperthyroidism, diabetes, high blood pressure, or low levels of potassium in your blood.

What is the usual dosage?
The information below is based on the dosage guidelines your doctor uses. Depending on your condition and medical history, your doctor may prescribe a different regimen. Do not change the dosage or stop taking your medication without your doctor's approval.

Adults and adolescents age 12 and older: The usual starting dose is 0.63 milligrams (mg) taken via a nebulizer 3 times a day (usually every 6-8 hours). Your doctor may increase your dose to 1.25 mg taken 3 times a day depending on your condition.

Children 6 to 11 years old: The usual dose is 0.31 mg taken via nebulizer 3 times a day.

How should I take Xopenex?
Xopenex foil pouches should be opened just enough to remove one unit dose. Carefully twist open the top of the unit dose and empty the contents into the nebulizer reservoir. Next, connect the nebulizer reservoir to the face mask, and then connect the nebulizer to the compressor. Sit in a comfortable, upright position, place the facemask on and then start the compressor. Breathe calmly and deeply until no more mist is produced from the reservoir (usually 5-15 minutes). Once the treatment is finished, clean and store the nebulizer for future use.

What should I avoid while taking Xopenex?

You should not take more Xopenex or increase the frequency of your Xopenex treatments without first checking with your doctor. You should also not take Xopenex within 2 weeks of taking MAOIs (monoamine oxidase inhibitors) or tricyclic antidepressants.

What are possible food and drug interactions associated with Xopenex?

If Xopenex is taken with certain other drugs, the effects of either could be increased, decreased, or altered. It is especially important to check with your doctor before combining Xopenex with the following: beta-adrenergic receptor blocking medicines (beta blockers), digoxin, nonpotassium-sparing diuretics, monoamine oxidase inhibitors (MAOIs), and tricyclic antidepressants.

What are the possible side effects of Xopenex?

Side effects cannot be anticipated. If any develop or change in intensity, tell your doctor as soon as possible. Only your doctor can determine if it is safe for you to continue taking this drug.

Side effects may include: palpitations, chest pain, rapid heart rate, accidental injury, weakness, fever, headache, viral infection, diarrhea, enlarged lymph nodes, muscle pain, asthma, sore throat, runny nose, eczema, rash, itching

Can I receive Xopenex if I am pregnant or breastfeeding?

The effects of Xopenex during pregnancy and breastfeeding are unknown. You should only take Xopenex during pregnancy if the benefits outweigh the risks to your unborn baby. Tell your doctor immediately if you are pregnant, plan to become pregnant, or are breastfeeding.

What should I do if I miss a dose of Xopenex?

If you forget to take Xopenex, take it as soon as you remember. If it is closer to your next scheduled dose, skip the dose you missed and take Xopenex according to your regular dosing schedule. Do not double your doses.

How should I store Xopenex?

Xopenex vials should be stored in the protective foil covering at room temperature, away from excessive heat and protected from light. Once the foil pouch is opened, the unopened vials inside should be used within 2 weeks. Vials that are removed from the foil pouch and not used immediately should be used within 1 week. Discard any vial if the solution is not colorless.

XOPENEX HFA

Generic name: Levalbuterol

What is Xopenex HFA?

Xopenex HFA is a medicine that treats airway tightness (bronchospasm) in adults, adolescents, and in children ages 4 years and older, who have reversible obstructive airway disease. Xopenex HFA helps to relax the muscles that surround the airway passages in your lungs, to help you breathe easier.

What is the most important information I should know about Xopenex HFA?

Rarely, instead of working the way it is intended, Xopenex HFA can cause a closing of the airway. This may occur with the first use of a new canister or vial. If this type of reaction occurs, stop using Xopenex HFA immediately and seek emergency medical attention.

If you notice that you need more Xopenex HFA than usual, this may be a sign of your asthma worsening. If you experience this, contact your doctor right away.

Use caution when taking this medication if you have high blood pressure, heart arrhythmias (irregular heartbeats), heart disease, or any other heart-related problems, due to the possible effects it may have on your heart or blood pressure.

Xopenex HFA overdoses may be life-threatening. Do not take more Xopenex HFA than your doctor has prescribed.

Xopenex HFA can sometimes cause an allergic reaction the first time you take it. Signs of this include rash, itching, trouble breathing, fluid buildup on the airway, or airway closure. Although rare, if this occurs, you should seek immediate emergency medical attention.

High doses of Xopenex HFA may worsen diabetes and lead to other diabetic complications. If you are a diabetic you should monitor your blood glucose and report any changes to your doctor while taking Xopenex.

Who should not take Xopenex HFA?

You should not take Xopenex HFA if you have ever had an allergic reaction or sensitivity to Xopenex or any of its ingredients.

What should I tell my doctor before I take the first dose of Xopenex HFA?

Mention all prescription, over-the-counter, and herbal medications you are taking before beginning treatment with Xopenex HFA. Also, talk to your doctor about your complete medical history, especially if you have a history of heart disease, heart arrhythmias (irregular heartbeats), convulsive disorders, hyperthyroidism, diabetes, high blood pressure, or low levels of potassium in your blood.

What is the usual dosage?
The information below is based on the dosage guidelines your doctor uses. Depending on your condition and medical history, your doctor may prescribe a different regimen. Do not change the dosage or stop taking your medication without your doctor's approval.

Adults, Adolescents, and Children ages 4 and older: 2 inhalations (90 mcg) repeated every 4-6 hours. To some patients, the use of 1 inhalation every 4 hours may be sufficient.

How should I take Xopenex HFA?
Shake well before using.
  You must prime the inhaler before using it for the first time or if it has not been used for more than 3 days, by releasing 4 test sprays into the air, away from the face. Remove the cap from the mouthpiece. Breathe out fully through your mouth. While breathing in deeply and slowly through your mouth, fully depress the top of the metal canister with your finger. Hold your breath for 10 seconds, or as long as you are comfortable. If the doctor has prescribed more than a single puff, wait 1 minute between inhalations. Shake well and repeat these steps.
  Keep the plastic actuator clean to maintain a good flow of medication, and prevent buildup or blockage. It should be washed by running warm water through the top and bottom for 30 seconds, shaken to remove excess water, and air dried at least once a week. Do not submerge the metal canister in water.
  Throw away the canister after you have used 200 inhalations.

What should I avoid while taking Xopenex HFA?
You should not take more Xopenex HFA or increase the frequency of your treatments without first checking with your doctor. Do not take Xopenex within 2 weeks of taking MAOIs (monoamine oxidase inhibitors) or tricyclic antidepressants.

What are possible food and drug interactions associated with Xopenex HFA?
If Xopenex HFA is taken with certain other drugs, the effects of either could be increased, decreased, or altered. It is especially important to check with your doctor before combining Xopenex with the following: beta-adrenergic receptor blocking medicines (beta blockers), digoxin, nonpotassium-sparing diuretics, monoamine oxidase inhibitors (MAOIs), and tricyclic antidepressants.

What are the possible side effects of Xopenex HFA?
Side effects cannot be anticipated. If any develop or change in intensity, tell your doctor as soon as possible. Only your doctor can determine if it is safe for you to continue taking this drug.

Side effects may include: accidental injury, weakness, fever, headache, viral infection, muscle pain, asthma, sore throat, runny nose, eczema, rash, itching, vomiting, palpitations, chest pain, rapid heartbeat, nervousness

Can I receive Xopenex HFA if I am pregnant or breastfeeding?
The effects of Xopenex HFA during pregnancy and breastfeeding are unknown. You should only take Xopenex HFA during pregnancy if the benefits outweigh the risks to your unborn baby. Tell your doctor immediately if you are pregnant, plan to become pregnant, or are breastfeeding.

What should I do if I miss a dose of Xopenex HFA?
If you forget to take Xopenex HFA, take it as soon as you remember. If it is closer to your next scheduled dose, skip the dose you missed and take Xopenex according to your regular dosing schedule. Do not double your doses.

The use of the inhaler is usually on an as-needed basis. If you do not need to use the inhaler to control your symptoms, then it is not necessary to use it at that exact dosing interval.

How should I store Xopenex HFA?
Store at room temperature, and protect from freezing and direct sunlight. Store the inhaler with the mouthpiece down.

XYZAL
Generic name: Levocetirizine

What is Xyzal?
Xyzal is an antihistamine used for the relief of symptoms associated with seasonal and perennial allergic rhinitis and chronic idiopathic urticaria.

What is the most important information I should know about Xyzal?
Xyzal may impair mental alertness. Do not engage in any hazardous activities requiring mental alertness, such as operating machinery, driving, etc.

Who should not take Xyzal?
Do not take Xyzal if you have a known hypersensitivity to levocetirizine or any of its ingredients. Do not use Xyzal if you have kidney problems.

What should I tell my doctor before I take the first dose of Xyzal?
Tell your doctor about all prescription, over-the-counter, and herbal medications you are taking before beginning treatment with Xyzal. Also talk

to your doctor about your complete medical history, especially if have kidney problems.

What is the usual dosage?
The information below is based on the dosage guidelines your doctor uses. Depending on your condition and medical history, your doctor may prescribe a different regimen. Do not change the dosage or stop taking your medication without your doctor's approval.

Adults: The usual dosage of Xyzal is 5 milligrams (mg) once daily.

Children: The usual dosage of Xyzal is 2.5 mg once daily.

How should I take Xyzal?
Take Xyzal as prescribed in the evening.

What should I avoid while taking Xyzal?
Avoid driving and operating machinery. Do not mix alcohol or any other central nervous system depressants with Xyzal.

What are possible food and drug interactions associated with Xyzal?
If Xyzal is used with certain other drugs, the effects of either could be increased, decreased, or altered. It is especially important to check with your doctor before combining Xyzal with the following: antipyrene, azithromycin, cimetidine, erythromycin, ketoconazole, theophylline, pseudoephedrine, and ritonavir.

What are the possible side effects of Xyzal?
Side effects cannot be anticipated. If any develop or change in intensity, tell your doctor as soon as possible. Only your doctor can determine if it is safe for you to continue taking this drug.

Side effects may include: allergic reactions, increased sleepiness, fatigue

Signs of severe allergic reactions may include hives, difficulty breathing, and swelling of the throat. If any of these events occur, seek immediate medical attention.

Can I receive Xyzal if I am pregnant or breastfeeding?
Xyzal is to be avoided during pregnancy and breastfeeding.

What should I do if I miss a dose of Xyzal?
If you miss a dose, take it as soon as you remember. If it is within 12 hours of your next dose, do not take the missed dose. Just take the next dose at your regular time. Do not take two doses at the same time to make up for a missed dose.

How should I store Xyzal?
Store at room temperature.

YAZ
Generic name: Drospirenone and ethinyl estradiol

What is YAZ?
YAZ is an oral contraceptive pill that is used by women to prevent pregnancy.

What is the most important information I should know about YAZ?
Smoking cigarettes increases your risk of serious heart problems while taking birth control pills. YAZ does not protect against HIV infection and other sexually transmitted diseases.

Who should not take YAZ?
You should not take YAZ if you have kidney, liver, or adrenal disease because this could cause serious heart and health problems. Also, YAZ should not be used if you are pregnant or think you may become pregnant. If you have a history of heart problems, blood clots, chest pain, unexplained vaginal bleeding, jaundice, diabetes, or high blood pressure, you should not use this type of contraception. If you are allergic to any of the ingredients in YAZ, do not begin using this contraception.

What should I tell my doctor before I take the first dose of YAZ?
Mention all prescription, over-the-counter, and herbal medications you are using, to prevent a potential interaction with YAZ. Also, talk to your doctor about your complete medical history, and be sure to inform your doctor if you smoke, recently had a baby or miscarriage, or are breastfeeding.

What is the usual dosage?
The information below is based on the dosage guidelines your doctor uses. Depending on your condition and medical history, your doctor may prescribe a different regimen. Do not change the dosage or stop taking your medication without your doctor's approval.

Take one pink "active" pill per day for 24 days, then 1 white "reminder" pill daily for 4 days. By this time the pack of YAZ should be completed.

Pediatric use: Safety and efficacy of YAZ has been established in women of reproductive age. Safety and efficacy are expected to be the same for postpubertal adolescents under the age of 16 and for users 16 years and older.

How should I take YAZ?
You can take YAZ without regard to meals. You should take the pills at the same time every day, so pick a time that is most convenient to you.

What should I avoid while taking YAZ?
Avoid smoking while on YAZ.

What are possible food and drug interactions associated with YAZ?
If YAZ is taken with certain other drugs, the effects of either could be increased, decreased, or altered. It is especially important to check with your doctor before combining this medication with any of the following: ACE inhibitors (captopril, enalapril, lisinopril, and others), aldosterone antagonists, angiotensin-II receptor antagonists (Cozaar, Diovan, Avapro, and others), heparin, NSAIDs (ibuprofen, naprosyn, and others), potassium-sparing diuretics (spironolactone and others), and potassium supplementation.

What are the possible side effects of YAZ?
Side effects cannot be anticipated. If any develop or change in intensity, tell your doctor as soon as possible. Only your doctor can determine if it is safe for you to continue taking this drug.

Side effects may include: nausea, vomiting, gastrointestinal symptoms (such as abdominal cramps and bloating), breakthrough bleeding, spotting, change in menstrual flow, amenorrhea, temporary infertility after discontinuation of treatment, edema, melasma that may persist, breast changes (tenderness, enlargement, secretion), change in weight or appetite, migraine, rash (allergic), mood changes (including depression)

An increased risk of the following serious adverse reactions has been associated with the use of oral contraceptives: thrombophlebitis, arterial thromboembolism, pulmonary embolism, myocardial infarction, cerebral thrombosis, hypertension, gallbladder disease, hepatic adenomas, benign liver tumor

Can I receive YAZ if I am pregnant or breastfeeding?
Pregnancy category X. Estrogens and progestins should not be used during pregnancy. Small amounts of oral contraceptive steroids have been identified in the milk of nursing mothers, and a few adverse effects on the child have been reported, including jaundice and breast enlargement.

What should I do if I miss a dose of YAZ?
If you miss a pink "active" pill, take it as soon as you remember, then continue on your regular schedule. This may mean taking 2 pills in one day.
  For additional information, see "Detailed Patient Labeling."

How should I store YAZ?
Store at room temperature.

ZADITOR
Generic name: Ketotifen fumarate

What is Zaditor?
Zaditor is a topical medicine that is applied to the eyes to relieve itching of the eyes due to allergies. Zaditor prevents the release of inflammation-causing substances in your eye, a process that often occurs in response to allergens.

**What is the most important information
I should know about Zaditor?**
To prevent eye infections and contamination of your Zaditor bottle, avoid letting the tip of the bottle touch any part of your eye.

Zaditor should not be used to treat redness or irritation to your eyes due to wearing contact lenses. Zaditor contains a preservative that may be absorbed by soft contact lenses. If you wear soft contact lenses, wait at least 10 minutes after instilling Zaditor before reinserting your contact lenses.

Zaditor should only be applied topically to the eyes and should not be ingested or injected.

Who should not take Zaditor?
You should not use Zaditor if you are allergic or sensitive to it or any of its ingredients.

**What should I tell my doctor before
I take the first dose of Zaditor?**
Mention all prescription, over-the-counter, and herbal medications you are taking before beginning treatment with Zaditor. Also, talk to your doctor about your complete medical history, especially if you have red or irritated eyes due to causes other than allergies, such as an infection or wearing contact lenses.

What is the usual dosage?
The information below is based on the dosage guidelines your doctor uses. Depending on your condition and medical history, your doctor may prescribe a different regimen. Do not change the dosage or stop taking your medication without your doctor's approval.

Adults: The usual dose is 1 drop instilled into the affected eye(s) twice a day (every 8-12 hours).

Pediatric Use: Safety and effectiveness in pediatric patients under the age of 3 have not been established.

How should I take Zaditor?
Remove any contact lenses or other eye inserts before instilling Zaditor drops.

What should I avoid while taking Zaditor?
Avoiding touching the tip of the Zaditor applicator to any part of your eye, so you will not contaminate the solution.

What are possible food and drug interactions associated with Zaditor?
If Zaditor is taken with certain other drugs, the effects of either could be increased, decreased, or altered. It is especially important to check with your doctor before combining Zaditor with other eye drops, including prescription or over-the-counter preparations.

What are the possible side effects of Zaditor?
Side effects cannot be anticipated. If any develop or change in intensity, tell your doctor as soon as possible. Only your doctor can determine if it is safe for you to continue taking this drug.

Side effects may include: eye infection, runny nose, headache

Can I receive Zaditor if I am pregnant or breastfeeding?
The effects of Zaditor during pregnancy and breastfeeding are unknown. Tell your doctor immediately if you are pregnant, plan to become pregnant, or are breastfeeding.

What should I do if I miss a dose of Zaditor?
If you forget to use Zaditor, instill the dose as soon as your remember. If it is closer to your next scheduled dose, skip the dose you missed and use Zaditor according to your regular dosing schedule. Do not double your doses.

How should I store Zaditor?
Store at room temperature with the top tightly closed.

Zafirlukast *See Accolate, page 4.*

Zaleplon *See Sonata, page 1206.*

ZANAFLEX
Generic name: Tizanidine

What is Zanaflex?
Zanaflex works inside your brain and spinal cord to act on receptors that help to control muscle spasticity (muscle spasms). It is used to treat muscle spasms that interfere with daily activities.

What is the most important information I should know about Zanaflex?
You should use caution when taking Zanaflex if you have any type of liver or kidney problems.

Contact your doctor right away if you experience any nausea, loss of appetite, vomiting, or yellowing of the skin or eyes.

Rarely, Zanaflex can also cause hallucinations or even psychosis. If you experience any type of hallucination while taking Zanaflex, tell your doctor right away.

Suddenly stopping treatment can cause certain medical problems; therefore, always talk to your doctor before deciding to stop Zanaflex therapy.

Zanaflex capsules and tablets are not interchangeable. If you have been taking one, make sure your doctor knows if you switch to another formulation.

The sedative effects of Zanaflex may be increased if you are also taking other medicines that cause tiredness or fatigue, or if you drink alcohol while taking Zanaflex.

Since this medication can decrease your spasticity, be careful when using Zanaflex if your spasticity helps you with posture or balance.

Who should not take Zanaflex?
You should not take Zanaflex if you are also taking ciprofloxacin or fluvoxamine. These medicines can greatly increase the level of Zanaflex in your body. You should also not take Zanaflex if you are allergic or sensitive to it or any of its ingredients.

What should I tell my doctor before I take the first dose of Zanaflex?
Mention all prescription, over-the-counter, and herbal medications you are taking before beginning treatment with Zanaflex. Also, talk to your doctor about your complete medical history, especially if you have a history of liver, kidney, or heart problems; if you are taking oral birth control pills or medicines to treat high blood pressure; or if you drink alcohol on a regular basis.

What is the usual dosage?

The information below is based on the dosage guidelines your doctor uses. Depending on your condition and medical history, your doctor may prescribe a different regimen. Do not change the dosage or stop taking your medication without your doctor's approval.

Adults: The usual starting dose is 4 milligrams (mg) taken every 6-8 hours as needed. Your doctor may increase your dose up to 6-8 mg taken every 6-8 hours depending on your condition.

How should I take Zanaflex?

Zanaflex should be taken at the same time every day, with or without food. However, food greatly affects the amount of Zanaflex your body absorbs. You should remain consistent in taking Zanaflex either with or without food throughout your Zanaflex therapy.

What should I avoid while taking Zanaflex?

You should not drive a car or operate heavy machinery until you know how Zanaflex will affect you. You should not take more Zanaflex than your doctor prescribes.

What are possible food and drug interactions associated with Zanaflex?

If Zanaflex is taken with certain other drugs, the effects of either could be increased, decreased, or altered. It is especially important to check with your doctor before combining Zanaflex with the following: acyclovir; alcohol; antiarrhythmics, including amiodarone, mexiletine, propafenone, and verapamil; cimetidine; ciprofloxacin; fluvoxamine; fluroquinolone-type antibiotics; famotidine; medicines used to treat high blood pressure, especially those known as alpha 2 agonists, such as clonidine; oral birth control pills; other medicines that cause tiredness or fatigue; and zileuton.

What are the possible side effects of Zanaflex?

Side effects cannot be anticipated. If any develop or change in intensity, tell your doctor as soon as possible. Only your doctor can determine if it is safe for you to continue taking this drug.

Side effects may include: dry mouth, weakness, tiredness, dizziness, light-headedness, urinary tract infection or other infections, constipation, liver damage, vomiting, trouble speaking, blurred vision, urinary frequency, flu-like symptoms, irregular muscle movements, nervousness, sore throat, runny nose, lowered blood pressure, slow heart rate

Can I receive Zanaflex if I am pregnant or breastfeeding?

The effects of Zanaflex during pregnancy and breastfeeding are unknown. Tizanidine should be given to pregnant women only if clearly needed. Tell your doctor immediately if you are pregnant, plan to become pregnant, or are breastfeeding.

It is not known whether Zanaflex is excreted in human milk, although as a lipid-soluble drug, it might be expected to pass into breast milk.

What should I do if I miss a dose of Zanaflex?
If you forget to take Zanaflex, take it as soon as you remember. If it is closer to your next scheduled dose, skip the dose you missed and take Zanaflex according to your regular dosing schedule. Do not double your doses.

How should I store Zanaflex?
Store at room temperature in a child-proof container.

Zanamivir *See Relenza, page 1127.*

ZANTAC
Generic name: Ranitidine

What is Zantac?
Zantac is a medicine that blocks certain receptors in your stomach known as H2 receptors, which leads to a decrease in the amount of acid secreted into your stomach.

Zantac is used to treat ulcers in the intestines and stomach. It is also used to prevent the occurrence of ulcers, to treat the erosion in the esophagus caused by acid, to reduce stomach acid in certain diseases where the stomach secretes too much acid, and to treat gastroesophageal reflux disease (GERD).

What is the most important information I should know about Zantac?
Even if Zantac relieves your stomach or ulcer-related symptoms, it is still important to finish Zantac therapy for the prescribed amount of time.

Use caution when taking Zantac if you have kidney or liver problems. If you have a blood disorder known as porphyria, do not take Zantac because it may increase your risk of experiencing an acute porphyric attack.

Who should not take Zantac?
You should not take Zantac if you are allergic or sensitive to it or any of its ingredients.

What should I tell my doctor before I take the first dose of Zantac?
Mention all prescription, over-the-counter, and herbal medications you are taking before beginning treatment with Zantac. Also, talk to your doc-

tor about your complete medical history, especially if you have a history of stomach or intestinal ulcers, or any type of kidney or liver problems.

What is the usual dosage?
The information below is based on the dosage guidelines your doctor uses. Depending on your condition and medical history, your doctor may prescribe a different regimen. Do not change the dosage or stop taking your medication without your doctor's approval.

Active Duodenal Ulcer, Benign Gastric Ulcer, GERD, or Maintenance of Healing of Erosive Esophagitis
Adults: The usual dose is 150 milligrams (mg) taken twice a day.

Maintenance of Healing of Duodenal and Gastric Ulcers
Adults: The usual dose is 150 mg taken once daily at bedtime.

Children ages 1 month to 16 years old: The usual dose is 2-4 mg per 2.2 pounds of body weight, up to a maximum of 150 mg per day.

*Pathological Hypersecretory Conditions
(such as Zollinger-Ellison Syndrome)*
Adults: The usual dose is 150 mg taken twice daily. Your doctor may increase your dose depending on your condition.

Erosive Esophagitis
Adults: The usual dose is 150 mg taken 4 times a day.

Treatment of Duodenal and Gastric Ulcers
Children ages 1 month to 16 years old: The usual dose is 2-4 mg per 2.2 pounds of body weight, up to a maximum of 300 mg per day.

Treatment of GERD and Erosive Esophagitis
Children ages 1 month to 16 years old: The usual dose is 5-10 mg per 2.2 pounds of body weight, given in 2 divided doses.

How should I take Zantac?
Zantac can be taken with or without food and should be taken at the same time every day. If you are an adult patient taking 150 mg twice a day, you may take 300 mg once a day at bedtime for easier dosing.

What should I avoid while taking Zantac?
You should not drink alcohol while taking Zantac.

What are possible food and drug interactions associated with Zantac?
If Zantac is taken with certain other drugs, the effects of either could be increased, decreased, or altered. It is especially important to check with your doctor before combining Zantac with warfarin or triazolam.

What are the possible side effects of Zantac?

Side effects cannot be anticipated. If any develop or change in intensity, tell your doctor as soon as possible. Only your doctor can determine if it is safe for you to continue taking this drug.

Side effects may include: headache, irregular heartbeats, dizziness, liver problems, rash, changes in the counts of blood cells in your blood, constipation, nausea, vomiting, possible allergic reaction including anaphylaxis (trouble breathing, swelling of airway)

Can I receive Zantac if I am pregnant or breastfeeding?

The effects of Zantac during pregnancy are unknown. Zantac is excreted in breast milk. You should use caution if you are nursing and taking Zantac. Tell your doctor immediately if you are pregnant, plan to become pregnant, or are breastfeeding.

What should I do if I miss a dose of Zantac?

If you forget to take Zantac, take it as soon as you remember. If it is closer to your next scheduled dose, skip the dose you missed and take Zantac according to your regular dosing schedule. Do not double your doses.

How should I store Zantac?

Store at room temperature in a light-resistant container.

ZAROXOLYN

Generic name: Metolazone

What is Zaroxolyn?

Zaroxolyn is used to treat fluid retention due to congestive heart failure, kidney problems, or a kidney disorder known as nephrotic syndrome. helps you form urine and get rid of excess body water.

Zaroxolyn is also used to treat high blood pressure; it may be used alone or in combination with other drugs that treat high blood pressure.

What is the most important information I should know about Zaroxolyn?

Zaroxolyn tablets are not interchangeable with other metolazone formulations.

Rarely, allergic reactions to Zaroxolyn can occur with the first dose. Seek medical attention immediately if you have trouble breathing, swelling of the throat or face, or any other allergic-type reaction after taking Zaroxolyn. You may be more likely to experience an allergy to Zaroxolyn if you are also allergic to sulfonamide-type medicines, thiazide-type diuretics, or quinethazone.

Take Zaroxolyn with caution if you are also currently taking other medicines to lower your blood pressure. Let your doctor know if you feel dizzy or light-headed when you take Zaroxolyn.

Zaroxolyn may cause dizziness, light-headedness, or fainting; alcohol, hot weather, exercise, or fever may increase these effects. To prevent them, sit up or stand slowly, especially in the morning. Sit or lie down at the first sign of any of these effects.

Do not drive or perform other possibly unsafe tasks until you know how you react to Zaroxolyn; this drug may cause drowsiness, dizziness, blurred vision, or light-headedness.

Zaroxolyn may cause you to become sunburned more easily. Avoid the sun, sunlamps, or tanning booths until you know how you react to Zaroxolyn. Use sunscreen or wear protective clothing if you must be outside for more than a short time.

Zaroxolyn may increase your blood sugar. If you are a diabetic, monitor your blood sugar and report any changes to your doctor.

Check with your doctor before you use a salt substitute or a product that has potassium in it.

Who should not take Zaroxolyn?
You should not take Zaroxolyn if you do not produce urine, are in a coma or pre-coma, or if you are allergic or sensitive to Zaroxolyn or any of its ingredients.

What should I tell my doctor before I take the first dose of Zaroxolyn?
Mention all prescription, over-the-counter, and herbal medications you are taking before beginning treatment with Zaroxolyn. Also, talk to your doctor about your complete medical history, especially if you have a history of kidney or liver problems, diabetes, gout, systemic lupus erythematosus, blood disorders, or electrolyte abnormalities in your blood.

What is the usual dosage?
The information below is based on the dosage guidelines your doctor uses. Depending on your condition and medical history, your doctor may prescribe a different regimen. Do not change the dosage or stop taking your medication without your doctor's approval.

Adults: The effective dosage of Zaroxolyn should be individualized according to what the medicine is being used for, as well as the patient's response. A single daily dose is recommended. Therapy with Zaroxolyn should be slowly increased to determine the minimal dose possible to maintain the desired response.

Edema of Cardiac Failure or Renal Disease
Adults: The usual dose is 5-20 milligrams (mg) taken once a day.

Mild to Moderate Hypertension (High Blood Pressure)
Adults: The usual dose is 2.5-5 mg taken once a day.

The time interval required for the initial dosage regimen to show effect may vary from three or four days to three to six weeks in the treatment of elevated blood pressure.

How should I take Zaroxolyn?

Zaroxolyn should be taken at the same time every day, with or without food. If stomach upset occurs, take it with food to reduce stomach irritation.

Zaroxolyn may increase the amount of urine or cause you to urinate more often when you first start taking it. To keep this from disturbing your sleep, try to take your dose before 6 pm.

What should I avoid while taking Zaroxolyn?

You should not drive a car or operate heavy machinery until you know how Zaroxolyn will affect you, especially after taking the first dose.

Do not stand or sit up quickly when taking Zaroxolyn, especially in the morning. Sit or lie down at the first sign of dizziness, light-headedness, or fainting.

Zaroxolyn may cause you to become sunburned more easily. Avoid the sun, sunlamps, or tanning booths until you know how you react to Zaroxolyn. Use sunscreen or wear protective clothing if you must be outside for more than a short time.

What are possible food and drug interactions associated with Zaroxolyn?

If Zaroxolyn is taken with certain other drugs, the effects of either could be increased, decreased, or altered. It is especially important to check with your doctor before combining Zaroxolyn with the following: alcohol; angiotensin-converting enzyme (ACE) inhibitors, such as enalapril; anticoagulants; antineoplastic agents, such as cyclophosphamide; barbiturates; corticosteroids or ACTH; curariform drugs; diazoxide; digitalis glycosides; diuretics, especially furosemide or other loop-type diuretics; insulin and oral antidiabetic agents; ketanserin; lithium; medications that lower your blood pressure; methenamine; narcotics; norepinephrine; and salicylates and other nonsteroidal anti-inflammatory drugs (NSAIDs).

What are the possible side effects of Zaroxolyn?

Side effects cannot be anticipated. If any develop or change in intensity, tell your doctor as soon as possible. Only your doctor can determine if it is safe for you to continue taking this drug.

Side effects may include: chest pain; low blood pressure, especially when rising from a seated position or lying down; fainting; dizziness; headache; fatigue; skin rashes; itching; diarrhea; constipation; stomach pain; loss of appetite; stomach bloating; electrolyte abnormalities in the blood; muscle cramps or spasms; dry mouth; chills

More serious side effects may include: sore throat with fever, unusual bleeding or bruising, severe skin rash with peeling skin, difficulty breathing or swallowing

Rarely, allergic reactions to Zaroxolyn can occur with the first dose. Seek medical attention immediately if you have trouble breathing, swelling of the throat or face, or any other allergic-type reaction after taking Zaroxolyn.

Can I receive Zaroxolyn if I am pregnant or breastfeeding?
Zaroxolyn should be used during pregnancy only if the anticipated benefit is weighed against possible hazards to the fetus. Zaroxolyn is excreted in breast milk. Because of the potential for serious adverse reactions in nursing infants from metolazone, a decision should be made whether to discontinue nursing or to discontinue the drug, taking into account the importance of the drug to the mother. Tell your doctor immediately if you are pregnant, plan to become pregnant, or are breastfeeding.

What should I do if I miss a dose of Zaroxolyn?
If you forget to take Zaroxolyn, take it as soon as you remember. If it is closer to your next scheduled dose, skip the dose you missed and take Zaroxolyn according to your regular dosing schedule. Do not double your doses.

How should I store Zaroxolyn?
Store at room temperature, between 68 and 77 degrees F (20 and 25 degrees C). Store away from heat, moisture, and light. Do not store in the bathroom. Keep Zaroxolyn out of the reach of children. .

ZEBETA
Generic name: Bisoprolol fumarate

What is Zebeta?
Zebeta is a beta-1 selective adrenergic blocker. It blocks a certain type of receptor found in the heart muscle. It is used to treat high blood pressure, alone or in combination with other medicines.

What is the most important information I should know about Zebeta?
Take Zebeta continuously as directed by your doctor. Suddenly stopping Zebeta therapy may lead to withdrawal symptoms, which may include chest pain, heart attack, and a fast or irregular heartbeat.

Zebeta may mask symptoms of low blood sugar. If you have diabetes, monitor your blood sugar frequently, especially when you first start taking Zebeta. Signs of low blood sugar may include a rapid heartbeat, anxiety, sweating, weakness, dizziness, drowsiness, faintness, vision changes, headache, chills, tremors, or an increase in appetite. Ask your doctor before you change the dose of your diabetes medicine.

Zebeta may mask the signs of an underlying thyroid disorder. Your doctor will likely check your thyroid function before you take Zebeta.

If you have a disease that makes it hard to breath, such as asthma or chronic obstructive pulmonary disease (COPD), Zebeta can worsen your condition. Tell your doctor immediately if you experience shortness of breath.

Do not drive or perform other possibly unsafe tasks until you know how you react to Zebeta; this medication may cause drowsiness, dizziness, or light-headedness. These effects may be worse if you take it with alcohol or certain medicines. Hot weather, exercise, or fever may also increase these effects. To prevent them, sit up or stand slowly, especially in the morning. Sit or lie down at the first sign of any of these effects.

Patients who take medicine for high blood pressure often feel tired or run down for a few weeks after starting treatment. Be sure to take your medicine even if you may not feel "normal." Tell your doctor if you develop any new symptoms.

If you have a disorder of the blood vessels in your feet, legs, and hands known as peripheral vascular disease, Zebeta may worsen your condition. Talk to your doctor about your condition before taking Zebeta.

Before undergoing any type of surgery, inform your physician or dentist that you are taking Zebeta.

Who should not take Zebeta?
You should not take Zebeta if you have been diagnosed with the following heart conditions: sinus bradycardia (a type of slow heartbeat), heart block greater than first degree, severe heart failure, or cardiogenic shock.

What should I tell my doctor before I take the first dose of Zebeta?
Mention all prescription, over-the-counter, and herbal medications you are taking before beginning treatment with Zebeta. Also, talk to your doctor about your complete medical history, especially if you have diabetes, overactive thyroid, asthma, COPD, or any other disease that makes it hard for you to breathe; peripheral vascular disease (PVD); or any type of liver, kidney, or heart problems. Tell your doctor if you have a history of anaphylactic reactions to allergens, because Zebeta may decrease the effectiveness of epinephrine.

What is the usual dosage?
The information below is based on the dosage guidelines your doctor uses. Depending on your condition and medical history, your doctor

may prescribe a different regimen. Do not change the dosage or stop taking your medication without your doctor's approval.

Adults: The usual starting dose is 2.5-5 milligrams (mg) taken once a day. Based on your condition, your doctor may increase your dose to 10-20 mg taken once a day. The dose of this medication should be individualized to the needs of the patient.

How should I take Zebeta?
Zebeta should be taken at the same time every day, with or without food. Continue to take Zebeta even if you feel well. Do not miss any doses.

What should I avoid while taking Zebeta?
You should avoid operating an automobile or heavy machinery, as well as engaging in other tasks that require mental alertness, until you know how Zebeta will affect you.

Do not stand or sit up quickly when taking Zebeta, especially in the morning. Sit or lie down at the first sign of dizziness, light-headedness, or fainting.

Do not stop taking this medication even if you feel well or change the dose without first speaking to your doctor.

What are possible food and drug interactions associated with Zebeta?
If Zebeta is taken with certain other drugs, the effects of either could be increased, decreased, or altered. It is especially important to check with your doctor before combining Zebeta with the following: bupivacaine; certain calcium channel blockers, such as diltiazem, verapamil, and mibefradil; cimetidine; clonidine; digoxin; diltiazem; disopyramide; flecainide; guanethidine; ketanserin; mefloquine; other beta-blocker medicines; reserpine; and verapamil.

What are the possible side effects of Zebeta?
Side effects cannot be anticipated. If any develop or change in intensity, tell your doctor as soon as possible. Only your doctor can determine if it is safe for you to continue taking this drug.

Side effects may include: cough, runny nose, urinary tract infection, fatigue, water retention, diarrhea, dizziness, drowsiness, headache, light-headedness, sleeplessness, weakness

Zebeta may mask symptoms of low blood sugar. Signs of low blood sugar may include a rapid heartbeat, anxiety, sweating, weakness, dizziness, drowsiness, faintness, vision changes, headache, chills, tremors, or an increase in appetite. Check blood sugar levels closely. Ask your doctor before you change the dose of your diabetes medicine; contact your doctor if any of these symptoms occur.

Can I receive Zebeta if I am pregnant or breastfeeding?

Zebeta should be used during pregnancy only if the potential benefit justifies the potential risk to the fetus. It is not known whether Zebeta is excreted in human milk. Caution should be exercised when Zebeta is administered to nursing women. Tell your doctor immediately if you are pregnant, plan to become pregnant, or are breastfeeding.

What should I do if I miss a dose of Zebeta?

If you forget to take Zebeta, take it as soon as you remember. If it is closer to your next scheduled dose, skip the dose you missed and take Zebeta according to your regular dosing schedule. Do not double your doses.

How should I store Zebeta?

Store at room temperature, between 59 and 86 degrees F (15 and 30 degrees C), and away from heat, moisture, and light. Do not store in the bathroom. Keep Zebeta out of the reach of children.

ZEGERID

Generic name: Omeprazole and sodium bicarbonate

What is Zegerid?

Zegerid is used to treat intestinal ulcers (duodenal ulcers), stomach ulcers (gastric ulcers), gastroesophageal reflux disease (GERD), and erosive esophagitis.

What is the most important information I should know about Zegerid?

Both the capsule and oral suspension forms of Zegerid can be taken with water and on an empty stomach. Do not substitute any other food or liquid in the place of water. Do not open the capsule and sprinkle the contents into food.

Who should not take Zegerid?

Do not take Zegerid if you are allergic to any of its ingredients.

What should I tell my doctor before I take the first dose of Zegerid?

Mention all prescription, over-the-counter, and herbal medications you are taking before beginning treatment with Zegerid. Also, talk to your doctor about your complete medical history, especially if you are on a sodium-restricted diet.

What is the usual dosage?

The information below is based on the dosage guidelines your doctor uses. Depending on your condition and medical history, your doctor

may prescribe a different regimen. Do not change the dosage or stop taking your medication without your doctor's approval.

Benign Gastric Ulcer
Adults: The recommended dosage is 40 milligrams (mg) once daily for 4-8 weeks.

Erosive Esophagitis
Adults: The recommended dosage is 20 mg once daily for 4-8 weeks. To maintain healing of erosive esophagitis, the daily dose is 20 mg for as long as the doctor prescribes Zegerid.

Short-Term Treatment of Active Duodenal Ulcer
Adults: The recommended dosage is 20 mg once daily for 4 weeks.

Symptomatic GERD
Adults: The recommended dosage is 20 mg once daily for up to 4 weeks.

Upper Gastrointestinal Bleeding
Adults: The recommended oral suspension dosage begins at 40 mg, followed by 40 mg 6-8 hours later and 40 mg daily for 14 days.

Zegerid has not been studied in patients under the age of 18.

How should I take Zegerid?
Zegerid capsules should be swallowed whole with water on an empty stomach 1 hour before a meal. Do not use any other liquid than water. Do not open the capsule and sprinkle on food.

Zegerid oral suspension should be emptied into a small cup with 1-2 tablespoons of water. Do not use any other liquid than water. Stir well and drink. Refill the cup with water and drink the remainder.

What should I avoid while taking Zegerid?
Avoid taking food simultaneously with Zegerid. Zegerid should be taken on an empty stomach at least 1 hour before a meal. Both 20 mg and 40 mg of Zegerid contain the same amount of one ingredient; therefore, do not substitute two 20-mg capsules or oral suspension packets for a 40-mg dose.

What are possible food and drug interactions associated with Zegerid?
If Zegerid is taken with certain other drugs, the effects of either could be increased, decreased, or altered. It is especially important to check with your doctor before combining Zegerid with the following: atazanavir, diazepam, other proton pump inhibitors, phenytoin, tacrolimus, or warfarin.

What are the possible side effects of Zegerid?

Side effects cannot be anticipated. If any develop or change in intensity, tell your doctor as soon as possible. Only your doctor can determine if it is safe for you to continue taking this drug.

Side effects may include: aches, back pain, constipation, cough, diarrhea, dizziness, headache, nausea, rash, upper respiratory infection, vomiting

Can I receive Zegerid if I am pregnant or breastfeeding?

The effects of Zegerid during pregnancy and breastfeeding are unknown. Tell your doctor immediately if you are pregnant, plan to become pregnant, or are breastfeeding. Zegerid is passed into breast milk.

What should I do if I miss a dose of Zegerid?

If you miss a dose of Zegerid, take it as soon as possible. If it is almost time for your next dose, skip the missed dose and go back to your regular dosing schedule. Do not take 2 doses at once.

How should I store Zegerid?

Store both the capsules and oral suspension at room temperature.

ZELAPAR

Generic name: Selegiline hydrochloride

What is Zelapar?

Zelapar is used in the management of patients with Parkinson's disease who are not responding to treatment with levodopa/carbidopa alone.

What is the most important information I should know about Zelapar?

Zelapar should not be taken with any type of tricyclic antidepressants, non-selective MAOIs, or selective MAO-B inhibitors. The interaction between these drugs may cause sweating, mental change/strange behavior, muscle stiffness, loss of consciousness, or death. Intake of food and liquid should be avoided 5 minutes before and after Zelapar administration.

Who should not take Zelapar?

Do not take Zelapar if you are allergic to selegiline or any of its other ingredients. Also, do not take Zelapar if you are taking meperidine; Zelapar should not be taken with this type of analgesic. It should also not be administered with the pain medicines: tramadol, methadone, and propoxyphene.

What should I tell my doctor before I take the first dose of Zelapar?
Mention all prescription, over-the-counter, and herbal medications you are taking before beginning treatment with Zelapar. Also, talk to your doctor about your complete medical history before beginning Parkinson's disease therapy.

What is the usual dosage?
The information below is based on the dosage guidelines your doctor uses. Depending on your condition and medical history, your doctor may prescribe a different regimen. Do not change the dosage or stop taking your medication without your doctor's approval.

Adults: The usual starting dose of Zelapar is 1.25 milligrams (mg) once per day for at least 6 weeks. After 6 weeks, the dosage of Zelapar may be increased to 2.5 mg once per day.

Safety and effectiveness in patients under the age of 16 have not been established.

How should I take Zelapar?
Zelapar should be taken in the morning, before breakfast and without any liquids.

Do not try to push Zelapar through the back foil of the container; instead, peel the back off the wrapper to remove the medication. With dry hands, immediately place the tablet(s) on the tongue which will rapidly disintegrate. Avoid any foods and liquid 5 minutes before and after taking Zelapar.

What should I avoid while taking Zelapar?
While being treated with Zelapar, avoid pregnancy, breastfeeding, and certain drugs.

What are possible food and drug interactions associated with Zelapar?
If Zelapar is taken with certain other drugs, the effects of either could be increased, decreased, or altered. It is especially important to check with your doctor before combining Zelapar with the following: dextromethorphan, MAOIs, meperidine, selective serotonin reuptake inhibitors, and tricyclic antidepressants.

What are the possible side effects of Zelapar?
Side effects cannot be anticipated. If any develop or change in intensity, tell your doctor as soon as possible. Only your doctor can determine if it is safe for you to continue taking this drug.

Side effects may include: back pain, dizziness, headache, nasal infection, nausea, pain, sleeplessness, swelling of the mouth, uncontrolled muscle movements, upset stomach, hallucinations

Can I receive Zelapar if I am pregnant or breastfeeding?
The effects of Zelapar during pregnancy and breastfeeding are unknown. Tell your doctor immediately if you are pregnant, plan to become pregnant, or are breastfeeding.

What should I do if I miss a dose of Zelapar?
Take the missed dose as soon as you remember it. If it is almost time for your next dose, skip the missed dose and return to your normal dosing schedule. Do not double the dose.

How should I store Zelapar?
Store at room temperature.

ZEMPLAR
Generic name: Paricalcitol

What is Zemplar?
Zemplar is used for the prevention and treatment of secondary hyperparathyroidism associated with chronic kidney disease (CKD) Stage 3 and 4.

What is the most important information I should know about Zemplar?
Taking too much vitamin D, as in Zemplar, can cause increased calcium levels, calcium in your urine, and bone disease.

Who should not take Zemplar?
Do not take Zemplar if you have elevated vitamin D levels, calcium levels, or you are allergic to any of its ingredients.

What should I tell my doctor before I take the first dose of Zemplar?
Mention all prescription, over-the-counter, and herbal medications you are taking before beginning treatment with Zemplar. Also, talk to your doctor about your complete medical history.

What is the usual dosage?
The information below is based on the dosage guidelines your doctor uses. Depending on your condition and medicay history, your doctor may prescribe a different regimen. Do not change the dosage or stop taking your medication without your doctor's approval.

Adults: Zemplar capsules may be taken daily or three times a week. When treated three times weekly, the dose should be given no more frequently than every other day.

How should I take Zemplar?
You should take Zemplar as directed by your doctor. Zemplar may be taken with or without food.

What should I avoid while taking Zemplar?
Avoid using even nonprescription/over-the-counter drugs without talking to your doctor first.

What are possible food and drug interactions associated with Zemplar?
If Zemplar is taken with certain other drugs, the effects of either could be increased, decreased, or altered. It is especially important to check with your doctor before combining Zemplar with the following: atazanavir, clarithromycin, indinavir, itraconazole, ketoconazole, nefazodone, nelfinavir, ritonavir, saquinavir, telithromycin, or voriconazole.

What are the possible side effects of Zemplar?
Side effects cannot be anticipated. If any develop or change in intensity, tell your doctor as soon as possible. Only your doctor can determine if it is safe for you to continue taking this drug.

Side effects may include: allergic reaction, back pain, chest pain, fever, flu, fungal/bacterial infections, headache, pain, stomach pain, viral infection

Symptoms of vitamin D overdose: Early signs and symptoms include bone pain, constipation, dry mouth, headache, nausea/vomiting, metallic taste, muscle pain, sleeplessness, weakness; late signs and symptoms include eye infection, itchiness, light sensitivity, nasal infection, weight loss/loss of appetite

Can I receive Zemplar if I am pregnant or breastfeeding?
The effects of Zemplar during pregnancy and breastfeeding are unknown. Tell your doctor immediately if you are pregnant, plan to become pregnant, or are breastfeeding.

What should I do if I miss a dose of Zemplar?
Take it as soon as you remember. If it is almost time for your next dose, skip the missed dose and return to your normal dosing schedule. Do not double the dose.

How should I store Zemplar?
Store at room temperature.

ZERIT
Generic name: Stavudine

What is Zerit?
Zerit is a medication used to treat HIV, the virus that causes AIDS. Zerit belongs to a class of drugs called nucleoside reverse transcriptase inhibitors. Zerit is taken in combination with other anti-HIV medications to reduce the amount of virus circulating in your blood, and to increase the number of disease-fighting cells in your blood.

What is the most important information I should know about Zerit?
Zerit will not cure your HIV infection. Even while taking Zerit, it is still possible to have HIV-related illnesses, including infections caused by other disease-producing organisms. See your doctor regularly and report any medical problems that occur.

Zerit does not prevent a person infected with HIV from passing the virus to others. It is important to practice safe sex and prevent others from coming in contact with your blood or body fluids.

Zerit may cause severe liver enlargement and injury. This can lead to a rise in the levels of lactic acid in your blood, causing a condition known as lactic acidosis. Fatal cases of lactic acidosis have been reported in pregnant women who took Zerit and didanosine along with other anti-HIV medicines.

Do not take zidovudine (AZT) while taking Zerit, because AZT may interfere with the actions of Zerit. Products containing AZT include Combivir, Retrovir, and Trizivir.

If you are taking ribaviron or interferon, your doctor may need to monitor your therapy more closely or may consider a change in your therapy.

Zerit and didanosine should only be taken together if the benefit outweighs the risk, a decision that your doctor will make. Fatal and nonfatal inflammation of the pancreas can occur if Zerit is taken with didanosine and/or hydroxyurea. Stop taking Zerit and tell your doctor immediately if you experience nausea, vomiting, or stomach pains. These may be a sign of injury to your pancreas.

Zerit may cause a disorder called peripheral neuropathy, which affects the nerves in the hands and feet, especially if you have advanced HIV disease, if you have ever had peripheral neuropathy, or if you are also taking other drugs that can cause neuropathies, such as didanosine.

Who should not take Zerit?
You should not take Zerit if you are allergic to any of its ingredients, including stavudine.

What should I tell my doctor before I take the first dose of Zerit?
Mention all prescription, over-the-counter, and herbal medications you are taking before beginning treatment with Zerit. Also, talk to your doctor about your complete medical history, especially if you have a history of kidney or liver problems, diabetes, peripheral neuropathies, or if you are pregnant, breastfeeding, or plan to become pregnant.

What is the usual dosage?
The information below is based on the dosage guidelines your doctor uses. Depending on your condition and medical history, your doctor may prescribe a different regimen. Do not change the dosage or stop taking your medication without your doctor's approval.

Your doctor will determine your dose based on your body weight, kidney and liver function, and any side effects that you may have had with other medicines.

Adults: The usual dose if you weigh 132 pounds or more is 40 milligrams (mg) taken twice a day (every 12 hours). If you weigh less than 132 pounds, the usual dose is 30 mg taken twice a day.

Children from birth to 13 days old: The usual dose is 0.5 mg per 2.2 pounds of body weight per dose, given once every 12 hours.

Children at least 14 days old and weighing less than 66 pounds: The usual dose is 1 mg per 2.2 pounds of body weight per dose, given once every 12 hours.

Note: Children weighing 66 pounds or more should receive the adult dose.

If you experience numbness, tingling, or pain in the feet or hands, Zerit should be stopped. In some cases, symptoms may worsen temporarily following discontinuation of therapy. If symptoms resolve completely, you should take one-half the recommended dose: 20 mg twice daily for patients weighing greater than or equal to 132 pounds of body weight and 15 mg twice daily for patients weighing less than 132 pounds of body weight.

How should I take Zerit?
Zerit may be taken with or without food. Each Zerit dose should be taken twice a day (12 hours apart) and should be taken at the same time every day. Take Zerit exactly as your doctor has prescribed. Do not skip doses.

What should I avoid while taking Zerit?
You should not breastfeed while taking Zerit. You should not take AZT while taking Zerit, because zidovudine may interfere with the actions of Zerit.

What are possible food and drug interactions associated with Zerit?

If Zerit is taken with certain other drugs, the effects of either could be increased, decreased, or altered. It is especially important to check with your doctor before combining Zerit with didanosine, doxorubicin, hydroxyurea, ribavirin, or zidovudine.

What are the possible side effects of Zerit?

Side effects cannot be anticipated. If any develop or change in intensity, tell your doctor as soon as possible. Only your doctor can determine if it is safe for you to continue taking this drug.

Side effects may include: headache, diarrhea, rash, nausea, vomiting, abdominal pain, muscle pain or weakness in the arms and legs, trouble sleeping (insomnia), loss of appetite, chills or fever, allergic reactions, blood disorders, changes in body fat, feeling weak and tired, shortness of breath

Can I receive Zerit if I am pregnant or breastfeeding?

The effects of Zerit during pregnancy are not known. Pregnant women have experienced serious side effects when taking Zerit in combination with didanosine or other HIV medicines. You should only take Zerit if you are pregnant, after discussing the risks and benefits with your doctor. Tell your doctor immediately if you are pregnant, plan to become pregnant, or are breastfeeding. The Centers for Disease Control and Prevention (CDC) recommends that HIV-infected mothers *not* breastfeed, to reduce the risk of passing HIV infection to their babies and the potential for serious adverse reactions in nursing infants. Therefore, do not nurse a baby while taking Zerit.

What should I do if I miss a dose of Zerit?

If you forget to take Zerit, take the missed dose right away. If it is almost time for your next dose, do not take the missed dose. Instead, follow your regular dosing schedule by taking the next dose at its regular time. Do not double your doses.

It is very important to not miss doses, as this may allow the HIV virus to multiply in your body.

How should I store Zerit?

Store Zerit capsules in a tightly closed container at room temperature away from heat. Do not store Zerit in a damp place, such as a bathroom medicine cabinet or near the kitchen sink. Store Zerit for oral solution in a tightly closed container in a refrigerator and throw away any unused portion after 30 days.

ZESTORETIC

Generic name: Lisinopril and hydrochlorothiazide

What is Zestoretic?

Zestoretic is a combination product that contains two medicines: Lisinopril, an angiotensin-converting enzyme (ACE) inhibitor, and hydrochlorothiazide, a diuretic. These two medications work together to lower blood pressure in patients who may not have experienced adequate blood pressure lowering from other medications. This should not be the first medication used to treat high blood pressure.

What is the most important information I should know about Zestoretic?

If taken during the second or third trimester of pregnancy, Zestoretic may cause serious harm or even death to an unborn baby. If you become pregnant while taking Zestoretic, you should immediately stop taking it and tell your doctor.

Zestoretic can cause a rare but serious allergic reaction leading to extreme swelling of the face, lips, tongue, throat, or gut (causing severe abdominal pain). You may have an increased risk of experiencing these symptoms if you have ever had an allergy to ACE inhibitor-type medicines or if you are African American. If you experience any of these symptoms, seek emergency medical attention.

Tell your doctor if you experience light-headedness, especially during the first few days of Zestoretic therapy. If you faint, stop taking Zestoretic until you have talked to your doctor.

Do not stand or sit up quickly when taking Zestoretic, especially in the morning. Sit or lie down at the first sign of dizziness, light-headedness, or fainting.

Vomiting, diarrhea, fever, exercise, hot weather, alcohol, excessive perspiration, and dehydration may lead to an excessive fall in blood pressure. Consult with your doctor if you experience these. Make sure to drink plenty of fluids when taking Zestoretic.

Zestoretic may decrease your blood levels of infection-fighting white blood cells, especially if you have a condition known as a collagen vascular disease (such as lupus) or kidney disease. Promptly report any indication of infection, such as sore throat or fever, to your doctor.

Zestoretic can also activate lupus or gout if you are susceptible.

Do not drive or perform other possibly unsafe tasks until you know how you react to Zestoretic; this drug may cause dizziness, light-headedness, or fainting. These effects may be worse if you take it with alcohol or certain medicines.

Zestoretic may raise your blood sugar. High blood sugar may make you feel confused, drowsy, or thirsty. It can also make you flush, breathe faster, or have a fruit-like breath odor. If these symptoms occur, tell your doctor right away.

Patients who take medicine for high blood pressure often feel tired or run down for a few weeks after starting treatment. Be sure to take your medicine even if you may not feel "normal." Tell your doctor if you develop any new symptoms.

Zestoretic may not work as well in black patients. They may also be at greater risk of side effects. Contact your doctor if your symptoms do not improve or if they become worse.

Zestoretic may cause you to become sunburned more easily. Avoid the sun, sunlamps, or tanning booths until you know how you react to Zestoretic. Use sunscreen or wear protective clothing if you must be outside for more than a short time.

Who should not take Zestoretic?
You should not take Zestoretic if you do not produce urine, you have a history of sensitivity or allergic reaction to ACE inhibitors, or you are allergic to sulfonamide-derived medications. You may be more at risk of experiencing sensitivity or an allergic reaction to Zestoretic if you have allergies or bronchial asthma. You should not take Zestoretic if you are allergic to lisinopril, hydrochlorothiazide, or any of the medication's other ingredients.

What should I tell my doctor before I take the first dose of Zestoretic?
Mention all prescription, over-the-counter, and herbal medications you are taking before beginning treatment with Zestoretic. Also, talk to your doctor about your complete medical history, especially if you are pregnant or plan on becoming pregnant. Also discuss this medication with your doctor if you have any of the following: diabetes; a history of liver or kidney problems, bone marrow suppression, heart disease, or scleroderma; severe immune system problems; lupus; asthma; are on a sodium-restricted diet, or if you have ever had an allergy or sensitivity to an ACE inhibitor or sulfonamide-derived medications.

What is the usual dosage?
The information below is based on the dosage guidelines your doctor uses. Depending on your condition and medical history, your doctor may prescribe a different regimen. Do not change the dosage or stop taking your medication without your doctor's approval.

Adults: The usual dose is 10/12.5 (10 milligrams [mg] of lisinopril and 12.5 mg of hydrochlorothiazide) or 20/12.5 (20 mg of lisinopril and 12.5 mg of hydrochlorothiazide). Your doctor may increase your dose to 20/25 mg depending on your condition and how you respond to the medication.

How should I take Zestoretic?

You should take Zestoretic with or without food at the same time every day. Continue to use Zestoretic even if you feel well. Do not miss any doses.

What should I avoid while taking Zestoretic?

You should avoid operating automobiles or heavy machinery until you know how Zestoretic will affect you. Also avoid becoming dehydrated; drink adequate fluids while taking Zestoretic. Do not take salt substitutes or supplements containing potassium unless otherwise directed by your doctor.

Do not stand or sit up quickly when taking Zebeta, especially in the morning. Sit or lie down at the first sign of dizziness, light-headedness, or fainting.

Avoid the sun, sunlamps, or tanning booths until you know how you react to Zestoretic. Use sunscreen or wear protective clothing if you must be outside for more than a short time.

What are possible food and drug interactions associated with Zestoretic?

If Zestoretic is taken with certain other drugs, the effects of either could be increased, decreased, or altered. It is especially important to check with your doctor before combining Zestoretic with the following: certain diuretics, such as thiazide-type diuretics and potassium-sparing diuretics such as spironolactone, amiloride, and triamterene; cholestyramine; colestipol; corticosteroids; insulin and oral antidiabetic medicines; lithium; methenamine; norepinephrine; nonsteroidal anti-inflammatory drugs (NSAIDs), such as ibuprofen or naproxen; potassium supplements; salt substitutes containing potassium; and skeletal muscle relaxants.

What are the possible side effects of Zestoretic?

Side effects cannot be anticipated. If any develop or change in intensity, tell your doctor as soon as possible. Only your doctor can determine if it is safe for you to continue taking this drug.

Side effects may include: dizziness, headache, low blood pressure (especially when rising from a seated position), fatigue, cough, nausea, tiredness, diarrhea

Zestoretic can cause a rare but serious allergic reaction leading to extreme swelling of the face, lips, tongue, throat, or gut (causing severe abdominal pain). You may have an increased risk of experiencing these symptoms if you have ever had an allergy to ACE inhibitor-type medicines or if you are African American. If you experience any of these symptoms, seek emergency medical attention.

Zestoretic may raise your blood sugar. High blood sugar may make you feel confused, drowsy, or thirsty. It can also make you flush, breathe faster, or have a fruit-like breath odor. If these symptoms occur, tell your doctor right away.

Can I receive Zestoretic if I am pregnant or breastfeeding?
Zestoretic should not be taken during pregnancy. Taking Zestoretic during your second or third trimesters of pregnancy could cause serious harm or even death to your unborn baby. Tell your doctor immediately if you are pregnant, plan to become pregnant, or are breastfeeding. Zestoretic is excreted in breast milk, and should not be taken if you are nursing unless you are directed to do so by your doctor.

What should I do if I miss a dose of Zestoretic?
If you miss a dose of Zestoretic, take it as soon as possible. If it is almost time for your next dose, skip the missed dose and go back to your regular dosing schedule. Do not take 2 doses at once.

How should I store Zestoretic?
Store at 77 degrees F (25 degrees C) in a tightly closed container. Brief storage at temperatures between 59 and 86 degrees F (15 and 30 degrees C) is permitted. Store away from heat, moisture, and light. Do not store in the bathroom. Keep Zestoretic out of the reach of children.

ZESTRIL
Generic name: Lisinopril

What is Zestril?
Zestril is a type of blood pressure lowering medication known as an angiotensin-converting enzyme (ACE) inhibitor. Zestril is used to lower your blood pressure when taken alone or in combination with other medications. Zestril may be used alone or with other medicines to manage heart failure or improve survival after a heart attack.

What is the most important information I should know about Zestril?
If taken during the second or third trimester of pregnancy, Zestril can cause serious harm or even death to an unborn baby. If you become pregnant while taking Zestril, stop taking Zestril immediately and tell your doctor right away.

Zestril can cause a rare but serious allergic reaction leading to extreme swelling of the face, lips, tongue, throat, or gut (causing severe abdominal pain). You may have an increased risk of experiencing these symptoms if you have ever had an allergy to ACE inhibitor-type medicines or if you are African American. If you experience any of these symptoms, seek emergency medical attention right away.

Zestril may rarely cause a yellowing of the skin or eyes, which can be a sign of liver injury. If this occurs tell your doctor immediately.

Zestril may cause light-headedness or fainting, especially upon standing from a lying or sitting position.

Zestril may decrease your blood levels of infection-fighting white blood cells, especially if you have lupus or kidney disease. If you have these diseases your doctor will most likely monitor you closely by taking regular blood samples.

If you get any type of infection (sore throat/fever) while taking Zestril you should report it to your doctor right away. Avoid contact with people who have colds or infections.

Zestril should be taken with caution if you have kidney disease or heart problems.

Zestril may increase the levels of an electrolyte known as potassium in your blood. You should not use salt substitutes or take potassium supplements unless otherwise directed by your doctor.

Zestril may increase your blood sugar and make medicines that treat diabetes less effective. If you have diabetes, you should monitor your blood sugar frequently and report any changes to your doctor.

Do not drive or perform other possibly unsafe tasks until you know how you react to Zestril; this drug may cause dizziness, light-headedness, or fainting. These effects may be worse if you take it with alcohol or certain medicines.

Zestril may not work as well in black patients. They may also be at greater risk of side effects. Contact your doctor if your symptoms do not improve or if they become worse.

Dehydration, excessive sweating, vomiting, or diarrhea may increase the risk of low blood pressure. Contact your healthcare provider at once if any of these occur.

Tell your doctor or dentist that you take Zestril before you receive any medical or dental care, emergency care, or surgery.

Patients who take medicine for high blood pressure often feel tired or run down for a few weeks after starting treatment. Be sure to take your medicine even if you may not feel "normal." Tell your doctor if you develop any new symptoms.

If you have high blood pressure, do not use nonprescription products that contain stimulants. These products may include diet pills or cold medicines. Contact your doctor if you have any questions or concerns.

Who should not take Zestril?

You should not take Zestril if you have had a previous allergic reaction to Zestril or any other ACE inhibitor, or if you were diagnosed with idiopathic or hereditary angioedema (swelling of the hands, face, lips, eyes, throat, or tongue; difficulty swallowing or breathing; or hoarseness). Do not take Zestril if you are allergic or sensitive to lisinopril or any other of its ingredients.

What should I tell my doctor before I take the first dose of Zestril?

Mention all prescription, over-the-counter, and herbal medications you are taking before beginning treatment with Zestril. Also, talk to your doctor about your complete medical history, especially if you have diabetes; liver, kidney, or heart disease; blood vessel problems; bone marrow problems; history of stroke, recent heart attack, or kidney transplant; autoimmune disease (rheumatoid arthritis, lupus, scleroderma); or if you have ever had an allergy or sensitivity to an ACE inhibitor such as Zestril. In addition, tell your doctor if you are pregnant or plan on becoming pregnant.

What is the usual dosage?

The information below is based on the dosage guidelines your doctor uses. Depending on your condition and medical history, your doctor may prescribe a different regimen. Do not change the dosage or stop taking your medication without your doctor's approval.

Acute Myocardial Infarction

Adults: The first dose following an acute myocardial infarction is 5 mg (milligrams), then 5 mg in the next 24 hours; 10 mg is usually given in 48 hours following this, then 10 mg taken once per day thereafter for 6 weeks. This is given to (hemodynamically) stable patients within 24 hours of onset of symptoms associated with a heart attack.

Heart Failure

Adults: The usual starting dose is 5 mg. Your doctor may increase your dose from 5-40 mg taken once a day depending on your individual response. The dose of Zestril can be increased by increments of no greater than 10 mg, at intervals of no less than 2 weeks to the highest tolerated dose, up to a maximum of 40 mg daily. Dose adjustment should be based on the patient's response.

Hypertension

Adults: The usual starting dosage is 10 mg taken once a day. Your individual dose may be increased to 20-40 mg taken as a once-daily dose or in divided doses, based on your response to the medication.

Children 6 years and older: The usual starting dose is .07 mg per 2.2 pounds of bodyweight (up to 5 mg) taken once daily. Dosage should be adjusted according to blood pressure response.

How should I take Zestril?

Zestril can be taken with or without food and should be taken at the same time every day.

What should I avoid while taking Zestril?

You should avoid operating automobiles or heavy machinery until you know how Zestril will affect you. You should avoid becoming very dehydrated because this could cause your blood pressure to drop too low. Drink adequate fluids while taking Zestril. You should not take salt substitutes or supplements containing potassium unless otherwise directed by your doctor.

Zestril may cause light-headedness or fainting, especially upon standing from a lying or sitting position.

Take this medication as prescribed by your doctor. Do not alter the dose or stop taking this medication without consulting your doctor.

Avoid taking any diet pills or cold medications without speaking to your doctor because they may alter the effectiveness of Zestril.

What are possible food and drug interactions associated with Zestril?

If Zestril is taken with certain other drugs, the effects of either could be increased, decreased, or altered. It is especially important to check with your doctor before combining Zestril with the following: aldosterone blockers, such as eplerenone; aspirin; gold-containing medicines, such as auranofin; lithium; nonsteroidal anti-inflammatory drugs (NSAIDs); oral antidiabetic medicines and insulin; potassium-sparing diuretics, such as spironolactone, amiloride, or triamterene; potassium supplements; salt substitutes containing potassium; and thiazide-type diuretics, such as hydrochlorothiazide.

What are the possible side effects of Zestril?

Side effects cannot be anticipated. If any develop or change in intensity, tell your doctor as soon as possible. Only your doctor can determine if it is safe for you to continue taking this drug.

Side effects may include: low blood pressure, dizziness, diarrhea, chest pain, headache

Zestril can cause a rare but serious allergic reaction leading to extreme swelling of the face, lips, tongue, throat, or gut (causing severe abdominal pain). Contact your doctor if you experience any of these symptoms.

If you get any type of infection (sore throat/fever) while taking Zestril you should report it to your doctor right away.

Can I receive Zestril if I am pregnant or breastfeeding?

Zestril should not be taken during pregnancy. Taking Zestril during the second or third trimesters of your pregnancy could cause serious harm or even death to your unborn baby. It is not known if Zestril is excreted in breast milk, so you should not take Zestril if you are nursing unless you are told to by your doctor. Tell your doctor immediately if you are pregnant, plan to become pregnant, or are breastfeeding.

What should I do if I miss a dose of Zestril?
If you miss a dose of Zestril take it as soon as possible. If it is almost time for your next dose, skip the missed dose and go back to your regular dosing schedule. Do not take 2 doses at once.

How should I store Zestril?
Store at room temperature away from heat, moisture, and light. Do not store in the bathroom.

ZETIA
Generic name: Ezetimibe

What is Zetia?
Zetia is a cholesterol-lowering medicine that works in your small intestines to block the absorption of cholesterol. Zetia, plus a low-saturated fat diet, is used to reduce your cholesterol either alone or in combination with other medicines, such as HMG-CoA reductase inhibitors or fenofibrates. Zetia may be prescribed for patients who have high cholesterol due to their diet, lifestyle, or if it runs in their family.

What is the most important information I should know about Zetia?
Zetia may cause injury to your liver, especially if you are taking Zetia along with other cholesterol-lowering medications. You should use caution when taking Zetia if you have any type of liver problems. Rarely, it may cause a serious muscle disorder. You should tell your doctor right away if you feel any muscle weakness, pain, or tenderness.

Zetia should not take the place of exercise and a healthy low-fat, low-cholesterol diet to lower your cholesterol. Follow the diet and exercise program given to you by your healthcare provider.

Do not drive or perform other possibly unsafe tasks until you know how you react to Zetia; this drug may cause dizziness. This effect may be worse if you take it with alcohol or certain medicines.

Who should not take Zetia?
You should not take Zetia if you are allergic or sensitive to any of its ingredients. You should also not take Zetia in combination with another cholesterol-lowering medication called a HMG-CoA reductase inhibitor if you have active liver disease, if you are pregnant, plan to become pregnant, or if you are nursing.

What should I tell my doctor before I take the first dose of Zetia?

Mention all prescription, over-the-counter, and herbal medications you are taking before beginning treatment with Zetia. Also, talk to your doctor about your complete medical history, especially if you have kidney or liver problems, hypothyroidism, a history of muscle weakness or tenderness after taking cholesterol-lowering medications, diabetes, or if you are pregnant, plan to become pregnant, or if you are nursing.

What is the usual dosage?

The information below is based on the dosage guidelines your doctor uses. Depending on your condition and medical history, your doctor may prescribe a different regimen. Do not change the dosage or stop taking your medication without your doctor's approval.

Adults: The usual dose is 10 milligrams (mg) taken once a day.

How should I take Zetia?

Zetia should be taken at the same time every day and can be taken with or without food. If you are also taking another cholesterol-lowering medication called a bile acid sequestrant, you should take your Zetia dose at least 2 hours before or 4 hours after it. Zetia may be taken at the same time as a statin or fenofibrate.

Continue to use Zetia even if you feel well. Do not miss any doses.

Take the medication as prescribed by your doctor. Do not change your dose or stop taking the medication without speaking to your doctor.

What should I avoid while taking Zetia?

You should avoid foods high in saturated fat or overall fat content while taking Zetia, to ensure you get the maximum cholesterol-lowering benefits from it.

Do not drive or perform other possibly unsafe tasks until you know how you react to Zetia; this drug may cause dizziness. This effect may be worse if you take it with alcohol or certain medicines.

Do not change your dose or stop taking the medication without speaking to your doctor.

What are possible food and drug interactions associated with Zetia?

If Zetia is taken with certain other drugs, the effects of either could be increased, decreased, or altered. It is especially important to check with your doctor before combining Zetia with the following: cholestyramine, cyclosporine, fibrates, fenofibrate, gemfibrozil, HMG-CoA reductase inhibitors, or warfarin.

What are the possible side effects of Zetia?

Side effects cannot be anticipated. If any develop or change in intensity, tell your doctor as soon as possible. Only your doctor can determine if it is safe for you to continue taking this drug.

Side effects may include: back pain, chest pain, diarrhea, headache, joint pain, muscle pain, upper respiratory tract infection, sinus inflammation, tiredness

You should tell your doctor right away if you feel any muscle weakness, pain, or tenderness. These may be symptoms of a more serious side effect of Zetia.

Can I receive Zetia if I am pregnant or breastfeeding?

The effects of Zetia during pregnancy and breastfeeding are unknown. Tell your doctor immediately if you are pregnant, plan to become pregnant, or are breastfeeding.

What should I do if I miss a dose of Zetia?

If you miss a dose of Zetia, take it as soon as possible. If it is almost time for your next dose, skip the missed dose and go back to your regular dosing schedule. Do not take 2 doses at once.

How should I store Zetia?

Store at room temperature away from heat, moisture, and light. Do not store in the bathroom.

ZIAC

Generic name: Bisoprolol fumarate and hydrochlorothiazide

What is Ziac?

Ziac is a blood pressure lowering product that contains two different medicines: bisoprolol fumarate and hydrochlorothiazide. Bisoprolol fumarate is a beta-1 selective adrenergic blocker, which means that it blocks a certain type of receptor found in the heart muscle. Hydrochlorothiazide is a medication that helps your body make urine, to get rid of excess fluid and lower your blood pressure. These two medications work together to lower blood pressure in patients who did not have enough blood pressure lowering from other medications.

What is the most important information I should know about Ziac?

You should take Ziac continuously—do not abruptly stop without first consulting your doctor. Suddenly stopping therapy may lead to withdrawal symptoms such as the worsening of chest pain, fast or irregular heartbeat, or even a heart attack. When stopping treatment with Ziac, your doctor will need to slowly decrease your dose over a period of 1 to 2 weeks and will watch you closely for side effects, especially if you have certain kinds of heart disease. If chest pain becomes more severe or a heart problem develops, Ziac should be restarted at once, at least temporarily, and other measures to help unstable chest pain should be taken. Because heart artery disease is common and you may not know you have it, it may be safer not to stop Ziac quickly even if you are only being treated for high blood pressure.

Ziac may mask the signs and symptoms of low blood sugar, especially in diabetics. If you have diabetes, monitor your blood sugar frequently, especially when you first start taking Ziac. Signs of low blood sugar may include a rapid heartbeat, anxiety, sweating, weakness, dizziness, drowsiness, faintness, vision changes, headache, chills, tremors, or an increase in appetite. Ask your doctor before you change the dose of your diabetes medicine.

Ziac may also mask the signs of an underlying thyroid disorder such as rapid heart rate.

This medication may cause alterations in the levels of electrolytes (important elements and minerals) in your blood. It is important to stay hydrated while taking Ziac.

Do not drive or perform other possibly unsafe tasks until you know how you react to Ziac; this drug may cause dizziness or light-headedness. These effects may be worse if you take it with alcohol or certain medicines.

Ziac may cause dizziness, light-headedness, or fainting; alcohol, hot weather, exercise, or fever may increase these effects. To prevent them, sit up or stand slowly, especially in the morning. Sit or lie down at the first sign of any of these effects.

Patients who take medicine for high blood pressure often feel tired or run down for a few weeks after starting treatment. Be sure to take your medicine even if you may not feel "normal." Tell your doctor if you develop any new symptoms.

Ziac may cause you to become sunburned more easily. Avoid the sun, sunlamps, or tanning booths until you know how you react to Ziac. Use sunscreen or wear protective clothing if you must be outside for more than a short time.

Tell your doctor or dentist that you take Ziac before you receive any medical or dental care, emergency care, or surgery.

If you have high blood pressure, do not use nonprescription products that contain stimulants. These products may include diet pills or cold medicines. Contact your doctor if you have any questions or concerns.

Who should not take Ziac?

You should not take Ziac if you have been diagnosed with heart conditions called sinus bradycardia (a type of slow heartbeat), heart block greater than first degree, severe heart failure, inability to produce urine, allergy to sulfonamide-derived medicines, or a life-threatening condition known as cardiogenic shock. You should not take Ziac if you are allergic or sensitive to Ziac or any of its ingredients.

What should I tell my doctor before I take the first dose of Ziac?

Mention all prescription, over-the-counter, and herbal medications you are taking before beginning treatment with Ziac. Also, talk to your doctor about your complete medical history, especially if you have diabetes, asthma, COPD or any other disease that can make it hard for you to breathe, gout, overactive thyroid, blood vessel problems, lupus, pheochromocytoma (a type of tumor found in the adrenal glands), or any type of liver, kidney, or heart problems. Tell your doctor if you have a history of anaphylactic reactions to allergens, because Ziac may decrease the effectiveness of epinephrine.

What is the usual dosage?

The information below is based on the dosage guidelines your doctor uses. Depending on your condition and medical history, your doctor may prescribe a different regimen. Do not change the dosage or stop taking your medication without your doctor's approval.

Adults: The usual starting dose is 2.5/6.25 milligrams (mg) taken once a day (equivalent to 2.5 mg of bisoprolol fumarate and 6.25 mg of hydrochlorothiazide). Your doctor may then increase your dose (usually every 14 days) up to 20/12.5 mg per day (given once daily or in 2 divided doses) depending on your condition.

If withdrawal of Ziac therapy is planned, it should be achieved gradually over a period of about 2 weeks. Patients should be carefully observed.

How should I take Ziac?

Ziac should be taken at the same time every day and can be taken with or without food.

Ziac may increase the amount of urine or cause you to urinate more often when you first start taking it. To keep this from disturbing your sleep, try to take your dose before 6 pm.

You should take Ziac continuously—do not abruptly stop without first consulting your doctor. Suddenly stopping therapy may lead to the worsening of chest pain or even cause a heart attack.

What should I avoid while taking Ziac?

You should avoid operating an automobile or heavy machinery, as well as engaging in other tasks that require mental alertness, until you know how Ziac will affect you. You should also avoid becoming dehydrated while taking Ziac, as this may cause your blood pressure to drop too low.

You should take Ziac continuously—do not abruptly stop without first consulting your doctor.

Avoid the sun, sunlamps, or tanning booths until you know how you react to Ziac. Use sunscreen or wear protective clothing if you must be outside for more than a short time.

Do not use nonprescription products that contain stimulants. These products may include diet pills or cold medicines. Contact your doctor if you have any questions or concerns.

Do not stand or sit up quickly when taking Ziac, especially in the morning. Sit or lie down at the first sign of dizziness, light-headedness, or fainting.

What are possible food and drug interactions associated with Ziac?

If Ziac is taken with certain other drugs, the effects of either could be increased, decreased, or altered. It is especially important to check with your doctor before combining Ziac with the following: alcohol, allopurinol, amantadine, barbiturates, beta-blockers or blood pressure lowering medicines, cimetidine, cholestyramine, clonidine, colestipol, corticosteroids or ACTH, diazoxide, digitalis, diltiazem, disopyramide, guanethidine, insulin or oral antidiabetic medicines, lithium, narcotics, nonsteroidal anti-inflammatory medications (such as ibuprofen or naproxen), norepinephrine, reserpine, and verapamil.

What are the possible side effects of Ziac?

Side effects cannot be anticipated. If any develop or change in intensity, tell your doctor as soon as possible. Only your doctor can determine if it is safe for you to continue taking this drug.

Side effects may include: diarrhea, fatigue, dizziness, light-headedness, headache

Ziac may mask the signs and symptoms of low blood sugar, especially in diabetics. Signs of low blood sugar may include a rapid heartbeat, anxiety, sweating, weakness, dizziness, drowsiness, faintness, vision changes, headache, chills, tremors, or an increase in appetite. Contact your doctor if any of these symptoms occur.

Suddenly stopping therapy with Ziac may lead to withdrawal symptoms such as the worsening of chest pain, fast or irregular heartbeat, or even a heart attack. Contact your doctor immediately if any of these symptoms occur.

Can I receive Ziac if I am pregnant or breastfeeding?

The effects of Ziac during pregnancy and breastfeeding are unknown. Tell your doctor immediately if you are pregnant, plan to become pregnant, or are breastfeeding.

What should I do if I miss a dose of Ziac?

If you forget to take Ziac, take it as soon as you remember. If it is closer to your next scheduled dose, skip the dose you missed and take Ziac according to your regular dosing schedule. Do not double your doses.

How should I store Ziac?

Store at room temperature away from heat, moisture, and light. Do not store in the bathroom.

ZIAGEN
Generic name: Abacavir sulfate

What is Ziagen?

Ziagen is a nucleoside analogue reverse transcriptase inhibitor (NRTI) used to treat HIV infection. It is always used in combination with other anti-HIV medicines to help lower the amount of the virus found in the blood. This helps to keep your immune system as healthy as possible so that it can help fight infection.

What is the most important information I should know about Ziagen?

Ziagen is not a cure for HIV infection and you may continue to experience illnesses associated with HIV infection, including opportunistic infections. It has not been shown to reduce the risk of transmission of HIV to others through sexual contact or blood contamination.

Serious and sometimes fatal allergic reactions have been associated with Ziagen, characterized by fever, rash, nausea, vomiting, diarrhea, or abdominal pain, generalized malaise, fatigue, or achiness, and shortness of breath, cough, or sore throat.

Prior to starting Ziagen, your doctor may want to take a series of blood tests to determine if you have a genetic component known as HLA B*5701 allele. There is an increased risk for experiencing a potentially fatal reaction to Ziagen if you carry the HLA-B*5701 allele.

As soon as an allergic reaction is suspected, discontinue the use of the medication and do not reuse or use other HIV medication that contains abacavir.

Other reported effects of this medication are lactic acidosis and severe enlarged, fatty liver, including fatal cases, and an inflammatory disease in response to certain bacterial infections with combination antiretroviral therapy within a few weeks to months after initiating therapy

Redistribution/accumulation of body fat (including central obesity and fat accumulation of the back known as a "buffalo hump"), peripheral and facial wasting, and breast enlargement have been observed in patients receiving antiretroviral therapy.

Who should not take Ziagen?
Do not take Ziagen if you are allergic to any of its components or medications that contain abacavir (such as Trizivir and Epzicom) or if you have moderate-to-severe liver impairment.

What should I tell my doctor before I take the first dose of Ziagen?
Tell your doctor about all your health conditions and all the medicines you take, including prescription and over-the-counter medicines, vitamins, supplements, and herbals. Be sure to tell your doctor if you have had an allergic reaction to this medication or other medications, if you smoke, have liver or cardiovascular problems, or have other chronic conditions that increase your risk of diabetes, high cholesterol, or high blood pressure

What is the usual dosage?
The information below is based on the dosage guidelines your doctor uses. Depending on your condition and medical history, your doctor may prescribe a different regimen. Do not change the dosage or stop taking your medication without your doctor's approval.

Adults >18 years: The usual dose is 600 milligrams (mg) daily, administered as either 300 mg twice daily or 600 mg once daily.

Children >3 months to older adolescents: The dose should be calculated on body weight (kg) and should not exceed 300 mg twice daily.

Patients with liver impairment: The adjusted dose for this population is 200 mg twice daily.

How should I take Ziagen?
Take this medication by mouth exactly as your doctor prescribes it. The usual dose is 1 tablet twice a day or 2 tablets once a day with or without food.

What should I avoid while taking Ziagen?
Avoid skipping or missing doses, because if you stop your anti-HIV drugs, even for a short time, the amount of virus in your blood may increase and the virus may become harder to treat.

Do not take this medication with other abacavir containing products such as Epzicom or Trizivir

Avoid activities that can spread HIV infection, as Ziagen does not stop you from passing the virus to others. Do not share needles or other injection equipment, do not share personal items that can have blood or body fluids on them, and do not have any kind of sex without protection.

What are possible food and drug interactions associated with Ziagen?

If Ziagen is taken with certain other drugs, the effects of either could be increased, decreased, or altered. It is especially important to check with your doctor before combining Ziagen with other medications including the following: abacavir-containing drugs (Epzicom or Trizivir), alcohol, methadone.

What are the possible side effects of Ziagen?

Side effects cannot be anticipated. If any develop or change in intensity, tell your doctor as soon as possible. Only your doctor can determine if it is safe for you to continue taking this drug.

Side effects may include: Nausea, headache, fatigue, vomiting, sleep/dream disturbances, chills, ear/nose/throat infections, rash, mood changes, muscle pain, and changes in your immune system and body fat

Can I receive Ziagen if I am pregnant or breastfeeding?

There have been no adequate trials to determine Ziagen's safety in pregnancy and breastfeeding. Taking this medication during pregnancy or breastfeeding should be discussed with you doctor to determine if benefits outweighs the risks. It is recommended to not breastfeed while using Ziagen.

What should I do if I miss a dose of Ziagen?

It is important not to run out of this medication or skip doses. If you miss a dose, take the missed dose right away. Then take the next dose at the usual time. Do not take 2 doses at once.

How should I store Ziagen?

Ziagen should be stored in room temperature away from light.

ZIANA GEL

Generic name: Clindamycin phosphate

What is Ziana Gel?

Ziana Gel is an antibiotic and retinoid combination prescription product used for the topical treatment of acne in patients 12 years and older.

What is the most important information I should know about Ziana Gel?

Ziana Gel may cause skin irritation such as dryness, redness, peeling, burning, or stinging. Stop Ziana Gel and call your doctor if your skin becomes very red, swollen, blistered, or crusted.

If you use Ziana Gel and you experience severe diarrhea or gastrointestinal (stomach and intestine) discomfort, you should discontinue using this medication and contact your physician.

Do not use more than the recommended dose.

A sunscreen should be applied every morning and reapplied over the course of the day as needed. You should avoid exposure to sunlight, sunlamp, UV light, and other medicines that may increase sensitivity to sunlight. If you have sunburn, you should discontinue the medication right away and contact your physician.

Important: Not for mouth, eye, or vaginal use.

Who should not take Ziana Gel?

Do not use Ziana Gel if you have Crohn's disease (inflammatory disease of the stomach and intestine), ulcerative colitis (inflammations of the large intestine), or if you have developed colitis (inflammation of the colon) with past antibiotic use.

What should I tell my doctor before I take the first dose of Ziana Gel?

Tell your doctor about all prescription, over-the-counter, and herbal medication you are taking before beginning treatment with Ziana Gel. Also, talk to your doctor about your complete medical history, especially if you are pregnant, planning to become pregnant, or if you are breastfeeding. Be sure your doctor knows about all the skin care products you use.

What is the usual dosage?

The information below is based on the dosage guidelines your doctor uses. Depending on your condition and medical history, your doctor may prescribe a different regimen. Do not change the dosage or stop taking your medication without your doctor's approval.

Adults and children 12 years and older: Apply a pea-sized amount to the face once a day at bedtime.

How should I take Ziana Gel?

Use Ziana Gel exactly as prescribed, even though it may take some time for your acne to improve. Your doctor will tell you how long to use Ziana Gel.

At bedtime: After washing your face gently with a mild soap and warm water, pat the skin dry. Apply a pea-size amount of Ziana Gel to your fingertip and spread it over your face. Gently, smooth it into your skin. Do not get Ziana Gel in your eyes or mouth, on your lips, on the corners of your nose, or on open wounds.

In the morning, apply a sunscreen and reapply during the day as needed.

Do not apply Ziana Gel more than once a day and do not use too much of it because it may irritate your skin.

Do not wash your face more than 2 to 3 times a day. Washing your face too often or scrubbing it may make your acne worse.

What should I avoid while taking Ziana Gel?

Avoid excessive exposure to the sun, cold, and wind. Weather extremes can dry and burn the skin. Always use a sunscreen on Ziana Gel-treated skin, even on cloudy days. Use other protective clothing such as a hat when you are in the sun.

Do not use sunlamps and tanning booths; medicated or rough soaps and cleansers; soaps and cosmetics that have a strong drying effect; and skin products that contain alcohol, astringents, spices, or lime. These products may cause increased skin irritation if used with Ziana Gel.

If your face becomes sunburned, stop Ziana Gel until your skin has healed.

What are possible food and drug interactions associated with Ziana Gel?

If Ziana Gel is taken with certain other drugs, the effects of either could be increased, decreased, or altered. It is especially important to check with your doctor before combining Ziana Gel with erythromycin-containing products.

What are the possible side effects of Ziana Gel?

Side effects cannot be anticipated. If any develop or change in intensity, tell your doctor as soon as possible. Only your doctor can determine if it is safe for you to continue taking this drug.

Side effects may include: change in skin color, diarrhea, skin dryness, redness, peeling, burning, stinging

Talk to your doctor about any side effect that bothers you or that does not go away. These are not all the side effects with Ziana Gel. Ask your doctor or pharmacist for more information.

Can I receive Ziana Gel if I am pregnant or breastfeeding?

The effects of Ziana Gel during pregnancy are unknown. Tell your doctor immediately if you are pregnant, plan to become pregnant, or are breastfeeding.

What should I do if I miss a dose of Ziana Gel?

Skip the dose you missed and resume treatment the following night.

How should I store Ziana Gel?

Store at room temperature away from heat and light. Keep the tube tightly closed.

Zidovudine (AZT) See Retrovir, page 1144.

Zileuton See Zyflo, page 1502.

Zileuton, extended-release See Zyflo CR, page 1504.

Ziprasidone hydrochloride See Geodon, page 611.

ZITHROMAX
Generic name: Azithromycin

What is Zithromax?
Zithromax is a macrolide antibiotic which treats the bacterial infections that can cause pneumonia, infections of chronic obstructive pulmonary disease, sinus infections, throat or tonsil infections, skin infections, infections of the urethra or cervix, genital ulcer disease, or ear infections.

What is the most important information I should know about Zithromax?
Zithromax can cause severe and life-threatening allergic reactions that require immediate medical attention. If you experience any difficulty breathing, swelling of the face or neck, as well as any type of rash or skin reaction, contact your doctor immediately. Taking antibiotics may increase your chances of getting another infection of the gut called pseudomembranous colitis. Tell your doctor right away if you experience any type of diarrhea or severe abdominal pain while taking Zithromax. You should use caution when taking Zithromax if you have kidney or liver problems. This drug may cause life-threatening irregular heartbeats.

Who should not take Zithromax?
You should not take Zithromax if you are allergic or sensitive to any other macrolide antibiotic or erythromycin.

It should also be avoided in any patients with pneumonia or those who cannot swallow or take medications orally due to moderate-to-severe illness or risk factors such as cystic fibrosis; patients with nosocomially acquired infections; patients with known or suspected bacteremia; patients requiring hospitalization; elderly or debilitated patients; or patients with significant underlying health problems that may compromise their ability to respond to their illness.

What should I tell my doctor before I take the first dose of Zithromax?
Tell your doctor about all prescription, over-the-counter, and herbal medications you are taking before beginning treatment with Zithromax. Also, talk to your doctor about your complete medical history, especially if you

have liver or severe kidney disease; heart problems, including irregular heartbeats; cystic fibrosis; an infection from a hospital or nursing home; an infection in your blood; or you are hospitalized, elderly, debilitated, or have a weakened immune system.

What is the usual dosage?
The information below is based on the dosage guidelines your doctor uses. Depending on your condition and medical history, your doctor may prescribe a different regimen. Do not change the dosage or stop taking your medication without your doctor's approval.

Acute Bacterial Exacerbations of Chronic Obstructive Pulmonary Disease (Mild to Moderate)
Adults: The usual dose is 500 milligrams (mg) taken once a day for 3 days, or 500 mg as a single dose on Day 1, followed by 250 mg once daily on Days 2 through 5.

Acute Bacterial Sinusitis
Adults: The usual dose is 500 mg taken once a day for 3 days.

Children (oral suspension): The usual dose is 10 mg per 2.2 pounds of bodyweight once daily for 3 days.

Acute Otitis Media
Children (oral suspension): The usual dose is 30 mg per 2.2 pounds of bodyweight given as a single dose, or 10 mg per 2.2 pounds of bodyweight given once daily for 3 days, or 10 mg per 2.2 pounds of bodyweight given as a single dose on the first day followed by 5 mg per 2.2 pounds of bodyweight per day on Days 2 through 5.

Community-Acquired Pneumonia (Mild Severity),
Pharyngitis/Tonsillitis (Second-Line Therapy),
or Skin/Skin Structure (Uncomplicated)
Adults: The usual dose is 500 mg as a single dose on Day 1, followed by 250 mg once daily on Days 2 through 5.

Children (oral suspension), for community-acquired pneumonia: The usual dose is 10 mg per 2.2 pounds of bodyweight as a single dose on the first day, followed by 5 mg per 2.2 pounds of bodyweight per day on Days 2 through 5.

Genital Ulcer Disease (Chancroid)
Adults: The usual dose is one single 1 gram (g) dose.

Gonococcal Urethritis and Cervicitis
Adults: The usual dose is one single 2 g dose.

Non-Gonoccocal Urethritis and Cervicitis
Adults: The usual dose is one single 1 g dose.

How should I take Zithromax?

Zithromax should be taken at the same time every day and can be taken with or without food.

What should I avoid while taking Zithromax?

You should not take aluminum- or magnesium-containing antacids with Zithromax.

What are possible food and drug interactions associated with Zithromax?

If Zithromax is taken with certain other drugs, the effects of either could be increased, decreased, or altered. It is especially important to check with your doctor before combining Zithromax with the following: cyclosporine, digoxin, ergotamine or dihydroergotamine, hexobarbital, nelfinavir, phenytoin, terfenadine, or warfarin.

What are the possible side effects of Zithromax?

Side effects cannot be anticipated. If any develop or change in intensity, tell your doctor as soon as possible. Only your doctor can determine if it is safe for you to continue taking this drug.

Side effects may include: abdominal pain, diarrhea, nausea

Can I receive Zithromax if I am pregnant or breastfeeding?

The effects of Zithromax during pregnancy and breastfeeding are unknown. Tell your doctor immediately if you are pregnant, plan to become pregnant, or are breastfeeding.

What should I do if I miss a dose of Zithromax?

If you forget to take Zithromax, take it as soon as your remember. If it is closer to your next scheduled dose, skip the dose you missed and take Zithromax according to your regular dosing schedule. Do not double your doses.

How should I store Zithromax?

Zithromax tablets and Zithromax suspension should both be stored at room temperature.

ZMAX

Generic name: Azithromycin, extended-release

What is Zmax?

Zmax is an antibiotic that kills bacteria. It is used in adults to treat sinus infections and certain kinds of pneumonia. It is also used to treat children 6 months and older with community-acquired pneumonia. Zmax only works against bacteria; it does not work against viruses like colds or the flu.

What is the most important information I should know about Zmax?

Zmax is dosed differently from other antibiotics. You take just one dose, one time. On Day 1, Zmax starts working. On Days 2 and 3, you may not feel better right away. After Day 3, Zmax continues to work over time. If your symptoms are not better, call your doctor.

Similar to other antibiotics, there is an increased chance of developing diarrhea while using this drug.

Who should not take Zmax?

Do not take Zmax if you are allergic to azithromycin, erythromycin, ketolide or any macrolide, or telithromycin. Also avoid this drug if you are allergic to any of its ingredients. Zmax has not been used in children under 6 months of age.

What should I tell my doctor before I take the first dose of Zmax?

Tell your doctor about all prescription, over-the-counter, and herbal medications you are taking before beginning treatment with Zmax, especially warfarin. Also, talk to your doctor about your complete medical history, especially if you have kidney or liver problems or myasthenia gravis.

What is the usual dosage?

Adults: Zmax should be taken in a single 2 gram (g) dose.

Children 6 months and older: Zmax should be given as a single dose of 60 mg/kg (equivalent to 27 mg/lb). If your child weighs 75 pounds or more, your doctor may prescribe the adult dose.

How should I take Zmax?

Shake well. It is recommended to take Zmax on an empty stomach (1 hour before or 2 hours after a meal). For adults, the entire contents of a bottle should be taken as one dose; for children, give the amount prescribed by your doctor. Take without regard to antacids containing magnesium and or aluminum hydroxide. To ensure accurate dosing for children, use a dosing spoon, medicine syringe, or cup.

If you receive Zmax in liquid form, it is ready to take. If you receive Zmax as dry powder, you must prepare it before taking your prescribed dose. Add ¼ cup of water to the Zmax bottle. Close tightly and shake thoroughly to mix it.

What should I avoid while taking Zmax?

You may not feel better right away after taking Zmax. In the meantime, to help improve your symptoms, avoid smoking, drinking alcohol or soda and coffee. Instead, get plenty of rest, drink lots of fluids (water or juice), and speak to your doctor before taking symptom-relief medicines (cough suppressants, pain-relievers, or fever reducers). If your child vomits within 1 hour of taking the medicine, avoid giving more Zmax to your child unless instructed to do so by your doctor.

What are possible food and drug interactions associated with Zmax?

If Zmax is taken with certain other drugs, the effects of either could be increased, decreased, or altered. It is especially important to check with your doctor before combining Zmax with the following: anti-HIV medication, anti-seizure medication, cyclosporines, digoxin, ergotamine or dihydroergotamine, migraine medication, phenytoin, or warfarin.

What are the possible side effects of Zmax?

Side effects cannot be anticipated. If any develop or change in intensity, tell your doctor as soon as possible. Only your doctor can determine if it is safe for you to continue taking this drug.

Side effects may include: abnormal heart rhythm, allergic reaction (hives, face/throat swelling, trouble swallowing, wheezing/trouble breathing), diarrhea, headache (common in adults), nausea/vomiting, stomach pain

Can I receive Zmax if I am pregnant or breastfeeding?

The effects of Zmax during pregnancy and breastfeeding are unknown. Tell your doctor immediately if you are pregnant, plan to become pregnant, or are breastfeeding.

What should I do if I miss a dose of Zmax?

Zmax requires only a single dose. If you forget to take your dose, take it as soon as you remember.

How should I store Zmax?

Store at room temperature. Once prepared, it should be used within 12 hours.

ZOCOR

Generic name: Simvastatin

What is Zocor?

Zocor works in your body to lower cholesterol. It is for people who are at risk for coronary heart disease (CHD) due to existing heart disease, diabetes, vascular disease, or a history of stroke. Zocor, along with a healthy diet and exercise, can reduce your risk of a heart attack or stroke, death from CHD, or the need for revascularization procedures. Zocor lowers high cholesterol and triglycerides while simultaneously increasing "good" high-density lipoprotein (HDL) cholesterol levels.

What is the most important information I should know about Zocor?

Zocor may cause a serious muscle condition that may lead to kidney damage, especially if you are taking a high dose or certain other medicines with it (see "What are possible food and drug interactions associated with this medication?"). You should tell your doctor right away if you feel any muscle weakness, pain, or tenderness, especially if you also have a fever or general body discomfort.

Zocor may cause liver injury if you have any pre-existing liver problems or drink large amounts of alcohol.

Zocor should not take the place of exercise and a healthy low-fat, low-cholesterol diet. Follow the diet and exercise program given to you by your health care provider.

Stop taking Zocor a few days prior to any elective major surgery or if you experience any sudden serious medical or surgical condition. Tell your doctor or dentist that you take Zocor before you receive any medical or dental care, emergency care, or surgery.

Who should not take Zocor?

Do not take Zocor if you are pregnant, plan to become pregnant, nursing, or have active liver disease or a damaged liver. Also avoid it if you are allergic or sensitive to any of its ingredients.

What should I tell my doctor before I take the first dose of Zocor?

Mention all prescription, over-the-counter, and herbal medications you are taking. Also, talk to your doctor about your complete medical history, especially if you have liver or kidney problems; have ever experienced muscle weakness or pain in the past (especially if due to a medication); if you drink alcohol or have a history of alcohol abuse; have low blood pressure, diabetes, a serious infection, a history of seizures, or problems with your metabolism, hormones, or electrolytes.

What is the usual dosage?
The information below is based on the dosage guidelines your doctor uses. Depending on your condition and medical history, your doctor may prescribe a different regimen. Do not change the dosage or stop taking your medication without your doctor's approval.

Adults: The usual dose ranges from 5 to 80 milligrams (mg) taken once daily. The recommended starting dose is 20 to 40 mg once a day. If you have a high risk for coronary heart disease, the recommended staring dose is 40 mg. Your doctor should check your lipids 4 weeks after therapy is initiated and periodically thereafter.

Adolescents 10 to 17 years old with a family history of high cholesterol: The recommended usual starting dose is 10 mg once a day in the evening. The recommended range is 10 to 40 mg/day, with a maximum of 40 mg/day. Adjustments should be made at intervals of 4 weeks or more.

How should I take Zocor?
Take it at the same time every day, usually in the evening, with or without food.
   Continue to take Zocor even if you feel well. Do not miss any doses.

What should I avoid while taking Zocor?
You should not drink grapefruit juice or large amounts of alcohol while taking Zocor. Eating grapefruit or drinking grapefruit juice may increase the amount of Zocor in your blood, which may increase your risk for serious side effects. Moreover, the risk may be greater with if you consume large amounts of grapefruit or grapefruit juice. (eg, more than one quart daily). Talk with your doctor or pharmacist if you have questions.

What are possible food and drug interactions associated with Zocor?
If Zocor is taken with certain other drugs, the effects of either could be increased, decreased, or altered. Check with your doctor before combining Zocor with the following: alcohol, amiodarone, anticoagulants such as warfarin, bosentan, carbamazepine, clarithromycin, cyclosporine, danazol, delavirdine, digoxin, diltiazem, erythromycin, fibrates such as niacin (greater than 1,000 mg or 1 gram per day), fluconazole, grapefruit juice (greater than 1 quart daily), itraconazole, ketoconazole, macrolide immunosuppressants such as tacrolimus, mibefradil, nefazodone, other cholesterol lowering medicines, rifampin, risperidone, ritonavir, spironolactone, streptogramins such as dalfopristin, St. John's wort, telithromycin, verapamil, and voriconazole.

What are the possible side effects of Zocor?
Side effects cannot be anticipated. If any develop or change in intensity, tell your doctor as soon as possible. Only your doctor can determine if it is safe for you to continue taking this drug.

Side effects may include: allergic reactions, blurred vision, constipation, diarrhea, gas, headaches, heartburn, liver or pancreas injury, muscle cramps/weakness/pain, rash, upset stomach

Tell your doctor right away if you feel any muscle weakness, pain, or tenderness, especially if you also have a fever or general body discomfort.

Rarely, changes to the skin, hair, and nails (such as discoloration, dryness, hair loss) may occur. Check with your doctor if these effects become bothersome or concern you.

Can I receive Zocor if I am pregnant or breastfeeding?
Do not take Zocor if you are pregnant, plan to become pregnant, or if you are nursing, due to the harmful effects it may have on your unborn or nursing baby. You should not take Zocor if you are of a child-bearing age unless it is highly unlikely that you will become pregnant. Check with your doctor if you have questions about using birth control in conjunction with Zocor.

What should I do if I miss a dose of Zocor?
Take the missed dose as soon as you remember it. However, if it almost time for your next dose, skip the one you missed and return to your regular dosing schedule. Do not double the dose.

How should I store Zocor?
Store at room temperature, away from heat, moisture, and light. Do not store Zocor in the bathroom.

ZOLADEX
Generic name: Goserelin acetate

What is Zoladex?
Zoladex is similar to a hormone chemical found in your body called gonadotropin releasing hormone (GnRH). This hormone is made by a gland in your brain that causes the release of several hormones, including testosterone. At first Zoladex may temporarily increase your levels of testosterone, but after a few weeks this drug will decrease them. Zoladex is used to treat advanced prostate cancer.

What is the most important information I should know about Zoladex?
Zoladex may temporarily increase your levels of testosterone, causing a short-term worsening of your symptoms, including additional signs or symptoms of prostate cancer, all which usually occur in the first few weeks of taking Zoladex. This drug can lead to a block in the outflow of urine from your bladder, or it may cause spinal cord compression. Zoladex may also cause an allergic reaction that can be life-threatening.

Who should not take Zoladex?
You should not take Zoladex if you are allergic or sensitive to any of its ingredients, or any luteinizing hormone-releasing hormone (LHRH) (also

called GnRH agonists) agonist medication. Zoladex should not be used by women who are pregnant, able to become pregnant, or breastfeeding.

What should I tell my doctor before I take the first dose of Zoladex?

Mention all prescription, over-the-counter, and herbal medications you are taking before beginning treatment with Zoladex. Also, talk to your doctor about your complete medical history, especially if you have difficulty urinating or have any type of urinary blockage.

What is the usual dosage?

The information below is based on the dosage guidelines your doctor uses. Depending on your condition and medical history, your doctor may prescribe a different regimen. Do not change the dosage or stop taking your medication without your doctor's approval.

Adults: The usual dose is 10.8 milligrams (mg) given subcutaneously every 12 weeks.

How should I take Zoladex?

Zoladex is usually given by a doctor or nurse, and is generally injected into the small layer of fat right under the skin in the front of the stomach.

What should I avoid while taking Zoladex?

You should receive a Zoladex injection every 12 weeks, so it is important not to miss any scheduled doses. While a delay of a few days is okay, every effort should be made to adhere to the 12-week schedule.

What are possible food and drug interactions associated with Zoladex?

No confirmed interactions have been reported between Zoladex and other drugs.

What are the possible side effects of Zoladex?

Side effects cannot be anticipated. If any develop or change in intensity, tell your doctor as soon as possible. Only your doctor can determine if it is safe for you to continue taking this drug.

Side effects may include: Breast enlargement, bone pain, hot flashes, pelvic pain, weakness, diarrhea, rectal bleeding, cystitis, anemia

Can I receive Zoladex if I am pregnant or breastfeeding?

This formulation of Zoladex is for use in men with prostate cancer. It should not be used by pregnant or breastfeeding women due to the possible harmful effects it can have on a developing or nursing baby.

What should I do if I miss a dose of Zoladex?

If you miss your Zoladex injection, contact your doctor right away. Depending on how much time has passed since your last injection, your doctor will determine the timing of your next dose.

How should I store Zoladex?

Store at room temperature.

Zolmitriptan nasal spray See Zomig Nasal Spray, page 1491.

ZOLOFT

Generic name: Sertraline hydrochloride

What is Zoloft?

Zoloft is an antidepressant medication known as a selective serotonin reuptake inhibitor (SSRI). It is used to treat major depression, obsessive-compulsive disorder, panic disorder, post-traumatic stress disorder, premenstrual dysphoric disorder, and social anxiety disorder.

What is the most important information I should know about Zoloft?

Antidepressants can increase the risk of suicidal thinking and behavior in children and teenagers. Adult and pediatric patients taking antidepressants should be watched closely for changes in moods or actions, especially when they first start therapy or when their dose is increased or decreased. Patients and their families should contact the doctor immediately if new symptoms develop or seem to get worse. Signs to watch for include anxiety, hostility, sleeplessness, restlessness, impulsive or dangerous behavior, and thoughts about suicide or dying.

Zoloft is not recommended in children and adolescents, except for the treatment of obsessive-compulsive disorder.

Who should not take Zoloft?

Do not take monoamine oxidase inhibitors (MAOIs) within 2 weeks before or after treatment with this medication. In some cases a serious, possibly fatal, reaction may occur. Examples of MAOIs include selegiline and the antidepressants phenelzine and tranylcypromine.

What should I tell my doctor before I take the first dose of Zoloft?

Tell your doctor about all prescription, over-the-counter, and herbal medications you are taking before beginning treatment with Zoloft. Also, talk to your doctor about your complete medical history, especially if you have liver or kidney problems, seizure or bleeding disorders, or a history of suicide or mental illness.

What is the usual dosage?

The information below is based on the dosage guidelines your doctor uses. Depending on your condition and medical history, your doctor may prescribe a different regimen. Do not change the dosage or stop taking your medication without your doctor's approval.

Major Depression

Adults: The usual starting dose is 50 milligrams (mg) once a day. If needed, your dose may be increased to up to 200 mg once a day.

Obsessive-Compulsive Disorder

Adults: The usual starting dose is 50 mg once a day. If needed, your dose may be increased to up to 200 mg once a day.

Children: For children 6-12 years old, the usual starting dose is 25 mg once a day. For children 13-17 years old, the usual starting dose is 50 mg once a day. Your child's dose may be increased up to a maximum of 200 mg per day depending on his or her condition.

Panic Disorder, Post-traumatic Stress Disorder, and Social Anxiety Disorder

Adults: The usual starting dose is 25 mg once a day. After 1 week, your dose may be increased to 50 mg once a day. If needed, your dose may be increased to 200 mg once a day.

Premenstrual Dysphoric Disorder

Adults: The usual starting dose is 50 mg once a day. If needed, your dose may be increased to 150 mg once a day.

How should I take Zoloft?

Zoloft should be taken once a day in the morning or in the evening. Take it at the same time every day. Zoloft may be taken with or without food.

What should I avoid while taking Zoloft?

You should not drink alcohol while taking Zoloft. You should also not drive a car or operate heavy machinery until you know how this drug affects you.

What are possible food and drug interactions associated with Zoloft?

If Zoloft is taken with certain other drugs, the effects of either could be increased, decreased, or altered. It is especially important to check with your doctor before combining Zoloft with the following: alcohol, aspirin, cimetidine, diazepam, digitoxin, flecainide, lithium, other antidepressants, MAOIs, nonsteroidal anti-inflammatory drugs (NSAIDs), phenytoin, pimozide, propafenone, sumatriptan, tolbutamide, valproate, and warfarin.

What are the possible side effects of Zoloft?
Side effects cannot be anticipated. If any develop or change in intensity, tell your doctor as soon as possible. Only your doctor can determine if it is safe for you to continue taking this drug.

Side effects may include: stomach pain, agitation, anxiety, changes in vision, constipation, decreased sexual drive, diarrhea, dizziness, dry mouth, fatigue, inability to sleep, increased sweating, loss of appetite/ upset stomach, nausea, ejaculation problems, shakiness, tiredness

Can I receive Zoloft if I am pregnant or breastfeeding?
The effects of Zoloft during pregnancy and breastfeeding are unknown. Tell your doctor immediately if you are pregnant, plan to become pregnant, or are breastfeeding.

What should I do if I miss a dose of Zoloft?
Take it as soon as your remember. If it is almost time for your next scheduled dose, skip the dose you missed and return to your regular schedule. Do not double your doses.

How should I store Zoloft?
Store at room temperature.

Zolpidem tartrate See Ambien, page 78.

Zolpidem tartrate, extended-release See Ambien CR, page 80.

ZOMIG NASAL SPRAY
Generic name: Zolmitriptan nasal spray

What is Zomig Nasal Spray?
Zomig nasal spray is used to treat migraine headaches in adults. Migraine headaches are severe and intense headaches that are often accompanied by throbbing pain on one or both sides of your head, nausea, vomiting, or sensitivity to light or sound. Zomig reduces the swelling of the blood vessels surrounding the brain, and it also blocks the actions of certain chemicals in your brain that lead to pain and sensitivity.

What is the most important information I should know about Zomig Nasal Spray?
Zomig nasal spray may cause an increase in your blood pressure, so you should not use it if you have uncontrolled high blood pressure. You

should not use Zomig within 24 hours of taking another 5-HT1 agonist, ergotamine, or ergotamine-derived medicines (ethysergide or dihydro-ergotamine). You should not use Zomig if you have a type of headache known as a hemiplegic or basilar migraine, or if you have heart conditions known as ischemic or vasospastic coronary artery disease. Do not use it if you are taking a medication called a MAO inhibitor (MAOI) or if you have taken an MAOI within the last 14 days.

Who should not take Zomig Nasal Spray?

Do not use Zomig nasal spray if you have heart disease or a history of heart disease; if you have uncontrolled high blood pressure; a type of headache known as a hemiplegic or basilar migraine; a history of stroke or blood circulation problems; serious liver problems; or if you have taken any triptans, dihydroergotamine, or MAOIs within the last 24 hours. Also, do not take Zomig nasal spray if you are allergic or sensitive to any of its ingredients.

What should I tell my doctor before I take the first dose of Zomig Nasal Spray?

Tell your doctor about all prescription, over-the-counter, and herbal medications you are taking before beginning treatment with Zomig nasal spray. Also talk to your doctor about your complete medical history, especially if you are taking antidepressants; have heart disease, shortness of breath, or irregular heartbeats; or you have risk factors for heart disease (such as high blood pressure, high cholesterol, obesity, diabetes, smoking, strong family history of heart disease, or you are postmenopausal or a male over the age of 40).

What is the usual dosage?

The information below is based on the dosage guidelines your doctor uses. Depending on your condition and medical history, your doctor may prescribe a different regimen. Do not change the dosage or stop taking your medication without your doctor's approval.

Adults: The usual dose is 5 milligrams (mg) or one spray into one nostril at the onset of a migraine. The dose may be repeated once in 2 hours if no relief is felt from the first dose. (Do not use more than two Zomig nasal spray canisters or 10 mg within 24 hours.)

How should I take Zomig Nasal Spray?

Before using Zomig nasal spray, gently blow your nose. Remove the canister's protective gray cap and place your middle and pointer fingers on the base of the plunger, and hold the bottom of the canister with your thumb. Do not prime the canister, otherwise you will lose your dose. Gently block one nostril with your free hand, and insert the tip of the canister into your other nostril. Press down on the plunger to release the dose into your nose and breathe in at the same time. The plunger may feel stiff and you may hear a click. Some of the Zomig medicine may drip down the back of your throat. This is normal and will subside within 10 to 15 minutes.

What should I avoid while taking Zomig Nasal Spray?
You should not use more than two Zomig doses in a 24-hour period.

What are possible food and drug interactions associated with Zomig Nasal Spray?
If Zomig nasal spray is taken with certain other drugs, the effects of either could be increased, decreased, or altered. It is especially important to check with your doctor before combining Zomig with the following: almotriptan, birth control, cimetidine, citalopram, dihydroergotamines such as methysergide, duloxetine, eletriptan, ergotamines, escitalopram, fluoxetine, fluvoxamine, frovatriptan, naratriptan, paroxetine, phenelzine sulfate, rizatriptan, sertraline, sumatriptan, tranylcypromine sulfate, and venlafaxine.

What are the possible side effects of Zomig Nasal Spray?
Side effects cannot be anticipated. If any develop or change in intensity, tell your doctor as soon as possible. Only your doctor can determine if it is safe for you to continue taking this drug.

Side effects may include: dizziness, drowsiness, dry mouth, nausea, pain, pressure/tightness of the nose/throat/chest, tingling sensation/skin sensitivity (especially around the nose), weakness

Can I receive Zomig Nasal Spray if I am pregnant or breastfeeding?
The effects of Zomig nasal spray during pregnancy and breastfeeding are unknown. Tell your doctor immediately if you are pregnant, plan to become pregnant, or are breastfeeding.

What should I do if I miss a dose of Zomig Nasal Spray?
If you miss a dose of Zomig, do not double your next dose. Use the nasal spray as soon as you remember, but do not use more than two doses in 24 hours.

How should I store Zomig Nasal Spray?
Store at room temperature.

ZONEGRAN

Generic name: Zonisamide

What is Zonegran?

Zonegran is taken with other medications to treat partial seizures in adults.

What is the most important information I should know about Zonegran?

Zonegran can cause serious reactions in some patients. Call your doctor right away if you experience any of the following: rash, fever, sore throat, sores in your mouth, bruising easily, sudden back pain, abdominal pain, pain when urinating, bloody or dark urine, decreased sweating or increased body temperature (especially if you are under 17 years old), depression, thoughts that are unusual for you, or speech or language problems. Zonegran may cause drowsiness or coordination problems. You should take it with caution if you have any type of kidney or liver problems.

Who should not take Zonegran?

Do not take Zonegran if you are allergic or sensitive to it or any of its ingredients. Also, you should not take Zonegran if you are allergic to sulfa-derived medications such as sulfamethoxazole/trimethoprim.

What should I tell my doctor before I take the first dose of Zonegran?

Mention all prescription, over-the-counter, and herbal medication you are taking before beginning treatment with Zonegran. Also, talk to your doctor about your complete medical history, especially if you have kidney or liver problems, if you are pregnant, plan to become pregnant, or if you are breastfeeding.

What is the usual dosage?

The information below is based on the dosage guidelines your doctor uses. Depending on your condition and medical history, your doctor may prescribe a different regimen. Do not change the dosage or stop taking your medication without your doctor's approval.

Adults 16 and older: The usual starting dose is 100 milligrams (mg) taken once a day for 2 weeks. The dose is usually increased to 200 mg per day for at least 2 additional weeks, after which the total daily dose may be increased to 300-600 mg per day depending on your condition.

How should I take Zonegran?

Zonegran should be taken exactly as prescribed. It is important to swallow the capsules whole; do not break or crush them. You should drink at least 6-8 glasses of water daily while taking Zonegran, which will help to prevent kidney stones. Do not suddenly stop taking it unless you are instructed by your doctor.

What should I avoid while taking Zonegran?
You should not drive a car or operate heavy machinery until you know how Zonegran will affect you.

What are possible food and drug interactions associated with Zonegran?
If Zonegran is taken with certain other drugs, the effects of either could be increased, decreased, or altered. It is especially important to check with your doctor before combining Zonegran with carbamazepine, phenobarbital, or phenytoin.

What are the possible side effects of Zonegran?
Side effects cannot be anticipated. If any develop or change in intensity, tell your doctor as soon as possible. Only your doctor can determine if it is safe for you to continue taking this drug.

Side effects may include: agitation, dizziness, drowsiness, headache, loss of appetite, nausea

Can I receive Zonegran if I am pregnant or breastfeeding?
The effects of Zonegran during pregnancy and breastfeeding are unknown. Tell your doctor immediately if you are pregnant, plan to become pregnant, or are breastfeeding.

What should I do if I miss a dose of Zonegran?
Talk to your doctor about what to do if you miss a dose. Depending on your condition, your doctor will decide when your next scheduled dose should be.

How should I store Zonegran?
Store at room temperature, in a dry place and protected from light.

Zonisamide *See Zonegran, page 1494.*

ZOSTAVAX
Generic name: Zoster vaccine, live

What is Zostavax?
Zostavax is a vaccine that is used for adults 60 years or older to prevent shingles (also known as zoster). It contains a weakened form of the chickenpox virus, which causes both chickenpox and shingles. Shingles

is a rash that usually occurs in one side of the body, which can blister and become painful. It can last for up to 30 days. Zostavax works by helping your immune system protect you from getting shingles and the associated pain and other serious complications.

If you do get shingles even though you have been vaccinated, this drug may help prevent the nerve pain that can follow shingles in some people.

What is the most important information I should know about Zostavax?

Zostavax may not protect everyone who receives the vaccine and it cannot be used to treat shingles once you have it. If you do get shingles, see your doctor within the first few days of getting the rash.

Who should not take Zostavax?

You should not receive Zostavax if you are allergic to any of its ingredients (including allergies to gelatin or neomycin); have a disease or condition that causes a weakened immune system, such as an immune deficiency (including leukemia, lymphoma, and HIV/AIDS); or you are taking high doses of steroids by injection or by mouth. Also, if you have active TB (tuberculosis) that is not being treated, or you are pregnant or may become pregnant, do not take Zostavax.

What should I tell my doctor before I take the first dose of Zostavax?

Mention all prescription, over-the-counter, and herbal medications you are taking before beginning treatment with the Zostavax injection. Also, talk to your doctor about your complete medical history, especially if you have had shingles before or are currently exposed to chicken pox. If you are pregnant or breastfeeding, you should inform your doctor.

What is the usual dosage?

The information below is based on the dosage guidelines your doctor uses. Depending on your condition and medical history, your doctor may prescribe a different regimen. Do not change the dosage or stop taking your medication without your doctor's approval.

Adults: Zostavax is given as a single dose by injection under the skin.

How should I take Zostavax?

Zostavax is given as an injection, directly under the skin, by your doctor.

What should I avoid while taking Zostavax?

Avoid receiving Zostavax if you already have shingles.

What are possible food and drug interactions associated with Zostavax?

No significant interactions have been reported at this time. However, always tell your doctor about any medicines you take, including over-the-counter drugs, vitamins, and herbal supplements.

What are the possible side effects of Zostavax?

Side effects cannot be anticipated. If any develop or change in intensity, tell your doctor as soon as possible. Only your doctor can determine if it is safe for you to continue taking this drug.

Side effects may include: bruising at the injection site, headache, itching, pain, redness, swelling, warmth

Can I receive Zostavax if I am pregnant or breastfeeding?

The effects of Zostavax during pregnancy and breastfeeding are unknown. Tell your doctor immediately if you are pregnant, plan to become pregnant, or are breastfeeding.

What should I do if I miss a dose of Zostavax?

Zostavax is administered as a single injection. Speak to your healthcare provider if you miss your scheduled vaccination with Zostavax.

How should I store Zostavax?

This medication will be stored by your healthcare provider.

Zoster vaccine, live See Zostavax, page 1495.

ZOVIRAX

Generic name: Acyclovir

What is Zovirax?

Zovirax is an antiviral medication that treats herpes infections caused by different types of herpes viruses. Zovirax is used to treat initial and recurrent genital herpes infections, chicken pox (varicella), and shingles (herpes zoster).

What is the most important information I should know about Zovirax?

Zovirax can cause injury to your kidneys and even death due to complete kidney failure. Take with caution if you have any type of kidney problems. Also, Zovirax may cause serious blood disorders if you have problems with your immune system. You should stay hydrated while taking Zovirax.

Who should not take Zovirax?
Do not take Zovirax if you are allergic to or sensitive to any of its ingredients.

What should I tell my doctor before I take the first dose of Zovirax?
Mention all prescription, over-the-counter, and herbal medications you are taking before beginning treatment with Zovirax. Also, talk to your doctor about your complete medical history, especially if you have kidney problems, a deficiency of your immune system, or if you are pregnant, plan to become pregnant, or are breastfeeding.

What is the usual dosage?
The information below is based on the dosage guidelines your doctor uses. Depending on your condition and medical history, your doctor may prescribe a different regimen. Do not change the dosage or stop taking your medication without your doctor's approval.

Acute Treatment of Herpes Zoster (shingles)
Adults: The usual dose is 800 milligrams (mg) taken every 4 hours, 5 times daily for 7 to 10 days.

Genital Herpes: Treatment of Initial Genital Herpes
Adults: The usual dose is 200 mg every 4 hours, taken 5 times a day for 10 days.

Chronic Suppressive Therapy for Recurrent Disease
Adults: The usual dose is 400 mg taken 2 times a day for up to 12 months, followed by a medical re-evaluation. Your doctor may vary your dose from 200 mg taken 3 times a day to 200 mg taken 5 times a day.

Intermittent Therapy
Adults: The usual dose is 200 mg taken every 4 hours, 5 times a day for 5 days. Therapy should be started at the earliest sign or symptom of herpes infection recurrence.

Treatment of Chickenpox
Adults: The usual dose is 800 mg taken 4 times a day for 5 days.

Children 2 years and older: The usual dose is 20 mg per 2.2 pounds of bodyweight per dose taken 4 times a day for 5 days.

Children over 88 pounds: The usual dose is 800 mg taken 4 times a day for 5 days.

How should I take Zovirax?
Zovirax doses should be taken at the same time every day, with or without food. Drink plenty of water.

What should I avoid while taking Zovirax?
Avoid becoming dehydrated.

**What are possible food and drug interactions
associated with Zovirax?**
If Zovirax is taken with certain other drugs, the effects of either could be
increased, decreased, or altered. It is especially important to check with
your doctor before combining Zovirax with probenecid.

What are the possible side effects of Zovirax?
Side effects cannot be anticipated. If any develop or change in intensity,
tell your doctor as soon as possible. Only your doctor can determine if it
is safe for you to continue taking this drug.

Side effects may include: diarrhea, flu-like symptoms, nausea, vomiting

Can I receive Zovirax if I am pregnant or breastfeeding?
The effects of Zovirax during pregnancy and breastfeeding are unknown.
Tell your doctor immediately if you are pregnant, plan to become preg-
nant, or are breastfeeding.

What should I do if I miss a dose of Zovirax?
If you forget to take Zovirax, take it as soon as you remember. If it is
closer to your next scheduled dose, skip the dose you missed and take
Zovirax according to your regular dosing schedule. Do not double your
doses.

How should I store Zovirax?
Store at room temperature.

ZYBAN

*Generic name: Bupropion hydrochloride
(for smoking cessation)*

What is Zyban?
Zyban is a nicotine-free medication used to help people quit smoking.

**What is the most important information
I should know about Zyban?**
About 1 person in 1,000 suffers a seizure while taking Zyban. For this
reason, people with epilepsy should never take this medication. Do not
share Zyban with your friends. Only a doctor can decide whether it's safe
for a particular individual to take this medication.

Zyban contains the same ingredient as the antidepressants Wellbutrin,
Wellbutrin SR, and Wellbutrin XL. Antidepressants can increase the risk

of suicidal thinking and behavior in children and teenagers. Adult and pediatric patients taking antidepressants should be watched closely for changes in moods or actions, especially when they first start therapy or when their dose is increased or decreased. Patients and their families should contact the doctor immediately if new symptoms develop or seem to get worse. Signs to watch for include anxiety, hostility, sleeplessness, restlessness, impulsive or dangerous behavior, and thoughts about suicide or dying.

Who should not take Zyban?

Do not take Zyban if you have a seizure disorder, anorexia or bulimia (eating disorders), or if you are going through alcohol recovery. In addition, you should not take Zyban if you are taking any other medicines that contain bupropion hydrochloride, such as Wellbutrin, Wellbutrin SR, or Wellbutrin XL, or if you have suddenly stopped taking sedatives.

Do not take monoamine oxidase inhibitors (MAOIs) within 2 weeks before or after treatment with this medication. In some cases a serious, possibly fatal, reaction may occur. Examples of MAOIs include selegiline and the antidepressants phenelzine and tranylcypromine.

Also, do not begin treatment with Zyban if you are allergic to any of its ingredients.

What should I tell my doctor before I take the first dose of Zyban?

Tell your doctor about all prescription, over-the-counter, and herbal medications you are taking before beginning treatment with Zyban. Also, talk to your doctor about your complete medical history, especially if you have ever had a seizure, eating disorders, liver or kidney problems, heart problems, high blood sugar, head injuries, or an addiction (eg, alcohol or drug abuse).

What is the usual dosage?

The information below is based on the dosage guidelines your doctor uses. Depending on your condition and medical history, your doctor may prescribe a different regimen. Do not change the dosage or stop taking your medication without your doctor's approval.

Adults: The recommended starting dose is 150 milligrams (mg) a day for the first 3 days. If needed, the doctor may increase your dose up to a maximum dose of 300 mg a day, given in two divided doses.

How should I take Zyban?

Take Zyban exactly as prescribed by your doctor. Swallow the tablets whole; do not chew, divide, or crush them. Take the tablets at the same time each day, at least 8 hours apart.

What should I avoid while taking Zyban?

Do not drink alcohol or smoke while taking Zyban. If you currently drink a lot of alcohol and suddenly stop, you should tell your doctor, since this may increase your risk of having a seizure. You should also not drive a car or operate heavy machinery until you know how this drug affects you.

What are possible food and drug interactions associated with Zyban?

If Zyban is taken with certain other drugs, the effects of either could be increased, decreased, or altered. It is especially important to check with your doctor before combining Zyban with any the following: alcohol, amantadine, antidepressants, blood pressure medications called beta-blockers, carbamazepine, cimetidine, cyclophosphamide, heart-stabilizing drugs, levodopa, major tranquilizers, MAOIs, orphenadrine, phenobarbital, phenytoin, steroids such as prednisone and hydrocortisone, theophylline, and warfarin.

What are the possible side effects of Zyban?

Side effects cannot be anticipated. If any develop or change in intensity, inform your doctor as soon as possible. Only your doctor can determine if it is safe for you to continue taking this drug.

Side effects include: dry mouth, difficulty sleeping

Can I receive Zyban if I am pregnant or breastfeeding?

Zyban has not been tested in pregnant women. If you are pregnant or plan to become pregnant, do your best to quit smoking with the aid of counseling and support before taking Zyban. You should avoid smoking or taking nicotine in any other form while pregnant.

Zyban appears in breast milk and could affect a nursing infant. Ask your doctor whether it will be better to discontinue the medication or to stop breastfeeding.

What should I do if I miss a dose of Zyban?

Do not double your next dose. Skip the dose you missed and return to your regular dosing schedule. This is very important because taking too much Zyban can increase your risk of having a seizure.

How should I store Zyban?

Store at room temperature away from light and moisture.

ZYFLO
Generic name: Zileuton

What is Zyflo?
Zyflo is a medicine that is used to prevent asthma attacks and for long-term management of asthma in adults and children 12 years and older. Zyflo blocks the production of leukotrienes. Leukotrienes are substances that may contribute to your asthma. Zyflo is not a rescue medicine (it is not a bronchodilator) and should not be used if you need relief right away for an asthma attack.

What is the most important information I should know about Zyflo?
Zyflo is not a bronchodilator and should not be used to relieve an asthma attack that has already started. The most serious side effect of Zyflo is potential elevation of liver enzymes and liver problems. While taking Zyflo, you must visit your doctor for liver enzyme tests on a regular basis.

Who should not take Zyflo?
You should not use Zyflo if you ever had an allergic reaction to any of its ingredients. Do not use Zyflo if you have active liver disease or if repeated blood tests show elevated liver enzymes.

What should I tell my doctor before I take the first dose of Zyflo?
Tell your doctor about all prescription, over-the-counter, and herbal medications you are taking before beginning treatment with Zyflo. Also, talk to your doctor about your complete medical history, especially if you have ever had liver problems, including hepatitis, jaundice (yellow eyes or skin), or dark urine; drink alcohol (tell your healthcare provider how much and how often you drink alcohol); are pregnant or planning to become pregnant; or you are breastfeeding

What is the usual dosage?
The information below is based on the dosage guidelines your doctor uses. Depending on your condition and medical history, your doctor may prescribe a different regimen. Do not change the dosage or stop taking your medication without your doctor's approval.

Adults and children 12 years and older: The usual dosage is one 600-milligram (mg) tablet four times a day, for a total daily dose of 2,400 mg.

How should I take Zyflo?
Take Zyflo exactly as prescribed by your healthcare provider. Do not decrease the dose of Zyflo or stop taking the medicine without talking to

your healthcare provider first, even if you have no asthma symptoms. For Zyflo to help control your asthma symptoms, it must be taken every day as directed by your doctor. While taking Zyflo, it is important to keep taking your other asthma medicines as directed and to follow all of your doctor's instructions.

Take Zyflo four times a day with or without food. It may be easier to remember to take your medication if you make it part of your daily routine such as with meals and at bedtime. When you take your dose of Zyflo, the tablets may be swallowed whole or split in half to make them easier to swallow.

What should I avoid while taking Zyflo?

Do not miss any doctor's appointments and be sure to follow all instructions. Have blood tests done as ordered by your doctor to check your liver enzymes.

What are possible food and drug interactions associated with Zyflo?

If Zyflo is taken with certain other drugs, the effects of either could be increased, decreased, or altered. It is especially important to check with your doctor before combining Zyflo with propranolol, theophylline, warfarin, or alcohol.

What are the possible side effects of Zyflo?

Side effects cannot be anticipated. If any develop or change in intensity, tell your doctor as soon as possible. Only your doctor can determine if it is safe for you to continue taking this drug.

Side effects may include: abdominal pain, upset stomach, nausea

Serious side effects include liver problems that may be associated with symptoms such as pain on the right side of your abdomen (stomach area), nausea, tiredness, lack of energy, itching, yellow skin or yellow color in the whites of your eyes, dark urine, or flu-like symptoms. Tell your doctor right away if you experience any of these symptoms.

Can I receive Zyflo if I am pregnant or breastfeeding?

The effects of Zyflo during pregnancy and breastfeeding are unknown. This medication should be used in pregnancy only if the potential benefit justifies the potential risk to the fetus. Tell your doctor immediately if you are pregnant or plan to become pregnant. It is not known if Zyflo passes into breast milk. You and your healthcare provider should decide if you will take Zyflo or breastfeed.

What should I do if I miss a dose of Zyflo?

If you miss a dose, take your next scheduled dose when it is due. Do not double the dose.

How should I store Zyflo?
Store at room temperature away from light.

ZYFLO CR
Generic name: Zileuton, extended-release

What is Zyflo CR?
Zyflo CR is a medicine that is used to prevent asthma attacks and for long-term management of asthma in adults and children 12 years of age and older. Zyflo CR blocks the production of leukotrienes. Leukotrienes are substances that may contribute to your asthma. Zyflo CR is not a rescue medicine (it is not a bronchodilator) and should not be used if you need relief right away for an asthma attack.

What is the most important information I should know about Zyflo CR?
Zyflo CR is not a bronchodilator and should not be used to relieve an asthma attack that has already started. The most serious side effect of Zyflo CR is potential elevation of liver enzymes and liver problems. While taking Zyflo CR, you must visit your doctor for liver enzyme tests on a regular basis.

Who should not take Zyflo CR?
You should not use Zyflo CR if you ever had an allergic reaction to any of its ingredients. Do not use Zyflo CR if you have active liver disease or if repeated blood tests show elevated liver enzymes.

What should I tell my doctor before I take the first dose of Zyflo CR?
Tell your doctor about all prescription, over-the-counter, and herbal medications you are taking before beginning treatment with Zyflo CR. Also, talk to your doctor about your complete medical history, especially if you have ever had liver problems, including hepatitis, jaundice (yellow eyes or skin), or dark urine; drink alcohol (tell your healthcare provider how much and how often you drink alcohol); have difficulty swallowing pills; are pregnant or planning to become pregnant; or you are breast-feeding

What is the usual dosage?
The information below is based on the dosage guidelines your doctor uses. Depending on your condition and medical history, your doctor may prescribe a different regimen. Do not change the dosage or stop taking your medication without your doctor's approval.

Adults and children 12 years and older: The usual dosage is two 600-milligram (mg) tablets two times daily, within 1 hour after your morning and evening meals, for a total daily dose of 2,400 mg.

How should I take Zyflo CR?

Take Zyflo CR exactly as prescribed by your healthcare provider. Do not decrease the dose of Zyflo CR or stop taking the medicine without talking to your healthcare provider first, even if you have no asthma symptoms. Swallow Zyflo CR whole. Do not chew, cut, or crush Zyflo CR tablets. Tell your healthcare provider if you cannot swallow the tablets whole. Follow your healthcare provider's instructions for what to do if you get sudden symptoms of an asthma attack. You can continue taking Zyflo CR during asthma attacks. Keep taking your other asthma medicines as directed while taking Zyflo CR.

What should I avoid while taking Zyflo CR?

Avoid chewing, cutting, or crushing Zyflo CR tablets.

Do not miss any doctor's appointments and be sure to follow all instructions. Have blood tests done as ordered by your doctor to check your liver enzymes.

What are possible food and drug interactions associated with Zyflo CR?

If Zyflo CR is taken with certain other drugs, the effects of either could be increased, decreased, or altered. It is especially important to check with your doctor before combining Zyflo CR with propranolol, theophylline, warfarin, or alcohol.

What are the possible side effects of Zyflo CR?

Side effects cannot be anticipated. If any develop or change in intensity, tell your doctor as soon as possible. Only your doctor can determine if it is safe for you to continue taking this drug.

Side effects may include: nose and throat irritation, sinusitis, upper respiratory infection, throat pain, headache, muscle aches, nausea, diarrhea

Serious side effects include liver problems that may be associated with symptoms such as pain on the right side of your abdomen (stomach area), nausea, tiredness, lack of energy, itching, yellow skin or yellow color in the whites of your eyes, dark urine, or flu-like symptoms. Tell your doctor right away if you experience any of these symptoms.

Can I receive Zyflo CR if I am pregnant or breastfeeding?

The effects of Zyflo CR during pregnancy and breastfeeding are unknown. This medication should be used in pregnancy only if the potential benefit justifies the potential risk to the fetus. Tell your doctor immediately if you are pregnant or plan to become pregnant. It is not known if Zyflo CR passes into breast milk. You and your healthcare provider should decide if you will take Zyflo CR or breastfeed.

What should I do if I miss a dose of Zyflo CR?
If you miss a dose, take your next scheduled dose when it is due. Do not double the dose.

How should I store Zyflo CR?
Store at room temperature away from light.

ZYMAR
Generic name: Gatifloxacin

What is Zymar?
Zymar is an antibiotic eye drop that is used to treat bacterial conjunctivitis (eye infection).

What is the most important information I should know about Zymar?
Zymar should only be used as a topical eye drop, and it should never be injected into the body. Stop using Zymar and contact your doctor immediately if you experience difficulty breathing, rash, itching of the skin, fainting, swelling of the face, throat or chest, or irregular heartbeats. You should not wear contact lenses if you have an infection in your eye. Contact your doctor if your condition gets worse, because this may be a sign of a different or more serious infection.

Who should not take Zymar?
Do not use Zymar eye drops if you are allergic or sensitive to other fluoroquinolone-type antibiotics or any of its ingredients.

What should I tell my doctor before I take the first dose of Zymar?
Tell your doctor about all prescription, over-the-counter, and herbal medication you are taking before beginning treatment with Zymar. Also, talk to your doctor about your complete medical history, especially if you have ever had an allergic reaction to fluoroquinolone-type antibiotics.

What is the usual dosage?
The information below is based on the dosage guidelines your doctor uses. Depending on your condition and medical history, your doctor may prescribe a different regimen. Do not change the dosage or stop taking your medication without your doctor's approval.

Bacterial Conjunctivitis
Adults: The usual dose is to instill one drop every two hours in the affected eye(s) while awake, up to 8 times daily on Days 1 and 2. On Days 3 through 7, instill one drop up to four times daily while awake.

How should I take Zymar?
Zymar drops should be instilled into the affected eye(s) around the same time every day. Do not let the tip of the bottle touch any part of your eye.

What should I avoid while taking Zymar?
You should not wear contact lenses in the affected(s) eyes.

What are possible food and drug interactions associated with Zymar?
If Zymar is taken with certain other drugs, the effects of either could be increased, decreased, or altered. It is especially important to check with your doctor before combining Zymar with the following: caffeine, cyclosporine, theophylline, and warfarin.

What are the possible side effects of Zymar?
Side effects cannot be anticipated. If any develop or change in intensity, tell your doctor as soon as possible. Only your doctor can determine if it is safe for you to continue taking this drug.

Side effects may include: eye irritation, increased tearing of the eye, swelling and redness of the eye lid or front part of the eye

Can I receive Zymar if I am pregnant or breastfeeding?
The effects of Zymar during pregnancy and breastfeeding are unknown. Tell your doctor immediately if you are pregnant, plan to become pregnant, or are breastfeeding.

What should I do if I miss a dose of Zymar?
If you forget to instill a dose of Zymar, administer it as soon as your remember. If it is closer to your next scheduled dose, skip the dose you missed and use Zymar according to your regular dosing schedule. Do not double your doses.

How should I store Zymar?
Zymar should be stored at room temperature with the cap securely closed.

ZYPREXA/ZYPREXA ZYDIS/ ZYPREXA INTRAMUSCULAR
Generic name: Olanzapine

What is Zyprexa/Zyprexa Zydis/Zyprexa Intramuscular?
Zyprexa is used to treat schizophrenia, bipolar disorder, and agitation associated with these disorders.

What is the most important information I should know about Zyprexa/Zyprexa Zydis/Zyprexa Intramuscular?
When you first start taking Zyprexa, you can develop very low blood pressure, increased heart rate, dizziness, and, in rare cases, a tendency to faint when first standing up. These problems are more likely to occur if you are dehydrated, have heart problems, or take blood pressure medications. To avoid such problems, your doctor may start with a low dose of Zyprexa and increase your dosage gradually.

Zyprexa and similar medications have been associated with an increased risk of developing high blood sugar, which on rare occasions has led to coma or death. See your doctor right away if you develop signs of high blood sugar, including dry mouth, unusual thirst, increased urination, and tiredness. If you have diabetes or have a high risk of developing it, see your doctor regularly for blood sugar testing.

Zyprexa should not be used to treat elderly patients who have dementia because the drug could increase the risk of stroke. In addition, Zyprexa has also been associated with swallowing and breathing problems in older people and those with Alzheimer's disease.

The safety and effectiveness of Zyprexa have not been studied in children.

Who should not take Zyprexa/Zyprexa Zydis/Zyprexa Intramuscular?
Do not take Zyprexa if you are allergic to any of its ingredients.

What should I tell my doctor before I take the first dose of Zyprexa/Zyprexa Zydis/Zyprexa Intramuscular?
Tell your doctor about all prescription, over-the-counter, and herbal medications you are taking before beginning treatment with Zyprexa. Also, talk to your doctor about your complete medical history, especially if you have liver or kidney disease or if you smoke.

What is the usual dosage?
The information below is based on the dosage guidelines your doctor uses. Depending on your condition and medical history, your doctor may prescribe a different regimen. Do not change the dosage or stop taking your medication without your doctor's approval.

Schizophrenia

Adults: The usual starting dose is 5-10 milligrams (mg) once a day. If you start at the lower dose, after a few days the doctor will increase it to 10 mg. After that, your dose will be increased no more than once a week, 5 mg at a time, up to a maximum of 20 mg a day. Once your condition is stabilized, your doctor may continue maintenance therapy at doses of 10-20 mg once a day.

Manic Episodes Associated with Bipolar Disorder

Adults: The usual starting dose is 10-15 mg once a day. If needed, your dose can be increased every 24 hours by 5 mg a day, up to a maximum daily dose of 20 mg. Once your condition is stabilized, your doctor may continue maintenance therapy at doses of 5-20 mg once a day. If Zyprexa is being combined with lithium or valproate, the usual starting dose is 10 mg once a day.

How should I take Zyprexa/Zyprexa Zydis/Zyprexa Intramuscular?

Take this medication exactly as prescribed by your doctor. Zyprexa comes in regular tablets, orally disintegrating tablets, and as an intramuscular injection. Regular Zyprexa tablets should be taken once a day with or without food.

Zyprexa Zydis is a tablet that will dissolve in your mouth. Immediately after opening the blister packet, use dry hands to remove the tablet and place it in your mouth. The tablet will dissolve quickly in your saliva so it can easily be swallowed with or without liquids.

Zyprexa Intramuscular is an injection that must be given by a doctor.

What should I avoid while taking Zyprexa/ Zyprexa Zydis/Zyprexa Intramuscular?

Avoid alcohol while taking Zyprexa. The combination can cause a sudden drop in blood pressure. Zyprexa sometimes causes drowsiness and can impair your judgment, thinking, and movements. Use caution while driving and don't operate dangerous machinery until you know how this drug affects you.

What are possible food and drug interactions associated with Zyprexa/Zyprexa Zydis/Zyprexa Intramuscular?

If Zyprexa is taken with certain other drugs, the effects of either could be increased, decreased, or altered. It is especially important to check with your doctor before combining Zyprexa with the following: blood pressure medications, benzodiazepines, carbamazepine, diazepam, drugs that boost the effect of dopamine such as Parkinson's medications, fluvoxamine, levodopa, omeprazole, and rifampin.

What are the possible side effects of Zyprexa/ Zyprexa Zydis/Zyprexa Intramuscular?

Side effects cannot be anticipated. If any develop or change in intensity, inform your doctor as soon as possible. Only your doctor can determine if it is safe for you to continue taking this drug.

Side effects may include: agitation, change in personality, constipation, dizziness, dry mouth, increased appetite, indigestion, low blood pressure upon standing, sleepiness, tremor, weakness, weight gain

Can I receive Zyprexa/Zyprexa Zydis/Zyprexa Intramuscular if I am pregnant or breastfeeding?

If you are pregnant or plan to become pregnant, inform your doctor immediately. Zyprexa should be used during pregnancy only if absolutely necessary. Zyprexa may appear in breast milk; do not breastfeed while taking this medication.

What should I do if I miss a dose of Zyprexa/ Zyprexa Zydis/Zyprexa Intramuscular?

Take it as soon as you remember. If it is almost time for your next dose, skip the one you missed and go back to your regular schedule. Do not take 2 doses at once.

How should I store Zyprexa/Zyprexa Zydis/ Zyprexa Intramuscular?

Store at room temperature away from light and moisture.

ZYRTEC

Generic name: Cetirizine hydrochloride

What is Zyrtec?

Zyrtec is an antihistamine used to treat the symptoms (eg, itching, redness, or inflammation) of allergies due to multiple causes such as pet dander, dust mites, pollen, ragweed, or grass. Zyrtec also treats chronic itching and hives of the skin.

What is the most important information I should know about Zyrtec?

Zytrec may make you drowsy or tired. You should not drive a car or engage in tasks that require mental alertness such as operating heavy machinery until you know how Zyrtec will affect you. You should avoid drinking alcohol or taking other medications that may make you drowsy or tired while taking Zyrtec. These medications may further decrease your mental alertness and can lead to impairment. You should take Zyrtec with caution if you have any type of liver or kidney problems.

Who should not take Zyrtec?
Do not take Zyrtec if you are allergic or sensitive to any of its ingredients.

What should I tell my doctor before I take the first dose of Zyrtec?
Tell your doctor about all prescription, over-the-counter, and herbal medication you are taking before beginning treatment with Zyrtec. Also, talk to your doctor about your complete medical history, especially if you are over the age of 77, or if you have kidney or liver problems.

What is the usual dosage?
The information below is based on the dosage guidelines your doctor uses. Depending on your condition and medical history, your doctor may prescribe a different regimen. Do not change the dosage or stop taking your medication without your doctor's approval.

Adults: The usual dose is 5-10 milligrams (mg) taken once a day.

Children 12 and older: The usual dose is 5-10 mg taken once a day.

Children 6 to 11 years old: The usual dose is 5-10 mg taken once a day.

Children 2 to 5 years old: The usual dose is 2.5 mg taken once a day (½ teaspoonful of the Zyrtec syrup).

Children 6 to 23 months: The usual dose is 2.5 mg taken once a day (½ teaspoonful of the Zyrtec syrup).

For children ages 12-23 months, your child's doctor may increase the dose to 5mg per day, taken as 2.5 mg twice a day.

How should I take Zyrtec?
Zyrtec doses should be taken at the same time every day and can be taken with or without food.

What should I avoid while taking Zyrtec?
You should not drink alcohol while taking Zyrtec. You should also not drive a car or operate heavy machinery until you know how Zyrtec will affect you.

What are possible food and drug interactions associated with Zyrtec?
If Zyrtec is taken with certain other drugs, the effects of either could be increased, decreased, or altered. It is especially important to check with your doctor before combining Zyrtec with the following: alcohol, other medications that may make you drowsy or tired, and theophylline.

What are the possible side effects of Zyrtec?

Side effects cannot be anticipated. If any develop or change in intensity, tell your doctor as soon as possible. Only your doctor can determine if it is safe for you to continue taking this drug.

Side effects may include: dry mouth, fatigue, headache, nausea, tiredness

Can I receive Zyrtec if I am pregnant or breastfeeding?

The effects of Zyrtec during pregnancy and breastfeeding are unknown. Tell your doctor immediately if you are pregnant, plan to become pregnant, or are breastfeeding.

What should I do if I miss a dose of Zyrtec?

If you forget to take Zyrtec, take it as soon as your remember. If it is closer to your next scheduled dose, skip the dose you missed and take Zyrtec according to your regular dosing schedule. Do not take two doses at once.

How should I store Zyrtec?

Store at room temperature. Zyrtec syrup may be stored at room temperature or under refrigeration.

ZYRTEC D

Generic name: Cetirizine hydrochloride and pseudoephedrine hydrochloride

What is Zyrtec D?

Zyrtec D is used to treat the nasal and non-nasal symptoms of seasonal and perennial allergies due to multiple causes in adults and children 12 years and older. Zyrtec D contains two different medications: cetirizine (an antihistamine) which stops itching, redness, or inflammation (heat) due to allergies or other causes; and pseudoephedrine (a decongestant) which relieves the nasal symptoms (stuffiness or runny nose) associated with allergies.

What is the most important information I should know about Zyrtec D?

Do not Zyrtec D if you have taken a medicine called an MAOI (monoamine oxidase inhibitor) within the last 14 days. Using Zyrtec D with an MAOI may reduce its antihypertensive effects.

Who should not take Zyrtec D?

You should not take Zyrtec D if you have taken a medicine called an MAOI (monoamine oxidase inhibitor) within the last 14 days, if you cannot completely empty your bladder, or if you have an eye condition called narrow-angle glaucoma, severe high blood pressure, or severe coronary artery disease. Also, you should not take Zyrtec D if you are allergic or sensitive any of its ingredients, or a similar medication called hydroxyzine.

What should I tell my doctor before I take the first dose of Zyrtec D?

Tell your doctor about all prescription, over-the-counter, and herbal medication you are taking before beginning treatment with Zyrtec D. Also, talk to your doctor about your complete medical history, especially if you have any type of liver or kidney problems, high blood pressure diabetes, ischemic heart disease, increased intraocular pressure (increase in the pressure inside the eye), narrow angle glaucoma, an overactive thyroid, trouble emptying your bladder, or an enlarged prostate.

What is the usual dosage?

The information below is based on the dosage guidelines your doctor uses. Depending on your condition and medical history, your doctor may prescribe a different regimen. Do not change the dosage or stop taking your medication without your doctor's approval.

Adults: The usual dose is one tablet (contains 5 milligrams (mg) of cetirizine and 120 mg of pseudoephedrine) taken twice a day.

Children age 12 and older: The usual dose is one tablet (contains 5 mg of cetirizine and 120 mg of pseudoephedrine) taken twice a day.

How should I take Zyrtec D?

Zyrtec D doses should be taken at the same time every day and can be taken with or without food. Zyrtec D tablets should be swallowed whole—do not break or chew the tablets.

What should I avoid while taking Zyrtec D?

You should not drink alcohol while taking Zyrtec D. Zyrtec D may cause drowsiness, therefore you should also not drive a car or operate heavy machinery until you know how it will affect you.

What are possible food and drug interactions associated with Zyrtec D?

If Zyrtec D is taken with certain other drugs, the effects of either could be increased, decreased, or altered. It is especially important to check with your doctor before combining Zyrtec D with the following: alcohol, mecamylamine, methyldopa, monoamine oxidase inhibitors (MAOIs), other medications that may make you drowsy or tired, reserpine, and theophylline.

What are the possible side effects of Zyrtec D?
Side effects cannot be anticipated. If any develop or change in intensity, tell your doctor as soon as possible. Only your doctor can determine if it is safe for you to continue taking this drug.

Side effects may include: dry mouth, fatigue, tiredness, trouble sleeping (insomnia)

Can I receive Zyrtec D if I am pregnant or breastfeeding?
The effects of Zyrtec D during pregnancy and breastfeeding are unknown. Tell your doctor immediately if you are pregnant, plan to become pregnant, or are breastfeeding.

What should I do if I miss a dose of Zyrtec D?
If you forget to take Zyrtec D, take it as soon as your remember. If it is closer to your next scheduled dose, skip the dose you missed and take Zyrtec D according to your regular dosing schedule. Do not double your doses.

How should I store Zyrtec D?
Store at room temperature.

ZYVOX
Generic name: Linezolid

What is Zyvox?
Zyvox is a strong antibiotic that treats infections untreatable by other common antibiotics. Under the direction of your physician, you may be prescribed Zyvox for one of the following: vancomycin-resistant *Enterococcus faecium,* multidrug-resistant or hospital-acquired pneumonia, community-acquired pneumonia, or complicated and uncomplicated skin and skin structure infections.

**What is the most important information
I should know about Zyvox?**
Zyvox should not be used to treat viral infections. To reduce the development of drug-resistant bacteria and maintain the effectiveness of Zyvox formulations and other antibacterial drugs, your prescriber should only use it treat or prevent certain infections.

Zyvox may decrease your blood cell count, and your doctor will do monitor your blood weekly, especially if you have current illnesses that put you at risk.

Similar to other antibiotics, Zyvox may disrupt normal bacteria found in the body, especially the stomach. This may increase your chances of getting mild to moderate diarrhea.

If you experience repeated episodes of nausea or vomiting, your doctor may take some tests to check the levels of acids and bases in your body to determine if you are developing lactic acidosis.

Changes in vision have been reported in some patients, especially those who are treated for longer than 28 days. If you experience any changes or if you are getting treated for 3 months or more, make regular visits to the eye doctor.

The use of this Zyvox with other medications, especially certain antidepressants, may increase your risk of experiencing a serious side effect known as serotonin syndrome. This is characterized by a very high fever, difficulty moving, and lack of coordination. If you experience any similar symptoms, seek immediate medical attention.

Convulsions have been reported in patients when treated with this drug and should be discussed with your doctor.

Zyvox is not approved for, and should not be used for, catheter-related bloodstream infections or catheter-site infections.

Who should not take Zyvox?

You should not take Zyvox if you have a known allergy to linezolid or any other of the drug's components, if you are taking medications that can increase your blood pressure, if you are taking monoamine oxidase inhibitors (such as phenelzine and isocarboxazid) and certain antidepressants.

You should not take this medication if you have uncontrolled high blood pressure or conditions that cause elevated blood pressure.

What should I tell my doctor before I take the first dose of Zyvox?

Tell your doctor about all prescription, over-the-counter, and herbal medications you are taking before beginning treatment with Zyvox. Also, talk to your doctor about your complete medical history, especially if you have high blood pressure, are taking cold medications that can increase your blood pressure, have had changes in vision due to a previous use of Zyvox, or have a history of seizures or convulsions.

What is the usual dosage?

The information below is based on the dosage guidelines your doctor uses. Depending on your condition and medical history, your doctor may prescribe a different regimen. Do not change the dosage or stop taking your medication without your doctor's approval.

Community-Acquired Pneumonia
Adults: The dose is 600 mg IV or orally every 12 hours for 10-14 days.

Children birth to 11 years old: 10mg/kg IV or orally every 8 hours for 10-14 days.

Hospital-Acquired Pneumonia
Adults: The dose is 600 mg IV or orally every 12 hours for 10-14 days.

Children birth to 11 years old: 10mg/kg IV or orally every 8 hours for 10-14 days.

Vancomycin-Resistant Enterococcus faecium
Adults: The dose is 600 mg IV or orally every 12 hours for 14-28 days.

Children birth to 11 years old: 10mg/kg IV or orally every 8 hours for 14-28 days.

Uncomplicated Skin and Skin Structure Infections
Adults: 400 mg orally every 12 hours for 10-14 days.

Adolescents: 600 mg orally every 12 hours for 10-14 days.

Children 5 to 11 years: 10 mg/kg orally every 12 hours for 10-14 days.

Children ≤5 years: 10 mg/kg orally every 8 hours for 10-14 days.

Complicated Skin and Skin Structure Infections
Adults: The dose is 600 milligrams (mg) IV or orally every 12 hours for 10-14 days.

Children birth to 11 years old: 10mg/kg IV or oral every 8 hours for 10-14 days.

Infection Due to Methicillin-resistant Staphylococcus aureus
Adults: The dose is 600 mg every 12 hours.

Neonates <7 days old: Your doctor will determine the dose of Zyvox that is more suitable for his or her age and weight.

How should I take Zyvox?

Take Zyvox exactly as directed. Skipping doses or not completing the full course of therapy may decrease treatment effectiveness and increase the likelihood that bacteria will develop resistance and will not be treatable by Zyvox or other antibacterial drugs in the future.

If you are in the hospital, the medication may be given to you by a healthcare professional intravenously. If you are taking it as a tablet or oral suspension, take it by mouth daily as directed. Before using the oral suspension, gently mix by inverting the bottle 3 to 5 times. DO NOT SHAKE.

What should I avoid while taking Zyvox?

Avoid eating large quantities (over 100 mg tyramine per meal) of foods or beverages with high tyramine content should be avoided while taking Zyvox. Foods high in tyramine content include those that may have undergone protein changes by aging, fermentation, pickling, or smoking to improve flavor, such as aged cheeses (0 to 15 mg tyramine per ounce); fermented or air-dried meats (0.1 to 8 mg tyramine per ounce); sauerkraut (8 mg tyramine per 8 ounces); soy sauce (5 mg tyramine per 1 teaspoon); tap beers (4 mg tyramine per 12 ounces); red wines (0 to 6 mg tyramine per 8 ounces). The tyramine content of any protein-rich food may be increased if stored for long periods or improperly refrigerated.

Avoid using the oral suspension formulation if you have problems breaking down amino acids as it contains about 20 mg of phenylalanine.

What are possible food and drug interactions associated with Zyvox?

If Zyvox is taken with certain food and other drugs, the effects of either could be increased, decreased, or altered. It is especially important to check with your doctor before combining Zyvox with the following: buspirone, dopamine, dobutamine, epinephrine, isocarboxazid, meperidine, norephinephrine, phenylpropanolamine, phenelzine, pseudoephedrine, serotonin 5-HT1 receptor antagonists (such as sumatriptan, zolmitriptan), serotonin reuptake inhibitors (such as citalopram, fluoxetine, paroxetine), tricyclic antidepressants, tyramine-rich foods (see "What should I avoid while taking Zyvox?")

What are the possible side effects of Zyvox?

Side effects cannot be anticipated. If any develop or change in intensity, tell your doctor as soon as possible. Only your doctor can determine if it is safe for you to continue taking this drug.

Side effects may include: diarrhea, headache, nausea, vomiting

Can I receive Zyvox if I am pregnant or breastfeeding?

The effects of Zyvox during pregnancy and breastfeeding are unknown. Tell your doctor immediately if you are pregnant, plan to become pregnant, or are breastfeeding as it should be used only if the benefits outweigh the risks.

What should I do if I miss a dose of Zyvox?

Take the missed dose as soon as you remember it. However, if it is almost time for your next dose, skip the one you missed and return to your regular dosing schedule. Do not double the dose.

How should I store Zyvox?

Store Zyvox infusion bags, tablets, and constituted suspension at room temperature away from light. Once reconstituted, the suspension should be used within 21 days.

Appendices

Disease and Disorder Index

APPENDIX 1
Safe Medication Use

Using medications safely is largely a matter of common sense and caution. The following are general guidelines to keep in mind:

You and your doctor

- Tell your doctor everything about your medical history, including reactions to medications you've used in the past.
- Tell the doctor about any medications you are using now, even if they are over-the-counter drugs, dietary supplements (such as glucosamine), or herbal medicines (such as St. John's wort).
- Keep track of your reactions to a medication and report them to your doctor.
- Ask your doctor what you can do when given a new drug. For example, are there any foods to avoid when taking the drug? Should you avoid alcohol? Should you avoid driving?
- Never change your dose schedule unless your doctor tells you to do so—and always finish all the medication unless instructed otherwise.

You and your pharmacist

- See if there are any written instructions that you can take with you.
- Ask the pharmacist to explain clearly when and how to take the drug.
- Ask about any possible interactions between the new prescription and any other drugs, dietary supplements, or herbals that you might be taking.
- Ask how long the medication remains effective. Don't take it after its expiration date.
- If you are going on a vacation, make sure your drug can be used in different climates—and make sure you have enough to get you through your trip. It's also a good idea to bring a copy of your prescriptions.

You and your medications

- Never take someone else's medication; and don't share your own medicines.
- Check the label each time you take a drug. Don't take—or dispense—a drug in the dark.

- Keep your medications in a dry, safe spot.
- Keep each medicine in the bottle from the drug store. Don't mix medicines together in a single bottle.
- If you think you are pregnant, consult with your doctor before using any medication.
- Destroy any unused portions of a drug and dispose of the bottle.
- Periodically check your medicine cabinet for expired medications. Toss them if they've expired.
- If you need a certain medicine (for instance, insulin) in case of emergency, carry the information with you.

Your medicines and your children

- Keep all medications in a locked cabinet or in a spot well out of the reach of children.
- Ask for child-proof safety bottles.
- Be alert and awake when giving a child medication.
- Make sure that children know medications can be dangerous if misused.
- Keep antidotes such as syrup of ipecac (which induces vomiting) on hand.
- Keep the numbers of your EMS and poison control centers handy.

APPENDIX 2
Poison Control Centers

The American Association of Poison Control Centers (AAPCC) uses a single, nationwide emergency number to automatically link callers with their regional poison center. This toll-free number, **800-222-1222**, also works for **teletype lines (TTY)** for the hearing-impaired and **telecommunication devices (TTD)** for individuals who are deaf. However, a few local poison centers and the ASPCA/Animal Poison Control Center are not part of this nationwide system and continue to use separate numbers.

Most of the centers listed below are certified by the AAPCC. **Certified centers are marked by an asterisk after the name**. Each has to meet certain criteria. It must, for example, serve a large geographic area; it must be open 24 hours a day and provide direct-dial or toll-free access; it must be supervised by a medical director; and it must have registered pharmacists or nurses available to answer questions from the public.

Within each state, centers are listed alphabetically by city. Some state poison centers also list their original emergency numbers (including TTY/TDD), which only work within that state. For these listings, callers may use either the state number or the nationwide 800 number.

ALABAMA

BIRMINGHAM
Regional Poison Control Center,
The Children's Hospital of Alabama (*)
1600 7th Ave. South
Birmingham, AL 35233-1711
Business: 205-939-9201
Emergency: 800-222-1222
www.chsys.org

TUSCALOOSA
Alabama Poison Center (*)
2503 Phoenix Dr.
Tuscaloosa, AL 35405
Business: 205-345-0600
Emergency: 800-222-1222
                  800-462-0800 (AL)
www.alapoisoncenter.org

ALASKA

JUNEAU
Alaska Poison Control System
Section of Injury Prevention
and EMS
410 Willoughby Ave., Room 103
Box 110616
Juneau, AK 99811-0616
Business: 907-465-3027
Emergency: 800-222-1222
www.chems.alaska.gov

(PORTLAND, OR)
Oregon Poison Center (*)
Oregon Health and Science
University
3181 SW Sam Jackson Park Rd.
Portland, OR 97239
Business: 503-494-8600
Emergency: 800-222-1222
www.oregonpoison.com

ARIZONA

PHOENIX
Banner Poison Control Center (*)
Banner Good Samaritan
Medical Center
901 E.Willetta St.
Suite 207-A
Phoenix, AZ 85006
Business: 602-253-3334
Emergency: 800-222-1222
www.bannerpoisoncontrol.com

TUCSON
Arizona Poison and Drug
Information Center
1295 N. Martin Ave.
Tucson, AZ 85724
Business: 520-626-7899
Emergency: 800-222-1222
www.pharmacy.arizona.edu/outreach/
poison/

ARKANSAS

LITTLE ROCK
Arkansas Poison and
Drug Information Center
College of Pharmacy—UAMS
4301 West Markham St.
Mail Slot 522-2
Little Rock, AR 72205-7122
Business: 501-686-6161
Emergency: 800-222-1222
             800-376-4766(AR)
TDD/TTY: 800-641-3805

ASPCA/ANIMAL POISON
CONTROL CENTER

1717 South Philo Rd.
Suite 36
Urbana, IL 61802
Business: 217-337-5030
Emergency: 888-426-4435
             800-548-2423
www.aspca.org/apcc

CALIFORNIA

FRESNO/MADERA
California Poison Control
System-Fresno/Madera Div.(*)
Valley Children's Hospital
9300 Valley Children's Place
MB15
Madera, CA 93638-8762
Business: 559-622-2300
Emergency: 800-222-1222
             800-876-4766 (CA)
TDD/TTY: 800-972-3323
www.calpoison.org

SACRAMENTO
California Poison Control
System-Sacramento Div.(*)
UC Davis Medical Center
2315 Stockton Blvd.
Sacramento, CA 95817
Business: 916-227-1400
Emergency: 800-222-1222
                     800-876-4766 (CA)
TDD/TTY: 800-972-3323
www.calpoison.org

SAN DIEGO
California Poison Control
System-San Diego Div. (*)
UC San Diego Medical Center
200 West Arbor Dr.
San Diego, CA 92103-8925
Business: 858-715-6300
Emergency: 800-222-1222
                     800-876-4766 (CA)
TDD/TTY: 800-972-3323
www.calpoison.org

SAN FRANCISCO
California Poison Control
System-San Francisco Div.(*)
San Francisco General Hospital
University of California
San Francisco
Box 1369
San Francisco, CA 94143-1369
Business: 415-502-6000
Emergency: 800-222-1222
                     800-876-4766 (CA)
TDD/TTY: 800-972-3323
www.calpoison.org

COLORADO

DENVER
Rocky Mountain Poison
and Drug Center (*)
777 Bannock St.
Mail Code 0180
Denver CO 80204-4028
Business: 303-739-1100
Emergency: 800-222-1222
TDD/TTY: 303-739-1127(CO)
www.RMPDC.org

CONNECTICUT

FARMINGTON
Connecticut Regional
Poison Control Center (*)
University of Connecticut
Health Center
263 Farmington Ave.
Farmington, CT 06030-5365
Business: 860-679-4540
Emergency: 800-222-1222
TDD/TTY: 866-218-5372
http://poisoncontrol.uchc.edu

DELAWARE

(PHILADELPHIA, PA)
The Poison Control Center (*)
Children's Hospital of Philadelphia
34th St. & Civic Center Blvd.
Philadelphia, PA 19104-4399
Business: 215-590-2100
Emergency: 800-222-1222
TDD/TTY: 215-590-8789
www.poisoncontrol.chop.edu

DISTRICT OF COLUMBIA

WASHINGTON, DC
National Capital
Poison Center (*)
3201 New Mexico Ave.
Suite 310
Washington, DC 20016
Business: 202-362-3867
Emergency: 800-222-1222
www.poison.org

FLORIDA

JACKSONVILLE
Florida Poison Information
Center-Jacksonville (*)
Shands Jacksonville Medical
Center
655 West 8th St.
Box C23
Jacksonville, FL 32209
Business: 904-244-4465
Emergency: 800-222-1222
http://fpicjax.org

MIAMI
Florida Poison Information
Center-Miami (*)
University of Miami-
Department of Pediatrics
P.O. Box 016960
Miami, FL 33101
Business: 305-585-5250
Emergency: 800-222-1222
www.miami.edu/poison-center

TAMPA
Florida Poison
Information Center-Tampa (*)
Tampa General Hospital
P.O. Box 1289
Tampa, FL 33601-1289
Business: 813-844-7044
Emergency: 800-222-1222
www.poisoncentertampa.org

GEORGIA

ATLANTA
Georgia Poison Center (*)
Hughes Spalding Children's
Hospital, Grady Health System
80 Jesse Hill Jr. Dr., SE
P.O. Box 26066
Atlanta, GA 30303-3050
Business: 404-616-9237
Emergency: 800-222-1222
                404-616-9000
                (Atlanta)
TDD: 404-616-9287
www.georgiapoisoncenter.org

HAWAII

(DENVER, CO)
Rocky Mountain Poison
and Drug Center (*)
777 Bannock St.
Mail Code 0180
Denver CO 80204-4028
Business: 303-739-1100
Emergency: 800-222-1222
www.RMPDC.org

IDAHO

(DENVER, CO)
Rocky Mountain Poison
and Drug Center (*)
777 Bannock St.
Mail Code 0180
Denver CO 80204-4028
Business: 303-739-1100
Emergency: 800-222-1222
www.RMPDC.org

ILLINOIS

CHICAGO
Illinois Poison Center (*)
222 South Riverside Plaza
Suite 1900
Chicago, IL 60606
Business: 312-906-6136
Emergency: 800-222-1222
TDD/TTY: 312-906-6185
www.illinoispoisoncenter.org

INDIANA

INDIANAPOLIS
Indiana Poison Control Center (*)
Clarian Health Partners
Methodist Hospital
I-65 at 21st St.
Indianapolis, IN 46206-1367
Business: 317-962-2335
Emergency: 800-222-1222
              800-382-9097
              317-962-2323
              (Indianapolis)
TTY: 317-962-2336
www.clarian.org/poisoncontrol

IOWA

SIOUX CITY
Iowa Statewide Poison
Control Center
Iowa Health System and the
University of Iowa Hospitals
and Clinics
401 Douglas St., Suite 402
Sioux City, IA 51101
Business: 712-279-3710
Emergency: 800-222-1222
              712-277-2222 (IA)
www.iowapoison.org

KANSAS

KANSAS CITY
University of Kansas
Poison Control Hospital Center
3901 Rainbow Blvd.
Room B400
Kansas City, KS 66160-7231
Business: 913-588-6638
Emergency: 800-222-1222
              800-332-6633(KS)
TDD: 866-238-0677
www.kumed.com/poison

KENTUCKY

LOUISVILLE
Kentucky Regional
Poison Center (*)
Kosair Children's Hospital
PO Box 35070
Louisville, KY 40232-5070
Business: 502-629-7264
Emergency: 800-222-1222
www.krpc.com

LOUISIANA

MONROE
Louisiana Drug and Poison
Information Center (*)
University of Louisiana at Monroe
700 University Ave.
Monroe, LA 71209-6430
Emergency: 800-222-1222

MAINE

PORTLAND
Northern New England
Poison Center
Maine Medical Center
22 Bramhall St.
Portland, ME 04102
Business: 207-662-0111
Emergency: 800-222-1222
               207-871-2879(ME)
TDD/TTY: 207-662-4900(ME)
www.nnepc.org

MARYLAND

BALTIMORE
Maryland Poison Center (*)
University of Maryland at
Baltimore
School of Pharmacy
220 Arch St.
Office Level 1
Baltimore, MD 21201
Business: 410-706-7604
Emergency: 800-222-1222
TDD: 410-706-1858
www.mdpoison.com

(WASHINGTON, DC)
National Capital
Poison Center (*)
3201 New Mexico Ave.
Suite 310
Washington DC 20016
Business: 202-362-3867
Emergency: 800-222-1222
TDD/TTY: 202-362-8563(MD)
www.poison.org

MASSACHUSETTS

BOSTON
Regional Center for Poison
Control and Prevention (*)
(Serving Massachusetts and
Rhode Island)
Children's Hospital Boston
300 Longwood Ave.
Boston, MA 02115
Business: 617-355-6609
Emergency: 800-222-1222
TDD/TTY: 888-244-5313
www.maripoisoncenter.com

MICHIGAN

DETROIT
Regional Poison
Control Center (*)
Children's Hospital of Michigan
4160 John R. Harper
Professional Office Bldg.
Suite 616
Detroit, MI 48201
Business: 313-745-5335
Emergency: 800-222-1222
TDD/TTY: 800-356-3232
www.mitoxic.org/pcc

GRAND RAPIDS
DeVos Children's Hospital
Regional Poison Center (*)
100 Michigan St., NE
Grand Rapids, MI 49503
Business: 616-391-3690
Emergency: 800-222-1222
http://poisoncenter.devoschildrens.org

MINNESOTA

MINNEAPOLIS
Minnesota Poison Control
System (*) Hennepin County
Medical Center
701 Park Ave.
Mail Code RL
Minneapolis, MN 55415
Business: 612-873-3144
Emergency: 800-222-1222
www.mnpoison.org

MISSISSIPPI

JACKSON
Mississippi Regional Poison
Control Center, University of
Mississippi Medical Center
2500 North State St.
Jackson, MS 39216
Business: 601-984-1680
Emergency: 800-222-1222
http://poisoncontrol.umc.edu

MISSOURI

ST. LOUIS
Missouri Regional
Poison Center (*)
Cardinal Glennon
Children's Hospital
7980 Clayton Rd.
Suite 200
St. Louis, MO 63117
Business: 314-772-5200
Emergency: 800-222-1222
TDD/TTY: 314-612-5705
www.cardinalglennon.com

MONTANA

(DENVER, CO)
Rocky Mountain Poison
and Drug Center (*)
777 Bannock St.
Mail Code 0180
Denver CO 80204-4028
Business: 303-739-1100
Emergency: 800-222-1222
TDD/TTY: 303-739-1127
www.RMPDC.org

NEBRASKA

OMAHA
The Poison Center (*)
Children's Hospital
8401 W. Dodge St., Suite 115
Omaha, NE 68114
Business: 402-955-5555
Emergency: 800-222-1222
www.nebraskapoison.com

NEVADA

(DENVER, CO)
Rocky Mountain Poison
and Drug Center (*)
777 Bannock St.
Mail Code 0180
Denver CO 80204-4028
Business: 303-739-1100
Emergency: 800-222-1222
www.RMPDC.org

(PORTLAND, OR)
Oregon Poison Center (*)
Oregon Health and
Science University
3181 SW Sam Jackson Park Rd.
Portland, OR 97239
Business: 503-494-8600
Emergency: 800-222-1222
www.oregonpoison.com

NEW HAMPSHIRE

(PORTLAND, ME)
Northern New England
Poison Center
Maine Medical Center
22 Bramhall St.
Portland, ME 04102
Business: 207-662-0111
Emergency: 800-222-1222
www.nnepc.org

NEW JERSEY

NEWARK
New Jersey Poison Information
and Education System (*)
UMDNJ
140 Bergen St. Suite G1600
Newark, NJ 07101
Business: 973-972-9280
Emergency: 800-222-1222
TDD/TTY: 973-926-8008
www.njpies.org

NEW MEXICO

ALBUQUERQUE
New Mexico Poison and
Drug Information Center (*)
MSC09/5080
1 University of New Mexico
Albuquerque, NM 87131-0001
Business: 505-272-4261
Emergency: 800-222-1222
http://HSC.UNM.edu/pharmacy/poison

NEW YORK

BUFFALO
Western New York Regional
Poison Control Center (*)
Women and Children's Hospital
of Buffalo
219 Bryant St.
Buffalo, NY 14222
Business: 716-878-7654
Emergency: 800-222-1222
www.wnypoison.org

MINEOLA
Long Island Regional Poison
and Drug Information Center (*)
Winthrop University Hospital
259 First St.
Mineola, NY 11501
Business: 516-663-2650
Emergency: 800-222-1222
TDD: 516-747-3323
               (Nassau)
               631-924-8811
               (Suffolk)
www.lirpdic.org

NEW YORK CITY
New York City
Poison Control Center (*)
NYC Dept. of Health
455 First Ave., Room 123
New York, NY 10016
Business: 212-447-8152
Emergency: 800-222-1222
(English)   212-340-4494
               212-POISONS
               (212-764-7667)
Emergency: 212-VENENOS
(Spanish)   (212-836-3667)
TDD: 212-689-9014
www.nyc.gov/html/
doh/html/poison/poison.shtml

ROCHESTER
Finger Lakes Regional Poison
and Drug Information Center (*)
University of Rochester
Medical Center
601 Elmwood Ave.
Box 321
Rochester, NY 14642
Business: 585-273-4155
Emergency: 800-222-1222
TTY: 585-273-3854
www.fingerlakespoison.org

SYRACUSE
Upstate New York
Poison Center (*)
SUNY Upstate Medical University
750 East Adams St.
Syracuse, NY 13210
Business: 315-464-7078
Emergency: 800-222-1222
TTY: 315-464-5424
www.upstatepoison.org

NORTH CAROLINA

CHARLOTTE
Carolinas Poison Center (*)
Carolinas Medical Center
PO Box 32861
Charlotte, NC 28232-2861
Business: 704-512-3795
Emergency: 800-222-1222
www.ncpoisoncenter.org

NORTH DAKOTA

BISMARK
ND Department of Health
Injury Prevention Program
North Dakota Poison Center
600 E. Boulevard Ave.
Bismark, ND 58505
Business: 612-873-3144
Emergency: 800-222-1222
www.ndpoison.org

OHIO

CINCINNATI
Cincinnati Drug and Poison
Information Center (*)
Cincinatti Children's Hospital
3333 Burnet Ave.
Cincinnati, OH 45229
Business: 513-636-5063
Emergency: 800-222-1222
TDD/TTY: 800-253-7955
www.cincinnatichildrens.org/dpic

CLEVELAND
Greater Cleveland
Poison Control Center
Rainbow Babies and Children's
Hospital
11100 Euclid Ave.
MP 6007
Cleveland, OH 44106-6007
Business: 216-844-1573
Emergency: 800-222-1222
www.uhhospitals.org/rainbowchildren/
tabid/195/Default.aspx

COLUMBUS
Central Ohio
Poison Center (*)
Nationwide Children's Hospital
700 Children's Dr.
Columbus, OH 43205-2696
Business: 614-355-0435
Emergency: 800-222-1222
TTY: 614-228-2272
www.bepoisonsmart.com

OKLAHOMA

OKLAHOMA CITY
Oklahoma Poison
Control Center (*)
College of Pharmacy at OU
Medical Center
940 Northeast 13th St.
Room 3N3510
Oklahoma City, OK 73104
Business: 405-271-5062
Emergency: 800-222-1222
www.oklahomapoison.org

OREGON

PORTLAND
Oregon Poison Center (*)
Oregon Health and Science
University
3181 S.W. Sam Jackson Park Rd.
Portland, OR 97239
Business: 503-494-8600
Emergency: 800-222-1222
www.ohsu.edu/poison

PENNSYLVANIA

PHILADELPHIA
The Poison Control Center (*)
Children's Hospital of
Philadelphia
34th Street & Civic Center Blvd.
Philadelphia, PA 19104-4399
Business: 215-590-2100
Emergency: 800-222-1222
                  215-386-2100 (PA)
TDD/TTY: 215-590-8789
www.poisoncontrol.chop.edu

PITTSBURGH
Pittsburgh Poison Center (*)
Children's Hospital of
Pittsburgh
3705 Fifth Ave.
Pittsburgh, PA 15213
Business: 412-390-3300
Emergency: 800-222-1222
                  412-681-6669
www.chp.edu/clinical/03a_poison.php

RHODE ISLAND

(BOSTON, MA)
Regional Center for Poison
Control and Prevention (*)
Children's Hospital Boston
(Serving Massachusetts and
Rhode Island)
300 Longwood Ave., IC Smith Bldg
Boston, MA 02115
Business: 617-355-6609
Emergency: 800-222-1222
TDD/TTY: 888-244-5313
www.maripoisoncenter.com

SOUTH DAKOTA

(MINNEAPOLIS, MN)
**Hennepin Regional Poison
Center (*) Hennepin County
Medical Center**
701 Park Ave., Mail Code RL
Minneapolis, MN 55415
Business: 612-873-3144
Emergency: 800-222-1222
www.mnpoison.org

SIOUX FALLS
Sanford Poison Center (*)
USD Medical Center
1305 W. 18th St.
Box 5039
Sioux Falls, SD 57117-5039
Business: 605-328-6670
Emergency: 800-222-1222
www.sdpoison.org

TENNESSEE

NASHVILLE
Tennessee Poison Center (*)
1161 21st Ave. South
501 Oxford House
Nashville, TN 37232-4632
Business: 615-936-0760
Emergency: 800-222-1222
www.poisonlifeline.org

TEXAS

AMARILLO
**Texas Panhandle
Poison Center (*)**
**Texas Tech University Health
Sciences Center**
1501 S. Coulter Dr.
Amarillo, TX 79106
Business: 806-354-1630
Emergency: 800-222-1222
www.poisoncontrol.org

DALLAS
North Texas Poison Center (*)
**Texas Poison Center Network
Parkland Health and Hospital
System**
5201 Harry Hines Blvd.
Dallas, TX 75235
Business: 214-589-0911
Emergency: 800-222-1222
www.poisoncontrol.org

EL PASO
**West Texas Regional
Poison Center (*)**
Thomason Hospital
4815 Alameda Ave.
El Paso, TX 79905
Business   915-534-3800
Emergency: 800-222-1222
www.poisoncontrol.org

GALVESTON
Southeast Texas Poison Center (*)
**The University of Texas
Medical Branch**
301 University Blvd.
Galveston, TX 77555-1175
Business: 409-772-9142
Emergency: 800-222-1222
www.poisoncontrol.org

SAN ANTONIO
South Texas
Poison Center (*)
The University of Texas Health
Science Center-San Antonio
7703 Floyd Curl Dr., MSC 7849
San Antonio, TX 78229-3900
Business: 210-567-5762
Emergency: 800-222-1222
www.poisoncontrol.org

TEMPLE
Central Texas Poison Center (*)
Scott & White Memorial Hospital
2401 South 31st St.
Temple, TX 76508
Business: 254-724-7401
Emergency: 800-222-1222
www.poisoncontrol.org

UTAH

SALT LAKE CITY
Utah Poison Control Center (*)
University of Utah
585 Komas Dr.
Salt Lake City, UT 84108
Business: 801-587-0600
Emergency: 800-222-1222
http://uuhsc.utah.edu/poison

VERMONT

(PORTLAND, ME)
Northern New England
Poison Center
Maine Medical Center
22 Bramhall St.
Portland, ME 04102
Business: 207-662-0111
Emergency: 800-222-1222
www.nnepc.org

VIRGINIA

CHARLOTTESVILLE
Blue Ridge Poison Center (*)
University of Virginia Health
System
PO Box 800774
Charlottesville, VA 22908-0774
Business: 434-924-0347
Emergency: 800-222-1222
www.healthsystem.virginia.edu/brpc

RICHMOND
Virginia Poison Center (*)
Virginia Commonwealth
University Medical Center
600 E. Broad St. Suite 640
P.O. Box 980522
Richmond, VA 23298-0522
Business: 804-828-4780
Emergency: 800-222-1222
                804-828-9123
www.poison.vcu.edu

WASHINGTON

SEATTLE
Washington Poison Center (*)
155 NE 100th St.
Seattle, WA 98125-8007
Business: 206-517-2359
Emergency: 800-222-1222
www.wapc.org

WEST VIRGINIA

CHARLESTON
West Virginia Poison Center (*)
WVU Charleston Division
3110 MacCorkle Ave. SE
Charleston, WV 25304
Business: 304-347-1212
Emergency: 800-222-1222
www.wvpoisoncenter.org

WISCONSIN

MILWAUKEE
Wisconsin Poison Center
Suite CC 660
P.O. Box 1997
Milwaukee, WI 53201
Business: 414-266-2952
Emergency: 800-222-1222
TDD/TTY: 414-266-2542
www.wisconsinpoison.org

WYOMING

(OMAHA, NE)
The Poison Center (*)
Children's Hospital
8401 W. Dodge St., Suite 115
Omaha, NE 68114
Business: 402-955-5555
Emergency: 800-222-1222
www.nebraskapoison.com

APPENDIX 3
Top 200 Brand-Name Drugs

The following list contains the top-selling brands prescribed during 2008, measured by the total number of prescriptions filled. The information was compiled by the market research group SDI Health based in Plymouth Meeting, Pa.

Rank	Product	Rank	Product
1.	Lipitor	34.	Concerta
2.	Nexium	35.	Levoxyl
3.	Lexapro	36.	Actonel
4.	Singulair	37.	Ambien CR
5.	Plavix	38.	Spiriva
6.	Synthroid	39.	Benicar
7.	Prevacid	40.	Xalatan
8.	Advair Diskus	41.	Benicar HCT
9.	Effexor XR	42.	Aricept
10.	Diovan	43.	Ortho Tri-Cyclen Lo
11.	Crestor	44.	Hyzaar
12.	Vytorin	45.	Tri-Sprintec
13.	Cymbalta	46.	Cialis
14.	ProAir HFA	47.	OxyContin
15.	Klor-Con	48.	Aciphex
16.	Diovan HCT	49.	Lunesta
17.	Levaquin	50.	Lamictal
18.	Actos	51.	Detrol LA
19.	Flomax	52.	Chantix
20.	Seroquel	53.	Avapro
21.	Zetia	54.	Proventil HFA
22.	Tricor	55.	Abilify
23.	Celebrex	56.	Yasmin 28
24.	Nasonex	57.	Budeprion XL
25.	Premarin Tabs	58.	Niaspan
26.	Lantus	59.	Combivent
27.	Viagra	60.	Januvia
28.	Yaz	61.	Boniva
29.	Lyrica	62.	Trinessa
30.	Adderall XR	63.	NuvaRing
31.	Valtrex	64.	Risperdal
32.	Cozaar	65.	Polymagma Plain
33.	Topamax	66.	Flovent HFA

Rank	Product	Rank	Product
67.	Imitrex Oral	111.	Prempro
68.	Evista	112.	Low-Ogestrel
69.	Avelox	113.	Patanol
70.	Depakote ER	114.	Lumigan
71.	Protonix	115.	Provigil
72.	Avalide	116.	Pulmicort Respules
73.	Lidoderm	117.	Altace
74.	Zyprexa	118.	Necon 1/35
75.	Namenda	119.	Micardis
76.	Tussionex	120.	Depakote
77.	Thyroid, Armour	121.	Fosamax Plus D
78.	Humalog	122.	Alphagan P
79.	Vigamox	123.	Geodon Oral
80.	Tamiflu	124.	Micardis HCT
81.	Budeprion SR	125.	Vesicare
82.	Suboxone	126.	Focalin XR
83.	Lanoxin	127.	Digitek
84.	Loestrin 24 Fe	128.	Sprintec
85.	Avodart	129.	Xopenex
86.	Coumadin Tabs	130.	Tobradex
87.	Wellbutrin XL	131.	Humulin N
88.	Endocet	132.	Clarinex
89.	Skelaxin	133.	Ciprodex Otic
90.	Nasacort AQ	134.	Coreg CR
91.	Keppra	135.	Apri
92.	Allegra-D 12 Hour	136.	Atacand
93.	Strattera	137.	Levothroid
94.	Lovaza	138.	Restasis
95.	Lotrel	139.	Ventolin HFA
96.	Avandia	140.	Rhinocort Aqua
97.	Ocella	141.	Prometrium
98.	Vyvanse	142.	Trivora-28
99.	Toprol XL	143.	Xyzal
100.	Levitra	144.	Ortho Evra
101.	Astelin	145.	Cosopt
102.	Vivelle-DOT	146.	Arimidex
103.	Glipizide XL	147.	Veramyst
104.	Xopenex HFA	148.	Requip
105.	Aviane	149.	Humulin 70/30
106.	Fosamax	150.	BenzaClin
107.	Caduet	151.	Differin
108.	Kariva	152.	Methylin
109.	Byetta	153.	Asacol
110.	Mirapex	154.	Dilantin

Rank	Product	Rank	Product
155.	Aggrenox	178.	Janumet
156.	Zymar	179.	Pataday
157.	Vagifem	180.	Travatan
158.	AndroGel	181.	Halflytely Bowel Prep
159.	Ethedent	182.	Travatan Z
160.	Lantus SoloSTAR	183.	Primacare One
161.	Fluvirin	184.	Bactroban
162.	Premarin Vaginal	185.	C-Phen DM
163.	ACTO*plus* met	186.	Trilyte
164.	Propecia	187.	Norvasc
165.	Exforge	188.	Welchol
166.	NovoLog Mix 70/30	189.	Lovenox
167.	Asmanex	190.	Junel FE
168.	Levora	191.	Novolin 70/30
169.	Uroxatral	192.	Sular
170.	Allegra-D 24 Hour	193.	Ultram ER
171.	Epipen	194.	Zovirax Topical
172.	Zyrtec	195.	Catapres-TTS
173.	Enablex	196.	Avandamet
174.	Levemir	197.	Maxalt
175.	Fluzone	198.	Jantoven
176.	Relpax	199.	Paxil CR
177.	Symbicort	200.	Femara

Disease and Disorder Index

Use this index to find out which drugs are available for a specific medical problem. Both brand and generic names are listed; *generic names are shown in italics*. Only brands and generics covered in the drug profiles are included.

Motrin, 850
Naprosyn, 860
Naproxen. See Anaprox and
   Naprosyn
Ponstel, 1039
Voltaren Gel, 1406

Menstrual periods, regulation of
Aygestin, 177
Medroxyprogesterone. See Provera
Norethindrone acetate. See Aygestin
Provera, 1099

Migraine headache
See Headache, migraine

Motion sickness
Antivert, 112
Meclizine. See Antivert
Promethazine, 1079

Mountain sickness
Acetazolamide, 13

Muscular discomfort due to sprain,
  strain, or injury
Carisoprodol. See Soma
Cyclobenzaprine. See Flexeril
Diazepam. See Valium
Flexeril, 559
Metaxalone. See Skelaxin
Methocarbamol. See Robaxin
Robaxin, 1167
Skelaxin, 1202
Soma, 1204
Tizanidine. See Zanaflex
Valium, 1366
Zanaflex, 1443

Narcolepsy
Adderall, 34
Amphetamines. See Adderall
Armodafinil. See Nuvigil
Methylphenidate. See Ritalin
Modafinil. See Provigil
Nuvigil, 929
Provigil, 1101
Ritalin/Ritalin-SR/Ritalin LA, 1162

Nasal polyps
Beclomethasone, 199
Mometasone. See Nasonex
Nasonex, 865

Nausea
See Vomiting and nausea

Obesity
Adipex-P, 39
Desoxyn, 403
Meridia, 797
Methamphetamine. See
   Desoxyn
Orlistat. See Xenical
Phentermine. See Adipex-P
Sibutramine. See Meridia
Xenical, 1428

Obsessive-compulsive disorder
Anafranil, 99
Clomipramine. See Anafranil
Fluoxetine. See Prozac
Fluvoxamine, extended-release. See
   Luvox CR
Luvox CR, 778
Paroxetine. See Paxil and Pexeva
Paxil, 981
Pexeva, 1014
Prozac, 1103
Sertraline. See Zoloft
Zoloft, 1489